Tuberculosis

A subject collection from *Cold Spring Harbor Perspectives in Medicine*

OTHER SUBJECT COLLECTIONS FROM *COLD SPRING HARBOR PERSPECTIVES IN MEDICINE*

The Biology of Heart Disease
The Skin and Its Diseases
MYC *and the Pathway to Cancer*
Bacterial Pathogenesis
Transplantation
Cystic Fibrosis: A Trilogy of Biochemistry, Physiology, and Therapy
Hemoglobin and Its Diseases
Addiction
Parkinson's Disease
Type 1 Diabetes
Angiogenesis: Biology and Pathology
HIV: From Biology to Prevention and Treatment
The Biology of Alzheimer Disease

SUBJECT COLLECTIONS FROM *COLD SPRING HARBOR PERSPECTIVES IN BIOLOGY*

The Genetics and Biology of Sexual Conflict
The Origin and Evolution of Eukaryotes
Endocytosis
Mitochondria
Signaling by Receptor Tyrosine Kinases
DNA Repair, Mutagenesis, and Other Responses to DNA Damage
Cell Survival and Cell Death
Immune Tolerance
DNA Replication
Endoplasmic Reticulum
Wnt Signaling
Protein Synthesis and Translational Control
The Synapse
Extracellular Matrix Biology
Protein Homeostasis
Calcium Signaling
The Golgi
Germ Cells
The Mammary Gland as an Experimental Model
The Biology of Lipids: Trafficking, Regulation, and Function
Auxin Signaling: From Synthesis to Systems Biology

Tuberculosis

A subject collection from *Cold Spring Harbor Perspectives in Medicine*

EDITED BY

Stefan H.E. Kaufmann
Max Planck Institute for Infection Biology

Eric J. Rubin
Harvard School of Public Health

Alimuddin Zumla
University College London

COLD SPRING HARBOR LABORATORY PRESS
Cold Spring Harbor, New York • www.cshlpress.org

Tuberculosis

A Subject Collection from *Cold Spring Harbor Perspectives in Medicine*
Articles online at www.perspectivesinmedicine.org

Printed in the United States of America

Executive Editor	Richard Sever
Managing Editor	Maria Smit
Senior Project Manager	Barbara Acosta
Permissions Administrator	Carol Brown
Production Editor	Kathleen Bubbeo and Diane Schubach
Production Manager/Cover Designer	Denise Weiss
Publisher	John Inglis

Front cover artwork: The image depicts murine bone marrow–derived macrophages infected with *Mycobacterium tuberculosis* (strain H37Rv) for 120 min. (Image kindly provided by Dr. Volker Brinkmann, Microscopy Core Facility, Max Planck Institute for Infection Biology, Berlin, Germany.)

Library of Congress Cataloging-in-Publication Data

Tuberculosis/edited by Stefan H. E. Kaufmann, Eric J. Rubin, and Alimuddin Zumla.
p. ; cm.
"A subject collection from Cold Spring Harbor perspectives in medicine."
Includes bibliographical references and index.
ISBN 978-1-62182-073-4 (hardcover : alk. paper)
I. Kaufmann, S. H. E. (Stefan H. E.), editor. II. Rubin, Eric J., editor. III. Zumla, Alimuddin, editor. IV. Cold Spring Harbor perspectives in medicine.
[DNLM: 1. Tuberculosis--Collected Works. 2. Mycobacterium tuberculosis--Collected Works. WF 200]

RC311
616.99'5--dc23

2014028231

10 9 8 7 6 5 4 3 2 1

All World Wide Web addresses are accurate to the best of our knowledge at the time of printing.

For a complete catalog of all Cold Spring Harbor Laboratory Press publications, visit our website at www.cshlpress.org.

Contents

SECTION 3. CLINICAL TUBERCULOSIS

Preface

IN JANUARY 1962, THE INTERNATIONAL UNION AGAINST TUBERCULOSIS declared its victory over tuberculosis (TB), "*If I had tuberculosis... this idea formerly terrifying, no longer makes anyone tremble... antibiotics have appeared, sanatoria have disappeared; as far as the public is concerned, the problem is solved, the disease has been conquered*" (Waksman 1964, p. 1). In the 1960s and 1970s, we, with our bias on the industrialized world, thought that the problem could and would be solved soon in the rest of the world.

Accordingly, research and development (R&D) on new diagnostics, drugs, and vaccines for TB dwindled from the 1970s on. This decline in interest in TB is reflected in the low number of publication hits in PubMed on TB, with numbers in the low thousands of hits annually in the years before 1990; this was followed by an increase leading to a doubling of publications on TB in 1995, 2 years after the WHO global emergency call for TB in 1993 (WHO 1993). The latest figures for 2013 are much more than 10,000 publications. The output of publications on TB follows the funding situation. In the 1980s, there was <US$10 million annually spent on TB (Kaufmann and Parida 2007). The beginning of this century has witnessed a clear increase, with ~US$500 million in funding since 2010 (Moran et al. 2013; WHO 2013). This increased financial investment in R&D activities for TB intervention measures is now starting to show signs of success. In recent years, we have witnessed introduction of a new rapid TB diagnostic test, the GeneXpert MTB-RIF Assay, the clinical evaluation of a dozen new TB drugs, and a portfolio of new TB vaccines in different stages of clinical trials.

However, this is only one side of the coin. TB remains a leading cause of illness and death worldwide and there is a worrying rise in the number of cases of multidrug-resistant (MDR)-TB and extensively drug-resistant (XDR)-TB in Asia, Eastern Europe, and Southern Africa. We are currently experiencing the emergence of drug-resistant strains of *Mycobacterium tuberculosis* that are totally resistant to all known first- and second-line TB drugs. Clearly, the misconception in the last quarter of the last century about TB, and the complacency that followed, has led to our failure to control this disease.

TB has been with humankind for tens of thousands of years. Originally, it was feared as phthisis, describing the wasting form of this disease, or scrofulosis, characterized by severe lymph node swellings. For centuries, these diseases were viewed as totally independent until the pathologist and anatomist Franciscus Deleboe Sylvius (1614–1672) became intrigued by the similarities of the "hidden" tubercles in the lungs of phthisis patients and the distracting swollen lymph nodes of scrofulosis patients (Deleboe 1679). In 1834, Johann Lukas Schönlein (1793–1864) used the term "tuberculosis" (tuberkulose) for the first time (Schönlein 1841) to describe diseases characterized by the formation of tubercles, as the characteristic granulomatous lesions were referred to, under a single heading. Even though he recognized the differences between scrofulosis and phthisis, the two polar forms of TB, he considered similarities more important and grouped them together in his scheme, analogous to the botanical system of Carl von Linné (1707–1778).

At the time when Schönlein introduced the term "tuberculosis," the anatomist Jakob Henle (1809–1885) was lecturing on anatomy at the University of Göttingen, Germany. He thought intensively about contagious diseases and postulated, without any experimental evidence, three crucial features of such an elusive type of illness: (1) the presence of a living organism (*contagium animatum*) in all affected tissues; (2) the isolation of the *contagium animatum* from these tissues; and

(3) experimental analysis of the *contagium animatum* outside of the body. Thus, the soil was prepared for his student Robert Koch (1843–1910), who ultimately proved the etiology of TB by elegant experiments published in 1882 (Koch 1882). True, Koch was not the first to transmit TB in experimental animal models, but his experiments were the first to provide formal proof of Henle's principles by the identification of *M. tuberculosis* in affected tissues in patient material, isolation and culture of *M. tuberculosis* in pure form as single colonies on solid plates, and elicitation of a similar disease in a large variety of experimental animals.

Although we now know the genome sequence of *M. tuberculosis* today, we remain puzzled by the tricks this pathogen plays. We hope that this book brings the reader closer to the most recent insights into at least some of the tricks and to new ways of harnessing these for novel intervention measures. There have been a number of textbooks on different aspects in the field of TB published in the past decade, notably, the *Handbook of Tuberculosis* (Kaufmann and Britton 2008; Kaufmann and Rubin 2008; Kaufmann and van Helden 2008), comprising three volumes that appeared in 2008, the treatise *Tuberculosis—A Comprehensive Clinical Reference* (Schaaf and Zumla 2009), and *Tuberculosis* (Zumla and Schaaf 2011). The book you have in hand is distinguished by being up to date and more concise, allowing researchers, clinicians, field-workers, students, patients, advocates, and the public ready access to state-of-the-art information about specific topics of interest, as well as more distant areas, across the entire field of TB.

We have divided the book into three sections of more than 10 chapters each: Section 1. Vaccines, Immunology, Host Cells, and Biomarkers, edited by Stefan H.E. Kaufmann; Section 2. Drugs and Biology of Tuberculosis, edited by Eric Rubin; and Section 3. Clinical Tuberculosis, edited by Alimuddin Zumla.

Section 1 covers all aspects of the host response to *M. tuberculosis*, ranging from basic research to medical application. The chapters by Srinivasan et al. and by Deretic describe the important role of cellular processes in host immunity—notably, in cell death caused by apoptosis and autophagy. Similarly, cell-autonomous effector mechanisms contribute to host defense against *M. tuberculosis*, as described by MacMicking. These mechanisms are probably the outcome of the intimate cross talk between pathogen and myeloid cells and participate in host immunity, as discussed by Lugo-Villarino and Neyrolles. Mayer-Barber and Barber provide an introduction to the highly intertwined cross talk between the innate and acquired immune responses in TB. Immunity against TB is mediated by T lymphocytes and effected by mononuclear phagocytes. In addition to conventional $CD4^+$ and $CD8^+$ T cells, nonclassical T cells participate in acquired immunity against TB, as discussed in chapters by Lindestam Arlehamn et al. and by De Libero et al. T cells stimulate various effector functions in macrophages, as described by MacMicking. These interactions are complex and in the in vivo setting, they are focused on the granuloma as the tissue site of both protection and pathology in TB (Pagán and Ramakrishnan). A concept that has long been championed by Casedevall and colleagues suggests that B lymphocytes and their products, antibodies, play a greater role in acquired immunity than thus far appreciated (Achkar et al.). TB is a highly complex disease; hence, in vitro studies need to be complemented by appropriate experimental animal models and human studies. The spectrum of the major animal models for TB with all their advantages and disadvantages is discussed in four chapters, which focus on mice (Cooper), guinea pigs (Clark et al.), zebrafish (van Leeuwen et al.), and nonhuman primates (Scanga and Flynn). The immune response in TB patients is covered by Walzl et al., with an emphasis on biomarkers indicative for disease and latent infection. This chapter is complemented by a description of state-of-the-art biomics approaches toward a better understanding of molecular mechanisms underlying TB (Maertzdorf et al.). Finally, the chapter by Andersen and Kaufmann describes how to best harness our increasing understanding of the immune response to *M. tuberculosis* for the development of novel vaccines against TB with an emphasis on those that have already entered the clinical pipeline.

Section 1 therefore spans the whole spectrum from basic cell biology and immunology to applied areas of biomarkers as a basis for novel diagnostic measures and vaccine candidates for prevention of this major health threat.

Section 2 describes the broad spectrum of the many unique biological characteristics of *M. tuberculosis* in a series of chapters. The cell wall of mycobacteria is made up of structures found in few other pathogens (Jackson and Alderwick et al.). Both this unusual structure and specific metabolic requirements (Warner) have led to cell division processes and regulation that, again, differ from those found in many other bacteria (Uhía et al.). Many of these critical processes are targeted by existing drugs, several of which, because of their molecular mechanisms of action, narrowly target *M. tuberculosis* (Chakraborty and Rhee). However, there is a substantial need for new antibiotics that are more rapidly effective and able to act against drug-resistant bacteria. These are being developed using newer approaches (Schnappinger and Mdluli et al.) with important pharmacologic considerations kept in mind (Davies). Given what we know about the mechanisms of host resistance described in other sections, therapies that influence the host–pathogen relationship can also potentially be manipulated (Tobin). But the genome is not just useful for drug discovery—it is also an important tool for tracking disease (Niemann and Supply) and understanding the evolution of the organism (Behr). All of these aspects of pathogen biology remain rich areas of inquiry with potential impact on disease in the very near future.

Section 3 contains 11 elegantly written chapters by a global authorship, providing the latest up-to-date information that will be useful to physicians and allied health-care workers dealing with TB worldwide. The epidemiology chapter (Glaziou et al.) shows that although there has been a steady, slow decline in total numbers of drug-sensitive TB, the emerging and alarming problems of MDR-TB and XDR-TB globally are worrying. The growing pipeline of new TB diagnostics and several evaluations of the GeneXpert MTB/RIF and urine LAM assays (Lawn) now enable missed TB cases to be detected at points of care. The highly illustrated chapter on imaging in TB (Bomanji et al.) includes PET scanning for localizing extrapulmonary TB and its potential use as a biomarker of disease activity. The chapter on TB treatment and drug regimens (Sotgiu et al.) details the current TB drug pipeline and recommended drug regimens for drug-sensitive and drug-resistant TB. With an estimated 2 billion people living with latent TB infection, the importance of screening for latent TB in migrants and in those who are immunosuppressed is highlighted in the chapter on latent TB (Muñoz et al.). Five chapters provide state-of-the-art coverage of clinical aspects of TB in adults (Loddenkemper et al.); children (Marais and Schaaf); management of drug-resistant TB (Seung et al.); TB HIV coinfection (Bruchfeld et al.); and TB and comorbid conditions (Bates et al.). The final chapter (Nardell) covers the importance of infection control and measures to reduce transmission in the community and in health-care facilities.

We want to thank the many people who helped make this book possible. Barbara Acosta, Senior Project Manager at Cold Spring Harbor Laboratory Press, supported us during the whole process of planning and preparation of the book. Mary Louise Grossman (Max Planck Institute for Infection Biology) supported Professor Kaufmann during editorial work, and Adam Zumla (UCL School of Pharmacy) kindly provided Professor Zumla with technical assistance.

STEFAN H.E. KAUFMANN
ERIC J. RUBIN
ALIMUDDIN ZUMLA

References

Deleboe FS. 1679. *Opera medica*. Danielum Elsevirium et Abrahamum Wolfgang, Amstelodami.

Kaufmann SH, Parida SK. 2007. Changing funding patterns in tuberculosis. *Nat Med* **13**: 299–303.

Kaufmann SHE, Britton WJ, eds. 2008. *Handbook of tuberculosis: Immunology and cell biology*, Vol. 2. Wiley-VCH, Weinheim, Germany.

Kaufmann SHE, Rubin E, eds. 2008. *Handbook of tuberculosis: Molecular biology and biochemistry*, Vol. 1. Wiley-VCH, Weinheim, Germany.

Kaufmann SHE, van Helden PD, eds. 2008. *Handbook of tuberculosis: Clinics, diagnostics, therapy, epidemiology*, Vol. 3. Wiley-VCH, Weinheim, Germany.

Koch R. 1882. Die Aetiologie der Tuberculose (Nach einem in der physiologischen Gesellschaft zu Berlin am 24.März gehaltenem Vortrage). *Berliner Klin Wochenschr* **19**: 221–230.

Moran M, Guzman J, Chapman N, Abela-Oversteegen L, Howard R, Farrell P, Luxford J, Finder JG. 2013. *Neglected disease research and development: The public divide. Global funding of innovation for neglected diseases.* Policy Cures, Sydney.

Schaaf HS, Zumla A. 2009. *Tuberculosis—A comprehensive clinical reference.* Saunders Elsevier, London.

Schönlein JL. 1841. *Allgemeine und specielle Pathologie und Therapie*, Vol. 3. Literatur-Comtoir, St. Gallen.

Waksman SA. 1964. *The conquest of tuberculosis.* University of California Press, Berkeley.

WHO. 1993. WHO declares tuberculosis a global emergency [press release]: 4-23-1993. *WHO/31.*

WHO. 2013. *Global tuberculosis report 2013.* WHO Press, Geneva.

Zumla A, Schaaf HS. 2011. *Tuberculosis.* Elsevier, London.

Cell-Autonomous Effector Mechanisms against *Mycobacterium tuberculosis*

John D. MacMicking

Department of Microbial Pathogenesis, Yale University School of Medicine, New Haven, Connecticut 06510
Correspondence: john.macmicking@yale.edu

Few pathogens run the gauntlet of sterilizing immunity like *Mycobacterium tuberculosis* (*Mtb*). This organism infects mononuclear phagocytes and is also ingested by neutrophils, both of which possess an arsenal of cell-intrinsic effector mechanisms capable of eliminating it. Here *Mtb* encounters acid, oxidants, nitrosylating agents, and redox congeners, often exuberantly delivered under low oxygen tension. Further pressure is applied by withholding divalent Fe^{2+}, Mn^{2+}, Cu^{2+}, and Zn^{2+}, as well as by metabolic privation in the form of carbon needed for anaplerosis and aromatic amino acids for growth. Finally, host E3 ligases ubiquinate, cationic peptides disrupt, and lysosomal enzymes digest *Mtb* as part of the autophagic response to this particular pathogen. It is a testament to the evolutionary fitness of *Mtb* that sterilization is rarely complete, although sufficient to ensure most people infected with this airborne bacterium remain disease-free.

Cells constitute the basic unit in biology. They safeguard and transmit genetic information, exchange gases, assimilate nutrients, and compartmentalize their enzymatic machinery to concentrate activities that share a common function. Beyond these servoregulatory duties, cells also deploy host defense factors to monitor their structural integrity and protect their inner sanctity from infection by the outside world. This universal system of self-defense is known as cell-autonomous immunity (Beutler et al. 2006; Kim et al. 2012a; MacMicking 2012; Randow et al. 2013).

Cell-autonomous immunity operates across all three domains of life where it defends against facultative and obligate intracellular pathogens (Randow et al. 2013). It is particularly effective against microorganisms engaged in accidental or fleeting interactions with their host; however, durable pathogens necessitate multiple intracellular defense programs to overcome microbial counterstrategies (Staskawicz et al. 2001). One such example is *Mycobacterium tuberculosis* (*Mtb*), the causative agent of tuberculosis (TB). It survives much of the microbicidal onslaught triggered inside human phagocytes via numerous adaptive and exaptative mechanisms (MacMicking 2008). These mechanisms reflect a close and long-standing association with its host. Indeed, paleogenetic evidence suggests *Mtb* has evolved alongside as well as within humans for at least 70,000 years (Comas et al. 2013).

Such tactics currently enable *Mtb* to persist within an estimated third of the world's populace. Here it causes disease in ~10% of people infected. For the remaining 90% of cases, how-

Cite this article as *Cold Spring Harb Perspect Med* doi: 10.1101/cshperspect.a018507

ever, host immunity likely contains and, in some cases, naturally eradicates *Mtb* (McKinney et al. 2001; Cobat et al. 2009). Autopsy studies conducted in the preantibiotic era, for example, found pulmonary lesions were often sterilized in latently infected individuals dying of nontuberculous causes (see McKinney et al. 2001 and references therein). Similar outcomes were recently reported for cynomolgus macaques (Lin et al. 2014), which together with Metchnikoff's original observations in rat macrophages and Lurie's classic studies of inbred rabbits encapsulate the idea that mycobactericidal activities may exist across several mammalian species (Metchnikoff 1905; Lurie 1964). How microbial killing is enacted and what molecular mechanisms are used for *Mtb* clearance or stasis remain central questions in mycobacterial pathogenesis. Potential antitubercular mechanisms are discussed below.

CELL-AUTONOMOUS DEFENSE AGAINST *Mtb*

Constitutive versus Inducible Programs

A basal repertoire of host defense factors provide some measure of protection against *Mtb*; however, resistance is often more effective in cells preactivated by cytokine or Toll-like receptor (TLR) signaling (Fig. 1). Here multiple defense genes are induced within 0.5–6 h of stimulation (MacMicking 2012). Notably, the order of activation and infection appears critical, because resting or naïve macrophages infected before immune stimulation allows *Mtb* time to interfere with host signaling events such as STAT1 binding its transcriptional coactivators, CBP and p300 (Ting et al. 1999), or blocking PI3K-dependent trafficking (Vergne et al. 2003). Both are needed to inhibit mycobacterial replication.

Likewise, the magnitude and success of cell-autonomous immunity depends on which immunoreceptor is engaged. Stimulating C-type lectin receptors dectin-1 or Mincle with *Mtb* mannosylated lipoarabinomannan or trehelose dimycolate, respectively, induces a limited defense repertoire that fails to control the pathogen (Ishikawa et al. 2009; Betz et al. 2011; Marakalala et al. 2011; Das et al. 2013; Heitmann et al. 2013). In contrast, activation with interferon-γ (IFN-γ) or tumor necrosis factor-α (TNF-α), elicits hundreds of genes that can curtail mycobacterial growth (Ehrt et al. 2001; Nau et al. 2002; Tailleux et al. 2008; Vogt and Nathan 2011).

Mtb-dependent signaling further enriches the host defense repertoire, either through direct transcription of effector genes by pattern-recognition receptor (PRR) ligation or after autocrine TNF-α and interleukin-1 beta (IL-1β) signaling (Ehrt et al. 2001; Nau et al. 2002; Vogt and Nathan 2011). Human monocytes and mouse macrophages regulate approximately 300–700 genes within 12–24 h of *Mtb* exposure (Ehrt et al. 2001; Ragno et al. 2001; Nau et al. 2002). Similar transcriptional plasticity occurs in human alveolar macrophages (AMs) and dendritic cells (Tailleux et al. 2008). This expression profile may reach as many as 1300 genes when IFN-γ is also present (Ehrt et al. 2001). Thus *Mtb* plus classical Th1 cytokines like IFN-γ are potent synergistic stimuli for remodeling the transcriptome of phagocytic cells. In combination they enlarge the suite of host proteins available for cell-autonomous defense, a recurring theme for many inducible programs directed against major human pathogens (MacMicking 2012). Indeed, resistance is most effective when multiple activating stimuli are present, consistent with the idea that a single stimulus may be necessary although not always sufficient to eradicate *Mtb* (Shi et al. 2003; Fabri et al. 2011; Vogt and Nathan 2011).

IFN-γR-Induced Programs

Discovery of IFN-γ as the principal macrophage-activating factor (Nathan et al. 1983, 1984; Pace et al. 1983) soon led to reports of its effectiveness against *Mtb* in monotypic cell culture (Rook et al. 1986a; Flesch and Kaufmann 1987). These in vitro activities likely operate in vivo given loss-of-function mutations in the IFN-γ signaling cascade confer profound susceptibility to *Mtb* and, more commonly, disseminated nontuberculous mycobacteriosis in both humans and mice (Cooper et al. 1993; Flynn et al. 1993; Casanova and Abel 2002). A congenital syndrome termed Mendelian sus-

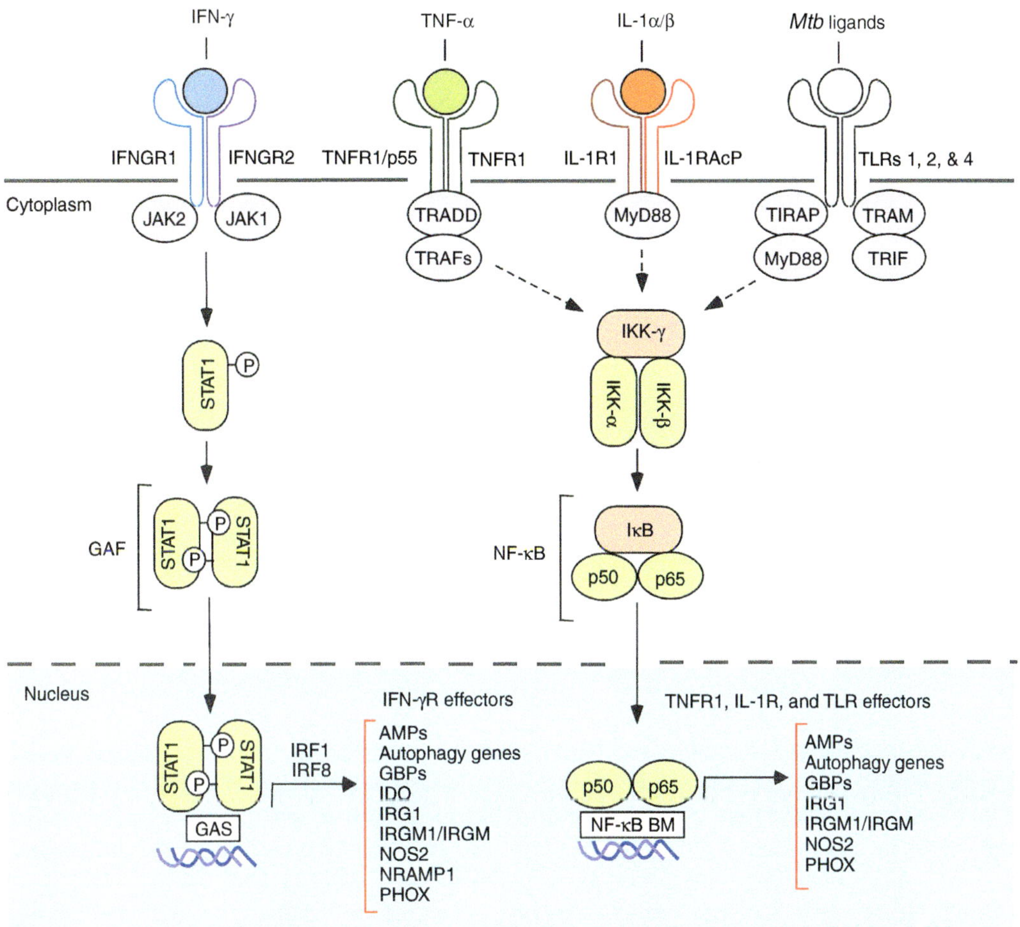

Figure 1. Immunoreceptor signaling for mobilizing the major cell-autonomous effector programs against *Mtb*. In addition, new NLR, VDR-, and P2XR-induced activities are emerging (see text). *Mtb* ligands that elicit TLR signaling include mannosylated lipoarabinomann, phosphatidylinositol mannosides (PIMs), and the 19-kDa lipoprotein. These pathways synergize to induce distinct as well as overlapping signatures of effector proteins for bacterial restriction as shown. For schematic simplicity, receptors are depicted as single chains instead of their trimeric, tetrameric, and heteromeric forms (especially in the case of the TLRs). Adaptor and transcription factor abbreviations: IRF, interferon regulatory factor; JAK, Janus kinase; NF-κB BM, NF-κB binding motif; STAT1, signal transducer and activator of transcription 1; TIRAP, toll-interleukin 1 receptor (TIR) domain containing adaptor protein; TRADD, tumor necrosis factor receptor type 1–associated DEATH domain; TRAF, TNF receptor–associated factor; TRAM, TRIF-related adaptor molecule; TRIF, TIR-domain-containing adapter-inducing interferon-β.

ceptibility to mycobacterial disease (MSMD) reveals impaired antimycobacterial immunity in patients with hypomorphic or nullizygous *IFNGR*, *STAT1*, and *IRF8* alleles, as do mutations in loci that encode IFN-induced effectors such as *ISG15* or *CYBB* (Zhang et al. 2008; Bustamante et al. 2011; Hambleton et al. 2011; Bogunovic et al. 2012).

Genetic lesions in the IFN-γ signaling cascade provide strong support for its role in antitubercular defense. Pharmacologic complementation further reinforces it. Here aerosolized recombinant IFN-γ can alleviate bacillary burdens in patients with antibiotic-resistant *Mtb* strains and mobilize bacteriostatic programs in human alveolar macrophages ex vivo

(Condos et al. 1997; Bonecini-Almeida et al. 1998). Concordant results are seen in long-term differentiated human PBMCs activated with IFN-γ under low physiologic oxygen (5%–10%) that may begin to approach hypoxic conditions found in some pulmonary and extrapulmonary tissue granulomas (Vogt and Nathan 2011). Importantly, the tuberculostatic activities of IFN-γ can be augmented by other stimuli. These include TNF superfamily members (TNF-α, CD40L), IL-1R/TLR, and NLR (NOD-like receptor) agonists or bioactive metabolites such as vitamin D_3 (Fabri et al. 2011; Vogt and Nathan 2011; Pilli et al. 2012; Jayaraman et al. 2013; Klug-Micu et al. 2013). Their synergistic effects are discussed below.

TNFR-Induced Programs

Besides their crucial role in granuloma formation (Flynn et al. 1995; Bean et al. 1999), members of the TNF superfamily directly stimulate cell-autonomous immunity to help contain *Mtb* (Chan et al. 1992; Klug-Micu et al. 2013). TNF-α enhances IFN-γ-induced macrophage programming for *Mtb* clearance, a synergy which provides several advantages: (1) diversifying the host gene repertoire through alternate transcription factor usage; (2) heightened gene expression from promoters harboring transcription factor-binding sites for both pathways; and (3) lowering the immune activation threshold, a change brought about by shared preexisting components (Fig. 1). This latter point is especially germane given the relative paucity of IFNGRs (4000–12,000/$cell^{-1}$) on the human macrophage surface (Pace et al. 1983; Finbloom et al. 1985). TNFR1 is likewise expressed at low levels for capturing soluble TNF-α to restrict *Mtb* growth rather than the nonprotective TNFR2 isoform that instead engages membrane-bound ligand (Jayaraman et al. 2013).

The other two benefits of this synergy emerge when regulation of the antitubercular enzyme, inducible nitric oxide synthase (NOS2), is considered (Chan et al. 1992; MacMicking et al. 1997a; Bekker et al. 2001; Nathan 2006). *NOS2* transcription requires IFN-γ-induced STAT1 binding to γ-activated sites (GASs) that is increased by NF-κB docking to its own sites within the *NOS2* promoter after TNF-α or lipoarabinomannan stimulation (MacMicking et al. 1997a; Chan et al. 2001. In addition, TNF-α elicits GTP cyclohydrolase 1 that furnishes tetrahydrobiopterin (BH_4) as an essential cofactor for NOS2 catalysis and induces argininosuccinate synthetase 1 and cationic amino acid transporter 2 (CAT-2) to regenerate and import the NOS2 substrate, L-arginine, respectively (Bogdan 2001; Qualls et al. 2012). Thus cooperation between TNF-α and IFN-γ regulates transcriptional and posttranslational events for antitubercular defense at the level of the individual cell.

Macrophage reprogramming by another TNF superfamily member, CD40L, also impacts *Mtb* survival. Human monocytes stimulated with CD40L, alone or in combination with IFN-γ, induce CYP27b1-hydroxylase, which converts the vitamin D_3 precursor, 25-hydroxyvitamin D_3 ($25D_3$), into bioactive 1,25-dihydroxyvitamin D ($1{,}25D_3$) (Klug-Micu et al. 2013). Subsequent 1,25D binding to the vitamin D receptor (VDR) elicits antimicrobial peptide expression and autophagy, both potent effector mechanisms targeting mycobacterial replication (Thoma-Uszynski et al. 2001; Gutierrez et al. 2004; Liu et al. 2006, 2007; Singh et al. 2006; Yuk et al. 2009; Ponpuak et al. 2010; Fabri et al. 2011; Pilli et al. 2012).

IL-1R-, TLR-, and NLR-Induced Programs

Members of the IL-1/TLR family stimulate distinct intracellular programs following cognate ligand interaction to combat TB. For IL-1 receptor (IL-1R) signaling, both IL-1β and IL-1α limit mycobacterial growth in murine macrophages via a MyD88-dependent pathway (Jayaraman et al. 2013). A similar IL-1β-dependent profile emerges within human monocyte-derived macrophages. Here IL-1β up-regulates TNFR1 and promotes autocrine signaling via TNF-α release, along with caspase 3–dependent apoptosis (Jayaraman et al. 2013). IL-1β can also elicit autophagic killing via a Tank-binding kinase-1 (TBK-1)-dependent pathway (Pilli et al. 2012), suggesting multiple effectors are deployed downstream of IL-1R to restrict *Mtb* growth. Such effects presumably operate within intact hosts because IL-1β- and IL-1R1-deficient mice display marked vulnerability to aerogenic *Mtb* challenge (Mayer-Barber et al. 2010).

Like the IL-1R cascade, TLRs 1, 2, and 4 mobilize multiple effectors as part of the antitubercular arsenal. Engagement of TLR1/TLR2 heterodimers with the 19-kDa *Mtb*-derived lipoprotein promotes a novel NOS2- and TNF-independent pathway in human macrophages, whereas the same lipopeptide induces a NOS2-dependent mechanism in mouse cells (Thoma-Uszynski et al. 2001). This novel human pathway involves CYP27b1-hydroxylase to produce $1,25D_3$ for binding the VDR, which in turn elicits cathelicidin (hCAP-18/LL-37) and defensin-4 (DEF4) antimicrobial peptides for tuberculostasis (Liu et al. 2006, 2007). Because the latter cascade also induces autophagy, it may overlap with signals provided by IFN-γ, CD40, and IL-1β at a common juncture downstream (Fabri et al. 2011; Klug-Micu et al. 2013).

Autophagic clearance of *Mtb* invoked by TLR4 stimulation in human and mouse macrophages requires TRIF (Toll-interleukin-1 receptor domain-containing adaptor-inducing interferon-β) adaptor signaling, unlike IL-1β that relies on MyD88 (Xu et al. 2007). Use of a different adaptor helps widen the TLR transcriptional response to encompass IRF3-dependent genes. In humans, genetic mapping has unearthed numerous *TLR4* SNPs that segregate with TB in ethnically diverse subjects, suggesting this TLR4-TRIF pathway operates across a broad swathe of the global population (Velez et al. 2009; Shah et al. 2012). Genetic TB associations have also been noted for TLRs 1 and 2 along with their signaling adaptors (Hawn et al. 2006; Thuong et al. 2007).

Recent studies have shown members of the NLR family may mobilize intracellular immunity to control *Mtb* growth. NOD2 detects muramyl dipeptide (MDP) that is *N*-glycolylated in mycobacteria to elicit TNF-α secretion as part of the defense profile in mouse macrophages (Coulombe et al. 2009). Human AMs stimulated with MDP also elicit IL-1β and TNF-α plus the antimicrobial peptide cathelicidin and autophagy-related defense protein, immunity-related GTPase M (IRGM) (Juárez et al. 2012). Here MDP promotes IRGM, ATG16L, and LC3B recruitment to *Mtb* phagosomes, suggesting NOD2 signaling governs both transcriptional and autophagic defense to this pathogen. Gain-of-function *NLRP3* and *CARD8* mutations cooperatively limit *Mtb* in human macrophages (Eklund et al. 2014). Hence several NLRs and related adaptors contribute to bacterial restriction within infected cells.

VDR- and P_2XR-Induced Programs

Besides classical cytokine and PRR signaling, two other inducible programs deserve mention within the context of cell-autonomous immunity to *Mtb*: VDR and purinergic receptor signaling. Early studies reported that $1,25D_3$ was crucial for IFN-γ-induced tuberculostasis in human macrophages; this effect was attributed to $1,25D_3$ promoting macrophage differentiation (Rook et al. 1986b; Crowle et al. 1987). Subsequent work, however, has delineated a circuitry whereby CYP27b1-hydroxylase expression and $1,25D_3$ production are induced by IL-15 following IFN-γ or TLR1/2 stimulation (Fabri et al. 2011). VDR signaling in turn elicits cathelicidin to activate Beclin-1 and Atg5 for autophagosomal capture of mycobacteria (Yuk et al. 2009). Such activities may impact TB outcomes in people because lower levels of serum 1,25D correlate with susceptibility, with *VDR* disease-related polymorphisms in linkage for some African and Asian populations (Bellamy et al. 1999; Wilkinson et al. 2000).

ATP-dependent stimulation of P2 purinergic receptor subtypes has likewise been strongly implicated in macrophage-mediated *Mtb* killing. In human macrophages, P2X7 activates cytosolic Ca^{2+} release and phospholipase D for maturation of *Mtb* phagosomes (Kusner and Adams 2000; Fairbairn et al. 2001; Kusner and Barton 2001). Subtypes other than P2X7, however, appear to stimulate NOS2-mediated killing in murine cells (Sikora et al. 1999). Because a number of *P2X7R* polymorphisms associate with TB susceptibility in the human population, this pathway likely influences disease development in its natural setting (Fernando et al. 2007; Sharma et al. 2010; Areeshi et al. 2013).

In sum, multiple receptors induce intracellular programs to protect the host cell from *Mtb* infection. These signals originate from IFN-γR, TNFR, IL-1R, TLR, NLR, VDR, and P2XR complexes after ligand binding primarily at the plasma membrane or in the cytosol. How their downstream effectors subsequently operate and the mechanisms they deploy are discussed below.

CELL-AUTONOMOUS ARSENAL FOR DEFENSE AGAINST *Mtb*

Cytotoxic Gases: Reactive Oxygen Species and Nitrogen-Centered Free-Radical Species

Production of cytotoxic gases is a major component of antimicrobial arsenals in all aerobic organisms (Nathan and Shiloh 2000). Reactive oxygen species (ROS) and nitrogen-centered free-radical species (RNS) show distinct chemical properties—oxidizing power, penetrative diffusion limits, lipophilicity—well-suited for killing a variety of facultative bacteria including *Mtb* (Klebanoff 1999; Nathan and Shiloh 2000). ROS and RNS typically possess low Stokes radii, are highly lipophilic, and electroneutral; thus they are small enough to bypass structural barriers that impede the access of larger host macromolecules and sufficiently permeable to diffuse across the bacterial membrane (Klebanoff 1999). Other chemical properties, notably extended diffusion limits for some RNS, allow them to protect neighboring cells (MacMicking 2012). Carbon monoxide (CO) has also been recently touted as an emerging bactericidal agent, although whether it is generated in sufficient amounts to act as a genuine mycobacterial poison in addition to its role as a sensory cue (Shiloh et al. 2008) has yet to be determined.

Oxidant Stress

Aerobic organisms use allotropic dioxygen as a substrate for generating superoxide $\left(O_2^-\right)$ via oxidoreductases and as a by-product of electron (e^-) transport in mitochondria to combat infection (Klebanoff 1999; MacMicking 2012). Single e^- additions yield, respectively, hydrogen peroxide (H_2O_2) and the hydroxyl radical (OH·), both powerful oxidants capable of damaging mycobacterial DNA, lipids, and hemoproteins (Chan et al. 1992; Nathan and Shiloh 2000; Vilchèze et al. 2013). Moreover, within phagolysosomes, elevated levels of O_2^- (Podinovskaia et al. 2013) undergo spontaneous dismutation at low pH to generate H_2O_2 that enhances lysosomal killing. Hypochlorous acid ($HOCl^-$) produced by myeloperoxidase-catalyzed oxidation of chloride by H_2O_2 in neutrophils could also target *Mtb* internalized from infected macrophages (Yang et al. 2012). Here *Mtb* expresses methionine sulfate reductases that may partly mitigate this damage (Lee et al. 2009). Indeed, *Mtb* detoxifying enzymes (e.g., catalases, SODs, peroxiredoxins) limit the overall effectiveness of ROS as a sole agent that could regain toxicity when other bactericidal agents help disable these antioxidant systems.

Large quantities of ROS are produced within phagocytic cells via the NADPH oxidase 2 (NOX2) isoform encoding the flavocytochrome$_{b558}$ heavy chain subunit (gp91^{phox}; *CYBB* gene) of the phagocyte oxidase, which generates the respiratory burst (Nathan and Shiloh 2000; MacMicking 2012) (Fig. 2). Congenital X-linked *CYBB* mutations lead to recurrent TB and "BCG-osis" in patients with defects preferentially manifest in macrophages rather than monocytes or granulocytes (Bustamante et al. 2011). Additional mutations in other NADPH oxidase subunits yield a collective syndrome—chronic granulomatous disease (CGD)—that also appears to predispose to TB (Lau et al. 1998). *Mtb* susceptibility is less pronounced in mice with targeted disruptions in either gp91^{phox} or gp47^{phox} subunits (Adams et al. 1997; Cooper et al. 2000); however, relative vulnerability increases when *Mtb* mutants lacking *KatG* are used, reinforcing the importance of pathogen detoxification systems (Ng et al. 2004).

NADPH oxidase is composed of two membrane-associated (gp91^{phox}, p22^{phox}) and three cytosolic subunits (p67^{phox}, p47^{phox}, p40^{phox}). IFN-γ increases gp91^{phox} and p22^{phox} mRNA transcription and promotes NADPH oxidase

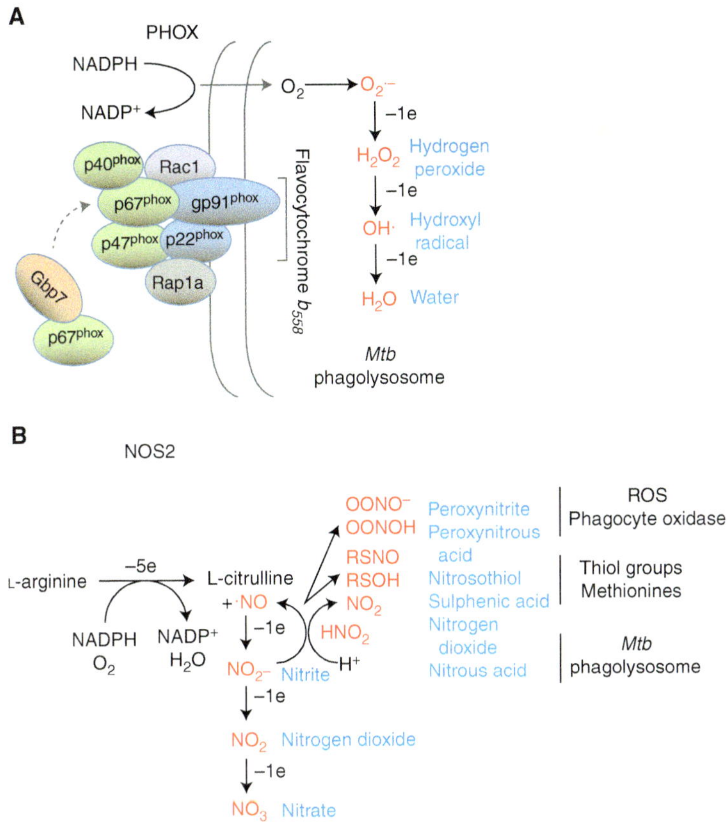

Figure 2. Oxidative and nitrosative defense against *Mtb.* (*A*) Multisubunit complex of the phagocyte oxidase (NADPH oxidase) depicting the core membrane (gp91^{phox}, p22^{phox}; known as flavocytochrome b_{558}) and cytosolic (p67^{phox}, p47^{phox}, p40^{phox}) components. Also shown are immune (Gbp7) and nonimmune GTPases (Rac1, Rap1a) that regulate trafficking to the *Mtb* phagosome for membrane anchorage as well as complex assembly. The product superoxide (O_2^-) and oxidant derivatives are shown in red font. (*B*) Enzymatic production of nitric oxide (·NO) via 5-electron oxidation of the guanidino nitrogen of L-arginine by inducible nitric oxide synthase 2. Downstream intermediates or congeners are shown in red font.

assembly on mycobacterial phagosomes (Kim et al. 2011). An IFN-γ-induced GTPase, guanylate binding protein 7 (Gbp7), facilitates this assembly by recruiting cytosolic p67^{phox}-p47^{phox} heterodimers to gp91^{phox}-p22^{phox} membrane complexes surrounding the pathogen compartment (Kim et al. 2011, 2012) (Fig. 2). Whether natural mutations in this or other members of the human GBP family induced during TB (Berry et al. 2010; Maertzdorf et al. 2011) are linked to disease is a topic for future investigation.

TNF-induced ROS has also recently emerged in zebrafish models of TB (Roca and Ramakrishnan 2013). RIP1-RIP3 signaling elicits its microbicidal activity that if left unabated can induce macrophage necroptosis for subsequent dissemination of bacilli. Notably, the primary source of ROS in this setting was mitochondria (Roca and Ramakrishnan 2013). It will therefore be interesting to see if mitochondrial ROS plays a defining role against *Mtb* like its reported anti-*Salmonella* activities (West et al. 2011).

Nitrosative Stress

RNS are a second class of oxidants capable of potent tuberculocidal activity. As little as 90 ppm of nitric oxide (·NO) gas—approaching the exhaled concentrations found for some TB patients (Wang et al. 1998)—kills >99% of plated organisms (Long et al. 1999). ·NO shows molar potencies approaching many of the current antibiotics used to treat TB, and the tuberculocidal activity of some new drugs like bicyclic nitroimidazoles are ascribed to release of ·NO (Singh et al. 2008). Because it is a water- and lipid-soluble diatomic gas, ·NO traverses biologic membranes to react with O_2^- or other ROS to yield stable nontoxic anions $\left(NO_2^-, NO_3^-\right)$ as well as intermediates with marked bactericidal properties. The latter include unstable dinitrogen oxides (N_2O_3, N_2O_4), compound peroxides ($ONOO^-$), and nitrosothiol adducts (RSNO) (Yu et al. 1999; Venketaraman et al. 2005) (Fig. 2).

Within acidified phagolysosomes, ·NO equivalents can be retrieved from stably oxidized forms (e.g., NO_2^-) by protonation to HNO_2 and subsequent dismutation (Nathan and Shiloh 2000) (Fig. 2). Indeed, acidified $NaNO_2$ was one of the earliest compounds used to show a tuberculostatic role for ·NO (Chan et al. 1992). Along with other RNS, ROS, and hypoxia, ·NO is sensed by *Mtb* to mobilize the dormancy regulon, underscoring the environmental pressure applied by both nitrosative and oxidative stress within tissue granulomas (Schnappinger et al. 2003; Voskuil et al. 2003). RNS-mediated growth arrest may also involve nitrogenous products from *Mtb* itself: Reduction of nitrate $\left(NO_3^-\right)$ by the bacterial *narG* system yields nitrite $\left(NO_2^-\right)$ that inhibits ATP consumption and induces a transcriptomic profile distinct from the ·NO dormancy regulon in human macrophages (Cunningham-Bussel et al. 2013).

The chief phagocytic source of RNS is the dimeric flavoenzyme, NOS2, which catalyzes the $5e^-$ oxidation of L-arginine to L-citrulline plus ·NO (MacMicking et al. 1997a) (Fig. 2). Robust NOS2 expression is elicited via cytokine (notably IFN-γ, TNF-α, IL-1β) and microbial-based PRR signals (e.g., lipopeptides), although its induction in human monocytes may be more complex. Some human cells require at least three combined stimuli—IFN-γ, TNF-α, and IL-1β—to produce a relatively weak response caused by STAT1 and NF-κB acting at some distance (~5–8 Kb) from the transcriptional start site (Ganster et al. 2001). Limited availability of the NOS2 cofactor, BH_4, may also contribute to the generally lower RNS production of human versus rodent phagocytes in cell culture (Bertholet et al. 1999).

Priming signals or cofactors that may be missing in vitro nonetheless appear present in vivo because robust NOS2 expression within *Mtb* granulomas is observed and macrophages isolated from inflamed lungs or peripheral blood of TB patients, or AMs from healthy donors subsequently infected with *Mtb*ex vivo, produce mycobactericidal amounts of ·NO (Nicholson et al. 1996; Fachetti et al. 1999; Dlugovitzky et al. 2000; Means et al. 2001; Wang et al. 2001; Choi et al. 2002; Mattila et al. 2013). Thus NOS2 is likely to be active under native TB settings. Other evidence supporting an in vivo role for RNS includes *NOS2* loss-of-function mutations or use of NOS inhibitors that lead to acute susceptibility in experimental mouse and zebrafish models (Chan et al. 1995; MacMicking et al. 1997b, 2003; Flynn et al. 1998; Mogues et al. 2001; Scanga et al. 2001; Cambier et al. 2014). Finally, the acquisition of *Mtb* resistance proteins, including NoxR1, NoxR3, alkyl hydroperoxide reductase (AhpC), peptidyl methionine sulphoxide reductase (MsrA), dihydrolipoamide dehydrogenase (Lpd), and dihydrolipoamide succinyl-transferase (SucB), also suggest RNS have impacted the evolutionary course of TB (Nathan and Shiloh 2000; St. John et al. 2001; Bryk et al. 2002; Nathan 2012).

Acid Exposure and Lysosomal Killing

Acid as an antimicrobial defense was first proposed by Metchnikoff using litmus dyes on infected guinea pig macrophages (Metchnikoff 1905) and gained credence from two early observations: (1) that activated phagocytes acidify their phagolysosomes (Rous 1925), and (2) that achlorhydric hosts permit colonization of the stomach (Giannella et al. 1973).

For *Mtb*, additional evidence came from its marked sensitivity to pH < 6.5 in axenic media with growth arrest at pH 5.0, especially when examined under hypoxic or microaerophilic conditions (Chapman and Bernard 1962; Tan et al. 2010). Whether protonation itself or other components (e.g., low divalent cation concentrations) contribute to this axenic attenuation is unknown (Jackett et al. 1978; Chan et al. 1992; Piddington et al. 2000; Vandal et al. 2008). *Mtb* has evolved periplasmic mechanisms such as Rv3176c encoding a serine protease (Vandal et al. 2008) and putative transporters that could exclude protons (H^+) acting directly on the bacterium (Pethe et al. 2004). Even so, because low pH embellishes both ROS and RNS (Fig. 2) coupled with the fact that lysosomal hydrolyses have pH optima in this range, acidification probably facilitates other tuberculocidal effectors to mediate killing inside the (auto)phagolysosomal compartment (Rohde et al. 2007).

IFN-γ- or TLR-stimulated macrophages rapidly acidify mycobacterial phagolysosomes to a pH of ~4.5–5.5, where it remains for at least 24 h (Schaible et al.1998; MacMicking et al. 2003; Vandal et al. 2008). Sustained acidification requires proton-pumping V-ATPases and enables processing of lysosomal cathepsins; both correlate with diminished *Mtb* growth (Schaible et al. 1998; Gomes et al. 1999; Ullrich et al. 1999; MacMicking et al. 2003). Agents that inhibit the V-ATPase (e.g., omeprezole) increase *Mtb* replication in human AMs and murine bone marrow–derived macrophages (Suzuki et al. 2000; MacMicking et al. 2003). Notably, the low luminal pH within phagolysosomes approaches the pK_a of nitrous acid (3.8), which may allow dismutation to ·NO and nitrogen dioxide (NO_2) as a way of reusing protonated nitrite (Vandal et al. 2009) (Fig. 2). This intraluminal RNS also overcomes phagosomal arrest normally imposed by *Mtb* and envelope lipids like trehalose dimycolate (Axelrod et al. 2008). Thus acidification cooperates with RNS to target intravacuolar *Mtb*. Low pH also promotes the activity of lysosomal proteases, lipases, glycosidases, and antimicrobial peptides—estimated at more than 200 in all (Trost et al. 2009)—that may disrupt and digest *Mtb* once it is delivered to this compartment.

Immune and Nonimmune GTPases

Delivery of *Mtb* to (auto)lysosomes relies on vesicular trafficking by immune and nonimmune GTPases. Members of the immunity-related GTPase (IRG) and GBP families orchestrate assembly of fusogenic SNARE proteins and autophagy components on mycobacterial phagosomes in IFN-γ-activated macrophages (MacMicking et al. 2003; Gutierrez et al. 2004; Singh et al. 2006; Tiwari et al. 2009; Kim et al. 2011, 2012a) (Fig. 3). Irgm1 targets the nascent phagocytic cup surrounding mycobacteria through carboxy-terminal amphipathic helical interactions with PI3,4,5P3 and PI3,4P2 generated by host lipid kinases on the plasma membrane (Tiwari et al. 2009). Once recruited, Irgm1 binds the SNARE and dynein motor adaptor, Snapin, for ATG14L-mediated endolysosomal fusion (MacMicking et al. 2003; Tiwari et al. 2009; Kim et al. 2012b). Human IRGM similarly facilitates trafficking of the autophagic machinery to *Mtb* vacuoles for lysosomal fusion and acidification (Singh et al. 2006). Such cell-autonomous activities also manifest in vivo: Irgm1$^{-/-}$ mice are profoundly susceptible to *Mtb* infection (MacMicking et al. 2003; Feng et al. 2004) (Fig. 3), and *IRGM* polymorphic variants associate with human TB in Ghanese, African American, Korean, and Chinese populations (Intemann et al. 2009; Che et al. 2010; King et al. 2011; Song et al. 2014).

For the GBPs, Gbp7 delivers antitubercular cargo in the form of NADPH oxidase to mycobacterial phagosomes for local ROS production (Kim et al. 2011) (Fig. 3). In addition, Gbp1 interacts with SQSTM1/p62 for transporting substrates that generate tuberculocidal peptides within lysosomes and Gbp1$^{-/-}$ mice are vulnerable to infection (Alonso et al. 2007; Kim et al. 2011). Last, RAB family proteins such as Rab20 recruit the Rab5 exchange factor Rabex-5 for transition to late endosomes in IFN- γ-activated macrophages infected with mycobacteria (Pei et al. 2014), and Rab8 directs TBK1-mediated autophagic clearance (Pilli et al. 2012). Together these different GTPase classes orchestrate lysosomal killing of *Mtb* following immune activation of host cells.

Ubiquitination and Autophagic Clearance

A second route to lysosomal degradation involves the detection of cytosolically exposed

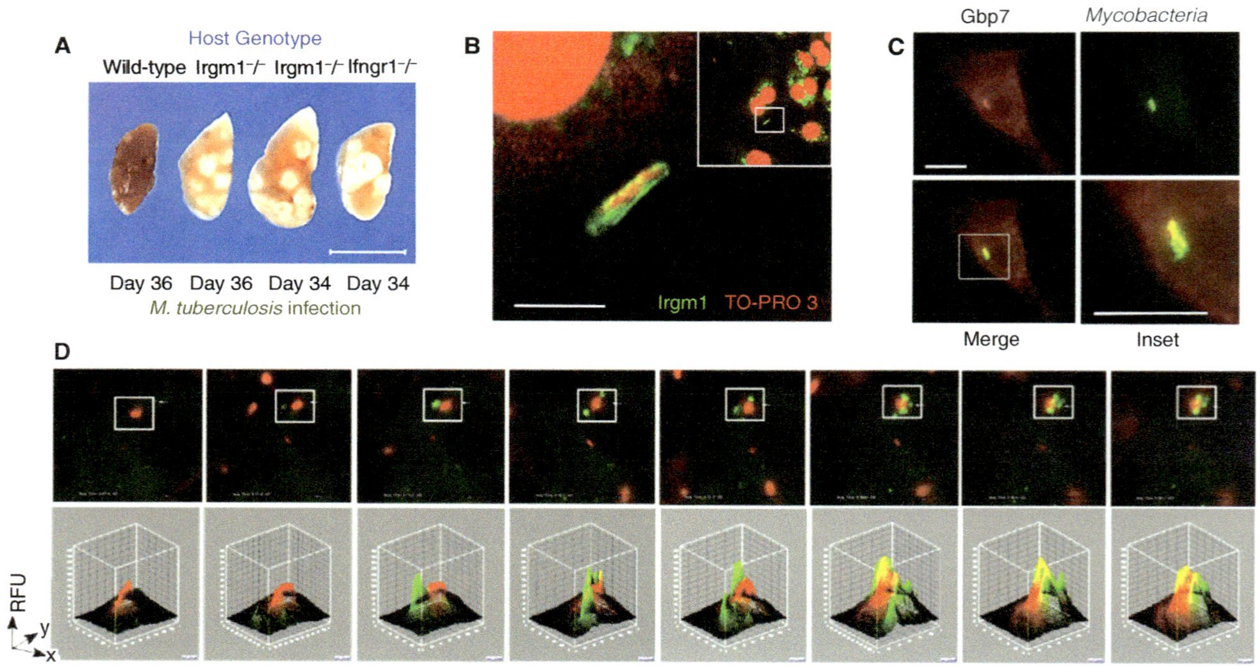

Figure 3. IFN-γ- and TLR-induced immune GTPases involved in autophagic trafficking of *Mtb* and antimicrobial cargo to lysosomes. (*A*) Deletion of the *Irgm1* gene leads to profound TB susceptibility after aerogenic challenge (MacMicking et al. 2003). Scale bar, 1.0 cm. (*B*) Targeting of endogenous Irgm1 to mycobacterial phagosomes in IFN-γ-activated macrophages. TO-PRO-3 detects nuclear and bacterial DNA. Original inset for higher magnification shown. Scale bar, 2 μm. (*C*) Recruitment of the 65-kDa guanylate binding protein, Gbp7, to mycobacterial phagosomes in IFN-γ-activated macrophages. Scale bar, 5 μm. Gbp7 helps recruit $p67^{phox}$ to assemble the phagocyte oxidase complex in this location (Kim et al. 2011). (*D*) Live imaging of Gbp7 vesicle recruitment (green) to internalized mycobacteria (red) over a 30.8-min data collection period. Image J software reveals fluorescence convergence within the chosen *inset* area (Kim et al. 2011).

Mtb and subsequent sequestration by autophagy (Stanley and Cox 2013) (Fig. 4). It has been known for some time that *Mtb* communicates with the cytosol (Myrvik et al. 1984; McDonough et al. 1993). Access to or escape into this compartment departs from the historical view of bacilli being exclusively phagosome-bound inside human macrophages (Armstrong and Hart 1971). In fact both fates probably operate within a given cell where most *Mtb* destined for lysosomal killing remain "trapped" inside vacuoles, whereas a smaller number (12%–25%) may enter the cytosol, most notably after several days of infection (see Stanley and Cox 2013 and references therein).

Rupture or permeabilization of phagosomal membranes appears to rely on the type VII secretion system ESX-1 as first shown by examining *Mtb* RD1 mutants via electron microscopy (van der Wel et al. 2007; Houben et al. 2012). Permeabilization leads to mycobacterial DNA leakage detected by cytosolic surveillance pathways including the DNA and cyclic dinucleotide sensor, STING (Manzinillo et al. 2012; Watson et al. 2012). STING activation initiates a cascade involving TBK1 that engages ubiquitin-binding receptors downstream (Watson et al. 2012) (Fig. 4). Cytosolic mycobacteria are ubiquitinated primarily on K63 chains for detection by p62/SQSTM1 and NDP52, both of which contain LC3-interacting regions (LIRs) for binding to the autophagic membrane proteins, LC3B and LC3C, respectively (von Muhlinen et al. 2012; Watson et al. 2012).

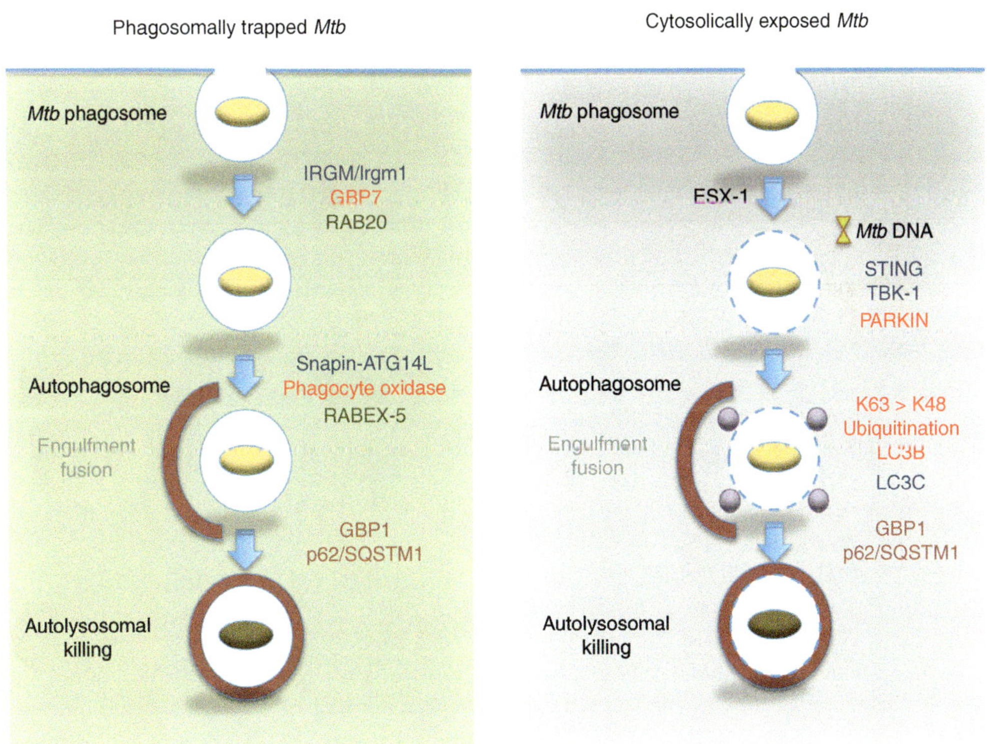

Figure 4. Differential recruitment of effectors to "trapped" and "escaped" *Mtb* in immunologically activated macrophages. (*Left*) Delivery of phagosomal bacilli to autolysosomes after autophagic capture requires both immune and nonimmune GTPases. Their position in the pathway and corresponding interacting partners are color matched. (*Right*) Cytosolically exposed bacilli following permeabilization of the phagosomal membrane by ESX-1 releases DNA for detection by STING. This recruits TBK-1 and probably LC3C for *Mtb* capture. The E3 ligase PARKIN also ubiquitinates *Mtb* directly or its surrounding membrane remnants for detection by the autophagic pathway. A preferential requirement for K63 over K48 ubiquitin linkage is reported (Manzanillo et al. 2013).

The E3 ligase, PARKIN, mediates ubiquitination and recruitment of downstream Ub receptors (Fig. 4) and PARK2-deficient mice are moderately susceptible to *Mtb* challenge (Manzanillo et al. 2013). This differs from the highly susceptible phenotype of $Atg5^{-}/^{-}$ animals, suggesting additional roles for some autophagy-related proteins (Watson et al. 2012). In this respect, SQSTM1/p62 also participates in delivering unbiquitinated substrates (e.g., ribosomal subunits) to autolysosomes for generating tuberculocidal peptides in IFN-γ-activated macrophages (Alonso et al. 2007; Ponpuak et al. 2010), a process that may require interaction with GBP1 (Kim et al. 2011). A human IRGMd isoform likewise induces mitochondrial Bax/Bak-dependent cell death during mycobacterial infection as an IFN-γ-induced mechanism distinct from its autophagic activities (Singh et al. 2010). Hence, unconventional roles may be subsumed by both autophagy-related and ubiquitin-binding proteins to confer antitubercular defense.

Antimicrobial Peptides

Antimicrobial peptides (AMPs) are evolutionarily ancient constituents of lysosomes, secretory granules, and inflammatory exudates (Ganz 2003; Zanetti 2004; Lai and Gallo 2009). At least 1700 AMPs exist in metazoans and unicellular organisms which show considerable sequence diversity (http://aps.unmc.edu/AP/). Nonetheless, AMPs share certain structural features, namely, an ∼15–30 amino acid amphipathic core composed largely of cationic and hydrophobic residues. Both features likely contribute to mycobacterial killing. Electrostatic interactions between positively charged amino acids and negatively charged *Mtb* cell wall phospholipids may provide initial contact, whereas hydrophobic residues integrate into the bacterial membrane for disruption (Ganz 2003). These features—size, amino acid composition, helical or extended loop conformations, and disulfide linkage—help classify the lytic intracellular AMPs into three major categories: α-defensins, β-defensins, and cathelicidins (Ganz 2003; Zanetti 2004; Lai and Gallo 2009).

More than 50 mammalian α-defensins, 90 β-defensins, and 30 cathelicidins are known. To date, evidence exists for β-defensins and cathelicidins in macrophage immunity to *Mtb* although neutrophil granules also kill bacilli via uncharacterized peptides (Tan et al. 2006). IFN-γ elicits β-defensin 4 and the single processed cathelicidin peptide, hCAP18/LL-37, in human macrophages to promote 1,25-dihydroxyvitamin D_3-dependent autophagic killing of tubercle bacilli (Fabri et al. 2011). In mice, IFN-γ elicits ubiquicidin-like peptides, which, when isolated from macrophage lysosomal fractions or synthetically reconstituted, kill *Mtb* at low micrometer concentrations (Alonso et al. 2007). Like the AMPs, Ub-like peptides (e.g., Ub2) have been shown to insert into the bacterial membrane to disrupt integrity and equilibrate the transmembrane potential (Foss et al. 2012).

Nutritional Immunity: Competition for Cations

Macrophages and other phagocytic cells constitute rich nutritional sources of amino acids, lipids, sugars, and transition metals. Competition for cations is one of the main contests fought between *Mtb* and its host cell with the pathogen coming well-equipped in terms of siderophores (e.g., mycobactins, exochelins) that sequester transition metals like iron (Schaible and Kaufmann 2004). Divalent zinc (Zn^{2+}), manganese (Mn^{2+}), magnesium (Mg^{2+}), and copper (Cu^{2+}) are other cations nutritionally contested within phagocytes.

Iron

Iron is essential for *Mtb* growth, although the labile pool of free ferrous form (Fe^{2+}) is low given that most Fe is complexed with transferrin, ferritin, lactoferrin, and other hemoproteins inside host cells (Schaible and Kaufmann 2004). Macrophage iron uptake proceeds via hemoglobin scavenger receptors (CD163) as well as capture via transferrin receptors (TFs) that internalize two Fe^{3+} moieties as part of the holoTF complex. Release of Fe^{3+} occurs in the endosome with which the *Mtb* phagosome intersects, thus allowing bacterial access to iron (Sturgill-Koszycki et al. 1996). IFN-γ-activated macrophages limit this availability by down-regulating TF expression and preventing accumulation of Fe^{2+} in its saturated storage form (as Fe^{3+}-holoferritin complex) within the cytosol (Byrd and Horwitz 1993; Schaible et al. 1998).

Phagosomal Fe^{2+} (as well as Mn^{2+}, Mg^{2+}, and Zn^{2+}) is concomittently lowered by approximately two- to sixfold in IFN-γ-activated macrophages infected with *Mtb* (Wagner et al. 2005), a reduction due in part to the proton-dependent Mn^{2+} and Fe^{2+} efflux pump, NRAMP1 (encoded by *SLC11A1*; Jabado et al. 2000). *Nramp1* was originally identified via positional cloning in inbred mouse strains harboring G169A variants of the *Bcg/Ity/Lsh* allele (denoting *Mycobacterium bovis* BCG, *Salmonella typhimurium*, and *Leishmania donovani* susceptibility), and *NRAMP1* polymorphisms are thought to predispose to human TB as well (see Fortin et al. 2007). NRAMP1 is a 12-transmembrane spanning protein found on lysosomes, tertiary granules (neutrophils), and phagosomes, where it aids mycobacterial killing (Jabado et al. 2000; Fortin et al. 2007). Genetic studies infer cationic competition between NRAMP1 and an *Mtb* homolog, Mramp, because Mn^{2+} and Fe^{2+} concentrations are elevated in phagosomes harboring Mramp-deficient *Mtb* (Wagner et al. 2005). Phagosomal recruitment of the Fe export protein ferriportin-1 also reduces intravacuolar iron after IFN-γ activation (Van Zandt et al. 2008), whereas lipocalin-2 directly sequesters iron to inhibit *Mtb* in macrophages, neutrophils, and airway epithelium (Martineau et al. 2007; Saiga et al. 2008; Johnson et al. 2010).

Other Cations

Magnesium, zinc, and copper are likewise sensed or used by *Mtb*; however, as with iron, high concentrations of these transitional metals are directly toxic or promote tuberculocidal ROS (Russell 2011; Samanovic et al. 2012). A requirement for Mg^{2+} in *Mtb* replication was identified under low cation and pH conditions akin to those found in the phagolysosome where bacterial growth was impaired (Piddington et al. 2000). This finding was reinforced by *Mtb* mutants lacking the *mgtC* (Mg^{2+} transporter) gene that perform poorly under the same conditions and are highly attenuated in human macrophages and mice (Buchmeier et al. 2000). For Zn^{2+}, intracellular stores are pumped into *Mtb* phagosomes via a ROS-dependent pathway to promote killing in TLR-activated macrophages (Botella et al. 2011). Here *Mtb* attempts to counter Zn^{2+} toxicity by expressing a P-type ATPase efflux transporter encoded in the *ctpC* locus (Botella et al. 2011). For Cu^{2+}, a host P-type ATPase pump ATP7A imports Cu^{2+} into the phagosome for generating intraluminal OH· radicals, which is countered to some extent by *Mtb* transport proteins CtpV and MctB (Ward et al. 2010; Wolschendorf et al. 2011; Samanovic et al. 2012). Divalent cations are thus selectively furnished or withheld to limit *Mtb* growth.

Nutritional Immunity: Carbon and Amino Acid Metabolism

ICLs and IRG1

Carbon catabolism is critical for *Mtb* survival and persistence (Muñoz-Elías and McKinney 2006). Conserving C_2 carbon during periods of nutrient restriction via anaplerosis helps maintain bacterial metabolism fueled by fatty acids. One metabolic target for cell-autonomous immunity is the *Mtb* glyoxylate shunt pathway that replenishes tricarboxylic acid (TCA) cycle intermediates normally diverted for biosynthetic purposes via successive carboxylation reactions (McKinney et al. 2000). Early work discovered a glycoxylate shunt enzyme, isocitrate lyase 1 (ICL1), was essential for *Mtb* persistence in IFN-γ-activated macrophages and mice (McKinney et al. 2000). Subsequent discovery of a second functional ICL isoform (ICL2) corroborates the strong metabolic pressure placed by cell-autonomous immunity on *Mtb* to use anaplerotic pathways (Muñoz-Elías and McKinney 2005).

The immune-responsive gene 1 (IRG1) has recently been identified as exerting part of that metabolic pressure in activated human and mouse macrophages (Michelucci et al. 2013) (Fig. 5). IRG1 is transcriptionally induced by autocrine IFN/STAT1 signaling in response to both virulent and environmental mycobacteria (Shi et al. 2005; Basler et al. 2006; Michelucci et al. 2013). Thereafter it localizes to mitochondria (DeGrandi et al. 2009), where it decarboxylates the TCA intermediate *cis*-aconitate needed for isocitrate synthesis, thus depriving ICL1 and ICL2 of their substrate to run the glyoxylate shunt (Michelucci et al. 2013) (Fig. 5). Decarboxylation of *cis*-aconitate also produces itaconic acid (alternatively known as methylenesuccinic acid) that may be directly toxic to bacilli (Michelucci et al. 2013). IRG1 could additionally promote β-oxidation-dependent mitochondrial ROS production for some of its bactericidal activities (Hall et al. 2013; Roca and Ramakrishnan 2013).

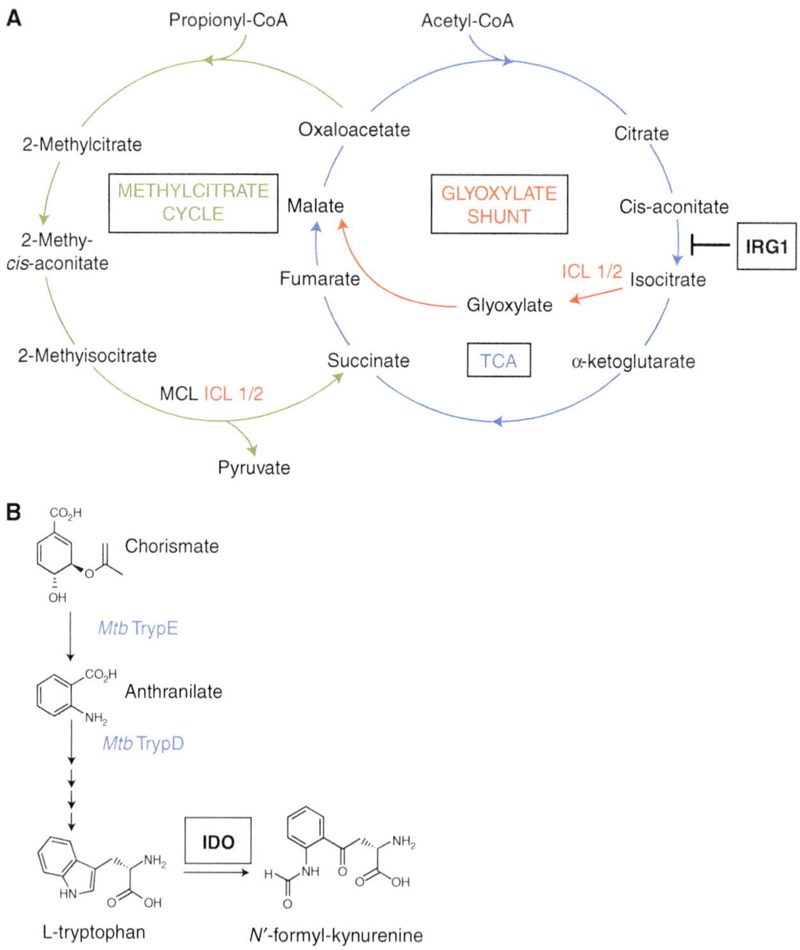

Figure 5. Nutritional immunity to *Mtb*. (*A*) Depletion of tricarboxylic acid (TCA) cycle and potential glyoxylate shunt substrates via a *cis*-aconitate decarboxylase known as immunoresponsive gene-1 (IRG1) that resides in mitochondria. Position at which IRG1 blocks anaplerotic substrate production for *Mtb* is shown. Isocitrate lyases 1 and 2 (ICL1/2) that serve as important *Mtb* anaplerotic enzymes in the glycoxylate shunt and that are the functional *Mtb* paralogs of methylcitrate lyases (MCLs) in the methylcitrate pathway (Muñoz-Elias et al. 2006) are also depicted. (Adapted from data in Michelucci et al. 2013.) (*B*) Tryptophan depletion by the IFN-γ-induced enzyme, indolamine-2,3-dioxygenase (IDO), in activated macrophages. *Mtb* genes encoding the enzymes known to be involved in generating precursors of tryptophan biosynthesis are shown in blue font.

IDO

Other effector mechanisms target the production of amino acids catabolized or assimilated by *Mtb* for its growth (Zhang and Rubin 2013). Tryptophan degradation is an effective defense against obligate bacterial pathogens like Chlamydia and protozoan parasites including *Toxoplasma* and *Leishmania* spp. (MacMicking 2012). IFN-γ induces indoleamine-2,3-dioxygenase (IDO), a heme-containing oxidoreductase responsible for the initial rate-limiting step of the kynurenine pathway in which it degrades L-tryptophan to generate *N*-formyl-kynurenine (MacMicking 2012) (Fig. 5).

Although most laboratory *Mtb* strains are not tryptophan auxotrophs and IDO inhibition does not impact their growth within IFN-γ-activated macrophages (MacMicking et al. 2003), recent use of *Mtb Trp*$^{-}$ mutants has revealed tryptophan degradation by the host does exert metabolic pressure on *Mtb* in macrophages and infected mice (Zhang et al. 2013). *Mtb* synthesizes L-tryptophan via an operon containing *TrpE*, encoding an enzyme that converts chorismate to anthranilate, and *TrpD*, which encodes a ribosylating enzyme for the substrate (Zhang et al. 2013) (Fig. 5). Deletion of *TrpE* greatly attenuates *Mtb* growth in IFN-γ-activated macrophages that is restored in IDO-1-deficient cells; a similar outcome occurs in vivo. Moreover, fluorinated anthranilate (5-FABA and 6-FABA) inhibitors that block *Mtb* tryptophan synthesis render the bacillus susceptible to IDO-mediated killing. Thus drugs targeting bacterial counterimmune mechanisms allow the corresponding host effector to regain functionality inside phagocytic cells.

CONCLUDING REMARKS

This perspective has outlined the major cell-autonomous effectors deployed against *Mtb*. Because apoptosis and autophagy are covered extensively elsewhere in this collection, they have been given limited coverage or omitted altogether in this particular article. Furthermore, the list of effectors is by no means complete. Cell-autonomous immunity typically uses all the tools at its disposal—proteins, peptides, nucleotides, cations, metabolites, and physiological gases—to defend the host against infection. Hence, it can be anticipated that new pathways and effector molecules will emerge with antitubercular defense functions. IFN-γ- or PRR-independent pathways like GM-CSF-mediated killing (Rothchild et al. 2014) and unconventional activities such as mitochondrial immunity (via ROS, IRGM1, and IRG1) or autophagic engulfment of cytosolically exposed bacilli will be fertile areas of future investigation. Once understood, these novel defense factors may join established mechanisms as a platform from which to design host-directed therapies or adjunctive treatments that more fully expose *Mtb* to killing by the human immune system (Nathan 2012; Hawn et al. 2013; Wilkinson 2014). Both offer hope for shortening treatment as well as for tackling the problem of bacterial multidrug resistance (Singh et al. 2008; Zhang et al. 2013; Stanley et al. 2014).

ACKNOWLEDGMENTS

The author acknowledges colleagues inside and outside of the laboratory plus the following funding sources for work highlighted in this perspective: National Institutes of Health/ National Institute of Allergy and Infectious Diseases (R01 AI068041–07), BWF Investigator in Pathogenesis of Infectious Disease Award (1007845), Cancer Research Institute Investigator Award Program (CRI06–10), Searle Foundation (05-F-114), and W.W. Winchester Award.

REFERENCES

Adams LB, Dinauer MC, Morgenstern DE, Krahenbuhl JL. 1997. Comparison of the roles of reactive oxygen and nitrogen intermediates in the host response to *Mycobacterium tuberculosis* using transgenic mice. *Tuber Lung Dis* **78:** 237–246.

Alonso S, Pethe K, Russell DG, Purdy GE. 2007. Lysosomal killing of *Mycobacterium* mediated by ubiquitin-derived peptides is enhanced by autophagy. *Proc Natl Acad Sci* **104:** 6031–6036.

Areeshi MY, Mandal RK, Panda AK, Haque S. 2013. Association of P2X7 A1513C (rs3751143) gene polymorphism with risk of tuberculosis: Evidence from a meta-analysis. *Genet Test Mol Biomarkers* **17:** 662–668.

Armstrong JA, Hart PD. 1971. Response of cultured macrophages to *Mycobacterium tuberculosis*, with observations on fusion of lysosomes with phagosomes. *J Exp Med* **134:** 713–740.

Axelrod S, Oschkinat H, Enders J, Schlegel B, Brinkmann V, Kaufmann SH, Haas A, Schaible UE. 2008. Delay of phagosome maturation by a mycobacterial lipid is reversed by nitric oxide. *Cell Microbiol* **10:** 1530–1545.

Basler T, Jeckstadt S, Valentin-Weigand P, Goethe R. 2006. *Mycobacterium paratuberculosis, Mycobacterium smegmatis*, and lipopolysaccharide induce different transcriptional and post-transcriptional regulation of the IRG1 gene in murine macrophages. *J Leukoc Biol* **79:** 628–638.

Bean AG, Roach DR, Briscoe H, France MP, Korner H, Sedgewick JD, Britton WJ. 1999. Structural deficiencies in granuloma formation in TNF gene-targeted mice underlie the heightened susceptibility to aerosol *Mycobacterium tuberculosis* infection, which is not compensated for by lymphotoxin. *J Immunol* **162:** 3504–3511.

Bekker LG, Freeman S, Murray PJ, Ryffel B, Kaplan G. 2001. TNF-α controls intracellular mycobacterial growth by both inducible nitric oxide synthase-dependent and inducible nitric oxide synthase-independent pathways. *J Immunol* **166:** 6728–6734.

Bellamy R, Ruwende C, Corrah R, McAdam KP, Whittle HC, Hill AV. 1999. Tuberculosis and chronic hepatitis B virus infection in Africans and variation in the vitamin D receptor gene. *J Infect Dis* **179:** 721–724.

Bertholet S, Tzeng E, Felley-Bosco E, Mauel J. 1999. Expression of inducible nitric oxide synthase in human monocytic U937 cells allows high output nitric oxide synthase. *J Leukoc Biol* **65:** 50–58

Berry MP, Graham CM, McNab FW, Xu Z, Bloch SA, Oni T, Wilkinson KA, Banchereau R, Skinner J, Wilkinson RJ, et al. 2010. An interferon-inducible neutrophil-driven blood transcriptional signature in human tuberculosis. *Nature* **466:** 973–977.

Betz BE, Azad AK, Morris JD, Rajaram MV, Schlesinger LS. 2011. β-Glucans inhibit intracellular growth of *Mycobacterium bovis* BCG but not virulent *Mycobacterium tuberculosis* in human macrophages. *Microb Pathog* **51:** 233–242.

Beutler B, Jiang Z, Georgel P, Crozat K, Croker B, Rutschmann S, Du X, Hoebe K. 2006. Genetic analysis of host resistance: Toll-like receptor signaling and immunity at large. *Annu Rev Immunol* **24:** 353–389.

Blumenthal A, Nagalingam G, Huch JH, Walker L, Guillemin GJ, Smythe GA, Ehrt S, Britton WJ, Saunders BM. 2012. *M. tuberculosis* induces potent activation of IDO-1, but this is not essential for the immunological control of infection. *PLoS ONE* **7:** e37314.

Bogdan C. 2001. Nitric oxide and the immune response. *Nat Immunol* **2:** 907–916.

Bogunovic D, Byun M, Durfee LA, Abhyankar A, Sanal O, Mansouri D, Salem S, Radovanovic I, Grant AV, Adimi P, et al. 2012. Mycobacterial disease and impaired IFN-γ immunity in humans with inherited *ISG15* deficiency. *Science* **337:** 1684–1688.

Bonecini-Almeida MG, Chitale S, Boutsikakis I, Geng J, Doo H, He S, Ho JL. 1998. Induction of *in vitro* human macrophage anti-*Mycobacterium tuberculosis* activity: Requirement for IFN-γ and primed lymphocytes. *J Immunol* **160:** 4490–4499.

Botella H, Peyron P, Levillain F, Poincloux R, Poquet Y, Brandli I, Wang C, Tailleux L, Tilleul S, Charrière GM, et al. 2011. Mycobacterial P_1-type ATPases mediate resistance to zinc poisoning in human macrophages. *Cell Host Microbe* **10:** 248–259.

Bryk R, Lima CD, Erdjument-Bromage H, Tempst P, Nathan C. 2002. Metabolic enzymes of mycobacteria linked to antioxidant defense by a thioredoxin-like protein. *Science* **295:** 1073–1077.

Byrd TF, Horwitz MA. 1993. Regulation of transferrin receptor expression and ferritin content in human mononuclear phagocytes. Coordinate upregulation by iron transferrin and downregulation by interferon γ. *J Clin Invest* **91:** 969–976.

Buchmeier N, Blanc-Polard A, Erht S, Piddington D, Riley L, Groisman EA. 2000. A parallel intraphagosomal survival strategy shared by *Mycobacterium tuberculosis* and *Salmonella enterica*. *Mol Microbiol* **35:** 1375–1382.

Bustamante J, Arias AA, Vogt G, Picard C, Galicia LB, Prando C, Grant AV, Marchal CC, Hubeau M, Chapgier A, et al. 2011. Germline *CYBB* mutations that selectively affect macrophages in kindreds with X-linked predisposition to tuberculous mycobacterial disease. *Nat Immunol* **12:** 213–221.

Cambier CJ, Takaki KK, Larson RP, Hernandez RE, Tobin DM, Urdahl KB, Cosma CL, Ramakrishnan L. 2014. Mycobacteria manipulate macrophage recruitment through coordinated use of membrane lipids. *Nature* **505:** 218–222.

Casanova J-L, Abel L. 2002. Genetic dissection of immunity to mycobacteria: The human model. *Ann Rev Immunol* **20:** 581–620.

Chan J, Xing Y, Magliozzo RS, Bloom BR. 1992. Killing of virulent *Mycobacterium tuberculosis* by reactive nitrogen intermediates produced by activated murine macrophages. *J Exp Med* **175:** 1111–1122.

Chan J, Tanaka K, Carroll D, Flynn J, Bloom BR. 1995. Effects of nitric oxide synthase inhibitors on murine infection with *Mycobacterium tuberculosis*. *Infect Immun* **63:** 736–740.

Chan ED, Morris KR, Belisle JT, Hill P, Remigio LK, Brennan PJ, Riches DW. 2001. Induction of inducible nitric oxide synthase-NO by lipoarabinomannan of *Mycobacterium tuberculosis* is mediated by MEK1-ERK, MKK7-JNK, and NFκB signaling pathways. *Infect Immun* **69:** 2001–2010.

Chapman J, Bernard J. 1962. The tolerances of unclassified mycobacteria. *Am Rev Respir Dis* **86:** 582–583.

Che N, Li S, Gao T, Zhang Z, Han Y, Zhang X, Sun Y, Liu Y, Sun Z, Zhang J, et al. 2010. Identification of a novel IRGM promoter single nucleotide polymorphism associated with tuberculosis. *Clin Chim Acta* **411:** 1645–1649.

Choi HS, Rai PR, Chu HW, Cool C, Chan ED. 2002. Analysis of nitric oxide synthase and nitrotyrosine expression in human pulmonary tuberculosis. *Am J Respir Crit Care Med* **166:** 178–186.

Cobat A, Gallant CJ, Simkin L, Black GF, Stanley K, Hughes J, Doherty TM, Hanekom WA, Eley B, Jaïs JP, et al. 2009. Two loci control tuberculin skin test reactivity in an area hyperendemic for tuberculosis. *J Exp Med* **206:** 2583–2591.

Comas I, Coscolla M, Luo T, Borrell S, Holt KE, Kato-Maeda M, Parkhill J, Malla B, Berg S, Thwaites G, et al. 2013. Out-of-Africa migration and Neolithic coexpansion of *Mycobacterium tuberculosis* with modern humans. *Nat Genet* **45:** 1176–1182.

Condos R, Rom WN, Schluger NW. 1997. Treatment of multi-drug-resistant pulmonary tuberculosis with interferon-γ via aerosol. *Lancet* **349:** 1513–1515.

Cooper AM, Dalton DK, Stewart TA, Griffin JP, Russell DG, Orme IM. 1993. Disseminated tuberculosis in interferon γ gene-disrupted mice. *J Exp Med* **178:** 2243–2247.

Cooper AM, Segal BH, Frank AA, Holland SM, Orme IM. 2000. Transient loss of resistance to pulmonary tuberculosis in $p47^{phox-/-}$ mice. *Infect Immun* **68:** 1231–1234.

Coulombe F, Divangahi M, Veyrier F, de Léséleuc L, Gleason JL, Yang Y, Kelliher MA, Pandey AK, Sassetti CM, Reed MB, et al. 2009. Increased NOD2-mediated recognition of *N*-glycolyl muramyl dipeptide. *J Exp Med* **206:** 1709–1716.

Crowle AJ, Ross EJ, May MH. 1987. Inhibition of 1,25(OH)2-vitamin D3 of the multiplication of virulent tubercle bacilli in cultured human macrophages. *Infect Immun* **55:** 2945–2950.

Cunningham-Bussel A, Zhang T, Nathan CF. 2013. Nitrite produced by *Mycobacterium tuberculosis* in human macrophages in physiologic oxygen impacts bacterial ATP consumption and gene expression. *Proc Natl Acad Sci* **110:** E4256–E4265.

Das R, Koo MS, Kim BH, Jacob ST, Subbian S, Yao J, Leng L, Levy R, Murchison C, Burman WJ, et al. 2013. Macrophage migration inhibitory factor (MIF) is a critical mediator of the innate immune response to *Mycobacterium tuberculosis*. *Proc Natl Acad Sci* **110:** E2997–E3006.

Degrandi D, Hoffmann R, Beuter-Gunia C, Pfeffer K. 2009. The proinflammatory cytokine-induced IRG1 protein associates with mitochondria. *J Interferon Cytokine Res* **29:** 55–67.

Dlugovitzky D, Bay ML, Rateni L, Fiorenza G, Vietti L, Farroni MA, Bottasso OA. 2000. Influence of disease severity on nitrite and cytokine production by peripheral blood monouclear cells (PBMC) from patients with pulmonary tuberculosis (TB). *Clin Exp Immunol* **122:** 343–349.

Eklund D, Welin A, Andersson H, Verma D, Söderkvist P, Stendahl O, Särndahl E, Lerm M. 2014. Human gene variants linked to enhanced NLRP3 activity limit intramacrophage growth of *Mycobacterium tuberculosis*. *J Infect Dis* **209:** 749–753.

Ehrt S, Schnappinger D, Bekiranov S, Drenkow J, Shi S, Gingeras TR, Gaasterland T, Schoolnik G, Nathan C. 2001. Reprogramming of the macrophage transcriptome in response to interferon-γ and *Mycobacterium tuberculosis*: Signaling roles of nitric oxide synthase-2 and phagocyte oxidase. *J Exp Med* **194:** 1123–1140.

Fabri M, Stenger S, Shin DM, Yuk JM, Liu PT, Realegeno S, Lee HM, Krutzik SR, Schenk M, Sieling PA, et al. 2011. Vitamin D is required for IFN-γ-mediated antimicrobial activity of human macrophages. *Sci Transl Med* **3:** 104ra102.

Fachetti F, Vermi W, Fiorentini S, Chilosi M, Caruso A, Duse M, Notarangelo LD, Badolato R. 1999. Expression of inducible nitric oxide synthase in human granulomas and histiocytic reactions. *Am J Path* **154:** 145–152.

Fairbairn IP, Stober CB, Kumararatne DS, Lammas DA. 2001. ATP-mediated killing of intracellular mycobacteria by macrophages is a $P2X_7$-dependent process inducing bacterial death by phagosome-lysosome fusion. *J Immunol* **167:** 3300–3307.

Feng CG, Collazo-Custodio CM, Eckhaus M, Hieny S, Belkaid Y, Elkins K, Jankovic D, Taylor GA, Sher A. 2004. Mice deficient in LRG-47 display increased susceptibility to mycobacterial infection associated with the induction of lymphopenia. *J Immunol* **172:** 1163–1168.

Fernando SL, Saunders BM, Sluyter R, Skarratt KK, Goldberg H, Marks GB, Wiley JS, Britton WJ. 2007. A polymorphism in the $P2X_7$ gene increases susceptibility to extrapulmonary tuberculosis. *Am J Respir Crit Care Med* **175:** 360–366.

Finbloom DS, Hoover DL, Wahl LM. 1985. The characteristics of binding of human recombinant interferon-γ to its receptor on human monocytes and human monocyte-like lines. *J Immunol* **135:** 300–305.

Flesch I, Kaufmann SH. 1987. Mycobacterial growth inhibition by interferon-γ activated bone marrow macrophages and differential susceptibility among strains of *Mycobacterium tuberculosis*. *J Immunol* **138:** 4408–4413.

Flynn J, Chan J, Triebold K, Dalton D, Stewart T, Bloom B. 1993. An essential role for interferon γ in resistance to *Mycobacterium tuberculosis* infection. *J Exp Med* **178:** 2249–2254.

Flynn JL, Goldstein MM, Chan J, Triebold KJ, Pfeffer K, Lowenstein CJ, Schreiber R, Mak TW, Bloom BR. 1995. Tumor necrosis factor-α is required in the protective immune response against *Mycobacterium tuberculosis* in mice. *Immunity* **2:** 561–572.

Flynn JL, Scanga CA, Tanaka KE, Chan J. 1998. Effects of aminoguanidine on latent murine tuberculosis. *J Immunol* **160:** 1796–1803.

Fortin A, Abel L, Casanova JL, Gros P. 2007. Host genetics of mycobacterial diseases in mice and men: Forward genetic studies of BCG-osis and tuberculosis. *Annu Rev Genomics Hum Genet* **8:** 163–192.

Foss MH, Powers KM, Purdy GE. 2012. Structural and functional characterization of mycobactericidal ubiquitin-derived peptides in model and bacterial membranes. *Biochemistry* **51:** 9922–9929.

Ganster RW, Taylor BS, Shao L, Geller DA. 2001. Complex regulation of human inducible nitric oxide synthase gene transcription by Stat 1 and NF-κB. *Proc Natl Acad Sci* **98:** 8638–8643.

Ganz T. 2003. Defensins: Antimicrobial peptides of innate immunity. *Nat Rev Immunol* **3:** 710–720.

Giannella RA, Broitman SA, Zamcheck N. 1973. Influence of gastric acidity on bacterial and parasitic enteric infections. *Ann Int Med* **78:** 271–276.

Gomes MS, Paul S, Moreira AL, Appelberg R, Rabinovitch M, Kaplan G. 1999. Survival of *Mycobacterium avium* and *Mycobacterium tuberculosis* in acidified vacuoles of murine macrophages. *Infect Immun* **67:** 3199–3206.

Gutierrez MG, Master SS, Singh SB, Taylor GA, Colombo MI, Deretic V. 2004. Autophagy is a defense mechanism inhibiting BCG and *Mycobacterium tuberculosis* survival in infected macrophages. *Cell* **119:** 753–766.

Hall CJ, Boyle RH, Astin JW, Flores MV, Oehlers SH, Sanderson LE, Ellett F, Lieschke GJ, Crosier KE, Crosier PS. 2013. Immunoresponsive gene 1 augments bactericidal activity of macrophage-lineage cells by regulating β-oxidation-dependent mitochondrial ROS production. *Cell Metab* **18:** 265–278.

Hambleton S, Salem S, Bustamante J, Bigley V, Boisson-Dupuis S, Azevedo J, Fortin A, Haniffa M, Ceron-Gutierrez L, Bacon CM, et al. 2011. *IRF8* mutations and human dendritic-cell immunodeficiency. *N Engl J Med* **365:** 127–138.

Hawn TR, Dunstan SJ, Thwaites GE, Simmons CP, Thuong NT, Lan NT, Quy HT, Chau TT, Hieu NT, Rodrigues S, et al. 2006. A polymorphism in Toll-interleukin 1 receptor domain containing adaptor protein is associated with susceptibility to meningeal tuberculosis. *J Infect Dis* **194:** 1127–1134.

Hawn TR, Matheson AI, Maley SN, Vandal O. 2013. Host-directed therapeutics for tuberculosis: Can we harness the host? *Microbiol Mol Biol Rev* **77:** 608–627.

Heitmann L, Schoenen H, Ehlers S, Lang R, Hölscher C. 2013. Mincle is not essential for controlling *Mycobacterium tuberculosis* infection. *Immunobiology* **218:** 506–516.

Houben D, Demangel C, van Ingen J, Perez J, Baldeón L, Abdallah AM, Caleechurn L, Bottai D, van Zon M, de Punder K, et al. 2012. ESX-1-mediated translocation to the cytosol controls virulence of mycobacteria. *Cell Microbiol* **14:** 1287–1298.

Intemann CD, Thye T, Niemann S, Browne EN, Amanua Chinbuah M, Enimil A, Gyapong J, Osei I, Owusu-Dabo E, Helm S, et al. 2009. Autophagy gene variant IRGM -261T contributes to protection from tuberculosis caused by *Mycobacterium tuberculosis* but not by *M. africanum* strains. *PLoS Pathog* **5:** e1000577.

Ishikawa E, Ishikawa T, Morita YS, Toyonaga K, Yamada H, Takeuchi O, Kinoshita T, Akira S, Yoshikai Y, Yamasaki S. 2009. Direct recognition of the mycobacterial glycolipid, trehalose dimycolate, by C-type lectin Mincle. *J Exp Med* **206:** 2879–2888.

Jabado N, Jankowski A, Dougaparsad S, Picard V, Grinstein S, Gros P. 2000. Natural resistance to intracellular infections: Natural resistance-associated macrophage protein 1 (Nramp1) functions as a pH-dependent manganese transporter at the phagosomal membrane. *J Exp Med* **192:** 1237–1248.

Jackett PS, Aber V, Lowrie DB. 1978. Virulence and resistance to superoxide, low pH and hydrogen peroxide among strains of *Mycobacterium tuberculosis*. *J Gen Microbiol* **107:** 37–45.

Jayaraman P, Sada-Ovalle I, Nishimura T, Anderson AC, Kuchroo VK, Remold HG, Behar SM. 2013. IL-1β promotes antimicrobial immunity in macrophages by regulating TNFR signaling and caspase-3 activation. *J Immunol* **190:** 4196–4204.

Johnson EE, Srikanth CV, Sandgren A, Harrington L, Trebicka E, Wang L, Borregaard N, Murray M, Cherayil BJ. 2010. Siderocalin inhibits the intracellular replication of *Mycobacterium tuberculosis* in macrophages. *FEMS Immunol Med Microbiol* **58:** 138–145.

Juárez E, Carranza C, Hernández-Sánchez F, León-Contreras JC, Hernández-Pando R, Escobedo D, Torres M, Sada E. 2012. NOD2 enhances the innate response of alveolar macrophages to *Mycobacterium tuberculosis* in humans. *Eur J Immunol* **42:** 880–889.

Kim BH, Shenoy AR, Kumar P, Das R, Tiwari S, MacMicking JD. 2011. A family of IFN-γ-inducible 65-kD GTPases protects against bacterial infection. *Science* **332:** 717–721.

Kim BH, Shenoy AR, Kumar P, Bradfield CJ, MacMicking JD. 2012a. IFN-inducible GTPases in host cell defense. *Cell Host Microbe* **12:** 432–444.

Kim HJ, Zhong Q, Sheng ZH, Yoshimori T, Liang C, Jung JU. 2012b. Beclin-1-interacting autophagy protein Atg14L targets the SNARE-associated protein Snapin to coordinate endocytic trafficking. *J Cell Sci* **125:** 4740–4750.

King KY, Lew JD, Ha NP, Lin JS, Ma X, Graviss EA, Goodell MA. 2011. Polymorphic allele of human IRGM1 is associated with susceptibility to tuberculosis in African Americans. *PLoS ONE* **6:** e16317.

Klebanoff S. 1999. Oxygen metabolites from phagocytes. In *Inflammation: Basic principles and clinical correlates*, 3rd ed (ed. Gallin JI, Snyderman R, Fearon DT, et al.), pp. 721–768. Lippincott Williams & Wilkins, Philadelphia.

Klug-Micu GM, Stenger S, Sommer A, Liu PT, Krutzik SR, Modlin RL, Fabri M. 2013. CD40 ligand and interferon-γ induce an antimicrobial response against *Mycobacterium tuberculosis* in human monocytes. *Immunology* **139:** 121–128.

Kusner DJ, Adams J. 2000. ATP-induced killing of virulent *Mycobacterium tuberculosis* within human macrophages requires phospholipase D. *J Immunol* **164:** 379–388.

Kusner DJ, Barton JA. 2001. ATP stimulates human macrophages to kill intracellular virulent *Mycobacterium tuberculosis* via calcium-dependent phagosome-lysosome fusion. *J Immunol* **167:** 3308–3315.

Lai Y, Gallo RL. 2009. AMPed up immunity: How antimicrobial peptides have multiple roles in immune defense. *Trends Immunol* **30:** 131–141.

Lau YL, Chan CF, Ha SY, Hui YF, Yuen KY. 1998. The role of phagocytic respiratory burst in host defense against *Mycobacterium tuberculosis*. *Clin Infect Dis* **26:** 226–227.

Lee WL, Gold B, Darby C, Brot N, Jiang X, de Carvalho LP, Wellner D, St John G, Jacobs WR Jr, Nathan C. 2009. *Mycobacterium tuberculosis* expresses methionine sulphoxide reductases A and B that protect from killing by nitrite and hypochlorite. *Mol Microbiol* **71:** 583–593.

Lin PL, Ford CB, Coleman MT, Myers AJ, Gawande R, Ioerger T, Sacchettini J, Fortune SM, Flynn JL. 2014. Sterilization of granulomas is common in active and latent tuberculosis despite within-host variability in bacterial killing. *Nat Med* **20:** 75–79.

Liu PT, Stenger S, Li H, Wenzel L, Tan BH, Krutzik SR, Ochoa MT, Schauber J, Wu K, Meinken C, et al. 2006. Toll-like receptor triggering of a vitamin D-mediated human antimicrobial response. *Science* **311:** 1770–1773.

Liu PT, Stenger S, Tang DH, Modlin RL. 2007. Cutting edge: Vitamin D-mediated human antimicrobial activity against *Mycobacterium tuberculosis* is dependent on the induction of cathelicidin. *J Immunol* **179:** 2060–2063.

Long R, Light B, Talbot JA. 1999. Mycobacteriocidal action of exogenous nitric oxide. *Antimicrob Agents Chemother* **43:** 403–405.

Lurie MB. 1964. *Resistance to tuberculosis: Experimental studies in native and acquired mechanisms.* Harvard University Press, Cambridge, MA.

MacMicking JD. 2008. *M. tuberculosis* passes the litmus test. *Nat Med* **14:** 809–810.

MacMicking JD. 2012. IFN-inducible effector mechanisms in cell-autonomous immunity. *Nat Rev Immunol* **12:** 367–382.

MacMicking J, Xie Qw, Nathan C. 1997a. Nitric oxide and macrophage function. *Ann Rev Immunol* **15:** 323–350.

MacMicking JD, North RJ, LaCourse R, Mudgett JS, Shah SK, Nathan CF. 1997b. Identification of nitric oxide synthase as a protective locus against tuberculosis. *Proc Natl Acad Sci* **94:** 5243–5248.

MacMicking JD, Taylor GA, McKinney JD. 2003. Immune control of tuberculosis by IFN-γ-inducible LRG-47. *Science* **302:** 654–659.

Maertzdorf J, Repsilber D, Parida SK, Stanley K, Roberts T, Black G, Walzl G, Kaufmann SH. 2011. Human gene expression profiles of susceptibility and resistance in tuberculosis. *Genes Immun* **12:** 15–22.

Manzanillo PS, Shiloh MU, Portnoy DA, Cox JS. 2012. *Mycobacterium tuberculosis* activates the DNA-dependent cytosolic surveillance pathway within macrophages. *Cell Host Microbe* **11:** 469–480.

Manzanillo PS, Ayres JS, Watson RO, Collins AC, Souza G, Rae CS, Schneider DS, Nakamura K, Shiloh MU, Cox JS. 2013. The ubiquitin ligase parkin mediates resistance to intracellular pathogens. *Nature* **501:** 512–516.

Marakalala MJ, Guler R, Matika L, Murray G, Jacobs M, Brombacher F, Rothfuchs AG, Sher A, Brown GD. 2011. The Syk/CARD9-coupled receptor Dectin-1 is not required for host resistance to *Mycobacterium tuberculosis* in mice. *Microbes Infect* **13:** 198–201.

Martineau AR, Newton SM, Wilkinson KA, Kampmann B, Hall BM, Nawroly N, Packe GE, Davidson RN, Griffiths CJ, Wilkinson RJ. 2007. Neutrophil-mediated innate immune resistance to mycobacteria. *J Clin Invest* **117:** 1894–1988.

Mattila JT, Ojo OO, Kepka-Lenhart D, Marino S, Kim JH, Eum SY, Via LE, Barry CE 3rd, Klein E, Kirschner DE, et al. 2013. Microenvironments in tuberculous granulomas are delineated by distinct populations of macrophage subsets and expression of nitric oxide synthase and arginase isoforms. *J Immunol* **191:** 773–784.

Mayer-Barber KD, Barber DL, Shenderov K, White SD, Wilson MS, Cheever A, Kugler D, Hieny S, Caspar P, Núñez G, et al. 2010. Caspase-1 independent IL-1β production is critical for host resistance to *Mycobacterium tuberculosis* and does not require TLR signaling in vivo. *J Immunol* **184:** 3326–3330.

McDonough KA, Kress Y, Bloom BR. 1993. Pathogenesis of tuberculosis: Interaction of *Mycobacterium tuberculosis* with macrophages. *Infect Immun* **61:** 2763–2773.

McKinney JD, Höner zu Bentrup K, Muñoz-Elías EJ, Miczak A, Chen B, Chan WT, Swenson D, Sacchettini JC, Jacobs WR Jr, Russell DG. 2000. Persistence of *Mycobacterium tuberculosis* in macrophages and mice requires the glyoxylate shunt enzyme isocitrate lyase. *Nature* **406:** 735–738.

McKinney JD, Bloom BR, Modlin RL. 2001. Tuberculosis and leprosy. In *Samter's immunologic diseases*, 6th ed (ed. Austen KF, Frank MM, Atkinson JP, et al.), pp. 985–1002. Lippincott Williams & Wilkins, Philadelphia.

Means TK, Jones BW, Schromm AB, Shurtleff BA, Smith JA, Keane J, Golenbock DT, Vogel SN, Fenton MJ. 2001. Differential effects of a Toll-like receptor antagonist on *Mycobacterium tuberculosis*-induced macrophage responses. *J Immunol* **166:** 4074–4082.

Metchnikoff E. 1905. *Immunity in the infectious diseases.* MacMillan, New York.

Michelucci A, Cordes T, Ghelfi J, Pailot A, Reiling N, Goldmann O, Binz T, Wegner A, Tallam A, Rausell A, et al. 2013. Immune-responsive gene 1 protein links metabolism to immunity by catalyzing itaconic acid production. *Proc Natl Acad Sci* **110:** 7820–7825.

Mogues T, Goodrich ME, Ryan L, LaCourse R, North RJ. 2001. The relative importance of T cell subsets in immunity and immunopathology of airborne *Mycobacterium tuberculosis* infection in mice. *J Exp Med* **193:** 271–280.

Muñoz-Elías EJ, McKinney JD. 2005. *Mycobacterium tuberculosis* isocitrate lyases 1 and 2 are jointly required for in vivo growth and virulence. *Nat Med* **11:** 638–644.

Muñoz-Elías EJ, McKinney JD. 2006. Carbon metabolism of intracellular bacteria. *Cell Microbiol* **8:** 10–22.

Muñoz-Elias EJ, Upton AM, Cherian J, McKinney JD. 2006. Role of the methylcitrate cycle in *Mycobacterium tuberculosis* metabolism, intracellular growth, and virulance. *Mol Microbiol* **60:** 1109–1122.

Myrvik QN, Leake ES, Wright MJ. 1984. Disruption of phagosomal membranes of normal alveolar macrophages by the H37Rv strain of *Mycobacterium tuberculosis.* A correlate of virulence. *Am Rev Respir Dis* **129:** 322–328.

Nathan C. 2006. Role of iNOS in human disease. *Science* **312:** 1874–1875.

Nathan C. 2012. Fresh approaches to anti-infective therapies. *Sci Transl Med* **4:** 140sr2.

Nathan C, Shiloh MU. 2000. Reactive oxygen and nitrogen intermediates in the relationship between mammalian hosts and microbial pathogens. *Proc Natl Acad Sci* **97:** 8841–8848.

Nathan CF, Murray HW, Wiebe ME, Rubin BY. 1983. Identification of interferon-γ as the lymphokine that activates human macrophage oxidative metabolism and antimicrobial activity. *J Exp Med* **158:** 670–89.

Nathan CF, Prendergast TJ, Wiebe ME, Stanley ER, Platzer E, Remold HG, Welte K, Rubin BY, Murray HW. 1984. Activation of human macrophages. Comparison of other cytokines with interferon-γ. *J Exp Med* **160:** 600–605.

Nau GJ, Richmond JF, Schlesinger A, Jennings EG, Lander ES, Young RA. 2002. Human macrophage activation programs induced by bacterial pathogens. *Proc Natl Acad Sci* **99:** 1503–1508.

Ng VH, Cox JS, Sousa AO, MacMicking JD, McKinney JD. 2004. Role of *KatG* catalase-peroxidase in mycobacterial pathogenesis: Countering the oxidative burst. *Mol Microbiol* **52:** 1291–1302.

Nicholson S, Bonecini-Almeida Mda G, Lapa e Silva JR, Nathan C, Xie QW, Mumford R, Weidner JR, Calaycay J, Geng J, et al. 1996. Inducible nitric oxide synthase in pulmonary alveolar macrophages from patients with tuberculosis. *J Exp Med* **183:** 2293–2302.

Pace JL, Russell SW, Schreiber RD, Altman A, Katz DH. 1983. Macrophage activation: Priming activity from a T-cell hybridoma is attributable to interferon-γ. *Proc Natl Acad Sci* **80:** 3782–3786.

Pei G, Repnik U, Griffiths G, Gutierrez MG. 2014. Identification of an immune regulated phagosomal Rab cascade in macrophages. *J Cell Sci* Feb 25. doi: 10.1242/jcs.144923.

Pethe K, Swenson DL, Alonso S, Anderson J, Wang C, Russell DG. 2004. Isolation of *Mycobacterium tuberculosis* mutants defective in the arrest of phagosome maturation. *Proc Natl Acad Sci* **101:** 13642–13647.

Piddington DL, Kashkouli A, Buchmeier NA. 2000. Growth of *Mycobacterium tuberculosis* in a defined medium is very restricted by acid pH and Mg^{2+} levels. *Infect Immun* **68:** 4518–4522.

Pilli M, Arko-Mensah J, Ponpuak M, Roberts E, Master S, Mandell MA, Dupont N, Ornatowski W, Jiang S, Bradfute SB, et al. 2012. TBK-1 promotes autophagy-mediated antimicrobial defense by controlling autophagosome maturation. *Immunity* **37:** 223–234.

Podinovskaia M, Lee W, Caldwell S, Russell DG. 2013. Infection of macrophages with *Mycobacterium tuberculosis* induces global modifications to phagosomal function. *Cell Microbiol* **15:** 589–843.

Ponpuak M, Davis AS, Roberts EA, Delgado MA, Dinkins C, Zhao Z, Virgin HW 4th, Kyei GB, Johansen T, Vergne I, et al. 2010. Delivery of cytosolic components by autophagic adaptor protein p62 endows autophagosomes with unique antimicrobial properties. *Immunity* **32:** 329–341.

Qualls JE, Subramanian C, Rafi W, Smith AM, Balouzian L, DeFreitas AA, Shirey KA, Reutterer B, Kernbauer E, Stockinger S, et al. 2012. Sustained generation of nitric oxide and control of mycobacterial infection requires argininosuccinate synthase 1. *Cell Host Microbe* **12:** 313–323.

Ragno S, Romano M, Howell S, Pappin DJ, Jenner PJ, Colston MJ. 2001. Changes in gene expression in macrophages infected with *Mycobacterium tuberculosis*: A combined transcriptomic and proteomic approach. *Immunology* **104:** 99–108.

Randow F, MacMicking JD, James LC. 2013. Cellular self-defense: How cell-autonomous immunity protects against pathogens. *Science* **340:** 701–706.

Roca FJ, Ramakrishnan L. 2013. TNF dually mediates resistance and susceptibility to mycobacteria via mitochondrial reactive oxygen species. *Cell* **153:** 521–534.

Rohde K, Yates RM, Purdy GE, Russell DG. 2007. *Mycobacterium tuberculosis* and the environment within the phagosome. *Immunol Rev* **219:** 37–54.

Rook GA, Steele J, Ainsworth M, Champion Br. 1986a. Activation of macrophages to inhibit proliferation of *Mycobacterium tuberculosis*: Comparison of the effects of recombinant γ interferon on human monocytes and murine peritoneal macrophages. *Immunology* **59:** 333–338.

Rook GA, Steele J, Fraher L, Barker S, Karmali R, O'Riordan J, Stanford J. 1986b. Vitamin D3, γ interferon, and control of the proliferation of *Mycobacterium tuberculosis* by human macrophages. *Immunology* **57:** 159–163.

Rothchild AC, Jayaraman P, Nunes-Alves C, Behar SM. 2014. iNKT cell production of GM-CSF controls *Mycobacterium tuberculosis*. *PLoS Pathog* **10:** e1003805.

Rous P. 1925. The relative reaction within living mammalian tissues. II. On the mobilization of acid material within cells, and the reaction as influenced by the cell state. *J Exp Med* **41:** 399–411.

Russell DG. 2011. The galvanizing of *Mycobacterium tuberculosis*: An antimicrobial mechanism. *Cell Host Microbe* **10:** 181–183.

Saiga H, Nishimura J, Kuwata H, Okuyama M, Matsumoto S, Sato S, Matsumoto M, Akira S, Yoshikai Y, Honda K, et al. 2008. Lipocalin 2-dependent inhibition of mycobacterial growth in alveolar epithelium. *J Immunol* **181:** 8521–8527.

Samanovic MI, Ding C, Thiele DJ, Darwin KH. 2012. Copper in microbial pathogenesis: Meddling with the metal. *Cell Host Microbe* **11:** 106–115.

Scanga CA, Mohan VP, Tanaka K, Alland D, Flynn JL, Chan J. 2001. The inducible nitric oxide synthase locus confers protection against aerogenic challenge of both clinical and laboratory strains of *Mycobacterium tuberculosis* in mice. *Infect Immun* **69:** 7711–7717.

Schaible UE, Kaufmann SH. 2004. Iron and microbial infection. *Nat Rev Microbiol* **2:** 946–953.

Schaible UE, Sturgill-Koszycki S, Schlesinger PH, Russell DG. 1998. Cytokine activation leads to acidification and increases maturation of *Mycobacterium avium*–containing phagosomes in murine macrophages. *J Immunol* **160:** 1290–1296.

Schnappinger D, Ehrt S, Voskuil MI, Liu Y, Mangan JA, Monahan IM, Dolganov G, Efron B, Butcher PD, Nathan C, et al. 2003. Transcriptional adaptation of *Mycobacterium tuberculosis* within macrophages: Insights into the phagosomal environment. *J Exp Med* **198:** 693–704.

Shah JA, Vary JC, Chau TT, Bang ND, Yen NT, Farrar JJ, Dunstan SJ, Hawn TR. 2012. Human TOLLIP regulates TLR2 and TLR4 signaling and its polymorphisms are associated with susceptibility to tuberculosis. *J Immunol* **189:** 1737–1746.

Sharma S, Kumar V, Khosla R, Kajal N, Sarin B, Sehajpal P. 2010. Association of P2X7 receptor +1513 (A→C) polymorphism with tuberculosis in a Punjabi population. *Int J Tuberc Lung Dis* **14:** 1159–1163.

Shi S, Nathan C, Schnappinger D, Drenkow J, Fuortes M, Block E, Ding A, Gingeras TR, Schoolnik G, Akira S, et al. 2003. MyD88 primes macrophages for full-scale activation by interferon-γ yet mediates few responses to *Mycobacterium tuberculosis*. *J Exp Med* **198:** 987–997.

Shi S, Blumenthal A, Hickey CM, Gandotra S, Levy D, Ehrt S. 2005. Expression of many immunologically important genes in *Mycobacterium tuberculosis*–infected macrophages is independent of both TLR2 and TLR4 but dependent on IFN-αβ receptor and STAT1. *J Immunol* **175:** 3318–3328.

Shiloh MU, Manzanillo P, Cox JS. 2008. *Mycobacterium tuberculosis* senses host-derived carbon monoxide during macrophage infection. *Cell Host Microbe* **3:** 323–330.

Sikora A, Lui J, Brosnan C, Buell G, Chessel I, Bloom BR. 1999. Purinergic signaling regulates radical-mediated bacterial killing mechanisms in macrophages through a P2X7-independent mechanism. *J Immunol* **163:** 558–561.

Singh SB, Davis AS, Taylor GA, Deretic V. 2006. Human IRGM induces autophagy to eliminate intracellular mycobacteria. *Science* **313:** 1438–1441.

Singh R, Manjunatha U, Boshoff HI, Ha YH, Niyomrattanakit P, Ledwidge R, Dowd CS, Lee IY, Kim P, Zhang L, et al. 2008. PA-824 kills nonreplicating *Mycobacterium tuberculosis* by intracellular NO release. *Science* **322:** 1392–1395.

Singh SB, Ornatowski W, Vergne I, Naylor J, Delgado M, Roberts E, Ponpuak M, Master S, Pilli M, White E, et al. 2010. Human IRGM regulates autophagy and cell-autonomous immunity functions through mitochondria. *Nat Cell Biol* **12:** 1154–1165.

Song JH, Kim SY, Chung KS, Moon CM, Kim SW, Kim EY, Jung JY, Park MS, Kim YS, Kim SK, et al. 2014. Association between genetic variants in the *IRGM* gene and tuberculosis in a Korean population. *Infection* doi: 10.1007/s15010-014-0604-6.

St. John G, Brot N, Ruan J, Erdjument-Bromage H, Tempst P, Weissbach H, Nathan C. 2001. Peptide methionine sulfoxide reductase from *Escherichia coli* and *Mycobacterium tuberculosis* protects bacteria against oxidative damage from reactive nitrogen intermediates. *Proc Natl Acad Sci* **98:** 9901–9906.

Stanley SA, Cox JS. 2013. Host–pathogen interactions during *Mycobacterium tuberculosis* infections. *Curr Top Microbiol Immunol* **374:** 211–241.

Stanley SA, Barczak AK, Silvis MR, Luo SS, Sogi K, Vokes M, Bray MA, Carpenter AE, Moore CB, Siddiqi N, et al. 2014. Identification of host-targeted small molecules that restrict intracellular *Mycobacterium tuberculosis* growth. *PLoS Pathog* **10:** e1003946.

Staskawicz BJ, Mudgett MB, Dangl JL, Galan JE. 2001. Common and contrasting themes of plant and animal diseases. *Science* **292:** 2285–2289.

Sturgill-Koszycki S, Schlesinger PH, Chakraborty P, Haddix PL, Collins HL, Fok AK, Allen RD, Gluck SL, Heuser J, Russell DG. 1994. Lack of acidification in mycobacterium phagosomes produced by exclusion of the vesicular proton-ATPase. *Science* **263:** 678–681.

Sturgill-Koszycki S, Schaible UE, Russell DG. 1996. Mycobacterium-containing phagosomes are accessible to early endosomes and reflect a transitional state in normal phagosome biogenesis. *EMBO J* **15:** 6960–6968.

Suzuki K, Tsuyuguchi K, Matsumoto H, Niimi A, Tanaka E, Amitani R. 2000. Effect of proton pump inhibitor alone or in combination with clathrinomycin on mycobacterial growth in human macrophages. *FEMS Microbiol Lett* **182:** 69–72.

Tailleux L, Waddell SJ, Pelizzola M, Mortellaro A, Withers M, Tanne A, Castagnoli PR, Gicquel B, Stoker NG, Butcher PD, et al. 2008. Probing host pathogen cross-talk by transcriptional profiling of both *Mycobacterium tuberculosis* and infected human dendritic cells and macrophages. *PLoS ONE* **3:** e1403.

Tan BH, Meinken C, Bastian M, Bruns H, Legaspi A, Ochoa MT, Krutzik SR, Bloom BR, Ganz T, Modlin RL, et al. 2006. Macrophages acquire neutrophil granules for antimicrobial activity against intracellular pathogens. *J Immunol* **177:** 1864–1871.

Tan MP, Sequeira P, Lin WW, Phong WY, Cliff P, Ng SH, Lee BH, Camacho L, Schnappinger D, Ehrt S, et al. 2010. Nitrate respiration protects hypoxic *Mycobacterium tuberculosis* against acid- and reactive nitrogen species stresses. *PLoS ONE* **5:** e13356.

Thuong NT, Hawn TR, Thwaites GE, Chau TT, Lan NT, Quy HT, Hieu NT, Aderem A, Hien TT, Farrar JJ, et al. 2007. A polymorphism in human TLR2 is associated with increased susceptibility to tuberculous meningitis. *Genes Immun* **8:** 422–428.

Ting LM, Kim AC, Cattamanchi A, Ernst JD. 1999. *Mycobacterium tuberculosis* inhibits IFN-γ transcriptional responses without inhibiting activation of STAT1. *J Immunol* **163:** 3898–3906.

Tiwari S, Choi HP, Matsuzawa T, Pypaert M, MacMicking JD. 2009. Targeting of the GTPase Irgm1 to the phagosomal membrane via PtdIns(3,4)P_2 and PtdIns(3,4,5)P_3 promotes immunity to mycobacteria. *Nat Immunol* **10:** 907–917.

Thoma-Uszynski S, Stenger S, Takeuchi O, Ochoa M, Engele MT, Sieling PA, Barnes PF, Rollinghoff M, Bolcskei PL, Wagner M, et al. 2001. Induction of direct antimicrobial activity through mammalian Toll-like receptors. *Science* **291:** 1544–1547.

Trost M, English L, Lemieux S, Courcelles M, Desjardins M, Thibault P. 2009. The phagosomal proteome in interferon-γ-activated macrophages. *Immunity* **30:** 143–154.

Ullrich H-J, Beatty WL, Russell DG. 1999. Direct delivery of procathepsin D to phagosomes: Implications for phagosome biogenesis and parasitism by mycobacterium. *Eur J Cell Biol* **78:** 739–748.

Vandal OH, Pierini LM, Schnappinger D, Nathan CF, Ehrt S. 2008. A membrane protein preserves intrabacterial pH in intraphagosomal *Mycobacterium tuberculosis*. *Nat Med* **14:** 849–854.

Vandal OH, Nathan CF, Ehrt S. 2009. Acid resistance in *Mycobacterium tuberculosis*. *J Bacteriol* **191:** 4714–4721.

van der Wel N, Hava D, Houben D, Fluitsma D, van Zon M, Pierson J, Brenner M, Peters PJ. 2007. *M. tuberculosis* and *M. leprae* translocate from the phagolysosome to the cytosol in myeloid cells. *Cell* **129:** 1287–1298.

Van Zandt KE, Sow FB, Florence WC, Zwilling BS, Satoskar AR, Schlesinger LS, Lafuse WP. 2008. The iron export protein ferroportin 1 is differentially expressed in mouse macrophage populations and is present in the mycobacterial-containing phagosome. *J Leukoc Biol* **84:** 689–700.

Velez DR, Hulme WF, Myers JL, Weinberg JB, Levesque MC, Stryjewski ME, Abbate E, Estevan R, Patillo SG, Gilbert JR, et al. 2009. *NOS2A*, *TLR4*, and *IFNGR1* interactions influence pulmonary tuberculosis susceptibility in African-Americans. *Hum Genet* **126:** 643–653.

Venketaraman V, Dayaram YK, Talaue MT, Connell ND. 2005. Glutathione and nitrosoglutathione in macrophage defense against *Mycobacterium tuberculosis*. *Infect Immun* **73:** 1886–1889.

Vergne I, Chua J, Deretic V. 2003. Tuberculosis toxin blocking phagosome maturation inhibits a novel Ca^{2+}/calmodulin-PI3K hVPS34 cascade. *J Exp Med* **198:** 653–659.

Vilchèze C, Hartman T, Weinrick B, Jacobs WR Jr. 2013. *Mycobacterium tuberculosis* is extraordinarily sensitive to killing by a vitamin C–induced Fenton reaction. *Nat Commun* **4:** 1881.

Vogt G, Nathan C. 2011. In vitro differentiation of human macrophages with enhanced antimycobacterial activity. *J Clin Invest* **121:** 3889–3901.

von Muhlinen N, Akutsu M, Ravenhill BJ, Foeglein Á, Bloor S, Rutherford TJ, Freund SM, Komander D, Randow F. 2012. LC3C, bound selectively by a noncanonical LIR motif in NDP52, is required for antibacterial autophagy. *Mol Cell* **48:** 329–342.

Voskuil MI, Schnappinger D, Visconti KC, Harrell MI, Dolganov GM, Sherman DR, Schoolnik GK. 2003. Inhibition of respiration by nitric oxide induces a *Mycobacterium tuberculosis* dormancy program. *J Exp Med* **198:** 705–713.

Wagner D, Maser J, Lai B, Cai Z, Barry CE 3rd, Höner Zu Bentrup K, Russell DG, Bermudez LE. 2005. Elemental analysis of *Mycobacterium avium*–, *Mycobacterium tuberculosis*–, and *Mycobacterium smegmatis*–containing phagosomes indicates pathogen-induced microenvironments within the host cell's endosomal system. *J Immunol* **174:** 1491–500.

Wang C-h, Lui C-Y, Lin H-C, Yu C-T, Chung K, Kuo H. 1998. Increased exhaled nitric oxide in active pulmonary tuberculosis due to inducible nitric oxide synthase upregulation in alveolar macrophages. *Eur J Respir* **11:** 809–815.

Wang C, Lin H, Lui C, Huang K, Huang T, Yu C, Kuo H. 2001. Upregulation of inducible nitric oxide synthase and cytokine secretion in peripheral blood monocytes from pulmonary tuberculosis patients. *Int J Tuberc Lung Dis* **5:** 283–291.

Ward SK, Abomoelak B, Hoye EA, Steinberg H, Talaat AM. 2010. CtpV: A putative copper exporter required for full virulence of *Mycobacterium tuberculosis*. *Mol Microbiol* **77:** 1096–1110.

Watson RO, Manzanillo PS, Cox JS. 2012. Extracellular *M. tuberculosis* DNA targets bacteria for autophagy by activating the host DNA-sensing pathway. *Cell* **150:** 803–815.

West AP, Brodsky IE, Rahner C, Woo DK, Erdjument-Bromage H, Tempst P, Walsh MC, Choi Y, Shadel GS, Ghosh S. 2011. TLR signalling augments macrophage bactericidal activity through mitochondrial ROS. *Nature* **472:** 476–480.

Wilkinson RJ. 2014. Host-directed therapies against tuberculosis. *Lancet Respir Med* 85–87.

Wilkinson RJ, Llewelyn M, Toossi Z, Patel P, Pasvol G, Lalvani A, Wright D, Latif M, Davidson RN. 2000. Influence of vitamin D deficiency and vitamin D receptor polymorphisms on tuberculosis among Gujarati Asians in west London: A case-control study. *Lancet* **355:** 618–621.

Wolschendorf F, Ackart D, Shrestha TB, Hascall-Dove L, Nolan S, Lamichhane G, Wang Y, Bossmann SH, Basaraba RJ, Niederweis M. 2011. Copper resistance is essential for virulence of *Mycobacterium tuberculosis*. *Proc Natl Acad Sci* **108:** 1621–1626.

Xu Y, Jagannath C, Liu XD, Sharafkhaneh A, Kolodziejska KE, Eissa NT. 2007. Toll-like receptor 4 is a sensor for autophagy associated with innate immunity. *Immunity* **27:** 135–144.

Yang CT, Cambier CJ, Davis JM, Hall CJ, Crosier PS, Ramakrishnan L. 2012. Neutrophils exert protection in the early tuberculous granuloma by oxidative killing of mycobacteria phagocytosed from infected macrophages. *Cell Host Microbe* **12:** 301–312.

Yu K, Mitchell C, Xing Y, Magliozzo RS, Bloom BR, Chan J. 1999. Toxicity of nitrogen oxides and related oxidants on mycobacteria: *M tuberculosis* is resistant to peroxynitrite anion. *Tuberc Lung Dis* **79:** 191–198.

Yuk JM, Shin DM, Lee HM, Yang CS, Jin HS, Kim KK, Lee ZW, Lee SH, Kim JM, Jo EK. 2009. Vitamin D3 induces autophagy in human monocytes/macrophages via cathelicidin. *Cell Host Microbe* **6:** 231–243.

Zanetti M. 2004. Cathelicidins, multifunctional peptides of the innate immunity. *J Leukoc Biol* **75:** 39–48.

Zhang YJ, Rubin EJ. 2013. Feast or famine: The host–pathogen battle over amino acids. *Cell Microbiol* **15:** 1079–1087.

Zhang SY, Boisson-Dupuis S, Chapgier A, Yang K, Bustamante J, Puel A, Picard C, Abel L, Jouanguy E, Casanova JL. 2008. Inborn errors of interferon (IFN)-mediated immunity in humans: Insights into the respective roles of IFN-α/β, IFN-γ, and IFN-λ in host defense. *Immunol Rev* **226:** 29–40.

Zhang YJ, Reddy MC, Ioerger TR, Rothchild AC, Dartois V, Schuster BM, Trauner A, Wallis D, Galaviz S, Huttenhower C, et al. 2013. Tryptophan biosynthesis protects mycobacteria from CD4 T-cell-mediated killing. *Cell* **155:** 1296–1308.

Manipulation of the Mononuclear Phagocyte System by *Mycobacterium tuberculosis*

Geanncarlo Lugo-Villarino[1,2] and Olivier Neyrolles[1,2]

[1]Centre National de la Recherche Scientifique (CNRS), Institut de Pharmacologie et de Biologie Structurale (IPBS), 31000 Toulouse, France

[2]Université de Toulouse, Université Paul Sabatier, Institut de Pharmacologie et de Biologie Structurale (IPBS), 31000 Toulouse, France

Correspondence: olivier.neyrolles@ipbs.fr

Over the past 20 years, there has been an emerging appreciation about the role of the mononuclear phagocyte system (MPS) to control and eradicate pathogens. Likewise, there have been significant advances in dissecting the mechanisms involved in the microbial subversion of MPS cells, mainly affecting their differentiation and effector functions. *Mycobacterium tuberculosis* is a chronic bacterial pathogen that represents an enigma to the field because of its remarkable ability to thrive in humans. One reason is that *M. tuberculosis* renders a defective MPS compartment, which is perhaps the most ingenious strategy for survival in the host given the prominence of these cells to modulate microenvironments, their function as sentinels and orchestrators of the immune response, and their pathogenic role as reservoirs for microbial persistence. In this article, the principal strategies used by *M. tuberculosis* to subvert the MPS compartment are presented along with emerging concepts.

As part of the constant evolutionary process taking place in all living organisms, microbes have evolved strategies to circumvent the host immune response. Among these, the ability of *Mycobacterium tuberculosis* to influence the differentiation, maturation, and activation programs of the mononuclear phagocyte system (MPS) is perhaps the best strategy to avoid challenges posed by a dedicated immune response. The main reason is that the MPS not only has a prominent role in maintaining body homeostasis, but it is also critical for multiple immune-related functions. This includes the monitoring of, and interaction with, the different local microenvironments, establishing symbiotic relationships between the host and local microbiota, recognition and capture of pathogens, activation of early defensive mechanisms of inflammation and innate effector cells, relay of innate information signals to the adaptive immune system resulting in immunological memory, and establishment of peripheral tolerance (van Furth and Cohn 1968; Gordon and Taylor 2005; Geissmann et al. 2010; Chow et al. 2011; Murray and Wynn 2011). Indeed, cells that compose the MPS, such as monocytes, macrophages, and dendritic cells, represent ideal targets of inhibition and modulation by

Cite this article as *Cold Spring Harb Perspect Med* doi: 10.1101/cshperspect.a018549

invading pathogens such as *M. tuberculosis* (Wiersma et al. 1996; Martino 2008; Serbina et al. 2008; Mege et al. 2011; Mihret 2012). This is a paradoxical situation because mononuclear phagocytes are immune cells specialized in the engulfment and clearance of microbes and cellular debris, and a better understanding of their subversion by *M. tuberculosis* is likely to yield substantial insights into microbe physiology and host defenses.

The purpose of this article is not to provide a comprehensive summary of the immune evasion strategies used by *M. tuberculosis*, as there are excellent reviews covering this subject (Engering et al. 2002; Flynn and Chan 2003; Alsultan et al. 2011; Dorhoi et al. 2011; Hajishengallis and Lambris 2011; Gupta et al. 2012; O'Garra et al. 2013; Russell 2013). Nor will it address in depth some of the subjects presented in this article, as other articles cover these issues in detail. Instead, this article will focus exclusively on the most important strategies and emerging concepts concerning the subversion of MPS cells by *M. tuberculosis*. This includes the bacillus' capacity to (i) interfere with vacuolar sorting and arrest phagosome maturation; (ii) avoid killing by natural phagocyte-derived products such as reactive oxygen and nitrogen species, antimicrobial peptides, and transition metals; and (iii) extract essential nutrients from its host's cells and tissues, thus ensuring its own metabolic demands. Moreover, the modulation of macrophage polarization intertwining hallmark metabolic processes and the manipulation of dendritic cell differentiation and activation via the subversion of receptor cross talk will be presented in this article as emerging concepts in the ability of *M. tuberculosis* to shape its local environments in a way that is both permissive and immunosuppressant.

PHAGOSOME MATURATION ARREST

Upon phagocytosis by macrophages, particles are engulfed within a membrane-bound vacuole, or phagosome, that progressively matures through a series of fusion events with intracellular endocytic organelles and ultimately coalesces with the host cell lysosomes, thus forming a so-called phagolysosome (Desjardins and Griffiths 2003). The phagolysosome is an acidic, hydrolase-enriched, and oxidative hostile environment in which particles are degraded. Intracellular pathogens have evolved multiple mechanisms to circumvent phagolysosomal degradation (Sarantis and Grinstein 2012). Chief among these strategies is the ability of the tubercle bacillus to arrest phagosome maturation (Russell 2001; Philips 2008), a process that was originally discovered more than 40 years ago through electron microscopy observation of *M. tuberculosis*–infected macrophages in which lysosomes were loaded with ferritin; in this experiment, the absence of colocalization between the bacilli and the electron-dense ferritin granules was interpreted as a natural reluctance of the mycobacterial vacuole to fuse with lysosomes and mature into a phagolysosome (Armstrong and Hart 1971). Since then, numerous reports using various technologies showed that the mycobacterial phagosome is characterized by an abnormal retention of early endosomal markers, such as the small GTPase Rab5 and other Rab proteins, transferrin, and its receptor, and by the exclusion of late endosomal and lysosomal markers, such as the small GTPase Rab7 and the vacuolar proton transporter v-ATPase (Sturgill-Koszycki et al. 1994). Central to the impaired ability of the *M. tuberculosis* phagosome to fuse with host cell lysosomes is the reduced accumulation of phosphatidylinositol-3-phosphate (PI3P) onto the phagosome membrane and the resulting diminished enrichment of the vacuole in PI3P-binding proteins early endosomal antigen 1 (EEA1) and hepatocyte growth factor–regulated tyrosine kinase substrate (Hrs), two molecules involved in protein sorting and required for phagosome fusion with late endosomes and lysosomes (Philips 2008).

How *M. tuberculosis* escapes lysosomal delivery inside macrophages is still an intensive area of research. Several mycobacterial lipids and glycolipids, such as lipoarabinomannan (LAM) and trehalose dimycolate (TDM), for instance, were early shown to play a part in the ability of the tubercle bacillus to avoid phagosome–lysosome fusion (Philips 2008; Russell

2011). Mycobacterial proteins and enzymes, such as the lipid phosphatase SapM and the tyrosine phosphatase PtpA, the lipoamide dehydrogenase LpdC, the metalloprotease Zmp1, the serine/threonine kinase PknG, and the PE-PGRS62 protein, among others, were also involved in this process (Walburger et al. 2004; Vergne et al. 2005; Deghmane et al. 2007; Bach et al. 2008; Thi et al. 2013). Additional microbial components identified through various genetic screening approaches are also involved in impaired intracellular trafficking of mycobacteria (Pethe et al. 2004; Stewart et al. 2005; Brodin et al. 2010). Distinguishing which of these factors directly contribute to phagosome maturation arrest from those required for bacterial fitness, and whose genetic alteration might result in an aberrant microbial trafficking inside host cells, is difficult. Recently, it was shown that the secreted tyrosine phosphatase PtpA directly binds to the H subunit of the v-ATPase, resulting in the dephosphorylation of vacuolar protein sorting protein 33B (VPS33B) and subsequent impairment of v-ATPase recruitment to the vacuole (Wong et al. 2011). It was also shown that *M. tuberculosis* uses its type VII secretion system ESX-3 to export two effector proteins—namely, EsxH and EsxG—that interact with Hrs and impair phagosome maturation through disrupting the endosomal sorting complex required for transport (ESCRT) (Mehra et al. 2013). Other mycobacterial secreted proteins are proposed to interfere with the host cell vacuolar sorting machinery, as suggested, for example, by the aberrant trafficking of a *M. tuberculosis* mutant inactivated in the alternative secretion system component SecA2 (Sullivan et al. 2012). This infers that PtpA, Esx proteins, and other mycobacterial proteins can translocate from the phagosomal lumen to the host cell cytosol, which remains to be elucidated.

RESISTANCE TO INTRACELLULAR KILLING BY ROI/RNI, ANTIMICROBIAL PEPTIDES, AND TRANSITION METAL OVERLOAD

Phagosome maturation blockade by pathogenic mycobacteria can be overcome by exogenous stimuli, including inflammatory cytokines (e.g., TNF-α, IFN-γ, and IL-1β) (Master et al. 2008), Toll-like receptor (TLR) ligands (Brightbill et al. 1999; Thoma-Uszynski et al. 2001), and vitamin D (Liu et al. 2006; Fabri et al. 2011), among others. Overall, these molecules result in forced maturation and acidification of the mycobacterial phagosome, enhancement of the production of reactive oxygen (ROI) and nitrogen (RNI) species, induction of the synthesis of antimicrobial peptides (e.g., cathelicidin), and promotion of autophagy, a process by which intracellular replication of the bacilli is impaired. Chemical manipulation of autophagy is considered a promising strategy to control mycobacterial infections (Deretic 2008; Bradfute et al. 2013). Another mechanism of microbial control by macrophages is the accumulation of transition metals (i.e., copper and zinc), up to potentially toxic levels within vacuoles. This was first reported in *Escherichia coli*–infected macrophages (White et al. 2009) and more recently in *M. tuberculosis*–infected cells (Wagner et al. 2005; Ward et al. 2010; Botella et al. 2011; Wolschendorf et al. 2011). Zinc and copper play vital functions in biological systems. The chemical properties of zinc (e.g., its Lewis acidity, coordination geometry, and rapid ligand exchange) allow it to form stable complexes with enzymes and proteins where it functions in catalysis or as a structural factor. The majority of zinc-containing enzymes catalyze hydrolysis or related transfer reactions, some of which are essential for cell viability. Regarding copper, because of its fast interconversion of Cu^{+} and Cu^{2+}, this metal species is involved in several essential biochemical processes, such as oxygen-dependent electron transport reactions. In *M. tuberculosis*, at least two enzymes require copper as cofactor, namely the SOD SodC and the cytochrome *c* oxidase subunits CtaC and CtaD.

To counteract intracellular intoxication by acid, reactive species, and transition metals, pathogenic mycobacteria have evolved a variety of sophisticated mechanisms. This includes the production of the acid resistance proteins Rv3671c, MgtC, and $OmpA_{Tb}$ (Vandal et al. 2008, 2009), the antioxidant mycothiol, the oxygen and nitrogen detoxification enzymes (i.e., superoxide dismutases SodA and SodC), the catalase KatG, and the NADH-dependent peroxidase and peroxynitrite reductase. SodA and KatG secretion depends on the SecA2 secretion machinery, which might partially account for the reduced ability of a Δ*secA2* mutant of *M. tuberculosis* to arrest phagosome maturation and replicate inside macrophages. Recently, transition metal efflux systems—namely, the P-type ATPases CtpC (Botella et al. 2011) and CtpV (Ward et al. 2010)—and the mycobacterial copper transporter MctB (Wolschendorf et al. 2011) were involved in mycobacterial virulence, indicating *M. tuberculosis* requires an intact transition metal detoxification system to thrive inside host cells. The requirement of P-ATPase-mediated copper resistance systems in bacterial virulence has been documented in several bacterial species (Hood and Skaar 2012), including *Listeria monocytogenes*, *Pseudomonas aeruginosa*, *Streptococcus pneumoniae*, and *Salmonella typhimurium*. Several mechanisms are proposed to explain copper ion toxicity. These mechanisms include (i) Fenton chemistry and generation of hydroxyl radicals, although this was challenged by data showing that there is no accumulation of hydroxyl radicals in copper-exposed *E. coli* (Macomber et al. 2007); (ii) degradation of iron–sulfur clusters in enzymes (Chillappagari et al. 2010); and (iii) replacement of other metal ion cofactors, such as zinc ions, in proteins. The exact mechanism(s) of copper toxicity in *M. tuberculosis* remain to be identified. The mechanism(s) of zinc ion toxicity may also include inactivation of iron–sulfur clusters (Xu and Imlay 2012) and inhibition of manganese uptake through transport competition in the bacterial perisplam (McDevitt et al. 2011). In addition, it was shown recently that P-ATPase-mediated copper export is required for copper supply to periplasmic Cu,Zn-SOD and resistance to oxidative stress in *Salmonella enterica* (Osman et al. 2013). Whether P-ATPases contribute to activation of the Fe^{2+}-cofactored, and maybe Mn^{2+}-cofactored, superoxide dismutase (SOD) SodA, and of the suggested periplasmic Cu,Zn-SOD SodC in *M. tuberculosis* (Padilla-Benavides et al. 2013), remains to be further investigated.

NUTRIENT ACQUISITION: IRON, CARBON, AND NITROGEN

In addition to resisting killing mechanisms by toxic compounds inside host cells, *M. tuberculosis* needs to acquire nutrients in order to sustain its own metabolic demands and to replicate. Considering that the mycobacterial phagosome is naturally a nutrient-poor environment, and that MPS cells are armed with nutrient deprivation machineries to further empty microbial vacuoles of nutrient sources to ultimately constrain microbial growth, the active nutrient acquisition systems described so far for *M. tuberculosis* are nothing short of remarkable.

One of the best examples illustrating the so-called field of nutritional immunity and nutritional virulence (i.e., the battle for nutrient acquisition between intracellular pathogens and host cells) is provided by iron. Phagocytes produce proteins that either efflux iron from intracellular microbial compartments (through the iron transporter NRAMP1/SLC11A1, for instance) or bind heme and hemoglobin (e.g., hemopexin and haptoglobin) and reduce the availability of heme as an iron source (Silva-Gomes et al. 2013). To overcome iron starvation, microbial pathogens evolved sophisticated high-affinity iron acquisition mechanisms (Hood and Skaar 2012). In the case of *M. tuberculosis*, the bacillus produces two siderophores: the cell-associated mycobactin and the soluble exported carboxymycobactin (Luo et al. 2005). Mycobacterial mutants unable to synthesize or export siderophores are strongly attenuated in a mouse model of tuberculosis infection, underscoring the importance of efficient iron acquisition for propagation of *M. tuberculosis*. In the extracellular environment, carboxymycobactin captures Fe^{3+} and transfers iron to mycobactin (Gobin and Horwitz 1996) or delivers iron via the iron-regulated ABC transporter IrtAB (Rodriguez and Smith 2006). It is likely siderophore-binding proteins in the *M. tuberculosis* envelope further facilitate Fe^{+3}-carboxymycobactin uptake. The mycobacterial type VII secretion system ESX-3 was shown to be necessary for growth of *M. tuberculosis* in

 Cite this article as *Cold Spring Harb Perspect Med* doi: 10.1101/cshperspect.a018549

iron-deficient medium and for utilization of exogenously added Fe^{+3}-carboxymycobactin (Siegrist et al. 2009), suggesting components of the ESX-3 system contribute to Fe^{+3}-carboxymycobactin uptake. Beyond siderophore-mediated iron uptake, *M. tuberculosis* captures iron from heme using a specialized hemophore (Tullius et al. 2011).

In addition to iron and other important nutritional elements, intracellular mycobacteria need to extract carbon, energy, and nitrogen from their host cells and tissues. Several studies showed how *M. tuberculosis* extracts carbon and energy from various sugars and fatty acids in host cells using key enzymes (e.g., the isocitrate lyases ICL1 and ICL2, the polyphosphate glucokinase PPGK, and the phosphoenolpyruvate carboxykinase PEPCK [McKinney et al. 2000; Munoz-Elias and McKinney 2005, 2006; de Carvalho et al. 2010; Marrero et al. 2010, 2013]) and how, like in other pathogens, carbon metabolism is intrinsically linked to virulence (Eisenreich et al. 2010). Moreover, *M. tuberculosis* can also exploit other lipids, such as cholesterol, to meet its carbon and energy demands (Pandey and Sassetti 2008; Griffin et al. 2012). Regarding nitrogen metabolism, we have recently reported that *M. tuberculosis* exploits the amino acid species aspartate and asparagine to acquire this essential element, and that the Asp and Asn exploitation machineries (i.e., the Asp transporter AnsP1, the Asn transporter AnsP2, and the asparaginase AnsA) are required for mycobacterial virulence (Gouzy et al. 2013, 2014). Whether immune defense mechanisms based on Asn and Asp deprivation exist in macrophages, as recently reported for another amino acid species (namely, tryptophan [Zhang et al. 2013]), will require further investigation.

MACROPHAGE POLARIZATION: MODULATION OF KEY METABOLISM PATHWAYS AND EFFECTOR FUNCTIONS

Alveolar macrophages are one of the first cell types to participate in the initial uptake of *M. tuberculosis* (O'Garra et al. 2013). Macrophages play a dual role in tuberculosis, as they are the primary host cell reservoir for *M. tuberculosis* and the major effector cells to eradicate this pathogen. The capacity of *M. tuberculosis* to modulate the host pro-inflammatory response and seize the anti-inflammatory mechanisms that ensure tissue integrity has awakened a strong interest to investigate how pathogenic infections manipulate the process of macrophage polarization (Benoit et al. 2008; Dorhoi et al. 2011; Lugo-Villarino et al. 2011; Mege et al. 2011; Murray and Wynn 2011). Macrophage polarization is a dynamic process governed by mechanisms dictating their abundance, tissue distribution, and function—in particular, the capacity to kill intracellular pathogens (Vogt and Nathan 2011; Sica and Mantovani 2012). Two programs broadly classify polarized macrophages: classical (M1) and alternative (M2). The M1 program arises from type-1 inflammatory conditions (e.g., IFN-γ). M1 macrophages are characterized by high production of pro-inflammatory signals and microbicidal molecules (e.g., nitric oxide, NO) and resistance against intracellular pathogens, among others. In contrast, the M2 program is a diverse response to type-2 immune signals such as IL-4 and IL-13 (M2a); immune complexes, TLR agonists, or IL-1 receptors (M2b); and immunosuppressants like IL-10 and TGF-β1 (M2c). M2 macrophage activity includes the suppression of inflammation, eradication of extracellular pathogens, and tissue repair, among others (Martinez et al. 2009). During infection, there is a frequent shift from M1 to M2 program of macrophage polarization at the sites of inflammation that is associated with the adaptive immune transition from acute to chronic phases. This shift is a common feature following pathogenic insult that causes tissue damage and may be essential for inflammation resolution and tissue reparation (Martinez et al. 2009; Mounier et al. 2013). However, an excessive or prolonged polarization of a given program may be detrimental to the host because of potential tissue injury or contribution to pathogenesis. In fact, there is increasing evidence that pathogens may have evolved strategies to take advantage of this polarization shift of macrophages to increase their fitness in the host (Benoit et al. 2008; Dorhoi et al. 2011; Lugo-Villarino et al. 2011; Mege et al. 2011; Murray and Wynn 2011). In the tuberculosis context, *M. tuberculosis* not only inhibits the pro-inflammatory activation of macrophages by secreting various virulence factors (Deretic et al. 2004; Benoit et al. 2008; Mege et al. 2011; Cambier et al. 2013), but it also promotes the shift toward M2 macrophages to ensure long-term intracellular survival (Kahnert et al. 2006; Benoit et al. 2008; Mege et al. 2011; Cambier et al. 2013). Implications stemming from the perceived ability of *M. tuberculosis* to influence the polarization process of macrophages are numerous, including direct contributions to the evasion strategies previously discussed. Yet, for the purpose of conciseness, we will focus exclusively on the capacity of this pathogen to modulate key metabolic pathways via the polarization of macrophages and, subsequently, influence the host production of NO and death modality of infected cells.

Beyond the established evidence supporting the ability of *M. tuberculosis* to influence and take advantage of the metabolic state of the host cell (McKinney et al. 2000; El Kasmi et al. 2008; Gallardo-Soler et al. 2008; Pandey and Sassetti 2008; Daniel et al. 2011; Mahajan et al. 2012; Gouzy et al. 2013; Marrero et al. 2013), an emerging theme within the field of macrophage polarization is to investigate how metabolic pathways are regulated to support or direct functional changes during pathological and pathogenic processes (Cairo et al. 2011; Chawla et al. 2011; McLaren et al. 2011; Biswas and Mantovani 2012; O'Neill and Hardie 2013; Odegaard and Chawla 2013; Pearce and Pearce 2013; Russell 2013). In general, M1 and M2 macrophages are characterized by distinct metabolic states in terms of amino acid and lipid utilization, among other types of metabolism (Fig. 1). Within the realm of amino acid metabolism, it has long been known that the differential use of arginine influences the functional capacity of polarized macrophages. A competition for this amino acid as a substrate between enzymes that drive M1 (inducible NO synthase, iNOS) or M2 (Arginase1, ARG1) polarization programs determines the NO production and, consequently, the microbicidal capacity of macrophages. From the host perspective, NO production is arguably one of the most important consequences mediated by IFN-γ polarization of macrophages, and mice deficient for NO production readily succumb to *M. tuberculosis* infection (Flynn et al. 1993). Moreover, M1 macrophages display a "fail-safe" mechanism to sustain NO production based on citrulline recycling via ASS1 (argininosuccinate synthase), which M2 macrophages lack (Qualls et al. 2012). Conversely, M2 macrophages with enhanced levels of ARG1 display a reduced NO production and increased of iron availability, arguing that the arginine metabolism influences nutrient deprivation mechanisms in place to limit microbial growth (Kahnert et al. 2006; Cairo et al. 2011). From the pathogen perspective, *M. tuberculosis* promotes its survival by inducing ARG1 expression through MyD88-dependent signaling pathways, supporting the concept that bacillus uses metabolic means to switch the macrophage polarization in its favor (El Kasmi et al. 2008) (Fig. 1). Furthermore, *M. tuberculosis* induces foam cell (macrophages rich in cholesterol and other carbon sources) formation via the production of mycobacterial lipids that trigger the activation of lipid-sensing nuclear receptors including PPARγ (peroxisome proliferator-activated receptor γ), the master regulator of M2 polarization and ARG1 (Gallardo-Soler et al. 2008; Mahajan et al. 2012). Interestingly, ARG1 is associated with M2 macrophages present in human and macaque tuberculous granuloma lesions (Pessanha et al. 2012; Mattila et al. 2013), arguing that the iNOS/ARG1 polarization axis may be pertinent beyond the murine context.

In terms of the metabolism of host lipids, there is an emerging interest on the role of eicosanoid production influencing the programmed macrophage death (Behar et al. 2010). This is partly owing to the fact that, as products of the arachidonic acid signaling cascade, eicosanoids are second messengers in tumor necrosis factor (TNF)-induced apoptosis (Wolf and Laster 1999) and modulators of the oxygen species production, which are also involved in cell death (Chang et al. 1992). Interestingly, M1 macrophages are characterized by the induction of prostaglandin-endoperoxide synthase 2

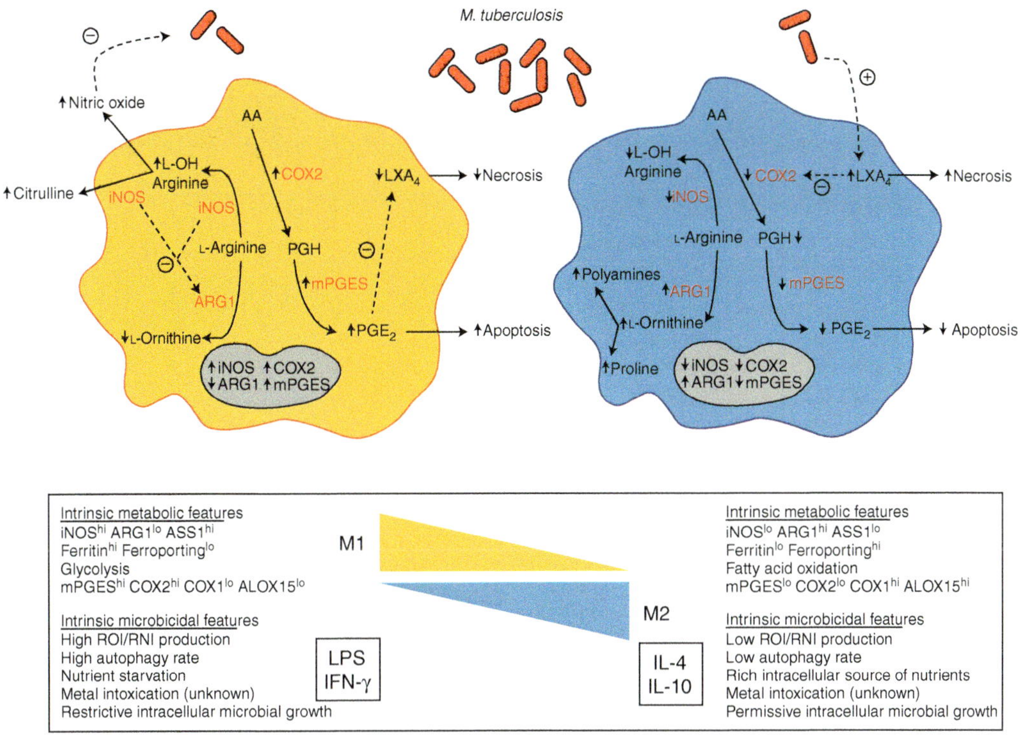

Figure 1. A model illustrating the modulation of key metabolism pathways via macrophage polarization by *M. tuberculosis*. On pathogenic challenge, a M1 macrophage (*left*) shifts its metabolic states in order to support microbicidal activities. Among these, the production of NO (nitric oxide) is an essential effector molecule to control microbial growth. To ensure an optimal NO production, M1 macrophages increase the expression ratio of iNOS (inducible NO synthase) to reduce the expression of ARG1 (arginase 1), and outcompete ARG1 for their common L-arginine substrate. In addition, as the death modality of infected macrophages is an innate immune mechanism, a M1 macrophage shifts the metabolism of arachidonic acid (AA) for the optimal production of PGE_2 (Prostaglandin E2) and favors the apoptosis process, which ultimately is thought to lead to the elimination of the pathogen. This is accomplished by the increase of COX2 (prostaglandin-endoperoxide synthase 2) expression that ensures a high ratio of PGE_2/LXA_4 (lipoxin4). In contrast, a M2 macrophage (*right*) displays different metabolic states to support different functional programs including tissue maintenance and repair, among others. Indeed, by increasing ARG1 expression and reciprocally diminishing that of iNOS, the metabolism of L-arginine is shifted toward the production of proline and polyamines, which foment collagen production and cell proliferation, respectively. Likewise, M2 macrophages decrease the production PGE_2 by arresting the expression of COX2. *M. tuberculosis* appears to have the capacity to modulate the process of macrophage polarization and influence the metabolic states of infected cells. Upon challenge with *M. tuberculosis*, the expression of ARG1 is augmented to outcompete the activity of iNOS for L-arginine and, as a consequence, diminish the production of NO. Similarly, *M. tuberculosis* also affects the AA metabolism by deliberately tilting a low ratio of PGE_2/LXA_4, driving infected macrophages toward the cell death process of necrosis, escaping intracellular defense mechanisms in a "timely" manner, and disseminating advantageously within the host.

(PTGS2, COX2) and PGE synthase (mPGES), leading to an enhanced pro-inflammatory potential exemplified by the production of prostaglandin E2 (PGE_2) (Fig. 1). Conversely, M2 macrophages display elevated levels of arachidonate 15-lipoxygenase (ALOX15) and PTGS1 (COX1), accompanied by the up-regulation of fatty acid uptake and oxidation, granting these cells an anti-inflammatory activity characterized by lipoxin A4 (LXA_4) production (Biswas and Mantovani 2012). Remarkably, the balance of the PGE_2/LXA_4 axis determines the cell death process of macrophages infected with *M. tuberculosis* (Behar et al. 2010; O'Garra et al. 2013). Indeed, driven by PTGS2 activity, the production of PGE_2 prevents necrosis of infected cells and, instead, promotes apoptosis by (1) protecting the mitochondria from inner-membrane damage and loss of membrane potential, (2) enabling the repair of the damage sustained by the plasma membrane, and (3) inhibiting the LXA_4 production. The macrophage response to attenuated *M. tuberculosis* strains, for example, is characterized by the strong expression of PTGS2 and PGE_2 production, consequently leading to high rates of apoptosis (Behar et al. 2010). In contrast, the strong production of LXA_4 is known to prevent the expression of PTGS2 and production of PGE_2, consequently leading to higher rates of necrosis, a situation that is reflected in the infection of macrophages with virulent strains of *M. tuberculosis* (Behar et al. 2010) (Fig. 1). In the field of host–pathogen interaction, the death modality of infected macrophages is considered an innate defense mechanism (Behar et al. 2010; Abebe et al. 2011; O'Garra et al. 2013). From the host perspective, a shift toward the M1 polarization program ensures the apoptosis of macrophages that is thought to enhance the containment of the infection, minimize tissue injury, promote the presentation of the pathogenic antigens via the cross-priming of $CD8^+$ T cells, and, ultimately, lead to the elimination of the pathogen. From the pathogen perspective, a shift toward the M2 polarization program promotes the necrosis of infected macrophage that consequently grants the pathogen to escape from intracellular defense mechanisms in a "timely" manner and disseminate advantageously within the host (Fig. 1).

Altogether, the iNOS/ARG1 and PGE_2/LXA_4 axes best illustrate the potential of macrophage polarization to modulate key metabolic processes during the immune response, a situation that, when not properly regulated, is detrimental to the host because of potential metabolic disorders contributing to obesity, insulin resistance, diabetes, and atherosclerosis (Biswas and Mantovani 2012). Indeed, the capacity to modulate macrophage polarization and influence its metabolic states may represent only the "tip of the iceberg" concerning microbial strategies to alter the macrophage response and enhance intracellular fitness.

DENDRITIC CELL DIFFERENTIATION AND ACTIVATION: MANIPULATION OF ANTI-INFLAMMATORY MEDIATORS THROUGH RECEPTOR CROSS TALK

Besides their crucial role as the "sentinels" of the immune system, dendritic cells are also considered the "orchestrators" of the immune response because of their remarkable ability to present antigen and prime naïve T cells. As the most potent professional antigen-presenting cell, dendritic cells are capable of delivering three different signals that ensure the establishment of a dedicated immune response resulting in immunological memory against a given pathogenic insult: signal 1, through the processing and loading of antigenic material to be presented in the context of MHC class I and class II; signal 2, through the specific up-regulation of costimulatory molecules (e.g., CD80, CD86); and signal 3, through the optimal secretion of cytokines (e.g., IL-12) and other signaling molecules. In the context of tuberculosis, however, the interaction of *M. tuberculosis* with dendritic cells is not fully understood (Mihret 2012). One reason is the contradictory studies in which dendritic cells either strengthen the cellular immune response against the bacillus or contribute to pathogenesis because of a poor stimulatory activity of antigen-specific $CD4^+$ T cells. Here, we will focus exclusively on the capacity of *M. tuberculosis* to induce anti-inflammation mediators via receptor cross talk and influence dendritic cell differentiation and functional capacity, with a particular emphasis on the immunosuppressive mediator IL-10.

As previously discussed, one of the ingenious ways to evade the host immune response is for a microbe to either prevent a dedicated pro-inflammatory response or hijack the anti-inflammatory mechanisms in place to ensure host tissue integrity. The manipulation of the host receptor talk in innate immunity is an efficient microbial strategy to accomplish this

(Hajishengallis and Lambris 2011). Receptor cross talk refers to the information that sentinel cells acquire from environmental clues through pattern recognition receptors (PRRs) and relay it intracellularly through nonlinear signaling cascades. In this manner, this information is integrated and processed to synergistically activate host defenses to clear infections or to antagonistically dampen unwarranted host defenses (Hajishengallis and Lambris 2011). The microbial manipulation of receptor cross talk takes place when the information to be processed is subverted or disrupted to tilt the final outcome to the microbe's favor. From the microbe perspective, subverting receptor cross talk in dendritic cells makes sense because they represent the first line of immune defense, and if properly performed, it can also undermine the overall adaptive immune response. In the context of tuberculosis, as well as with other clinical infections caused by other pathogens (e.g., *Mycobacterium leprae*, *Helicobacter pylori*, *Candida albicans*), the subversion of the cross talk between TLRs and the C-type lectin receptor (CLR) is thought to play a crucial role during pathogenesis (van Kooyk and Geijtenbeek 2003). By targeting the DC-SIGN (dendritic cell–specific intercellular adhesion molecule-3-grabbing nonintegrin) receptor in human dendritic cells (Tailleux et al. 2003), *M. tuberculosis* induces the production of the immunosuppressive mediator IL-10 and, at the same time, counteracts the pro-inflammatory response driven by TLR-4 (Geijtenbeek et al. 2003). This is accomplished by mycobacterial mannosylated lipoarabinomannan (ManLAM), which binds to DC-SIGN in an autocrine or paracrine manner and foments a complex signaling cascade that leads to the phosphorylation of the p65 subunit of the transcription factor NF-κB. In fact, this posttranscriptional modification prolongs the presence of NF-κB in the nucleus and, as a direct consequence, the augmentation of the transcription of the IL-10 gene (Geijtenbeek et al. 2003). The enhanced production of IL-10 grants multiple advantages to the invading microbe, including the inhibition of costimulatory molecules and down-regulation of IL-12 in dendritic cells, ultimately tilting the adaptive immunity in its favor from a T helper 1 (Th1) to a Th2 response (Redford et al. 2011; O'Garra et al. 2013).

Beyond the direct effect on dendritic cells, the modulation of anti-inflammatory mediators via receptor cross talk may also allow *M. tuberculosis* to shift the local environment in its favor and create a "bystander" effect on immune effector cells being recruited to the site of infection. For instance, it is well annotated that *M. tuberculosis* modulates the local environments favoring HIV-1 replication and systemic HIV-1 heterogeneity (Pawlowski et al. 2012). This bystander effect in turn leads to higher viral loads, $CD4^+$ T-cell destruction, and higher mortality in coinfected patients. Besides the overproduction of IL-10, *M. tuberculosis* also promotes an environment composed of other immunosuppressive mediators such as TGF-β, Th2 cytokines (e.g., IL-4, IL-5, IL-13), deregulation of inflammatory lipids (e.g., PGE_2), overproduction of acute-phase proteins (e.g., α1-acid glycoprotein), and low production of β-defensins, among others (Cooper 2009; Hernandez-Pando et al. 2009; Cooper et al. 2011; Sundareshan et al. 2011). Together, the modulation of these factors may be responsible for a bystander effect that allows *M. tuberculosis* to subvert the differentiation of monocytes into dendritic cells that are deficient in priming naïve T cells and, instead, contribute to pathogenic dissemination (Mariotti et al. 2002; Skold and Behar 2008; Rajashree et al. 2009). This premise is in line with the imbalance in the relative proportions of blood-circulating monocytes observed in tuberculosis patients, in which the abundance of the $CD14^+CD16^+$ subset is accentuated and shown to have a defective differentiation program toward functional dendritic cells (Vanham et al. 1996; Balboa et al. 2013). In the case of IL-10, it was shown to be part of the bystander effect induced by *M. tuberculosis* to inhibit the differentiation of human monocytes into $CD1c^+$ DCs, suggesting it plays an important role in the recruitment of dendritic cell precursors that may be incapable to activate efficiently the adaptive immune response (Remoli et al. 2011). Supporting the concept that *M. tuberculosis* modulates its environment and the functional capacity of antigen-presenting cells in its favor, a recent study in zebrafish shows that its close pathogenic relative, *Mycobacterium marinum*, is able to avoid immune recognition by using cell surface–associated phthiocerol dymycoceroserate (PDIM) lipids, and at the same time, to promote the recruitment of permissive macrophages to site of infection via phenolic glycolipids (PGLs) (Cambier et al. 2013). Although the description of this study does not include the modulation of monocytes or dendritic cells by *M. marinum*, it can be inferred that PGLs may also be responsible for the induction of anti-inflammatory factors that modulate the recruitment of monocytes that differentiate poorly into effective antigen-presenting dendritic cells, as shown recently for *M. tuberculosis* and *M. leprae* (Goulart et al. 2000; Hashimoto et al. 2002).

CONCLUDING REMARKS

A tenet of this article is that further progress in the identification and characterization of microbial and host factors that are involved in macrophage polarization and key metabolic pathways during the context of microbial infection will foment a better understanding of how these processes are intertwined to influence the immune response to, and pathogenesis of, *M. tuberculosis*. It is anticipated that molecules that facilitate such processes are potential targets for preventive and therapeutic agents against tuberculosis. Indeed, several options are being explored for the rational design of host-directed therapies that could either reduce the destructive inflammatory responses against *M. tuberculosis* or augment the inadequate immunity due to virulence factors, without further fomenting the occurrence of multiple-drug resistant mycobacterial strains. To accomplish this, future studies must also include efforts to bridge the knowledge obtained in the human context and from all experimental animal models, ranging from zebrafish, mouse, and guinea pig to rabbit and nonhuman primate. In addition, these studies could go along with more sophisticated "omics" global approaches to correlate transcript, protein, and metabolic content of host cells under different pathogenic contexts. Finally, it is expected that cellular and molecular mechanisms involved in preserving the tissue integrity and establishing peripheral tolerance (Medzhitov et al. 2012) might represent new venues to further investigate the ability of *M. tuberculosis* to evade and subvert the MPS compartment. Indeed, the ability of the host to tolerate a pathogen's presence is a new concept being integrated in the host–pathogen field, and one that is completely different from the host defense strategies.

REFERENCES

Abebe M, Kim L, Rook G, Aseffa A, Wassie L, Zewdie M, Zumla A, Engers H, Andersen P, Doherty TM. 2011. Modulation of cell death by *M. tuberculosis* as a strategy for pathogen survival. *Clin Dev Immunol* **2011:** 678570.

Alsultan A, Giller RH, Gao D, Bathurst J, Hild E, Gore L, Foreman NK, Keating A, Quinones RR. 2011. GVHD after unrelated cord blood transplant in children: Characteristics, severity, risk factors and influence on outcome. *Bone Marrow Transplant* **46:** 668–675.

Armstrong JA, Hart PD. 1971. Response of cultured macrophages to *Mycobacterium tuberculosis*, with observations on fusion of lysosomes with phagosomes. *J Exp Med* **134:** 713–740.

Bach H, Papavinasasundaram KG, Wong D, Hmama Z, Av-Gay Y. 2008. *Mycobacterium tuberculosis* virulence is mediated by PtpA dephosphorylation of human vacuolar protein sorting 33B. *Cell Host Microbe* **3:** 316–322.

Balboa L, Romero MM, Laborde E, Sabio YGCA, Basile JI, Schierloh P, Yokobori N, Musella RM, Castagnino J, de la Barrera S, et al. 2013. Impaired dendritic cell differentiation of CD16-positive monocytes in tuberculosis: Role of p38 MAPK. *Eur J Immunol* **43:** 335–347.

Behar SM, Divangahi M, Remold HG. 2010. Evasion of innate immunity by *Mycobacterium tuberculosis*: Is death an exit strategy? *Nat Rev Microbiol* **8:** 668–674.

Benoit M, Desnues B, Mege JL. 2008. Macrophage polarization in bacterial infections. *J Immunol* **181:** 3733–3739.

Biswas SK, Mantovani A. 2012. Orchestration of metabolism by macrophages. *Cell Metab* **15:** 432–437.

Botella H, Peyron P, Levillain F, Poincloux R, Poquet Y, Brandli I, Wang C, Tailleux L, Tilleul S, Charriere GM, et al. 2011. Mycobacterial P_1-type ATPases mediate resistance to zinc poisoning in human macrophages. *Cell Host Microbe* **10:** 248–259.

Bradfute SB, Castillo EF, Arko-Mensah J, Chauhan S, Jiang S, Mandell M, Deretic V. 2013. Autophagy as an immune effector against tuberculosis. *Curr Opin Microbiol* **16:** 355–365.

Brightbill HD, Libraty DH, Krutzik SR, Yang RB, Belisle JT, Bleharski JR, Maitland M, Norgard MV, Plevy SE, Smale ST, et al. 1999. Host defense mechanisms triggered by microbial lipoproteins through Toll-like receptors. *Science* **285:** 732–736.

Brodin P, Poquet Y, Levillain F, Peguillet I, Larrouy-Maumus G, Gilleron M, Ewann F, Christophe T, Fenistein D, Jang J, et al. 2010. High content phenotypic cell-based visual screen identifies *Mycobacterium tuberculosis* acyltrehalose-containing glycolipids involved in phagosome remodeling. *PLoS Pathog* **6:** e1001100.

Cairo G, Recalcati S, Mantovani A, Locati M. 2011. Iron trafficking and metabolism in macrophages: Contribution to the polarized phenotype. *Trends Immunol* **32:** 241–247.

Cambier CJ, Takaki KK, Larson RP, Hernandez RE, Tobin DM, Urdahl KB, Cosma CL, Ramakrishnan L. 2013. Mycobacteria manipulate macrophage recruitment through coordinated use of membrane lipids. *Nature* **505:** 218–222.

Chang DJ, Ringold GM, Heller RA. 1992. Cell killing and induction of manganous superoxide dismutase by tumor necrosis factor-α is mediated by lipoxygenase metabolites of arachidonic acid. *Biochem Biophys Res Commun* **188:** 538–546.

Chawla A, Nguyen KD, Goh YP. 2011. Macrophage-mediated inflammation in metabolic disease. *Nat Rev Immunol* **11:** 738–749.

Chillappagari S, Seubert A, Trip H, Kuipers OP, Marahiel MA, Miethke M. 2010. Copper stress affects iron homeostasis by destabilizing iron-sulfur cluster formation in *Bacillus subtilis*. *J Bacteriol* **192:** 2512–2524.

Chow A, Brown BD, Merad M. 2011. Studying the mononuclear phagocyte system in the molecular age. *Nat Rev Immunol* **11:** 788–798.

Cooper AM. 2009. Cell-mediated immune responses in tuberculosis. *Annu Rev Immunol* **27:** 393–422.

Cooper AM, Mayer-Barber KD, Sher A. 2011. Role of innate cytokines in mycobacterial infection. *Mucosal Immunol* **4:** 252–260.

Daniel J, Maamar H, Deb C, Sirakova TD, Kolattukudy PE. 2011. *Mycobacterium tuberculosis* uses host triacylglycerol to accumulate lipid droplets and acquires a dormancy-like phenotype in lipid-loaded macrophages. *PLoS Pathog* **7:** e1002093.

de Carvalho LP, Fischer SM, Marrero J, Nathan C, Ehrt S, Rhee KY. 2010. Metabolomics of *Mycobacterium tuberculosis* reveals compartmentalized co-catabolism of carbon substrates. *Chem Biol* **17:** 1122–1131.

Deghmane AE, Soualhine H, Bach H, Sendide K, Itoh S, Tam A, Noubir S, Talal A, Lo R, Toyoshima S, et al. 2007. Lipoamide dehydrogenase mediates retention of coronin-1 on BCG vacuoles, leading to arrest in phagosome maturation. *J Cell Sci* **120:** 2796–2806.

Deretic V. 2008. Autophagy, an immunologic magic bullet: *Mycobacterium tuberculosis* phagosome maturation block and how to bypass it. *Future Microbiol* **3:** 517–524.

Deretic V, Vergne I, Chua J, Master S, Singh SB, Fazio JA, Kyei G. 2004. Endosomal membrane traffic: Convergence point targeted by *Mycobacterium tuberculosis* and HIV. *Cell Microbiol* **6:** 999–1009.

Desjardins M, Griffiths G. 2003. Phagocytosis: Latex leads the way. *Curr Opin Cell Biol* **15:** 498–503.

Dorhoi A, Reece ST, Kaufmann SH. 2011. For better or for worse: The immune response against *Mycobacterium tuberculosis* balances pathology and protection. *Immunol Rev* **240:** 235–251.

Eisenreich W, Dandekar T, Heesemann J, Goebel W. 2010. Carbon metabolism of intracellular bacterial pathogens and possible links to virulence. *Nat Rev Microbiol* **8:** 401–412.

El Kasmi KC, Qualls JE, Pesce JT, Smith AM, Thompson RW, Henao-Tamayo M, Basaraba RJ, Konig T, Schleicher U, Koo MS, et al. 2008. Toll-like receptor-induced arginase 1 in macrophages thwarts effective immunity against intracellular pathogens. *Nat Immunol* **9:** 1399–1406.

Engering A, Geijtenbeek TB, van Kooyk Y. 2002. Immune escape through C-type lectins on dendritic cells. *Trends Immunol* **23:** 480–485.

Fabri M, Stenger S, Shin DM, Yuk JM, Liu PT, Realegeno S, Lee HM, Krutzik SR, Schenk M, Sieling PA, et al. 2011. Vitamin D is required for IFN-γ-mediated antimicrobial activity of human macrophages. *Sci Transl Med* **3:** 104ra102.

Flynn JL, Chan J. 2003. Immune evasion by *Mycobacterium tuberculosis*: Living with the enemy. *Curr Opin Immunol* **15:** 450–455.

Flynn JL, Chan J, Triebold KJ, Dalton DK, Stewart TA, Bloom BR. 1993. An essential role for interferon γ in resistance to *Mycobacterium tuberculosis* infection. *J Exp Med* **178:** 2249–2254.

Gallardo-Soler A, Gomez-Nieto C, Campo ML, Marathe C, Tontonoz P, Castrillo A, Corraliza I. 2008. Arginase I induction by modified lipoproteins in macrophages: A peroxisome proliferator-activated receptor-γ/δ-mediated effect that links lipid metabolism and immunity. *Mol Endocrinol* **22:** 1394–1402.

Geijtenbeek TB, Van Vliet SJ, Koppel EA, Sanchez-Hernandez M, Vandenbroucke-Grauls CM, Appelmelk B, Van Kooyk Y. 2003. Mycobacteria target DC-SIGN to suppress dendritic cell function. *J Exp Med* **197:** 7–17.

Geissmann F, Manz MG, Jung S, Sieweke MH, Merad M, Ley K. 2010. Development of monocytes, macrophages, and dendritic cells. *Science* **327:** 656–661.

Gobin J, Horwitz MA. 1996. Exochelins of *Mycobacterium tuberculosis* remove iron from human iron-binding proteins and donate iron to mycobactins in the *M. tuberculosis* cell wall. *J Exp Med* **183:** 1527–1532.

Gordon S, Taylor PR. 2005. Monocyte and macrophage heterogeneity. *Nat Rev Immunol* **5:** 953–964.

Goulart IM, Mineo JR, Foss NT. 2000. Production of transforming growth factor-β 1 (TGF-β1) by blood monocytes from patients with different clinical forms of leprosy. *Clin Exp Immunol* **122:** 330–334.

Gouzy A, Larrouy-Maumus G, Wu T-D, Peixoto A, Levillain F, Gerquin-Kern J-L, de Carvalho LPS, Poquet Y, Neyrolles O. 2013. *Mycobacterium tuberculosis* nitrogen assimilation and host colonization require aspartate. *Nat Chem Biol* **9:** 674–676.

Gouzy A, Larrouy-Maumus G, Bottai D, Levillain F, Wallach JB, Caire-Brandli I, de Chastellier C, Wu T-D, Poincloux R, Brosch R, et al. 2014. *Mycobacterium tuberculosis* exploits asparagine to assimilate nitrogen and resist acid stress during infection. *PLoS Pathog* **10:** e1003928.

Griffin JE, Pandey AK, Gilmore SA, Mizrahi V, McKinney JD, Bertozzi CR, Sassetti CM. 2012. Cholesterol catabolism by *Mycobacterium tuberculosis* requires transcriptional and metabolic adaptations. *Chem Biol* **19:** 218–227.

Gupta A, Kaul A, Tsolaki AG, Kishore U, Bhakta S. 2012. *Mycobacterium tuberculosis*: immune evasion, latency and reactivation. *Immunobiology* **217:** 363–374.

Hajishengallis G, Lambris JD. 2011. Microbial manipulation of receptor crosstalk in innate immunity. *Nat Rev Immunol* **11:** 187–200.

Hashimoto K, Maeda Y, Kimura H, Suzuki K, Masuda A, Matsuoka M, Makino M. 2002. *Mycobacterium leprae* infection in monocyte-derived dendritic cells and its influence on antigen-presenting function. *Infect Immun* **70:** 5167–5176.

Hernandez-Pando R, Orozco H, Aguilar D. 2009. Factors that deregulate the protective immune response in tuberculosis. *Arch Immunol Ther Exp* **57:** 355–367.

Hood MI, Skaar EP. 2012. Nutritional immunity: Transition metals at the pathogen–host interface. *Nat Rev Microbiol* **10:** 525–537.

Kahnert A, Seiler P, Stein M, Bandermann S, Hahnke K, Mollenkopf H, Kaufmann SH. 2006. Alternative activation deprives macrophages of a coordinated defense program to *Mycobacterium tuberculosis*. *Eur J Immunol* **36:** 631–647.

Liu PT, Stenger S, Li H, Wenzel L, Tan BH, Krutzik SR, Ochoa MT, Schauber J, Wu K, Meinken C, et al. 2006. Toll-like receptor triggering of a vitamin D–mediated human antimicrobial response. *Science* **311:** 1770–1773.

Lugo-Villarino G, Verollet C, Maridonneau-Parini I, Neyrolles O. 2011. Macrophage polarization: Convergence point targeted by mycobacterium tuberculosis and HIV. *Front Immunol* **2:** 43.

Luo M, Fadeev EA, Groves JT. 2005. Mycobactin-mediated iron acquisition within macrophages. *Nat Chem Biol* **1:** 149–153.

Macomber L, Rensing C, Imlay JA. 2007. Intracellular copper does not catalyze the formation of oxidative DNA damage in *Escherichia coli*. *J Bacteriol* **189:** 1616–1626.

Mahajan S, Dkhar HK, Chandra V, Dave S, Nanduri R, Janmeja AK, Agrewala JN, Gupta P. 2012. *Mycobacterium tuberculosis* modulates macrophage lipid-sensing nuclear receptors PPARγ and TR4 for survival. *J Immunol* **188:** 5593–5603.

Mariotti S, Teloni R, Iona E, Fattorini L, Giannoni F, Romagnoli G, Orefici G, Nisini R. 2002. *Mycobacterium tuberculosis* subverts the differentiation of human monocytes into dendritic cells. *Eur J Immunol* **32:** 3050–3058.

Marrero J, Rhee KY, Schnappinger D, Pethe K, Ehrt S. 2010. Gluconeogenic carbon flow of tricarboxylic acid cycle intermediates is critical for *Mycobacterium tuberculosis* to establish and maintain infection. *Proc Natl Acad Sci* **107:** 9819–9824.

Marrero J, Trujillo C, Rhee KY, Ehrt S. 2013. Glucose phosphorylation is required for *Mycobacterium tuberculosis* persistence in mice. *PLoS Pathog* **9:** e1003116.

Martinez FO, Helming L, Gordon S. 2009. Alternative activation of macrophages: An immunologic functional perspective. *Annu Rev Immunol* **27:** 451–483.

Martino A. 2008. Mycobacteria and innate cells: Critical encounter for immunogenicity. *J Biosci* **33:** 137–144.

Master SS, Rampini SK, Davis AS, Keller C, Ehlers S, Springer B, Timmins GS, Sander P, Deretic V. 2008. *Mycobacterium tuberculosis* prevents inflammasome activation. *Cell Host Microbe* **3:** 224–232.

Mattila JT, Ojo OO, Kepka-Lenhart D, Marino S, Kim JH, Eum SY, Via LE, Barry CE III, Klein E, Kirschner DE, et al. 2013. Microenvironments in tuberculous granulomas are delineated by distinct populations of macrophage subsets and expression of nitric oxide synthase and arginase isoforms. *J Immunol* **191:** 773–784.

McDevitt CA, Ogunniyi AD, Valkov E, Lawrence MC, Kobe B, McEwan AG, Paton JC. 2011. A molecular mechanism for bacterial susceptibility to zinc. *PLoS Pathog* **7:** e1002357.

McKinney JD, Honer zu Bentrup K, Munoz-Elias EJ, Miczak A, Chen B, Chan WT, Swenson D, Sacchettini JC, Jacobs WR Jr, Russell DG. 2000. Persistence of *Mycobacterium tuberculosis* in macrophages and mice requires the glyoxylate shunt enzyme isocitrate lyase. *Nature* **406:** 735–738.

McLaren JE, Michael DR, Ashlin TG, Ramji DP. 2011. Cytokines, macrophage lipid metabolism and foam cells: Implications for cardiovascular disease therapy. *Prog Lipid Res* **50:** 331–347.

Medzhitov R, Schneider DS, Soares MP. 2012. Disease tolerance as a defense strategy. *Science* **335:** 936–941.

Mege JL, Mehraj V, Capo C. 2011. Macrophage polarization and bacterial infections. *Curr Opin Infect Dis* **24:** 230–234.

Mehra A, Zahra A, Thompson V, Sirisaengtaksin N, Wells A, Porto M, Koster S, Penberthy K, Kubota Y, Dricot A, et al. 2013. *Mycobacterium tuberculosis* type VII secreted effector EsxH targets host ESCRT to impair trafficking. *PLoS Pathog* **9:** e1003734.

Mihret A. 2012. The role of dendritic cells in *Mycobacterium tuberculosis* infection. *Virulence* **3:** 654–659.

Mounier R, Theret M, Arnold L, Cuvellier S, Bultot L, Goransson O, Sanz N, Ferry A, Sakamoto K, Foretz M, et al. 2013. AMPKα1 regulates macrophage skewing at the time of resolution of inflammation during skeletal muscle regeneration. *Cell Metab* **18:** 251–264.

Munoz-Elias EJ, McKinney JD. 2005. *Mycobacterium tuberculosis* isocitrate lyases 1 and 2 are jointly required for in vivo growth and virulence. *Nat Med* **11:** 638–644.

Munoz-Elias EJ, McKinney J.D. 2006. Carbon metabolism of intracellular bacteria. *Cell Microbiol* **8:** 10–22.

Murray PJ, Wynn TA. 2011. Protective and pathogenic functions of macrophage subsets. *Nat Rev Immunol* **11:** 723–737.

O'Garra A, Redford PS, McNab FW, Bloom CI, Wilkinson RJ, Berry MP. 2013. The immune response in tuberculosis. *Annu Rev Immunol* **31:** 475–527.

O'Neill LA, Hardie DG. 2013. Metabolism of inflammation limited by AMPK and pseudo-starvation. *Nature* **493:** 346–355.

Odegaard JI, Chawla A. 2013. The immune system as a sensor of the metabolic state. *Immunity* **38:** 644–654.

Osman D, Patterson CJ, Bailey K, Fisher K, Robinson NJ, Rigby SE, Cavet JS. 2013. The copper supply pathway to a salmonella Cu,Zn-superoxide dismutase (SodCII) involves P_{1B}-type ATPase copper efflux and periplasmic CueP. *Mol Microbiol* **87:** 466–477.

Padilla-Benavides T, Long JE, Raimunda D, Sassetti CM, Arguello JM. 2013. A novel P_{1B}-type Mn^{2+}-transporting ATPase is required for secreted protein metallation in mycobacteria. *J Biol Chem* **288:** 11334–11347.

Pandey AK, Sassetti CM. 2008. Mycobacterial persistence requires the utilization of host cholesterol. *Proc Natl Acad Sci* **105:** 4376–4380.

Pawlowski A, Jansson M, Skold M, Rottenberg ME, Kallenius G. 2012. Tuberculosis and HIV co-infection. *PLoS Pathog* **8:** e1002464.

Pearce EL, Pearce EJ. 2013. Metabolic pathways in immune cell activation and quiescence. *Immunity* **38:** 633–643.

Pessanha AP, Martins RA, Mattos-Guaraldi AL, Vianna A, Moreira LO. 2012. Arginase-1 expression in granulomas of tuberculosis patients. *FEMS Immunol Med Microbiol* **66:** 265–268.

Pethe K, Swenson DL, Alonso S, Anderson J, Wang C, Russell DG. 2004. Isolation of *Mycobacterium tuberculosis* mutants defective in the arrest of phagosome maturation. *Proc Natl Acad Sci* **101:** 13642–13647.

Philips JA. 2008. Mycobacterial manipulation of vacuolar sorting. *Cell Microbiol* **10:** 2408–2415.

Qualls JE, Subramanian C, Rafi W, Smith AM, Balouzian L, DeFreitas AA, Shirey KA, Reutterer B, Kernbauer E, Stockinger S, et al. 2012. Sustained generation of nitric oxide and control of mycobacterial infection requires argininosuccinate synthase 1. *Cell Host Microbe* **12:** 313–323.

Rajashree P, Krishnan G, Das SD. 2009. Impaired phenotype and function of monocyte derived dendritic cells in pulmonary tuberculosis. *Tuberculosis* **89:** 77–83.

Redford PS, Murray PJ, O'Garra A. 2011. The role of IL-10 in immune regulation during *M. tuberculosis* infection. *Mucosal Immunol* **4:** 261–270.

Remoli ME, Giacomini E, Petruccioli E, Gafa V, Severa M, Gagliardi MC, Iona E, Pine R, Nisini R, Coccia EM. 2011. Bystander inhibition of dendritic cell differentiation by *Mycobacterium tuberculosis*–induced IL-10. *Immunol Cell Biol* **89:** 437–446.

Rodriguez GM, Smith I. 2006. Identification of an ABC transporter required for iron acquisition and virulence in *Mycobacterium tuberculosis*. *J Bacteriol* **188:** 424–430.

Russell DG. 2001. *Mycobacterium tuberculosis*: Here today, and here tomorrow. *Nat Rev Mol Cell Biol* **2:** 569–577.

Russell DG. 2011. *Mycobacterium tuberculosis* and the intimate discourse of a chronic infection. *Immunol Rev* **240:** 252–268.

Russell DG. 2013. The evolutionary pressures that have molded *Mycobacterium tuberculosis* into an infectious adjuvant. *Curr Opin Microbiol* **16:** 78–84.

Sarantis H, Grinstein S. 2012. Subversion of phagocytosis for pathogen survival. *Cell Host Microbe* **12:** 419–431.

Serbina NV, Jia T, Hohl TM, Pamer EG. 2008. Monocyte-mediated defense against microbial pathogens. *Annu Rev Immunol* **26:** 421–452.

Sica A, Mantovani A. 2012. Macrophage plasticity and polarization: In vivo veritas. *J Clin Invest* **22:** 787–795.

Siegrist MS, Unnikrishnan M, McConnell MJ, Borowsky M, Cheng TY, Siddiqi N, Fortune SM, Moody DB, Rubin EJ. 2009. Mycobacterial Esx-3 is required for mycobactin-mediated iron acquisition. *Proc Natl Acad Sci* **106:** 18792–18797.

Silva-Gomes S, Vale-Costa S, Appelberg R, Gomes MS. 2013. Iron in intracellular infection: To provide or to deprive? *Front Cell Infect Microbiol* **3:** 96.

Skold M, Behar SM. 2008. Tuberculosis triggers a tissue-dependent program of differentiation and acquisition of effector functions by circulating monocytes. *J Immunol* **181:** 6349–6360.

Stewart GR, Patel J, Robertson BD, Rae A, Young DB. 2005. Mycobacterial mutants with defective control of phagosomal acidification. *PLoS Pathog* **1:** 269–278.

Sturgill-Koszycki S, Schlesinger PH, Chakraborty P, Haddix PL, Collins HL, Fok AK, Allen RD, Gluck SL, Heuser J, Russell DG. 1994. Lack of acidification in *Mycobacterium phagosomes* produced by exclusion of the vesicular proton-ATPase. *Science* **263:** 678–681.

Sullivan JT, Young EF, McCann JR, Braunstein M. 2012. The *Mycobacterium tuberculosis* SecA2 system subverts phagosome maturation to promote growth in macrophages. *Infect Immun* **80:** 996–1006.

Sundareshan V, Modi J, Khardori NM. 2011. Mycobacteria and biological response modifiers: Two sides of the relationship. *Infect Dis Clin North Am* **25:** 865–893.

Tailleux L, Schwartz O, Herrmann JL, Pivert E, Jackson M, Amara A, Legres L, Dreher D, Nicod LP, Gluckman JC, et al. 2003. DC-SIGN is the major *Mycobacterium tuberculosis* receptor on human dendritic cells. *J Exp Med* **197:** 121–127.

Thi EP, Hong CJ, Sanghera G, Reiner NE. 2013. Identification of the *Mycobacterium tuberculosis* protein PE-PGRS62 as a novel effector that functions to block phagosome maturation and inhibit iNOS expression. *Cell Microbiol* **15:** 795–808.

Thoma-Uszynski S, Stenger S, Takeuchi O, Ochoa MT, Engele M, Sieling PA, Barnes PF, Rollinghoff M, Bolcskei PL, Wagner M, et al. 2001. Induction of direct antimicrobial activity through mammalian Toll-like receptors. *Science* **291:** 1544–1547.

Tullius MV, Harmston CA, Owens CP, Chim N, Morse RP, McMath LM, Iniguez A, Kimmey JM, Sawaya MR, Whitelegge JP, et al. 2011. Discovery and characterization of a unique mycobacterial heme acquisition system. *Proc Natl Acad Sci* **108:** 5051–5056.

van Furth R, Cohn ZA. 1968. The origin and kinetics of mononuclear phagocytes. *J Exp Med* **128:** 415–435.

van Kooyk Y, Geijtenbeek TB. 2003. DC-SIGN: Escape mechanism for pathogens. *Nat Rev Immunol* **3:** 697–709.

Vandal OH, Nathan CF, Ehrt S. 2009. Acid resistance in *Mycobacterium tuberculosis*. *J Bacteriol* **191:** 4714–4721.

Vandal OH, Pierini LM, Schnappinger D, Nathan CF, Ehrt S. 2008. A membrane protein preserves intrabacterial pH in intraphagosomal *Mycobacterium tuberculosis. Nat Med* **14:** 849–854.

Vanham G, Edmonds K, Qing L, Hom D, Toossi Z, Jones B, Daley CL, Huebner B, Kestens L, Gigase P, et al. 1996. Generalized immune activation in pulmonary tuberculosis: Co-activation with HIV infection. *Clin Exp Immunol* **103:** 30–34.

Vergne I, Chua J, Lee HH, Lucas M, Belisle J, Deretic V. 2005. Mechanism of phagolysosome biogenesis block by viable *Mycobacterium tuberculosis. Proc Natl Acad Sci* **102:** 4033–4038.

Vogt G, Nathan C. 2011. In vitro differentiation of human macrophages with enhanced antimycobacterial activity. *J Clin Invest* **121:** 3889–3901.

Wagner D, Maser J, Lai B, Cai Z, Barry CE 3rd, Honer Zu Bentrup K, Russell DG, Bermudez LE. 2005. Elemental analysis of *Mycobacterium avium-*, *Mycobacterium tuberculosis-*, and *Mycobacterium smegmatis*-containing phagosomes indicates pathogen-induced microenvironments within the host cell's endosomal system. *J Immunol* **174:** 1491–1500.

Walburger A, Koul A, Ferrari G, Nguyen L, Prescianotto-Baschong C, Huygen K, Klebl B, Thompson C, Bacher G, Pieters J. 2004. Protein kinase G from pathogenic mycobacteria promotes survival within macrophages. *Science* **304:** 1800–1804.

Ward SK, Abomoelak B, Hoye EA, Steinberg H, Talaat AM. 2010. CtpV: A putative copper exporter required for full virulence of *Mycobacterium tuberculosis. Mol Microbiol* **77:** 1096–1110.

White C, Lee J, Kambe T, Fritsche K, Petris MJ. 2009. A role for the ATP7A copper-transporting ATPase in macrophage bactericidal activity. *J Biol Chem* **284:** 33949–33956.

Wiersma T, Mol SS, Thomas S. 1996. [Bone density measurement and prevention of fractures: Who should be eligible?]. *Ned Tijdsch Geneeskd* **140:** 1622.

Wolf LA, Laster SM. 1999. Characterization of arachidonic acid–induced apoptosis. *Cell Biochem Biophys* **30:** 353–368.

Wolschendorf F, Ackart D, Shrestha TB, Hascall-Dove L, Nolan S, Lamichhane G, Wang Y, Bossmann SH, Basaraba RJ, Niederweis M. 2011. Copper resistance is essential for virulence of *Mycobacterium tuberculosis. Proc Natl Acad Sci* **108:** 1621–1626.

Wong D, Bach H, Sun J, Hmama Z, Av-Gay Y. 2011. *Mycobacterium tuberculosis* protein tyrosine phosphatase (PtpA) excludes host vacuolar-H^+-ATPase to inhibit phagosome acidification. *Proc Natl Acad Sci* **108:** 19371–19376.

Xu FF, Imlay JA. 2012. Silver(I), mercury(II), cadmium(II), and zinc(II) target exposed enzymic iron-sulfur clusters when they toxify *Escherichia coli. Appl Environ Microbiol* **78:** 3614–3621.

Zhang YJ, Reddy MC, Ioerger TR, Rothchild AC, Dartois V, Schuster BM, Trauner A, Wallis D, Galaviz S, Huttenhower C, et al. 2013. Tryptophan biosynthesis protects mycobacteria from CD4 T-cell-mediated killing. *Cell* **155:** 1296–1308.

Interaction of *Mycobacterium tuberculosis* with Host Cell Death Pathways

Lalitha Srinivasan, Sarah Ahlbrand, and Volker Briken

Department of Cell Biology and Molecular Genetics, University of Maryland, College Park, Maryland 20742

Correspondence: vbriken@umd.edu

Mycobacterium tuberculosis (*Mtb*) has coevolved with humans for tens of thousands of years. It is thus highly adapted to its human host and has evolved multiple mechanisms to manipulate host immune responses to its advantage. One central host pathogen interaction modality is host cell death pathways. Host cell apoptosis is associated with a protective response to *Mtb* infection, whereas a necrotic response favors the pathogen. Consistently, *Mtb* inhibits host cell apoptosis signaling but promotes induction of programmed necrosis. The molecular mechanisms involved in *Mtb*-mediated host cell death manipulation, the consequences for host immunity, and the potential for therapeutic and preventive approaches will be discussed.

The death of eukaryotic cells is an extremely diverse and complex event that has been categorized into multiple cell death types according to morphological features and unique cell signaling and effector molecules involved (Galluzzi et al. 2012b). Here we will give a brief overview of apoptosis, necroptosis, and pyroptosis, as these are the cell death modalities that are the most relevant in regard to interac tion of pathogens with their host cell (Lamkanfi and Dixit 2010).

Apoptosis is morphologically characterized by cell shrinking, fragmentation of the nucleus, formation of membrane blebs, and apoptotic bodies. The apoptotic bodies contain cell cytoplasm and other cellular organelles and they are taken up by macrophages via receptor-mediated phagocytosis. In a process defined as efferocytosis, a macrophage phagocytoses a whole apoptotic cell. In both cases the cytoplasm and other cellular components never leave the dying cell, and hence apoptosis is immunologically silent. Important biochemical and cell signaling events that are often used to measure cellular apoptosis are the loss of mitochondrial outer membrane permeability (MOMP), cleavage and activation of members of the caspase protease family, fragmentation of chromosomal DNA, and externalization of phosphatidylserine at the cell membrane. The extrinsic apoptosis signaling pathway is activated by ligand binding to a death receptor (DR) such as TNF-receptor or Fas. Intracellular signaling events are complex but lead to the activation of caspase 8, which will then activate the executioner caspase 3, 6, and 7. The intrinsic apoptosis signaling pathway can be engaged by an increase in cytosolic reactive oxygen species (ROS), UV exposure, genotoxic stress, growth factor withdrawal, and others. These events will change the equilibrium of pro- and

Cite this article as *Cold Spring Harb Perspect Med* doi: 10.1101/cshperspect.a022459

antiapoptotic Bcl-2 family members toward a majority of proapoptotic proteins being activated. Two of these are Bax and Bak, which after activation form a pore that results in MOMP and release of cytochrome *c* into the cytosol. Here it associates with the apoptosis protease activating factor-1 (Apaf-1) to form the apoptosome complex, which will cleave and activate procaspase 9. Just like caspase 8, caspase 9 also cleaves and activates the executioner caspases 3, 6, and 7. The activated executioner caspase target and activate a wide array of cellular proteins, which are responsible for the morphological changes associated with apoptosis, such as caspase-activated DNases that cleave chromosomal DNA (Lamkanfi and Dixit 2010; Galluzzi et al. 2012a) (Fig. 1).

Historically, it was assumed that all cellular necrosis is accidental but it is now evident that most necrotic events are highly regulated by a multitude of pathways (Vanlangenakker et al. 2012). DRs and Toll-like receptors (TLRs) can induce the formation of an intracellular signaling complex containing Fas-associated death domain (FADD), caspase 8, rest in peace 1 (RIPK1), and rest in peace 3 (RIPK3). This complex can either induce apoptosis via activated caspase 8 or necroptosis via activated RIPK3, depending on other regulatory proteins. RIPK3 leads, via activation of other signaling proteins, to the disruption of mitochondrial function and necrosis. RIPK1 knockout mice are not viable and so necrostatin-1, a very specific inhibitor of RIPK1, is commonly used to investigate RIPK1-mediated necroptosis induction. Another important modulator of a necrotic cell death pathway, referred to as parthanatos, is the poly(ADP-ribose) polymerase 1 (PARP1). PARP1 upon short-term activation actually helps to prevent apoptotic cell death via its DNA repair function. Nevertheless, continuous activation leads to massive ATP consumption that triggers mitochondrial malfunction and necrosis. PARP1 may also be activated by RIPK1, highlighting a connection with DR and TLR signaling (Vanlangenakker et al. 2012; Sridharan and Upton 2014).

Finally, pyroptosis can be regarded as a mixture between apoptosis and programmed necrosis because, like the latter, pyroptosis leads to cell membrane rupture and no membrane blebs or apoptotic bodies are produced but, similar to apoptosis, genomic DNA is degraded and caspase activation is required (Kepp et al. 2010; Aachoui et al. 2013). In contrast to apoptosis, pyroptosis leads to inflammation caused by the leakage of cytosolic content via damaged cell membranes and because of the caspase 1–mediated generation of the secreted inflammatory cytokines IL-1β and IL-18. The caspase 1–mediated pyroptosis can be dependent on the adaptor ASC in the cases of NLRP3 and AIM2 activation or independent of ASC in the case of NLRC4-mediated activation. Caspase 11 transcription can be induced via TLR signaling after bacterial infection, and then it can either lead to stimulation of caspase 1 activity or directly induce pyroptosis. In contrast to caspase 1, caspase 11 is unable to cleave proIL-1β and proIL-18 cytokines. The mechanism of caspase 11 activation and its downstream targets for pyroptosis induction are unknown (Miao et al. 2011; Aachoui et al. 2013; Broz and Monack 2013; Ng and Monack 2013).

HOST CELL APOPTOSIS AND CONSEQUENCES TO *Mtb* PATHOGENESIS

The induction of host cell apoptosis was reported to have some direct bactericidal effects on intracellular bacterial viability (Molloy et al. 1994; Duan et al. 2002). Nevertheless, recent reports show that this is probably not a major factor during in vivo infections; instead, uptake of apoptotic cells by bystander macrophages and/or neutrophils, a process defined as efferocytosis, can lead to killing of *Mtb* (Fratazzi et al. 1997; Blomgran et al. 2012; Briken 2012; Martin et al. 2012; Yang et al. 2012). The killing of the bacteria inside the phagocytosed dead cell depends on recruitment and activation of the phagosomal NADPH oxidase complex, NOX2, to generate ROS (Yang et al. 2012). Another mechanism for the increased killing after efferocytosis is that *Mtb*, contained within double membrane phagosomes, is unable to inhibit phagosome maturation, and consequently lyso-

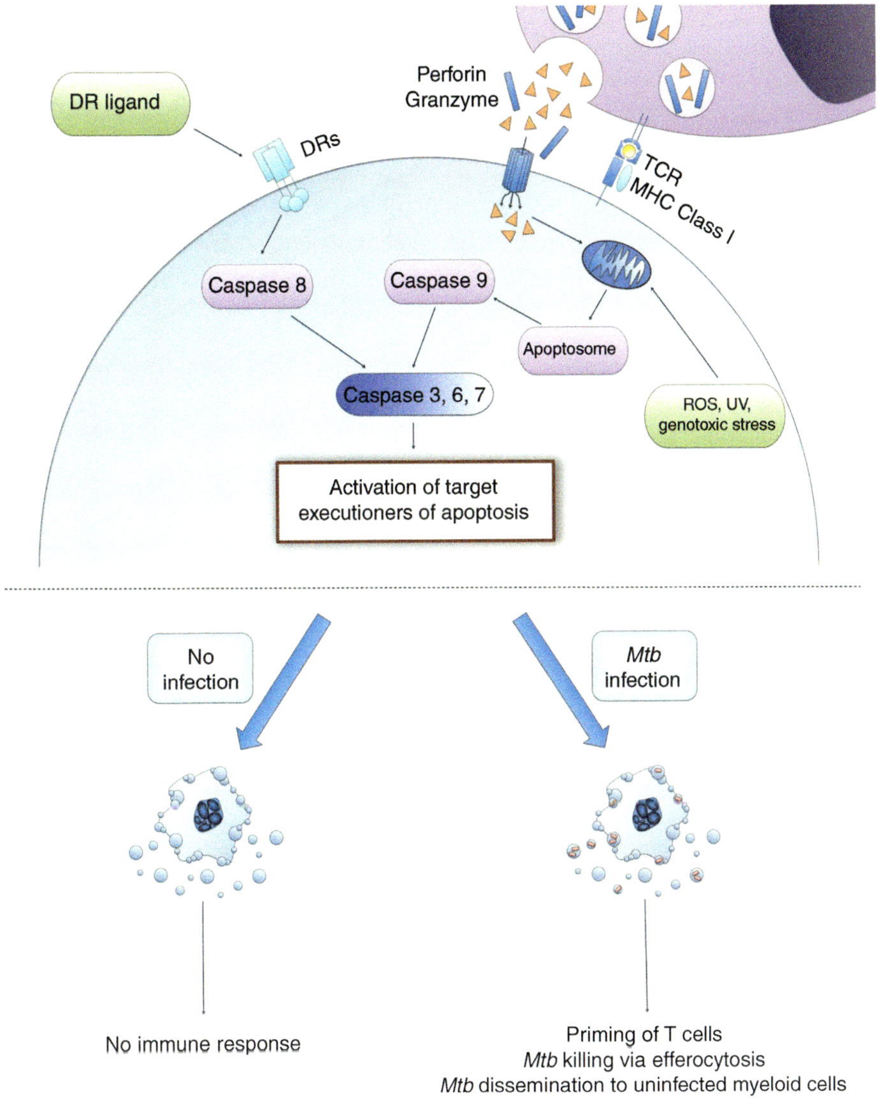

Figure 1. Host cell apoptosis pathways are classified into two main categories—extrinsic and intrinsic pathways. The extrinsic pathway of cell death is triggered by the interaction of death receptors (DRs) with specific death ligands and involves activation of caspase 8. Intrinsic pathways are triggered by stimuli that target mitochondria and result in release of cytochrome *c*, which participates in apoptosome formation, a platform for caspase 9 activation. In addition, $CD8^+$ T cells engage the extrinsic pathway via the Fas death receptor and the intrinsic pathway via perforin/granzyme secretion. Caspase 8 and 9 activate downstream effector caspases (caspase 3, 6, and 7), which leads to the characteristic features of apoptotic cells via activation of multiple targets. Apoptosis is immunologically silent as cellular material is enclosed within apoptotic bodies. Apoptosis of *Mtb*-infected cells results in packaging of mycobacterial antigens within apoptotic bodies that, when phagocytosed by dendritic cells, allow for antigen presentation to $CD8^+$ T cells via cross-presentation and the induction of a robust adaptive immune response. Additionally, uptake of dying apoptotic cells by healthy macrophages or neutrophils (efferocytosis) leads to killing of bacteria. However, *Mtb*-mediated apoptosis induction was also reported to help in dissemination of bacteria during early phase of infection.

somes and their bactericidal enzymes will fuse with the *Mtb* phagosome (Martin et al. 2012).

Granuloma formation is a hallmark feature of tuberculosis lung pathology (Ramakrishnan 2012; Reece and Kaufmann 2012). Compelling evidence from the zebrafish model shows that the ESX-1 secretion system, via secretion of EsxA (ESAT-6), is involved in the up-regulation of MMP9 on epithelial cells surrounding the granuloma, leading to recruitment of uninfected macrophages (Volkman et al. 2010), and that this, together with apoptosis induction of infected macrophages, helps in the dissemination of the bacteria (Davis and Ramakrishnan 2009). The beneficial effect of host cell apoptosis in the spread of bacteria and its dependence on the ESX-1 system were supported by evidence from *Mtb* in mouse lung infections showing a correlation between strains that induce increased lung cell apoptosis and bacterial growth (Aguilo et al. 2013). Consistently, the proapoptotic *nuoG Mtb* mutant was present in a larger number of diverse lung myeloid cells, albeit with fewer bacteria per cell, compared with wild-type *Mtb* during the early phase of aerosol mouse infection (Blomgran et al. 2012).

It is difficult to reconcile the contradictory observations of host cell apoptosis on *Mtb* pathology during the innate phase of the immune response. One explanation is that maybe during this phase both features (protective and permissive) of host cell apoptosis come into play. This may explain why proapoptotic *Mtb* mutants do not have a virulence defect during the early phase of in vivo infections, as one would expect if only the defense features of host cell apoptosis are in effect (Hinchey et al. 2007; Velmurugan et al. 2007; Blomgran et al. 2012). Consequently, proapoptosis mutants may induce better innate immune defense responses, but they may also be more efficient in attracting uninfected macrophages, neutrophils, and dendritic cells, and hence disseminate better according to the results obtained in the zebrafish model (Davis and Ramakrishnan 2009) and by comparing dissemination of wild-type and the proapoptotic *nuoG* mutant *Mtb* in mouse lungs (Blomgran et al. 2012).

In contrast, the long-term in vivo survival studies using proapoptosis *Mtb* mutants show that host cell apoptosis induction is beneficial to host survival overall (Edwards et al. 2001; Velmurugan et al. 2007; Sun et al. 2013). Mice infected with the *nuoG Mtb* mutant survive longer and have lower bacterial burden in the lungs during the persistent phase of the infection (Velmurugan et al. 2007). The knockdown of superoxide dismutase A (SodA) resulted in increased apoptosis of host cells in mouse lungs and decreased virulence of the bacteria (Edwards et al. 2001). SodA is secreted via the SecA2 secretion system in *Mtb*, and a *secA2* deletion mutant was attenuated in mice (Braunstein et al. 2003) and has a proapoptosis phenotype because of its defect in SodA secretion (Hinchey et al. 2007). However, the SecA2 system also affects other responses of the host cell and consequently these pleiotropic effects of the mutant make the interpretation of the cause of the in vivo attenuation difficult (Ligon et al. 2012). For example, the early growth defect of the *secA2* mutant is not caused by a lack in SodA export, because expressing a SodA protein secreted via the SecA1 pathway could not reverse the phenotype (Sullivan et al. 2012). This suggests that it is not the proapoptotic feature of the *SecA2* mutant that mediates that phenotype but rather the defect in the secretion of another effector (Sullivan et al. 2012). Recently, an antisense knockdown approach was successful in reducing expression of the nucleoside diphosphate kinase (*Ndk*) gene in *Mtb* and showed its importance for host cell apoptosis inhibition and virulence (Sun et al. 2013).

Another line of evidence supporting the role of host cell apoptosis in host defense is provided by studies using mouse mutants that lack genes important for either induction or repression of host cell apoptosis and their changes in susceptibility to *Mtb* infections. The Intracellular pathogen resistance 1 (*Ipr1*) gene is crucial for mediating host cell apoptosis instead of necrosis on *Mtb* infections ex vivo (Pan et al. 2005). The *Ipr1* knockout mice are more susceptible to *Mtb* infections and induce less host cell apoptosis (Pan et al. 2005). Mice deficient in the 5-lipoxygenase gene (*Alox5*$^{-/-}$) cannot produce the lipoxin A_4 (LXA_4) and therefore infected macrophages undergo apoptosis instead of necrosis after *Mtb* infections (Chen et al. 2008). The *Alox5*$^{-/-}$ mice are also more resistant to *Mtb* infection (Bafica et al. 2005; Divangahi et al. 2010). Finally, mice deficient in the protein kinase R (*Pkr*) gene are more resistant to *Mtb* infections, and this correlates with higher levels of apoptosis in infected macrophages (Wu et al. 2012).

During tissue homeostasis the apoptosis of cells is immunologically silent. Nevertheless, in the context of an infection, microbial components within apoptotic bodies can, after phagocytosis, activate dendritic cells in order to induce antigen presentation and acquired immunity (Winau et al. 2004). This was first shown for a bacterial pathogen in the context of *Salmonella* infection (Yrlid and Wick 2000) and subsequently also for mycobacterial infection (Schaible et al. 2003). The uptake of *Mtb* antigens via phagocytosis of apoptotic bodies by DCs allowed for the presentation of extracellular antigens to CD8^{+} T cells, a process defined as cross-presentation (Schaible et al. 2003). Interestingly, the apoptotic bodies purified from mycobacteria-infected cells can be used to vaccinate mice and induce a protective immune response (Winau et al. 2006). This indirect pathway of generating CD8^{+} T-cell responses via uptake of antigen-containing apoptotic bodies by DCs was defined as the detour pathway (Winau et al. 2004). Additional evidence for the importance of host cell apoptosis induction for priming of *Mtb*-specific CD8^{+} T cells was provided by an analysis of the immune response after infection of mice with the proapoptotic *secA2 Mtb* mutant (Hinchey et al. 2007). The increase in CD8^{+} T-cell priming by the *secA2* mutant was abolished by overexpression of SodA, which reversed the proapoptotic phenotype of the *secA2* mutant (Hinchey et al. 2007). In an elegant system, adoptive transfer of wild-type or *Alox5*$^{-/-}$ macrophages was used to study the impact of increased apoptosis on the induction of CD8^{+} T cells (Divangahi et al. 2010). Transfer of the *Mtb*-infected *Alox5*$^{-/-}$ macrophages (which show higher rates of apoptosis than wild-type macrophages) results in an increased and more rapid CD8^{+} T-cell response against the mycobacterial antigen TB10.4 (Divangahi et al. 2010). The depletion of endogenous DCs abrogates the increase in antigen presentation after adoptive transfer of the macrophages, thus showing the need for cross-presentation of *Mtb* antigens from apoptotic macrophages by DCs (Divangahi et al. 2010). Finally, aerosol infection of mice with *Mtb* and the *nuoG Mtb* mutant showed an increase of lung neutrophil apoptosis after mutant infection that led to an increase in acquisition of bacteria by myeloid DCs (Blomgran et al. 2012). This resulted in a quicker and more robust priming of *Mtb* antigen 85–specific CD4^{+} T cells (Blomgran et al. 2012), thus highlighting the impact of host cell apoptosis induction not only on CD8^{+} but also CD4^{+} T-cell priming. In conclusion, there is strong evidence that host cell apoptosis is an important pathway for increased host resistance to *Mtb* infection via induction of an improved acquired immune response.

MANIPULATION OF APOPTOSIS PATHWAYS BY *Mtb*

The literature on the inhibition of host cell apoptosis by *Mtb* has been reviewed recently (Abebe et al. 2011; Behar et al. 2011; Briken 2013). The mechanisms of inhibition include the up-regulation of host cell antiapoptosis signaling proteins such as the Bcl-2 family member Mcl-1 (Sly et al. 2003) or the Bfl-1 protein (Kausalya et al. 2001). The *Mtb*-induced secretion of soluble host cell TNF-receptor 2 to inhibit TNF signaling has also been described (Balcewicz-Sablinska et al. 1998). In addition, virulent *Mtb* H37Rv strains, but not attenuated *Mtb* H37Ra, can inhibit TNF-mediated cell death signaling in infected cells (Keane et al. 1997). The Fas–FasL interaction is one pathway for a CD8^{+} T cell to induce death of target cells. *Mtb* infection leads to a reduction of Fas expression at the cell surface to inhibit T-cell-mediated killing (Oddo et al. 1998) and activates intracellular signaling pathways to suppress FasL-induced apoptosis signaling (Loeuillet et al. 2006). Finally, the neutralization of phagosomal ROS by bacterial defense mechanisms detailed below is important in suppressing TNF-mediated host cell apoptosis (Miller et al. 2010).

Mtb GENES INVOLVED IN HOST CELL APOPTOSIS INHIBITION

The *Mtb nuoG* gene is part of a 14-gene operon (NDH-1) encoding for a type I NADH dehydrogenase whose function is important for the capacity of *Mtb* to inhibit host cell apoptosis (Velmurugan et al. 2007; Miller et al. 2010). In cells infected with the *nuoG Mtb* mutant, ROS accumulates in the phagosome, which leads to an increase in apoptosis (Miller et al. 2010). The detailed mechanism of how the NDH-1 system neutralizes and/or inhibits the ROS generated by the phagocyte NADPH oxidase system, NOX2, is still unknown. Catalases and superoxide dismutases are enzymes important for the detoxification of superoxides. The deletion mutant of the *Mtb* superoxide dismutase, *SodA*, is not viable but it was shown that the proapoptotic phenotype of the secretion mutant *SecA2* is dependent on the secretion defect of SodA (Hinchey et al. 2007). It is thus likely that the mutants deficient in secretion of SodA lead to an increase in phagosomal ROS similar to the *nuoG* mutant, which results in increased apoptosis. Another *Mtb* protein that targets host cell ROS is the enhanced intracellular survival (eis) protein. Nevertheless, it can inhibit not only NOX2-generated phagosomal ROS but also mitochondrial ROS via inhibition of the intracellular kinase JNK (Kim et al. 2012). eis is a secreted protein that reaches the host cell cytosol and, via its acetyltransferase activity, acetylates the phosphatase DUSP16/MKP-7 that increases its activity to dephosphorylate and hence inactivate JNK (Kim et al. 2012). The *eis Mtb* mutant induces caspase-independent apoptosis and autophagy that is different from the *nuoG* mutant that induces caspase-dependent apoptosis and no autophagy (Miller et al. 2010; L Srinivasan, unpubl.). Besides ROS, reactive nitrogen intermediates (RNIs) are generated in the phagosome to kill bacteria. The serine/threonine protein kinase E (PknE) of *Mtb* is up-regulated by an increase in RNIs, and without PknE there is an increase in the expression of proapoptotic members of the Bcl-2 family (Bax and Bid), a down-regulation of the antiapoptotic members such as Mcl-1, and a dephosphorylation of the prosurvival kinase Akt (Jayakumar et al. 2008; Kumar and Narayanan 2012).

A "loss-of-function" genetic screen for proapoptotic transposon mutants of *Mtb* identified the importance of two operons for host cell death inhibition (Danelishvili et al. 2010). The first operon (*Rv3654c-Rv3660c*) encompasses four genes that have homology with type IV pili. Interestingly, Rv3654c is secreted into the host cell cytosol, where it binds to and cleaves the protein-associated splice factor (PSF), which is important for splicing of caspase 8 pre-mRNA (Danelishvili et al. 2010). The consequence of this interaction is that there are lower levels of caspase 8 in cells infected with wild-type *Mtb* compared with a *Rv3654c* deletion mutant (Danelishvili et al. 2010). The other antiapoptotic operon is Rv3361c-Rv3365c, which is implicated in the inhibition of cell death dependent on the inflammatory caspase 1 (Danelishvili et al. 2011). After *Mtb* infection, Rv3364c enters the host cell cytosol and binds to and inactivates the host cell protease cathepsin G (Danelishvili et al. 2011). How cathepsin G regulates caspase 1 activity is not known but it was hypothesized that the effect might be mediated via cathepsin G cleavage and activation of the protease activated receptor-4, which then can induce caspase 1 activation via a NOD (nucleotide-binding oligomerization domain)-dependent pathway (Danelishvili et al. 2011) (for a detailed review, see Briken 2013).

HOST CELL PROGRAMMED NECROSIS AND CONSEQUENCES TO *Mtb* PATHOGENESIS

Host cell programmed necrosis is not detrimental to viability of intracellular *Mtb* (Molloy et al. 1994; Duan et al. 2002; Gan et al. 2008). Instead *Mtb*, after infection and multiplication, induces programmed necrosis to escape the cell (Chen et al. 2006; Lee et al. 2006; Behar et al. 2010).

The host cell production of the eicosanoids, PGE_2 versus LXA_4, is of critical importance for the induction of apoptosis or necrosis, respectively (Behar et al. 2010). Mice deficient in 5-

lipoxygenase cannot make LXA_4 and thus are more resistant to *Mtb* infections (Bafica et al. 2005). On the other hand, mice deficient in prostaglandin E synthase (PTGES) cannot produce PGE_2, and these animals are more susceptible to *Mtb* infections (Divangahi et al. 2009). Mutations in zebrafish and humans in the leukotriene A4 hydrolase (LTA4H) are associated with hypersusceptibility state to mycobacterial infections (Tobin et al. 2010). This is due to the increase in LXA_4 in the absence of LTA4H, leading to increased necrosis and decreased TNF production, which favors mycobacterial replication and leads to host cell programmed necrosis and increased bacterial virulence (Tobin et al. 2010). Interestingly, the overexpression of LTA4H and subsequent high levels of the leukotriene B4 (LTB4) and low levels of LXA_4 also leads to an increase in host cell programmed necrosis and increased susceptibility to mycobacterial infections (Tobin et al. 2012). This is due to the induction of excessive TNF production by LTB4, which keeps bacterial replication low, but favors induction of host cell necrosis and excessive inflammation leading to tissue damage and pathology (Tobin et al. 2012; Roca and Ramakrishnan 2013). Hence at both extreme ends of the spectrum, high LXA_4/no LTB4 and high LTB4/no LXA_4, the outcomes for the host are very similar with high levels of host cell necrosis, host tissue pathology, and host susceptibility (Tobin et al. 2012; Roca and Ramakrishnan 2013). This is despite the fact that the bacterial numbers are quite different in the two scenarios. High LXA_4 levels result in high bacterial numbers, and high LTB4 levels result in a low bacterial burden (Tobin et al. 2012; Roca and Ramakrishnan 2013). In conclusion, the Goldilocks principle applies to levels of LXA_4 and LTB4 in order to produce a successful host immune response (Tobin and Ramakrishnan 2013).

MANIPULATION OF PROGRAMMED NECROSIS PATHWAYS BY *Mtb*

A correlation between virulence of *Mtb* and its capacity to induce mitochondrial-dependent necrosis was first proposed by studies comparing the capacities of *Mtb* H37Rv and the attenuated *Mtb* H37Ra strains to disrupt mitochondrial function (Chen et al. 2006; Behar et al. 2011). Indeed only *Mtb* H37Rv led to an early mitochondrial transmembrane potential loss caused by mitochondrial permeability transition (MPT) pore complex. Inhibitors of MPT and mitochondrial Ca^{2+} influx both abrogated *Mtb* H37Rv-mediated programmed necrosis induction (Duan et al. 2002; Chen et al. 2006). Other reports showed caspase-independent, programmed necrotic cell death induction after infection of cells with high bacterial numbers that did not lead to bactericidal activity (Lee et al. 2006). The threshold for host cells to undergo necrosis was determined to be between 20 and 40 bacteria per phagocyte as determined in ex vivo and in vivo studies (Lee et al. 2006; Repasy et al. 2013). This death pathway was independent of Ca^{2+} flux and MPT and did not require lysosomal cathepsin protease activity (Lee et al. 2006, 2011; Welin et al. 2011; Wong and Jacobs 2011). One report showed that this high bacterial burden, programmed necrosis pathway is independent of ESX-1 secretion system but requires the presence of the PhoPR two-component system for the activation of lysosomal lipases that mediate cell necrosis (Lee et al. 2011). This is in contrast to other studies, which showed that cell death induction of *Mtb*-infected cells was dependent on bacterial expression of EsxA, one protein of the ESX-1 system that is involved in function of the system but is also a secreted effector itself (Welin et al. 2011; Wong and Jacobs 2011; Simeone et al. 2012). The function of the ESX-1 system was linked to escape of *Mtb* out of the phagosome at later stages of the infection, which coincided with host cell necrosis induction (Simeone et al. 2012). The *Mtb* EsxA protein is important in forming pores in the phagosomal membrane (Wong and Jacobs 2011), which is essential for subsequent NLRP3-inflammasome activation, because *esxA Mtb* mutants are deficient in activation of this inflammasome (Koo et al. 2008; Kurenuma et al. 2009; Wong and Jacobs 2011; Abdalla et al. 2012; Dorhoi et al. 2012). The activation of NLRP3 inflammasome in *Mtb*-infected cells is dependent on the tyrosine kinase Syk, and this activation is essential for cell lysis, hence showing a necroptotic host cell death pathway (Wong and Jacobs 2011) (Fig. 2). This is consistent with a previous report showing the activation of the NLRP3 inflammasome by Syk during a fungal infection (Gross et al. 2009). Another intriguing aspect of host cell programmed necrosis during mycobacterial infections was recently revealed by studies in the zebrafish model, which showed that too low as well as too high levels of host TNF production resulted in increased necrosis and host susceptibility to infection (Roca and Ramakrishnan 2013). At too low levels of TNF, the high intracellular bacterial burden led to necrosis, whereas at too high levels of TNF the burden of bacterial per cell was actually reduced but cells were sensitized by TNF to undergo RIPK1/3-dependent necroptosis (Roca and Ramakrishnan 2013).

Virulent *Mtb* induces the production of LXA_4 that inhibits cyclooxygenase 2 (COX2) expression, which is an essential enzyme in the PGE_2 synthesis pathway, and thus increased LXA_4 levels result in decreased PGE_2 (Chen et al. 2008). PGE_2 is a central inhibitor of host cell programmed necrosis via two potentially related mechanisms. First, high levels of PGE_2 limit the mitochondrial membrane damage, which leads to less ROS leakage into the cytosol and hence less programmed necrosis induction (Chen et al. 2008). This effect is mediated via PGE_2 binding to the E-prostanoid (EP) 2 receptor leading to protein kinase A activation and increased cAMP production (Chen et al. 2008). Second, PGE_2 induces the recruitment of Lamp-1-positive vesicles of lysosomal origin to the cell surface to repair damaged cell membranes (Divangahi et al. 2009). On the basis of susceptibility to PI3(K) inhibitors it was proposed that the mechanism involves binding of PGE_2 to the EP4 receptor leading to PI(3)K activation. In the same study it was clearly shown that PGE_2 leads to increased expression of the calcium sensor synaptotagmin 7 (Syt-7) and reduced necrosis and, vice versa, that reduction of Syt-7 via siRNA approaches inhibited plasma membrane repair (Divangahi et al. 2009). These data show that regulation of Syt-7 by PGE_2 is central to suppression of host cell necrosis during infection with avirulent *Mtb* strains.

Another pathway through which LXA_4 facilitates programmed necrosis is via inhibition of the formation of the apoptotic cell envelope (Gan et al. 2008). The primary target of LXA_4 in these events is the serine protease inhibitor, plasminogen activator inhibitor type 2 (PAI2), which is down-regulated by increasing LXA_4 levels (Gan et al. 2008). During the apoptotic envelope formation, phosphatidylserine (PS) and annexin-1 levels at the cell membrane are augmented. Annexin-1 binds to PS and is the target for the tissue transglutaminase (tTG), which cross-links annexin-1 to form a matrix that stabilizes the apoptotic envelope. Nevertheless, annexin-1 can be cleaved by an unknown cellular serine protease, which will result in a truncated annexin-1 that binds to PS but cannot be cross-linked and hence fails to support the formation of a stable apoptotic envelope (Gan et al. 2008). The result will be the induction of cellular lysis. PAI2 is a serine protease inhibitor that can inhibit the protease cleaving annexin-1. Thus, *Mtb*, by inhibiting PAI2 expression, facilitates programed necrosis induction (Gan et al. 2008).

As mentioned above, *Mtb* inhibits the lysosomal cell membrane repair pathway via down-regulation of the calcium sensor Syt-7. There is a second cell membrane repair pathway that is not controlled by PGE_2 and is dependent on Golgi-derived vesicles (Divangahi et al. 2009). Interestingly, only this pathway shuttles PS and annexin-1 to the cell membrane in order to inhibit cell necrosis and support induction of apoptosis (Divangahi et al. 2009). Hence, by targeting the PAI2 protease inhibitor, *Mtb* has evolved to find a way to functionally inhibit also this second cell membrane repair mechanism. It is fascinating that this is achieved via targeting of one central cellular signaling molecule the eicosanoid LXA_4 (for review, see Behar et al. 2011). A precise programmed necrosis pathway using the available hallmark inhibitors or knockout mice (Fig. 2) has not been defined by these studies involving LXA_4 and consequently it was referred to here just as programmed necrosis.

 Cite this article as *Cold Spring Harb Perspect Med* doi: 10.1101/cshperspect.a022459

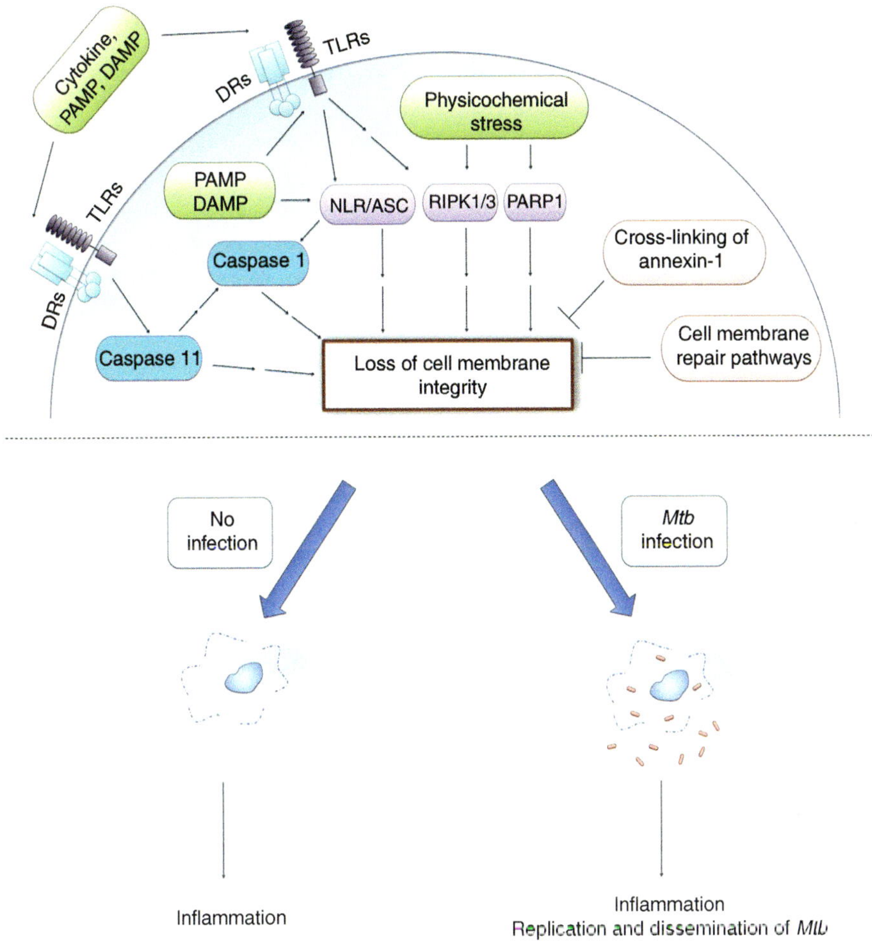

Figure 2. Necroptosis and pyroptosis both lead to the loss of cell membrane integrity. Necroptosis can be initiated by extracellular ligands interacting with their cognate cell surface receptors (DRs, death receptors; TLR, Toll-like receptors) or by varied intracellular stress signals (physicochemical stress). One pathway involves activation of RIPK1 and RIPK3, which leads to mitochondrial malfunction. Intracellular stress can also activate PARP1, which can signal for mitochondrial dysfunction potentially involving RIPK1 (sometimes referred to as the parthanatos death pathway). The inflammasome (NLR/ASC) may signal directly for necroptosis induction or indirectly via caspase 1 leading to pyroptosis, which also results in cell lysis but induces DNA degradation similar to apoptotic cell death. Caspase 11 can signal directly for a pyroptosis-like cell death or indirectly via NLR/ASC to activate caspase 1–dependent pyroptosis signaling. The cell may attempt to inhibit cell membrane lysis either by recruitment of lysosomal membranes to the cell surface to repair the cell membrane or by cross-linking annexin-1 on the cell surface and thus leading to formation of a stable apoptotic envelope. Necrotic cell death is inflammatory as it leads to spilling of the intracellular contents into the extracellular milieu. *Mtb* has been associated with both the induction of necrosis pathways and the inhibition of the inhibitory mechanisms. Programmed necrosis of *Mtb*-infected host cells leads to bacterial escape, whereas the associated inflammatory response recruits new host cells for extracellular *Mtb* to infect and replicate in, thus leading to dissemination of infection.

Mtb GENES INVOLVED IN HOST CELL PROGRAMMED NECROSIS INDUCTION

There are several *Mtb* genes that are involved in the induction of host cell death (Briken 2013). Nevertheless, it is still not determined which of these or other, yet to be discovered, genes are the mediators of the *Mtb* necrotic cell death induction during the final stage of the bacterial intracellular replication cycle. An interesting candidate for a major role is the heparin-binding hemaglutinin (HBHA) protein, which is secreted into the host cell cytosol and targeted to the mitochondria to induce activation of the Bax protein (Sohn et al. 2011). This leads to the creation of a mitochondrial membrane channel resulting in the loss of membrane potential (Sohn et al. 2011). It is noteworthy that inhibition of mitochondrial membrane damage is one of the key features of PGE2 to inhibit host cell necrosis (Chen et al. 2008). Nevertheless, the *Mtb* HBHA protein does not seem to induce necrotic cell death but instead leads to caspase 9–dependent apoptotic cell death (Sohn et al. 2011).

The ancestral mycobacterial type VII secretion system ESX-4 has been duplicated four times during the evolution of mycobacterial species to yield ESX-1 to ESX-5 (Gey van Pittius et al. 2006; Houben et al. 2013). The EsxA protein of the ESX-1 system can form homo- and heterodimers that can insert into the host cell membrane to induce necrosis (Hsu et al. 2003; de Jonge et al. 2007; Smith et al. 2008; Welin et al. 2011). In contrast, other reports show that ectopic expression of EsxA and/or the incubation of cells with purified EsxA induce host cell apoptosis (Derrick and Morris 2007; Choi et al. 2010). There is a clear consensus though in the literature that *Mtb* or Mm mutants deficient in *esxA* induce less cell death and that these mutants are also severely attenuated in the mouse and zebrafish model of tuberculosis (Abdallah et al. 2007; DiGiuseppe Champion and Cox 2007; Ramakrishnan 2012). The interpretation of results with the *esxA* mutants in regard to the bacterial effector mediating the phenotype is difficult because deletion of *esxA* not only affects secretion of EsxA but also of all the other ESX-1 secretion system substrates.

A functional ESX-1 system is also essential for full activation of the NLRP3-inflammasome after mycobacterial infection (Koo et al. 2008; Mayer-Barber et al. 2010; McElvania Tekippe et al. 2010; Mishra et al. 2010; Walter et al. 2010; Abdalla et al. 2012; Dorhoi et al. 2012). One report shows that this activation of NLRP3 leads to the induction of necroptosis (Wong and Jacobs 2011). The *Mtb* Rv3364c protein is an inhibitor of host cell cathepsin G and this inhibition led to less caspase 1–dependent pyroptosis (Danelishvili et al. 2011). The ESX-5 system has also been implicated in the induction of host cell necrosis and inflammasome activation (Abdallah et al. 2011). According to the proposed model, the ESX-1 system helps *Mtb* to escape the phagosome following which ESX-5-secreted effector proteins participate in the induction of programmed necrosis to allow bacteria to leave the infected cell (Abdallah et al. 2011). The ESX-5 system is crucial for the secretion of the *Mtb* PE/PPE family of proteins (Abdallah et al. 2006, 2009). Interestingly, the PE_PGRS33 protein is transported to host cell mitochondria and induces programmed necrosis when expressed ectopically in mammalian cells (Cadieux et al. 2011). It remains to be determined what the function of this protein is in the context of live *Mtb* infection.

POTENTIAL FOR THERAPEUTIC AND PREVENTIVE APPROACHES

The fact that increased host cell apoptosis resulted in improved $CD8^+$ and $CD4^+$ T-cell priming as discussed above obviously led to efforts to improve the current vaccine, BCG (Bacillus Calmette–Guérin), by increasing its apoptosis-inducing potential. The first evidence that this strategy might be successful was provided by a BCG vaccine modified to express the *Listeria monocytogenes* toxin Listeriolysin O (LLO). The toxin is not secreted outside the infected cell but inserts into the phagosomal membrane to generate pores that allow better access of BCG proteins to the host cell cytosol, which should result in improved $CD8^+$ T-cell priming. This BCG-LLO strain also induces increased host cell apoptosis compared with wild-type BCG (Grode et al. 2005). Indeed, apoptotic vesicles derived from macrophages infected with this vaccine strain led to increased $CD8^+$ and $CD4^+$ T-cell priming (Farinacci et al. 2012). Overall the BCG-LLO strain offered better protection to mice from virulent *Mtb* challenge (Grode et al. 2005), and this vaccine is now in phase IIa human clinical trials (Kaufmann 2013). The *secA2* deletion mutant in the background of an auxotroph *Mtb* vaccine strain also increases protection of mice to virulent *Mtb* challenge when compared with the original auxotroph *Mtb* vaccine strain or to BCG-vaccinated animals (Hinchey et al. 2007, 2011).

Immunotherapeutic approaches to treatment of tuberculosis are one additional approach besides traditional chemotherapy and vaccine prevention. The hypersusceptibility of zebrafish with a specific LTA4H genotype resulting in high TNF levels could be reversed by using inhibitors of the TNF-induced programmed necrosis pathway (Tobin et al. 2010; Roca and Ramakrishnan 2013). Indeed, alisporvir is an inhibitor of cyclophilin D that is released by the mitochondria via the MPT pore and is currently in phase III human trial to treat hepatitis C (Quarato et al. 2012). The other drug used in the study is desipramine, which is an antidepressant that has been given to humans for half a century. Desipramine inhibits the production of ceramides, which, at sufficiently high levels, may induce host cell necroptosis (Roca and Ramakrishnan 2013). The combination of both drugs results in synergy in suppressing virulence of mycobacterial infection in zebrafish (Roca and Ramakrishnan 2013). Human patients with a variant of the LTA4H promoter that resulted in high LXA_4 levels could be successfully treated with dexamethasone, a TNF-suppressive drug (Tobin et al. 2012). Hence, inhibition of host cell necroptosis holds a lot of promise as one part of a multipronged approach to tuberculosis treatment (Tobin and Ramakrishnan 2013).

CONCLUDING REMARKS

The interaction of *Mtb* with the host in regard to cell death is complex. Currently, the research is at a stage that does not allow designing a model that explains all of the data available. For example, more time and effort is needed to elucidate the ambiguous role of host cell apoptosis in *Mtb* pathogenesis. Also, how does *Mtb* regulate the induction of host cell necrosis in order to escape the cell and what are the bacterial effectors involved? Identifying these effectors may provide excellent novel drug targets because inhibiting the necrotic property of *Mtb* during the later stages of active pulmonary disease should be able to provide clear therapeutic benefits. It is now well established that *Mtb* infection of host cells involves interaction with the three major cell death pathways: apoptosis, pyroptosis, and necroptosis. It is quite likely that we will be able to gain many insights into these cell death pathways by studying a pathogen that has coevolved with humans for more than 50,000 years (Hershberg et al. 2008).

ACKNOWLEDGMENTS

Research in the Briken laboratory was supported by National Institutes of Health grant AI072584.

REFERENCES

Aachoui Y, Sagulenko V, Miao EA, Stacey KJ. 2013. Inflammasome-mediated pyroptotic and apoptotic cell death, and defense against infection. *Curr Opin Microbiol* **16:** 319–326.

Abdallah AM, Verboom T, Hannes F, Safi M, Strong M, Eisenberg D, Musters RJ, Vandenbroucke-Grauls CM, Appelmelk BJ, Luirink J, et al. 2006. A specific secretion system mediates PPE41 transport in pathogenic mycobacteria. *Mol Microbiol* **62:** 667–679.

Abdallah AM, Gey van Pittius NC, Champion PA, Cox J, Luirink J, Vandenbroucke-Grauls CM, Appelmelk BJ, Bitter W. 2007. Type VII secretion–mycobacteria show the way. *Nat Rev Microbiol* **5:** 883–891.

Abdallah AM, Verboom T, Weerdenburg EM, Gey van Pittius NC, Mahasha PW, Jimenez C, Parra M, Cadieux N, Brennan MJ, Appelmelk BJ, et al. 2009. PPE and PE_PGRS proteins of *Mycobacterium marinum* are transported via the type VII secretion system ESX-5. *Mol Microbiol* **73:** 329–340.

Abdallah AM, Bestebroer J, Savage ND, de Punder K, van Zon M, Wilson L, Korbee CJ, van der Sar AM, Ottenhoff TH, van der Wel NN, et al. 2011. Mycobacterial secretion systems ESX-1 and ESX-5 play distinct roles in host cell death and inflammasome activation. *J Immunol* **187:** 4744–4753.

Abdalla H, Srinivasan L, Shah S, Mayer-Barber KD, Sher A, Sutterwala FS, Briken V. 2012. *Mycobacterium tuberculosis* infection of dendritic cells leads to partially caspase-1/11-independent IL-1β and IL-18 secretion but not to pyroptosis. *PLoS ONE* **7:** e40722.

Abebe M, Kim L, Rook G, Aseffa A, Wassie L, Zewdie M, Zumla A, Engers H, Andersen P, Doherty TM. 2011. Modulation of cell death by *M. tuberculosis* as a strategy for pathogen survival. *Clin Dev Immunol* **2011:** 678570.

Aguilo JI, Alonso H, Uranga S, Marinova D, Arbues A, de Martino A, Anel A, Monzon M, Badiola J, Pardo J, et al. 2013. ESX-1-induced apoptosis is involved in cell-to-cell spread of *Mycobacterium tuberculosis*. *Cell Microbiol* **15:** 1994–2005.

Bafica A, Scanga CA, Serhan C, Machado F, White S, Sher A, Aliberti J. 2005. Host control of *Mycobacterium tuberculosis* is regulated by 5-lipoxygenase-dependent lipoxin production. *J Clin Invest* **115:** 1601–1606.

Balcewicz-Sablinska MK, Keane J, Kornfeld H, Remold HG. 1998. Pathogenic *Mycobacterium tuberculosis* evades apoptosis of host macrophages by release of TNF-R2, resulting in inactivation of TNF-α. *J Immunol* **161:** 2636–2641.

Behar SM, Divangahi M, Remold HG. 2010. Evasion of innate immunity by *Mycobacterium tuberculosis*: Is death an exit strategy? *Nat Rev Microbiol* **8:** 668–674.

Behar SM, Martin CJ, Booty MG, Nishimura T, Zhao X, Gan HX, Divangahi M, Remold HG. 2011. Apoptosis is an innate defense function of macrophages against *Mycobacterium tuberculosis*. *Mucosal Immunol* **4:** 279–287.

Blomgran R, Desvignes L, Briken V, Ernst JD. 2012. *Mycobacterium tuberculosis* inhibits neutrophil apoptosis, leading to delayed activation of naive CD4 T cells. *Cell Host Microbe* **11:** 81–90.

Braunstein M, Espinosa BJ, Chan J, Belisle JT, Jacobs WR Jr. 2003. SecA2 functions in the secretion of superoxide dismutase A and in the virulence of *Mycobacterium tuberculosis*. *Mol Microbiol* **48:** 453–464.

Briken V. 2012. "With a little help from my friends": Efferocytosis as an antimicrobial mechanism. *Cell Host Microbe* **12:** 261–263.

Briken V. 2013. *Mycobacterium tuberculosis* genes involved in regulation of host cell death. *Adv Exp Med Biol* **783:** 93–102.

Broz P, Monack DM. 2013. Noncanonical inflammasomes: Caspase-11 activation and effector mechanisms. *PLoS Pathog* **9:** e1003144.

Cadieux N, Parra M, Cohen H, Maric D, Morris SL, Brennan MJ. 2011. Induction of cell death after localization to the host cell mitochondria by the *Mycobacterium tuberculosis* PE_PGRS33 protein. *Microbiology* **157:** 793–804.

Chen M, Gan H, Remold HG. 2006. A mechanism of virulence: Virulent *Mycobacterium tuberculosis* strain H37Rv, but not attenuated H37Ra, causes significant mitochondrial inner membrane disruption in macrophages leading to necrosis. *J Immunol* **176:** 3707–3716.

Chen M, Divangahi M, Gan H, Shin DS, Hong S, Lee DM, Serhan CN, Behar SM, Remold HG. 2008. Lipid mediators in innate immunity against tuberculosis: Opposing roles of PGE2 and LXA4 in the induction of macrophage death. *J Exp Med* **205:** 2791–2801.

Choi HH, Shin DM, Kang G, Kim KH, Park JB, Hur GM, Lee HM, Lim YJ, Park JK, Jo EK, et al. 2010. Endoplasmic reticulum stress response is involved in *Mycobacterium tuberculosis* protein ESAT-6-mediated apoptosis. *FEBS Lett* **584:** 2445–2454.

Danelishvili L, Yamazaki Y, Selker J, Bermudez LE. 2010. Secreted *Mycobacterium tuberculosis* Rv3654c and Rv3655c proteins participate in the suppression of macrophage apoptosis. *PLoS ONE* **5:** e10474.

Danelishvili L, Everman JL, McNamara MJ, Bermudez LE. 2011. Inhibition of the plasma-membrane-associated serine protease cathepsin G by *Mycobacterium tuberculosis* Rv3364c suppresses caspase-1 and pyroptosis in macrophages. *Front Microbiol* **2:** 281.

Davis JM, Ramakrishnan L. 2009. The role of the granuloma in expansion and dissemination of early tuberculous infection. *Cell* **136:** 37–49.

de Jonge MI, Pehau-Arnaudet G, Fretz MM, Romain F, Bottai D, Brodin P, Honore N, Marchal G, Jiskoot W, England P, et al. 2007. ESAT-6 from *Mycobacterium tuberculosis* dissociates from its putative chaperone CFP-10 under acidic conditions and exhibits membrane-lysing activity. *J Bacteriol* **189:** 6028–6034.

Derrick SC, Morris SL. 2007. The ESAT6 protein of *Mycobacterium tuberculosis* induces apoptosis of macrophages by activating caspase expression. *Cell Microbiol* **9:** 1547–1555.

DiGiuseppe Champion PA, Cox JS. 2007. Protein secretion systems in mycobacteria. *Cell Microbiol* **9:** 1376–1384.

Divangahi M, Chen M, Gan H, Desjardins D, Hickman TT, Lee DM, Fortune S, Behar SM, Remold HG. 2009. *Mycobacterium tuberculosis* evades macrophage defenses by inhibiting plasma membrane repair. *Nat Immunol* **10:** 899–906.

Divangahi M, Desjardins D, Nunes-Alves C, Remold HG, Behar SM. 2010. Eicosanoid pathways regulate adaptive immunity to *Mycobacterium tuberculosis*. *Nat Immunol* **11:** 751–758.

Dorhoi A, Nouailles G, Jorg S, Hagens K, Heinemann E, Pradl L, Oberbeck-Muller D, Duque-Correa MA, Reece ST, Ruland J, et al. 2012. Activation of the NLRP3 inflammasome by *Mycobacterium tuberculosis* is uncoupled from susceptibility to active tuberculosis. *Eur J Immunol* **42:** 374–384.

Duan L, Gan H, Golan DE, Remold HG. 2002. Critical role of mitochondrial damage in determining outcome of macrophage infection with *Mycobacterium tuberculosis*. *J Immunol* **169:** 5181–5187.

Edwards KM, Cynamon MH, Voladri RKR, Hager CC, Destefano MS, Tham KT, Lakey DL, Bochan MR, Kernodle DS. 2001. Iron-cofactored superoxide dismutase inhibits host responses to *Mycobacterium tuberculosis*. *Am J Respir Crit Care Med* **164:** 2213–2219.

Farinacci M, Weber S, Kaufmann SH. 2012. The recombinant tuberculosis vaccine rBCG ΔureC::hly$^+$ induces apoptotic vesicles for improved priming of CD4$^+$ and CD8$^+$ T cells. *Vaccine* **30:** 7608–7614.

Fratazzi C, Arbeit RD, Carini C, Remold HG. 1997. Programmed cell death of *Mycobacterium avium serovar* 4-infected human macrophages prevents the mycobacteria from spreading and induces mycobacterial growth inhibition by freshly added, uninfected macrophages. *J Immunol* **158:** 4320–4327.

Galluzzi L, Kepp O, Kroemer G. 2012a. Mitochondria: Master regulators of danger signalling. *Nat Rev Mol Cell Biol* **13:** 780–788.

Galluzzi L, Vitale I, Abrams JM, Alnemri ES, Baehrecke EH, Blagosklonny MV, Dawson TM, Dawson VL, El-Deiry WS, Fulda S, et al. 2012b. Molecular definitions of cell death subroutines: Recommendations of the Nomenclature Committee on Cell Death 2012. *Cell Death Differ* **19:** 107–120.

Gan H, Lee J, Ren F, Chen M, Kornfeld H, Remold HG. 2008. *Mycobacterium tuberculosis* blocks crosslinking of annexin-1 and apoptotic envelope formation on infected macrophages to maintain virulence. *Nat Immunol* **9:** 1189–1197.

Gey van Pittius NC, Sampson SL, Lee H, Kim Y, van Helden PD, Warren RM. 2006. Evolution and expansion of the *Mycobacterium tuberculosis* PE and PPE multigene families and their association with the duplication of the ESAT-6 (*esx*) gene cluster regions. *BMC Evol Biol* **6:** 95.

Grode L, Seiler P, Baumann S, Hess J, Brinkmann V, Eddine AN, Mann P, Goosmann C, Bandermann S, Smith D, et al. 2005. Increased vaccine efficacy against tuberculosis of recombinant *Mycobacterium bovis* bacille Calmette–Guérin mutants that secrete listeriolysin. *J Clin Invest* **115:** 2472–2479.

Gross O, Poeck H, Bscheider M, Dostert C, Hannesschlager N, Endres S, Hartmann G, Tardivel A, Schweighoffer E, Tybulewicz V, et al. 2009. Syk kinase signalling couples to the Nlrp3 inflammasome for anti-fungal host defence. *Nature* **459:** 433–436.

Hershberg R, Lipatov M, Small PM, Sheffer H, Niemann S, Homolka S, Roach JC, Kremer K, Petrov DA, Feldman MW, et al. 2008. High functional diversity in *Mycobacterium tuberculosis* driven by genetic drift and human demography. *PLoS Biol* **6:** e311.

Hinchey J, Lee S, Jeon BY, Basaraba RJ, Venkataswamy MM, Chen B, Chan J, Braunstein M, Orme IM, Derrick SC, et al. 2007. Enhanced priming of adaptive immunity by a proapoptotic mutant of *Mycobacterium tuberculosis*. *J Clin Invest* **117:** 2279–2288.

Hinchey J, Jeon BY, Alley H, Chen B, Goldberg M, Derrick S, Morris S, Jacobs WR Jr, Porcelli SA, Lee S. 2011. Lysine auxotrophy combined with deletion of the *SecA2* gene results in a safe and highly immunogenic candidate live attenuated vaccine for tuberculosis. *PLoS ONE* **6:** e15857.

Houben EN, Korotkov KV, Bitter W. 2013. Take five—Type VII secretion systems of mycobacteria. *Biochim Biophys Acta* doi: 10.1016/j.bbamcr.2013.11.003.

Hsu T, Hingley-Wilson SM, Chen B, Chen M, Dai AZ, Morin PM, Marks CB, Padiyar J, Goulding C, Gingery M, et al. 2003. The primary mechanism of attenuation of bacillus Calmette–Guérin is a loss of secreted lytic function required for invasion of lung interstitial tissue. *Proc Natl Acad Sci* **100:** 12420–12425.

Jayakumar D, Jacobs WR Jr, Narayanan S. 2008. Protein kinase E of *Mycobacterium tuberculosis* has a role in the nitric oxide stress response and apoptosis in a human macrophage model of infection. *Cell Microbiol* **10:** 365–374.

Kaufmann SH. 2013. Tuberculosis vaccines: Time to think about the next generation. *Semin Immunol* **25:** 172–181.

Kausalya S, Somogyi R, Orlofsky A, Prystowsky MB. 2001. Requirement of A1-a for bacillus Calmette–Guèrin–mediated protection of macrophages against nitric oxide-induced apoptosis. *J Immunol* **166:** 4721–4727.

Keane J, Balcewicz-Sablinska MK, Remold HG, Chupp GL, Meek BB, Fenton MJ, Kornfeld H. 1997. Infection by *Mycobacterium tuberculosis* promotes human alveolar macrophage apoptosis. *Infect Immun* **65:** 298–304.

Kepp O, Galluzzi L, Zitvogel L, Kroemer G. 2010. Pyroptosis—A cell death modality of its kind? *Eur J Immunol* **40:** 627–630.

Kim KH, An DR, Song J, Yoon JY, Kim HS, Yoon HJ, Im HN, Kim J, Kim do J, Lee SJ, et al. 2012. *Mycobacterium tuberculosis* Eis protein initiates suppression of host immune responses by acetylation of DUSP16/MKP-7. *Proc Natl Acad Sci USA* **109:** 7729–7734.

Koo IC, Wang C, Raghavan S, Morisaki JH, Cox JS, Brown EJ. 2008. ESX-1-dependent cytolysis in lysosome secretion and inflammasome activation during mycobacterial infection. *Cell Microbiol* **10:** 1866–1878.

Kumar D, Narayanan S. 2012. pknE, a serine/threonine kinase of *Mycobacterium tuberculosis*, modulates multiple apoptotic paradigms. *Infect Genet Evol* **12:** 737–747.

Kurenuma T, Kawamura I, Hara H, Uchiyama R, Daim S, Dewamitta SR, Sakai S, Tsuchiya K, Nomura T, Mitsuyama M. 2009. The RD1 locus in the *Mycobacterium tuberculosis* genome contributes to activation of caspase-1 via induction of potassium ion efflux in infected macrophages. *Infect Immun* **77:** 3992–4001.

Lamkanfi M, Dixit VM. 2010. Manipulation of host cell death pathways during microbial infections. *Cell Host Microbe* **8:** 44–54.

Lee J, Remold HG, Ieong MH, Kornfeld H. 2006. Macrophage apoptosis in response to high intracellular burden of *Mycobacterium tuberculosis* is mediated by a novel caspase-independent pathway. *J Immunol* **176:** 4267–4274.

Lee J, Repasy T, Papavinasasundaram K, Sassetti C, Kornfeld H. 2011. *Mycobacterium tuberculosis* induces an atypical cell death mode to escape from infected macrophages. *PLoS ONE* **6:** e18367.

Ligon LS, Hayden JD, Braunstein M. 2012. The ins and outs of *Mycobacterium tuberculosis* protein export. *Tuberculosis (Edinb)* **92:** 121–132.

Loeuillet C, Martinon F, Perez C, Munoz M, Thome M, Meylan PR. 2006. *Mycobacterium tuberculosis* subverts innate immunity to evade specific effectors. *J Immunol* **177:** 6245–6255.

Martin CJ, Booty MG, Rosebrock TR, Nunes-Alves C, Desjardins DM, Keren I, Fortune SM, Remold HG, Behar SM. 2012. Efferocytosis is an innate antibacterial mechanism. *Cell Host Microbe* **12:** 289–300.

Mayer-Barber KD, Barber DL, Shenderov K, White SD, Wilson MS, Cheever A, Kugler D, Hieny S, Caspar P, Nunez G, et al. 2010. Caspase-1 independent IL-1β production is critical for host resistance to *Mycobacterium tuberculosis* and does not require TLR signaling in vivo. *J Immunol* **184:** 3326–3330.

McElvania Tekippe E, Allen IC, Hulseberg PD, Sullivan JT, McCann JR, Sandor M, Braunstein M, Ting JP. 2010.

Granuloma formation and host defense in chronic *Mycobacterium tuberculosis* infection requires PYCARD/ASC but not NLRP3 or caspase-1. *PLoS ONE* **5:** e12320.

Miao EA, Rajan JV, Aderem A. 2011. Caspase-1-induced pyroptotic cell death. *Immunol Rev* **243:** 206–214.

Miller JL, Velmurugan K, Cowan MJ, Briken V. 2010. The type I NADH dehydrogenase of *Mycobacterium tuberculosis* counters phagosomal NOX2 activity to inhibit TNF-alpha-mediated host cell apoptosis. *PLoS Pathog* **6:** e1000864.

Mishra BB, Moura-Alves P, Sonawane A, Hacohen N, Griffiths G, Moita LF, Anes E. 2010. *Mycobacterium tuberculosis* protein ESAT-6 is a potent activator of the NLRP3/ASC inflammasome. *Cell Microbiol* **12:** 1046–1063.

Molloy A, Laochumroonvorapong P, Kaplan G. 1994. Apoptosis, but not necrosis, of infected monocytes is coupled with killing of intracellular bacillus Calmette–Guèrin. *J Exp Med* **180:** 1499–1509.

Ng TM, Monack DM. 2013. Revisiting caspase-11 function in host defense. *Cell Host Microbe* **14:** 9–14.

Oddo M, Renno T, Attinger A, Bakker T, MacDonald HR, Meylan PR. 1998. Fas ligand-induced apoptosis of infected human macrophages reduces the viability of intracellular *Mycobacterium tuberculosis*. *J Immunol* **160:** 5448–5454.

Pan H, Yan BS, Rojas M, Shebzukhov YV, Zhou H, Kobzik L, Higgins DE, Daly MJ, Bloom BR, Kramnik I. 2005. *Ipr1* gene mediates innate immunity to tuberculosis. *Nature* **434:** 767–772.

Quarato G, D'Aprile A, Gavillet B, Vuagniaux G, Moradpour D, Capitanio N, Piccoli C. 2012. The cyclophilin inhibitor alisporivir prevents hepatitis C virus-mediated mitochondrial dysfunction. *Hepatology* **55:** 1333–1343.

Ramakrishnan L. 2012. Revisiting the role of the granuloma in tuberculosis. *Nat Rev Immunol* **12:** 352–366.

Reece ST, Kaufmann SH. 2012. Floating between the poles of pathology and protection: Can we pin down the granuloma in tuberculosis? *Curr Opin Microbiol* **15:** 63–70.

Repasy T, Lee J, Marino S, Martinez N, Kirschner DE, Hendricks G, Baker S, Wilson AA, Kotton DN, Kornfeld H. 2013. Intracellular bacillary burden reflects a burst size for *Mycobacterium tuberculosis* in vivo. *PLoS Pathog* **9:** e1003190.

Roca FJ, Ramakrishnan L. 2013. TNF dually mediates resistance and susceptibility to mycobacteria via mitochondrial reactive oxygen species. *Cell* **153:** 521–534.

Schaible UE, Winau F, Sieling PA, Fischer K, Collins HL, Hagens K, Modlin RL, Brinkmann V, Kaufmann SH. 2003. Apoptosis facilitates antigen presentation to T lymphocytes through MHC-I and CD1 in tuberculosis. *Nat Med* **9:** 1039–1046.

Simeone R, Bobard A, Lippmann J, Bitter W, Majlessi L, Brosch R, Enninga J. 2012. Phagosomal rupture by *Mycobacterium tuberculosis* results in toxicity and host cell death. *PLoS Pathog* **8:** e1002507.

Sly LM, Hingley-Wilson SM, Reiner NE, McMaster WR. 2003. Survival of *Mycobacterium tuberculosis* in host macrophages involves resistance to apoptosis dependent upon induction of antiapoptotic Bcl-2 family member Mcl-1. *J Immunol* **170:** 430–437.

Smith J, Manoranjan J, Pan M, Bohsali A, Xu J, Liu J, McDonald KL, Szyk A, LaRonde-LeBlanc N, Gao LY. 2008. Evidence for pore formation in host cell membranes by ESX-1-secreted ESAT-6 and its role in *Mycobacterium marinum* escape from the vacuole. *Infect Immun* **76:** 5478–5487.

Sohn H, Kim JS, Shin SJ, Kim K, Won CJ, Kim WS, Min KN, Choi HG, Lee JC, Park JK, et al. 2011. Targeting of *Mycobacterium tuberculosis* heparin-binding hemagglutinin to mitochondria in macrophages. *PLoS Pathog* **7:** e1002435.

Sridharan H, Upton JW. 2014. Programmed necrosis in microbial pathogenesis. *Trends Microbiol.* DOI: 10.1016/j.tim.2014.01.005

Sullivan JT, Young EF, McCann JR, Braunstein M. 2012. The *Mycobacterium tuberculosis* SecA2 system subverts phagosome maturation to promote growth in macrophages. *Infect Immun* **80:** 996–1006.

Sun J, Singh V, Lau A, Stokes RW, Obregon-Henao A, Orme IM, Wong D, Av-Gay Y, Hmama Z. 2013. *Mycobacterium tuberculosis* nucleoside diphosphate kinase inactivates small GTPases leading to evasion of innate immunity. *PLoS Pathog* **9:** e1003499.

Tobin DM, Ramakrishnan L. 2013. TB: The yin and yang of lipid mediators. *Curr Opin Pharmacol* **13:** 641–645.

Tobin DM, Vary JC Jr, Ray JP, Walsh GS, Dunstan SJ, Bang ND, Hagge DA, Khadge S, King MC, Hawn TR, et al. 2010. The lta4 h locus modulates susceptibility to mycobacterial infection in zebrafish and humans. *Cell* **140:** 717–730.

Tobin DM, Roca FJ, Oh SF, McFarland R, Vickery TW, Ray JP, Ko DC, Zou Y, Bang ND, Chau TT, et al. 2012. Host genotype-specific therapies can optimize the inflammatory response to mycobacterial infections. *Cell* **148:** 434–446.

Vanlangenakker N, Vanden Berghe T, Vandenabeele P. 2012. Many stimuli pull the necrotic trigger, an overview. *Cell Death Differ* **19:** 75–86.

Velmurugan K, Chen B, Miller JL, Azogue S, Gurses S, Hsu T, Glickman M, Jacobs WR Jr, Porcelli SA, Briken V. 2007. *Mycobacterium tuberculosis nuoG* is a virulence gene that inhibits apoptosis of infected host cells. *PLoS Pathogens* **3:** e110.

Volkman HE, Pozos TC, Zheng J, Davis JM, Rawls JF, Ramakrishnan L. 2010. Tuberculous granuloma induction via interaction of a bacterial secreted protein with host epithelium. *Science* **327:** 466–469.

Walter K, Holscher C, Tschopp J, Ehlers S. 2010. NALP3 is not necessary for early protection against experimental tuberculosis. *Immunobiology* **215:** 804–811.

Welin A, Eklund D, Stendahl O, Lerm M. 2011. Human macrophages infected with a high burden of ESAT-6-expressing *M. tuberculosis* undergo caspase-1- and cathepsin B-independent necrosis. *PLoS ONE* **6:** e20302.

Winau F, Kaufmann SH, Schaible UE. 2004. Apoptosis paves the detour path for CD8 T cell activation against intracellular bacteria. *Cell Microbiol* **6:** 599–607.

Winau F, Weber S, Sad S, de Diego J, Hoops SL, Breiden B, Sandhoff K, Brinkmann V, Kaufmann SH, Schaible UE.

2006. Apoptotic vesicles crossprime CD8 T cells and protect against tuberculosis. *Immunity* **24:** 105–117.

Wong KW, Jacobs WR Jr. 2011. Critical role for NLRP3 in necrotic death triggered by *Mycobacterium tuberculosis*. *Cell Microbiol* **13:** 1371–1384.

Wu K, Koo J, Jiang X, Chen R, Cohen SN, Nathan C. 2012. Improved control of tuberculosis and activation of macrophages in mice lacking protein kinase R. *PLoS ONE* **7:** e30512.

Yang CT, Cambier CJ, Davis JM, Hall CJ, Crosier PS, Ramakrishnan L. 2012. Neutrophils exert protection in the early tuberculous granuloma by oxidative killing of mycobacteria phagocytosed from infected macrophages. *Cell Host Microbe* **12:** 301–312.

Yrlid U, Wick MJ. 2000. Salmonella-induced apoptosis of infected macrophages results in presentation of a bacteria-encoded antigen after uptake by bystander dendritic cells. *J Exp Med* **191:** 613–624.

Autophagy in Tuberculosis

Vojo Deretic

Department of Molecular Genetics and Microbiology, University of New Mexico Health Sciences Center, Albuquerque, New Mexico 87131

Correspondence: vderetic@salud.unm.edu

Autophagy as an immune mechanism controls inflammation and acts as a cell-autonomous defense against intracellular microbes including *Mycobacterium tuberculosis*. An equally significant role of autophagy is its anti-inflammatory and tissue-sparing function. This combination of antimicrobial and anti-inflammatory actions prevents active disease in animal models. In human populations, genetic links between autophagy, inflammatory bowel disease, and susceptibility to tuberculosis provide further support to these combined roles of autophagy. The autophagic control of *M. tuberculosis* and prevention of progressive disease provide novel insights into physiological and immune control of tuberculosis. It also offers host-based therapeutic opportunities because autophagy can be pharmacologically modulated.

Autophagy in a broader sense is a collection of homeostatic processes (macroautophagy, chaperone mediate autophagy, microautophagy) in the eukaryotic cell that deliver cytoplasmic portions or specific cytosolic targets to lysosomes for degradation or removal (Mizushima et al. 2011). Macroautophagy, commonly referred to as autophagy (and in this text), is a pathway defined in genetic terms as dependent on autophagy-related (Atg) genes (Mizushima et al. 2011) and in morphological terms as the appearance in the cytoplasm of double-membrane organelles termed autophagosomes that capture cytosolic cargo and fuse with lysosomes (Deter and De Duve 1967; Deter et al. 1967). Autophagy affects human health and diseases including aging, neurodegeneration, cancer, and metabolic disorders (Mizushima et al. 2008). The recognition that autophagy plays an antimicrobial role against pathogens (Deretic 2005) when they invade the mammalian cell interior came from two nearly simultaneous reports in 2004 (Gutierrez et al. 2004; Nakagawa et al. 2004). One of these studies reported on the autophagic elimination of virulent *Mycobacterium tuberculosis* and the vaccine strain *Mycobacterium bovis* BCG (Bacillus Calmette–Guérin) in infected murine and human macrophages (Gutierrez et al. 2004). These and additional studies have established that autophagy is a bona fide immunological process (Deretic 2005; Levine et al. 2011). Today we recognize that autophagy is widely integrated with immunity starting from cell-autonomous defense against invading bacteria and viruses to regulation of innate and adaptive immunity in general (Deretic et al. 2013). The initial observations uncovering the role of autophagy against *M. tuberculosis* (Gutierrez et al. 2004; Singh et al. 2006) have been followed by a gradual increase in

Cite this article as *Cold Spring Harb Perspect Med* doi: 10.1101/cshperspect.a018481

studies supporting and extending these early findings (Alonso et al. 2007; Harris et al. 2007; Xu et al. 2007; Biswas et al. 2008; Jagannath et al. 2009; Yuk et al. 2009; Ghadimi et al. 2010; Kumar et al. 2010; Ponpuak et al. 2010; Shin et al. 2010b; Singh et al. 2010; Fabri et al. 2011a,b; Campbell and Spector 2012; Juarez et al. 2012; Petruccioli et al. 2012; Watson et al. 2012; Zullo and Lee 2012; Anandaiah et al. 2013; Klug-Micu et al. 2013; Manzanillo et al. 2013). In this article we briefly cover autophagy as a pathway and its broad roles in immunity and summarize what has been learned about autophagy in tuberculosis thus far.

AUTOPHAGY PATHWAY

Autophagy is a cytoplasmic quality and quantity control pathway ubiquitous in eukaryotes. The core autophagy pathway is depicted in its minimalistic rendition in Figure 1. The membranes forming autophagic organelles come primarily from the endoplasmic reticulum, but additional compartments provide sources of membrane or lipids for the growing autophagosomal isolation membrane (phagophore) (Fig. 1). Autophagosome formation is dependent on a suite of Atg factors, which are consecutively numbered: for example, Atg1–Atg35 in yeast, with alternative names in mammals such as the Atg1 paralogs in mammals ULK1 and 2 (ULK1 being more studied) and the Atg6 ortholog Beclin 1. Autophagy is often equated with the emergence or modifications of endomembranes decorated with "LC3" (LC3B), which is one of six mammalian Atg8s (LC3A, LC3B, LC3C, GABARAP, GABARAPL1, and GABRAPL2) (Mizushima et al. 2011), with a key event being the carboxy-terminal lipidation of LC3 to generate LC3-II (LC3-phosphatidylethanolamine). Autophagosomes capture cytosolic or cytoplasmic cargo destined for elimination, most commonly through lysosomal degradation (Deter and De Duve 1967; Deter et al. 1967; Itakura et al. 2012), although other modes of cargo disposal have been observed (Jiang et al. 2013). Autophagy can be modulated by metabolic, physiological, immunological (cytokines and innate immunity signaling), and pharmacological (e.g., rapamycin) agonists and antagonists. There are two forms of autophagy—nonselective (bulk or generalized) autophagic degradation of the cytoplasm, usually as a response to starvation, and selective autophagy, whereby specific targets in the cytosol are recognized by autophagic receptors and captured by autophagosomes (Birgisdottir et al. 2013).

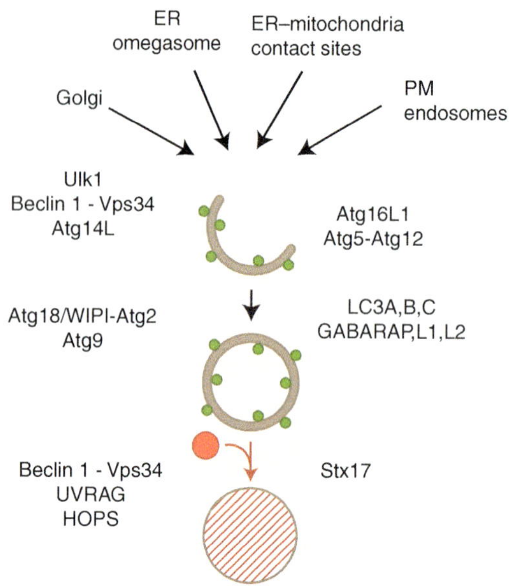

Figure 1. Autophagy pathway. Shown are a simplified macroautophagy pathway, protein factors, and membrane sources for the formation of autophagosomes in mammalian cells. (*Top*) Different sources of membranes contributing to the formation of autophagosomes. ER, endoplasmic reticulum; PM, plasma membrane. Within the cartoon: Crescent, autophagic phagophore or isolation membrane; double-membrane, closed autophagosome; red circle, lysosome; hatched circle delimited by a single membrane, autolysosome; green dots, LC3B (one of six mammalian Atg8s listed on the *right* side; typically used as a marker for autophagosomes). Other key factors are shown using their mammalian nomenclature.

INDUCTION OF BULK AUTOPHAGY BY NUTRITIONAL SIGNALS

The classical signal for generalized autophagy is starvation, which can be caused by low levels of amino acids, low energy, or absence of growth factors. Starvation can induce autophagy to kill virulent *M. tuberculosis* in macrophages (Fig. 2A) (Gutierrez et al. 2004). During starvation, portions of the cytosol are corralled into autophagosomes to generate amino acids (Lum et al. 2005) and energy sources, for example, via lipolysis (Settembre et al. 2013). These upstream metabolic events leading to autophagy activation are controlled via mTOR (mammalian target of rapamycin) and AMPK (AMP-activated Ser/Thr protein kinase). The mTOR Ser/Thr protein kinase negatively controls the most upstream of the Atg factors, ULK1, by phosphorylating it at inactivating sites (e.g., Ser 757), whereas AMPK positively regulates ULK1 by phosphorylating ULK1 at activating sites (e.g.,

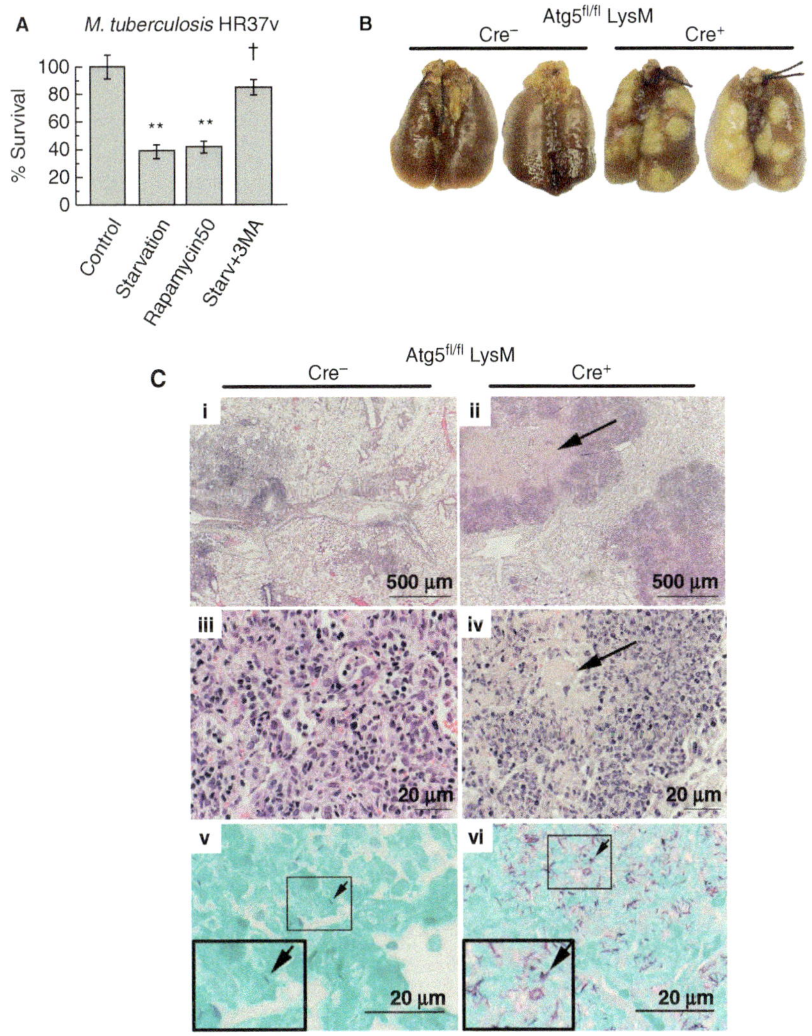

Figure 2. Autophagy protects against *M. tuberculosis* infection and pathogenesis. (*A*) Autophagy induction by starvation or rapamycin kills virulent *M. tuberculosis* in macrophages. (*B*) Increased gross lung pathology in mice defective for autophagy in the myeloid lineage (Cre^{+}) relative to autophagy-competent (Cre^{-}) mice infected with *M. tuberculosis* H37Rv. (*C*) Increased lung tissue necrosis and bacillary load in the lungs of mice defective for autophagy in the myeloid lineage (Cre^{+}) relative to their autophagy-competent (Cre^{-}) littermates. (Bottom panels) Acid-fast stain. Arrows, *M. tuberculosis* H37Rv bacilli. (*A*, Reprinted, with permission, from Gutierrez et al. 2004; *B*,*C*, reprinted, with permission, from Castillo et al. 2012.)

Ser 317 and Ser 777) (Egan et al. 2011; Kim et al. 2011). ULK1 phosphorylates a number of key substrates, most pertinently Beclin 1 (mammalian Atg6) at Ser 15 (Russell et al. 2013). Beclin 1 works with other subunits of class III phosphatidylinositol 3 kinase hVPS34 to generate phosphatidylinositol 3-phosphate (PI3P) on donor (e.g., ER [Axe et al. 2008]) membranes. PI3P marks the spot for initiation of autophagic phagophore formation. A phagophore expands into a full autophagosome. This is concomitant with or preceding the acquisition of SNARE Syntaxin 17 (Itakura et al. 2012; Hamasaki et al. 2013), which promotes fusion with lysosomes whereby a terminal degradative organelle, autolysosome, is formed where the captured cargo is degraded.

SELECTIVE AUTOPHAGY

Selective autophagy is driven by the recognition of cargos for selective autophagy via autophagic receptors (Fig. 3). The spectrum of selective autophagy targets includes defunct organelles such as depolarized mitochondria, protein aggregates, and intracellular microbes in contact with the cytosol. A subset of autophagic receptors involved in antimicrobial defense is termed

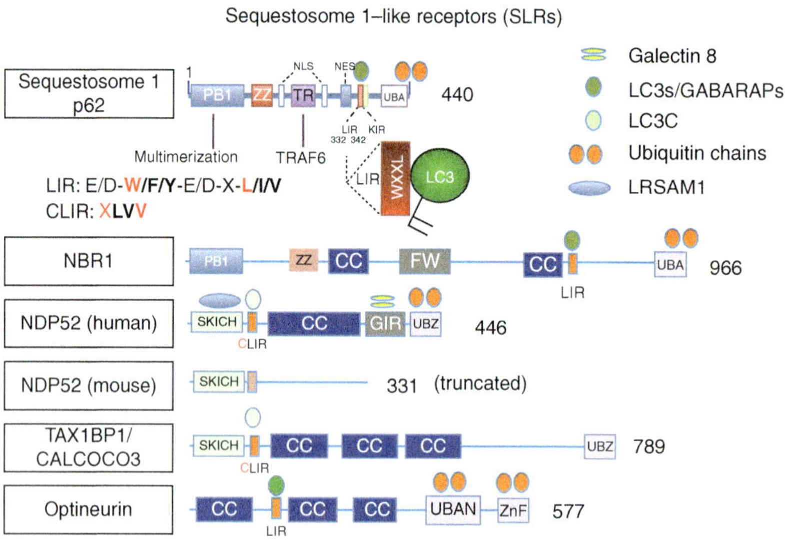

Figure 3. Sequestosome 1/p62–like receptors (SLRs), a new class of pattern-recognition receptors involved in autophagic elimination of intracellular microbes. LIR, LC3-interacting region (consensus sequence shown and key positions in red); aromatic pocket-filling W (or F/Y) and aliphatic pocket-filling L (or I/V) form an intermolecular parallel β sheet with LC3s or GABARAPs, at the interface between the amino-terminal α-helical domain and ubiquitin-like fold of LC3s/GABARAPs. CLIR, a LIR specific for LC3C, whereby aromatic residue is not present (X) to fill in the aromatic pocket and instead the interactions are stabilized by compensatory hydrophobic contacts provided by additional aliphatic residues located between the W and L position anchors. KIR, KAEP1-interacting region; NES, nuclear export signal; NLS, nuclear localization signal; PB1, protein-binding domain (homopolymerization of p62 hetero-oligomerization between p62 and NBR1, or interactions with other partners); TR, TRAF6-interacting region (also a multipartner binding region); ZZ, ZZ-type zinc finger (ZnF) domain; FW, four-Trp domain, also known as the NBR1 box; UBAN, a parallel coiled-coiled dimer UBD with specificity for linear ubiquitin chains; CC, coiled coil; UBA, a three-helix bundle UBD (ubiquitin-binding domain) with affinity for monoubiquitin and the more open conformation of K63 ubiquitin linkages; UBZ, a Zn finger ββα fold UBD binding mono- and polyubiquitin; SKICH, skeletal muscle and kidney enriched inositol phosphatase carboxyl homology domain; GIR, galectin-interacting region. Sequestosome 1/p62 has been shown to affect *M. tuberculosis* clearance (Ponpuak et al. 2010). NDP52 has been implicated in elimination of *M. tuberculosis* in murine macrophages (Watson et al. 2012); note, however, that NDP52 is severely truncated in this species. (Image modified from Deretic et al. 2013.)

SLRs, for Sequestosome 1/p62-like receptors (Fig. 3). The cargo, such as a cytosolic bacterium or a depolarized mitochondrion (bacteria and mitochondria share recognition machinery [Deretic 2010]), is often tagged by ubiquitin (Bjorkoy et al. 2005; Kirkin et al. 2009), galectins (Thurston et al. 2012; Li et al. 2013), and possibly other modifications (Deretic et al. 2013). Ubiquitin is placed on or around bacteria via specific E3 ligases such as LRSAM1, which possesses a leucine-rich repeat characteristic of pattern recognition receptors and a RING domain conferring its E3 ubiquitin ligase activity (Huett et al. 2012), or another E3 ligase, Parkin (Manzanillo et al. 2013). Parkin is well known for ubiquitination of depolarized or damaged mitochondria en route for autophagic elimination via mitophagy (Youle and Narendra 2011). Ubiquitin and other earmarks are recognized by autophagic receptors that bind the tags at one end and interact at the other end with mammalian Atg8s via an LC3-interacting region (LIR) (Birgisdottir et al. 2013). Whether and how cargo capture triggers signaling and execution of membrane growth during selective autophagy are not well understood, but many of the factors participating in generalized/nonselective autophagy are engaged.

LC3-ASSOCIATED PHAGOCYTOSIS

An example of a known exception to using all parts of the autophagy pathway is a process called LC3-associated autophagy (LAP), which is a merger between conventional phagocytosis and autophagy (Cemma and Brumell, 2012). LAP appears to be a modification of the conventional phagocytic pathway distinguished by the recruitment of LC3, which enhances phagosomal fusogenicity with lysosomes (Fig. 4). LAP does not require ULK1 but needs Beclin 1-hVPS34 and LC3-conjugation systems (Henault et al. 2012). LAP occurs following uptake of various extracellular targets: bacteria or particles coated with Toll-like receptor (TLR) agonists (Sanjuan et al. 2007; Xu et al. 2007; Lee et al. 2010), phagocytosed dead cells (Martinez et al. 2011), live epithelial cells engulfed via entotisis by neighboring cells (Florey et al. 2011),

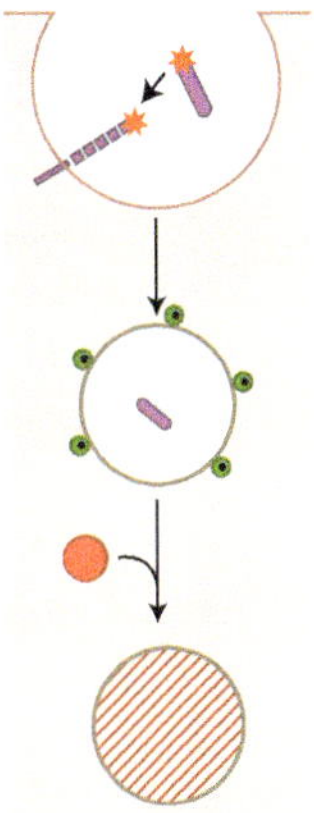

Figure 4. LC3-associated phagocytosis (LAP) as an intersection between autophagy and phagocytosis. Autophagy is frequently morphologically described as formation of double-membrane autophagosomes in the cytoplasm. This is requisite when an internal phagosome is derived from intracellular membranes such as the endoplasmic reticulum (ER). One important exception in the context of the role of autophagy during infection is the formation of conventional phagosomes that are also decorated with LC3 (green dots). Note that LC3 is only on the cytofacial side of the phagosomal membrane, and that this is a single membrane as in the case of conventional phagosomes. Depicted also is a Toll-like receptor molecule recognizing pathogen-associated molecular patterns (asterisks), involved in the induction of LAP and capable of concomitantly inducing conventional autophagy in the cell. The presence of LC3 on these phagosomes promotes maturation of the standard phagosome into autolysosomes. LAP depends on Beclin 1-hVPS34, LC3-conjugation systems, and other parts of autophagy pathway but is independent of ULK1, which is needed to generate double-membrane autophagosomes during starvation from internal ER membranes. The role of LC3 may be a manifestation of the tethering and fusogenic properties of LC3; furthermore, concomitantly generated autolysosomes are enriched in their bactericidal properties, whereas other immunologically active compartments such as those involved in antigen presentation and TLR signaling (e.g., TLR9) can enhance or exacerbate a variety of immune responses. (Image modified from Deretic et al. 2013.)

rod outer segments phagocytosed by retinal pigment epithelial cells (Kim et al. 2013), and FcγR-dependent uptake of immune complexes (Henault et al. 2012). *M. tuberculosis* and

M. bovis BCG bacilli that reside inside the phagosome can be subjected to LAP on induction of autophagy by physiological, immunological, or pharmacological means (Gutierrez et al. 2004; Harris et al. 2007; Xu et al. 2007; Jagannath et al. 2009; Pilli et al. 2012). LAP enhances conventional phagosomes by conferring improved lytic properties, enhanced bactericidal functions (Gutierrez et al. 2004; Harris et al. 2007; Sanjuan et al. 2007; Cemma and Brumell 2012; Pilli et al. 2012), better antigen presentation (Jagannath et al. 2009; Lee et al. 2010), and enhanced intracellular trafficking of pathogen-associated molecular patterns (PAMPs) or damage-associated molecular patterns (DAMPs) complexed with pattern-recognition receptors (PRRs) (Chaturvedi et al. 2008; Lee et al. 2010; Henault et al. 2012). The recapitulation of phagosomal/autophagosomal maturation steps in LAP is linked to PI3P generation, long known to be key for phagosomal maturation (Vergne et al. 2004), whereas the role of LC3 may be a manifestation of the tethering and fusogenic properties of LC3 (Nakatogawa et al. 2007; Weidberg et al. 2011).

IMMUNE SIGNALING AND AUTOPHAGY AS AN ANTI-*M. tuberculosis* EFFECTOR

In addition to being controlled globally by starvation, autophagy responds to innate immunity signals and cytokine stimulation during immune responses (Deretic et al. 2013). Autophagy can be induced via PRRs. TLR ligands and TLRs activate autophagy (Xu et al. 2007; Delgado et al. 2008) via TRAF6 (Shi and Kehrl 2010), which activates or stabilizes Beclin 1 (Shi and Kehrl 2010) and ULK1 (Nazio et al. 2013). NOD2 can activate autophagy via RIPK2 and ULK1 (Lupfer et al. 2013). Second messenger 2′-5′ cyclic GMP-AMP (cGAMP) generated by mammalian cGAMP synthase in response to the presence of cytosolic DNA (viral, mitochondrial, or bacterial, including mycobacterial) or secreted bacterial 3′-5′ cyclic-di-GMP or cyclic-di-AMP can stimulate autophagy and ULK1 (Watson et al. 2012; Konno et al. 2013). IL-1β stimulates autophagy (Pilli et al. 2012), which is of high relevance for *M. tuberculosis* control. MyD88 signaling is key to early protection against *M. tuberculosis,* although TLRs, which act via MyD88, appear not to be essential for protection (Fremond et al. 2004, 2007; Scanga et al. 2004; Holscher et al. 2008). In contrast, IL-1 receptor signaling, which also relies on MyD88 as an adapter, is key to early control of *M. tuberculosis* (Mayer-Barber et al. 2010, 2011; Guler et al. 2011). IL-1β eliminates *M. tuberculosis* through autophagy (Pilli et al. 2012). Th1 cytokines activate autophagy to kill intracellular *M. tuberculosis* (Harris et al. 2007). Stimulation of autophagy mediated through P2X purinergic receptors can eliminate intracellular *M. tuberculosis* (Biswas et al. 2008). Activation of anti-*M. tuberculosis* autophagy has also been reported via direct cell–cell contacts between specific T cells and *M. tuberculosis*–infected macrophages (Petruccioli et al. 2012).

MECHANISMS OF INTRACELLULAR KILLING OF *M. tuberculosis* BY AUTOPHAGY

Autophagy eliminates intracellular *M. tuberculosis* through lytic and antimicrobial properties unique to autolysosomes, which are much more robust antimicrobial compartments than conventional phagosomes (Ponpuak et al. 2010). A step-by-step analysis of autophagy factors, starting with an SLR, Sequestosome 1/p62, has established that the entire pathway is important for anti–*M. tuberculosis* action of autophagy (Ponpuak et al. 2010). Another SLR, NDP52, has been reported as being necessary for elimination of *M. tuberculosis* in mouse macrophages (Watson et al. 2012), but this cannot be the case, at least in murine cells, because *Mus musculus* lacks a functional NDP52 gene (Fig. 3) (Deretic et al. 2013). Induction of autophagy promotes maturation and acidification of *M. tuberculosis* phagosomes and their conversion into mycobactericidal organelles (Gutierrez et al. 2004; Harris et al. 2007; Fabri et al. 2011b) via processes akin to LAP (Cemma and Brumell 2012). Thus, induction of autophagy overcomes the classical *M. tuberculosis* virulence determinant known as inhibition of phagosome-lysosome (Hart et al. 1987; Vergne et al. 2004). Among the constituents delivered via these enhanced trafficking pathways are conventional anti–*M. tuberculosis* antimicrobial peptides including cathelicidin potentially through autophagy-stimulated fusion with lysosomes where cathelicidin is stored (Yuk et al. 2009; Fabri et al. 2011b). Moreover, autophagy captures cytosolic proteins and partially digests them. These autophagosomal contents, which have enhanced antimycobacterial properties (Ponpuak et al. 2010), are delivered to the *M. tuberculosis* phagosome in cells induced for autophagy. A specific manifestation of this is that induction of autophagy generates and delivers to *M. tuberculosis* a mixture of neo-antimicrobial peptides (known as cryptides [Ponpuak and Deretic 2011]) produced through autophagic proteolysis of otherwise innocuous cytosolic proteins such as ribosomal proteins (Ponpuak et al. 2010) and ubiquitin (Alonso et al. 2007). A certain fraction of intracellular *M. tuberculosis* bacilli escape from phagosomes into the cytoplasm or are in contact with the cytosol (van der Wel et al. 2007). The bacilli that are in contact with the cytosol represent a minor proportion of the total intracellular *M. tuberculosis*, but are nevertheless subject to a cleanup through selective autophagy (Watson et al. 2012).

An unexpected link between action of the frontline antituberculosis chemotherapeutics and autophagy has been reported (Kim et al. 2012a). The key antituberculosis drugs, isoniazid and pyrazinamide, express their full potency in cooperation with a functional autophagy (Kim et al. 2012a). During treatment of *M. tuberculosis* with isoniazid or pyrazinamide, the release of bacterial products induces autophagy in infected macrophages in association with a generation of reactive oxygen species (ROS) from mitochondrial and NADPH oxidase sources (Kim et al. 2012a). This is in keeping with induction of autophagy by ROS released by mitochondria and NADPH oxidase (Scherz-Shouval et al. 2007; Huang et al. 2009). The enhanced effectiveness of these antibiotics in synergy with autophagy may explain the sterilizing properties of pyrazinamide. Furthermore, several compounds that can induce autophagy have been shown to inhibit *M. tuberculosis* (Floto et al. 2007; Lam et al. 2012; Sundaramurthy et al. 2013), raising the possibility of host-based therapies based on autophagy-inducing drugs.

M. tuberculosis POSSESSES COUNTERMEASURES AGAINST AUTOPHAGY

Mycobacterial infections show evidence of mTOR activation (mTOR inhibits autophagy) or autophagy induction, correlating with the species or strain virulence (Zullo and Lee 2012). Furthermore, metabolic reprogramming of host macrophages by *M. tuberculosis* (Russell et al. 2009; Singh et al. 2012) leads to an increase in lipid droplets, the cytoplasmic stores of neutral lipids such as triglycerides and cholesterol esters. Lipid droplets are dynamic organelles (Fujimoto and Parton 2011) that are known to intersect with the autophagic pathway (Singh et al. 2009; Velikkakath et al. 2012). The host cell reprogramming by *M. tuberculosis* reduces autophagic capacity of the cell and protects intracellular *M. tuberculosis* from autophagic elimination (Singh et al. 2012).

A number of candidate antiautophagy factors encoded by *M. tuberculosis* have been reported. An *M. tuberculosis* protein termed Eis (enhanced intracellular survival) (Shin et al. 2010a; Ganaie et al. 2011; Kim et al. 2012b) may interact with specific autophagy factors or affect upstream signaling regulators. Eis is an ε-aminoacetyltransferase that acetylates Lys-55 in a JNK-specific phosphatase (Kim et al. 2012b). JNK action is important for activation of the key autophagy regulator Beclin 1, and thus Eis may modulate autophagy (Shin et al. 2010a; Ganaie et al. 2011; Kim et al. 2012b). A mycobacterial glycolipid lipoarabinomannan has also been reported as inhibiting autophagy (Shui et al. 2011). ESX-1, a type VII secretion system of *M. tuberculosis*, releases a 6-kDa protein ESAT-6 to block *M. tuberculosis* phagosomal maturation into degradative autolysosomal organelles (Romagnoli et al. 2012; Zhang et al. 2012). Pharmacological agonists of autophagy can overcome the ESAT-6-based block (Romagnoli et al. 2012), in keeping with the observations that physiological or immunological stimulation of autophagy (e.g., by starvation or IFN-γ) (Gutierrez et al. 2004; Harris et al. 2007) can kill *M. tuberculosis* overpowering antiautophagy mechanisms of *M. tuberculosis.*

IFN-γ, TH1 VERSUS TH2 CYTOKINES, AND VITAMIN D IN ANTI-*M. tuberculosis* AUTOPHAGY

Response of autophagy, as an antimicrobial effector, to Th1 and Th2 cytokines correlates with the general association of Th1 versus Th2 cytokines with their restriction versus permissiveness to intracellular pathogens. IFN-γ, a key Th1 cytokine, can turn on autophagy (Gutierrez et al. 2004; Harris et al. 2007). Th2 cytokines IL-4 and IL-13 inhibit IFN-γ-dependent autophagy in a dominant fashion; that is, they can trump IFN-γ effects during simultaneous exposure (Harris et al. 2007; Ghadimi et al. 2010). Th2 cytokines can also override other physiological inducers of autophagy, although the inhibitory signaling pathways differ in terms of interference with IFN-γ or, for example, starvation as inducers of autophagy (Harris et al. 2007). IL-4 and IL-13 inhibit IFN-γ-induced autophagy via a pathway dependent on STAT6, whereas they inhibit starvation-induced autophagy via Akt signaling. IL-10 can also be inhibitory to autophagy (Van Grol et al. 2010; Park et al. 2011).

There are important hormonal agonists of IFN-γ activation of autophagy, including sterol-derived vitamin D metabolite calcitriol, also known by various names as 1,25-dihydroxyvitamin D3, 1,25-dihydroxycholecalciferol, or 1,25(OH)D3. Calcitriol circulates at very low concentrations in the serum and is generated in the kidney. However, calcitriol can additionally be generated in human macrophages from its precursor calcidiol (25-hydroxy vitamin D3; present at much higher concentrations in the serum) by a specific 1-α hydroxylase induced in macrophages in response to TLR activation (Liu et al. 2006), stimulation with IFN-γ (Reichel et al. 1987), or exposure to other stimuli (Evans et al. 2006). Low levels of calcitriol and its precursor calcidiol in the serum have been associated with susceptibility to tuberculosis (Nnoaham and Clarke 2008). Of note, lower calcidiol and calcitriol levels also factor in HIV–*M. tuberculosis* coinfections (Campbell and Spector 2012). Recent studies have indicated a strong synergistic role between calcitriol with IFN-γ during induction of autophagy in human macrophages as a contributing mechanism to *M. tuberculosis* killing (Yuk et al. 2009; Shin et al. 2010b; Fabri et al. 2011a,b; Campbell and Spector 2012; Anandaiah et al. 2013; Klug-Micu et al. 2013). Calcitriol induces autophagy via Ca^{2+} and Ca^{2+}/calmodulin-dependent kinase kinase-β (CaMKKβ) (Hoyer-Hansen et al. 2007), which in turn activates AMPK (AMP-activated protein kinase) (Mihaylova and Shaw 2011). Studies outside of the tuberculosis field have shown that CaMKKβ, which responds to calcitriol via Ca^{2+}, promotes induction of autophagy in a manner sensitive to membrane-permeant Ca^{2+} chelators (Hoyer-Hansen et al. 2007) by activating a phosphorylation cascade involving ULK1 and then Beclin 1, as discussed above in the section Autophagy Pathway (Egan et al. 2011; Kim et al. 2011; Russell et al. 2013). The phosphorylation of AMPK by CaMKKβ occurs on the same critical Thr 172 residue as with other key kinases that control AMPK activation (Mihaylova and Shaw 2011). The aforementioned cathelicidin has also been reported to play a role in induction of autophagy by calcitriol (Yuk et al. 2009). However, the proposed activation of autophagy by cathelicidin has no defined mechanism in contrast to its documented effector functions of an antimicrobial peptide with enhanced delivery to intracellular *M. tuberculosis* through autophagy (Fabri et al. 2011b). Whereas in human macrophages calcitriol is required for IFN-γ-induced autophagy (Fabri et al. 2011b), it is not necessary in human macrophages when autophagy is induced by nutritional (starvation) or pharmacological (rapamycin) means (Fabri et al. 2011b). Calcidiol and calcitriol levels appear not to be a determinant of autophagy induction by IFN-γ in murine macrophages (Gutierrez et al. 2004; Singh et al. 2006; Harris et al. 2007). This is in keeping with the notion that expression of antimicrobial peptides (e.g., cathelcidin) in murine cells is not controlled

 Cite this article as *Cold Spring Harb Perspect Med* doi: 10.1101/cshperspect.a018481

by vitamin D response elements (Fabri et al. 2011b).

GENETIC PREDISPOSITIONS TO TUBERCULOSIS AND AUTOPHAGY

In keeping with the above role of calcitriol in autophagy, human genetic polymorphisms in the gene encoding vitamin D receptor are associated with susceptibility to tuberculosis when combined with low serum levels of calcidiol, a precursor to calcitriol (Wilkinson et al. 2000). There are further genetic links between autophagy and risks for active tuberculosis. A recent genome-wide association study (GWAS) shows a widespread overlap between genetic risks for inflammatory bowel disease (IBD) and tuberculosis (Jostins et al. 2012). As a subset of these overlaps, genetic polymorphisms in autophagy genes affect both IBD and tuberculosis. For example, polymorphisms in *ATG16L1* and *IRGM*, have been initially identified through GWASs as autophagy risk loci for Crohn's disease (Wellcome Trust Case Control Consortium 2007), a common form of IBD. Subsequent human population studies have shown that *IRGM*, encoding an autophagy-modulating factor (Singh et al. 2006, 2010), is also a risk factor for tuberculosis (Intemann et al. 2009; Che et al. 2010; King et al. 2011; Bahari et al. 2012).

AUTOPHAGY PROTECTS AGAINST *M. tuberculosis* INFECTION IN VIVO

Autophagy protects in vivo against bacillary burden, inflammation, lung pathology (Fig. 2B,C), and death in transgenic mouse models of *M. tuberculosis* infection (Castillo et al. 2012; Watson et al. 2012). This has been shown with virulent *M. tuberculosis* strains, H37Rv (Castillo et al. 2012) and Erdman (Watson et al. 2012), using Atg5$^{fl/fl}$ LysM-Cre transgenic mice with autophagy defective in myeloid cells. Atg7$^{fl/fl}$ LysM-Cre mice with a similar autophagy defect in myeloid cells show increased pathology when challenged with *M. bovis* BCG, whereas higher numbers of bacilli are taken up by Atg7$^{fl/fl}$ LysM-Cre^{+} macrophages ex vivo ascribed in part to changes in phagocytic receptors (Bonilla et al. 2013). Although the details of respiratory infection and strains used varied, all studies observed higher bacillary load, exacerbated lung involvement, and increased lung pathology relative to autophagy-competent mice (Castillo et al. 2012; Watson et al. 2012; Bonilla et al. 2013). The two studies with virulent *M. tuberculosis* strains showed increased mortality of Atg5$^{fl/fl}$ LysM-Cre^{+} mice (Castillo et al. 2012; Watson et al. 2012).

AUTOPHAGY PROTECTS AGAINST EXCESSIVE INFLAMMATION AND TUBERCULOSIS PATHOGENESIS

Most prominently, IL-1 has been found elevated in the infected Atg5$^{fl/fl}$ LysM-Cre^{+} mice relative to their Atg5$^{fl/fl}$ LysM-Cre^{-} littermates (Castillo et al. 2012; Watson et al. 2012). In contrast, IFN-γ or IL-4 responses are equal in autophagy-proficient and autophagy-deficient mice (Castillo et al. 2012). Of IL-1s, IL-1α has turned out to be the dominant cytokine in the infected Atg5$^{fl/fl}$ LysM-Cre^{+} lung. IL-1β, albeit increased in autophagy-deficient mice, is present at low absolute levels in the lung challenged with disparate pathogens (Castillo et al. 2012; Lupfer et al. 2013). Although inflammasome is hyperactivated in autophagy-defective mice (Saitoh et al. 2008; Nakahira et al. 2011; Zhou et al. 2011), the lung environment may suppress excess IL-1β (Castillo et al. 2012; Lupfer et al. 2013). Nevertheless, the lung immune cells from mice with autophagic defect in myeloid cells show propensity towards extended Th17 polarization (Castillo et al. 2012). This is attributable to a cell-autonomous defect in autophagy-deficient macrophages, which secrete excess IL-1α (Castillo et al. 2012). IL-1α, just like IL-1β, promotes Th17 polarization leading to extended IL-17 response during *M. tuberculosis* infection of Atg5$^{fl/fl}$ LysM-Cre^{+} mice (Castillo et al. 2012). This scenario makes it impossible for IFN-γ, one of the functions of which is a suppression of excessive and pathology-inducing IL-1β responses by inhibiting inflammasome activation (Mishra et al. 2013), to overcome the alternative IL-1 responses via IL-1α. Unlike IL-1β, which depends on inflammasome activation, IL-1α can be activated independently of inflammasome via calpain (Castillo et al. 2012; Gross et al. 2012).

The above anti-inflammatory action of autophagy may not stop at direct control of intracellular *M. tuberculosis* and tempering of the IL-1 response (see Fig. 5 for an overall model). We propose a model that extends to potential effects on type I IFN responses. Type I interferon (IFN) is a key biosignature of active tuberculosis (Berry et al. 2010; Maertzdorf et al. 2012; Ottenhoff et al. 2012; Teles et al. 2013). *M. tuberculosis*–mediated induction of type I IFN requires the ESX-1 system (Stanley et al. 2007; Pandey et al. 2009; Novikov et al. 2011; Manzanillo et al. 2012), and this signaling has been shown to be induced by *M. tuberculosis* extracellular DNA through IRF3 (Manzanillo et al. 2012). Mice lacking IRF3 (or lacking IFNAR) survive *M. tuberculosis* infection longer than wild-type mice (Manca et al. 2005; Manzanillo et al. 2012). Because autophagy clears *M. tuber-*

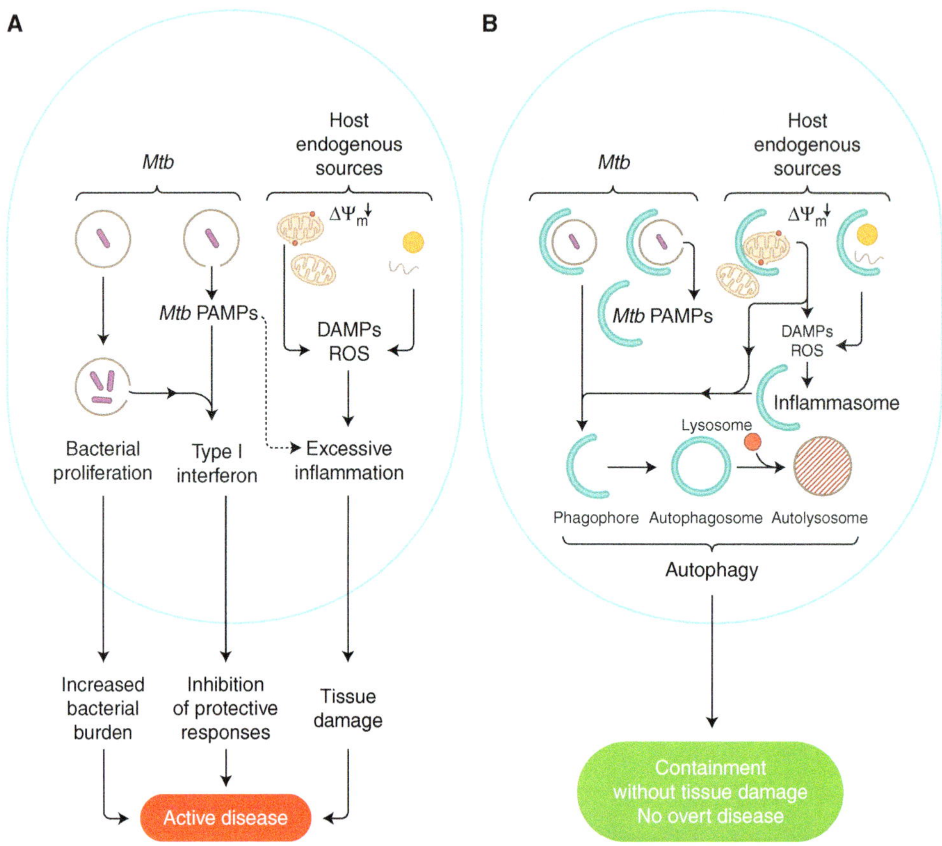

Figure 5. Proposed model of how autophagy interferes with progression to active disease during *M. tuberculosis* infection. (*A*) Proposed processes contributing to progression into active disease pertinent to the role of autophagy: uncontrolled *M. tuberculosis* growth; endogenous sources of excessive inflammation (e.g., damaged organelles such as depolarized mitochondria, which are the source of reactive oxygen species [ROS] and mitochondrial DNA released into the cytosol) acting as damage-associated molecular patterns (DAMPs) that amplify inflammatory responses to the point of causing excessive tissue damage; *M. tuberculosis* pathogen-associated molecular patterns (PAMPs; e.g., mycobacterial *N*-glycolyl muramyl dipeptide or bacterial DNA released from or associated with the bacilli) inducing type I IFN, which is a biomarker of active disease and suppresses measured host responses that inhibit *M. tuberculosis* proliferation and thus curtails their protective effectiveness. (*B*) Autophagy (represented by crescents) eliminates the above promoters of active disease and thus acts as an antibacterial and tissue-sparing process.

culosis along with its extracellular DNA (Watson et al. 2012), it is possible that removal of this PAMP (bacterial extracellular DNA) prevents activation of now well-delineated pathways of induction of type I IFN via dicyclic nucleotide second messengers and STING (Ablasser et al. 2013; Civril et al. 2013; Wu et al. 2013). Specific molecular intersections between autophagy (e.g., ULK1) and these systems (e.g., STING) have been recently uncovered (Konno et al. 2013). It is possible that autophagic removal of other type I IFN-inducing products, such as the *M. tuberculosis* peptidoglycan *N*-glycolyl MDP (Pandey et al. 2009), may also act to prevent excess type I IFN production.

CONCLUSIONS AND OUTLOOK

Autophagy is a cell-autonomous innate immunity defense that enables host cells to capture intracellular pathogens and kill them in lysosomal organelles that during autophagy acquire enhanced bactericidal properties. Equally or perhaps more importantly, autophagy can suppress excessive inflammatory responses that contribute to progression to active disease. This occurs via autophagic elimination of endogenous cellular agonists of inflammasome or calpain activation, thus preventing excess IL-1 response, and may also remove mycobacterial products eliciting other pathogenesis-associated responses such as type I IFN linked to active disease. When balanced, both IL-1 and type I IFN may have their role in protection but without autophagy to remove the contributing agonists, these important cytokine responses may be out of alignment and cause pathology and active disease. Consequently, pharmacological activation of autophagy may offer therapeutic host-targeted options for better control of *M. tuberculosis* infection.

ACKNOWLEDGMENTS

Work in V. Deretic's laboratory is supported by grants AI042999 and AI111935 from the National Institutes of Health and a Bill and Melinda Gates Grand Challenge Explorations grant.

REFERENCES

Ablasser A, Goldeck M, Cavlar T, Deimling T, Witte G, Rohl I, Hopfner KP, Ludwig J, Hornung V. 2013. cGAS produces a 2′-5′-linked cyclic dinucleotide second messenger that activates STING. *Nature* **498:** 380–384.

Alonso S, Pethe K, Russell DG, Purdy GE. 2007. Lysosomal killing of *Mycobacterium* mediated by ubiquitin-derived peptides is enhanced by autophagy. *Proc Natl Acad Sci* **104:** 6031–6036.

Anandaiah A, Sinha S, Bole M, Sharma SK, Kumar N, Luthra K, Li X, Zhou X, Nelson B, Han X, et al. 2013. Vitamin D rescues impaired *Mycobacterium tuberculosis*–mediated tumor necrosis factor release in macrophages of HIV-seropositive individuals through an enhanced Toll-like receptor signaling pathway in vitro. *Infect Immun* **81:** 2–10.

Axe EL, Walker SA, Manifava M, Chandra P, Roderick HL, Habermann A, Griffiths G, Ktistakis NT. 2008. Autophagosome formation from membrane compartments enriched in phosphatidylinositol 3-phosphate and dynamically connected to the endoplasmic reticulum. *J Cell Biol* **182:** 685–701.

Bahari G, Hashemi M, Taheri M, Naderi M, Eskandari-Nasab E, Atabaki M. 2012. Association of IRGM polymorphisms and susceptibility to pulmonary tuberculosis in Zahedan, Southeast Iran. *Scientific World Journal* **2012:** 950801.

Berry MP, Graham CM, McNab FW, Xu Z, Bloch SA, Oni T, Wilkinson KA, Banchereau R, Skinner J, Wilkinson RJ, et al. 2010. An interferon-inducible neutrophil-driven blood transcriptional signature in human tuberculosis. *Nature* **466:** 973–977.

Birgisdottir AB, Lamark T, Johansen T. 2013. The LIR motif—Crucial for selective autophagy. *J Cell Sci* **126:** 3237–3247.

Biswas D, Qureshi OS, Lee WY, Croudace JE, Mura M, Lammas DA. 2008. ATP-induced autophagy is associated with rapid killing of intracellular mycobacteria within human monocytes/macrophages. *BMC Immunol* **9:** 35.

Bjorkoy G, Lamark T, Brech A, Outzen H, Perander M, Overvatn A, Stenmark H, Johansen T. 2005. p62/SQSTM1 forms protein aggregates degraded by autophagy and has a protective effect on huntingtin-induced cell death. *J Cell Biol* **171:** 603–614.

Bonilla DL, Bhattacharya A, Sha Y, Xu Y, Xiang Q, Kan A, Jagannath C, Komatsu M, Eissa NT. 2013. Autophagy regulates phagocytosis by modulating the expression of scavenger receptors. *Immunity* **39:** 537–547.

Campbell GR, Spector SA. 2012. Vitamin D inhibits human immunodeficiency virus type 1 and *Mycobacterium tuberculosis* infection in macrophages through the induction of autophagy. *PLoS Pathog* **8:** e1002689.

Castillo EF, Dekonenko A, Arko-Mensah J, Mandell MA, Dupont N, Jiang S, Delgado-Vargas M, Timmins GS, Bhattacharya D, Yang H, et al. 2012. Autophagy protects against active tuberculosis by suppressing bacterial burden and inflammation. *Proc Natl Acad Sci* **109:** E3168–E3176.

Cemma M, Brumell JH. 2012. Interactions of pathogenic bacteria with autophagy systems. *Curr Biol* **22:** R540–R545.

Chaturvedi A, Dorward D, Pierce SK. 2008. The B cell receptor governs the subcellular location of Toll-like receptor 9 leading to hyperresponses to DNA-containing antigens. *Immunity* **28:** 799–809.

Che N, Li S, Gao T, Zhang Z, Han Y, Zhang X, Sun Y, Liu Y, Sun Z, Zhang J, et al. 2010. Identification of a novel IRGM promoter single nucleotide polymorphism associated with tuberculosis. *Clin Chim Acta* **411:** 1645–1649.

Civril F, Deimling T, de Oliveira Mann CC, Ablasser A, Moldt M, Witte G, Hornung V, Hopfner KP. 2013. Structural mechanism of cytosolic DNA sensing by cGAS. *Nature* **498:** 332–337.

Delgado MA, Elmaoued RA, Davis AS, Kyei G, Deretic V. 2008. Toll-like receptors control autophagy. *EMBO J* **27:** 1110–1121.

Deretic V. 2005. Autophagy in innate and adaptive immunity. *Trends Immunol* **26:** 523–528.

Deretic V. 2010. Autophagy of intracellular microbes and mitochondria: Two sides of the same coin? *F1000 Biol Rep* **2:** 45.

Deretic V, Saitoh T, Akira S. 2013. Autophagy in infection, inflammation, and immunity. *Nat Rev Immunol* **13:** 722–737.

Deter RL, De Duve C. 1967. Influence of glucagon, an inducer of cellular autophagy, on some physical properties of rat liver lysosomes. *J Cell Biol* **33:** 437–449.

Deter RL, Baudhuin P, De Duve C. 1967. Participation of lysosomes in cellular autophagy induced in rat liver by glucagon. *J Cell Biol* **35:** C11–C16.

Egan DF, Shackelford DB, Mihaylova MM, Gelino S, Kohnz RA, Mair W, Vasquez DS, Joshi A, Gwinn DM, Taylor R, et al. 2011. Phosphorylation of ULK1 (hATG1) by AMP-activated protein kinase connects energy sensing to mitophagy. *Science* **331:** 456–461.

Evans CE, Mylchreest S, Mee AP, Berry JL, Andrew JG. 2006. Cyclic hydrostatic pressure and particles increase synthesis of 1,25-dihydroxyvitamin D3 by human macrophages in vitro. *Int J Biochem Cell Biol* **38:** 1540–1546.

Fabri M, Realegeno SE, Jo EK, Modlin RL. 2011a. Role of autophagy in the host response to microbial infection and potential for therapy. *Curr Opin Immunol* **23:** 65–70.

Fabri M, Stenger S, Shin DM, Yuk JM, Liu PT, Realegeno S, Lee HM, Krutzik SR, Schenk M, Sieling PA, et al. 2011b. Vitamin D is required for IFN-γ-mediated antimicrobial activity of human macrophages. *Sci Transl Med* **3:** 104ra102.

Florey O, Kim SE, Sandoval CP, Haynes CM, Overholtzer M. 2011. Autophagy machinery mediates macroendocytic processing and entotic cell death by targeting single membranes. *Nat Cell Biol* **13:** 1335–1343.

Floto RA, Sarkar S, Perlstein EO, Kampmann B, Schreiber SL, Rubinsztein DC. 2007. Small molecule enhancers of rapamycin-induced TOR inhibition promote autophagy, reduce toxicity in Huntington's disease models and enhance killing of mycobacteria by macrophages. *Autophagy* **3:** 620–622.

Fremond CM, Yeremeev V, Nicolle DM, Jacobs M, Quesniaux VF, Ryffel B. 2004. Fatal *Mycobacterium tuberculosis* infection despite adaptive immune response in the absence of MyD88. *J Clin Invest* **114:** 1790–1799.

Fremond CM, Togbe D, Doz E, Rose S, Vasseur V, Maillet I, Jacobs M, Ryffel B, Quesniaux VF. 2007. IL-1 receptor-mediated signal is an essential component of MyD88-dependent innate response to *Mycobacterium tuberculosis* infection. *J Immunol* **179:** 1178–1189.

Fujimoto T, Parton RG. 2011. Not just fat: The structure and function of the lipid droplet. *Cold Spring Harb Perspect Biol* **3:** a004838.

Ganaie AA, Lella RK, Solanki R, Sharma C. 2011. Thermostable hexameric form of Eis (Rv2416c) protein of *M. tuberculosis* plays an important role for enhanced intracellular survival within macrophages. *PLoS ONE* **6:** e27590.

Ghadimi D, de Vrese M, Heller KJ, Schrezenmeir J. 2010. Lactic acid bacteria enhance autophagic ability of mononuclear phagocytes by increasing Th1 autophagy-promoting cytokine (IFN-γ) and nitric oxide (NO) levels and reducing Th2 autophagy-restraining cytokines (IL-4 and IL-13) in response to *Mycobacterium tuberculosis* antigen. *Int Immunopharmacol* **10:** 694–706.

Gross O, Yazdi AS, Thomas CJ, Masin M, Heinz LX, Guarda G, Quadroni M, Drexler SK, Tschopp J. 2012. Inflammasome activators induce interleukin-1α secretion via distinct pathways with differential requirement for the protease function of caspase-1. *Immunity* **36:** 388–400.

Guler R, Parihar SP, Spohn G, Johansen P, Brombacher F, Bachmann MF. 2011. Blocking IL-1α but not IL-1β increases susceptibility to chronic *Mycobacterium tuberculosis* infection in mice. *Vaccine* **29:** 1339–1346.

Gutierrez MG, Master SS, Singh SB, Taylor GA, Colombo MI, Deretic V. 2004. Autophagy is a defense mechanism inhibiting BCG and *Mycobacterium tuberculosis* survival in infected macrophages. *Cell* **119:** 753–766.

Hamasaki M, Furuta N, Matsuda A, Nezu A, Yamamoto A, Fujita N, Oomori H, Noda T, Haraguchi T, Hiraoka Y, et al. 2013. Autophagosomes form at ER-mitochondria contact sites. *Nature* **495:** 389–393.

Harris J, De Haro SA, Master SS, Keane J, Roberts EA, Delgado M, Deretic V. 2007. T helper 2 cytokines inhibit autophagic control of intracellular *Mycobacterium tuberculosis*. *Immunity* **27:** 505–517.

Hart PD, Young MR, Gordon AH, Sullivan KH. 1987. Inhibition of phagosome-lysosome fusion in macrophages by certain mycobacteria can be explained by inhibition of lysosomal movements observed after phagocytosis. *J Exp Med* **166:** 933.

Henault J, Martinez J, Riggs JM, Tian J, Mehta P, Clarke L, Sasai M, Latz E, Brinkmann MM, Iwasaki A, et al. 2012. Noncanonical autophagy is required for type I interferon secretion in response to DNA-immune complexes. *Immunity* **37:** 986–997.

Holscher C, Reiling N, Schaible UE, Holscher A, Bathmann C, Korbel D, Lenz I, Sonntag T, Kroger S, Akira S, et al. 2008. Containment of aerogenic *Mycobacterium tuberculosis* infection in mice does not require MyD88 adaptor function for TLR2, -4 and -9. *Eur J Immunol* **38:** 680–694.

Hoyer-Hansen M, Bastholm L, Szyniarowski P, Campanella M, Szabadkai G, Farkas T, Bianchi K, Fehrenbacher N, Elling F, Rizzuto R, et al. 2007. Control of macroautophagy by calcium, calmodulin-dependent kinase kinase-β, and Bcl-2. *Mol Cell* **25:** 193–205.

Huang J, Canadien V, Lam GY, Steinberg BE, Dinauer MC, Magalhaes MA, Glogauer M, Grinstein S, Brumell JH. 2009. Activation of antibacterial autophagy by NADPH oxidases. *Proc Natl Acad Sci* **106:** 6226–6231.

Huett A, Heath RJ, Begun J, Sassi SO, Baxt LA, Vyas JM, Goldberg MB, Xavier RJ. 2012. The LRR and RING domain protein LRSAM1 is an E3 ligase crucial for ubiquitin-dependent autophagy of intracellular *Salmonella typhimurium*. *Cell Host Microbe* **12:** 778–790.

Intemann CD, Thye T, Niemann S, Browne EN, Amanua Chinbuah M, Enimil A, Gyapong J, Osei I, Owusu-Dabo E, Helm S, et al. 2009. Autophagy gene variant IRGM -261T contributes to protection from tuberculosis caused by *Mycobacterium tuberculosis* but not by *M. africanum* strains. *PLoS Pathog* **5:** e1000577.

Itakura E, Kishi-Itakura C, Mizushima N. 2012. The hairpin-type tail-anchored SNARE syntaxin 17 targets to autophagosomes for fusion with endosomes/lysosomes. *Cell* **151:** 1256–1269.

Jagannath C, Lindsey DR, Dhandayuthapani S, Xu Y, Hunter RL Jr, Eissa NT. 2009. Autophagy enhances the efficacy of BCG vaccine by increasing peptide presentation in mouse dendritic cells. *Nat Med* **15:** 267–276.

Jiang S, Dupont N, Castillo EF, Deretic V. 2013. Secretory versus degradative autophagy: Unconventional secretion of inflammatory mediators. *J Innate Immun* **5:** 474–479.

Jostins L, Ripke S, Weersma RK, Duerr RH, McGovern DP, Hui KY, Lee JC, Schumm LP, Sharma Y, Anderson CA, et al. 2012. Host-microbe interactions have shaped the genetic architecture of inflammatory bowel disease. *Nature* **491:** 119–124.

Juarez E, Carranza C, Hernandez-Sanchez F, Leon-Contreras JC, Hernandez-Pando R, Escobedo D, Torres M, Sada E. 2012. NOD2 enhances the innate response of alveolar macrophages to *Mycobacterium tuberculosis* in humans. *Eur J Immunol* **42:** 880–889.

Kim J, Kundu M, Viollet B, Guan KL. 2011. AMPK and mTOR regulate autophagy through direct phosphorylation of Ulk1. *Nat Cell Biol* **13:** 132–141.

Kim JJ, Lee HM, Shin DM, Kim W, Yuk JM, Jin HS, Lee SH, Cha GH, Kim JM, Lee ZW, et al. 2012a. Host cell autophagy activated by antibiotics is required for their effective antimycobacterial drug action. *Cell Host Microbe* **11:** 457–468.

Kim KH, An DR, Song J, Yoon JY, Kim HS, Yoon HJ, Im HN, Kim J, Kim do J, Lee SJ, et al. 2012b. *Mycobacterium tuberculosis* Eis protein initiates suppression of host immune responses by acetylation of DUSP16/MKP-7. *Proc Natl Acad Sci* **109:** 7729–7734.

Kim JY, Zhao H, Martinez J, Doggett TA, Kolesnikov AV, Tang PH, Ablonczy Z, Chan CC, Zhou Z, Green DR, et al. 2013. Noncanonical autophagy promotes the visual cycle. *Cell* **154:** 365–376.

King KY, Lew JD, Ha NP, Lin JS, Ma X, Graviss EA, Goodell MA. 2011. Polymorphic allele of human IRGM1 is associated with susceptibility to tuberculosis in African Americans. *PLoS ONE* **6:** e16317.

Kirkin V, McEwan DG, Novak I, Dikic I. 2009. A role for ubiquitin in selective autophagy. *Mol Cell* **34:** 259–269.

Klug-Micu GM, Stenger S, Sommer A, Liu PT, Krutzik SR, Modlin RL, Fabri M. 2013. CD40 ligand and interferon-γ induce an antimicrobial response against *Mycobacterium tuberculosis* in human monocytes. *Immunology* **139:** 121–128.

Konno H, Konno K, Barber GN. 2013. Cyclic dinucleotides trigger ULK1 (ATG1) phosphorylation of STING to prevent sustained innate immune signaling. *Cell* **155:** 688–698.

Kumar D, Nath L, Kamal MA, Varshney A, Jain A, Singh S, Rao KV. 2010. Genome-wide analysis of the host intracellular network that regulates survival of *Mycobacterium tuberculosis*. *Cell* **140:** 731–743.

Lam KK, Zheng X, Forestieri R, Balgi AD, Nodwell M, Vollett S, Anderson HJ, Andersen RJ, Av-Gay Y, Roberge M. 2012. Nitazoxanide stimulates autophagy and inhibits mTORC1 signaling and intracellular proliferation of *Mycobacterium tuberculosis*. *PLoS Pathog* **8:** e1002691.

Lee HK, Mattei LM, Steinberg BE, Alberts P, Lee YH, Chervonsky A, Mizushima N, Grinstein S, Iwasaki A. 2010. In vivo requirement for Atg5 in antigen presentation by dendritic cells. *Immunity* **32:** 227–239.

Levine B, Mizushima N, Virgin HW. 2011. Autophagy in immunity and inflammation. *Nature* **469:** 323–335.

Li S, Wandel MP, Li F, Liu Z, He C, Wu J, Shi Y, Randow F. 2013. Sterical hindrance promotes selectivity of the autophagy cargo receptor NDP52 for the danger receptor galectin-8 in antibacterial autophagy. *Sci Signal* **6:** ra9.

Liu PT, Stenger S, Li H, Wenzel L, Tan BH, Krutzik SR, Ochoa MT, Schauber J, Wu K, Meinken C, et al. 2006. Toll-like receptor triggering of a vitamin D–mediated human antimicrobial response. *Science* **311:** 1770–1773.

Lum JJ, Bauer DE, Kong M, Harris MH, Li C, Lindsten T, Thompson CB. 2005. Growth factor regulation of autophagy and cell survival in the absence of apoptosis. *Cell* **120:** 237–248.

Lupfer C, Thomas PG, Anand PK, Vogel P, Milasta S, Martinez J, Huang G, Green M, Kundu M, Chi H, et al. 2013. Receptor interacting protein kinase 2–mediated mitophagy regulates inflammasome activation during virus infection. *Nat Immunol* **14:** 480–488.

Maertzdorf J, Weiner J, 3rd, Mollenkopf HJ, Bauer T, Prasse A, Muller-Quernheim J, Kaufmann SH. 2012. Common patterns and disease related signatures in tuberculosis and sarcoidosis. *Proc Natl Acad Sci* **109:** 7853–7858.

Manca C, Tsenova L, Freeman S, Barczak AK, Tovey M, Murray PJ, Barry C, Kaplan G. 2005. Hypervirulent *M. tuberculosis* W/Beijing strains upregulate type I IFNs and increase expression of negative regulators of the Jak-Stat pathway. *J Interferon Cytokine Res* **25:** 694–701.

Manzanillo PS, Shiloh MU, Portnoy DA, Cox JS. 2012. *Mycobacterium tuberculosis* activates the DNA-dependent cytosolic surveillance pathway within macrophages. *Cell Host Microbe* **11:** 469–480.

Manzanillo PS, Ayres JS, Watson RO, Collins AC, Souza G, Rae CS, Schneider DS, Nakamura K, Shiloh MU, Cox JS. 2013. The ubiquitin ligase parkin mediates resistance to intracellular pathogens. *Nature* **501:** 512–516.

Martinez J, Almendinger J, Oberst A, Ness R, Dillon CP, Fitzgerald P, Hengartner MO, Green DR. 2011. Microtubule-associated protein 1 light chain 3 α (LC3)-associated phagocytosis is required for the efficient clearance of dead cells. *Proc Natl Acad Sci* **108:** 17396–17401.

Mayer-Barber KD, Barber DL, Shenderov K, White SD, Wilson MS, Cheever A, Kugler D, Hieny S, Caspar P, Nunez G, et al. 2010. Caspase-1 independent IL-1β production is critical for host resistance to *Mycobacterium tuberculosis* and does not require TLR signaling in vivo. *J Immunol* **184:** 3326–3330.

Mayer-Barber KD, Andrade BB, Barber DL, Hieny S, Feng CG, Caspar P, Oland S, Gordon S, Sher A. 2011. Innate and adaptive interferons suppress IL-1α and IL-1β production by distinct pulmonary myeloid subsets during *Mycobacterium tuberculosis* infection. *Immunity* **35:** 1023–1034.

Mihaylova MM, Shaw RJ. 2011. The AMPK signalling pathway coordinates cell growth, autophagy and metabolism. *Nat Cell Biol* **13:** 1016–1023.

Mishra BB, Rathinam VA, Martens GW, Martinot AJ, Kornfeld H, Fitzgerald KA, Sassetti CM. 2013. Nitric oxide controls the immunopathology of tuberculosis by inhibiting NLRP3 inflammasome-dependent processing of IL-1β. *Nat Immunol* **14:** 52–60.

Mizushima N, Levine B, Cuervo AM, Klionsky DJ. 2008. Autophagy fights disease through cellular self-digestion. *Nature* **451:** 1069–1075.

Mizushima N, Yoshimori T, Ohsumi Y. 2011. The role of atg proteins in autophagosome formation. *Annu Rev Cell Dev Biol* **27:** 107–132.

Nakagawa I, Amano A, Mizushima N, Yamamoto A, Yamaguchi H, Kamimoto T, Nara A, Funao J, Nakata M, Tsuda K, et al. 2004. Autophagy defends cells against invading group A streptococcus. *Science* **306:** 1037–1040.

Nakahira K, Haspel JA, Rathinam VA, Lee SJ, Dolinay T, Lam HC, Englert JA, Rabinovitch M, Cernadas M, Kim HP, et al. 2011. Autophagy proteins regulate innate immune responses by inhibiting the release of mitochondrial DNA mediated by the NALP3 inflammasome. *Nat Immunol* **12:** 222–230.

Nakatogawa H, Ichimura Y, Ohsumi Y. 2007. Atg8, a ubiquitin-like protein required for autophagosome formation, mediates membrane tethering and hemifusion. *Cell* **130:** 165–178.

Nazio F, Strappazzon F, Antonioli M, Bielli P, Cianfanelli V, Bordi M, Gretzmeier C, Dengjel J, Piacentini M, Fimia GM, et al. 2013. mTOR inhibits autophagy by controlling ULK1 ubiquitylation, self-association and function through AMBRA1 and TRAF6. *Nat Cell Biol* **15:** 406–416.

Nnoaham KE, Clarke A. 2008. Low serum vitamin D levels and tuberculosis: A systematic review and meta-analysis. *Int J Epidemiol* **37:** 113–119.

Novikov A, Cardone M, Thompson R, Shenderov K, Kirschman KD, Mayer-Barber KD, Myers TG, Rabin RL, Trinchieri G, Sher A, et al. 2011. *Mycobacterium tuberculosis* triggers host type I IFN signaling to regulate IL-1β production in human macrophages. *J Immunol* **187:** 2540–2547.

Ottenhoff TH, Dass RH, Yang N, Zhang MM, Wong HE, Sahiratmadja E, Khor CC, Alisjahbana B, van Crevel R, Marzuki S, et al. 2012. Genome-wide expression profiling identifies type 1 interferon response pathways in active tuberculosis. *PLoS ONE* **7:** e45839.

Pandey AK, Yang Y, Jiang Z, Fortune SM, Coulombe F, Behr MA, Fitzgerald KA, Sassetti CM, Kelliher MA. 2009. NOD2, RIP2 and IRF5 play a critical role in the type I interferon response to *Mycobacterium tuberculosis*. *PLoS Pathog* **5:** e1000500.

Park HJ, Lee SJ, Kim SH, Han J, Bae J, Kim SJ, Park CG, Chun T. 2011. IL-10 inhibits the starvation induced autophagy in macrophages via class I phosphatidylinositol 3-kinase (PI3K) pathway. *Mol Immunol* **48:** 720–727.

Petruccioli E, Romagnoli A, Corazzari M, Coccia EM, Butera O, Delogu G, Piacentini M, Girardi E, Fimia GM, Goletti D. 2012. Specific T cells restore the autophagic flux inhibited by *Mycobacterium tuberculosis* in human primary macrophages. *J Infect Dis* **205:** 1425–1435.

Pilli M, Arko-Mensah J, Ponpuak M, Roberts E, Master S, Mandell MA, Dupont N, Ornatowski W, Jiang S, Bradfute SB, et al. 2012. TBK-1 promotes autophagy-mediated antimicrobial defense by controlling autophagosome maturation. *Immunity* **37:** 223–234.

Ponpuak M, Deretic V. 2011. Autophagy and p62/sequestosome 1 generate neo-antimicrobial peptides (cryptides) from cytosolic proteins. *Autophagy* **7:** 336–337.

Ponpuak M, Davis AS, Roberts EA, Delgado MA, Dinkins C, Zhao Z, Virgin HWt, Kyei GB, Johansen T, Vergne I, et al. 2010. Delivery of cytosolic components by autophagic adaptor protein p62 endows autophagosomes with unique antimicrobial properties. *Immunity* **32:** 329–341.

Reichel H, Koeffler HP, Norman AW. 1987. Synthesis in vitro of 1,25-dihydroxyvitamin D3 and 24,25-dihydroxyvitamin D3 by interferon-γ-stimulated normal human bone marrow and alveolar macrophages. *J Biol Chem* **262:** 10931–10937.

Romagnoli A, Etna MP, Giacomini E, Pardini M, Remoli ME, Corazzari M, Falasca L, Goletti D, Gafa V, Simeone R, et al. 2012. ESX-1 dependent impairment of autophagic flux by *Mycobacterium tuberculosis* in human dendritic cells. *Autophagy* **8:** 1357–1370.

Russell DG, Cardona PJ, Kim MJ, Allain S, Altare F. 2009. Foamy macrophages and the progression of the human tuberculosis granuloma. *Nat Immunol* **10:** 943–948.

Russell RC, Tian Y, Yuan H, Park HW, Chang YY, Kim J, Kim H, Neufeld TP, Dillin A, Guan KL. 2013. ULK1 induces autophagy by phosphorylating Beclin-1 and activating VPS34 lipid kinase. *Nat Cell Biol* **15:** 741–750.

Saitoh T, Fujita N, Jang MH, Uematsu S, Yang BG, Satoh T, Omori H, Noda T, Yamamoto N, Komatsu M, et al. 2008. Loss of the autophagy protein Atg16L1 enhances endotoxin-induced IL-1β production. *Nature* **456:** 264–268.

Sanjuan MA, Dillon CP, Tait SW, Moshiach S, Dorsey F, Connell S, Komatsu M, Tanaka K, Cleveland JL, Withoff S, et al. 2007. Toll-like receptor signalling in macrophages links the autophagy pathway to phagocytosis. *Nature* **450:** 1253–1257.

Scanga CA, Bafica A, Feng CG, Cheever AW, Hieny S, Sher A. 2004. MyD88-deficient mice display a profound loss in resistance to *Mycobacterium tuberculosis* associated with partially impaired Th1 cytokine and nitric oxide synthase 2 expression. *Infect Immun* **72:** 2400–2404.

Scherz-Shouval R, Shvets E, Fass E, Shorer H, Gil L, Elazar Z. 2007. Reactive oxygen species are essential for autophagy and specifically regulate the activity of Atg4. *EMBO J* **26:** 1749–1760.

Settembre C, Fraldi A, Medina DL, Ballabio A. 2013. Signals from the lysosome: A control centre for cellular clearance and energy metabolism. *Nat Rev Mol Cell Biol* **14:** 283–296.

Shi CS, Kehrl JH. 2010. TRAF6 and A20 regulate lysine 63-linked ubiquitination of Beclin-1 to control TLR4-induced autophagy. *Sci Signal* **3:** ra42.

Shin DM, Jeon BY, Lee HM, Jin HS, Yuk JM, Song CH, Lee SH, Lee ZW, Cho SN, Kim JM, et al. 2010a. *Mycobacterium tuberculosis* eis regulates autophagy, inflammation, and cell death through redox-dependent signaling. *PLoS Pathog* **6:** e1001230.

Shin DM, Yuk JM, Lee HM, Lee SH, Son JW, Harding CV, Kim JM, Modlin RL, Jo EK. 2010b. Mycobacterial lipoprotein activates autophagy via TLR2/1/CD14 and a functional vitamin D receptor signalling. *Cell Microbiol* **12:** 1648–1665.

Shui W, Petzold CJ, Redding A, Liu J, Pitcher A, Sheu L, Hsieh TY, Keasling JD, Bertozzi CR. 2011. Organelle membrane proteomics reveals differential influence of mycobacterial lipoglycans on macrophage phagosome maturation and autophagosome accumulation. *J Proteome Res* **10:** 339–348.

Singh SB, Davis AS, Taylor GA, Deretic V. 2006. Human IRGM induces autophagy to eliminate intracellular mycobacteria. *Science* **313:** 1438–1441.

Singh R, Kaushik S, Wang Y, Xiang Y, Novak I, Komatsu M, Tanaka K, Cuervo AM, Czaja MJ. 2009. Autophagy regulates lipid metabolism. *Nature* **458:** 1131–1135.

Singh SB, Ornatowski W, Vergne I, Naylor J, Delgado M, Roberts E, Ponpuak M, Master S, Pilli M, White E, et al. 2010. Human IRGM regulates autophagy and cell-autonomous immunity functions through mitochondria. *Nat Cell Biol* **12:** 1154–1165.

Singh V, Jamwal S, Jain R, Verma P, Gokhale R, Rao KV. 2012. *Mycobacterium tuberculosis*-driven targeted recalibration of macrophage lipid homeostasis promotes the foamy phenotype. *Cell Host Microbe* **12:** 669–681.

Stanley SA, Johndrow JE, Manzanillo P, Cox JS. 2007. The Type I IFN response to infection with *Mycobacterium tuberculosis* requires ESX-1-mediated secretion and contributes to pathogenesis. *J Immunol* **178:** 3143–3152.

Sundaramurthy V, Barsacchi R, Samusik N, Marsico G, Gilleron J, Kalaidzidis I, Meyenhofer F, Bickle M, Kalaidzidis Y, Zerial M. 2013. Integration of chemical and RNAi multiparametric profiles identifies triggers of intracellular mycobacterial killing. *Cell Host Microbe* **13:** 129–142.

Teles RM, Graeber TG, Krutzik SR, Montoya D, Schenk M, Lee DJ, Komisopoulou E, Kelly-Scumpia K, Chun R, Iyer SS, et al. 2013. Type I interferon suppresses type II interferon-triggered human anti-mycobacterial responses. *Science* **339:** 1448–1453.

Thurston TL, Wandel MP, von Muhlinen N, Foeglein A, Randow F. 2012. Galectin 8 targets damaged vesicles for autophagy to defend cells against bacterial invasion. *Nature* **482:** 414–418.

van der Wel N, Hava D, Houben D, Fluitsma D, van Zon M, Pierson J, Brenner M, Peters PJ. 2007. *M. tuberculosis* and *M. leprae* translocate from the phagolysosome to the cytosol in myeloid cells. *Cell* **129:** 1287–1298.

Van Grol J, Subauste C, Andrade RM, Fujinaga K, Nelson J, Subauste CS. 2010. HIV-1 inhibits autophagy in bystander macrophage/monocytic cells through Src-Akt and STAT3. *PLoS ONE* **5:** e11733.

Velikkakath AK, Nishimura T, Oita E, Ishihara N, Mizushima N. 2012. Mammalian Atg2 proteins are essential for autophagosome formation and important for regulation of size and distribution of lipid droplets. *Mol Biol Cell* **23:** 896–909.

Vergne I, Chua J, Singh SB, Deretic V. 2004. Cell biology of *Mycobacterium tuberculosis* phagosome. *Annu Rev Cell Dev Biol* **20:** 367–394.

Watson RO, Manzanillo PS, Cox JS. 2012. Extracellular *M. tuberculosis* DNA targets bacteria for autophagy by activating the host DNA-sensing pathway. *Cell* **150:** 803–815.

Weidberg H, Shpilka T, Shvets E, Abada A, Shimron F, Elazar Z. 2011. LC3 and GATE-16 N termini mediate membrane fusion processes required for autophagosome biogenesis. *Dev Cell* **20:** 444–454.

Wellcome Trust Case Control Consortium. 2007. Genome-wide association study of 14,000 cases of seven common diseases and 3,000 shared controls. *Nature* **447:** 661–678.

Wilkinson RJ, Llewelyn M, Toossi Z, Patel P, Pasvol G, Lalvani A, Wright D, Latif M, Davidson RN. 2000. Influence of vitamin D deficiency and vitamin D receptor polymorphisms on tuberculosis among Gujarati Asians in west London: A case-control study. *Lancet* **355:** 618–621.

Wu J, Sun L, Chen X, Du F, Shi H, Chen C, Chen ZJ. 2013. Cyclic GMP-AMP is an endogenous second messenger in innate immune signaling by cytosolic DNA. *Science* **339:** 826–830.

Xu Y, Jagannath C, Liu XD, Sharafkhaneh A, Kolodziejska KE, Eissa NT. 2007. Toll-like receptor 4 is a sensor for autophagy associated with innate immunity. *Immunity* **27:** 135–144.

Youle RJ, Narendra DP. 2011. Mechanisms of mitophagy. *Nat Rev Mol Cell Biol* **12:** 9–14.

Yuk JM, Shin DM, Lee HM, Yang CS, Jin HS, Kim KK, Lee ZW, Lee SH, Kim JM, Jo EK. 2009. Vitamin D3 induces autophagy in human monocytes/macrophages via cathelicidin. *Cell Host Microbe* **6:** 231–243.

Zhang L, Zhang H, Zhao Y, Mao F, Wu J, Bai B, Xu Z, Jiang Y, Shi C. 2012. Effects of *Mycobacterium tuberculosis* ESAT-6/CFP-10 fusion protein on the autophagy function of mouse macrophages. *DNA Cell Biol* **31:** 171–179.

Zhou R, Yazdi AS, Menu P, Tschopp J. 2011. A role for mitochondria in NLRP3 inflammasome activation. *Nature* **469:** 221–225.

Zullo AJ, Lee S. 2012. Mycobacterial induction of autophagy varies by species and occurs independently of mammalian target of rapamycin inhibition. *J Biol Chem* **287:** 12668–12678.

Innate and Adaptive Cellular Immune Responses to *Mycobacterium tuberculosis* Infection

Katrin D. Mayer-Barber[1] and Daniel L. Barber[2]

[1]Immunobiology Section, Laboratory of Parasitic Diseases, National Institute of Allergy and Infectious Diseases, National Institutes of Health, Bethesda, Maryland 20892

[2]T Lymphocyte Biology Unit, Laboratory of Parasitic Diseases, National Institute of Allergy and Infectious Diseases, National Institutes of Health, Bethesda, Maryland 20892

Correspondence: barberd@niaid.nih.gov

Host resistance to *Mycobacterium tuberculosis* (*Mtb*) infection requires the coordinated efforts of innate and adaptive immune cells. Diverse pulmonary myeloid cell populations respond to *Mtb* with unique contributions to both host-protective and potentially detrimental inflammation. Although multiple cell types of the adaptive immune system respond to *Mtb* infection, CD4 T cells are the principal antigen-specific cells responsible for containment of *Mtb* infection, but they can also be major contributors to disease during *Mtb* infection in several different settings. Here, we will discuss the role of different myeloid populations as well as the dual nature of CD4 T cells in *Mtb* infection with a primary focus on data generated using in vivo cellular immunological studies in experimental animal models and in humans when available.

Unlike many less-virulent microorganisms that are readily cleared by phagocytes or soluble innate effector molecules, *Mycobacterium tuberculosis* (*Mtb*) establishes a chronic infection primarily in the lungs. The activation of bacilli-laden macrophages by effector T-helper 1 (Th1) cells is the key cell-to-cell interaction in immunological control of *Mtb* infection. Although this classic paradigm is essentially correct, it is now clear that the diversity of myeloid cells and CD4 T cells responding to *Mtb* infection is far more complex. Multiple populations of innate immune cells with distinct functions cooperate for control of *Mtb* infection. CD4 T cells are indeed critical for host resistance, but the mechanisms of CD4 T-cell-dependent control are poorly understood. Moreover, CD4 T cells can also play a major role in driving tissue damage during tuberculosis. Here, we will review the current knowledge of the functional heterogeneity of myeloid cells, and the role of CD4 T cells in both host protection and immunopathology during *Mtb* infection with a focus on data generated from single-cell analysis of in vivo studies.

ESTABLISHMENT OF INFECTION

Infection with *Mtb* occurs via the aerosol route, and consequently, lung resident myeloid cells are the primary cells initiating "first contact" with the bacilli. Alveolar macrophages (AMs)

Cite this article as *Cold Spring Harb Perspect Med* doi: 10.1101/cshperspect.a018424

are long-lived, specialized innate immune cells that reside in pulmonary alveoli and ingest the inhaled bacteria, and therefore, AMs are critical in setting the stage for the subsequent immune response against *Mtb* (Murphy et al. 2008; Guilliams et al. 2013a). Lung resident myeloid cells, in particular AMs, have been recognized to play a dual role in *Mtb* control. Whereas they can contribute to host resistance, they are also key to establishment of infection in the first place.

Role of Alveolar Macrophages in Early Events of *Mtb* Infection

Situated at an important barrier site, AMs perform critical sentinel tasks to both preserve proper lung function and avoid collateral damage from exposure to harmless antigens. This is achieved by their great capacity for phagocytosis while being able to maintain a relatively low-cellular activation state and low-migratory potential (Guilliams et al. 2013b). Phagocytosis of *Mtb* is facilitated by binding to complement receptors, mannose receptor (MR), surfactant molecules, and DC-SIGN (dendritic cell-specific intracellular adhesion molecule-3–grabbing nonintegrin) (Berrington and Hawn 2007; Jo 2008). In addition, AMs express a large array of pattern recognition receptors (PRR), including Toll-like receptors (TLRs), C-type lectin receptors (CLRs), and Nod-like receptors (NLRs), all of which have been shown to participate in *Mtb* recognition. Among the TLRs, TLR-2, -4, and -9 are of particular importance in sensing *Mtb*, with NOD2, Mincle, Dectin-1, MR, and DC-SIGN contributing to PRR-driven macrophage activation (Jo et al. 2007; Jo 2008; Reiling et al. 2008; Kleinnijenhuis et al. 2011). Once activation has been sufficiently elicited, AMs in murine experimental systems as well as TB patients can produce nitric oxide and reactive oxygen species, two antimycobacterial effector molecules shown to be able to kill *Mtb* (Nicholson et al. 1996; Jo et al. 2007). Therefore, it is not clear why AMs are not be able to eliminate the bacilli before infection is established.

Macrophage depletion studies around the time of aerosol challenge, however, revealed that lung-resident AMs and not CCR2-dependent myeloid cells, such as inflammatory monocytes/macrophages (IMs), play an important role in establishment of infection and initial growth of bacteria (Leemans et al. 2001; 2005; Samstein et al. 2013). Moreover, elegant studies using adoptive transfer approaches of *Mtb*-infected AMs exposed an important early role for these cells not only in establishment of infection, but also in influencing initiation and priming of T-cell responses 2–3 wk later (Divangahi et al. 2010). When *Mtb*-infected AMs that had a predisposition for apoptotic cell death caused by Alox5 deficiency were adoptively transferred into naïve wild-type mice, a greater CD4 and CD8 T-cell response was observed compared with transfer of wild-type AMs. This data highlights the importance of AMs in early stages of infection and their ability to set the stage for the ensuing immune response to *Mtb* infection, including adaptive immunity.

Spread of *Mtb* from Macrophages to Other Myeloid Cells

The cellular events that immediately follow infection of AMs in the airways are not well understood. Once engulfed by the macrophage, *Mtb* potently inhibits macrophage activation and becomes highly resistant to clearance. Virulent *Mtb* manipulates the response of infected cells to avoid detection and elimination through a variety of immune evasion strategies, including inhibition of phago-lysosome fusion and detoxification of nitrogen and oxygen radicals and dormancy (Flynn and Chan 2003; Pieters 2008; Gengenbacher and Kaufmann 2012; Mariotti et al. 2013). When the cell-intrinsic response to *Mtb* proves inadequate and/or the bacilli replicate to sufficient numbers within AMs, the infected cells burst. Release of bacteria from infected cells allows for infection of neighboring cells, and the cell death modalities of infected macrophages play an important role in dissemination of *Mtb* infection (Keane et al. 1997; Chen et al. 2006; Lee et al. 2009). Apoptotic cell death is associated with bacterial containment, enhanced antigen-cross presentation by dendritic cells (DCs), and efferocytosis, all processes important for controlling infection

(Chen et al. 2006; Behar et al. 2010; Divangahi et al. 2010; Martin et al. 2012, 2014). In contrast, death of macrophages resulting in cytolysis (e.g., necrosis) allows the bacilli to spread and disseminate (Fratazzi et al. 1999; Divangahi et al. 2009; Lee et al. 2011). Importantly, for replicating bacteria to cause cytolysis of the cell, the bacilli need to reach a particular threshold termed burst-size, estimated to be 25 bacteria per cell (Lee et al. 2006; Repasy et al. 2013), which may take several days to achieve given the slow replication time of *Mtb*. During this time, it is possible that the infection goes largely undetected by other host cells. It is not clear what signals trigger the recruitment of circulating myeloid effector cells, but the cell death outcome of infected AMs is likely a critical determinant.

Initially the predominant myeloid cell within the airways, eventually the proportion of AMs among myeloid cells decreases as newly recruited myeloid effector cells arrive in the lung within the first 2 wk after low-dose aerosol challenge (Wolf et al. 2007; Garcia-Romo et al. 2013).

HETEROGENEITY OF INNATE EFFECTOR CELLS

Macrophages and DCs are by far the most studied innate effector cells in murine models of tuberculosis. Most of our knowledge regarding the antimycobacterial myeloid response to *Mtb* infection in the lungs, however, has been extrapolated from in vitro studies using bone-marrow-derived macrophages and DCs. Nonetheless, immunohistochemical techniques clearly established that macrophages are the primary cell type laden with *Mtb* bacilli and present in pulmonary tuberculous granulomas. Although DC responses and functions have been more examined in vivo, most studies have used CD11c as a single definitive marker to identify conventional DCs (cDCs) in the lungs.

Nonetheless, DCs have been shown to be critically important to generate *Mtb*-specific T-cell responses, findings consistent with their known function in priming naïve T cells (Banchereau and Steinman 1998; Tian et al. 2005; Khader et al. 2006).

Identifying Myeloid Subset Diversity In Vivo

Recent advances in multicolor flow cytometry have revealed that pulmonary myeloid effector cells are vastly heterogeneous, with lung resident pulmonary DCs and macrophage subsets in addition to a plethora of effector populations, such as neutrophils, IMs, inflammatory monocyte-derived dendritic cells (mDCs), plasmacytoid DCs and cDCs being recruited to the site of infection (de Heer et al. 2005; Mayer-Barber et al. 2011; Guilliams et al. 2013b). Based on CD11c and CD11b expression, most pulmonary myeloid effector cell types, including granulocyte receptor (Gr-1)-expressing neutrophils, have been reported to harbor live bacteria (Wolf et al. 2007). These diverse myeloid cells express a number of effector molecules and cytokines, such as inducible nitric oxide synthase (iNOS), tumor necrosis factor-α (TNF-α), interleukin-12 (IL-12)/23p40, IL-1α, and IL-1β, that are each critical for control of the infection (Cooper et al. 1997, 2007, 2011; Yamada et al. 2000; Saunders et al. 2004; Sköld and Behar 2008; Mayer-Barber et al. 2010, 2011). Indeed, in the lungs of *Mtb*-infected mice, at least five different myeloid cell types express CD11c, and most of them in addition CD11b, a surface molecule often considered as a pan-myeloid marker (Gonzalez-Juarrero and Orme 2001; Mayer-Barber et al. 2011; Guilliams et al. 2013b). Even more concerning then is that natural killer (NK) cells, which can up-regulate both CD11b and CD11c on activation, can comprise up to 40% of all CD11b-expressing cells in the lungs of *Mtb*-infected mice (Mayer-Barber et al. 2011). These studies highlight the importance of using sufficient numbers of flow cytometric parameters together with CD68, a macrophage/DC-restricted molecule (Rabinowitz and Gordon 1991), to accurately identify desired populations of interest.

Conventional Dendritic Cells

Arguably, the most in vivo work has been performed regarding the role of CD11c-expressing cells, presumably cDCs, which are required for priming of naïve CD4 and CD8 T-cell responses against *Mtb* (Gonzalez-Juarrero and Orme 2001; Tian et al. 2005; Khader 2006; Wolf et al. 2007; Samstein et al. 2013). Pulmonary cDCs ($CD11b^+$/dim, $Ly6C^{neg}$) express high levels of CD11c and various degrees of CD103 after *Mtb* infection (Mayer-Barber et al. 2011). $CD103^+$ DCs are present exclusively in the lung airways and parenchyma after *Mtb* infection and are considered lung resident DCs, with migratory capacity to the draining lymph node (Geurts-vanKessel et al. 2008; Geissmann et al. 2010; Guilliams et al. 2013b; Leepiyasakulchai et al. 2013; Anderson et al. 2014). cDCs and $CD103^+$ cDCs represent a functionally and phenotypically distinct pulmonary DC subset after *Mtb* infection and produce predominantly IL-12/23p40 (Mayer-Barber et al. 2011; Leepiyasakulchai et al. 2013). They express all the classical DC surface molecules (high levels of major histocompatibility complex class II (MHC-II), CD80, and CD86) as well as additional markers associated with antigen presentation and antigen-presenting cell (APC)-T-cell interactions, such as CD40, CD70, DEC-205, CD83, and PD-L2 (Mayer-Barber et al. 2011; KD Mayer-Barber, unpubl.).

Inflammatory Monocytes and Macrophages

IMs are characterized by their high Ly6C and little CD11c expression (within $CD68^+$, $CD11b^+$ myeloid cells) and are recruited to the lungs after low-dose aerosol infection (Mayer-Barber et al. 2011). They do express MHC-II as well as costimulatory markers, such as CD80 and CD86, albeit to a lesser extent when compared with $CD11c^+$ DC subsets (Mayer-Barber et al. 2011). In addition, they display phenotypic markers corresponding to the IMs described in nonlymphoid tissue (e.g., 7/4, F4/80, CD14 high, and CD115 low) (Dunay et al. 2008; Sköld and Behar 2008; Varol et al. 2009; Geissmann et al. 2010; Mayer-Barber et al. 2011). They were found to be multifunctional and produce predominantly IL-1α, IL-1β, and TNF-α, proinflammatory cytokines important for bacterial control (Mayer-Barber et al. 2011). They also share functional properties, e.g., IL-10 and iNOS production, similar to myeloid-derived suppressor cells (MDSCs) that have been described under unresolved pathological conditions such as chronic infections, inflammation, and cancer (Biswas and Mantovani 2010). IMs are very responsive to regulatory cytokines in vivo, in particular they preferentially express high levels of IL-10 and IFN-γ receptor, and IFN-γ from CD4 T cells is able to directly modulate their inflammatory cytokine production in the lungs of *Mtb*-infected mice (Mayer-Barber et al. 2011). Although IFN-γ is important for induction of iNOS, it potently suppresses IL-1α, IL-1β, and IL-10 expression by pulmonary IMs. In addition to adaptive interferon (IFN), innate-derived type I IFNs are also able to potently limit proinflammatory IL-1 cytokine production by IMs while inducing anti-inflammatory IL-10 production, reflecting perhaps an important checkpoint in limiting excessive inflammation and/or immune evasion strategies triggered by *Mtb* itself (Stanley et al. 2007; Mayer-Barber et al. 2011). Based on a large array of phenotypic markers assessed by single-cell analysis, IMs seem to represent a single homogeneous cell population (Mayer-Barber et al. 2011). Interestingly, use of an intravascular staining technique using flow-cytometry to examine the distribution of IMs in the lung parenchyma and pulmonary blood vasculature revealed that IMs are primarily located inside the lung-associated vasculature and that only a small fraction of IMs were actually present inside the lung tissue itself (Mayer-Barber et al. 2011; Anderson et al. 2014).

Despite their uniform appearance, IMs can thus be separated into two subsets based on their localization within the lung, and future studies need to determine the functional role of tissue resident IMs, perhaps representing true macrophages versus vasculature-associated monocytes.

Inflammatory Dendritic Cells

Inflammatory mDCs comprise the most functionally diverse pulmonary innate effector cell type in response to *Mtb* infection. They are identified based on their high CD11c, CD13, and high Ly6C, 7/4 and TLR2 expression (within CD68$^+$, CD11b$^+$ myeloid cells) (Mayer-Barber et al. 2011). They also express high levels of MHC-II, CD80, and CD86 and are primarily located in the lung parenchyma, rather than the lung vasculature (Mayer-Barber et al. 2011; Anderson et al. 2014), suggesting that these cells have potent antigen-presentation capacity. Inflammatory mDCs are highly polyfunctional and are able to coexpress IL-1α, IL-1β, IL-10, TNF-α, and iNOS at the single-cell level in vivo, where they are recruited to the lungs between 2 and 3 wk after *Mtb* infection. Based on their functional profile, they resemble an iNOS and TNF-α-producing DC subset that has been previously implicated in murine resistance to intracellular bacteria, parasites, or viruses as well as human psoriasis (Serbina et al. 2003; Lowes et al. 2005; Lin et al. 2008; De Trez et al. 2009). Similar to IMs, their effector functions are directly regulated during infection by cell-intrinsic type I IFN receptor signaling (Mayer-Barber et al. 2011). Whereas IL-1α, IL-1β, and iNOS expression are negatively regulated, type I IFNs induce anti-inflammatory IL-10 production in mDCs. However, in contrast to IMs, CD4 T-cell-derived IFN-γ is unable to limit the proinflammatory cytokine production by mDCs in vivo. Unraveling the functional heterogeneity of inflammatory mDCs, their antimicrobial properties, and whether these diverse characteristics can be attributed to multiple functionally distinct subsets within mDCs will be important in our understanding of their role in tuberculosis control and pathogenesis.

Neutrophils

Although neutrophils are the cell type predominantly infected in the airways of active tuberculosis patients, their role in host resistance against *Mtb* in experimental models remains poorly understood and controversial at best (Eum 2010; Lowe et al. 2012). The short-lived nature of these cells has made it difficult to isolate them and perform functional studies in vitro. Gr-1$^+$ staining was thought to be specific for neutrophils, but the Gr-1 monoclonal antibody (mAb) recognizes both Ly6C and Ly6G, antigens expressed also by monocytes/macrophages and DCs. Therefore, its use for accurately identifying neutrophils in vivo has proven problematic, and the use of a Ly6G-specific mAb instead of Gr-1 has made it possible to more accurately distinguish these cells in vivo. Along these lines, neutrophil depletion studies targeting Gr-1 must be interpreted with some caution, because Ly6C expressing monocytes, mDCs, as well as effector CD4 and CD8 T cells, express Ly6C. Studies in which neutrophils were experimentally recruited to the airways before infection showed a decrease in bacterial loads, whereas depletion of neutrophils shortly after infection increases bacterial burden (Pedrosa et al. 2000; Sugawara et al. 2004; Blomgran and Ernst 2011). Therefore, neutrophils can contribute to host resistance. Potential antimycobacterial effector functions of neutrophils involve TNF-α, reactive oxygen species, antimicrobial peptides, extracellular traps (NETs), efferocytosis of infected myeloid cells, and boosting the ability of DCs to prime T-cell responses (Blomgran and Ernst 2011; Blomgran et al. 2012; Lowe et al. 2012). In contrast, neutrophils have also been suggested to adapt a regulatory IL-10 producing, anti-inflammatory phenotype that limits antimycobacterial control (Zhang et al. 2009). Moreover, there is mounting evidence including association studies in humans that neutrophils during later stages of infection could mediate pathological changes and disease progression (Berry et al. 2010; Dorhoi et al. 2014). It is possible that neutrophils directly contribute to mortality by promoting necrotic lung pathology, liquefaction of granulomas, and collapse of lung functions. In this context, IFN-γ has been suggested to regulate neutrophil recruitment and function (Nandi and Behar 2011), perhaps via inhibition of IL-1 and IL-17 (Desvignes and Ernst 2009; Mayer-Barber et al. 2011), and depletion of Ly6G expressing cells via administration of 1A8 mAb has extended the survival of susceptible IFN-γ, CARD9, and microRNA-223-deficient animals (Dorhoi et al. 2010, 2013; Nandi and Behar 2011). Indeed, the influx of a large number of GR-1$^+$ and Ly6G$^+$ cells into the lungs could be considered a general hallmark of highly susceptible mice that undergo cachexia as well as uncontrolled bacterial replication, regardless of their genetic make-up (Eruslanov et al. 2005; Lyadova et al. 2010). It is possible, however, that during these late stages of lethal *Mtb* infection, the Ly6G and Gr-1 expressing population might not reflect true neutrophils (Antonelli et al. 2010; Lyadova et al. 2010). Moreover, these cells share characteristics of immature myeloid-derived suppressor cells, and future studies have to determine their role in tuberculosis pathogenesis (Obregón-Henao et al. 2013; Tsiganov et al. 2014).

PRIMING OF *Mtb*-SPECIFIC T-CELL RESPONSES

HIV infection induced CD4 T-cell depletion, and mice or nonhuman primates experimentally depleted of CD4 T cells are highly susceptible to *Mtb* infection (Müller et al. 1987; Orme 1988; Leveton et al. 1989; Flory et al. 1992; Lin et al. 2012; Pawlowski et al. 2012; Yao et al. 2014). Indeed, it is well established that T helper cells are critical for containment of *Mtb*.

Delay in T-Cell Priming Following *Mtb* Exposure

The initiation of the CD4 T-cell response to *Mtb* is notoriously slow, as CD4 T cells first arrive in the lungs of infected mice several weeks after exposure. This lag time between the establishment of infection and the arrival of T cells at the site of infection likely contributes to the inability of the host to clear the organism by allowing the bacteria to increase significantly in number before adaptive immune cells can mediate their protective effects.

More recently, the use of *Mtb*-specific T-cell receptor (TCR) transgenic (Tg) CD4 T cells has allowed the visualization of the earliest events of CD4 T-cell priming in *Mtb* infection. This is typically performed by adoptively transferring congenically marked TCR Tg CD4 T cells into naïve mice that are then infected with *Mtb*, thereby dramatically increasing the precursor frequency of antigen-specific CD4 T cells so that they can be visualized in vivo without the need for expansion. Using CD4 T cells that are specific for Ag85b (Wolf et al. 2008) or ESAT-6 (Gallegos et al. 2008; Reiley et al. 2008), it was definitively shown that initial recognition of *Mtb* by naïve CD4 T cells (read out by the first appearance of the activation marker CD69) occurs in the lung-draining lymph nodes. Interestingly, delivery of bacilli and subsequent T-cell priming is not accelerated by increased bacterial inoculum size, but once the bacteria reach the lymph node, the CD4 T-cell response is directly proportional to the number of viable organisms present in the lymph node (Wolf et al. 2008). The mechanisms leading to the delay in *Mtb*-specific T-cell priming are not known, but there is evidence that infected myeloid cells, not free bacteria or soluble antigens, must traffic to the lung-associated lymph nodes to initiate the T-cell response.

Role of Dendritic Cells in Priming of CD4 T Cells during *Mtb* Infection

Mtb-infected bone marrow–derived dendritic cells but not macrophages instilled into the trachea of mice can migrate into the lymph node and prime CD4 T cells (Bhatt et al. 2004). Indeed, dendritic cells are well understood to be essential in the induction of T-cell responses, and transient depletion of CD11c$^+$ cells impairs CD4 T-cell priming during intravenous *Mtb* infection (Tian et al. 2005). Moreover, autocrine production of IL-12p40 homodimers has also been shown to play a major role in the migration of instilled bone marrow–derived dendritic cells from the lungs to the lymph nodes following *Mtb* infection (Khader 2006). Dissemination of viable bacilli from the lung to secondary lymphoid organs always precedes the first evidence of adaptive T-cell response against *Mtb* between days 9 and 12, indicating that T-cell priming requires bacteria in the lymph node (Chackerian et al. 2002). *Plt/plt* mice that are deficient in the CCR7 ligands, CCL19, and CCL21, develop high levels of bacteria in their lungs, but very few bacteria are found in the draining lymph nodes, indicating that activated myeloid cells are essential for bacteria to arrive in the lymph node (Wolf et al. 2007). Because most innate effector cell types are infected with *Mtb*, it is possible that multiple cell types contribute either directly or indirectly to the delivery of bacteria to the lymph node. For example, depletion of neutrophils decreases the migration of dendritic cells to the lymph node and delays the priming of CD4 T-cell responses (Blomgran and Ernst 2011). Moreover, infection of mice with a *nuoG* mutant *Mtb* that cannot suppress neutrophil apoptosis leads to more rapid trafficking of bacteria to the lymph nodes and CD4 T-cell priming (Blomgran et al. 2012). Therefore, it has been suggested that apoptotic neutrophils play an important role in facilitating activation of *Mtb*-specific CD4 T cells by modulating the migratory capacity of dendritic cells.

Cooperation between Migratory CCR2$^+$ Monocytes and Conventional Dendritic Cells in Priming T Cells during *Mtb* Infection

A recent study has shown that depletion of CCR2$^+$ cells with injection of diphtheria toxin into CCR2-DTR mice dramatically reduces the appearance of bacteria in the lymph node and delays CD4 T-cell priming (Samstein et al. 2013). Adoptive transfer of wild-type (WT) CCR2$^+$ cells into MHC-II KO mice depleted of endogenous CCR2$^+$ monocytes, completely restored trafficking of bacteria to the lymph node but not CD4 T-cell priming. These data indicate that CCR2$^+$ myeloid cells are required for delivering viable bacilli to the lymph node but themselves do not present antigen to CD4 T cells. In contrast, depletion of conventional dendritic cells using zbtb46-DTR mice had no impact on bacterial trafficking to the lymph node, but dramatically decreased CD4 T-cell priming. Therefore, it is likely that CCR2$^+$ myeloid cells are essential for trafficking bacteria to the lymph node where conventional dendritic cells then uptake bacteria and directly present antigen to prime naïve CD4 T-cell responses. Ultimately, it is very likely that a complex orchestration of diverse myeloid effector cells acting together is required for optimal priming of *Mtb*-specific CD4 T cells.

PROTECTIVE CD4 T-CELL RESPONSES DURING *Mtb* INFECTION

Although a few key pathways have been elucidated, much is unknown about the mechanisms of CD4 T-cell-dependent control. Moreover, it should be emphasized that the main protective outcome of the T-cell response against *Mtb* is the containment of bacterial growth as the bacilli are not cleared.

Th1 Immunity Is Required for Host Resistance to *Mtb*

Early studies found that mice with defects in IFN-γ expression are extremely susceptible to *Mtb* infection (Cooper et al. 1993; Flynn et al. 1993). A recent study found that RAG KO mice reconstituted with a mixture of IFN-γKO CD4 T cells + WT CD4-depleted splenocytes died earlier than RAG KO mice reconstituted with WT CD4 T cells + WT CD4-depleted splenocytes, supporting the hypothesis that IFN-γ production by CD4 T cells themselves is important for survival of *Mtb* infection (Green et al. 2013). Moreover, mice deficient in the Th1-polarizing cytokine IL-12 (Cooper et al. 1997) or, albeit to a lesser extent, the Th1 lineage-specifying transcription factor Tbet (Sullivan et al. 2005) succumb early following *Mtb* exposure. Therefore, CD4 T cells polarized toward the Th1 phenotype are likely critical for host resistance to *Mtb* infection, and there is evidence in humans that the IL-12/IFN-γ axis is also critical for control of *Mtb* infection. Individuals with inborn errors in IL-12/23p40, IL-12Rβ1, IL-12Rβ2, IFNγR1, IFNγR2, or STAT1 are highly susceptible to even avirulent nontuberculosis mycobacteria (Filipe-Santos et al. 2006; Vosse et al. 2013). Moreover, individuals who develop neutralizing autoantibodies against IFN-γ become very susceptible to both tuberculosis and opportunistic nontuberculous mycobacterial infections (Browne and Holland 2010). Indeed, given the severity of disease in its absence, it may appear that IFN-γ is the most important T-cell-derived protective effector molecule described to date in *Mtb* infection.

IFN-γ-Independent Mechanisms of Protection

Despite the critical role of IFN-γ in host resistance to *Mtb* infection, it is not the only mechanism of CD4 T-cell-dependent control. In fact, in *Mtb*-infected individuals IFN-γ levels positively correlate with the severity of pulmonary disease, fever, and weight loss (Tsao et al. 2002). MHC-II-deficient mice eventually develop normal levels of IFN-γ in their lungs (Caruso et al. 1999), and depletion of CD4 T cells at late time points following *Mtb* infection has no effect on IFN-γ message levels in the lung (Scanga et al. 2000), yet in both settings, loss of CD4 T cells leads to the death of the host. Reconstitution of RAG KO mice with T cells showed that TNF-α KO CD4 T cells are not as protective as WT CD4 T cells against *Mtb* infection, but the effect was minor, indicating that TNF-α production does not account for the IFN-γ independent effects of CD4 T cells against *Mtb* (Saunders et al. 2004). In a CD4 T cell:macrophage coculture system, it was found that primed CD4 T cells suppressed the growth of *Mtb* in IFN-γR KO WT macrophages almost as well as WT macrophages (Cowley and Elkins 2003). Importantly, adoptive transfer of in vitro Th1 polarized ESAT-6-specific TCR Tg CD4 T cells into WT mice leads to dramatically decreased bacterial loads (Gallegos et al. 2008), but a comparison of WT and IFN-γTNF-α double-KO TCR Tg cells found that the majority of the host protective effect mediated by the adoptively transferred effector cells was independent of these two cytokines (Gallegos et al. 2011). Finally, whereas increasing numbers of *Mtb*-specific CD4 T cells through vaccination or through adoptive transfer of TCR Tg T cells leads to enhanced bacterial control, injection of recombinant IFN-γ into WT *Mtb*-infected mice is not protective (Moreira et al. 2002). Therefore, there is clear evidence that CD4 T cells can induce the control of *Mtb* infection in vitro and in vivo via mechanisms independent of both IFN-γ and TNF-α.

IL-17 is another major inflammatory cytokine that can be produced by subsets of *Mtb*-specific CD4 T cells. In humans, Ag-specific Th17 responses can be detected in individuals that are BCG (Bacillus Calmette–Guérin)-immunized and were found to be recalled by boosting with an Ag85a-expressing viral vector (Tameris et al. 2013), but Th17 responses are almost absent in individuals with active tuberculosis (Perreau et al. 2013). Interestingly, in mice, a similar phenomenon is observed. Ag-specific Th17 cells are readily generated by immunization with complete Freund's adjuvant which contains dead *Mtb* (Shenderov et al. 2013) but are relatively rare during *Mtb* infection when compared with Th1 responses. In fact, it appears that Th17 cells do not have a major role in control of *Mtb* infection. Mice deficient in the Th17-promoting cytokine IL-23p19 completely lack IL-17-producing CD4 T cells but display only small increases in bacterial burden at very late time point postinfection (Khader et al. 2005; 2011). Likewise, mice deficient in the IL-17 receptor display normal control of bacterial growth after a typical 100 colony-forming units (CFU) aerosol exposure to *Mtb* (Aujla et al. 2007; Khader et al. 2011). However, there is evidence that vaccine-elicited Th17 cells may contribute to protection by driving the expression of Th1-cell-recruiting chemokines (Khader et al. 2007).

IL-22 is often associated with Th17 cells and is found in the bronchiolar lavage fluid of tuberculosis patients at higher levels than IL-17 (Scriba et al. 2008; Matthews et al. 2011). Interestingly, IL-22 is predominantly produced by a subset of CD4 T cells distinct from the IL-17-producing cells in both humans (Scriba et al. 2008) and mice (Behrends et al. 2013). However, Th22 cells are unlikely to play a major role in host defense against *Mtb* as IL-22 blockade (Khader et al. 2007; Wilson et al. 2010) of WT mice has no apparent effect on control of *Mtb* infection, and IL-22-deficient mice also display normal bacterial loads (Khader et al. 2007) and long-term survival of *Mtb* infection (Behrends et al. 2013).

Role of CD4 T-Cell Migration

It was recently found that CD4 T cells must directly recognize MHC-II on *Mtb*-infected cells to suppress intracellular growth of the bacilli. This study used bone marrow chimeric mice reconstituted with congenically marked WT and MHC-II KO bone marrow, to evaluate the role of direct recognition of infected cells by CD4 T cells in bacterial control by myeloid cells (Srivastava and Ernst 2013). It was found that similar frequencies of WT and MHC-II KO cells were infected in the lung, but the KO cells contained higher numbers of bacilli in each infected cell. Moreover, depletion of CD4 T cells resulted in identical frequency distributions of bacteria/infected cell between the WT and KO macrophages. This clearly shows that for CD4 T cells to induce myeloid cells to limit replication of ingested bacteria, they must directly interact with the infected cells and recognize antigen. Therefore, the ability of CD4 T cells to enter the lung and interact with infected cells is another critical aspect of CD4 T-cell-dependent control of *Mtb* infection.

A recent study used an intravascular staining technique (Anderson et al. 2014) to examine the distribution of pulmonary CD4 T cells among the airways, the lung parenchyma, the lung-associated blood vasculature, and the peripheral circulating blood of *Mtb*-infected mice (Sakai et al. 2014). Surprisingly, it was found that Ag-specific CD4 T cells are present in similar numbers in both the lung parenchyma and blood vasculature. Interestingly, the parenchymal *Mtb*-specific CD4 T cells expressed high levels of the activation marker CD69 and PD-1, whereas the intravascular effector CD4 T cells expressed high levels of KLRG1, indicating a terminally differentiated phenotype. The intravascular *Mtb*-specific CD4 T cells expressed higher levels of Tbet and produced much higher levels of IFN-γ in vivo and on peptide restimulation in vitro. Moreover, adoptively transferred parenchymal CD4 T cells were able to rapidly migrate back into the lungs of infection matched mice, whereas intravascular donor CD4 T cells entered lung tissue poorly and were instead retained in the blood vasculature. Importantly, it was found that purified parenchymal CD4 T cells were able to protect *Mtb*-infected T-cell-deficient recipient mice much better than equal numbers of intravascular T cells. Therefore, *Mtb*-specific CD4 T cells dramatically vary in their ability to enter the lung parenchyma, and control of *Mtb* infection correlates with the ability of the CD4 T cell to enter the lung parenchyma rather than secrete high levels of IFN-γ. The mechanisms that regulate CD4 T-cell differentiation into a parenchyma-homing phenotype, however, are not understood.

PATHOGENIC CD4 T-CELL RESPONSES DURING *Mtb* INFECTION

Immune-mediated damage accounts for a large amount of the pathology of tuberculosis. Although the critical role for CD4 T cells in host resistance to *Mtb* is clear, there is also evidence that these cells can contribute to immunopathology associated with mycobacterial infections in both humans and experimental animal models.

Pathology Associated with Therapeutic Vaccination during *Mtb* Infection

In the late 1800s, Robert Koch performed experiments to promote the diagnostic and therapeutic value of preparations containing killed *Mtb* or bacterial extracts. He found that injection of naïve guinea pigs with dead bacilli had little effect on the animals, even when high doses were administered. However, when he inoculated *Mtb*-infected guinea pigs with preparations of dead bacteria, the animals succumbed, and the time to death depended on the dose he gave (Koch 1891). Some people may have even suffered lethal reactions on inoculations with Koch's intended remedy (Virchow 1891). The exacerbation of tuberculosis on therapeutic vaccination is now referred to as the Koch phenomenon, and has been observed in several animal models. For example, repeated injections of nonvirulent BCG into *Mtb*-infected mice leads to severe tissue damage (Turner et al. 2000a; Moreira et al. 2002). Although the mechanisms of the Koch reaction are not well understood, one study indicated that the induction of Th17 cells may promote disease in the model of repeated BCG injection–induced tuberculosis exacerbation (Cruz et al. 2010).

Interestingly, in the 1950s and 1960s, a large number of studies by Yamamura and colleagues explored the observation that in rabbits, prophylactic vaccination followed by multiple rounds of boosting with avirulent mycobacteria results in a dramatic increase in pulmonary cavities following a challenge with virulent mycobacteria. Prophylactic immunization of guinea pigs (Turner et al. 2000b) or mice (Taylor et al.

2003) with certain protein antigens or DNA vaccine constructs can predispose to necrotic lung damage when those animals are later challenged with *Mtb*. Although the role of CD4 T cells themselves has not formally been tested, this is consistent with observations in CD4 T-cell-deficient HIV/*Mtb* coinfected individuals, where the pathology of tuberculosis is altered.

Evidence for CD4 T-Cell-Mediated Immunopathology from Studies of HIV/*Mtb* Coinfection

As mentioned above, CD4 deficiency in HIV-coinfected individuals leads to an inability to control *Mtb* infection, but it has also been recognized since the early days of the HIV epidemic that HIV coinfection alters the radiographic patterns of tuberculosis lung lesions. Consistent with poor bacterial control, CD4-deficient HIV coinfected individuals with low CD4 T-cell counts are more likely to have miliary tuberculosis (large numbers of unusually small lesions visible on chest X-ray), lymphadenopathy caused by dissemination of the bacilli to the lung-draining lymph nodes and pleural effusion (Long et al. 1991; Batungwanayo et al. 1992; Mukadi et al. 1993; Pastores et al. 1993; Keiper et al. 1995; Awil et al. 1997; Jones et al. 1997; Perlman et al. 1997; Busi Rizzi et al. 2004; Geng et al. 2005; Chamie et al. 2010). In contrast, HIV-negative individuals are more likely to develop upper lung disease and, importantly, lung cavities. In fact, a large cohort study of HIV/tuberculosis coinfection found strong positive correlations between increasing numbers of CD4 T cells and the likelihood of cavitary tuberculosis (Chamie et al. 2010), indicating that CD4 T cells may contribute to cavity formation. HIV-infected individuals with extremely low numbers of CD4 T cells are even much more likely to have a completely normal chest X-ray. It has been suggested that cavitation is beneficial to *Mtb*. Individuals with cavitary tuberculosis are more infectious compared with individuals with active disease who do not display cavities (Rodrigo et al. 1997), indicating that cavities facilitate the transmission of *Mtb* from one host to the next, a critical step in the life cycle of this obligate human pathogen. Consistent with the lack of cavities in HIV patients, CD4-deficient HIV patients are less likely to produce bacteria in their sputum. Moreover, a recent study found that human T-cell epitopes are hyperconserved in the tuberculosis genome (Comas et al. 2010), again supporting the hypothesis that *Mtb* benefits from T-cell recognition and may be under strong selective pressure to actually induce T-cell responses. Therefore, the phenotype of tuberculosis in CD4-depleted HIV-infected individuals, that is, the inability to control *Mtb* growth and lack of lung cavities, indicates that CD4 T-cell responses in HIV-negative individuals may be both required for host resistance and responsible for severe tissue immunopathology.

Immune Reconstitution Inflammatory Syndrome

Another scenario in which CD4 T-cell responses can mediate pathology during mycobacterial infection occurs in the context of CD4 T-cell reconstitution of lymphopenic HIV-infected individuals during therapy. Although the treatment of HIV infection with antiretroviral therapy (ART) usually leads to clinical improvement, some individuals experience a rapid deterioration in symptoms within the first few weeks of beginning ART, termed immune reconstitutive inflammatory syndrome (IRIS) (French 2012). This paradoxical worsening of disease occurs most frequently in individuals with severe T-cell deficiency and a concurrent microbial coinfection, which is often *Mtb*. The symptoms of the IRIS event depend on the site of infection and the particular microbe, but in *Mtb*-coinfected individuals, the pathology often manifests as extreme lymphadenopathy, the worsening or formation of new pulmonary lesions, or meningitis. Some studies have found that HIV/*Mtb*-coinfected individuals who develop IRIS display increased frequencies of *Mtb*-specific or -activated CD4 T cells at the time of the IRIS event, whereas those who do not develop IRIS lack this T-cell expansion at a similar time point posttreatment (Bourgarit et al. 2006; 2009; Meintjes et al. 2008). The mechanisms of

IRIS are not understood, but the prevailing hypothesis concerning the development of IRIS is that when CD4 T-cell numbers begin to recover as viral replication is suppressed with ART, the reconstituting T cells drive dysregulated inflammatory responses against the microbial coinfection leading to destructive tissue pathology.

A murine model of IRIS has been developed by reproducing the underlying immunological scenario preceding the development of immune reconstitution disease; that is, CD4 T-cell reconstitution of a mycobacterial-infected, T-cell-deficient host (Barber et al. 2010). In this model, TCRαKO mice are first inoculated with *Mycobacterium avium*, and after several months, the chronically infected mice are injected with CD4 T cells. Although it may be expected that CD4 T-cell reconstitution would lead to enhanced control of the established mycobacterial infection, instead, it leads to a rapid wasting disease, and most of the animals succumb to fatal immunopathology within a few weeks after the T-cell infusion (Barber et al. 2014, 2010). IFN-γ production by the reconstituting CD4 T cells, which is normally required for containment of mycobacterial infection, is a major mediator of the disease in this setting. Models of IRIS associated with other microbial infections (Roths et al. 1990; Roths and Sidman 1992, 1993; Bhagwat et al. 2006; Mutnal et al. 2013) have also found that in the setting of immune reconstitution, CD4 T cells can mediate severe immunopathology. Collectively, the data from studies of IRIS in HIV-coinfected individuals and the experimental animal model data strongly support the hypothesis that IRIS in humans is mediated by CD4 T cells and provide another example of CD4 T-cell-mediated pathology in mycobacterial infection.

Negative Regulation of T-Cell Responses during Tuberculosis

Most of the work on CD4 T-cell immunity and host resistance to *Mtb* infection has focused on the inductive signals that lead to the priming and differentiation of antigen-specific Th1 responses. Negative regulatory pathways play a major role in immune homeostasis, in controlling immune responses against self-antigens, tumors, and pathogens. Although bacterial evasion strategies certainly play a major role in the inability to the host to clear *Mtb* infection, inhibitory pathways may also contribute to the persistence of the bacilli. On the other hand, proper negative regulation of inflammatory responses is also important for preventing immunopathology. Several major negative regulatory pathways and cell types have been examined, primarily in the context of *Mtb* infection in mice, which serve to either limit control of the infection or prevent immune-mediated tissue damage.

IL-10 is an anti-inflammatory pleiotropic cytokine that, among other things, can suppress IL-1 and IL-12 production by dendritic cells and macrophages, so there has been much interest in the role of IL-10 in *Mtb* infection. During the past 15 years, multiple studies have examined and reexamined the role of IL-10 in resistance to *Mtb* infection. These studies have found that IL-10 either has a minor role in suppressing Th1 responses and limiting control of *Mtb* infection (Roach et al. 2001; Turner et al. 2002; Beamer et al. 2008; Redford et al. 2010) or has no discernible role at all (North 1998; Jung et al. 2003). Although the factors that contributed to the different outcomes observed in these studies are not clear, collectively, they show that this inhibitory cytokine is not a major factor leading to the inability of the host to control *Mtb* infection and may have a minor role in limiting immunopathology at very late stages of the infection (Higgins et al. 2009).

$Foxp3^+$ regulatory CD4 T cells are essential in maintaining peripheral tolerance to self-antigens, but they also contribute to the inhibition of pathogen-specific immune responses (Josefowicz et al. 2012). During inflammatory conditions, Tregs (regulatory T cells) can functionally specialize to match the contemporaneous class of effector CD4 T-cell responses (Campbell and Koch 2011). In one of the earliest demonstrations of Treg specialization, it was found that Tregs up-regulate the Th1 lineage-specifying transcription factor Tbet during *Mtb* infection, and Tbet expression by Tregs is required for their normal expansion (Koch et al.

2009). Moreover, it has been shown that Ag-specific Foxp3$^+$ regulatory CD4 T cells are generated during *Mtb* infection (Shafiani et al. 2013) and that depletion of Tregs enhances Th1 priming, resulting in ~1 log lower bacterial loads (Scott-Browne et al. 2007). Conversely, injection of Ag85b TCR Tg Foxp3$^+$ CD4 T cells delays T-cell priming, resulting in ~1 log increased bacterial loads (Shafiani et al. 2010). The role of Foxp3$^+$ regulatory T cells may be even more pronounced during infection with hypervirulent strains of *Mtb* such as the W-Beijing strains (Shang et al. 2011). There is also evidence that the hyperinduction of Tregs during infections with W-Beijing strains of *Mtb* may overcome much of the protective effects of BCG vaccination (Ordway et al. 2011). Therefore, signals from regulatory T cells inhibit the priming of *Mtb*-specific CD4 T cells and may limit their function in the periphery, and they directly contribute to the inability of the host to clear *Mtb* infection.

Apart from anti-inflammatory cytokines and cell types described above, inhibitory receptors expressed by the activated T cells themselves are also critical in controlling T-cell function. Killer-cell lectin-like receptor G1 (KLRG1) is an inhibitory receptor widely expressed on natural killer (NK) cells, and when expressed on CD4 and CD8 T cells, it is often associated with a terminally differentiated or senescent phenotype (Akbar and Henson 2011). In *Mtb* infection, a subpopulation of T cells with high cytokine producing potential up-regulate KLRG1 (Reiley et al. 2010), and KLRG1-deficient mice display slightly increased T-cell responses and survive for extremely long periods following *Mtb* infection, albeit on a genetic background that is already capable of surviving for ~1 yr following infection (Cyktor et al. 2013).

Programmed death-1 (PD-1) is a cell surface inhibitory receptor that is highly expressed on activated CD4 and CD8 T cells. On binding to either of its ligands, PD-L1 or PD-L2, SHP-2 is recruited to an ITSM (immunoreceptor tyrosine-based switch motif) domain in the cytoplasmic tail of PD-1, which then blocks several components of the proximal TCR signal transduction machinery (Keir et al. 2008). PD-1 is important for maintaining peripheral tolerance as older PD-1 knockout mice spontaneously develop autoimmune disease that varies in severity depending on the genetic background of the mouse. PD-1 also plays a major role in the regulation of immune responses to pathogens. The first evidence that PD-1 plays a role during infection was observed in chronic lymphocytic choriomeningitis virus infection in which it was found that blockade of PD-1/PD-L1 interactions boosts the function of the "exhausted" CD8 T cell and enhances viral control (Barber et al. 2006). It is now widely recognized that PD-1 is a major inhibitor of pathogen-specific T cells in mice, nonhuman primates, and humans. Moreover, PD-1 blockade also dramatically improves tumor-specific immunity and is one of the most promising new developments in cancer therapy (Topalian et al. 2012; Brahmer et al. 2012).

The major success of PD-1 immunotherapy in other model systems created much interest in the possibility of also targeting the PD-1 pathway in *Mtb* infection, and several recent studies have examined the expression of PD-1 on T cells in human tuberculosis and tested its role in murine models *Mtb* infection. Patients with active tuberculosis have higher numbers of PD-1-expressing T cells, and PD-1 blockade in vitro can enhance responses of cultured T cells to *Mtb* antigens (Jurado et al. 2008). Moreover, infection of PD-1 KO mice with BCG leads to enhanced T-cell responses and bacterial control rather than immunopathology (Sakai et al. 2010). However, rather than displaying enhanced protection, PD-1 knockout mice succumb rapidly on exposure to low doses of virulent *Mtb* (Lázár-Molnár et al. 2010; Barber et al. 2011; Tousif et al. 2011). It was found that PD-1 KO mice have greatly increased numbers of I-A^{b}ESAT-6$_{1-20}$ tetramer-binding CD4 T cells in their lungs and that transient depletion of CD4 T cells in the first month of infection prevented the severe tissue destruction and death of the PD-1 KO mice (Barber et al. 2011). Moreover, whereas injection of TCRαKO mice with WT CD4 T cells rescues them from early mortality, reconstituting TCRαKO with a mixture of WT and PD-1 KO CD4 T cells leads to the rapid death of the animals. This indicates that in the absence of PD-1-mediated inhibition, CD4 T-cell responses are greatly enhanced, but this drives lethal immunopathology in *Mtb* infection instead of enhanced protection. Therefore, CD4 T-cell-mediated pathology in *Mtb* infection can also be revealed by removal of a single negative regulatory pathway. Thus, although CD4 T cells are clearly essential for containment for *Mtb* infection, these cells can also promote lung tissue destruction during *Mtb* monoinfection, during IRIS after antiretroviral therapy of HIV patients, and when certain negative regulatory pathways are perturbed.

CONCLUSIONS

With the advent of novel immunological tools and techniques for studying immune responses at the single-cell level in vivo, the classical paradigm of the T-cell macrophage interaction at the core of antituberculous immunity has now been expanded to include a large number of functionally diverse innate and adaptive effector cells with multiple cellular interactions. Whereas many of the effector functions of inflammatory myeloid cells as well as CD4 T cells are required for host protection, each of these cell types also has potential for mediating tissue damage, and a major goal should be to understand the factors that determine the balance between detrimental and protective cellular immunity. The dual nature of inflammation in *Mtb* infection underscores a major challenge of vaccine development as well as immunomodulatory host-directed treatment strategies for tuberculosis.

REFERENCES

Akbar AN, Henson SM. 2011. Are senescence and exhaustion intertwined or unrelated processes that compromise immunity? *Nat Rev Immunol* **11:** 289–295.

Anderson KG, Mayer-Barber K, Sung H, Beura L, James BR, Taylor JJ, Qunaj L, Griffith TS, Vezys V, Barber DL, et al. 2014. Intravascular staining for discrimination of vascular and tissue leukocytes. *Nat Protoc* **9:** 209–222.

Antonelli LRV, Gigliotti Rothfuchs A, Gonçalves R, Roffê E, Cheever AW, Bafica A, Salazar AM, Feng CG, Sher A. 2010. Intranasal poly-IC treatment exacerbates tuberculosis in mice through the pulmonary recruitment of a pathogen-permissive monocyte/macrophage population. *J Clin Invest* **120:** 1674–1682.

Aujla SJ, Dubin PJ, Kolls JK. 2007. Th17 cells and mucosal host defense. *Semin Immunol* **19:** 377–382.

Awil PO, Bowlin SJ, Daniel TM. 1997. Radiology of pulmonary turberculosis and human immunodeficiency virus infection in Gulu, Uganda. *Eur Respir J* **10:** 615–618.

Banchereau J, Steinman RM. 1998. Dendritic cells and the control of immunity. *Nature (London)* **392:** 245.

Barber DL, Wherry EJ, Masopust D, Zhu B, Allison JP, Sharpe AH, Freeman GJ, Ahmed R. 2006. Restoring function in exhausted CD8 T cells during chronic viral infection. *Nature* **439:** 682–687.

Barber DL, Mayer-Barber KD, Antonelli LRV, Wilson MS, White S, Caspar P, Hieny S, Sereti I, Sher A. 2010. Th1-driven immune reconstitution disease in *Mycobacterium avium*-infected mice. *Blood* **116:** 3485–3493.

Barber DL, Mayer-Barber KD, Feng CG, Sharpe AH, Sher A. 2011. CD4 T cells promote rather than control tuberculosis in the absence of PD-1-mediated inhibition. *J Immunol* **186:** 1598–1607.

Barber DL, Andrade BB, McBerry C, Sereti I, Sher A. 2014. Role of IL-6 in *Mycobacterium avium*-associated immune reconstitution inflammatory syndrome. *J Immunol* **192:** 676–682.

Batungwanayo J, Taelman H, Dhote R, Bogaerts J, Allen S, Van de Perre P. 1992. Pulmonary tuberculosis in Kigali, Rwanda. Impact of human immunodeficiency virus infection on clinical and radiographic presentation. *Am Rev Respir Dis* **146:** 53–56.

Beamer GL, Flaherty DK, Assogba BD, Stromberg P, Gonzalez-Juarrero M, de Waal Malefyt R, Vesosky B, Turner J. 2008. Interleukin-10 promotes *Mycobacterium tuberculosis* disease progression in CBA/J mice. *J Immunol* **181:** 5545–5550.

Behar SM, Divangahi M, Remold HG. 2010. Evasion of innate immunity by *Mycobacterium tuberculosis*: Is death an exit strategy? *Nat Rev Microbiol* **8:** 668–674.

Behrends J, Renauld J-C, Ehlers S, Hölscher C. 2013. IL-22 is mainly produced by IFNγ-secreting cells but is dispensable for host protection against *Mycobacterium tuberculosis* infection. *PLoS ONE* **8:** e57379.

Berrington WR, Hawn TR. 2007. *Mycobacterium tuberculosis*, macrophages, and the innate immune response: Does common variation matter? *Immunol Rev* **219:** 167–186.

Berry MPR, Graham CM, McNab FW, Xu Z, Bloch SAA, Oni T, Wilkinson KA, Banchereau R, Skinner J, Wilkinson RJ, et al. 2010. An interferon-inducible neutrophil-driven blood transcriptional signature in human tuberculosis. *Nature* **466:** 973–977.

Bhagwat SP, Gigliotti F, Xu H, Wright TW. 2006. Contribution of T cell subsets to the pathophysiology of pneumocystis-related immunorestitution disease. *Am J Physiol Lung Cell Mol Physiol* **291:** L1256–L1266.

Bhatt K, Hickman SP, Salgame P. 2004. Cutting edge: A new approach to modeling early lung immunity in murine tuberculosis. *J Immunol* **172:** 2748–2751.

Biswas SK, Mantovani A. 2010. Macrophage plasticity and interaction with lymphocyte subsets: Cancer as a paradigm. *Nat Immunol* **11:** 889–896.

Blomgran R, Ernst JD. 2011. Lung neutrophils facilitate activation of naive antigen-specific CD4$^+$ T cells during *Mycobacterium tuberculosis* infection. *J Immunol* **186:** 7110–7119.

Blomgran R, Desvignes L, Briken V, Ernst JD. 2012. *Mycobacterium tuberculosis* inhibits neutrophil apoptosis, leading to delayed activation of naive CD4 T cells. *Cell Host Microbe* **11:** 81–90.

Bourgarit A, Carcelain G, Martinez V, Lascoux C, Delcey V, Gicquel B, Vicaut E, Lagrange PH, Sereni D, Autran B. 2006. Explosion of tuberculin-specific Th1-responses induces immune restoration syndrome in tuberculosis and HIV co-infected patients. *AIDS* **20:** F1–F7.

Bourgarit A, Carcelain G, Samri A, Parizot C, Lafaurie M, Abgrall S, Delcey V, Vicaut E, Sereni D, Autran B, et al. 2009. Tuberculosis-associated immune restoration syndrome in HIV-1-infected patients involves tuberculin-specific CD4 Th1 cells and KIR-negative γδ T cells. *J Immunol* **183:** 3915–3923.

Brahmer JR, Tykodi SS, Chow LQM, Hwu W-J, Topalian SL, Hwu P, Drake CG, Camacho LH, Kauh J, Odunsi K, et al. 2012. Safety and activity of anti-PD-L1 antibody in patients with advanced cancer. *N Engl J Med* **366:** 2455–2465.

Browne SK, Holland SM. 2010. Anticytokine autoantibodies in infectious diseases: Pathogenesis and mechanisms. *Lancet Infect Dis* **10:** 875–885.

Busi Rizzi E, Schininà V, Palmieri F, Girardi E, Bibbolino C. 2004. Cavitary pulmonary tuberculosis HIV-related. *Eur J Radiol* **52:** 170–174.

Campbell DJ, Koch MA. 2011. Phenotypical and functional specialization of FOXP3$^+$ regulatory T cells. *Nat Rev Immunol* **11:** 119–130.

Caruso AM, Serbina N, Klein E, Triebold K, Bloom BR, Flynn JL. 1999. Mice deficient in CD4 T cells have only transiently diminished levels of IFN-γ, yet succumb to tuberculosis. *J Immunol* **162:** 5407–5416.

Chackerian AA, Alt JM, Perera TV, Dascher CC, Behar SM. 2002. Dissemination of *Mycobacterium tuberculosis* is influenced by host factors and precedes the initiation of T-cell immunity. *Infect Immun* **70:** 4501–4509.

Chamie G, Luetkemeyer A, Walusimbi-Nanteza M, Okwera A, Whalen CC, Mugerwa RD, Havlir DV, Charlebois ED. 2010. Significant variation in presentation of pulmonary tuberculosis across a high resolution of CD4 strata. *Int J Tuberc Lung Dis* **14:** 1295–1302.

Chen M, Gan H, Remold HG. 2006. A mechanism of virulence: Virulent *Mycobacterium tuberculosis* strain H37Rv, but not attenuated H37Ra, causes significant mitochondrial inner membrane disruption in macrophages leading to necrosis. *J Immunol* **176:** 3707–3716.

Comas I, Chakravartti J, Small PM, Galagan J, Niemann S, Kremer K, Ernst JD, Gagneux S. 2010. Human T cell epitopes of *Mycobacterium tuberculosis* are evolutionarily hyperconserved. *Nat Genet* **42:** 498–503.

Cooper AM, Dalton DK, Stewart TA, Griffin JP, Russell DG, Orme IM. 1993. Disseminated tuberculosis in interferon γ gene-disrupted mice. *J Exp Med* **178:** 2243–2247.

Cooper AM, Magram J, Ferrante J, Orme IM. 1997. Interleukin 12 (IL-12) is crucial to the development of protective immunity in mice intravenously infected with *Mycobacterium tuberculosis*. *J Exp Med* **186:** 39–45.

Cooper AM, Solache A, Khader SA. 2007. Interleukin-12 and tuberculosis: An old story revisited. *Curr Opin Immunol* **19:** 441–447.

Cooper AM, Mayer-Barber KD, Sher A. 2011. Role of innate cytokines in mycobacterial infection. *Mucosal Immunol* **4:** 252–260.

Cowley SC, Elkins KL. 2003. CD4$^+$ T cells mediate IFN-γ-independent control of *Mycobacterium tuberculosis* infection both in vitro and in vivo. *J Immunol* **171:** 4689–4699.

Cruz A, Fraga AG, Fountain JJ, Rangel-Moreno J, Torrado E, Saraiva M, Pereira DR, Randall TD, Pedrosa J, Cooper AM, et al. 2010. Pathological role of interleukin 17 in mice subjected to repeated BCG vaccination after infection with *Mycobacterium tuberculosis*. *J Exp Med* **207:** 1609–1616.

Cyktor JC, Carruthers B, Stromberg P, Flaño E, Pircher H, Turner J. 2013. Killer cell lectin-like receptor G1 deficiency significantly enhances survival after *Mycobacterium tuberculosis* infection. *Infect Immun* **81:** 1090–1099.

de Heer HJ, Hammad H, Kool M, Lambrecht BN. 2005. Dendritic cell subsets and immune regulation in the lung. *Semin Immunol* **17:** 295–303.

De Trez C, Magez S, Akira S, Ryffel B, Carlier Y, Muraille E. 2009. iNOS-producing inflammatory dendritic cells constitute the major infected cell type during the chronic *Leishmania major* infection phase of C57BL/6 resistant mice. *PLoS Pathog* **5:** e1000494.

Desvignes L, Ernst JD. 2009. Interferon-γ-responsive nonhematopoietic cells regulate the immune response to *Mycobacterium tuberculosis*. *Immunity* **31:** 974–985.

Divangahi M, Chen M, Gan H, Desjardins D, Hickman TT, Lee DM, Fortune S, Behar SM, Remold HG. 2009. *Mycobacterium tuberculosis* evades macrophage defenses by inhibiting plasma membrane repair. *Nat Immunol* **10:** 899–906.

Divangahi M, Desjardins D, Nunes-Alves C, Remold HG, Behar SM. 2010. Eicosanoid pathways regulate adaptive immunity to *Mycobacterium tuberculosis*. *Nat Immunol* **11:** 751–758.

Dorhoi A, Desel C, Yeremeev V, Pradl L, Brinkmann V, Mollenkopf H-J, Hanke K, Gross O, Ruland J, Kaufmann SHE. 2010. The adaptor molecule CARD9 is essential for tuberculosis control. *J Exp Med* **207:** 777–792.

Dorhoi A, Iannaccone M, Farinacci M, Faé KC, Schreiber J, Moura-Alves P, Nouailles G, Mollenkopf H-J, Oberbeck-Müller D, Jörg S, et al. 2013. MicroRNA-223 controls susceptibility to tuberculosis by regulating lung neutrophil recruitment. *J Clin Invest* **123:** 4836–4848.

Dorhoi A, Iannaccone M, Maertzdorf J, Nouailles G, Weiner J 3rd, Kaufmann SHE. 2014. Reverse translation in tuberculosis: Neutrophils provide clues for understanding development of active disease. *Frontiers Immunol* **5:** 36.

Dunay IR, Damatta RA, Fux B, Presti R, Greco S, Colonna M, Sibley LD. 2008. Gr1(+) inflammatory monocytes are required for mucosal resistance to the pathogen *Toxoplasma gondii*. *Immunity* **29:** 306–317.

Eruslanov EB, Lyadova IV, Kondratieva TK, Majorov KB, Scheglov IV, Orlova MO, Apt AS. 2005. Neutrophil responses to *Mycobacterium tuberculosis* infection in genetically susceptible and resistant mice. *Infect Immun* **73:** 1744–1753.

Eum S-Y. 2010. Neutrophils are the predominant infected phagocytic cells in the airways of patients with active pulmonary TB. *Chest* **137:** 122–128.

Filipe-Santos O, Bustamante J, Chapgier A, Vogt G, de Beaucoudrey L, Feinberg J, Jouanguy E, Boisson Dupuis S, Fieschi C, Picard C, et al. 2006. Inborn errors of IL-12/23- and IFN-γ-mediated immunity: Molecular, cellular, and clinical features. *Semin Immunol* **18:** 347–361.

Flory CM, Hubbard RD, Collins FM. 1992. Effects of in vivo T lymphocyte subset depletion on mycobacterial infections in mice. *J Leukoc Biol* **51:** 225–229.

Flynn JL, Chan J. 2003. Immune evasion by *Mycobacterium tuberculosis*: Living with the enemy. *Curr Opin Immunol* **15:** 450–455.

Flynn JL, Chan J, Triebold KJ, Dalton DK, Stewart TA, Bloom BR. 1993. An essential role for interferon γ in resistance to *Mycobacterium tuberculosis* infection. *J Exp Med* **178:** 2249–2254.

Fratazzi C, Arbeit RD, Carini C, Balcewicz-Sabliska MK, Keane J, Kornfeld H, Remold HG. 1999. Macrophage apoptosis in mycobacterial infection. *J Leukoc Biol* **66:** 763–764.

French MAH. 2012. Immune reconstitution inflammatory syndrome: Immune restoration disease 20 years on. *Med J Aust* **196:** 318–321.

Gallegos AM, Pamer EG, Glickman MS. 2008. Delayed protection by ESAT-6-specific effector CD4$^+$ T cells after airborne *M. tuberculosis* infection. *J Exp Med* **205:** 2359–2368.

Gallegos AM, van Heijst JWJ, Samstein M, Su X, Pamer EG, Glickman MS. 2011. A γ interferon independent mechanism of CD4 T cell mediated control of *M. tuberculosis* infection in vivo. *PLoS Pathog* **7:** e1002052.

Garcia-Romo GS, Pedroza-Gonzalez A, Lambrecht BN, Aguilar-Leon D, Estrada-Garcia I, Hernandez-Pando R, Flores-Romo L. 2013. *Mycobacterium tuberculosis* manipulates pulmonary APCs subverting early immune responses. *Immunobiology* **218:** 393–401.

Geissmann F, Gordon S, Hume DA, Mowat AM, Randolph GJ. 2010. Unravelling mononuclear phagocyte heterogeneity. *Nat Rev Immunol* **10:** 453–460.

Geng E, Kreiswirth B, Burzynski J, Schluger NW. 2005. Clinical and radiographic correlates of primary and reactivation tuberculosis: A molecular epidemiology study. *JAMA* **293:** 2740–2745.

Gengenbacher M, Kaufmann SHE. 2012. *Mycobacterium tuberculosis*: Success through dormancy. *FEMS Microbiol Rev* **36:** 514–532.

GeurtsvanKessel CH, Willart MAM, van Rijt LS, Muskens F, Kool M, Baas C, Thielemans K, Bennett C, Clausen BE, Hoogsteden HC, et al. 2008. Clearance of influenza virus from the lung depends on migratory langerin+CD11b- but not plasmacytoid dendritic cells. *J Exp Med* **205:** 1621–1634.

Gonzalez-Juarrero M, Orme IM. 2001. Characterization of murine lung dendritic cells infected with *Mycobacterium tuberculosis*. *Infect Immun* **69:** 1127–1133.

Green AM, Difazio R, Flynn JL. 2013. IFN-γ from CD4 T cells is essential for host survival and enhances CD8 T cell function during *Mycobacterium tuberculosis* infection. *J Immunol* **190:** 270–277.

Guilliams M, De Kleer I, Henri S, Post S, Vanhoutte L, De Prijck S, Deswarte K, Malissen B, Hammad H, Lambrecht BN. 2013a. Alveolar macrophages develop from fetal monocytes that differentiate into long-lived cells in the first week of life via GM-CSF. *J Exp Med* **210:** 1977–1992.

Guilliams M, Lambrecht BN, Hammad H. 2013b. Division of labor between lung dendritic cells and macrophages in the defense against pulmonary infections. *Mucosal Immunol* **6:** 464–473.

Higgins DM, Sanchez-Campillo J, Rosas-Taraco AG, Lee EJ, Orme IM, Gonzalez-Juarrero M. 2009. Lack of IL-10 alters inflammatory and immune responses during pulmonary *Mycobacterium tuberculosis* infection. *Tuberculosis* **89:** 149–157.

Jo E-K. 2008. Mycobacterial interaction with innate receptors: TLRs, C-type lectins, and NLRs. *Curr Opin Infect Dis* **21:** 279–286.

Jo EK, Yang CS, Choi CH, Harding CV. 2007. Intracellular signalling cascades regulating innate immune responses to mycobacteria: Branching out from Toll-like receptors. *Cell Microbiol* **9:** 1087–1098.

Jones BE, Ryu R, Yang Z, Cave MD, Pogoda JM, Otaya M, Barnes PF. 1997. Chest radiographic findings in patients with tuberculosis with recent or remote infection. *Am J Resp Crit Care Med* **156:** 1270–1273.

Josefowicz SZ, Lu L-F, Rudensky AY. 2012. Regulatory T cells: Mechanisms of differentiation and function. *Annu Rev Immunol* **30:** 531–564.

Jung Y-J, Ryan L, LaCourse R, North RJ. 2003. Increased interleukin-10 expression is not responsible for failure of T helper 1 immunity to resolve airborne *Mycobacterium tuberculosis* infection in mice. *Immunology* **109:** 295–299.

Jurado JO, Alvarez IB, Pasquinelli V, Martínez GJ, Quiroga MF, Abbate E, Musella RM, Chuluyan HE, García VE. 2008. Programmed death (PD)-1:PD-ligand 1/PD-ligand 2 pathway inhibits T cell effector functions during human tuberculosis. *J Immunol* **181:** 116–125.

Keane J, Balcewicz-Sablinska MK, Remold HG, Chupp GL, Meek BB, Fenton MJ, Kornfeld H. 1997. Infection by *Mycobacterium tuberculosis* promotes human alveolar macrophage apoptosis. *Infect Immun* **65:** 298–304.

Keiper MD, Beumont M, Elshami A, Langlotz CP, Miller WT. 1995. CD4 T lymphocyte count and the radiographic presentation of pulmonary tuberculosis. A study of the relationship between these factors in patients with human immunodeficiency virus infection. *Chest* **107:** 74–80.

Keir ME, Butte MJ, Freeman GJ, Sharpe AH. 2008. PD-1 and its ligands in tolerance and immunity. *Annu Rev Immunol* **26:** 677–704.

Khader SA. 2006. Interleukin 12p40 is required for dendritic cell migration and T cell priming after *Mycobacterium tuberculosis* infection. *J Exp Med* **203:** 1805–1815.

Khader SA, Pearl JE, Sakamoto K, Gilmartin L, Bell GK, Jelley-Gibbs DM, Ghilardi N, deSauvage F, Cooper AM. 2005. IL-23 compensates for the absence of IL-12p70 and is essential for the IL-17 response during tuberculosis but is dispensable for protection and antigen-specific IFN-γ responses if IL-12p70 is available. *J Immunol* **175:** 788–795.

Khader SA, Partida-Sanchez S, Bell G, Jelley-Gibbs DM, Swain S, Pearl JE, Ghilardi N, Desauvage FJ, Lund FE, Cooper AM. 2006. Interleukin 12p40 is required for dendritic cell migration and T cell priming after *Mycobacterium tuberculosis* infection. *J Exp Med* **203:** 1805–1815.

Khader SA, Bell GK, Pearl JE, Fountain JJ, Rangel-Moreno J, Cilley GE, Shen F, Eaton SM, Gaffen SL, Swain SL, et al. 2007. IL-23 and IL-17 in the establishment of protective pulmonary CD4$^+$ T cell responses after vaccination and during *Mycobacterium tuberculosis* challenge. *Nat Immunol* **8:** 369–377.

Khader SA, Guglani L, Rangel-Moreno J, Gopal R, Junecko BAF, Fountain JJ, Martino C, Pearl JE, Tighe M, Lin Y-Y, et al. 2011. IL-23 is required for long-term control of *Mycobacterium tuberculosis* and B cell follicle formation in the infected lung. *J Immunol* **187:** 5402–5407.

Kleinnijenhuis J, Oosting M, Joosten LAB, Netea MG, Van Crevel R. 2011. Innate immune recognition of *Mycobacterium tuberculosis*. *Clin Dev Immunol* **2011:** 405310–405312.

Koch R. 1891. Professor Koch's remedy for tuberculosis. *Br Med J* **1:** 21–26.

Koch MA, Tucker-Heard G, Perdue NR, Killebrew JR, Urdahl KB, Campbell DJ. 2009. The transcription factor T-bet controls regulatory T cell homeostasis and function during type 1 inflammation. *Nat Immunol* **10:** 595–602.

Lázár-Molnár E, Chen B, Sweeney KA, Wang EJ, Liu W, Lin J, Porcelli SA, Almo SC, Nathenson SG, Jacobs WR. 2010. Programmed death-1 (PD-1)-deficient mice are extraordinarily sensitive to tuberculosis. *Proc Natl Acad Sci* **107:** 13402–13407.

Lee J, Remold HG, Ieong MH, Kornfeld H. 2006. Macrophage apoptosis in response to high intracellular burden of *Mycobacterium tuberculosis* is mediated by a novel caspase-independent pathway. *J Immunol* **176:** 4267–4274.

Lee J, Hartman M, Kornfeld H. 2009. Macrophage apoptosis in tuberculosis. *Yonsei Med J* **50:** 1–11.

Lee J, Repasy T, Papavinasasundaram K, Sassetti C, Kornfeld H. 2011. *Mycobacterium tuberculosis* induces an atypical cell death mode to escape from infected macrophages. *PLoS ONE* **6:** e18367.

Leemans JC, Juffermans NP, Florquin S, van Rooijen N, Vervoordeldonk MJ, Verbon A, van Deventer SJ, van der Poll T. 2001. Depletion of alveolar macrophages exerts protective effects in pulmonary tuberculosis in mice. *J Immunol* **166:** 4604–4611.

Leemans JC, Thepen T, Weijer S, Florquin S, van Rooijen N, van de Winkel JG, van der Poll T. 2005. Macrophages play a dual role during pulmonary tuberculosis in mice. *J Infect Dis* **191:** 65–74.

Leepiyasakulchai C, Taher C, Chuquimia OD, Mazurek J, Söderberg-Naucler C, Fernández C, Sköld M. 2013. Infection rate and tissue localization of murine IL-12p40-producing monocyte-derived CD103(+) lung dendritic cells during pulmonary tuberculosis. *PLoS ONE* **8:** e69287.

Leveton C, Barnass S, Champion B, Lucas S, De Souza B, Nicol M, Banerjee D, Rook G. 1989. T-cell-mediated protection of mice against virulent *Mycobacterium tuberculosis*. *Infect Immun* **57:** 390–395.

Lin KL, Suzuki Y, Nakano H, Ramsburg E, Gunn MD. 2008. CCR2$^+$ monocyte-derived dendritic cells and exudate macrophages produce influenza-induced pulmonary immune pathology and mortality. *J Immunol* **180:** 2562–2572.

Lin PL, Rutledge T, Green AM, Bigbee M, Fuhrman C, Klein E, Flynn JL. 2012. CD4 T cell depletion exacerbates acute *Mycobacterium tuberculosis* while reactivation of latent infection is dependent on severity of tissue depletion in cynomolgus macaques. *AIDS Res Hum Retroviruses* **28:** 1693–1702.

Long R, Maycher B, Scalcini M, Manfreda J. 1991. The chest roentgenogram in pulmonary tuberculosis patients seropositive for human immunodeficiency virus type 1. *Chest* **99:** 123–127.

Lowe DM, Redford PS, Wilkinson RJ, O'Garra A, Martineau AR. 2012. Neutrophils in tuberculosis: Friend or foe? *Trends Immunol* **33:** 14–25.

Lowes MA, Chamian F, Abello MV, Fuentes-Duculan J, Lin S-L, Nussbaum R, Novitskaya I, Carbonaro H, Cardinale I, Kikuchi T, et al. 2005. Increase in TNF-α and inducible nitric oxide synthase-expressing dendritic cells in psoriasis and reduction with efalizumab (anti-CD11a). *Proc Natl Acad Sci* **102:** 19057–19062.

Lyadova IV, Tsiganov EN, Kapina MA, Shepelkova GS, Sosunov VV, Radaeva TV, Majorov KB, Shmitova NS, van den Ham H-J, Ganusov VV, et al. 2010. In mice, tuberculosis progression is associated with intensive inflammatory response and the accumulation of Gr-1 cells in the lungs. *PLoS ONE* **5:** e10469.

Mariotti S, Pardini M, Gagliardi MC, Teloni R, Giannoni F, Fraziano M, Lozupone F, Meschini S, Nisini R. 2013. Dormant *Mycobacterium tuberculosis* fails to block phagosome maturation and shows unexpected capacity to stimulate specific human T lymphocytes. *J Immunol* **191:** 274–282.

Martin CJ, Booty MG, Rosebrock TR, Nunes-Alves C, Desjardins DM, Keren I, Fortune SM, Remold HG, Behar SM. 2012. Efferocytosis is an innate antibacterial mechanism. *Cell Host Microbe* **12:** 289–300.

Martin CJ, Peters KN, Behar SM. 2014. Macrophages clean up: Efferocytosis and microbial control. *Curr Opin Microbiol* **17C:** 17–23.

Matthews K, Wilkinson KA, Kalsdorf B, Roberts T, Diacon A, Walzl G, Wolske J, Ntsekhe M, Syed F, Russell J, et al. 2011. Predominance of interleukin-22 over interleukin-17 at the site of disease in human tuberculosis. *Tuberculosis* **91:** 587–593.

Mayer-Barber KD, Barber DL, Shenderov K, White SD, Wilson MS, Cheever A, Kugler D, Hieny S, Caspar P, Núñez G, et al. 2010. Caspase-1 independent IL-1beta production is critical for host resistance to *Mycobacterium tuberculosis* and does not require TLR signaling in vivo. *J Immunol* **184:** 3326–3330.

Mayer-Barber KD, Andrade BB, Barber DL, Hieny S, Feng CG, Caspar P, Oland S, Gordon S, Sher A. 2011. Innate and adaptive interferons suppress IL-1α and IL-1β production by distinct pulmonary myeloid subsets during *Mycobacterium tuberculosis* infection. *Immunity* **35:** 1023–1034.

Meintjes G, Wilkinson KA, Rangaka MX, Skolimowska K, van Veen K, Abrahams M, Seldon R, Pepper DJ, Rebe K, Mouton P, et al. 2008. Type 1 helper T cells and FoxP3-positive T cells in HIV-tuberculosis-associated immune reconstitution inflammatory syndrome. *Am J Resp Crit Care Med* **178:** 1083–1089.

Moreira AL, Tsenova L, Aman MH, Bekker L-G, Freeman S, Mangaliso B, Schröder U, Jagirdar J, Rom WN, Tovey MG, et al. 2002. Mycobacterial antigens exacerbate disease manifestations in *Mycobacterium tuberculosis*-infected mice. *Infect Immun* **70:** 2100–2107.

Mukadi Y, Perriëns JH, St Louis ME, Brown C, Prignot J, Willame JC, Pouthier F, Kaboto M, Ryder RW, Portaels F. 1993. Spectrum of immunodeficiency in HIV-1-infected patients with pulmonary tuberculosis in Zaire. *Lancet* **342:** 143–146.

Müller I, Cobbold SP, Waldmann H, Kaufmann SH. 1987. Impaired resistance to *Mycobacterium tuberculosis* infection after selective in vivo depletion of L3T4^{+} and Lyt-2^{+} T cells. *Infect Immun* **55:** 2037–2041.

Murphy J, Summer R, Wilson AA, Kotton DN, Fine A. 2008. The prolonged life-span of alveolar macrophages. *Am J Respir Cell Mol Biol* **38:** 380–385.

Mutnal MB, Schachtele SJ, Hu S, Lokensgard JR. 2013. T-cell reconstitution during murine acquired immunodeficiency syndrome (MAIDS) produces neuroinflammation and mortality in animals harboring opportunistic viral brain infection. *J Neuroinflammation* **10:** 98.

Nandi B, Behar SM. 2011. Regulation of neutrophils by interferon-γ limits lung inflammation during tuberculosis infection. *J Exp Med* **208:** 2251–2262.

Nicholson S, Bonecini-Almeida Mda G, Lapa e Silva JR, Nathan C, Xie QW, Mumford R, Weidner JR, Calaycay J, Geng J, Boechat N, et al. 1996. Inducible nitric oxide synthase in pulmonary alveolar macrophages from patients with tuberculosis. *J Exp Med* **183:** 2293–2302.

North RJ. 1998. Mice incapable of making IL-4 or IL-10 display normal resistance to infection with *Mycobacterium tuberculosis*. *Clin Exp Immunol* **113:** 55–58.

Obregón-Henao A, Henao-Tamayo M, Orme IM, Ordway DJ. 2013. Gr1^{int}CD11b^{+} myeloid-derived suppressor cells in *Mycobacterium tuberculosis* infection. *PLoS ONE* **8:** e80669.

Ordway DJ, Shang S, Henao-Tamayo M, Obregon-Henao A, Nold L, Caraway M, Shanley CA, Basaraba RJ, Duncan CG, Orme IM. 2011. *Mycobacterium bovis* BCG-mediated protection against W-Beijing strains of *Mycobacterium tuberculosis* is diminished concomitant with the emergence of regulatory T cells. *Clin Vaccine Immunol* **18:** 1527–1535.

Orme IM. 1988. Characteristics and specificity of acquired immunologic memory to *Mycobacterium tuberculosis* infection. *J Immunol* **140:** 3589–3593.

Pastores SM, Naidich DP, Aranda CP, McGuinnes G, Rom WN. 1993. Intrathoracic adenopathy associated with pulmonary tuberculosis in patients with human immunodeficiency virus infection. *Chest* **103:** 1433–1437.

Pawlowski A, Jansson M, Sköld M, Rottenberg ME, Källenius G. 2012. Tuberculosis and HIV co-infection. *PLoS Pathog* **8:** e1002464.

Pedrosa J, Saunders BM, Appelberg R, Orme IM, Silva MT, Cooper AM. 2000. Neutrophils play a protective, nonphagocytic, role in systemic *Mycobacterium* tuberculosis infection of mice. *Infect Immun* **68:** 577–583.

Perlman DC, el-Sadr WM, Nelson ET, Matts JP, Telzak EE, Salomon N, Chirgwin K, Hafner R. 1997. Variation of chest radiographic patterns in pulmonary tuberculosis by degree of human immunodeficiency virus-related immunosuppression. The Terry Beirn Community Programs for Clinical Research on AIDS (CPCRA). The AIDS Clinical Trials Group (ACTG). *Clin Infect Dis* **25:** 242–246.

Perreau M, Rozot V, Welles HC, Belluti-Enders F, Vigano S, Maillard M, Dorta G, Mazza-Stalder J, Bart P-A, Roger T, et al. 2013. Lack of *Mycobacterium tuberculosis*-specific interleukin-17A-producing CD4^{+} T cells in active disease. *Eur J Immunol.* **43:** 939–948.

Pieters J. 2008. *Mycobacterium tuberculosis* and the macrophage: Maintaining a balance. *Cell Host Microbe* **3:** 399–407.

Rabinowitz SS, Gordon S. 1991. Macrosialin, a macrophage-restricted membrane sialoprotein differentially glycosylated in response to inflammatory stimuli. *J Exp Med* **174:** 827–836.

Redford PS, Boonstra A, Read S, Pitt J, Graham C, Stavropoulos E, Bancroft GJ, O'Garra A. 2010. Enhanced protection to *Mycobacterium tuberculosis* infection in IL-10-deficient mice is accompanied by early and enhanced Th1 responses in the lung. *Eur J Immunol* **40:** 2200–2210.

Reiley WW, Calayag MD, Wittmer ST, Huntington JL, Pearl JE, Fountain JJ, Martino CA, Roberts AD, Cooper AM, Winslow GM, et al. 2008. ESAT-6-specific CD4 T cell responses to aerosol *Mycobacterium tuberculosis* infection are initiated in the mediastinal lymph nodes. *Proc Natl Acad Sci* **105:** 10961–10966.

Reiley WW, Shafiani S, Wittmer ST, Tucker Heard G, Moon JJ, Jenkins MK, Urdahl KB, Winslow GM, Woodland DL. 2010. Distinct functions of antigen-specific CD4 T cells during murine *Mycobacterium tuberculosis* infection. *Proc Natl Acad Sci* **107:** 19408–19413.

Reiling N, Ehlers S, Hölscher C. 2008. MyDths and un-TOLLed truths: Sensor, instructive and effector immunity to tuberculosis. *Immunol Lett* **116:** 15–23.

Repasy T, Lee J, Marino S, Martinez N, Kirschner DE, Hendricks G, Baker S, Wilson AA, Kotton DN, Kornfeld H. 2013. Intracellular bacillary burden reflects a burst size for *Mycobacterium tuberculosis* in vivo. *PLoS Pathog* **9:** e1003190.

Roach DR, Martin E, Bean AG, Rennick DM, Briscoe H, Britton WJ. 2001. Endogenous inhibition of antimycobacterial immunity by IL-10 varies between mycobacterial species. *Scand J Immunol* **54:** 163–170.

Rodrigo T, Caylà JA, García de Olalla P, Galdós-Tangüis H, Jansà JM, Miranda P, Brugal T. 1997. Characteristics of tuberculosis patients who generate secondary cases. *Int J Tuberc Lung Dis* **1:** 352–357.

Roths JB, Sidman CL. 1992. Both immunity and hyperresponsiveness to *Pneumocystis carinii* result from transfer of CD4^{+} but not CD8^{+} T cells into severe combined immunodeficiency mice. *J Clin Invest* **90:** 673–678.

Roths JB, Sidman CL. 1993. Single and combined humoral and cell-mediated immunotherapy of *Pneumocystis carinii* pneumonia in immunodeficient scid mice. *Infect Immun* **61:** 1641–1649.

Roths JB, Marshall JD, Allen RD, Carlson GA, Sidman CL. 1990. Spontaneous *Pneumocystis carinii* pneumonia in immunodeficient mutant scid mice. Natural history and pathobiology. *Am J Pathol* **136:** 1173–1186.

Sakai S, Kawamura I, Okazaki T, Tsuchiya K, Uchiyama R, Mitsuyama M. 2010. PD-1-PD-L1 pathway impairs Th1 immune response in the late stage of infection with *Mycobacterium bovis* bacillus Calmette-Guerin. *Int Immunol* **22:** 915–925.

Sakai S, Kauffman KD, Schenkel JM, McBerry CC, Mayer-Barber KD, Masopust D, Barber DL. 2014. Cutting edge: Control of *Mycobacterium tuberculosis* infection by a subset of lung parenchyma-homing CD4 T cells. *J Immunol* **192:** 2965–2969.

Samstein M, Schreiber HA, Leiner IM, Susac B, Glickman MS, Pamer EG. 2013. Essential yet limited role for $CCR2^{+}$ inflammatory monocytes during *Mycobacterium tuberculosis*-specific T cell priming. *eLife* **2:** e01086.

Saunders BM, Briscoe H, Britton WJ. 2004. T cell-derived tumour necrosis factor is essential, but not sufficient, for protection against *Mycobacterium tuberculosis* infection. *Clin Exp Immunol* **137:** 279–287.

Scanga CA, Mohan VP, Yu K, Joseph H, Tanaka K, Chan J, Flynn JL. 2000. Depletion of CD4(+) T cells causes reactivation of murine persistent tuberculosis despite continued expression of interferon γ and nitric oxide synthase 2. *J Exp Med* **192:** 347–358.

Scott-Browne JP, Shafiani S, Tucker-Heard G, Ishida-Tsubota K, Fontenot JD, Rudensky AY, Bevan MJ, Urdahl KB. 2007. Expansion and function of Foxp3-expressing T regulatory cells during tuberculosis. *J Exp Med* **204:** 2159–2169.

Scriba TJ, Kalsdorf B, Abrahams D-A, Isaacs F, Hofmeister J, Black G, Hassan HY, Wilkinson RJ, Walzl G, Gelderbloem SJ, et al. 2008. Distinct, specific IL-17- and IL-22-producing $CD4^{+}$ T cell subsets contribute to the human anti-mycobacterial immune response. *J Immunol* **180:** 1962–1970.

Serbina NV, Salazar-Mather TP, Biron CA, Kuziel WA, Pamer EG. 2003. TNF/iNOS-producing dendritic cells mediate innate immune defense against bacterial infection. *Immunity* **19:** 59–70.

Shafiani S, Tucker-Heard G, Kariyone A, Takatsu K, Urdahl KB. 2010. Pathogen-specific regulatory T cells delay the arrival of effector T cells in the lung during early tuberculosis. *J Exp Med* **207:** 1409–1420.

Shafiani S, Dinh C, Ertelt JM, Moguche AO, Siddiqui I, Smigiel KS, Sharma P, Campbell DJ, Way SS, Urdahl KB. 2013. Pathogen-specific Treg cells expand early during *Mycobacterium tuberculosis* infection but are later eliminated in response to Interleukin-12. *Immunity* **38:** 1261–1270.

Shang S, Harton M, Tamayo MH, Shanley C, Palanisamy GS, Caraway M, Chan ED, Basaraba RJ, Orme IM, Ordway DJ. 2011. Increased Foxp3 expression in guinea pigs infected with W-Beijing strains of *M. tuberculosis*. *Tuberculosis* **91:** 378–385.

Shenderov K, Barber DL, Mayer-Barber KD, Gurcha SS, Jankovic D, Feng CG, Oland S, Hieny S, Caspar P, Yamasaki S, et al. 2013. Cord factor and peptidoglycan recapitulate the Th17-promoting adjuvant activity of mycobacteria through mincle/CARD9 signaling and the inflammasome. *J Immunol* **190:** 5722–5730.

Sköld M, Behar SM. 2008. Tuberculosis triggers a tissue-dependent program of differentiation and acquisition of effector functions by circulating monocytes. *J Immunol* **181:** 6349–6360.

Srivastava S, Ernst JD. 2013. Cutting edge: Direct recognition of infected cells by CD4 T cells is required for control of intracellular *Mycobacterium tuberculosis* in vivo. *J Immunol* **191:** 1016–1020.

Stanley SA, Johndrow JE, Manzanillo P, Cox JS. 2007. The Type I IFN response to infection with *Mycobacterium tuberculosis* requires ESX-1-mediated secretion and contributes to pathogenesis. *J Immunol* **178:** 3143–3152.

Sugawara I, Udagawa T, Yamada H. 2004. Rat neutrophils prevent the development of tuberculosis. *Infect Immun* **72:** 1804–1806.

Sullivan BM, Jobe O, Lazarevic V, Vasquez K, Bronson R, Glimcher LH, Kramnik I. 2005. Increased susceptibility of mice lacking T-bet to infection with *Mycobacterium tuberculosis* correlates with increased IL-10 and decreased IFN-γ production. *J Immunol* **175:** 4593–4602.

Tameris MD, Hatherill M, Landry BS, Scriba TJ, Snowden MA, Lockhart S, Shea JE, McClain JB, Hussey GD, Hanekom WA, et al. 2013. Safety and efficacy of MVA85A, a new tuberculosis vaccine, in infants previously vaccinated with BCG: A randomised, placebo-controlled phase 2b trial. *Lancet* **381:** 1021–1028.

Taylor JL, Turner OC, Basaraba RJ, Belisle JT, Huygen K, Orme IM. 2003. Pulmonary necrosis resulting from DNA vaccination against tuberculosis. *Infect Immun* **71:** 2192–2198.

Tian T, Woodworth J, Sköld M, Behar SM. 2005. In vivo depletion of $CD11c^{+}$ cells delays the $CD4^{+}$ T cell response to *Mycobacterium tuberculosis* and exacerbates the outcome of infection. *J Immunol* **175:** 3268–3272.

Topalian SL, Hodi FS, Brahmer JR, Gettinger SN, Smith DC, McDermott DF, Powderly JD, Carvajal RD, Sosman JA, Atkins MB, et al. 2012. Safety, activity, and immune correlates of anti–PD-1 antibody in cancer. *N Engl J Med* **366:** 2443–2454.

Tousif S, Singh Y, Prasad DVR, Sharma P, Van Kaer L, Das G. 2011. T cells from Programmed Death-1 deficient mice respond poorly to *Mycobacterium tuberculosis* infection. *PLoS ONE* **6:** e19864.

Tsao TCY, Huang CC, Chiou WK, Yang PY, Hsieh MJ, Tsao KC. 2002. Levels of interferon-γ and interleukin-2 receptor-alpha for bronchoalveolar lavage fluid and serum were correlated with clinical grade and treatment of pulmonary tuberculosis. *Int J Tuberc Lung Dis* **6:** 720–727.

Tsiganov EN, Verbina EM, Radaeva TV, Sosunov VV, Kosmiadi GA, Nikitina IY, Lyadova IV. 2014. $Gr\text{-}1^{dim}CD11b^{+}$ immature myeloid-derived suppressor cells but not neutrophils are markers of lethal tuberculosis infection in mice. *J Immunol* **192:** 4718–4727.

Turner J, Rhoades ER, Keen M, Belisle JT, Frank AA, Orme IM. 2000a. Effective preexposure tuberculosis vaccines fail to protect when they are given in an immunotherapeutic mode. *Infect Immun* **68:** 1706–1709.

Turner OC, Roberts AD, Frank AA, Phalen SW, McMurray DM, Content J, Denis O, D'Souza S, Tanghe A, Huygen K, et al. 2000b. Lack of protection in mice and necrotizing bronchointerstitial pneumonia with bronchiolitis in guinea pigs immunized with vaccines directed against the hsp60 molecule of *Mycobacterium tuberculosis*. *Infect Immun* **68:** 3674–3679.

Turner J, Gonzalez-Juarrero M, Ellis DL, Basaraba RJ, Kipnis A, Orme IM, Cooper AM. 2002. In vivo IL-10 production reactivates chronic pulmonary tuberculosis in C57BL/6 mice. *J Immunol* **169:** 6343–6351.

Varol C, Yona S, Jung S. 2009. Origins and tissue-context-dependent fates of blood monocytes. *Immunol Cell Biol* **87:** 30–38.

Virchow R. 1891. Remarks on the effect of Koch's remedy on the internal organs of tuberculous patients. *Br Med J* **1:** 127–132.

Vosse E, Haverkamp MH, Ramirez Alejo N, Martinez Gallo M, Blancas Galicia L, Metin A, Garty BZ, Sun Tan Ç, Broides A, Paus RA, et al. 2013. IL-12Rβ1 Deficiency: Mutation update and description of the IL12RB1 variation database. *Hum Mutat* **34:** 1329–1339.

Wilson MS, Feng CG, Barber DL, Yarovinsky F, Cheever AW, Sher A, Grigg M, Collins M, Fouser L, Wynn TA. 2010. Redundant and pathogenic roles for IL-22 in mycobacterial, protozoan, and helminth infections. *J Immunol* **184:** 4378–4390.

Wolf AJ, Linas B, Trevejo-Nuñez GJ, Kincaid E, Tamura T, Takatsu K, Ernst JD. 2007. *Mycobacterium tuberculosis* infects dendritic cells with high frequency and impairs their function in vivo. *J Immunol* **179:** 2509–2519.

Wolf AJ, Desvignes L, Linas B, Banaiee N, Tamura T, Takatsu K, Ernst JD. 2008. Initiation of the adaptive immune response to *Mycobacterium tuberculosis* depends on antigen production in the local lymph node, not the lungs. *J Exp Med* **205:** 105–115.

Yamada H, Mizumo S, Horai R, Iwakura Y, Sugawara I. 2000. Protective role of interleukin-1 in mycobacterial infection in IL-1 α/β double-knockout mice. *Lab Invest* **80:** 759–767.

Yao S, Huang D, Chen CY, Halliday L, Wang RC, Chen ZW. 2014. $CD4^+$ T Cells contain early extrapulmonary tuberculosis (TB) dissemination and rapid TB progression and sustain multieffector functions of $CD8^+$ T and $CD3^-$ lymphocytes: Mechanisms of $CD4^+$ T cell immunity. *J Immunol* **192:** 2120–2132.

Zhang X, Majlessi L, Deriaud E, Leclerc C, Lo-Man R. 2009. Coactivation of Syk kinase and MyD88 adaptor protein pathways by bacteria promotes regulatory properties of neutrophils. *Immunity* **31:** 761–771.

Antigens for CD4 and CD8 T Cells in Tuberculosis

Cecilia S. Lindestam Arlehamn[1], David Lewinsohn[2,3], Alessandro Sette[1], and Deborah Lewinsohn[2]

[1]La Jolla Institute for Allergy and Immunology, La Jolla, California 92037

[2]Oregon Health and Science University, Portland, Oregon 97239

[3]Portland VA Medical Center, Portland, Oregon 97239

Correspondence: lewinsde@ohsu.edu

Tuberculosis (TB), caused by infection with *Mycobacterium tuberculosis* (MTB), represents an important cause of morbidity and mortality worldwide for which an improved vaccine and immunodiagnostics are urgently needed. CD4$^+$ and CD8$^+$ T cells play an important role in host defense to TB. Definition of the antigens recognized by these T cells is critical for improved understanding of the immunobiology of TB and for development of vaccines and diagnostics. Herein, the antigens and epitopes recognized by classically HLA class I– and II–restricted CD4$^+$ and CD8$^+$ T cells in humans infected with MTB are reviewed. Immunodominant antigens and epitopes have been defined using approaches targeting particular TB proteins or classes of proteins and by genome-wide discovery approaches. Antigens and epitopes recognized by classically restricted CD4$^+$ and CD8$^+$ T cells show extensive breadth and diversity in MTB-infected humans.

Mycobacterium tuberculosis (MTB), the intracellular bacterium that causes tuberculosis (TB), was discovered in 1882 by Robert Koch and is responsible for more human deaths than any other single pathogen today (WHO 2011). One-third of the world's population is infected by MTB, each year more than 1.5 million people die of TB, and more than 9 million develop TB (WHO 2011). Conquering this staggering problem is further complicated by the increasing prevalence of multidrug-resistant (MDR) and extensively drug-resistant (XDR) MTB strains (Gandhi et al. 2010) and recently virtually untreatable totally drug-resistant (TDR) strains (Velayati et al. 2009).

T-cell responses are essential for TB immunity, primarily because of the intracellular lifestyle of MTB. Both CD4$^+$ Th1 cells and CD8$^+$ T cells produce IFN-γ, which has been shown to be critical for protection in the murine TB model and for immune control in MTB-infected humans (Grotzke and Lewinsohn 2005; Flynn 2006; Winslow et al. 2008). A key role for IFN-γ in the control of TB is also clearly shown by increased susceptibility to TB in mice with a disrupted IFN-γ gene and in humans with mutations in genes involved in the IFN-γ and IL-12 pathways (Cooper et al. 1993; Flynn et al. 1993; de Jong et al. 1998; Dorman and Holland 2000). Because of this, IFN-γ production by T

Cite this article as *Cold Spring Harb Perspect Med* doi: 10.1101/cshperspect.a018465

cells has been a critical criterion for antigen discovery.

Many antigens have been identified and characterized, both classically HLA class I– and II–restricted (Blythe et al. 2007), as well as restricted by nonclassical molecules CD1 (Sieling et al. 1995), MR1 (Gold et al. 2010; Gold and Lewinsohn 2013), and HLA-E (Heinzel et al. 2002). MTB has evolved many strategies that subvert and evade the host adaptive response (Baena and Porcelli 2009). Because of the complexity of TB disease and diversity of donors, it is challenging to find antigens that are recognized by the majority of MTB-infected humans.

Defining the repertoire of antigenic targets is central to understanding the immune response against TB, and it has been vigorously pursued. Identification of novel epitopes and antigens from MTB is important because they can be used for identification and design of new vaccine candidates, diagnostics (including diagnostics to assess vaccine take), and markers to follow treatment response. Here we discuss discovery approaches and describe TB antigens and epitopes recognized by human classically restricted CD4$^+$ and CD8$^+$ T cells.

ROLE OF CD4$^+$ T CELLS IN CONTROLLING TUBERCULOSIS

Early murine studies and evidence from HIV infection have proved an essential role for CD4$^+$ T cells in the control of MTB infection. This was shown by antibody depletion of CD4$^+$ T cells (Muller et al. 1987), by adoptive transfer of CD4$^+$ T cells (Orme and Collins 1983, 1984), and in gene-disrupted mice (Caruso et al. 1999). In the case of HIV infection, loss of CD4$^+$ T cells results in progressive primary TB infection, reactivation of latent TB infection (LTBI), and enhanced susceptibility to reinfection (Barnes et al. 1991; Hopewell 1992; Raviglione et al. 1995). Strikingly, the risk for HIV$^+$TST$^+$ (tuberculin skin test) subjects to develop TB disease is 8%–10% annually compared with a 10% lifetime risk for HIV$^-$TST$^+$ individuals (Selwyn et al. 1989). Because these early experiments showed a dominant role for CD4$^+$ T cells in controlling TB infection, CD4 antigens have been more extensively characterized than CD8 antigens (Skjot et al. 2001; Reed and Lobet 2005).

PROTEIN-BASED ANTIGEN DISCOVERY

In the early 1990s attempts were made to dissect the secreted MTB proteome (Nagai et al. 1991). Traditional biochemical methods for separation and antigen discovery identified many immunodominant antigens from complex mycobacterial protein mixtures, abundant or easily purified proteins (Boesen et al. 1995; Covert et al. 2001; Andersen and Doherty 2005). A short-term culture filtrate was defined that was enriched in secreted antigens (Andersen et al. 1991). These secreted antigens were shown to offer a CD4$^+$ T-cell-dependent protective effect following vaccination in mice and guinea pigs (Hubbard et al. 1992; Pal and Horwitz 1992; Andersen 1994). This in turn led to a focus on antigen discovery in culture filtrates also strengthened by the notion that in contrast to live BCG (Bacillus Calmette–Guérin) vaccine, immunization with killed BCG confers little or no protection against infection with MTB, thus giving rise to the theory that active secretion of antigenic proteins induces appropriate protective T-cell responses (Orme et al. 1993; Horwitz et al. 1995). Recently it was shown that mycobacteria secrete membrane vesicles rich in antigens (Prados-Rosales et al. 2011). It is now clear, however, that T-cell antigens are also found among nonsecreted antigens. Several of the antigens identified early are now pursued as candidates for a TB vaccine, such as one of the most studied antigens from the mycobacterial secretome, antigen 85A, part of the antigen 85 complex of proteins (Ag85 A, B, and C) (Andersen and Doherty 2005).

Traditional methods rely on isolation of antigens from protein mixtures, offer limited proteome coverage, and depend on relative quantity and amenability to standard purification techniques. The completion of the MTB genome sequence (Cole et al. 1998) made more rational antigen discovery methods possible. Several studies have used bioinformatical approaches to select a subset of genes as antigen candidates (Bertholet et al. 2008; Chegou et al.

2012) or have screened MTB expression libraries in *Escherichia coli* with T-cell clones derived from individuals with LTBI (Coler et al. 2009). In only a few cases have techniques allowing ex vivo detection and/or characterization of MTB-specific T cells before any in vitro expansion and manipulations been used (Lalvani et al. 2001; Pathan et al. 2001; Lindestam Arlehamn et al. 2012, 2013).

EPITOPE DISCOVERY BY TARGETED APPROACHES

Several studies have reported the identification of T-cell epitopes from MTB in a wide variety of cohorts including individuals with TB disease, LTBI, BCG vaccination, or exposure to MTB and/or nontuberculosis mycobacteria (NTM, also known as environmental mycobacteria, atypical mycobacteria, and mycobacteria other than tuberculosis) (Vordermeier et al. 2003; Hammond et al. 2005; McMurry et al. 2005, 2007; Mustafa and Shaban 2006; Vani et al. 2006; Roupie et al. 2007; Lindestam Arlehamn et al. 2012). These studies have used either a classical approach using overlapping peptide pools covering a specific protein (Brock et al. 2004; Mustafa et al. 2005; Axelsson-Robertson et al. 2012) or reverse immunology based on bioinformatics tools followed by in vitro confirmation by demonstration of peptide-epitope-expanded T cells (Hammond et al. 2005; McMurry et al. 2007). However, similarly to antigen discovery efforts, these studies are restricted to a limited number of genes or HLA molecules resulting in a limited coverage of the MTB proteome (Blythe et al. 2007; Axelsson-Robertson et al. 2012). For the majority of antigens only very limited number of epitopes have been identified, whereas for others, such as ESAT-6 and CFP10 (Arend et al. 2000; Mustafa et al. 2000), a large number (>20) of epitopes have been described (Blythe et al. 2007; Axelsson-Robertson et al. 2012).

PROTEIN CATEGORIES OF DESCRIBED ANTIGENS

T-cell antigens have been described from all main MTB protein categories, indicating that protein function or cellular location per se does not determine which proteins can be recognized. Two important protein categories are the PE/PPE proteins and the Esx protein family, which have both been shown to elicit humoral and cellular immune responses (Akhter et al. 2011; Sampson 2011). PE/PPE proteins are found exclusively in pathogenic mycobacteria. The function(s) of PE/PPE proteins are not fully understood, but data indicates that they influence bacterial attachment to host cells, immunomodulation, antigen presentation, and host cell apoptosis (Akhter et al. 2011; Sampson 2011). The PE/PPE genes encode almost 200 proteins and constitute almost 10% of the TB genome coding capacity (Cole et al. 1998). They are categorized based on their proline-glutamic acid (PE) and proline-proline-glutamic acid (PPE) motifs near their amino termini (Sampson 2011). PE/PPE proteins are mainly located within the bacterial cell wall and cell surface; however, some are also secreted, thus readily accessible to the immune system (Abdallah et al. 2009).

The PE/PPE genes are closely related to the Esx regions. Esx regions encode Type VII secretion systems (or ESX systems) and include well-known antigens such as ESAT-6 (early secretory antigenic target-6, EsxA) and CFP10 (culture filtrate protein 10, EsxB) (Gey van Pittius et al. 2006). Secretion of some PE/PPE proteins is dependent on ESX systems. All ESX systems, five complete and six incomplete systems in TB, carry a pair of genes that encode homologs of ESAT-6 and CFP10, and most of them also encode PE/PPE proteins (Gey van Pittius et al. 2001). Despite these similarities these systems do not complement each other and play distinct roles in TB virulence and physiology (Gey van Pittius et al. 2001).

Attenuation of BCG resulted in major deletions of 129 open reading frames (ORFs), among which were the RD1 region containing ESAT-6 and CFP10. The genes in this region play an important role in virulence, as shown by attenuation of TB with a knockout in the RD1 region (Andersen and Doherty 2005). The antigens from RD1 are strongly recognized by a majority of MTB-infected individuals, and commercial tests for LTBI (QuantiFERON and T-SPOT.TB) use ESAT-6 and CFP10 as antigens (Lalvani et al. 1998, 2001; Ulrichs et al. 1998; Ravn et al. 1999; Arend et al. 2000; Mustafa et al. 2000; Olsen et al. 2000; Pathan et al. 2000; van Pinxteren et al. 2000; Aagaard et al. 2004; Brock et al. 2004; Mori et al. 2004; Shams et al. 2004). These tests marked a major advance in diagnosis of LTBI compared with the classically used TST, which is not able to distinguish between LTBI and BCG vaccination. In addition to BCG, ESAT-6 and CFP10 are also absent from the majority of NTM, providing an ability to distinguish LTBI not only from BCG vaccination but also some of the NTM diseases (Harboe et al. 1996; Lalvani et al. 1998; Behr et al. 1999).

METABOLIC STATE–SPECIFIC ANTIGENS

During infection, MTB alters its metabolic state from active replication to slow or nonreplication, which is accompanied by changes in the gene expression profile and thus protein expression and antigens available to the immune system (Schnappinger et al. 2003). Expression of early secreted antigens decrease, whereas antigens encoded during starvation and dormancy increase (Leyten et al. 2006; Rustad et al. 2008; Schuck et al. 2009). Furthermore, the MTB genome encodes a large number of regulatory proteins (Cole et al. 1998), which indicates an ability to adapt to different environments by altered gene expression (Yuan et al. 1996; Triccas and Gicquel 2000; Florczyk et al. 2001; Honer zu Bentrup and Russell 2001; Mehrotra and Bishai 2001). Other antigens have been described as "resuscitation antigens" (Commandeur et al. 2011b), which are small bacterial proteins that promote proliferation of dormant mycobacteria, and are therefore believed to be involved in the reactivation of MTB. The discovery of these metabolic state–specific antigens provided the hypothesis that these might be preferentially recognized by certain stages of infection.

DISEASE STAGE–SPECIFIC ANTIGENS

The identification of disease stage–specific antigens is difficult (Honer zu Bentrup and Russell 2001), but there is evidence of stage-specific antigens in humans (Wilkinson et al. 1998; Leyten et al. 2006). Initial studies used MTB grown under conditions that mimic the environmental stresses believed to be encountered in granulomas such as hypoxia, low pH, NO, nutrient deprivation, and host immune pressure (Yuan et al. 1996; Florczyk et al. 2001; Monahan et al. 2001). Under these conditions MTB is believed to be in a dormant state and genes encoded by the DosR regulon are up-regulated. Several antigens encoded by this regulon have been described as preferentially recognized by individuals with LTBI (Black et al. 2009; Schuck et al. 2009), but other studies failed to detect this correlation (Gideon et al. 2010). The resuscitation antigens also do not distinguish LTBI from TB disease. The difficulty in identifying disease stage–specific antigens is complicated by the spectrum of infection ranging from sterilizing immunity, to subclinical active disease to fulminant active disease (Young et al. 2009). Furthermore, hypoxic lesions are found in both LTBI and TB disease (Barry III et al. 2009; Young et al. 2009). The relative scarcity of data relating to disease stage–specific antigens may also be related to the lack of a genome-wide screen of MTB reactivity in individuals with different stages of MTB infection and disease.

GENOME-WIDE ANTIGEN DISCOVERY

MTB has a very large genome with around 4000 ORFs (Cole et al. 1998), and identification of T-cell antigens/epitopes from such a large genome is especially challenging, yet necessary for vaccine development, vaccine trials, and disease monitoring. Several investigations have tried to identify immunodominant antigens through genomics and proteomics (Covert et al. 2001; Malen et al. 2008; Deenadayalan et al. 2010), comparative genomics (Cockle et al. 2002), or bioinformatics (Zvi et al. 2008), none of which covered the entire genome. The majority of the MTB genome was covered in an investigation for in vivo expression of MTB genes during MTB infection in the lungs of mice (Commandeur et al. 2013). Identified antigens were confirmed in humans with TB disease and may represent antigen candidates for vaccine development.

Advances in high-throughput peptide synthesis had made it possible to perform a genome-wide analysis for MTB antigens (Lindestam Arlehamn et al. 2013). Taking advantage of computational prediction methods and high-throughput assays to identify immunodominant epitopes and antigens, a synthetic peptide library was constructed following predictions for binding affinity to common DR, DP, and DQ HLA class II alleles representative of those most commonly expressed in the general population, using a consensus approach based on three prediction methods (Wang et al. 2008). The advantage of this approach is that it identifies the optimal set of peptide candidates for immunogenicity testing, eliminating the necessity of synthesizing a large number of overlapping peptides and, more importantly, circumvents the need to test each one of them for binding to numerous HLA class II molecules in vitro. Circulating T cells from individuals with LTBI were then directly tested against the peptide library using high-throughput IFN-γ ELISPOT (enzyme-linked immunosorbent spot [assay]), which is in contrast to other studies in which in vitro expansion is typically preformed. The results published recently identified hundreds of new CD4 epitopes and several antigens. Analysis of responses revealed that natural immunity to MTB is multiantigenic and enriched for responses to secreted and cell wall–associated proteins such as PE/PPE and ESX-associated proteins, consistent with earlier studies as described above. However, both secreted and nonsecreted proteins were shown to induce a strong immune response. A large fraction of the identified PE/PPE proteins were novel, which implies that there is still a lot to discover. The prevalence of responses to PE/PPE and ESX proteins could represent cross-reactive epitopes shared by multiple homologous family members (Sayes et al. 2012). It has been shown that T-cell responses were greater to peptide pools representing the conserved amino-terminal region of PE/PPE proteins than to peptide pools representing other regions of the protein (Vordermeier et al. 2012). The same phenomenon has not yet been shown for ESX proteins. In addition, the genome-wide screen identified three distinct antigenic regions all containing Esx protein pairs and two containing type VII secretion systems ESX-1 and ESX-3.

High-throughput approaches do not capture all immunodominant antigens. In this respect, it is important to highlight that a number of studies have shown that many peptides with highly promiscuous binding capacity are frequently recognized by immune individuals (Alexander et al. 1994; Lamonaca et al. 1999; Doolan et al. 2000; Wilson et al. 2001; Tangri et al. 2005), and that promiscuous recognition in the context of multiple HLA class II molecules may be a mechanism significantly contributing to epitope immunodominance (Lindestam Arlehamn et al. 2012). Studies have showed that bioinformatics predictions directed toward selection of the most promiscuous binding peptides can allow identification of a dominant fraction of the pathogen-specific response (Assarsson et al. 2008; Oseroff et al. 2010, 2012a,b).

Two studies have used analysis of serum antibody responses, as a surrogate for $CD4^+$ T-cell responses, to interrogate the entire MTB proteome for antigens (Kunnath-Velayudhan et al. 2010; Li et al. 2010). These studies relied on the assumption that there is a strong linkage between targets of antibodies and of the $CD4^+$ Th cells involved in their generation (Sette et al. 2008). In these studies ~6%–10% of the proteome was found to be immunogenic and also enriched for secreted and cell wall–associated proteins. In particular these studies also identified a prominence of responses to PE/PPE and ESX protein families, emphasizing the immunodominance of these proteins.

The comprehensive proteome-wide screens for epitopes and serum antibody responses revealed striking levels of heterogeneity of responses to MTB in humans. This might reflect differences in MTB strains, bacillary load, and metabolic state, resulting in qualitative or quantitative differences in antigen expression.

Once defined, T-cell epitope responses can be characterized by several different approaches, including determination of the secreted cytokine patterns by intracellular cytokine staining, characterization of the specific T-cell subsets generated in response to the epitopes by the use of tetramer staining reagents, and characterization of memory phenotypes. Importantly, definition of T-cell epitopes allows in-depth characterization and tracking of responding T-cell subsets. The genome-wide screen for $CD4^+$ T-cell epitopes documented the novel observation that T cells in individuals with LTBI are confined to a recently described $CXCR3^+$ $CCR6^+$ phenotype (Acosta-Rodriguez et al. 2007; Gosselin et al. 2010; Lindestam Arlehamn et al. 2013).

ROLE OF $CD8^+$ T CELLS IN TB HOST DEFENSE

As discussed above, control of MTB infection relies heavily on the cellular immune system—that is, the interaction of lymphocytes and MTB-infected macrophages and dendritic cells (DCs) (Flynn and Chan 2001; North and Jung 2004). Although the essential role of $CD4^+$ T cells in TB host defense was defined first, ample experimental evidence in the mouse TB model now suggests a protective role for $CD8^+$ T cells as well. Adoptive transfer or in vivo depletion of $CD8^+$ cells showed that this subset could confer protection against subsequent challenge (Muller et al. 1987; Orme 1987; Silva et al. 1994). β2-microglobulin-deficient mice, deficient in expression of major histocompatibility complex (MHC) class I (Flynn et al. 1992), and CD8-deficient mice (Sousa et al. 2000) are more susceptible to MTB infection than their wild-type littermates. As reviewed above, because IFN-γ is an important TB host defense effector molecule and $CD8^+$ T cells represent a cellular source of this cytokine, this set of experimental evidence also supports the importance of $CD8^+$ T cells. Finally, evidence in both mice and non-human primates suggests that $CD8^+$ T cells may play a unique role in the immune surveillance of chronic infection (Cooper 2009). In humans, MTB-specific $CD8^+$ T cells have been identified in MTB-infected individuals and include $CD8^+$ T cells that are classically, HLA class Ia–restricted, and nonclassically, HLA class Ib, restricted by HLA-E (Lewinsohn et al. 1998; Heinzel et al. 2002) and by CD1 (Beckman et al. 1996; Rosat et al. 1999; Moody et al. 2000). $CD8^+$ T cells share some redundant effector mechanisms with $CD4^+$ T cells, such as IFN-γ secretion and cytolytic functions (Lewinsohn et al. 2011). However, $CD8^+$ T cells can also play a unique role in TB host defense. $CD8^+$ T cells preferentially recognize and destroy heavily infected macrophages (Lewinsohn et al. 2003). This ability to distinguish heavily infected cells suggests that the magnitude of the $CD8^+$ T-cell response may represent a sensor of intracellular burden. In support of this, the magnitude of the $CD8^+$ T-cell response decreased in adults effectively treated for pulmonary TB (Nyendak et al. 2013), Rosat et al. showed higher $CD8^+$ T-cell response in adults with pulmonary TB than with extrapulmonary TB and with extrapulmonary TB than with LTBI (Rosat et al. 1999), and the presence of detectable $CD8^+$ T-cell responses in young children distinguished those with pulmonary TB from asymptomatic household contacts of adults with infectious TB (Lancioni et al. 2012). $CD8^+$ T cells are also able to eliminate infected HLA class II–negative cells such as epithelial cells, endothelial cells, and fibroblasts, as well as inhibit mycobacterial growth and induce apoptosis in infected cells (Lazarevic and Flynn 2002). The role of apoptosis as a host defense mechanism has been highlighted by Behar and colleagues (Behar et al. 2010; Divangahi et al. 2010). Furthermore, components of the cytotoxic granule, such as granulysin, may play a direct role in the inhibition of MTB growth (Stenger et al. 1998). Taken together, studies of mice and humans support an important role for $CD8^+$ T cells in TB immunity.

PROCESSING AND PRESENTATION OF TB ANTIGENS TO CLASSICALLY RESTRICTED $CD8^+$ T CELLS

$CD8^+$ T cells typically recognize short peptides of 9–11 amino acids in length derived from cytosolic proteins, such as viral proteins, that are presented by HLA class I molecules. That MTB antigen does get into the class I processing pathway is evidenced by the induction of classically restricted CD8$^+$ T cells in MTB-infected individuals. Yet how this occurs is not straightforward. Rather, MTB antigen likely accesses the class I processing pathway through multiple mechanisms, which include both pathways that include and do not include trafficking of antigenic peptide through the cytosol. Noncytosolic pathways include a TAP (transporter for antigen presentation)- and proteasome-independent MHC-I recycling pathway (Pfeifer et al. 1993; Song and Harding 1996) and cross-presentation through the uptake of exosomes including MTB lipids and proteins (Beatty et al. 2000, 2001; Beatty and Russell 2000) or of apoptotic bodies (Schaible et al. 2003). However, most evidence supports that antigenic peptide accesses the cytosol (Behar 2013). Specifically, evidence suggests that in primary human DCs, MTB phagosomes contain class I processing machinery, and antigens contained in the phagosome are retrotranslocated into the cytosol, processed in a proteasome- and TAP-dependent manner, and egress to the cell surface through the endoplasmic reticulum Golgi apparatus (Grotzke et al. 2009, 2010).

DEFINITION OF CD8 TB ANTIGENS

As described above, substantial effort has been dedicated to the definition of TB CD4 antigens and, more recently, epitopes. In contrast, much less effort has been expended to date on TB CD8 antigens, perhaps because the importance of CD8$^+$ T cells in host defense to TB has been more recently defined. In fact, many investigations defining CD8 antigens have focused on MTB proteins already well characterized as CD4 antigens (Smith et al. 2000; Lewinsohn et al. 2007; Commandeur et al. 2011a). For example, Smith et al. investigated recognition of CD4 antigens Ag85A, Ag85B, and ESAT-6 by CD8$^+$ T cells. Peripheral blood mononuclear cells (PBMCs) from BCG-vaccinated individuals or individuals with TB disease were expanded in vitro with MTB and then CD8$^+$ T cells responding to antigen-presenting cells (APCs) expressing Ag85A, Ag85B, or ESAT-6 were measured using intracellular cytokine staining (ICS) with analysis by flow cytometry (Smith et al. 2000). CD8$^+$ T cells from individuals with TB disease recognized all three antigens, whereas CD8$^+$ T cells from healthy BCG-vaccinated individuals recognized only Ag85A and Ag85B. Lewinsohn et al. (2007) compared ex vivo CD8$^+$ T-cell responses in individuals with LTBI, TB disease, or no infection using autologous DC displaying overlapping 15-mers representing each protein and CD8$^+$ T cells positively selected from PBMC in an IFN-γ ELISPOT assay. In this study, CD8$^+$ T cells recognizing known CD4 antigens Mtb39, CFP10, ESAT-6, Ag85, EsxG, 19 kDa, and Mtb 9.9a were detected only in MTB-infected individuals (LTBI and TB disease). Commandeur et al. (2011a) focused on another TB protein group of interest, proteins expressed from the DosR-regulon (Rv1733 and Rv2029c), and compared the CD8$^+$ T-cell responses with those directed toward Ag85B and HspX (hsp 16, a-crystallin, Rv 2031c) in a unique group of elderly individuals with LTBI who had never received TB therapy. Using ICS with analysis by flow cytometry and overlapping 20-mers as a source of antigen, they showed stronger IFN-γ/TNF-α producing CD8$^+$ T cells to the DosR-regulon encoded proteins and HspX as compared with Ag85, and no CD8$^+$ T-cell responses in MTB-uninfected individuals. In summary, study of CD8$^+$ T-cell responses to entire MTB proteins has been fairly limited and shows that both BCG and MTB infection can induce CD8$^+$ T cells to proteins shared by BCG and TB, and, as might be expected, only MTB infection induces CD8$^+$ T-cell responses to proteins found only in MTB, such as CFP10 and ESAT-6.

DEFINITION OF CD8 TB EPITOPES: TARGETING MTB PROTEINS OF INTEREST

By far the preponderance of studies defining CD8 epitopes focus on MTB proteins of interest and use a "reverse immunogenetics" approach—that is, the MTB protein of interest is interrogated for peptides predicted to bind to a particular HLA allele, and then a CD8$^+$ T-cell response restricted by this HLA allele is shown in MTB-infected individuals. In these studies MHC restriction is showed using tetramers or, as in the case of HLA-A*02:01, by recognition of T2 cells or THP-1 cells only expressing A*02:01. In fact, perhaps because of the availability of these reagents, and that A*02 is a commonly expressed allele with a well-defined motif, HLA-A*02:01 has been the most thoroughly studied. HLA-A*02:01-restricted CD8$^+$ T-cell responses within MTB-infected individuals have been shown in epitopes contained within a variety of proteins including secreted proteins Ag85B (Weichold et al. 2007), ESAT-6 (Lalvani et al. 1998; Axelsson-Robertson et al. 2013), TB10.4 (Axelsson-Robertson et al. 2010), Mtb19 (Mohagheghpour et al. 1998), SodA (Dong et al. 2004), AlaDH (Dong et al. 2004), Glns (Dong et al. 2004), 38-kDa antigen (Shams et al. 2003), and 28-kDa hemolysin (Shams et al. 2003); PE/PPE family members PE_PGRS33, PE_PGRS62, and PPE46 (Chaitra et al. 2008); and proteins expressed during hypoxia, the 16-kDa antigen (Caccamo et al. 2002), and Rv1733c (Commandeur et al. 2011a). Additional HLA-A alleles have been interrogated for MTB proteins of interest and CD8 epitopes defined. These include A*24:02, A*30:01, A*30:02, A*68:01, and A*68:02-restricted epitopes in ESAT-6 (Pathan et al. 2000; Axelsson-Robertson et al. 2013), A*01:01, A*03:01, A*11:01, A*24:02, A*30:01, A*30:02, and A*68:01-restricted epitopes in TB10.4 (Axelsson-Robertson et al. 2011, 2013), and A*01:01, A*11:01, A*24:02, A*30:01, A*30:02, and A*68:01-restricted epitopes in Ag85B (Weichold et al. 2007; Axelsson-Robertson et al. 2013). HLA-B alleles have been less frequently interrogated by this approach. However, several HLA-B-restricted CD8 epitopes have been defined, including B*52, B*07:02, and B*58:01-restricted epitopes in ESAT-6 (Lalvani et al. 1998; Axelsson-Robertson et al. 2013), B*07:02, B*08:01, B*15:01, and B*58:01-restricted epitopes in TB10.4 (Axelsson-Robertson et al. 2010, 2013), and B*07:02, B*08:01, B*15:01, and B*58:01-restricted epitopes in Ag85B (Weichold et al. 2007; Axelsson-Robertson et al. 2013).

One measure of immunodominance is the detection of strong (high-magnitude) CD8$^+$ T-cell responses directly ex vivo in MTB-infected individuals. In this regard, using the "reverse immunogenetics" approach, several studies report strong ex vivo CD8$^+$ T-cell responses as have been observed for common viruses (Yewdell and Bennink 1999), in MTB-infected individuals using IFN-γ ELISPOT (Lalvani et al. 1998; Pathan et al. 2000), ICS with analysis by flow cytometry (Caccamo et al. 2002), or tetramer analysis (Weichold et al. 2007; Axelsson-Robertson et al. 2010, 2011, 2013). However, in many studies ex vivo CD8$^+$ T-cell responses were not performed (Mohagheghpour et al. 1998; Shams et al. 2003; Dong et al. 2004; Chaitra et al. 2008) requiring establishment of T-cell lines or clones in vitro to define the epitope, suggesting that these do not represent immunodominant epitopes.

Although all studies reported here isolated CD8$^+$ T cells recognizing these epitopes from MTB-infected individuals, only a few studies looked at specificity—that is, whether or not epitope-specific T cells could be detected in individuals without MTB infection—and all showed the absence of epitope-specific CD8$^+$ T-cell responses in uninfected individuals (Mohagheghpour et al. 1998; Pathan et al. 2000; Caccamo et al. 2002; Dong et al. 2004). However, the majority of studies only looked at MTB-infected individuals. This is especially problematic for the interpretation of the studies by Axelsson-Robertson et al. (2011, 2012, 2013) who reported particularly broad and numerous epitopes within a few MTB proteins, some of which were detected at relatively low frequencies. Using tetramer analysis, these studies did not look at uninfected individuals, and either did not study MTB-infected individuals with HLA-type mismatched for the tetramer HLA allele, or when MTB-infected individuals with mismatched HLA alleles were investigated, reactivity in these HLA-mismatched individuals was detected, although attributed to promiscuous epitopes. Nonetheless, when taking the literature in aggregate, CD8$^+$ T cells are readily detected in MTB-infected individuals and CD8 epitopes are present in almost every MTB protein investigated.

DEFINITION OF CD8 TB EPITOPES: GENOME-WIDE APPROACH

With the sequencing of the MTB genome completed (Cole et al. 1998), two more recent studies have interrogated the entire MTB genome for CD8 epitopes. Caccamo et al. (2009) evaluated the MTB genome for 9-mer peptide sequences predicted to bind to A2*01 and then showed binding of peptides predicted to bind with the highest affinity. Six peptides showing the highest binding affinity for A2*01 were tested using tetramers in individuals with TB and LTBI. Using this approach they reported two new CD8 epitopes restricted by A*02:01 in Rv1490 and Rv1614. Moreover, these epitopes were observed in those with TB and LTBI but not in uninfected individuals. In addition, Tang et al. (2011) screened the entire H37Rv genome for 9-mers predicted to bind to A*02:01, A*03:01, and B*07:02, evaluating predicted affinity as well as processing and presentation. Screening more than 400 peptides in individuals with LTBI, the highest frequencies of responses were found within secreted proteins and within MTB proteins commonly used in TB vaccines. From these data 18 tetramers were selected and 16 of 18 tetramers detected epitope-specific $CD8^+$ T cells in 16 distinct MTB proteins, many of which have unknown function.

DEFINITION OF CD8 TB EPITOPES: USING T CELLS RECOGNIZING THE MTB-INFECTED CELL

An alternative approach to CD8 epitope discovery uses $CD8^+$ T cells derived from MTB-infected individuals that recognize an MTB-infected cell. The advantage of this approach is that it is unbiased with regard to the HLA restricting allele. First, to identify the MTB protein recognized, $CD8^+$ T-cell clones, derived from individuals with LTBI and isolated using MTB-infected DC, were screened against either a limited synthetic peptide library comprised of 15-mers overlapping by 11 amino acids representing known CD4 antigens (Lewinsohn et al. 2001, 2007) or a more comprehensive peptide library representing 10% of the MTB proteome selected for potential antigenicity (Lewinsohn et al. 2013). Peptide pools were deconvoluted to identify the 15-mer recognized, and then nested peptides within the 15-mer were used to identify the minimal epitope. Using this approach, 17 epitopes were defined located in several previously defined CD4 antigens (CFP10, EsxG, Mtb8.4, and Ag85), as well as in EsxJ and members of the PE/PPE family of MTB proteins (PE9 and PE_PGRS). Strikingly, using this approach unbiased for HLA alleles, all but one of these epitopes are restricted by a diverse set of HLA-B alleles. Thus, further delineation of TB epitopes will require careful evaluation of HLA-B alleles. Finally, these epitopes were recognized at high frequency in individuals from whom they were recognized, suggesting that this approach was efficient at identifying immunodominant epitopes.

CONCLUDING REMARKS

For both $CD4^+$ and $CD8^+$ T-cell responses in TB, there is extensive diversity of immunodominant responses in infected individuals. For both CD4 and CD8 antigens, secreted antigens are important. Moreover, there is extensive overlap between defined CD4 and CD8 antigens. However, this is likely biased by the CD8 discovery process, which at least initially, focused on previously defined CD4 antigens.

Several important gaps remain to be addressed in the definition of CD4 and CD8 TB antigens, particularly in regard to the spectrum, magnitude, and phenotypes of T-cell responses elicited by different disease stages and vaccination strategies. First, given the breadth and diversity of immunodominant antigens defined thus far, and the relatively limited number of studies using genome-wide approaches, there likely remain more CD4 and CD8 TB antigens and epitopes to be defined. In addition, studies comparing the antigenic specificity, magnitude, and phenotype of T-cell responses in different stages of MTB infection, from LTBI to subclinical disease to advanced TB disease, remain limited. Thus far, neither CD4 nor CD8 antigen recognition can distinguish those with LTBI from those with TB disease. In this regard, there may be antigens and/or epitopes that are specifically recognized in a particular disease stage or a particular phenotype associated with a disease stage. Moreover, different disease stages may show distinct composite immunologic signatures. Regardless, more extensive definition of T-cell antigens and epitopes are likely to inform immunologic definition of disease stages and may be used to develop accurate correlates of protective immunity to use in TB vaccine studies and/or immunodiagnostics to identify individuals who may benefit from early therapy.

ACKNOWLEDGMENTS

Aeras TB Vaccine Foundation, a nonprofit organization, has licensed technology from Oregon Health and Science University (OHSU) of which Dr. David Lewinsohn and Dr. Deborah Lewinsohn are inventors. Published literature related to this technology is reviewed herein. In addition, OHSU, Dr. David Lewinsohn, and Dr. Deborah Lewinsohn have a financial interest in ViTi, Inc., a company that may have a commercial interest in some research results reported in the published literature that is reviewed herein. This potential individual and institutional conflict of interest has been reviewed and managed by OHSU.

REFERENCES

Aagaard C, Brock I, Olsen A, Ottenhoff THM, Weldingh K, Andersen P. 2004. Mapping immune reactivity toward Rv2653 and Rv2654: Two novel low-molecular-mass antigens found specifically in the *Mycobacterium tuberculosis* complex. *J Infect Dis* **189:** 812–819.

Abdallah AM, Verboom T, Weerdenburg EM, Gey van Pittius NC, Mahasha PW, Jiménez C, Parra M, Cadieux N, Brennan MJ, Appelmelk BJ, et al. 2009. PPE and PE_PGRS proteins of *Mycobacterium marinum* are transported via the type VII secretion system ESX-5. *Mol Microbiol* **73:** 329–340.

Acosta-Rodriguez EV, Rivino L, Geginat J, Jarrossay D, Gattorno M, Lanzavecchia A, Sallusto F, Napolitani G. 2007. Surface phenotype and antigenic specificity of human interleukin 17-producing T helper memory cells. *Nat Immunol* **8:** 639–646.

Akhter Y, Ehebauer MT, Mukhopadhyay S, Hasnain SE. 2011. The PE/PPE multigene family codes for virulence factors and are a possible source of mycobacterial antigenic variation: Perhaps more? *Biochimie* **94:** 110–116.

Alexander J, Sidney J, Southwood S, Ruppert J, Oseroff C, Maewal A, Snoke K, Serra HM, Kubo RT, Sette A, et al. 1994. Development of high potency universal DR-restricted helper epitopes by modification of high affinity DR-blocking peptides. *Immunity* **1:** 751–761.

Andersen P. 1994. The T cell response to secreted antigens of *Mycobacterium tuberculosis*. *Immunobiology* **191:** 537–547.

Andersen P, Doherty TM. 2005. TB subunit vaccines—Putting the pieces together. *Microbes Infect* **7:** 911–921.

Andersen P, Askgaard D, Ljungqvist L, Bennedsen J, Heron I. 1991. Proteins released from *Mycobacterium tuberculosis* during growth. *Infect Immun* **59:** 1905–1910.

Arend SM, Geluk A, van Meijgaarden KE, van Dissel JT, Theisen M, Andersen P, Ottenhoff THM. 2000. Antigenic equivalence of human T-cell responses to *Mycobacterium tuberculosis*-specific RD1-encoded protein antigens ESAT-6 and culture filtrate protein 10 and to mixtures of synthetic peptides. *Infect Immun* **68:** 3314–3321.

Assarsson E, Bui H-H, Sidney J, Zhang Q, Glenn J, Oseroff C, Mbawuike IN, Alexander J, Newman MJ, Grey H, et al. 2008. Immunomic analysis of the repertoire of T-cell specificities for influenza A virus in humans. *J Virol* **82:** 12241–12251.

Axelsson-Robertson R, Weichold F, Sizemore D, Wulf M, Skeiky YA, Sadoff J, Maeurer MJ. 2010. Extensive major histocompatibility complex class I binding promiscuity for *Mycobacterium tuberculosis* TB10.4 peptides and immune dominance of human leucocyte antigen (HLA)-B*0702 and HLA-B*0801 alleles in TB10.4 CD8 T-cell responses. *Immunology* **129:** 496–505.

Axelsson-Robertson R, Ahmed RK, Weichold FF, Ehlers MM, Kock MM, Sizemore D, Sadoff J, Maeurer M. 2011. Human leukocyte antigens A*3001 and A*3002 show distinct peptide-binding patterns of the *Mycobacterium tuberculosis* protein TB10.4: Consequences for immune recognition. *Clin Vaccine Immunol* **18:** 125–134.

Axelsson-Robertson R, Magalhaes I, Parida SK, Zumla A, Maeurer M. 2012. The immunological footprint of *Mycobacterium tuberculosis* T-cell epitope recognition. *J Infect Dis* **205:** S301–S315.

Axelsson-Robertson R, Loxton AG, Walzl G, Ehlers MM, Kock MM, Zumla A, Maeurer M. 2013. A broad profile of co-dominant epitopes shapes the peripheral *Mycobacterium tuberculosis* specific $CD8^+$ T-cell immune response in South African patients with active tuberculosis. *PLoS ONE* **8:** e58309.

Baena A, Porcelli SA. 2009. Evasion and subversion of antigen presentation by *Mycobacterium tuberculosis*. *Tissue Antigens* **74:** 189–204.

Barnes PF, Bloch AB, Davidson PT, Snider DE Jr. 1991. Tuberculosis in patients with human immunodeficiency virus infection. *N Engl J Med* **324:** 1644–1650.

Barry CE 3rd, Boshoff HI, Dartois V, Dick T, Ehrt S, Flynn J, Schnappinger D, Wilkinson RJ, Young D. 2009. The spectrum of latent tuberculosis: Rethinking the biology and intervention strategies. *Nat Rev Microbiol* **7:** 845–855.

Beatty WL, Russell DG. 2000. Identification of mycobacterial surface proteins released into subcellular compartments of infected macrophages. *Infect Immun* **68:** 6997–7002.

Beatty WL, Rhoades ER, Ullrich HJ, Chatterjee D, Heuser JE, Russell DG. 2000. Trafficking and release of mycobacterial lipids from infected macrophages. *Traffic* **1:** 235–247.

Beatty WL, Ullrich HJ, Russell DG. 2001. Mycobacterial surface moieties are released from infected macrophages by a constitutive exocytic event. *Eur J Cell Biol* **80:** 31–40.

Beckman EM, Melian A, Behar SM, Sieling PA, Chatterjee D, Furlong ST, Matsumoto R, Rosat JP, Modlin RL, Porcelli SA. 1996. CD1c restricts responses of mycobacteria-specific T cells. Evidence for antigen presentation by a second member of the human CD1 family. *J Immunol* **157:** 2795–2803.

Behar SM. 2013. Antigen-specific $CD8^+$ T cells and protective immunity to tuberculosis. *Adv Exp Med Biol* **783:** 141–163.

Behar SM, Divangahi M, Remold HG. 2010. Evasion of innate immunity by Mycobacterium tuberculosis: Is death an exit strategy? *Nat Rev Microbiol* **8:** 668–674.

Behr M, Wilson M, Gill W, Salamon H, Schoolnik G, Rane S, Small P. 1999. Comparative genomics of BCG vaccines by whole-genome DNA microarray. *Science* **284:** 1520–1523.

Bertholet S, Ireton GC, Kahn M, Guderian J, Mohamath R, Stride N, Laughlin EM, Baldwin SL, Vedvick TS, Coler RN, et al. 2008. Identification of human T cell antigens for the development of vaccines against *Mycobacterium tuberculosis*. *J Immunol* **181:** 7948–7957.

Black GF, Thiel BA, Ota MO, Parida SK, Adegbola R, Boom WH, Dockrell HM, Franken KL, Friggen AH, Hill PC, et al. 2009. Immunogenicity of novel DosR regulon-encoded candidate antigens of *Mycobacterium tuberculosis* in three high-burden populations in Africa. *Clin Vaccine Immunol* **16:** 1203–1212.

Blythe M, Zhang Q, Vaughan K, de Castro R, Salimi N, Bui H-H, Lewinsohn D, Ernst J, Peters B, Sette A. 2007. An analysis of the epitope knowledge related to Mycobacteria. *Immunome Res* **3:** 10.

Boesen H, Jensen B, Wilcke T, Andersen P. 1995. Human T-cell responses to secreted antigen fractions of *Mycobacterium tuberculosis*. *Infect Immun* **63:** 1491–1497.

Brock I, Weldingh K, Leyten EMS, Arend SM, Ravn P, Andersen P. 2004. Specific T-cell epitopes for immunoassay-based diagnosis of *Mycobacterium tuberculosis* infection. *J Clin Microbiol* **42:** 2379–2387.

Caccamo N, Milano S, Di Sano C, Cigna D, Ivanyi J, Krensky AM, Dieli F, Salerno A. 2002. Identification of epitopes of *Mycobacterium tuberculosis* 16-kDa protein recognized by human leukocyte antigen-A*0201 $CD8^+$ T lymphocytes. *J Infect Dis* **186:** 991–998.

Caccamo N, Guggino G, Meraviglia S, Gelsomino G, Di Carlo P, Titone L, Bocchino M, Galati D, Matarese A, Nouta J, et al. 2009. Analysis of *Mycobacterium tuberculosis*-specific CD8 T-cells in patients with active tuberculosis and in individuals with latent infection. *PLoS ONE* **4:** e5528.

Caruso AM, Serbina N, Klein E, Triebold K, Bloom BR, Flynn JL. 1999. Mice deficient in CD4 T cells have only transiently diminished levels of IFN-γ, yet succumb to tuberculosis. *J Immunol* **162:** 5407–5416.

Chaitra MG, Shaila MS, Chandra NR, Nayak R. 2008. HLA-A*0201-restricted cytotoxic T-cell epitopes in three PE/PPE family proteins of *Mycobacterium tuberculosis*. *Scand J Immunol* **67:** 411–417.

Chegou N, Black G, Loxton A, Stanley K, Essone P, Klein M, Parida S, Kaufmann S, Doherty TM, Friggen A, et al. 2012. Potential of novel *Mycobacterium tuberculosis* infection phase-dependent antigens in the diagnosis of TB disease in a high burden setting. *BMC Infect Dis* **12:** 10.

Cockle PJ, Gordon SV, Lalvani A, Buddle BM, Hewinson RG, Vordermeier HM. 2002. Identification of novel *Mycobacterium tuberculosis* antigens with potential as diagnostic reagents or subunit vaccine candidates by comparative genomics. *Infect Immun* **70:** 6996–7003.

Cole S, Brosch R, Parkhill J, Garnier T, Churcher C, Harris D, Gordon S, Eiglmeier K, Gas S, Barry C, et al. 1998. Deciphering the biology of *Mycobacterium tuberculosis* from the complete genome sequence. *Nature* **393:** 537–544.

Coler RN, Dillon DC, Skeiky YAW, Kahn M, Orme IM, Lobet Y, Reed SG, Alderson MR. 2009. Identification of *Mycobacterium tuberculosis* vaccine candidates using human $CD4^+$ T-cells expression cloning. *Vaccine* **27:** 223–233.

Commandeur S, Lin MY, van Meijgaarden KE, Friggen AH, Franken KL, Drijfhout JW, Korsvold GE, Oftung F, Geluk A, Ottenhoff TH. 2011a. Double- and monofunctional $CD4^+$ and $CD8^+$ T-cell responses to *Mycobacterium tuberculosis* DosR antigens and peptides in long-term latently infected individuals. *Eur J Immunol* **41:** 2925–2936.

Commandeur S, van Meijgaarden KE, Lin MY, Franken KLMC, Friggen AH, Drijfhout JW, Oftung F, Korsvold GE, Geluk A, Ottenhoff THM. 2011b. Identification of human T-cell responses to *Mycobacterium tuberculosis* resuscitation promoting factors in long-term latently infected individuals. *Clin Vaccine Immunol* **41:** 2925–2936.

Commandeur S, van Meijgaarden KE, Prins C, Pichugin AV, Dijkman K, van den Eeden SJ, Friggen AH, Franken KL, Dolganov G, Kramnik I, et al. 2013. An unbiased genome-wide *Mycobacterium tuberculosis* gene expression approach to discover antigens targeted by human T cells expressed during pulmonary infection. *J Immunol* **190:** 1659–1671.

Cooper AM. 2009. Cell-mediated immune responses in tuberculosis. *Annu Rev Immunol* **27:** 393–422.

Cooper AM, Dalton DK, Stewart TA, Griffin JP, Russell DG, Orme IM. 1993. Disseminated tuberculosis in interferon γ gene-disrupted mice. *J Exp Med* **178:** 2243–2247.

Covert BA, Spencer JS, Orme IM, Belisle JT. 2001. The application of proteomics in defining the T cell antigens of *Mycobacterium tuberculosis*. *Proteomics* **1:** 574–586.

de Jong R, Altare F, Haagen IA, Elferink DG, Boer T, van Breda Vriesman PJ, Kabel PJ, Draaisma JM, van Dissel JT, Kroon FP, et al. 1998. Severe mycobacterial and salmonella infections in interleukin-12 receptor-deficient patients. *Science* **280:** 1435–1438.

Deenadayalan A, Heaslip D, Rajendiran AA, Velayudham BV, Frederick S, Yang HL, Dobos K, Belisle JT, Raja A. 2010. Immunoproteomic identification of human T cell antigens of *Mycobacterium tuberculosis* that differentiate healthy contacts from tuberculosis patients. *Mol Cell Proteomics* **9:** 538–549.

Divangahi M, Desjardins D, Nunes-Alves C, Remold HG, Behar SM. 2010. Eicosanoid pathways regulate adaptive immunity to *Mycobacterium tuberculosis. Nat Immunol* **11:** 751–758.

Dong Y, Demaria S, Sun X, Santori FR, Jesdale BM, De Groot AS, Rom WN, Bushkin Y. 2004. HLA-A2-restricted CD8^{+}-cytotoxic-T-cell responses to novel epitopes in *Mycobacterium tuberculosis* superoxide dismutase, alanine dehydrogenase, and glutamine synthetase. *Infect Immun* **72:** 2412–2415.

Doolan DL, Southwood S, Chesnut R, Appella E, Gomez E, Richards A, Higashimoto YI, Maewal A, Sidney J, Gramzinski RA, et al. 2000. HLA-DR-promiscuous T cell epitopes from *Plasmodium falciparum* pre-erythrocytic-stage antigens restricted by multiple HLA Class II alleles. *J Immunol* **165:** 1123–1137.

Dorman SE, Holland SM. 2000. Interferon-γ and interleukin-12 pathway defects and human disease. *Cytokine Growth Factor Rev* **11:** 321–333.

Florczyk MA, McCue LA, Stack RF, Hauer CR, McDonough KA. 2001. Identification and characterization of mycobacterial proteins differentially expressed under standing and shaking culture conditions, including Rv2623 from a novel class of putative ATP-binding proteins. *Infect Immun* **69:** 5777–5785.

Flynn JL. 2006. Lessons from experimental *Mycobacterium tuberculosis* infections. *Microbes Infect* **8:** 1179–1188.

Flynn JL, Chan J. 2001. Immunology of tuberculosis. *Annu Rev Immunol* **19:** 93–129.

Flynn JL, Goldstein MM, Triebold KJ, Koller B, Bloom BR. 1992. Major histocompatibility complex class I-restricted T cells are required for resistance to *Mycobacterium tuberculosis* infection. *Proc Natl Acad Sci* **89:** 12013–12017.

Flynn JL, Chan J, Triebold KJ, Dalton DK, Stewart TA, Bloom BR. 1993. An essential role for interferon γ in resistance to *Mycobacterium tuberculosis* infection. *J Exp Med* **178:** 2249–2254.

Gandhi NR, Nunn P, Dheda K, Schaaf HS, Zignol M, van Soolingen D, Jensen P, Bayona J. 2010. Multidrug-resistant and extensively drug-resistant tuberculosis: A threat to global control of tuberculosis. *Lancet* **375:** 1830–1843.

Gey van Pittius N, Gamieldien J, Hide W, Brown G, Siezen R, Beyers A. 2001. The ESAT-6 gene cluster of *Mycobacterium tuberculosis* and other high G + C Gram-positive bacteria. *Genome Biol* **2:** research0044.0041–research0044.0018.

Gey van Pittius N, Sampson S, Lee H, Kim Y, van Helden P, Warren R. 2006. Evolution and expansion of the *Mycobacterium tuberculosis* PE and PPE multigene families and their association with the duplication of the ESAT-6 (*esx*) gene cluster regions. *BMC Evol Biol* **6:** 95.

Gideon HP, Wilkinson KA, Rustad TR, Oni T, Guio H, Kozak RA, Sherman DR, Meintjes G, Behr MA, Vordermeier HM, et al. 2010. Hypoxia induces an immunodominant target of tuberculosis specific T cells absent from common BCG vaccines. *PLoS Pathog* **6:** e1001237.

Gold MC, Lewinsohn DM. 2013. Co-dependents: MR1-restricted MAIT cells and their antimicrobial function. *Nat Rev Microbiol* **11:** 14–19.

Gold MC, Cerri S, Smyk-Pearson S, Cansler ME, Vogt TM, Delepine J, Winata E, Swarbrick GM, Chua WJ, Yu YY, et al. 2010. Human mucosal associated invariant T cells detect bacterially infected cells. *PLoS Biol* **8:** e1000407.

Gosselin A, Monteiro P, Chomont N, Diaz-Griffero F, Said EA, Fonseca S, Wacleche V, El-Far M, Boulassel MR, Routy JP, et al. 2010. Peripheral blood CCR4^{+}CCR6^{+} and CXCR3^{+}CCR6^{+}CD4^{+} T cells are highly permissive to HIV-1 infection. *J Immunol* **184:** 1604–1616.

Grotzke JE, Lewinsohn DM. 2005. Role of CD8^{+} T lymphocytes in control of *Mycobacterium tuberculosis* infection. *Microbes Infect* **7:** 776–788.

Grotzke JE, Harriff MJ, Siler AC, Nolt D, Delepine J, Lewinsohn DA, Lewinsohn DM. 2009. The *Mycobacterium tuberculosis* phagosome is a HLA-I processing competent organelle. *PLoS Pathog* **5:** e1000374.

Grotzke JE, Siler AC, Lewinsohn DA, Lewinsohn DM. 2010. Secreted immunodominant *Mycobacterium tuberculosis* antigens are processed by the cytosolic pathway. *J Immunol* **185:** 4336–4343.

Hammond AS, Klein MR, Corrah T, Fox A, Jaye A, McAdam KP, Brookes RH. 2005. *Mycobacterium tuberculosis* genome-wide screen exposes multiple CD8^{+} T cell epitopes. *Clin Exp Immunol* **140:** 109–116.

Harboe M, Oettinger T, Wiker HG, Rosenkrands I, Andersen P. 1996. Evidence for occurrence of the ESAT-6 protein in *Mycobacterium tuberculosis* and virulent *Mycobacterium bovis* and for its absence in *Mycobacterium bovis* BCG. *Infect Immun* **64:** 16–22.

Heinzel AS, Grotzke JE, Lines RA, Lewinsohn DA, McNabb AL, Streblow DN, Braud VM, Grieser HJ, Belisle JT, Lewinsohn DM. 2002. HLA-E-dependent presentation of *Mtb*-derived antigen to human CD8^{+} T cells. *J Exp Med* **196:** 1473–1481.

Honer zu Bentrup K, Russell DG. 2001. Mycobacterial persistence: Adaptation to a changing environment. *Trends Microbiol* **9:** 597–605.

Hopewell PC. 1992. Impact of human immunodeficiency virus infection on the epidemiology, clinical features, management, and control of tuberculosis. *Clin Infect Dis* **15:** 540–547.

Horwitz MA, Lee BW, Dillon BJ, Harth G. 1995. Protective immunity against tuberculosis induced by vaccination with major extracellular proteins of *Mycobacterium tuberculosis. Proc Natl Acad Sci* **92:** 1530–1534.

Hubbard RD, Flory CM, Collins FM. 1992. Immunization of mice with mycobacterial culture filtrate proteins. *Clin Exp Immunol* **87:** 94–98.

Kunnath-Velayudhan S, Salamon H, Wang H-Y, Davidow AL, Molina DM, Huynh VT, Cirillo DM, Michel G, Talbot EA, Perkins MD, et al. 2010. Dynamic antibody responses to the *Mycobacterium tuberculosis* proteome. *Proc Natl Acad Sci* **107:** 14703–14708.

Lalvani A, Brookes R, Wilkinson RJ, Malin AS, Pathan AA, Andersen P, Dockrell H, Pasvol G, Hill AVS. 1998. Human cytolytic and interferon γ-secreting CD8^{+} T lymphocytes specific for *Mycobacterium tuberculosis. Proc Natl Acad Sci* **95:** 270–275.

Lalvani A, Nagvenkar P, Udwadia Z, Pathan AA, Wilkinson KA, Shastri JS, Ewer K, Hill AVS, Mehta A, Rodrigues C. 2001. Enumeration of T cells specific for RD1-encoded antigens suggests a high prevalence of latent *Mycobacterium tuberculosis* infection in healthy urban Indians. *J Infect Dis* **183:** 469–477.

Lamonaca V, Missale G, Urbani S, Pilli M, Boni C, Mori C, Sette A, Massari M, Southwood S, Bertoni R, et al. 1999.

Conserved hepatitis C virus sequences are highly immunogenic for CD4$^+$ T cells: Implications for vaccine development. *Hepatology* **30:** 1088–1098.

Lancioni C, Nyendak M, Kiguli S, Zalwango S, Mori T, Mayanja-Kizza H, Balyejusa S, Null M, Baseke J, Mulindwa D, et al. 2012. CD8$^+$ T cells provide an immunologic signature of tuberculosis in young children. *Am J Respir Crit Care Med* **185:** 206–212.

Lazarevic V, Flynn J. 2002. CD8$^+$ T cells in tuberculosis. *Am J Respir Crit Care Med* **166:** 1116–1121.

Lewinsohn DM, Alderson MR, Briden AL, Riddell SR, Reed SG, Grabstein KH. 1998. Characterization of human CD8$^+$ T cells reactive with *Mycobacterium tuberculosis*-infected antigen-presenting cells. *J Exp Med* **187:** 1633–1640.

Lewinsohn DM, Zhu L, Madison VJ, Dillon DC, Fling SP, Reed SG, Grabstein KH, Alderson MR. 2001. Classically restricted human CD8$^+$ T lymphocytes derived from *Mycobacterium tuberculosis*-infected cells: Definition of antigenic specificity. *J Immunol* **166:** 439–446.

Lewinsohn DA, Heinzel AS, Gardner JM, Zhu L, Alderson MR, Lewinsohn DM. 2003. *Mycobacterium tuberculosis*-specific CD8$^+$ T cells preferentially recognize heavily infected cells. *Am J Respir Crit Care Med* **168:** 1346–1352.

Lewinsohn DA, Winata E, Swarbrick GM, Tanner KE, Cook MS, Null MD, Cansler ME, Sette A, Sidney J, Lewinsohn DM. 2007. Immunodominant tuberculosis CD8 antigens preferentially restricted by HLA-B. *PLoS Pathog* **3:** 1240–1249.

Lewinsohn DA, Gold MC, Lewinsohn DM. 2011. Views of immunology: Effector T cells. *Immunol Rev* **240:** 25–39.

Lewinsohn DM, Swarbrick GM, Cansler ME, Null MD, Rajaraman V, Frieder MM, Sherman DR, McWeeney S, Lewinsohn DA. 2013. Human CD8 T cell antigens/epitopes identified by a proteomic peptide library. *PLoS ONE* **8:** e67016.

Leyten EMS, Lin MY, Franken KLMC, Friggen AH, Prins C, van Meijgaarden KE, Voskuil MI, Weldingh K, Andersen P, Schoolnik GK, et al. 2006. Human T-cell responses to 25 novel antigens encoded by genes of the dormancy regulon of *Mycobacterium tuberculosis*. *Microbes Infect* **8:** 2052–2060.

Li Y, Zeng J, Shi J, Wang M, Rao M, Xue C, Du Y, He ZG. 2010. A proteome-scale identification of novel antigenic proteins in *Mycobacterium tuberculosis* toward diagnostic and vaccine development. *J Proteome Res* **9:** 4812–4822.

Lindestam Arlehamn CS, Sidney J, Henderson R, Greenbaum JA, James EA, Moutaftsi M, Coler R, McKinney DM, Park D, Taplitz R, et al. 2012. Dissecting mechanisms of immunodominance to the common tuberculosis antigens ESAT-6, CFP10, Rv2031c (hspX), Rv2654c (TB7.7), and Rv1038c (EsxJ). *J Immunol* **188:** 5020–5031.

Lindestam Arlehamn CS, Gerasimova A, Mele F, Henderson R, Swann J, Greenbaum JA, Kim Y, Sidney J, James EA, Taplitz R, et al. 2013. Memory T cells in latent *Mycobacterium tuberculosis* infection are directed against three antigenic islands and largely contained in a CXCR3$^+$ CCR6$^+$ Th1 subset. *PLoS Pathog* **9:** e1003130.

Malen H, Berven F, Softeland T, Arntzen M, D'Santos C, De Souza G, Wiker H. 2008. Membrane and membrane-associated proteins in Triton X-114 extracts of *Mycobacterium bovis* BCG identified using a combination of gel-based and gel-free fractionation strategies. *Proteomics* **8:** 1859–1870.

McMurry J, Sbai H, Gennaro ML, Carter EJ, Martin W, De Groot AS. 2005. Analyzing *Mycobacterium tuberculosis* proteomes for candidate vaccine epitopes. *Tuberculosis (Edinb)* **85:** 95–105.

McMurry JA, Kimball S, Lee JH, Rivera D, Martin W, Weiner DB, Kutzler M, Sherman DR, Kornfeld H, De Groot AS. 2007. Epitope-driven TB vaccine development: A streamlined approach using immuno-informatics, ELISpot assays, and HLA transgenic mice. *Curr Mol Med* **7:** 351–368.

Mehrotra J, Bishai WR. 2001. Regulation of virulence genes in *Mycobacterium tuberculosis*. *Int J Med Microbiol* **291:** 171–182.

Mohagheghpour N, Gammon D, Kawamura LM, van Vollenhoven A, Benike CJ, Engleman EG. 1998. CTL response to *Mycobacterium tuberculosis*: Identification of an immunogenic epitope in the 19-kDa lipoprotein. *J Immunol* **161:** 2400–2406.

Monahan IM, Betts J, Banerjee DK, Butcher PD. 2001. Differential expression of mycobacterial proteins following phagocytosis by macrophages. *Microbiology* **147:** 459–471.

Moody DB, Ulrichs T, Muhlecker W, Young DC, Gurcha SS, Grant E, Rosat JP, Brenner MB, Costello CE, Besra GS, et al. 2000. CD1c-mediated T-cell recognition of isoprenoid glycolipids in *Mycobacterium tuberculosis* infection. *Nature* **404:** 884–888.

Mori T, Sakatani M, Yamagishi F, Takashima T, Kawabe Y, Nagao K, Shigeto E, Harada N, Mitarai S, Okada M, et al. 2004. Specific detection of tuberculosis infection: An interferon-γ-based assay using new antigens. *Am J Respir Crit Care Med* **170:** 59–64.

Muller I, Cobbold SP, Waldmann H, Kaufmann SH. 1987. Impaired resistance to *Mycobacterium tuberculosis* infection after selective in vivo depletion of L3T4$^+$ and Lyt-2$^+$ T cells. *Infect Immun* **55:** 2037–2041.

Mustafa AS, Shaban FA. 2006. ProPred analysis and experimental evaluation of promiscuous T-cell epitopes of three major secreted antigens of *Mycobacterium tuberculosis*. *Tuberculosis* **86:** 115–124.

Mustafa AS, Oftung F, Amoudy HA, Madi NM, Abal AT, Shaban F, Rosen Krands I, Andersen P. 2000. Multiple epitopes from the *Mycobacterium tuberculosis* ESAT-6 antigen are recognized by antigen-specific human T cell lines. *Clin Infect Dis* **30:** S201–S205.

Mustafa AS, Abal AT, Shaban F, El-Shamy AM, Amoudy HA. 2005. HLA-DR binding prediction and experimental evaluation of T-cell epitopes of mycolyl transferase 85B (Ag85B), a major secreted antigen of *Mycobacterium tuberculosis*. *Med Princ Pract* **14:** 140–146.

Nagai S, Wiker HG, Harboe M, Kinomoto M. 1991. Isolation and partial characterization of major protein antigens in the culture fluid of *Mycobacterium tuberculosis*. *Infect Immun* **59:** 372–382.

North RJ, Jung YJ. 2004. Immunity to tuberculosis. *Annu Rev Immunol* **22:** 599–623.

Nyendak MR, Park B, Null MD, Baseke J, Swarbrick G, Mayanja-Kizza H, Nsereko M, Johnson DF, Gitta P, Okwera A, et al. 2013. *Mycobacterium tuberculosis* specific

CD8^{+} T cells rapidly decline with antituberculosis treatment. *PLoS ONE* **8:** e81564.

Olsen AW, Hansen PR, Holm A, Andersen P. 2000. Efficient protection against *Mycobacterium tuberculosis* by vaccination with a single subdominant epitope from the ESAT-6 antigen. *Eur J Immunol* **30:** 1724–1732.

Orme IM. 1987. The kinetics of emergence and loss of mediator T lymphocytes acquired in response to infection with *Mycobacterium tuberculosis. J Immunol* **138:** 293–298.

Orme IM, Collins FM. 1983. Protection against *Mycobacterium tuberculosis* infection by adoptive immunotherapy. Requirement for T cell-deficient recipients. *J Exp Med* **158:** 74–83.

Orme IM, Collins FM. 1984. Adoptive protection of the *Mycobacterium tuberculosis*-infected lung. Dissociation between cells that passively transfer protective immunity and those that transfer delayed-type hypersensitivity to tuberculin. *Cellular Immunol* **84:** 113–120.

Orme IM, Andersen P, Boom WH. 1993. T cell response to *Mycobacterium tuberculosis. J Infect Dis* **167:** 1481–1497.

Oseroff C, Sidney J, Kotturi MF, Kolla R, Alam R, Broide DH, Wasserman SI, Weiskopf D, McKinney DM, Chung JL, et al. 2010. Molecular determinants of T cell epitope recognition to the common Timothy grass allergen. *J Immunol* **185:** 943–955.

Oseroff C, Sidney J, Tripple V, Grey H, Wood R, Broide DH, Greenbaum J, Kolla R, Peters B, Pomes A, et al. 2012a. Analysis of T cell responses to the major allergens from German cockroach: Epitope specificity and relationship to IgE production. *J Immunol* **189:** 679–688.

Oseroff C, Sidney J, Vita R, Tripple V, McKinney DM, Southwood S, Brodie TM, Sallusto F, Grey H, Alam R, et al. 2012b. T cell responses to known allergen proteins are differently polarized and account for a variable fraction of total response to allergen extracts. *J Immunol* **189:** 1800–1811.

Pal PG, Horwitz MA. 1992. Immunization with extracellular proteins of *Mycobacterium tuberculosis* induces cell-mediated immune responses and substantial protective immunity in a guinea pig model of pulmonary tuberculosis. *Infect Immun* **60:** 4781–4792.

Pathan AA, Wilkinson KA, Wilkinson RJ, Latif M, McShane H, Pasvol G, Hill AVS, Lalvani A. 2000. High frequencies of circulating IFN-γ-secreting CD8 cytotoxic T cells specific for a novel MHC class I-restricted *Mycobacterium tuberculosis* epitope in *M. tuberculosis*-infected subjects without disease. *Eur J Immunol* **30:** 2713–2721.

Pathan AA, Wilkinson KA, Klenerman P, McShane H, Davidson RN, Pasvol G, Hill AVS, Lalvani A. 2001. Direct ex vivo analysis of antigen-specific IFN-γ-secreting CD4 T cells in *Mycobacterium tuberculosis*-infected individuals: Associations with clinical disease state and effect of treatment. *J Immunol* **167:** 5217–5225.

Pfeifer JD, Wick MJ, Roberts RL, Findlay K, Normark SJ, Harding CV. 1993. Phagocytic processing of bacterial antigens for class I MHC presentation to T cells. *Nature* **361:** 359–362.

Prados-Rosales R, Baena A, Martinez LR, Luque-Garcia J, Kalscheuer R, Veeraraghavan U, Camara C, Nosanchuk JD, Besra GS, Chen B, et al. 2011. Mycobacteria release active membrane vesicles that modulate immune responses in a TLR2-dependent manner in mice. *J Clin Invest* **121:** 1471–1483.

Raviglione MC, Snider DE Jr, Kochi A. 1995. Global epidemiology of tuberculosis. Morbidity and mortality of a worldwide epidemic. *JAMA* **273:** 220–226.

Ravn P, Demissie A, Eguale T, Wondwosson H, Lein D, Amoudy Hanady A, Mustafa Abu S, Jensen Axel K, Holm A, Rosenkrands I, et al. 1999. Human T cell responses to the ESAT-6 antigen from *Mycobacterium tuberculosis. J Infect Dis* **179:** 637–645.

Reed S, Lobet Y. 2005. Tuberculosis vaccine development; from mouse to man. *Microbes Infect* **7:** 922–931.

Rosat JP, Grant EP, Beckman EM, Dascher CC, Sieling PA, Frederique D, Modlin RL, Porcelli SA, Furlong ST, Brenner MB. 1999. CD1-restricted microbial lipid antigen-specific recognition found in the CD8^{+} αβ T cell pool. *J Immunol* **162:** 366–371.

Roupie V, Romano M, Zhang L, Korf H, Lin MY, Franken KLMC, Ottenhoff THM, Klein MR, Huygen K. 2007. Immunogenicity of eight dormancy regulon-encoded proteins of *Mycobacterium tuberculosis* in DNA-vaccinated and tuberculosis-infected mice. *Infect Immun* **75:** 941–949.

Rustad TR, Harrell MI, Liao R, Sherman DR. 2008. The enduring hypoxic pesponse of *Mycobacterium tuberculosis. PLoS ONE* **3:** e1502.

Sampson SL. 2011. Mycobacterial PE/PPE proteins at the host–pathogen interface. *Clin Dev Immunol* **2011:** 497203.

Sayes F, Sun L, Di Luca M, Simeone R, Degaiffier N, Fiette L, Esin S, Brosch R, Bottai D, Leclerc C, et al. 2012. Strong immunogenicity and cross-reactivity of *Mycobacterium tuberculosis* ESX-5 Type VII secretion-encoded PE-PPE proteins predicts vaccine potential. *Cell Host Microbe* **11:** 352–363.

Schaible UE, Winau F, Sieling PA, Fischer K, Collins HL, Hagens K, Modlin RL, Brinkmann V, Kaufmann SH. 2003. Apoptosis facilitates antigen presentation to T lymphocytes through MHC-I and CD1 in tuberculosis. *Nat Med* **9:** 1039–1046.

Schnappinger D, Ehrt S, Voskuil MI, Liu Y, Mangan JA, Monahan IM, Dolganov G, Efron B, Butcher PD, Nathan C, et al. 2003. Transcriptional adaptation of *Mycobacterium tuberculosis* within macrophages: Insights into the phagosomal environment. *J Exp Med* **198:** 693–704.

Schuck SD, Mueller H, Kunitz F, Neher A, Hoffmann H, Franken KLCM, Repsilber D, Ottenhoff THM, Kaufmann SHE, Jacobsen M. 2009. Identification of T-cell antigens specific for latent *Mycobacterium tuberculosis* infection. *PLoS ONE* **4:** e5590.

Selwyn PA, Hartel D, Lewis VA, Schoenbaum EE, Vermund SH, Klein RS, Walker AT, Friedland GH. 1989. A prospective study of the risk of tuberculosis among intravenous drug users with human immunodeficiency virus infection. *N Engl J Med* **320:** 545–550.

Sette A, Moutaftsi M, Moyron-Quiroz J, McCausland MM, Davies DH, Johnston RJ, Peters B, Rafii-El-Idrissi Benhnia M, Hoffmann J, Su H-P, et al. 2008. Selective CD4^{+} T cell help for antibody responses to a large viral pathogen: Deterministic linkage of specificities. *Immunity* **28:** 847–858.

Shams H, Barnes PF, Weis SE, Klucar P, Wizel B. 2003. Human CD8$^+$ T cells recognize epitopes of the 28-kDa hemolysin and the 38-kDa antigen of *Mycobacterium tuberculosis*. *J Leukocyte Biol* **74:** 1008–1014.

Shams H, Klucar P, Weis SE, Lalvani A, Moonan PK, Safi H, Wizel B, Ewer K, Nepom GT, Lewinsohn DM, et al. 2004. Characterization of a *Mycobacterium tuberculosis* peptide that is recognized by human CD4$^+$ and CD8$^+$ T cells in the context of multiple HLA alleles. *J Immunol* **173:** 1966–1977.

Sieling PA, Chatterjee D, Porcelli SA, Prigozy TI, Mazzaccaro RJ, Soriano T, Bloom BR, Brenner MB, Kronenberg M, Brennan PJ, et al. 1995. CD1-restricted T cell recognition of microbial lipoglycan antigens. *Science* **269:** 227–230.

Silva CL, Silva MF, Pietro RC, Lowrie DB. 1994. Protection against tuberculosis by passive transfer with T-cell clones recognizing mycobacterial heat-shock protein 65. *Immunology* **83:** 341–346.

Skjot RLV, Agger EM, Andersen P. 2001. Antigen discovery and tuberculosis vaccine development in the post-genomic era. *Scand J Infect Dis* **33:** 643–647.

Smith SM, Klein MR, Malin AS, Sillah J, Huygen K, Andersen P, McAdam KP, Dockrell HM. 2000. Human CD8$^+$ T cells specific for *Mycobacterium tuberculosis* secreted antigens in tuberculosis patients and healthy BCG-vaccinated controls in The Gambia. *Infect Immun* **68:** 7144–7148.

Song R, Harding CV. 1996. Roles of proteasomes, transporter for antigen presentation (TAP), and β 2-microglobulin in the processing of bacterial or particulate antigens via an alternate class I MHC processing pathway. *J Immunol* **156:** 4182–4190.

Sousa AO, Mazzaccaro RJ, Russell RG, Lee FK, Turner OC, Hong S, Van Kaer L, Bloom BR. 2000. Relative contributions of distinct MHC class I-dependent cell populations in protection to tuberculosis infection in mice. *Proc Nat Acad Sci* **97:** 4204–4208.

Stenger S, Hanson DA, Teitelbaum R, Dewan P, Niazi KR, Froelich CJ, Ganz T, Thoma-Uszynski S, Melian A, Bogdan C, et al. 1998. An antimicrobial activity of cytolytic T cells mediated by granulysin. *Science* **282:** 121–125.

Tang ST, van Meijgaarden KE, Caccamo N, Guggino G, Klein MR, van Weeren P, Kazi F, Stryhn A, Zaigler A, Sahin U, et al. 2011. Genome-based in silico identification of new *Mycobacterium tuberculosis* antigens activating polyfunctional CD8$^+$ T cells in human tuberculosis. *J Immunol* **186:** 1068–1080.

Tangri S, Mothe BR, Eisenbraun J, Sidney J, Southwood S, Briggs K, Zinckgraf J, Bilsel P, Newman M, Chesnut R, et al. 2005. Rationally engineered therapeutic proteins with reduced immunogenicity. *J Immunol* **174:** 3187–3196.

Triccas JA, Gicquel B. 2000. Life on the inside: Probing *Mycobacterium tuberculosis* gene expression during infection. *Immunol Cell Biol* **78:** 311–317.

Ulrichs T, Munk ME, Mollenkopf H, Behr-Perst S, Colangeli R, Gennaro ML, Kaufmann SHE. 1998. Differential T cell responses to *Mycobacterium tuberculosis* ESAT6 in tuberculosis patients and healthy donors. *Eur J Immunol* **28:** 3949–3958.

van Pinxteren LAH, Ravn P, Agger EM, Pollock J, Andersen P. 2000. Diagnosis of tuberculosis based on the two specific antigens ESAT-6 and CFP10. *Clin Diagn Lab Immunol* **7:** 155–160.

Vani J, Shaila MS, Chandra NR, Nayak R. 2006. A combined immuno-informatics and structure-based modeling approach for prediction of T cell epitopes of secretory proteins of *Mycobacterium tuberculosis*. *Microbes Infect* **8:** 738–746.

Velayati AA, Masjedi MR, Farnia P, Tabarsi P, Ghanavi J, Ziazarifi AH, Hoffner SE. 2009. Emergence of new forms of totally drug-resistant tuberculosis bacilli: Super extensively drug-resistant tuberculosis or totally drug-resistant strains in Iran. *Chest* **136:** 420–425.

Vordermeier M, Whelan AO, Hewinson RG. 2003. Recognition of mycobacterial epitopes by T cells across mammalian species and use of a program that predicts human HLA-DR binding peptides to predict bovine epitopes. *Infect Immun* **71:** 1980–1987.

Vordermeier HM, Hewinson RG, Wilkinson RJ, Wilkinson KA, Gideon HP, Young DB, Sampson SL. 2012. Conserved immune recognition hierarchy of mycobacterial PE/PPE proteins during infection in natural hosts. *PLoS ONE* **7:** e40890.

Wang P, Sidney J, Dow C, Mothe B, Sette A, Peters B. 2008. A systematic assessment of MHC Class II peptide binding predictions and evaluation of a consensus approach. *PLoS Comput Biol* **4:** e1000048.

Weichold FF, Mueller S, Kortsik C, Hitzler WE, Wulf MJ, Hone DM, Sadoff JC, Maeurer MJ. 2007. Impact of MHC class I alleles on the M. tuberculosis antigen-specific CD8$^+$ T-cell response in patients with pulmonary tuberculosis. *Genes Immun* **8:** 334–343.

WHO. 2011. *World Health Organization report 2011: Global tuberculosis control*. WHO, Geneva.

Wilkinson RJ, Wilkinson KA, De Smet KAL, Haslov K, Pasvol G, Singh M, Svarcova I, Ivanyi J. 1998. Human T- and B-cell reactivity to the 16 kDa α-crystallin protein of *Mycobacterium tuberculosis*. *Scand J Immunol* **48:** 403–409.

Wilson CC, Palmer B, Southwood S, Sidney J, Higashimoto Y, Appella E, Chesnut R, Sette A, Livingston BD. 2001. Identification and antigenicity of broadly cross-reactive and conserved human immunodeficiency virus Type 1-derived helper T-lymphocyte epitopes. *J Virol* **75:** 4195–4207.

Winslow GM, Cooper A, Reiley W, Chatterjee M, Woodland DL. 2008. Early T-cell responses in tuberculosis immunity. *Immunol Rev* **225:** 284–299.

Yewdell JW, Bennink JR. 1999. Immunodominance in major histocompatibility complex class I-restricted T lymphocyte responses. *Annu Rev Immunol* **17:** 51–88.

Young DB, Gideon HP, Wilkinson RJ. 2009. Eliminating latent tuberculosis. *Trends Microbiol* **17:** 183–188.

Yuan Y, Crane DD, Barry CE. 1996. Stationary phase-associated protein expression in *Mycobacterium tuberculosis*: Function of the mycobacterial α-crystallin homolog. *J Bacteriol* **178:** 4484–4492.

Zvi A, Ariel N, Fulkerson J, Sadoff JC, Shafferman A. 2008. Whole genome identification of *Mycobacterium tuberculosis* vaccine candidates by comprehensive data mining and bioinformatic analyses. *BMC Med Genomics* **1:** 18.

Nonclassical T Cells and Their Antigens in Tuberculosis

Gennaro De Libero[1,2], Amit Singhal[1], Marco Lepore[2], and Lucia Mori[1,2]

[1]SIgN (Singapore Immunology Network), A*STAR (Agency for Science, Technology and Research), 138648 Singapore

[2]Experimental Immunology, Department of Biomedicine, University Hospital Basel, CH-4031 Basel, Switzerland

Correspondence: gennaro_delibero@immunol.a-star.edu.sg

T cells that recognize nonpeptidic antigens, and thereby are identified as nonclassical, represent important yet poorly characterized effectors of the immune response. They are present in large numbers in circulating blood and tissues and are as abundant as T cells recognizing peptide antigens. Nonclassical T cells exert multiple functions including immunoregulation, tumor control, and protection against infections. They recognize complexes of nonpeptidic antigens such as lipid and glycolipid molecules, vitamin B_2 precursors, and phosphorylated metabolites of the mevalonate pathway. Each of these antigens is presented by antigen-presenting molecules other than major histocompatibility complex (MHC), including CD1, MHC class I–related molecule 1 (MR1), and butyrophilin 3A1 (BTN3A1) molecules. Here, we discuss how nonclassical T cells participate in the recognition of mycobacterial antigens and in the mycobacterial-specific immune response.

The recognition by T lymphocytes of antigenic complexes formed by antigens and antigen-presenting molecules is a hallmark of the adaptive immune system. A wide range of exogenous and endogenous antigenic molecules reflecting a variety of chemical structures have been identified and are represented by proteins, lipids, phosphorylated metabolites, or vitamin B_2 pathway metabolites. The role of classical T cells, which recognize peptidic antigens associated with MHC-encoded molecules, during *Mycobacterium tuberculosis* (MTB) infection is well documented and studied for a long time (Cooper 2009). On the contrary, nonclassical T cells recognizing nonpeptidic antigens associated with non-MHC antigen-presenting molecules have been described more recently. They have also been identified as important contributors to host defense against infections, although many aspects of their physiological role still remain to be discovered. Based on the restriction molecule, antigen specificity, and T-cell receptor (TCR) structure, non-MHC-restricted T cells can be grouped into three categories: lipid- and glycolipid-specific CD1-restricted T cells, mucosal-associated invariant T (MAIT) MR1-restricted cells, and TCR γδ BTN3A1-restricted T cells. In this article, we review critical issues of the basic immunobiology of non-MHC-restricted T cells related to recognition of

Cite this article as *Cold Spring Harb Perspect Med* doi: 10.1101/cshperspect.a018473

mycobacterial antigens and discuss their roles during MTB infection.

LIPID-SPECIFIC CD1-RESTRICTED T CELLS

Lipid-specific T cells recognize lipid antigens as complexes formed with the CD1 antigen-presenting molecules. The human CD1a, CD1b, CD1c, and CD1d proteins bind and present lipid antigens (De Libero and Mori 2006), whereas CD1e behaves as a lipid chaperone, which participates in lipid antigen presentation without interacting with the TCR (Garcia-Alles et al. 2011). The CD1–lipid antigen complexes are mostly formed within antigen-presenting cells (APCs) in compartments where CD1 molecules recycle. Each CD1 molecule has unique modes of intracellular trafficking and thus can intersect with lipids, which also have different trafficking modes within APCs. Several studies have shown how CD1 structure, trafficking, and loading influence lipid antigen presentation, thereby directly contributing to lipid immunogenicity during immune responses (De Libero and Mori 2012). CD1-presented antigens are represented by amphipathic molecules characterized by a hydrophobic moiety, instrumental for binding within the CD1 pockets, and by a polar part, which in most of the cases directly interacts with the TCR.

Structure, Expression, and Intracellular Trafficking of CD1 Molecules

During mycobacterial infection the activation of lipid-specific T cells occurs upon the generation of stable CD1-lipid antigen complexes, which are formed within APCs. The immunogenicity of mycobacterial lipids is influenced by the type of cell that internalizes the lipid antigen and by the intersection of the lipid antigen with individual CD1 isoforms that recycle in different endosomal compartments.

All CD1 molecules show general structural features similar to MHC class I molecules, including two α helices in the distal α1 and α2 domains and a α3 domain that noncovalently associates with β_2 microglobulin. The antigen-binding groove of CD1 molecules allows insertion of the hydrophobic moieties of lipid antigens, whereas the antigenic polar moieties usually remain outside the groove and, along with CD1 key amino acids, interact with the TCRs (Moody et al. 2005; Rossjohn et al. 2012). Among different CD1 molecules, lipid-binding pockets vary in number, shape, and total volume. Together, these structural properties allow selective binding of lipid antigens differing in the number and length of alkyl chains. An important difference between CD1 and MHC molecules is a very limited sequence diversity and thus almost absence of functional polymorphism (Han et al. 1999; Porcelli and Modlin 1999). Two examples of *CD1* gene polymorphisms were described that influence the response to lipid antigens. The first example concerns CD1d in congenic mice in which CD1d alleles influence development and presentation of endogenous and exogenous ligands to CD1d-restricted T cells (Zimmer et al. 2009). The second example applies to CD1e in humans. *CD1e* gene is the most polymorphic gene of the CD1 family, with six allelic variants reported so far. CD1e is necessary for processing of mycobacterial hexamannosylated phosphatidylinositol mannosides (PIM_6) (de La Salle et al. 2005) and controls the generation and persistence of complexes formed by different lipid antigens and all other CD1 molecules (Facciotti et al. 2011). The CD1e allele 4 is unable to participate in the presentation of PIM_6 to CD1b-restricted specific T cells (Tourne et al. 2008), suggesting that homozygous individuals might display altered immune responses to microbial glycolipid antigens.

A different mechanism controlling the presentation of lipid antigens in the population is represented by regulation of *CD1* gene expression. Indeed, a unique SNP in the 5′ untranslated region of the human *CD1a* gene is associated with altered expression of CD1a and antigen presentation (Seshadri et al. 2013).

The immunological relevance of lipid-specific recognition during mycobacterial infections is also determined by the constitutive or inducible expression of CD1a, b, and c isoforms on unique cell types, indicating distinct roles during immune responses in tissues (Porcelli

 Cite this article as *Cold Spring Harb Perspect Med* doi: 10.1101/cshperspect.a018473

1995; Dougan et al. 2007). CD1d expression is distributed on almost all types of hematopoietic cells (Brossay et al. 1997; Roark et al. 1998) and also on some cells of nonhematopoietic origin, including epithelial cells and adipocytes. Whether CD1d-expressing epithelial cells present mycobacterial antigens at the foci of infection remains to be investigated.

The third important feature of CD1 isoforms is their intracellular trafficking route that determines the encounter with different mycobacterial lipids. CD1 molecules use different trafficking pathways, mainly governed by motifs present in their cytoplasmic tails, which interact with various adaptor protein complexes. Although CD1b, CD1c, and CD1d molecules bind to the adaptor protein 2 and recycle through late endosomes where lipid antigens are loaded (Barral and Brenner 2007), CD1a localizes in membrane rafts and recycles through early endosomes (Barral et al. 2008; Sloma et al. 2008). Mouse CD1d and human CD1b also interact with the adaptor protein 3, responsible for lysosomal trafficking. Lysosomal route is instrumental for binding complex mycobacterial lipids, which require processing and low pH environment for CD1b loading.

Mycobacterial Lipid Antigens Presented by CD1 Molecules

Because of their abundance in mycobacterial cell envelope, several mycobacterial lipids are antigenic (Fig. 1; Table 1) (De Libero et al. 2009). Among all CD1 molecules, CD1b binds lipids of different size ranging from C12 to C80 (Beckman et al. 1994; Batuwangala et al. 2004; Guiard et al. 2009; Layre et al. 2009; Garcia-Alles et al. 2011). CD1b-restricted MTB-derived mycolic acid (MA) having α-branched β-hydroxy long chain fatty acid was the first lipid antigen found to stimulate CD1-specific T cells (Beckman et al. 1994). Glucose monomycolate (GMM), an MA with a single glucose molecule, is another CD1b-restricted immunogenic lipid, which is synthesized by pathogenic MTB upon use of glucose derived from its host (Moody et al. 2000a). Recently, a conserved T-cell population expressing TCR α chain with limited junctional variability and with biased selection of TCR β chains was detected in the blood of some MTB-infected individuals. This type of conserved TCR has high affinity to mycolyl lipid-CD1b complexes and might be an example of "public" TCR expanding in response to mycobacterial antigen (Van Rhijn et al. 2013).

Glycerol monomycolate (GroMM), a MA with a glycerol, stimulates CD1-restricted lipid-specific T lymphocytes from TB patients (Layre et al. 2009). Chemical characterization of this antigen showed that it exists as two stereoisomers, one synthetic isomer being more stimulatory than the other. The hydroxyl groups of glycerol and mycolic acid length are critical for triggering T-cell responses. GroMM is presented by MTB-infected dendritic cells (DCs), showing that it is available for presentation during natural infection. Evidence from ex vivo experiments that GroMM stimulates T cells from vaccinated or latently infected donors but not cells from patients with active TB suggests that GroMM-specific T cells are primed during infection and their detection correlates with lack of clinical active disease (Layre et al. 2009). Other CD1b-restricted immunogenic mycobacterial lipids are glycosylphosphatidylinositols. They include phosphatidylinositol mannosides (PIMs) with varying numbers of mannose residues (Sieling et al. 1995; de La Salle et al. 2005), and further extensions of glycosylations like lipomannan (LM) (Ernst et al. 1998) and lipoarabinomannan (LAM) (Sieling et al. 1995). Of particular interest, diacylsulfoglycolipid (Ac_2SGL), found exclusively in the cell envelope of virulent MTB, is a potent antigen that stimulates CD1b- (Gilleron et al. 2004; Layre et al. 2009) and CD1c-restricted immune responses in TB (Lepore et al. 2014). The length of the linear acyl chain at position 2, the stereochemistry of the methyl-branched fatty acid chain at position 3, and the number of C-methyl-branched acyl groups influence antigenicity. A direct correlation was observed between the T-cell stimulatory capacities of the analogs and the number of methyl-branched groups, suggesting that the most abundant sulfoglycolipid form naturally produced by MTB is the most stimulatory one

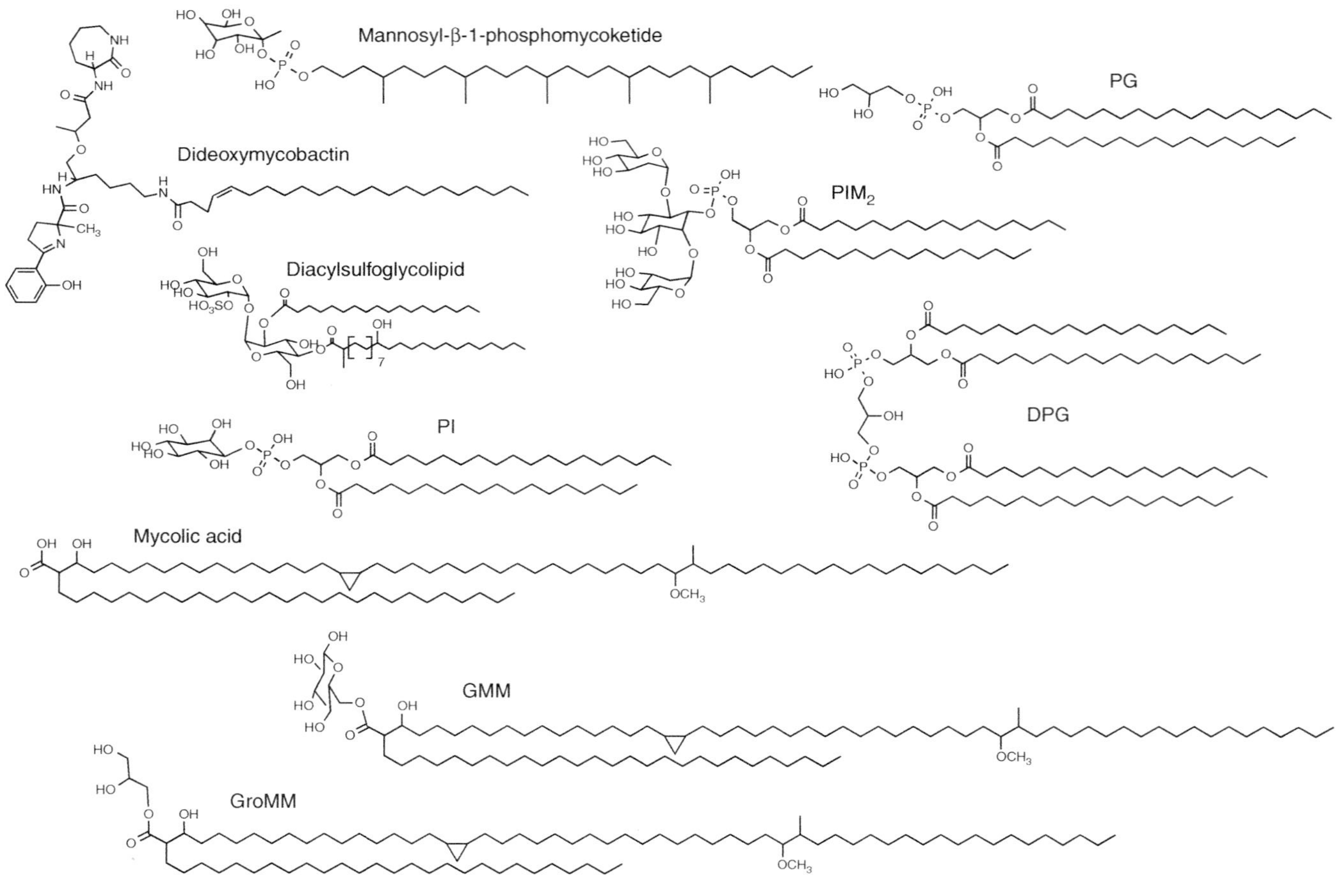

Figure 1. Structure of mycobacterial lipid antigens. The structures of representative mycobacterial lipid antigens are illustrated. Diacylsulfoglycolipid is illustrated in the natural form found in MTB. DPG, diphosphatidylglycerol; GMM, glucose monomycolate; GroMM, glycerol monomycolate; PG, phosphatidylglycerol; PI, phosphatidylinositol; PIM_2, phosphatidylinositoldimannoside.

Table 1. Mycobacterial lipid antigens with CD1 restriction

Antigen	CD1	Reference(s)
Dideoxymycobactin	CD1a	Moody et al. 2004; Kasmar et al. 2013
Diacylsulfoglycolipid	CD1b	Gilleron et al. 2004
Glucose monomycolate	CD1b	Sieling et al. 1995
Glycerol monomycolate	CD1b	Layre et al. 2009
Mycolic acid	CD1b	Beckman et al. 1994
LAM	CD1b	Sieling et al. 1995
LM	CD1b	Sieling et al. 1995
PIMs	CD1b	Sieling et al. 1995
Mannosyl-β-1-phosphomycoketide	CD1c	Moody et al. 2000a; Matsunaga et al. 2004; Ly et al. 2013
PIM	CD1d	Fischer et al. 2004
Phosphoglycerolipids: PG, DPG, PI	CD1d	Tatituri et al. 2013

LAM, lipoarabinomannan; LM, lipomannan; PIMs, phosphatidylinositolmannosides; PG, phosphatidylglycerol; DPG, diphosphatidylglycerol; PI, phosphatidylinositol.

for T cells (Gau et al. 2013; Geerdink et al. 2013).

A unique mode of binding lipid antigens is that of CD1a. This CD1 isoform shows a quite large and open F′ pocket and a deep A′ pocket, which bind and present mycobacterial dideoxymycobactin, a single chain lipopeptide precursor in the biosynthesis of mycobactin (Moody et al. 2004; Zajonc et al. 2005; Madigan et al. 2012). Mycobactin being essential in mycobacterial iron acquisition and survival of MTB in vivo (De Voss et al. 2000; Siegrist et al. 2009), the existence of T lymphocytes targeting cells presenting this type of antigen might represent an important protective mechanism. Another mycobacterial lipid antigen, mannosyl-β-1-phosphomycoketide (MPM) is stimulatory in association with CD1c and its tail is composed of a single saturated alkane with methyl branches on every fourth carbon (Moody et al. 2000b; Matsunaga et al. 2004). CD1c-restricted T cells recognizing synthetic mycoketide expand in the blood of TB patients as compared with uninfected controls (Moody et al. 2000b). Furthermore, an organism-wide survey has identified C32-phosphomycoketide (PM) from MTB as another CD1c-restricted lipid antigen (Ly et al. 2013).

Mycobacterial antigens that stimulate CD1d-restricted T cells, which are not invariant natural killer (NK) T cells, have been identified (Tatituri et al. 2013). These lipid antigens comprised several phospholipids, such as phosphatidylglycerol, diphosphatidylglycerol (or cardiolipin), and phosphatidylinositol. The response to these antigens required antigen internalization and engagement of the TCR with the CD1d-lipid complex. Two important aspects of this type of antigen specificity remain to be clarified: (i) the role of these responses in patients with mycobacterial infections, because only mouse hybridoma cells were studied, and (ii) the potential reactivity with self-phospholipids that show identical structures to the bacterial ones.

Functions of CD1-Restricted T Cells during Mycobacterial Infection

The absence of group 1 CD1 genes in mice and rats and the limited availability of reliable tools to directly visualize ex vivo antigen-specific CD1-restricted T cells has severely hampered the progress in the study of lipid-specific T cells. However, in vivo and ex vivo data on the presentation of mycobacterial lipids in humans and other animal species have provided direct evidence of the function of CD1-specific T cells during mycobacterial infections. These studies showed that group 1 CD1-restricted T cells have effector functions typical of T helper 1 (Th1), T helper 2 (Th2), and T helper 17 (Th17) cells, and that these functions increase during infection with MTB, suggesting their role in protection (Cohen et al. 2009). Experiments conducted with guinea pigs, which have an extended family of CD1 molecules, showed development of CD1b- and CD1c-restricted proliferative and cytolytic T-cell responses on immunization either by *Mycobacterium bovis* Bacillus Calmette–Guérin (BCG) or with partially purified lipid extracts of MTB (Hiromatsu et al. 2002; Watanabe et al. 2006). MTB-lipid-immunized guinea pigs had smaller lung lesions on challenge with MTB than vehicle-only-immunized animals (Dascher et al. 2003). In the cattle, which have *cd1a* and *cd1b* genes, a CD1b-restricted T-cell response could be detected after immunization with GMM (Nguyen et al. 2009). Studies conducted in TB patients suggested that CD1-restricted T cells are not infrequent and represent an important fraction of circulating T cells. We have shown the presence of cytolytic Ac_2SGL-specific CD1b-restricted T cells in latent TB individuals and active TB patients, but not in healthy donors (Gilleron et al. 2004). Ex vivo analysis of peripheral T cells has shown a CD1b-restricted response against GroMM in latent TB and BCG-vaccinated individuals, but not in active TB patients or healthy donors (Layre et al. 2009). In contrast, GMM was recognized ex vivo by T cells from latent TB individuals only (Ulrichs et al. 2003). More recently, using GMM-loaded CD1b tetramers a small $CD4^+$ CD1b-restricted population was detected in TB patients (Kasmar et al. 2011). MA-specific CD1b-restricted T cells have been detected in the periphery and lungs of TB patients (Montamat-Sicotte et al. 2011). These T cells produced IFN-γ and IL-2, showed effector and central memory phenotypes and were absent in BCG-vaccinated individuals. Upon anti-TB therapy, MA-specific T cells contracted, became undetectable at 6 months post-initiation of treatment and exhibited recall expansion on antigen reencounter in vitro long after successful treatment, indicating persistence of lipid-specific memory T cells. The role of CD1-restricted responses in in vivo immune response was further strengthened by demonstration of the expansion of phosphomycoketide-specific CD1c-restricted T cells (Moody et al. 2000b) and detection of DDM-specific CD1a-restricted T cells (Kasmar et al. 2013) in TB patients. The use of CD1 tetramers loaded with different lipid antigens has revealed that the number of circulating CD1-restricted T cells is in the same range of peptide-specific T cells, at least for tested CD1-antigen complexes. It remains to be investigated whether CD1-restricted T cells accumulate within tissues in which lipid-specific responses occur (i.e., skin, lung, gut, and liver), which might represent niches of preferential accumulation.

CD1d-restricted iNKT cells acquire an effector/memory phenotype and rapidly secrete large amounts of Th1 and Th2 cytokines on primary stimulation (Bendelac et al. 2007). iNKT cells contain preformed IFN-γ mRNA in their cytoplasm, which promotes immediate secretion of this cytokine on TCR stimulation at levels 200 times higher than conventional MHC-restricted $CD4^+$ T cells (Stetson et al. 2003). This secretion of cytokines is controlled by the strength of TCR signal received during antigen recognition (Wang et al. 2008), which depends on the number of CD1 complexes as well as their persistence on the surface of APCs. In addition, human NKT cells express granulysin (Gansert et al. 2003) that participates in killing intracellular bacteria resident within target cells. The effector capacities of iNKT cells contribute to the activation of other cells including DCs, NK cells, and $CD4^+$ and $CD8^+$ T cells (Hermans et al. 2003), and thus iNKT cells can be considered as regulatory cells of adaptive immune responses. This function is important during mycobacterial infection for the expansion of $CD8^+$ T cells that participate in protective immunity (Behar et al. 1999). Further, iNKT cells express a variety of chemokine receptors that may drive their traffic to inflamed tissues (Thomas et al. 2003). Intriguingly, iNKT cells display poor expression of the lymphoid homing receptors, CCR7 and CXCR5, suggesting that their function is mostly exerted in peripheral tissues rather than in peripheral lymphoid organs. Studies performed in mice infected with live mycobacteria or injected with purified MTB lipids provided evidence for the expansion, recruitment, and activation of iNKT cells (Ryll et al. 2001; Dieli et al. 2003) and suggested the importance of iNKT cells in the formation of granulomas (Gilleron et al. 2001). The importance of iNKT cells in anti-mycobacterial protective immunity has been further shown in experimental models using knockout animals with deletions in *cd1d* or TCR *Jα18* genes (Chen et al. 1997; Sousa et al. 2000; Kawakami et al. 2002; Sugawara et al. 2002). The role of iNKT cells in controlling

MTB infection in humans is indirectly suggested by phenotypic observations showing variations as compared with healthy individuals (Snyder-Cappione et al. 2007; Im et al. 2008; Montoya et al. 2008). Thus, clear evidence of the role of iNKT cells in protection against TB is still formally lacking.

Modulation of CD1 Expression and Evasion of CD1-Mediated Detection by MTB

MTB has evolved a series of strategies to modulate the expression of CD1 molecules and to prevent CD1-restricted responses. MTB infection of human monocytes inhibits the expression of CD1 molecules and induces the generation of CD1a$^-$, CD1b$^-$, and CD1c$^-$ DCs in the presence of IFN-α (Mariotti et al. 2002, 2004). This is attributed to cell wall–associated α-glucans of MTB that through CR3 activate the p38 MAPK pathway, and in turn the ATF-2 transcription factor (Gagliardi et al. 2007), leading to the inhibition of *cd1* gene transcription. MTB-infected monocytes differentiate into macrophage-like host cells and have reduced capacities to stimulate CD1-restricted T cells, thus representing an immunoprivileged niche for mycobacterial persistence. Other studies performed with CD1-expressing and mature DCs showed down-regulation of *cd1* gene transcription by MTB (Stenger et al. 1998), which was ascribed to engagement of Toll-like receptor 2 (TLR2) (Roura-Mir et al. 2005). Another important mechanism with potential effects on CD1-restricted lipid presentation is the inhibition of apoptosis of infected cells by MTB. As apoptosis is required for release of mycobacterial lipids and subsequent cross-presentation by CD1-expressing APCs (Schaible et al. 2003), its inhibition may also have indirect inhibitory effects on presentation of mycobacterial lipid antigens. The evolution of these evasion mechanisms suggests a protective role of CD1-restricted T-cell responses during MTB infection. Despite these in vitro compelling data, the physiological significance of CD1 protein down-regulation in vivo during mycobacterial infections remains to be investigated.

MAIT CELLS

MAIT cells are innate-like T lymphocytes present at high frequency in human blood (Martin et al. 2009). They were originally found enriched in the mucosal lamina propria, from where their name was derived (Treiner et al. 2003). Recently they also have been found to be a major population of liver-resident T cells (Dusseaux et al. 2011; Tang et al. 2013). MAIT cells express an evolutionarily conserved TCR-α chain characterized by the semi-invariant rearrangement Vα7.2-Jα33 in human and Vα19-Jα33 in mice paired with a limited set of Vβ chains, mainly Vβ2 and Vβ13 in humans and Vβ6 and Vβ8 in mice (Porcelli et al. 1993; Tilloy et al. 1999; Treiner et al. 2003; Kawachi et al. 2006; Goldfinch et al. 2010).

Antigens Stimulating MAIT Cells

MAIT cells recognize pterin-containing compounds generated during the synthesis of riboflavin (vitamin B_2) by bacteria and yeasts (Kjer-Nielsen et al. 2012) (Fig. 2A) and presented by nonpolymorphic MR1, which is the restriction element for these T lymphocytes (Treiner et al. 2003; Huang et al. 2005). MAIT cells react to APCs infected with a broad array of microbes able to synthesize riboflavin, whereas they are not stimulated by microbes that lack this capacity (Kjer-Nielsen et al. 2012). The responsiveness to a wide group of microorganisms suggests an important function of MAIT cells in antimicrobial immunity (Gold et al. 2010; Le Bourhis et al. 2010). Furthermore, MAIT cells are absent in the periphery of germ-free mice and their peripheral expansion depends on bacterial colonization (Treiner et al. 2005), thus further suggesting that they participate in the control of infections.

Structural studies have shown how the pterin-containing metabolites are inserted within the antigen-binding pocket of MR1 (Lopez-Sagaseta et al. 2013; Patel et al. 2013). The pocket is very large and delimited by hydrophilic and hydrophobic amino acids. Furthermore, the cocrystallized antigens showed a minimal occupancy of the groove, suggesting that additional

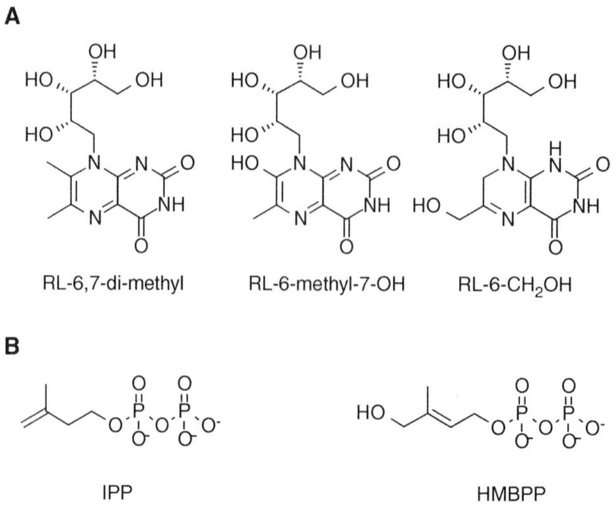

Figure 2. Structure of antigenic metabolites. (*A*) Structures of three different ribityl lumazines (RL), which bind MR1 and stimulate MAIT cells. (*B*) Structures of isopentenyl pyrophosphate (IPP) and (E)-4-hydroxy-3-methyl-but-2-enyl pyrophosphate (HMBPP) metabolite antigens, which stimulate Vγ9-Vδ2 T cells.

large hydrophobic or hydrophilic molecules might also bind to MR1. There is no evidence so far that MR1 molecules can present other antigens to non-MAIT T cells.

Role of MR1-Restricted T Cells in Mycobacterial Infections

Mycobacteria, including MTB, *Mycobacterium smegmatis*, *Mycobacterium abscessus*, and BCG are potent stimulators of human and mouse MAIT cells (Gold et al. 2010; Le Bourhis et al. 2010; Chua et al. 2012). A recent work showed that MAIT cells are reduced in blood of pulmonary TB patients compared with individuals with latent TB and healthy controls (Gold et al. 2010). In this study the percentage of MTB-reactive T-cell clones restricted to MR1 was higher in healthy donors and LTB individuals compared with patients with active disease. These studies were performed by analyzing the ex vivo frequency of MAIT cells measuring TNF-α release in response to MTB-infected epithelial cells. The reduction of MR1-restricted T cells in blood of patients with active TB was possibly attributed to migration of MAIT cells into the lung, the natural site of MTB infection. The same study showed that a small percentage of lung-infiltrating T cells expressing the TCR Vα7.2 from two donors released TNF-α in response to MTB-infected APCs in an MR1-dependent manner. As MTB-infected primary lung epithelial cells stimulate MAIT cells, they might be involved in the activation of MAIT cells in the lung (Gold et al. 2010). Another study described a reduction of MAIT cells in blood of patients with pulmonary bacterial infections, including TB, compared with healthy individuals (Le Bourhis et al. 2010). Here, MAIT cells were identified ex vivo by flow cytometry according to the coexpression of their specific markers TCR Vα7.2 and CD161. The drawback of this alternative approach is the known down-modulation of CD161 marker following antigen recognition, which limits the number of cells identified as true MAIT. However, it is not biased by the intrinsic differential capacity of individual T cells to adapt and grow in vitro following cloning. Despite the intrinsic limitations of used techniques, both studies confirmed that the MAIT cell compartment is impaired in blood of TB patients (Gold et al. 2010; Le Bourhis et al. 2010). As MAIT cells disappear from circulating blood on infection, they might accumulate at the site of infection. If this is the case, these findings raise the question of whether

MAIT cells accumulating in the lung are protective in the context of TB infection.

Effector Functions of MAIT Cells

Upon recognition of bacteria, including MTB, MAIT cells released large amounts of IFN-γ and TNF-α (Dusseaux et al. 2011; Chua et al. 2012; Gold et al. 2013), which are crucial cytokines for an effective immune response against MTB (reviewed in O'Garra et al. 2013). Furthermore, they killed in vitro APCs infected with *Escherichia coli* and BCG (Chua et al. 2012; Gold et al. 2013), thus contributing to control of intracellular infection and to limiting of pathogen spreading. Indications of a putative protective function of MAIT cells are also being investigated using MR1-deficient mice ($MR1^{-/-}$), which lack MAIT cells. These mice mounted a less efficient immune response at early time points than wild-type (WT) mice following intraperitoneal infection with *Klebsiella pneumoniae* (Georgel et al. 2011). It is of note that, in the same study, no differences between WT and $MR1^{-/-}$ mice were observed when the animals were infected with *E. coli*, *Shigella dysenteriae*, and *Yersinia enterocolitica* (Georgel et al. 2011), although these bacteria can stimulate MAIT cells (Kjer-Nielsen et al. 2012). A transient impaired ability to clear aerosol-administered BCG was also described in mice lacking MAIT cells, as highlighted by the higher bacterial counts in the lung of $MR1^{-/-}$ animals compared with WT ones (Chua et al. 2012). In keeping with this, MR1-deficient Vα19-Jα33 transgenic mice, intravenously injected with *M. abscessus*, showed an increased bacterial burden in the spleen compared with their MR1-sufficient counterpart (Le Bourhis et al. 2010). In another study, purified human MAIT cells were reprogrammed into induced pluripotent stem cells and redifferentiated back in vitro into MAIT cells (re-MAIT) (Wakao et al. 2013). Re-MAIT showed MAIT-like phenotype and properties in vitro and, when adoptively transferred into immune-compromised NOD/SCID mice challenged with *M. abscessus*, elicited a protective function via a granulysin-dependent mechanism (Wakao et al. 2013). In all these studies the protective activity of MAIT cells was noticed only at the early stage of infection, in line with the innate-like properties of these T lymphocytes. Nevertheless, a more recent work showed that MAIT cells can also elicit long-term bacterial control in a mouse model of pulmonary infection with the live vaccine strain of *Francisella tularensis* (Meierovics et al. 2013). The investigators found that $CD4^+$ and $CD8^+$ T-cell-depleted WT mice were resistant to a sublethal dose of *F. tularensis*, whereas MR1-deficient animals devoid of $CD4^+$ and $CD8^+$ T cells succumbed to the infection. These data represented, to our knowledge, the first report of an effective long-lasting antimicrobial role of MAIT cells in vivo. Importantly, the same study showed that MAIT cells accumulated in the lung of *F. tularensis*–challenged mice and induced a prompt recruitment of IFN-γ-producing $CD4^+$ and $CD8^+$ T cells to the infected site. Indeed MR1-deficient animals showed no MAIT accumulation in the lung and a significant delay in the recruitment of adaptive conventional T cells, resulting in a lower efficiency in the clearing of the bacteria (Meierovics et al. 2013). Such characteristics resemble those of CD1d-restricted iNKT cells, which have been defined as a "bridge" between innate and adaptive immunity (reviewed in Brennan et al. 2013).

It is still unclear whether the accumulation of MAIT cells in inflamed tissues resulted from the migration of circulating MAIT cells or from the expansion of the tissue-resident MAIT cell pool. In some instances, human MAIT cells do not proliferate in vitro after antigen stimulation (Dusseaux et al. 2011; Cosgrove et al. 2013), which instead induces an apoptotic program in these T lymphocytes (Cosgrove et al. 2013). However, in other laboratories MAIT cells have been successfully expanded and cloned (Gold et al. 2010; Lepore et al. 2014), showing that they survive in vitro when provided with the right culture conditions. Furthermore, they express high levels of tissue homing markers and chemokine receptors and display a marked tropism for solid organs (Kawachi et al. 2006; Dusseaux et al. 2011; Gold et al. 2013; Tang et al. 2013; Wakao et al. 2013). According to these findings, tissue-resident MAIT cells might be crucial as the first line of defense against invading pathogens. The prompt reactivity of "tissue-patrolling" MAIT cells to microbes might be important in containing the initial phase of local infections, further sustained by the fast influx of MAIT cells from blood, driven by chemotactic signals. The inflammatory environment resulting from MAIT cell activation would be important for the rapid recruitment of the effectors of the adaptive immunity. Further studies will be needed to challenge this model and to better characterize the potential protective activity of MAIT cells in TB. The definition of their role in the orchestrated mucosal immune response in the lung, their ability to modulate and regulate the function of other immune cells, such as macrophages and neutrophils, important in the early immune response against MTB (O'Garra et al. 2013), and the molecular mechanisms governing their antibacterial capacity remain unsolved and debated issues.

GAMMA-DELTA T CELLS

T cells expressing the gamma-delta (γδ) TCR represent the third population of nonclassical T cells in humans. The main characteristic of human γδ T cells is their expression of unique TCR heterodimers. Three main populations of γδ T cells are detected: The most abundant population in circulating blood and secondary lymphoid organs expresses the Vδ2 chain almost always paired with the Vγ9 chain. These TCR heterodimers are disulphide linked as they use the Cγ1 constant region and are polyclonal. Junctional diversity is present in the CDR3 regions of both the TCR γ and δ chains. The second main population expresses the Vδ1 chain, which is paired with different Vγ chains, mostly belonging to the VγI family (Vγ2, 3, 4, 5, and 8). This population of γδ T cells is polyclonal and the TCR is not disulphide linked, as in most of the cases the Cγ2 constant region is used. The Vδ1-expressing cells are abundant in the lamina propria of the gut and in the intraepithelial spaces. Noteworthy, these cells are also found in the lung and in the skin. The third population of γδ T cells expresses the Vδ3 chain, which usually pairs with Vγ chains of the VγI family.

Antigen Recognition by γδ Cells

Although we know a lot about TCR gene use, tissue localization, and effector functions of γδ T cells, we remain quite unaware of the antigens that stimulate human γδ T cells. In addition, we have only partial information on the function of this T-cell population in TB.

The population expressing the TCR Vγ9-Vδ2 heterodimer recognizes phosphorylated metabolites, such as isopentenyl pyrophosphate (IPP) and (E)-4-hydroxy-3-methyl-but-2-enyl pyrophosphate (HMBPP), which are produced in the mevalonate and methyl erythritol pathways, respectively (Fig. 2B). IPP is made by eukaryotic and prokaryotic cells, whereas HMBPP is made only by some microorganisms, including MTB. IPP and HMBPP are very small molecules (245 and 262 Da, respectively) and require appropriate antigen presentation. Recently, it was reported that Butyrophilin 3A1 (BTN3A1) is required for activation of Vγ9-Vδ2 cells (Harly et al. 2012) and that this molecule is involved in the presentation of both phosphorylated metabolites to the TCR Vγ9-Vδ2 (Vavassori et al. 2013). Surface plasmon resonance and surface-enhanced Raman scattering showed a direct interaction of the TCR Vγ9-Vδ2 with BTN3A1, and the presence of IPP increased the binding (Vavassori et al. 2013). Studies performed with site-directed mutagenesis of TCR chains indicated that the TCR becomes activated only when several amino acids present in the CDR regions of both the TCR γ and δ chains interact with the antigen-presenting molecule (Wang et al. 2010).

Interestingly, BCG-infected cells stimulated only a subset of Vγ9-Vδ2 cells, and only a fraction of Vγ9-Vδ2 cells expanded in vitro with synthetic HMBPP was reactive to infected cells (Spencer et al. 2008). Whether the differential response results from recognition of additional mycobacterial antigens or reflects differences in TCR avidity or variable expression of co-stimulatory/inhibitory molecules remains to be investigated.

 Cite this article as *Cold Spring Harb Perspect Med* doi: 10.1101/cshperspect.a018473

The antigens stimulating γδ cells expressing non-Vγ9 chains and non-Vδ2 chains remain poorly characterized. These cells can be activated during CMV infections, and one clone expressing a Vδ5-Vγ4 TCR was activated by the endothelial protein C receptor (Willcox et al. 2012). Vδ1-expressing cells were also found to interact with the bacterial phycoerythrin protein in a manner resembling antigen–antibody recognition, without requirements for antigen processing or presentation by dedicated presenting molecules (Zeng et al. 2012).

A small number of non-Vδ2 cells recognize glycolipids presented by CD1c and CD1d molecules (Faure et al. 1990; Spada et al. 2000; Bai et al. 2012). The structure of the TCR γδ-CD1-lipid complex showed a MHC-like recognition (Luoma et al. 2013; Uldrich et al. 2013), disclosing the enormous plasticity of antigen recognition by TCR γδ. So far, there is no evidence of recognition of mycobacterial lipid antigens by γδ cells. Recent studies reported the identification of two mycobacterial proteins, namely of 1-deoxy-D-xylulose 5-phosphate synthase 2 and Rv2272 protein, which activated γδ T cells from pulmonary TB patients (Xi et al. 2013). Responding γδ cells secreted IFN-γ and monocyte chemoattractant protein 1 implicating an important role of these cells in protection and stimulation of monocyte chemotaxis toward the site of infection.

Role of γδ Cells in TB

In TB patients many changes in γδ cell populations have been detected for many years. However, molecular mechanisms and implications in protection and disease progression remain poorly characterized. Only in the recent past have novel mechanisms begun to be carefully investigated. In patients with active TB it was observed a decrease of circulating Vγ9Vδ2 cells and in particular of central memory cells and of effector memory and terminally differentiated cells, which exert immediate effector functions (Meraviglia et al. 2010). These changes reversed after antimycobacterial therapy, suggesting an indirect correlation with antigen burden. In severe TB patients, an increase of γδ cells with enhanced interleukin-10 production was also described (Pinheiro et al. 2012), indicating changes associated with disease progression. This plasticity in T-cell function was confirmed in another study conducted in acute TB patients, in which a progressive reduction of the cytolytic activity of αβ cells was described. However, in the same patients, γδ cells remained perforin$^+$ and capable of killing intracellular bacteria (De La Barrera et al. 2003).

The implication of γδ cells in the immune response within MTB-infected lungs is supported by a series of investigations. Vγ9Vδ2 cells accumulate within lung granulomas (Huang et al. 2012), and in a macaque model of BCG and MTB infection they rapidly expanded upon second exposure to mycobacteria (Shen et al. 2002). This behavior resembles that of adaptive immunity cells and suggests that Vγ9Vδ2 cells may contribute to adaptive immunity to mycobacterial infections. In pleural effusions of TB patients, two populations of γδ cells were identified as TCR^{low} Vδ2$^+$ and TCR^{high} Vδ1$^+$ (Yokobori et al. 2009). The Vδ2 cells were CD45RA$^{+/-}$CCR7$^+$CXCR3$^+$, released large amounts of IFN-γ, and expressed the CD107a marker, indicating a status of activated cells within the tissue.

Finally, in a mouse model of lung infection with MTB, γδ cells were instrumental to activate DCs in the lung and facilitate subsequent priming of lung CD8 cytotoxic T cells (Caccamo et al. 2006), thus representing important protagonists of the early response during infection.

CONCLUDING REMARKS

All together these studies depict nonclassical T cells as major players of the immune response during MTB infection. The capacity of these cells to recognize unique nonpeptidic antigens, together with their memory phenotype and effector capacities, represent good indications that they participate in protective mechanisms, alongside with MHC-restricted and peptide-specific T cells. Therefore, mycobacterial lipid antigens stimulating protective CD1-restricted T cells may be considered as candidate constituents of subunit anti-TB vaccines.

A second important feature of other main populations of nonclassical T cells (MAIT and γδ cells) is their recognition of small metabolites produced by most bacteria and their activation following TCR interaction with dedicated presenting molecules, such as MR1 and BTN3A1, which are both nonpolymorphic and almost ubiquitously expressed. These characteristics indicate a common strategy of tissue-resident nonclassical T-cell activation during early infection, which prompts immediate release of proinflammatory cytokines. This feature has not been exploited in animal models of TB and might represent a novel approach to facilitate early protection and efficient priming of adaptive T cells during MTB infection.

ACKNOWLEDGMENTS

We thank SIgN, University Hospital Basel, Swiss National Science Foundation, and European Union (NEWTBVAC) for support.

REFERENCES

Bai L, Picard D, Anderson B, Chaudhary V, Luoma A, Jabri B, Adams EJ, Savage PB, Bendelac A. 2012. The majority of CD1d-sulfatide-specific T cells in human blood use a semiinvariant Vδ1 TCR. *Eur J Immunol* **42:** 2505–2510.

Barral DC, Brenner MB. 2007. CD1 antigen presentation: How it works. *Nat Rev Immunol* **7:** 929–941.

Barral DC, Cavallari M, McCormick PJ, Garg S, Magee AI, Bonifacino JS, De Libero G, Brenner MB. 2008. CD1a and MHC class I follow a similar endocytic recycling pathway. *Traffic* **9:** 1446–1457.

Batuwangala T, Shepherd D, Gadola SD, Gibson KJ, Zaccai NR, Fersht AR, Besra GS, Cerundolo V, Jones EY. 2004. The crystal structure of human CD1b with a bound bacterial glycolipid. *J Immunol* **172:** 2382–2388.

Beckman EM, Porcelli SA, Morita CT, Behar SM, Furlong ST, Brenner MB. 1994. Recognition of a lipid antigen by CD1-restricted αβ+ T cells. *Nature* **372:** 691–694.

Behar SM, Dascher CC, Grusby MJ, Wang CR, Brenner MB. 1999. Susceptibility of mice deficient in CD1D or TAP1 to infection with *Mycobacterium tuberculosis*. *J Exp Med* **189:** 1973–1980.

Bendelac A, Savage PB, Teyton L. 2007. The biology of NKT cells. *Annu Rev Immunol* **25:** 297–336.

Brennan PJ, Brigl M, Brenner MB. 2013. Invariant natural killer T cells: An innate activation scheme linked to diverse effector functions. *Nat Rev Immunol* **13:** 101–117.

Brossay L, Jullien D, Cardell S, Sydora BC, Burdin N, Modlin RL, Kronenberg M. 1997. Mouse CD1 is mainly expressed on hemopoietic-derived cells. *J Immunol* **159:** 1216–1224.

Caccamo N, Sireci G, Meraviglia S, Dieli F, Ivanyi J, Salerno A. 2006. γδ T cells condition dendritic cells in vivo for priming pulmonary CD8 T cell responses against *Mycobacterium tuberculosis*. *Eur J Immunol* **36:** 2681–2690.

Chen YH, Chiu NM, Mandal M, Wang N, Wang CR. 1997. Impaired NK1$^+$ T cell development and early IL-4 production in CD1-deficient mice. *Immunity* **6:** 459–467.

Chua WJ, Truscott SM, Eickhoff CS, Blazevic A, Hoft DF, Hansen TH. 2012. Polyclonal mucosa-associated invariant T cells have unique innate functions in bacterial infection. *Infect Immun* **80:** 3256–3267.

Cohen NR, Garg S, Brenner MB. 2009. Antigen presentation by CD1 lipids, T cells, and NKT cells in microbial immunity. *Adv Immunol* **102:** 1–94.

Cooper AM. 2009. Cell-mediated immune responses in tuberculosis. *Annu Rev Immunol* **27:** 393–422.

Cosgrove C, Ussher JE, Rauch A, Gartner K, Kurioka A, Huhn MH, Adelmann K, Kang YH, Fergusson JR, Simmonds P, et al. 2013. Early and nonreversible decrease of CD161^{++}/MAIT cells in HIV infection. *Blood* **121:** 951–961.

Dascher CC, Hiromatsu K, Xiong X, Morehouse C, Watts G, Liu G, McMurray DN, LeClair KP, Porcelli SA, Brenner MB. 2003. Immunization with a mycobacterial lipid vaccine improves pulmonary pathology in the guinea pig model of tuberculosis. *Int Immunol* **15:** 915–925.

De La Barrera SS, Finiasz M, Frias A, Aleman M, Barrionuevo P, Fink S, Franco MC, Abbate E, del C Saslain M. 2003. Specific lytic activity against mycobacterial antigens is inversely correlated with the severity of tuberculosis. *Clin Exp Immunol* **132:** 450–461.

de La Salle H, Mariotti S, Angenieux C, Gilleron M, Garcia-Alles LF, Malm D, Berg T, Paoletti S, Maître B, Mourey L, et al. 2005. Assistance of microbial glycolipid antigen processing by CD1e. *Science* **310:** 1321–1324.

De Libero G, Mori L. 2006. Mechanisms of lipid-antigen generation and presentation to T cells. *Trends Immunol* **27:** 485–492.

De Libero G, Mori L. 2012. Novel insights into lipid antigen presentation. *Trends Immunol* **33:** 103–111.

De Libero G, Collmann A, Mori L. 2009. The cellular and biochemical rules of lipid antigen presentation. *Eur J Immunol* **39:** 2648–2656.

De Voss JJ, Rutter K, Schroeder BG, Su H, Zhu Y, Barry CE III. 2000. The salicylate-derived mycobactin siderophores of *Mycobacterium tuberculosis* are essential for growth in macrophages. *Proc Natl Acad Sci* **97:** 1252–1257.

Dieli F, Taniguchi M, Kronenberg M, Sidobre S, Ivanyi J, Fattorini L, Iona E, Orefici G, De Leo G, Russo D, et al. 2003. An anti-inflammatory role for V α 14 NK T cells in *Mycobacterium bovis* bacillus Calmette–Guérin-infected mice. *J Immunol* **171:** 1961–1968.

Dougan SK, Kaser A, Blumberg RS. 2007. CD1 expression on antigen-presenting cells. *Curr Top Microbiol Immunol* **314:** 113–141.

Dusseaux M, Martin E, Serriari N, Peguillet I, Premel V, Louis D, Milder M, Le Bourhis L, Soudais C, Treiner E, et al. 2011. Human MAIT cells are xenobiotic-resistant, tissue-targeted, CD161hi IL-17-secreting T cells. *Blood* **117:** 1250–1259.

Ernst WA, Maher J, Cho S, Niazi KR, Chatterjee D, Moody DB, Besra GS, Watanabe Y, Jensen PE, Porcelli SA, et al. 1998. Molecular interaction of CD1b with lipoglycan antigens. *Immunity* **8:** 331–340.

Facciotti F, Cavallari M, Angenieux C, Garcia-Alles LF, Signorino-Gelo F, Angman L, Gilleron M, Prandi J, Puzo G, Panza L, et al. 2011. Fine tuning by human CD1e of lipid-specific immune responses. *Proc Natl Acad Sci* **108:** 14228–14233.

Faure F, Jitsukawa S, Miossec C, Hercend T. 1990. CD1c as a target recognition structure for human T lymphocytes: Analysis with peripheral blood γ/δ cells. *Eur J Immunol* **20:** 703–706.

Fischer K, Scotet E, Niemeyer M, Koebernick H, Zerrahn J, Maillet S, Hurwitz R, Kursar M, Bonneville M, Kaufmann SH, et al. 2004. Mycobacterial phosphatidylinositol mannoside is a natural antigen for CD1d-restricted T cells. *Proc Natl Acad Sci* **101:** 10685–10690.

Gagliardi MC, Lemassu A, Teloni R, Mariotti S, Sargentini V, Pardini M, Daffe M, Nisini R. 2007. Cell wall–associated α-glucan is instrumental for *Mycobacterium tuberculosis* to block CD1 molecule expression and disable the function of dendritic cell derived from infected monocyte. *Cell Microbiol* **9:** 2081–2092.

Gansert JL, Kiessler V, Engele M, Wittke F, Rollinghoff M, Krensky AM, Porcelli SA, Modlin RL, Stenger S. 2003. Human NKT cells express granulysin and exhibit antimycobacterial activity. *J Immunol* **170:** 3154–3161.

Garcia-Alles LF, Giacometti G, Versluis C, Maveyraud L, de Paepe D, Guiard J, Tranier S, Gilleron M, Prandi J, Hanau D, et al. 2011. Crystal structure of human CD1e reveals a groove suited for lipid-exchange processes. *Proc Natl Acad Sci* **108:** 13230–13235.

Gau B, Lemetais A, Lepore M, Garcia-Alles LF, Bourdreux Y, Mori L, Gilleron M, De Libero G, Puzo G, Beau JM, et al. 2013. Simplified deoxypropionate acyl chains for *Mycobacterium tuberculosis* sulfoglycolipid analogues: Chain length is essential for high antigenicity. *Chembiochem* **14:** 2413–2417.

Geerdink D, ter Horst B, Lepore M, Mori L, Puzo G, Hirsch AKH, Gilleron M, de Libero G, Minnaard AJ. 2013. Total synthesis, stereochemical elucidation and biological evaluation of Ac_2SGL; a 1,3-methyl branched sulfoglycolipid from *Mycobacterium tuberculosis*. *Chem Sci* **4:** 709–716.

Georgel P, Radosavljevic M, Macquin C, Bahram S. 2011. The non-conventional MHC class I MR1 molecule controls infection by *Klebsiella pneumoniae* in mice. *Mol Immunol* **48:** 769–775.

Gilleron M, Ronet C, Mempel M, Monsarrat B, Gachelin G, Puzo G. 2001. Acylation state of the phosphatidylinositol mannosides from *Mycobacterium bovis* bacillus Calmette–Guérin and ability to induce granuloma and recruit natural killer T cells. *J Biol Chem* **276:** 34896–34904.

Gilleron M, Stenger S, Mazorra Z, Wittke F, Mariotti S, Bohmer G, Prandi J, Mori L, Puzo G, De Libero G. 2004. Diacylated sulfoglycolipids are novel mycobacterial antigens stimulating CD1-restricted T cells during infection with *Mycobacterium tuberculosis*. *J Exp Med* **199:** 649–659.

Gold MC, Cerri S, Smyk-Pearson S, Cansler ME, Vogt TM, Delepine J, Winata E, Swarbrick GM, Chua WJ, Yu YY, et al. 2010. Human mucosal associated invariant T cells detect bacterially infected cells. *PLoS Biol* **8:** e1000407.

Gold MC, Eid T, Smyk-Pearson S, Eberling Y, Swarbrick GM, Langley SM, Streeter PR, Lewinsohn DA, Lewinsohn DM. 2013. Human thymic MR1-restricted MAIT cells are innate pathogen-reactive effectors that adapt following thymic egress. *Mucosal Immunol* **6:** 35–44.

Goldfinch N, Reinink P, Connelley T, Koets A, Morrison I, Van Rhijn I. 2010. Conservation of mucosal associated invariant T (MAIT) cells and the MR1 restriction element in ruminants, and abundance of MAIT cells in spleen. *Vet Res* **41:** 62.

Guiard J, Collmann A, Garcia-Alles LF, Mourey L, Brando T, Mori L, Gilleron M, Prandi J, De Libero G, Puzo G. 2009. Fatty acyl structures of *Mycobacterium tuberculosis* sulfoglycolipid govern T cell response. *J Immunol* **182:** 7030–7037.

Han M, Hannick LI, DiBrino M, Robinson MA. 1999. Polymorphism of human CD1 genes. *Tissue Antigens* **54:** 122–127.

Harly C, Guillaume Y, Nedellec S, Peigne CM, Monkkonen H, Monkkonen J, Li J, Kuball J, Adams EJ, Netzer S, et al. 2012. Key implication of CD277/butyrophilin-3 (BTN3A) in cellular stress sensing by a major human γδ T-cell subset. *Blood* **120:** 2269–2279.

Hermans IF, Silk JD, Gileadi U, Salio M, Mathew B, Ritter G, Schmidt R, Harris AL, Old L, Cerundolo V. 2003. NKT cells enhance $CD4^+$ and $CD8^+$ T cell responses to soluble antigen in vivo through direct interaction with dendritic cells. *J Immunol* **171:** 5140–5147.

Hiromatsu K, Dascher CC, LeClair KP, Sugita M, Furlong ST, Brenner MB, Porcelli SA. 2002. Induction of CD1-restricted immune responses in guinea pigs by immunization with mycobacterial lipid antigens. *J Immunol* **169:** 330–339.

Huang S, Gilfillan S, Cella M, Miley MJ, Lantz O, Lybarger L, Fremont DH, Hansen TH. 2005. Evidence for MR1 antigen presentation to mucosal-associated invariant T cells. *J Biol Chem* **280:** 21183–21193.

Huang D, Chen CY, Zhang M, Qiu L, Shen Y, Du G, Zhou K, Wang R, Chen ZW. 2012. Clonal immune responses of mycobacterium-specific γδ T cells in tuberculous and non-tuberculous tissues during *M. tuberculosis* infection. *PloS ONE* **7:** e30631.

Im JS, Kang TJ, Lee SB, Kim CH, Lee SH, Venkataswamy MM, Serfass ER, Chen B, Illarionov PA, Besra GS, et al. 2008. Alteration of the relative levels of iNKT cell subsets is associated with chronic mycobacterial infections. *Clin Immunol* **127:** 214–224.

Kasmar AG, van Rhijn I, Cheng TY, Turner M, Seshadri C, Schiefner A, Kalathur RC, Annand JW, de Jong A, Shires J, et al. 2011. CD1b tetramers bind αβ T cell receptors to identify a mycobacterial glycolipid-reactive T cell repertoire in humans. *J Exp Med* **208:** 1741–1747.

Kasmar AG, Van Rhijn I, Magalhaes KG, Young DC, Cheng TY, Turner MT, Schiefner A, Kalathur RC, Wilson IA, Bhati M, et al. 2013. Cutting edge: CD1a tetramers and dextramers identify human lipopeptide-specific T cells ex vivo. *J Immunol* **191:** 4499–4503.

Kawachi I, Maldonado J, Strader C, Gilfillan S. 2006. MR1-restricted V α 19i mucosal-associated invariant T cells are innate T cells in the gut lamina propria that provide a rapid and diverse cytokine response. *J Immunol* **176:** 1618–1627.

Kawakami K, Kinjo Y, Uezu K, Yara S, Miyagi K, Koguchi Y, Nakayama T, Taniguchi M, Saito A. 2002. Minimal contribution of Vα14 natural killer T cells to Th1 response and host resistance against mycobacterial infection in mice. *Microbiol Immunol* **46:** 207–210.

Kjer-Nielsen L, Patel O, Corbett AJ, Le Nours J, Meehan B, Liu L, Bhati M, Chen Z, Kostenko L, Reantragoon R, et al. 2012. MR1 presents microbial vitamin B metabolites to MAIT cells. *Nature* **491:** 717–723.

Layre E, Collmann A, Bastian M, Mariotti S, Czaplicki J, Prandi J, Mori L, Stenger S, De Libero G, Puzo G, et al. 2009. Mycolic acids constitute a scaffold for mycobacterial lipid antigens stimulating CD1-restricted T cells. *Chem Biol* **16:** 82–92.

Le Bourhis L, Martin E, Peguillet I, Guihot A, Froux N, Core M, Levy E, Dusseaux M, Meyssonnier V, Premel V, et al. 2010. Antimicrobial activity of mucosal-associated invariant T cells. *Nat Immunol* **11:** 701–708.

Lepore M, Kalinicenko A, Colone A, Paleja B, Singhal A, Tschumi A, Lee B, Poidinger M, Zolezzi F, Quagliata L, et al. 2014. Parallel T-cell cloning and deep sequencingof human MAIT cells reveal stable oligoclonal TCRβ répertoire. *Nat Comm* (in press).

Lopez-Sagaseta J, Dulberger CL, Crooks JE, Parks CD, Luoma AM, McFedries A, Van Rhijn I, Saghatelian A, Adams EJ. 2013. The molecular basis for mucosal-associated invariant T cell recognition of MR1 proteins. *Proc Natl Acad Sci* **110:** E1771–E1778.

Luoma AM, Castro CD, Mayassi T, Bembinster LA, Bai L, Picard D, Anderson B, Scharf L, Kung JE, Sibener LV, et al. 2013. Crystal structure of Vδ1 T cell receptor in complex with CD1d-sulfatide shows MHC-like recognition of a self-lipid by human γδ T cells. *Immunity* **39:** 1032–1042.

Ly D, Kasmar AG, Cheng TY, de Jong A, Huang S, Roy S, Bhatt A, van Summeren RP, Altman JD, Jacobs WR Jr, et al. 2013. CD1c tetramers detect ex vivo T cell responses to processed phosphomycoketide antigens. *J Exp Med* **210:** 729–741.

Madigan CA, Cheng TY, Layre E, Young DC, McConnell MJ, Debono CA, Murry JP, Wei JR, Barry CE III, Rodriguez GM, et al. 2012. Lipidomic discovery of deoxysiderophores reveals a revised mycobactin biosynthesis pathway in *Mycobacterium tuberculosis*. *Proc Natl Acad Sci* **109:** 1257–1262.

Mariotti S, Teloni R, Iona E, Fattorini L, Giannoni F, Romagnoli G, Orefici G, Nisini R. 2002. *Mycobacterium tuberculosis* subverts the differentiation of human monocytes into dendritic cells. *Eur J Immunol* **32:** 3050–3058.

Mariotti S, Teloni R, Iona E, Fattorini L, Romagnoli G, Gagliardi MC, Orefici G, Nisini R. 2004. *Mycobacterium tuberculosis* diverts α interferon-induced monocyte differentiation from dendritic cells into immunoprivileged macrophage-like host cells. *Infect Immun* **72:** 4385–4392.

Martin E, Treiner E, Duban L, Guerri L, Laude H, Toly C, Premel V, Devys A, Moura IC, Tilloy F, et al. 2009. Stepwise development of MAIT cells in mouse and human. *PLoS Biol* **7:** e54.

Matsunaga I, Bhatt A, Young DC, Cheng TY, Eyles SJ, Besra GS, Briken V, Porcelli SA, Costello CE, Jacobs WR Jr, et al. 2004. *Mycobacterium tuberculosis* pks12 produces a novel polyketide presented by CD1c to T cells. *J Exp Med* **200:** 1559–1569.

Meierovics A, Yankelevich WJ, Cowley SC. 2013. MAIT cells are critical for optimal mucosal immune responses during in vivo pulmonary bacterial infection. *Proc Natl Acad Sci* **110:** E3119–E3128.

Meraviglia S, Caccamo N, Salerno A, Sireci G, Dieli F. 2010. Partial and ineffective activation of Vγ9Vδ2 T cells by *Mycobacterium tuberculosis*-infected dendritic cells. *J Immunol* **185:** 1770–1776.

Montamat-Sicotte DJ, Millington KA, Willcox CR, Hingley-Wilson S, Hackforth S, Innes J, Kon OM, Lammas DA, Minnikin DE, Besra GS, et al. 2011. A mycolic acid-specific CD1-restricted T cell population contributes to acute and memory immune responses in human tuberculosis infection. *J Clin Invest* **121:** 2493–2503.

Montoya CJ, Catano JC, Ramirez Z, Rugeles MT, Wilson SB, Landay AL. 2008. Invariant NKT cells from HIV-1 or *Mycobacterium tuberculosis*-infected patients express an activated phenotype. *Clin Immunol* **127:** 1–6.

Moody DB, Guy MR, Grant E, Cheng TY, Brenner MB, Besra GS, Porcelli SA. 2000a. CD1b-mediated T cell recognition of a glycolipid antigen generated from mycobacterial lipid and host carbohydrate during infection. *J Exp Med* **192:** 965–976.

Moody DB, Ulrichs T, Muhlecker W, Young DC, Gurcha SS, Grant E, Rosat JP, Brenner MB, Costello CE, Besra GS, et al. 2000b. CD1c-mediated T-cell recognition of isoprenoid glycolipids in *Mycobacterium tuberculosis* infection. *Nature* **404:** 884–888.

Moody DB, Young DC, Cheng TY, Rosat JP, Roura-Mir C, O'Connor PB, Zajonc DM, Walz A, Miller MJ, Levery SB, et al. 2004. T cell activation by lipopeptide antigens. *Science* **303:** 527–531.

Moody DB, Zajonc DM, Wilson IA. 2005. Anatomy of CD1-lipid antigen complexes. *Nat Rev Immunol* **5:** 387–399.

Nguyen TK, Koets AP, Santema WJ, van Eden W, Rutten VP, Van Rhijn I. 2009. The mycobacterial glycolipid glucose monomycolate induces a memory T cell response comparable to a model protein antigen and no B cell response upon experimental vaccination of cattle. *Vaccine* **27:** 4818–4825.

O'Garra A, Redford PS, McNab FW, Bloom CI, Wilkinson RJ, Berry MP. 2013. The immune response in tuberculosis. *Annu Rev Immunol* **31:** 475–527.

Patel O, Kjer-Nielsen L, Le Nours J, Eckle SB, Birkinshaw R, Beddoe T, Corbett AJ, Liu L, Miles JJ, Meehan B, et al. 2013. Recognition of vitamin B metabolites by mucosal-associated invariant T cells. *Nat Commun* **4:** 2142.

Pinheiro MB, Antonelli LR, Sathler-Avelar R, Vitelli-Avelar DM, Spindola-de-Miranda S, Guimaraes TM, Teixeira-Carvalho A, Martins-Filho OA, Toledo VP. 2012. CD4-CD8-αβ and γδ T cells display inflammatory and regulatory potentials during human tuberculosis. *PloS ONE* **7:** e50923.

Porcelli SA. 1995. The CD1 family: A third lineage of antigen-presenting molecules. *Adv Immunol* **59:** 1–98.

Porcelli SA, Modlin RL. 1999. The CD1 system: Antigen-presenting molecules for T cell recognition of lipids and glycolipids. *Annu Rev Immunol* **17:** 297–329.

Porcelli S, Yockey CE, Brenner MB, Balk SP. 1993. Analysis of T cell antigen receptor (TCR) expression by human peripheral blood CD4−8- α/β T cells demonstrates preferential use of several V β genes and an invariant TCR α chain. *J Exp Med* **178:** 1–16.

Roark JH, Park SH, Jayawardena J, Kavita U, Shannon M, Bendelac A. 1998. CD1.1 expression by mouse antigen-presenting cells and marginal zone B cells. *J Immunol* **160:** 3121–3127.

Rossjohn J, Pellicci DG, Patel O, Gapin L, Godfrey DI. 2012. Recognition of CD1d-restricted antigens by natural killer T cells. *Nat Rev Immunol* **12:** 845–857.

Roura-Mir C, Wang L, Cheng TY, Matsunaga I, Dascher CC, Peng SL, Fenton MJ, Kirschning C, Moody DB. 2005. *Mycobacterium tuberculosis* regulates CD1 antigen presentation pathways through TLR-2. *J Immunol* **175:** 1758–1766.

Ryll R, Watanabe K, Fujiwara N, Takimoto H, Hasunuma R, Kumazawa Y, Okada M, Yano I. 2001. Mycobacterial cord factor, but not sulfolipid, causes depletion of NKT cells and upregulation of CD1d1 on murine macrophages. *Microbes Infect* **3:** 611–619.

Schaible UE, Winau F, Sieling PA, Fischer K, Collins HL, Hagens K, Modlin RL, Brinkmann V, Kaufmann SH. 2003. Apoptosis facilitates antigen presentation to T lymphocytes through MHC-I and CD1 in tuberculosis. *Nat Med* **9:** 1039–1046.

Seshadri C, Shenoy M, Wells RD, Hensley-McBain T, Andersen-Nissen E, McElrath MJ, Cheng TY, Moody DB, Hawn TR. 2013. Human CD1a deficiency is common and genetically regulated. *J Immunol* **191:** 1586–1593.

Shen Y, Zhou D, Qiu L, Lai X, Simon M, Shen L, Kou Z, Wang Q, Jiang L, Estep J, et al. 2002. Adaptive immune response of Vγ2Vδ2^{+} T cells during mycobacterial infections. *Science* **295:** 2255–2258.

Siegrist MS, Unnikrishnan M, McConnell MJ, Borowsky M, Cheng TY, Siddiqi N, Fortune SM, Moody DB, Rubin EJ. 2009. Mycobacterial Esx-3 is required for mycobactin-mediated iron acquisition. *Proc Natl Acad Sci* **106:** 18792–18797.

Sieling PA, Chatterjee D, Porcelli SA, Prigozy TI, Mazzaccaro RJ, Soriano T, Bloom BR, Brenner MB, Kronenberg M, Brennan PJ, et al. 1995. CD1-restricted T cell recognition of microbial lipoglycan antigens. *Science* **269:** 227–230.

Sloma I, Zilber MT, Vasselon T, Setterblad N, Cavallari M, Mori L, De Libero G, Charron D, Mooney N, Gelin C. 2008. Regulation of CD1a surface expression and antigen presentation by invariant chain and lipid rafts. *J Immunol* **180:** 980–987.

Snyder-Cappione JE, Nixon DF, Loo CP, Chapman JM, Meiklejohn DA, Melo FF, Costa PR, Sandberg JK, Rodrigues DS, Kallas EG. 2007. Individuals with pulmonary tuberculosis have lower levels of circulating CD1d-restricted NKT cells. *J Infect Dis* **195:** 1361–1364.

Sousa AO, Mazzaccaro RJ, Russell RG, Lee FK, Turner OC, Hong S, Van Kaer L, Bloom BR. 2000. Relative contributions of distinct MHC class I-dependent cell populations in protection to tuberculosis infection in mice. *Proc Natl Acad Sci* **97:** 4204–4208.

Spada FM, Grant EP, Peters PJ, Sugita M, Melian A, Leslie DS, Lee HK, van Donselaar E, Hanson DA, Krensky AM, et al. 2000. Self-recognition of CD1 by γ/δ T cells: Implications for innate immunity. *J Exp Med* **191:** 937–948.

Spencer CT, Abate G, Blazevic A, Hoft DF. 2008. Only a subset of phosphoantigen-responsive γ9δ2 T cells mediate protective tuberculosis immunity. *J Immunol* **181:** 4471–4484.

Stenger S, Niazi KR, Modlin RL. 1998. Down-regulation of CD1 on antigen-presenting cells by infection with *Mycobacterium tuberculosis*. *J Immunol* **161:** 3582–3588.

Stetson DB, Mohrs M, Reinhardt RL, Baron JL, Wang ZE, Gapin L, Kronenberg M, Locksley RM. 2003. Constitutive cytokine mRNAs mark natural killer (NK) and NK T cells poised for rapid effector function. *J Exp Med* **198:** 1069–1076.

Sugawara I, Yamada H, Mizuno S, Li CY, Nakayama T, Taniguchi M. 2002. Mycobacterial infection in natural killer T cell knockout mice. *Tuberculosis (Edinb)* **82:** 97–104.

Tang XZ, Jo J, Tan AT, Sandalova E, Chia A, Tan KC, Lee KH, Gehring AJ, De Libero G, Bertoletti A. 2013. IL-7 licenses activation of human liver intrasinusoidal mucosal-associated invariant T cells. *J Immunol* **190:** 3142–3152.

Tatituri RVV, Watts GFM, Bhowruth V, Barton N, Rothchild A, Hsu FF, Almeida CF, Cox LR, Eggeling L, Cardell S, et al. 2013. Recognition of microbial and mammalian phospholipid antigens by NKT cells with diverse TCRs. *Proc Natl Acad Sci* **110:** 1827–1832.

Thomas SY, Hou R, Boyson JE, Means TK, Hess C, Olson DP, Strominger JL, Brenner MB, Gumperz JE, Wilson SB, et al. 2003. CD1d-restricted NKT cells express a chemokine receptor profile indicative of Th1-type inflammatory homing cells. *J Immunol* **171:** 2571–2580.

Tilloy F, Treiner E, Park SH, Garcia C, Lemonnier F, de la Salle H, Bendelac A, Bonneville M, Lantz O. 1999. An invariant T cell receptor α chain defines a novel TAP-independent major histocompatibility complex class Ib-restricted α/β T cell subpopulation in mammals. *J Exp Med* **189:** 1907–1921.

Tourne S, Maitre B, Collmann A, Layre E, Mariotti S, Signorino-Gelo F, Loch C, Salamero J, Gilleron M, Angenieux C, et al. 2008. Cutting edge: A naturally occurring mutation in CD1e impairs lipid antigen presentation. *J Immunol* **180:** 3642–3646.

Treiner E, Duban L, Bahram S, Radosavljevic M, Wanner V, Tilloy F, Affaticati P, Gilfillan S, Lantz O. 2003. Selection of evolutionarily conserved mucosal-associated invariant T cells by MR1. *Nature* **422:** 164–169.

Treiner E, Duban L, Moura IC, Hansen T, Gilfillan S, Lantz O. 2005. Mucosal-associated invariant T (MAIT) cells: An evolutionarily conserved T cell subset. *Microbes Infect* **7:** 552–559.

Uldrich AP, Le Nours J, Pellicci DG, Gherardin NA, McPherson KG, Lim RT, Patel O, Beddoe T, Gras S, Rossjohn J, et al. 2013. CD1d-lipid antigen recognition by the γδ TCR. *Nat Immunol* **14:** 1137–1145.

Ulrichs T, Moody DB, Grant E, Kaufmann SH, Porcelli SA. 2003. T-cell responses to CD1-presented lipid antigens in humans with *Mycobacterium tuberculosis* infection. *Infect Immun* **71**, 3076–3087.

Van Rhijn I, Kasmar A, de Jong A, Gras S, Bhati M, Doorenspleet ME, de Vries N, Godfrey DI, Altman JD, de Jager W, et al. 2013. A conserved human T cell population targets mycobacterial antigens presented by CD1b. *Nat Immunol* **14:** 706–713.

Vavassori S, Kumar A, Wan GS, Ramanjaneyulu GS, Cavallari M, El Daker S, Beddoe T, Theodossis A, Williams NK, Gostick E, et al. 2013. Butyrophilin 3A1 binds phosphorylated antigens and stimulates human γδ T cells. *Nat Immunol* **14:** 908–916.

Wakao H, Yoshikiyo K, Koshimizu U, Furukawa T, Enomoto K, Matsunaga T, Tanaka T, Yasutomi Y, Yamada T, Minakami H, et al. 2013. Expansion of functional human mucosal-associated invariant T cells via reprogramming to pluripotency and redifferentiation. *Cell Stem Cell* **12:** 546–558.

Wang X, Chen X, Rodenkirch L, Simonson W, Wernimont S, Ndonye RM, Veerapen N, Gibson D, Howell AR, Besra GS, et al. 2008. Natural killer T-cell autoreactivity leads to a specialized activation state. *Blood* **112:** 4128–4138.

Wang H, Fang Z, Morita CT. 2010. Vγ2Vδ2 T cell receptor recognition of prenyl pyrophosphates is dependent on all CDRs. *J Immunol* **184:** 6209–6222.

Watanabe Y, Watari E, Matsunaga I, Hiromatsu K, Dascher CC, Kawashima T, Norose Y, Shimizu K, Takahashi H, Yano I, et al. 2006. BCG vaccine elicits both T-cell mediated and humoral immune responses directed against mycobacterial lipid components. *Vaccine* **24:** 5700–5707.

Willcox CR, Pitard V, Netzer S, Couzi L, Salim M, Silberzahn T, Moreau JF, Hayday AC, Willcox BE, Dechanet-Merville J. 2012. Cytomegalovirus and tumor stress surveillance by binding of a human γδ T cell antigen receptor to endothelial protein C receptor. *Nat Immunol* **13:** 872–879.

Xi X, Han X, Li L, Zhao Z. 2013. Identification of a new tuberculosis antigen recognized by γδ T cell receptor. *Clin Vaccine Immunol* **20:** 530–539.

Yokobori N, Schierloh P, Geffner L, Balboa L, Romero M, Musella R, Castagnino J, De Stefano G, Aleman M, de la Barrera S, et al. 2009. CD3 expression distinguishes two γδT cell receptor subsets with different phenotype and effector function in tuberculous pleurisy. *Clin Exp Immunol* **157:** 385–394.

Zajonc DM, Crispin MD, Bowden TA, Young DC, Cheng TY, Hu J, Costello CE, Rudd PM, Dwek RA, Miller MJ, et al. 2005. Molecular mechanism of lipopeptide presentation by CD1a. *Immunity* **22:** 209–219.

Zeng X, Wei YL, Huang J, Newell EW, Yu H, Kidd BA, Kuhns MS, Waters RW, Davis MM, Weaver CT, et al. 2012. γδ T cells recognize a microbial encoded B cell antigen to initiate a rapid antigen-specific interleukin-17 response. *Immunity* **37:** 524–534.

Zimmer MI, Nguyen HP, Wang B, Xu H, Colmone A, Felio K, Choi HJ, Zhou P, Alegre ML, Wang CR. 2009. Polymorphisms in CD1d affect antigen presentation and the activation of CD1d-restricted T cells. *Proc Natl Acad Sci* **106:** 1909–1914.

Role of B Cells and Antibodies in Acquired Immunity against *Mycobacterium tuberculosis*

Jacqueline M. Achkar[1], John Chan[1,2], and Arturo Casadevall[1,2]

[1]Department of Medicine, Albert Einstein College of Medicine, Bronx, New York 10461

[2]Departments of Microbiology and Immunology, Albert Einstein College of Medicine, Bronx, New York 10461

Correspondence: jacqueline.achkar@einstein.yu.edu

Accumulating evidence has documented a role for B cells and antibodies (Abs) in the immunity against *Mycobacterium tuberculosis* (*Mtb*). Passive transfer studies with monoclonal antibodies (mAbs) against mycobacterial antigens have shown protection against the tubercle bacillus. B cells and Abs are believed to contribute to an enhanced immune response against *Mtb* by modulating various immunological components in the infected host including the T-cell compartment. Nevertheless, the extent and contribution of B cells and Abs to protection against *Mtb* remains uncertain. In this article we summarize the most relevant findings supporting the role of B cells and Abs in the defense against *Mtb* and discuss the potential mechanisms of protection.

Approximately one-third of the world's population is infected with *M. tuberculosis* (*Mtb*). It is generally thought that the majority of this population harbors latent bacilli, of which only ~10% develop the disease active tuberculosis (TB) during their lifetime. The interplay of immunological components resulting in contained and stable latent *Mtb* infection (LTBI) is incompletely understood. Cell-mediated immunity (CMI) plays a key role in the defense against *Mtb* (Lewinsohn et al. 2011; Ottenhoff 2012; Ottenhoff and Kaufmann 2012), but increasing evidence suggests that CMI is not the sole defense mechanism against the tubercle bacillus. In humans, an intact CMI does not consistently protect against disease, and in *Mtb*-infected nonhuman primates, cell-mediated responses do not significantly correlate with the outcome of infection (Lin et al. 2009). Furthermore, not all individuals with LTBI and impaired CMI develop TB. Current and newly developed TB vaccines targeting CMI have limited efficacy in humans, and vaccine-induced cell-mediated responses often lack significant correlation with efficacy (Colditz et al. 1994; Fletcher et al. 2013; Tameris et al. 2013). These findings support a role for additional immune components in the protection against *Mtb* beyond that contributed by CMI.

The strong evidence for CMI as the main defense mechanism against TB has historically set up a false dichotomy that posited no role for humoral immunity (Maglione and Chan 2009; Achkar and Casadevall 2013). The general belief that, because of their extracellular location, antibodies (Abs) are not involved in the

Cite this article as *Cold Spring Harb Perspect Med* doi: 10.1101/cshperspect.a018432

protection against intracellular pathogens further limits an open view for the role of B cells and Ab-mediated immunity against *Mtb*. However, this view has been largely discredited and abandoned based on abundant evidence from many systems (reviewed in Casadevall 2003). We note that although immunoglobulins are a major product of B cells, these lymphocytes can contribute to the host immune response to *Mtb* via Ab-independent mechanisms (Bosio et al. 2000; Maglione et al. 2007; Maglione and Chan 2009; Russo and Mariano 2010; Almeida et al. 2011; Zhang et al. 2012). Whereas Ab-independent B-cell effects are largely accepted by the field, the historical controversy revolving around the role for B cells and the humoral immune response in the defense against *Mtb* typically relates solely to that of Abs. Therefore, in this review, we refer to B cells and Abs as distinct immunological elements simply to stay within the currently operating intellectual framework in the *Mtb* field.

Abs have many mechanisms by which they can modify the outcome of bacterial intracellular pathogenesis, ranging from opsonization to signaling through Fc receptors (FcRs) (reviewed in Casadevall 1998, 2003; Nimmerjahn and Ravetch 2008). Furthermore, just as for other facultative intracellular pathogens, there is plenty of evidence for an extracellular phase of *Mtb* during which it can be directly targeted by Abs (Smith et al. 2000; Casadevall 2003; Grosset 2003; Karakousis et al. 2004; Kim et al. 2010; Ahmad et al. 2011; Hoff et al. 2011; Driver et al. 2012). Importantly, Abs have been shown to play an important role in the defense against other intracellular pathogens such as *Salmonella*, *Chlamydia*, *Cryptococcus*, and *Histoplasma* spp. (reviewed in Casadevall 2003), and for some of these pathogens such as *Salmonella*, vaccines protecting through Ab-mediated immunity have ultimately been developed and licensed (Collins 1974).

A classic example for a paradigm shift from an exclusive CMI-centric view toward acceptance of an important role for Ab-mediated immunity occurred in the field of mycology, in which B cells and Abs were also once considered to have no protective role. As in TB, it was not possible to establish a consisted protective role for humoral immunity with polyclonal sera against fungi such as *Candida albicans* and *Cryptococcus neoformans* (reviewed in Casadevall 1995). However, the implementation of hybridoma technology produced immunoglobulins that revealed the existence of protective monoclonal antibodies (mAbs) and challenged this dogma (reviewed in Casadevall 1995; Casadevall and Pirofski 2012a). Also like *Mtb*, many of the medically relevant fungi such as *C. neoformans* and *Histoplasma capsulatum* are facultative intracellular pathogens, and the control of infection with these fungi requires vigorous granuloma formation indicative of CMI. The breakthrough in medical mycology came from the work of Françoise Dromer and colleagues who identified a protective Ab against *C. neoformans*, a finding that suggested the notion that humoral immunity could mediate protection if the right Ab response was elicited (Dromer et al. 1987). Two decades later humoral immunity had been shown to be protective against numerous fungi (reviewed in Casadevall and Pirofski 2012a), and two vaccines against *C. albicans* are currently in clinical trials, both of which are believed to mediate protection by eliciting a protective Ab response (reviewed in Cassone and Casadevall 2012). Parallel developments appear to be occurring in the TB field. In the following sections we discuss the complexity of humoral immunity in TB, the evidence for a role of Abs and B cells in the protection against TB, and the potential mechanisms for Ab-mediated immunity. Based on the discussed findings we posit a role for B cells and Abs in the protection against TB and suggest that an effective immunity against *Mtb* includes a humoral component.

COMPLEXITY OF THE HUMORAL IMMUNE RESPONSES AGAINST *Mtb*

TB serological studies provide abundant data that *Mtb* induces a humoral immune response to a wide variety of mycobacterial antigens (Ags) in humans and animals. Although humans and nonhuman primates show considerable heterogeneity in Ab responses against *Mtb*

(Lyashchenko et al. 1998; Ireton et al. 2010; Kunnath-Velayudhan et al. 2010, 2012), Ab responses in other animal species such as elephants or deer are more homogeneous (Lyashchenko et al. 2008, 2012). Animal and human serum transfer studies have provided inconsistent and sometimes contradictory data regarding a role of Abs in the protection against TB (reviewed in Glatman-Freedman and Casadevall 1998). Several observations suggest explanations for these inconsistent results. Just as in other diseases such as fungal infections in which the Ab response is complex and involves both protective and nonprotective Abs (reviewed in Casadevall and Pirofski 2012a), interstudy inconsistencies might have been due to the variability typically found in polyclonal preparations. Nonprotective or even disease-enhancing Abs can also negatively or positively influence the efficacy of protective Abs when these act in combinations (Nussbaum et al. 1996; Chow et al. 2013), further highlighting the difficulty when evaluating polyclonal preparations. The discovery that fungal Ags targeted by protective mAbs do not always elicit an Ab response during a natural infection (Nosanchuk et al. 2003), could be another explanation for negative results when transferring immune sera from vaccine studies. On the other hand, little is known about the role and complexity of protective Abs in *Mtb* infection models that mimic human infection by developing both natural LTBI and TB without modification of immunity. And last, Ab responses against *Mtb* can be species-specific (Lyashchenko et al. 2007, 2008), and thus the transfer of Ab preparations obtained from a species different than the one studied would also result in considerable variability.

EVIDENCE FOR A ROLE OF HUMORAL IMMUNITY IN THE PROTECTION AGAINST TB

The efficacy of Ab-mediated immunity against a microbe can be established by the three general approaches as proposed by Casadevall (2004): (1) Establish that passive administration of a microbe-specific Ab modifies the course of infection to the benefit of the host; (2) ascertain that the presence of microbe-specific Abs in a host is associated with decreased susceptibility to infection and disease; and (3) establish that increased susceptibility to disease exists in hosts with deficits in humoral immunity and/or B cell function. For TB evidence for all three criteria has now been documented (Table 1).

Passive transfer studies with Abs against mycobacterial Ags. Evidence that passive Ab transfer can improve the outcome of experimental mycobacterial infection in mice was documented by eight independent groups for mAbs against mycobacterial Ags (Teitelbaum et al. 1998; Pethe et al. 2001; Chambers et al. 2004; Hamasur et al. 2004; Williams et al. 2004; Buccheri et al. 2009; Lopez et al. 2009; Balu et al. 2011) and three recent studies with polyclonal IgG or serum within the same species (mice) or from humans to mice (Roy et al. 2005; Guirado et al. 2006; Olivares et al. 2006) (Table 2). Depending on the study design and the types and targets of mAbs evaluated, the measures of protection used included significantly increased survival times (Teitelbaum et al. 1998; Chambers et al. 2004; Hamasur et al. 2004), reduction of disease dissemination (Pethe et al. 2001), reduction of organ pathology (Chambers et al. 2004; Lopez et al. 2009; Balu et al. 2011), and/or reduced organ colony forming units (CFU) (Hamasur et al. 2004; Williams et al. 2004; Buccheri et al. 2009; Lopez et al. 2009; Balu et al. 2011). Of note, one study also compared the effect of mAb with IFN-γ and the combination of both (Balu et al. 2011). Although a significant reduction of lung CFU was seen with the combination of mAb and IFN-γ, and a borderline effect for mAb alone, no significant CFU reduction was seen with IFN-γ alone, pointing toward a potentially important interplay between Ab and cytokine in the protection against TB. Furthermore, three recent passive polyclonal IgG or serum transfer studies within the same species (mice) or from humans to mice have shown protection against TB (Roy et al. 2005; Guirado et al. 2006; Olivares et al. 2006). Of note, none of the Ab transfer studies included a comparison to BCG (Bacille Calmette–Guérin)-vaccinated mice. In comparison to vaccination studies with BCG substrains that induce

Table 1. Evidence of antibody-mediated protection against *Mycobacterium tuberculosis* infection

Criterion	Evidence	References
Passive Ab transfer studies	Eight independent groups have shown protection and/or modification of the course of mycobacterial infection in mice with passive transfer of mAbs to mycobacterial antigens (Table 2).	Teitelbaum et al. 1998; Pethe et al. 2001; Chambers et al. 2004; Hamasur et al. 2004; Williams et al. 2004; Buccheri et al. 2009; Lopez et al. 2009; Balu et al. 2011
	Three independent groups have recently shown protection in mice with passive transfer of immune polyclonal sera.	Roy et al. 2005; Guirado et al. 2006; Olivares et al. 2006
High Ab titer associated with reduced susceptibility	AM-containing conjugate vaccine elicits Ab response that reduces susceptibility to infection.	Hamasur et al. 2003; Glatman-Freedman et al. 2004
	BCG as well as *Mtb* antigen-containing conjugate and DNA/RNA vaccines elicit cellular and humoral immune responses and improve outcome of infection.	Huygen et al. 1996; Hamasur et al. 2003; Glatman-Freedman et al. 2004; Xue et al. 2004; de Valliere et al. 2005; Giri et al. 2006; Grover et al. 2006; Teixeira et al. 2006; Chang-hong et al. 2008; Kohama et al. 2008; Palma et al. 2008; Niu et al. 2011
Increased susceptibility in hosts with Ab deficits	Peak of childhood TB is temporally correlated with nadir in maternal Ab.	Beyazova et al. 1995; Cruz and Starke 2007; Donald et al. 2010
	Lack of Abs against certain mycobacterial antigens is associated with TB dissemination in children and adults.	Sada et al. 1990; Costello et al. 1992; Boggian et al. 1996; Gupta et al. 1997; Dayal et al. 2008
	Lack of early humoral immune response in *Mtb*-infected nonhuman primates predicts high likelihood for reactivation disease.	Kunnath-Velayudhan et al. 2012
	B-cell-deficient mice are more susceptible to TB.	Vordermeier et al. 1996; Maglione et al. 2007, 2008
	Polymeric IgR-deficient mice loose mycobacterial antigen-specific IgA response in saliva and are more susceptible to respiratory BCG infection.	Tjarnlund et al. 2006
	IgA deficiency increases susceptibility to mycobacterial infection in mice.	Rodriguez et al. 2005; Buccheri et al. 2007
Other	Existence of mycobactericidal Abs	Conti et al. 1998
	FcR-mediated phagocytosis promotes phagolysosomal fusion.	Armstrong and Hart 1975
	FcR-mediated phagocytosis increases macrophage Ca^{2+} signaling and intracellular killing.	Malik et al. 2000
	Higher FcγRIA expression in (i) subjects with TB compared with LTBI, and (ii) subjects before compared with after antituberculous treatment.	Sutherland et al. 2013; Cliff et al. 2013
	IgG bound to BCG enhances oxygen release in phagosomes and antimycobacterial activity of alveolar macrophages.	Suga et al. 1996

Data in table modified with permission from Achkar and Casadevall 2013.

mAb, monoclonal Ab; AM, arabinomannan; BCG, Bacillus Calmette–Guérin; *Mtb*, *M. tuberculosis*; TB, tuberculosis; FcR, Fc receptor; LTBI, latent *Mtb* infection.

Table 2. Passive transfer studies with monoclonal antibodies showing protective effects against experimental mycobacterial infection

mAb (isotype)	Target antigen (type)	Model	Organism/antigen challenge (route)	mAb administration (timing to infection)	Change in CFU	Biological effect	Quantitative effect	Reference
9d8 (IgG3)	AM (capsular polysaccharide)	Mouse (BALB/c and C57BL/6)	*Mtb* (ae and i.t.)	i.t. (simultaneous/preincubated mAb with *Mtb*)	↔ Lungs, spleen and liver	Prolonged survival and enhanced containment of *Mtb* within granuloma centers	30%–60% of mAb-treated mice survived >75 d (33% for >220 d) vs. death in control mice within 30 d ($p < 0.01$)	Teitelbaum et al. 1998
4057 (IgG3)	HBHA (surface-exposed protein)	Mouse (BALB/c)	BCG (i.n.)	i.n. (simultaneous/preincubated mAb with BCG)	↔ Lungs ↓ Spleen	Reduction of disease dissemination	Reduced spleen colonization by ~3 log(10) CFUs 3 wk postinfection in mAb-treated mice compared with controls (p value not stated)	Pethe et al. 2001
TBA61 (IgA)	16-kDa α-crystallin (intracellular and cell wall protein)	Mouse (BALB/c)	*Mtb* (ae and i.n.)	i.n. (3 h before and 3 or 6 d after)	↓ Lungs	CFU reduction in early disease	Reduced lung colonization by ~1 log(10) CFU 9 d postinfection in mAb-treated mice compared with controls ($p < 0.01$)	Williams et al. 2004
SMITH14 (IgG1)	AM portion of LAM (cell wall glycolipid)	Mouse (BALB/c)	*Mtb* (i.v.)	i.v. (simultaneous/preincubated mAb with *Mtb* or 1 h prior)	↓ Lungs ↓ Liver ↓ Spleen	CFU reduction and prolonged survival	Reduced lung, liver, and spleen colonization by ~1–2 log(10) CFU 14 d postinfection in mAb-treated mice 1 h before infection compared with controls ($p < 0.05$ lungs and $p < 0.01$ liver and spleen) and survival of 7–8/10 (75%) mAb-treated mice versus 4/10 (40%) controls at 70 d ($p < 0.01$)	Hamasur et al. 2004

Continued

Table 2. *Continued*

mAb (isotype)	Target antigen (type)	Model	Organism/ antigen challenge (route)	mAb administration (timing to infection)	Change in CFU	Biological effect	Quantitative effect	Reference
MBS43 (IgG2b)	MPB83 (cell wall and CF protein)	Mouse (BALB/c)	*Mycobacterium bovis* (i.v.)	i.n. (simultaneous/pre-incubated mAb with *M. bovis*)	↔ Lungs ↔ Spleen ↔ Liver	Reduced lung pathology and prolonged survival	Twice the estimated amount of normal lung tissue in mAb-treated mice compared with controls ($p < 0.05$) and 8/8 (100%) of mAb-treated mice survived >38 d (end of experiment) versus 0/8 (0%) of control mice (death within 30–34 d) ($p < 0.005$)	Chambers et al. 2004
TBA61 (IgA) and TBA84 (IgA)	16 kDa α-crystallin (intracellular and cell wall protein) and 38-kDa PstS-1 (CF protein)	Mouse (BALB/c)	*Mtb* (i.t.)	i.t. (mAb given 30 min before infection)	↓ Lungs (only for TBA61)	Reduced lung pathology (only for TBA61)	Reduced lung colonization by ~200×10^3 CFU 21 d postinfection in mAb TBA61-treated mice compared with controls and TBA84-treated mice ($p < 0.05$) and reduced peribronchial inflammation in TBA61-treated mice compared with controls 21 d post-infection ($p < 0.05$)	Lopez et al. 2009

TBA61 (IgA)	16-kDa α-crystallin (intracellular and cell wall protein)	Mouse (BALB/c, C57BL/6, C3H/HeJ)	*Mtb* (i.v.)	i.n. and i.v. given at 3, 5, or 7 wk as CIT with INF-γ, polyclonal Ab against IL-4, and mAbTBA61 in mice treated for 4 wk with INH/R	↓ Lungs in CIT-treated mice	Prevention of TB relapse in mice treated with CIT together with ↑ granuloma formation and ↑ cyto- and chemokine levels	Reduced lung colonization by ∼3–4 log(10) CFU 8 wk postinfection in CIT-treated mice compared with controls; strongest protection when CIT given 5 wk postinfection ($p = 0.001$)	Buccheri et al. 2009
2E9 (IgA1)	16-kDa α-crystallin (intracellular and cell wall protein)	Mouse (CD89tg)	*Mtb* (i.n.)	i.n. with and without INF-γ (2 h prior and 1 or 21 d post)	↓ Lungs ↓ Spleen	Reduced lung pathology	Reduced lung colonization by <1 log(10) CFU 4 wk postinfection in mAb plus INF-γ-treated mice compared with controls ($p < 0.05$) and significantly reduced lung granuloma formation in mAb-treated mice (<10%) compared with controls (∼45%; $p < 0.001$)	Balu et al. 2011

Data in table reproduced with permission from Achkar and Casadevall 2013.

mAb, monoclonal Ab; CFU, colony-forming units; INF-γ, interferon-γ; IL, interleukin. AM, arabinomannan; LAM, lipoarabinomannan; HBHA, heparin-binding hemaglutinin; *Mtb*, *M. tuberculosis*; CF, culture filtrate; CIT, combined immunotherapy; INH/R, isoniazid and rifampin; ae, aerosol; i.n., intranasal; i.v., intravenous; i.t., intratracheal.

variable CFU reduction ranging from $\frac{1}{2}$ to $1\frac{1}{2}$ mean log(10) organ CFU reduction 30 d after experimental *Mtb* infection in mice (Keyser et al. 2011), the quantitative effects of some mAbs were less than, some similar to, and some superior to those described for BCG vaccines (reviewed in Achkar and Casadevall 2013).

Association of the presence of Abs against Mtb with decreased susceptibility to infection and disease. Mice immunized with conjugate vaccines, containing arabinomannan (AM), a mycobacterial capsular, and cell wall polysaccharide, develop high IgG titers against AM and are more TB-resistant than control mice (Hamasur et al. 2003; Glatman-Freedman et al. 2004; R Prados-Rosales, unpubl.). In fact, two of these AM conjugate vaccines showed prolonged survival and reduced histopathological findings comparable to BCG vaccine (Hamasur et al. 2003; R Prados-Rosales, unpubl.). Furthermore, BCG, subunit, and DNA/RNA vaccines elicit humoral immune responses and improve the outcome of TB infection, although most of these vaccine studies conclude that protection against TB was based solely on cell-mediated immunity (reviewed in Achkar and Casadevall 2013). In contrast to most TB vaccine studies, de Valliere et al. (2005) investigated the role of Abs induced after BCG vaccination. They showed that BCG-induced Abs enhance effects of both the innate and cell-mediated immune responses against mycobacteria.

Association of increased susceptibility to disease with deficits in humoral immunity and B-cell function. The peak of vulnerability to TB in early childhood coincides with a nadir in Ab (Beyazova et al. 1995; Fairchok et al. 1995; Cruz and Starke 2007; Donald et al. 2010). This association is supported by a study showing that the lack of Abs against the mycobacterial cell wall glycolipid lipoarabinomannan (LAM) correlates significantly with disseminated TB in age-matched children (Costello et al. 1992). Also of note is that patients with HIV-associated TB, which tends to progress faster and frequently disseminates, also have lower Ab titers against LAM or AM (Boggian et al. 1996; Yu et al. 2012), although this association warrants further investigation. Furthermore, serological studies have found lower Ab levels against mycobacterial Ags in both children and adults with miliary or disseminated, meningeal and pleural TB in contrast to localized pulmonary TB (Sada et al. 1990; Gupta et al. 1997; Dayal et al. 2008; Ziegenbalg et al. 2013). These findings suggest that Abs against certain Ags could reduce the risk of TB dissemination in humans. Such a hypothesis is supported by studies in animal models. For example, the mycobacterial surface protein heparin-binding hemagglutinin adhesin (HBHA) promotes *Mtb* dissemination in mice, whereas passive transfer with a mAb against HBHA reduces extrapulmonary dissemination (Pethe et al. 2001) (Table 2). Furthermore, our group has recently shown that an AM-conjugate vaccine prevented *Mtb* dissemination in mice, an effect that was not observed with BCG vaccination (R Prados-Rosales, unpubl.).

Perhaps the closest to a state of pure B-cell-related deficiency in humans is the clinical entity of hypogamaglobulinemia (Bruton 1952; Good and Zak 1956; Conley et al. 2009). Although clinical studies have reported TB in persons with immunoglobulin (Ig) deficiency, these patients typically present with infections caused by bacteria commonly associated with human diseases such as *Streptococcus pneumonia* (Good and Zak 1956; Conley et al. 2009). On diagnosis of hypogammaglobulinemia, sustained periodic IVIG therapy is required for preventing infection-associated mortality (Bruton 1952; Good and Zak 1956). Such therapies can obscure the potential significance of Ab deficiency in the defense against *Mtb*. Patients not receiving this standard Ig therapy will likely succumb to "endogenous" colonizing pathogens and not *Mtb*. Therapy with Rituximab, which depletes $CD20^+$ B cells and has been used widely in the treatment of B-cell malignancies and autoimmune diseases (Czuczman and Gregory 2010; Townsend et al. 2010), has not been associated with increased susceptibility to *Mtb*. In contrast, it has been amply showed that anti-TNF therapies enhances the risk for developing reactivation TB (Keane et al. 2001). Of note, however, is that studies including individuals receiving Rituximab have not revealed an increased risk for infection to bacterial pathogens (reviewed in Rubbert-Roth 2012; Ruderman 2012; Schoels et al. 2012; Isaacs 2013) including those that are known colonizers of the host, and which defense has been shown to be highly B-cell-dependent (Bruton 1952; Good and Zak 1956). Hence, the absence of increased susceptibility to TB with these therapies cannot be used to argue against a role for Ab-mediated immunity. The mechanisms underlying this observation are likely multifactorial and remain to be determined. It is conceivable that they could be due to specific pharmacokinetic property of Rituximab or the inability of this monoclonal antibody to deplete the long-lived $CD20^-$ plasma cells.

In animal models, IgA-deficient mice are more susceptible to BCG infection than wild-type controls (Rodriguez et al. 2005). Polymeric IgR-deficient mice vaccinated with the mycobacterial protein PstS-1 had lower PstS-1-specific IgA levels in their saliva and were more susceptible to BCG infection than vaccinated wild-type mice (Tjarnlund et al. 2006), and IgA administration in the setting of interleukin-4 (IL-4) and interferon-γ (IFN-γ) administration conferred protection against *Mtb* in mice (Buccheri et al. 2007). Furthermore, mice lacking the γ-chain of an activating receptor for the Fc portion of Abs (FcγR) are more susceptible to *Mtb* infection and advanced pulmonary disease than wild-type mice (Maglione et al. 2008).

Studies with B-cell-deficient mice mostly support the role of B cells in TB immunity but some have also provided inconsistent results. Two of four published studies report that B-cell-deficient mice are more susceptible to experimental infection (Vordermeier et al. 1996; Maglione et al. 2007). A different study challenging with *Mtb* after isoniazid therapy found no difference between B-cell-deficient and wild-type mice (Johnson et al. 1997). One study found that the pulmonary histopathology was more pronounced in B-cell-knockout compared with wild-type mice after low-dose *Mtb* infection (Bosio et al. 2000). Of note is that humans with pulmonary TB were also found to have lower percentages of peripheral blood B cells compared with asymptomatic individuals with and without presumed *Mtb* infection (Corominas et al. 2004; Hernandez et al. 2010). These findings, together with the observation that an infected host mounts a robust Ab response against *Mtb*, provide strong support for the notion that B cells actively participate in the immune response to *Mtb*.

INFLUENCE OF B CELLS ON OTHER IMMUNE CELLS IN *Mtb* INFECTION

There is ample evidence that T cells and macrophages play a critical role in the defense against *Mtb* infection and disease. However, B cells, just as T cells, interact with various immune cells, thus contributing to the defense mechanisms. We note that the extent of cellular interactions renders it challenging to quantify the amount of protection contributed by a single specific immune cell population. Studies involving various animal TB models have provided compelling evidence that T-cell deficiency produces strong susceptibility phenotypes (Flynn and Chan 2001; Cooper 2009; Ernst 2012). A recent report showing that T cells play a central role in coordinating the antimycobacterial effects of a variety of immune cells during the innate phase of the host response further underscores the significance of this lymphocyte population in defense against *Mtb* (Yao et al. 2014). The importance of T cells in defense against the tubercle bacillus is further supported by enhanced susceptibility of humans defective in T-cell-activating elements as a result of mutation in the receptors of IFN-γ and IL-12 (Abel and Casanova 2000; Casanova and Abel 2002; Fortin et al. 2007). It is curious that in these naturally occurring human models, the genotypes are mostly associated with infection with relatively weakly virulent mycobacteria such as environmental bacilli and BCG. This observation could be due to the higher probability of exposure to environmental mycobacteria than to *Mtb*, and that BCG-osis is the result of direct inoculation of the vaccine during immunization.

Although macrophages play an important role in initiating IL-12/IFN-γ-related antimycobacterial functions, it was reported that nonselective depletion of this immune cell in a murine TB model resulted in enhanced protection against pulmonary TB, whereas selective ablation of activated macrophages increased susceptibility (Leemans et al. 2001, 2005). In addition, although it was shown that mutations at or near the Scl11a1 (Nramp1) locus, a gene that confers macrophage resistance to mycobacteria, resulted in susceptibility to *Mtb* in certain human populations (Fortin et al. 2007), this allele appears to play no role in the control of the tubercle bacillus in mice (North et al. 1999). These results suggest that valid testing of the significance of specific immunological factors in defense against *Mtb* may require an appropriate host, adding yet another layer of complexity to studies aimed at deciphering protective antituberculous response.

B cells, in addition to being a rich source of Abs, can modulate the immune response by virtue of their ability to present Ags and produce a wide variety of cytokines. These modulating functions play important roles in affecting the development of immune cells including T cells, neutrophils, macrophages, and dendritic cells (reviewed in Maglione and Chan 2009; Kozakiewicz et al. 2013b). B-cell-deficient mice are more susceptible to *Mtb* infection, and this deficiency results in enhanced lung immunopathology and increased pulmonary neutrophil infiltration and IL-10 production (Maglione et al. 2007). The importance of B cells in the regulation of neutrophil influx at the site of infection is supported by another study showing an abnormally rapid neutrophil migration in B-cell-deficient mice, and demonstrating the capacity of B cells to down-regulate neutrophil motility (Kondratieva et al. 2010). The capacity of B cells to down-regulate neutrophil motility appears critical for the effectiveness of BCG vaccination in mice (Kondratieva et al. 2010). The B-cell-deficient phenotypes are reversible by adoptive transfer of B cells from infected wild-type (WT) C57BL/6 mice, establishing B-cell specificity. Reversal of these lung phenotypes is associated with the presence of Ig in serum of recipient mice without a requirement for pulmonary homing of transferred cells (Maglione et al. 2007). These observations suggest that the rescue effect of transferred B cells is at least partially caused by Ab-mediated immune regulation and indicate that humoral immunity plays a significant role in the defense against *Mtb*. This notion is further supported by our recent observations that tissue neutrophilia in B-cell-deficient mice can be reversed by administration of sera from tuberculous mice (Kozakiewicz et al. 2013a).

A role for B cells regulating T cells in immune responses to *Mtb* is supported by our finding that in chronic infection, CD4 T-cell proliferation and IFN-γ production in B-cell-deficient mice are significantly different than that in WTs (Maglione and Chan 2009). Mice deficient for the inhibitory FcγRIIB (FcyRIIB$^{-/-}$) are more resistant to *Mtb* compared with WT controls (Maglione et al. 2008). These findings correlated with enhanced pulmonary Th1 responses, evidenced by increased IFN-γ-producing CD4^{+} T cells, and suggests that Abs can regulate CD4 Th1 response in acute TB through engagement of FcR by Ab-Ag complexes. Furthermore, in mice and humans, features of germinal center B cells suggest that they are immunologically active (Ulrichs et al. 2004; Maglione et al. 2007). We and others have shown that B cells are a conspicuous cellular component in lung granuloma of humans, nonhuman primates, and mice with TB (Gonzalez-Juarrero et al. 2001; Ulrichs et al. 2004; Tsai et al. 2006; Flynn 2010). It has recently been shown in both human and mouse models that B-cell nodules in tuberculous lung tissues are populated with CXCR5^{+} T cells (Slight et al. 2013). This T-cell population, which is directed to infected lungs via expression of CXCR5, plays a role in the control of *Mtb* by promoting macrophage activation and lymphoid nodule formation (Slight et al. 2013).

Accumulating experimental evidence has revealed the significance of the interaction between B and T lymphocytes in the germinal center in an immune response, including that developed against microbial pathogens (Vinuesa et al. 2005; Ma et al. 2012). The clinical relevance of this interaction was shown recently in the qualitative and quantitative analysis of the germinal center reaction in HIV (human immunodeficiency virus) models (Vinuesa 2012;

 Cite this article as *Cold Spring Harb Perspect Med* doi: 10.1101/cshperspect.a018432

Cubas et al. 2013; Locci et al. 2013; Pillai 2013; Schmitt and Ueno 2013). The results of these studies revealed that the nature of the B-cell humoral immunity in response to antigens, particularly as it related to the generation of broadly neutralizing antibodies, was highly dependent on the T follicular helper cells, whose development occurs in the germinal center (Vinuesa 2012; Cubas et al. 2013; Locci et al. 2013; Pillai 2013; Schmitt and Ueno 2013). Indeed, abnormalities of the B-cell and humoral immune response in individuals infected with HIV have been documented (Moir and Fauci 2009). Thus, it remains possible that the aberrant B-cell compartment of the host immune response contributes to the susceptibility of HIV-infected individuals to the tubercle bacillus. Similarly, because of this B:T interaction, it is not straightforward to determine the relative contribution of these two lymphocyte populations in the defense against *Mtb*. It is possible that B cells and humoral immunity could account, at least in part, for the enhanced susceptibility to *Mtb* in individuals afflicted with T-cell-deficient states other than that associated with HIV infection. Together, these observations indicate that protective mechanisms against the tubercle bacillus are complex and most certainly involve redundancy, rendering quantification of the relative contribution to the overall host resistance to *Mtb* by specific immunological factors difficult. This difficulty is further compounded by the highly interactive nature of immune cells.

MECHANISMS OF Ab-MEDIATED PROTECTION AGAINST *Mtb*

Despite being a facultative intracellular pathogen, *Mtb* is potentially susceptible to various mechanisms of Ab-mediated immunity (Fig. 1). Opsonization of *Mtb* through FcγR promotes phagolysosomal fusion (Armstrong and Hart 1975) and increases macrophage Ca^{2+} signaling and intracellular killing (Malik et al. 2000). IgG bound to BCG increased the release of oxygen in the phagosomes of alveolar macrophages, suggesting the enhancement of antimycobacterial macrophage activity by Ab (Suga et al. 1996). Immune complexes that stimulate FcεRII-CD23 receptors triggered cellular changes that promote the killing of *Toxoplasma gondii*, another intracellular pathogen (Vouldoukis et al. 2011), and stimulation of the same receptor was associated with antimycobacterial activity (Mossalayi et al. 2009). Furthermore, the existence of potentially synergistic functions between humoral and cell-mediated immunity against TB is suggested by the observation that Abs to mycobacterial Ags in BCG-vaccinated persons enhance both innate and cell-mediated immune responses against mycobacteria (de Valliere et al. 2005), and that sera from TB contacts with high, but not low IgG titers against tuberculin, can block proliferation of PBMC cultures with tuberculin (Encinales et al. 2010). Moreover, a robust T-cell response against intracellular pathogens such a *Chlamydia* spp. and mycobacteria is enhanced by specific Ab responses that can augment Th1 activation via FcR by facilitating a rapid uptake, processing, and presentation of Ags (Igietseme et al. 2004). In addition, there is also clear evidence for an extracellular phase of *Mtb* during which it can be directly targeted by Abs (Smith et al. 2000; Casadevall 2003; Grosset 2003; Karakousis et al. 2004; Kim et al. 2010; Ahmad et al. 2011; Hoff et al. 2011; Driver et al. 2012).

Engagement of distinct FcγRs can divergently affect the susceptibility for TB, suggesting that targeting FcγRs can be a means to enhance TB immunity (Maglione et al. 2008). In contrast to the inhibitory $FcγRIIB^{-/-}$ strain, mice lacking the γ-chain of activating FcγRs are more susceptible to *Mtb* infection with exacerbated immunopathology and increased production of the anti-inflammatory cytokine IL-10 (Maglione et al. 2008). Because different isotypes and IgG subclasses engage different types of FcγR, the class of the Ab response is likely to be important in resistance. This is consistent with the well-established data that Ag-Ab interactions with FcR can modulate the immune response, which has been exploited in the treatment of a variety of diseases, most notably neoplastic and autoimmune disorders (Kalergis and Ravetch 2002; Rafiq et al. 2002; Clynes 2005; Dhodapkar et al. 2005). In fact, a recent

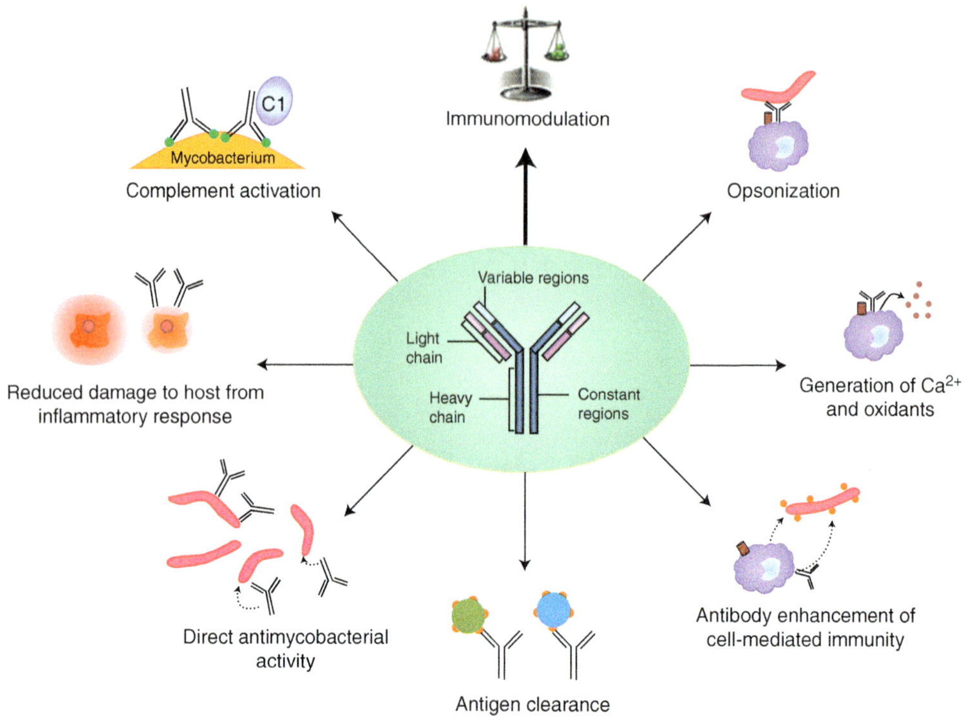

Figure 1. Illustration of the various reported mechanisms of antibody-mediated protection against *Mycobacterium tuberculosis* such as opsonization (Armstrong and Hart 1975), increase of macrophage Ca^{2+} signaling (Malik et al. 2000), and release of oxidants (Suga et al. 1996; Mossalayi et al. 2009) enhancing intracellular killing, other mechanisms enhancing cell-mediated immunity (de Valliere et al. 2005; Encinales et al. 2010), clearance of immunomodulatory mycobacterial antigens (Glatman-Freedman et al. 2000), direct antimycobacterial activity (Conti et al. 1998), and activation of complement (Hetland et al. 1998; Carroll et al. 2009; Manivannan et al. 2012).

multisite human gene expression study found that expression of FcγRIA was significantly and consistently higher in subjects with TB compared with those with LTBI, regardless of HIV coinfection (Sutherland et al. 2013). These findings were consistent with another study showing a significant reduction in FcγRIA expression in TB cases after antituberculous treatment when compared with pretreatment expression (Cliff et al. 2013). FcγRIA is predominantly expressed by monocytes and macrophages, is induced by IFN-γ, promotes Ab-dependent cytotoxicity, mediates the clearance of immune complexes, and may have been responsible for the control of *Mtb* after Ab-mediated phagocytosis observed in earlier studies (Armstrong and Hart 1971). Overall, these study results of FcγRs in both humans and animals further support a protective role of the humoral immune component against *Mtb*.

Abs can also contribute to host defense against *Mtb* by promoting the clearance of immunomodulatory Ags such as LAM (Glatman-Freedman et al. 2000). In addition, there are mechanisms shown for other intracellular pathogens that could also apply to *Mtb*. Protective and nonprotective mAbs mediate differences in gene expression for *Cryptococcus neoformans* (McClelland et al. 2010), and agglutinating nonopsonic Abs have been shown to mediate bactericidal effects against *Streptococcus pneumoniae* through quorum-sensing-related mechanisms (Yano et al. 2011). Finally, Abs that mimic the action of fungal killer toxin have been shown to be bactericidal to *Mtb* (Conti et al. 1998). Although such Abs are unlikely to be present in *Mtb* infection, the fact that mycobacteria can be killed directly by certain Abs provides a precedent for such a mechanism of Ab-mediated protection.

In addition to the direct mechanisms, Abs can influence the outcome of mycobacterial infection through their ability to modulate inflammation. Some Abs, such as IgM, mediate proinflammatory properties through their ability to activate complement (Ciurana et al. 2004), whereas other Abs, such as IgG, can produce pro- or anti-inflammatory effects depending on the antigen and FcR receptor engaged (Lux et al. 2010; Ballow 2011). Ab-mediated activation of complement in mycobacterial infection was shown in several studies by various groups. Human IgG, and to a lesser extent IgM, enhanced complement binding to BCG (Carroll et al. 2009). In TB patients, serum IgG2 levels, but not IgM, to LAM correlated positively with classical complement activation induced by BCG (Hetland et al. 1998). Furthermore, human IgG against mycobacterial Ags in bacterial sonicates enhanced complement activation by *Mtb* and increased phagocytosis of *Mtb* by macrophages (Manivannan et al. 2012).

When the action of Abs is analyzed from the context of the damage–response framework it is apparent how the pro- or anti-inflammatory properties can be protective or deleterious depending on the immune status of the host. *Mtb* is pathogenic in hosts with either too much or too little of an inflammatory response, as evidenced by disease states characterized by caseous necrosis or widespread dissemination, such as miliary TB, respectively (Casadevall and Pirofski 2003; Achkar and Jenny-Avital 2011). In contrast, hosts that mount an intermediate response can presumably control infection through granuloma formation. The need for the right balance of inflammatory response to control *Mtb* infection is further supported by a recent study showing that although the proinflammatory cytokine tumor necrosis factor (TNF) is critical in the host defense against TB, its excess leads to enhanced disease in zebrafish and humans (Roca and Ramakrishnan 2013). Taking the importance of the right balance of the combined immune responses to *Mtb* into consideration, Abs that are proinflammatory could help hosts that respond with too little inflammation, whereas those that are anti-inflammatory could help hosts with exuberant inflammatory responses that result in tissue destructions (Fig. 2).

CHARACTERISTICS OF PROTECTIVE Abs AGAINST *Mtb*

The Ab parameters that contribute to protection include amount, specificity, affinity, and isotype. For *Mtb*, very few mAbs have been characterized in detail and consequently the difficulty to identify trends in the characteristics of protective Abs to *Mtb*. However, it is possible to discern some themes. Protective Abs to *Mtb* recognize at least six different antigenic determinants. The murine isotypes IgM, IgG1, IgG3, and IgA have each been shown to protect against TB (Table 2). The finding that an IgG3 to AM lost protective efficacy when converted to IgG2a provides additional support for the notion that the constant region type has an important role in the activity of the Ab against *Mtb*. (Schwebach 2002). An additional example of this phenomenon is the observation an IgA against the 16-kDa α-cristallin was active against *Mtb*, whereas an IgG1 mAb to the same epitope had no protective efficacy (Williams et al. 2004). Intranasal administration of an IgA1 combined with IFN-γ significantly ameliorated lung H37Rv infection in mice transgenic for human CD89m but not in CD89-negative littermate controls, providing evidence that IgA-mediated protection required CD89 (Balu et al. 2011). The fact that IgA can protect against pulmonary *Mtb* infection is important given the role of this isotype in mucosal immunity. Evidence that the amount of Ab is critical for protection comes from the observation of prozone-like effects in passive experiments in mice (Schwebach 2002).

PERSPECTIVE ON IMPACT OF Abs AT THE VARIOUS *Mtb* INFECTION STATES

Based on the known functions of Abs and the results of various studies we envision that Ab-mediated immunity can serve a protective role

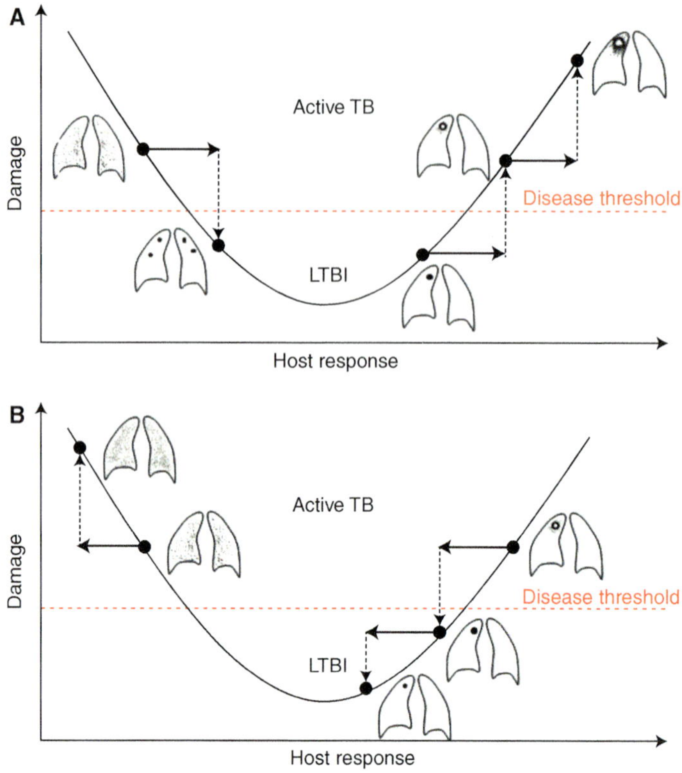

Figure 2. Interpretation of the potential function of pro- and anti-inflammatory antibodies against *Mtb* in the context of the damage–response framework. (*A*) Potential effects of a proinflammatory antibody with enhanced inflammation leading, on the one hand, to the improvement from disseminated/miliary TB in an immunocompromised host (*left*) to localized granuloma formation and, on the other hand, to progression from granuloma to caseous necrosis in the more immunocompetent host (*right*). (*B*) Potential effects of an anti-inflammatory antibody leading to worsening TB dissemination in the immunocompromised host who has already reduced inflammation (*left*), but improved containment of local disease from caseous necrosis to granuloma formation in the more immunocompetent host with a strong inflammatory response (*right*). LTBI, latent TB infection. (Figure reproduced with permission from Achkar and Casadevall 2013.)

against *Mtb* at various states of infection. Early in infection Abs could enhance host defenses by promoting phagocytosis through FcR, a process that is known to increase intracellular killing and rapid uptake and processing of mycobacterial Ags. Similarly, Abs could activate complement, a process that would further promote phagocytosis and cellular recruitment to the site of infection. Given that mycobacterial polysaccharides and lipopolysaccharides are powerful immunomodulators that can interfere with the development of effective immune response, the presence of Ab to these Ags could contribute to host defense by promoting their clearance. Abs can function as pro- and anti-inflammatory molecules depending on their ability to activate FcR, and this effect could be beneficial by heightening an effective inflammatory response or down-modulating runaway granuloma formation, which has the capacity to destroy tissues. We anticipate that Ab could have different roles depending on the immunological state of the host. For example, the proinflammatory effects of Ab-mediated immunity may help protect immunologically naïve hosts during initial infection. In this regards, naturally occurring Ab, in particular IgM, is critical for defense against many infectious diseases (Casadevall and Pirofski 2012b) and could have an important role in protection against *Mtb* by promoting an early inflammatory response. In contrast, IgG elicited by vaccines would be expected to function primarily through FcR engagement. At this time the relative importance of these mechanisms is unknown, and it is possible that they differ from host to host. However, given that Abs have the capacity to modulate practically all aspects of the interaction between *Mtb* and its host, there is a high likelihood that this arm of the adaptive immune response can make a major contribution to host defense. Hence, there is a need for additional studies of Ab function and its potential role on both defense against and pathogenesis of mycobacterial infections.

PERSPECTIVE FOR A ROLE OF Abs IN TB VACCINE EFFICACY AND TB TREATMENT

Vaccines based solely on induction of T cells have not been successful to date. One possible explanation is that immunity requires a layered defense including a multipronged approach to obtain effective protection by a TB vaccine. In mice, as discussed above, B cells and Ig are important components of anti-TB immunity capable of modulating various aspects of host response against *Mtb* (Maglione and Chan 2009; Achkar and Casadevall 2013; Kozakiewicz et al. 2013b). In view of these observations, it would be prudent to explore the possibility that B cells or Abs may play a role in engendering protection during vaccination against *Mtb*, regardless of the importance of humoral immunity in optimal control of a natural tuberculous infection in humans. Indeed, BCG has been shown to be ineffective in engendering protection in B-cell-deficient CBA/xid mice against *Mtb* challenge (Kondratieva et al. 2010) and BCG immunization in B-cell-deficient μMT mice elicits a CD4 Th1 response that is inferior to that in the wild types (Kozakiewicz et al. 2013a). Understanding the B-cell and humoral immunity during *Mtb* infection and immunization and harnessing such responses might lead to strategies and protocols required for the development of a much needed effective TB vaccine.

The ideal role of vaccine-induced neutralizing Abs would be the prevention of both infection in naïve individuals and progression to disease in *Mtb*-infected individuals. Whether this is an achievable goal, and to what extent humoral immunity with specific isotypes would be required, is unclear with the current state of knowledge. Given the heterogeneity of human hosts and their humoral immune response, as well as the complexity of TB pathogenesis, it is possible that a cocktail of induced Abs against various targets and with various functions would provide higher protective efficacy than a single type of Ab. One of the likely most promising targets would include the *Mtb* capsular polysaccharide AM, as our group has recently shown that immunization with a conjugate vaccine containing this antigen protects mice better against *Mtb* infection than immunization with BCG.

An additional promising role of Abs would lie in their use as adjunctive treatment of TB, especially in the setting of drug resistance. Such treatment could potentially shorten treatment duration and improve cure rates. Ab therapy against TB would likely have to be based on mAbs given the unpredictable heterogeneity of polyclonal serum preparations. Ab-based therapies have revolutionized the treatment of certain malignancies and autoimmune diseases (reviewed in Chan and Carter 2010; Weiner et al. 2010), and two mAbs have been approved for the treatment of infectious diseases (reviewed in Casadevall et al. 2004; Saylor et al. 2009). Furthermore, recent data, generated by our group and others, provide evidence that a combination of mAbs against different epitopes can enhance protective effects against infectious pathogens (Chow et al. 2013; Pohl et al. 2013). Thus, just as for vaccines, Ab-based therapy against TB will also be likely most effective if targeting multiple epitopes and/or antigens. Furthermore, for a beneficial impact on the disease, pro- versus anti-inflammatory mAbs might have to be selected taking the level of host inflammatory response to TB into account (Fig. 2). To move the field of therapeutic Abs ahead, various mAbs will need to be generated, characterized, optimized, and tested individually and in combination in vitro before being evaluated for their protection against experimental TB in animal models.

SUMMARY

When taking into account the older data (Glatman-Freedman and Casadevall 1998; Glatman-Freedman 2006), the fact that for other facultative intracellular pathogens such as fungi and *Salmonella* spp. Ab-mediated immunity has been shown to be important, the complexity of Ab responses to mycobacteria and more recent studies (Table 1), it is difficult to avoid the conclusion that humoral immunity has an important role in the protection against TB. When weighing the evidence, positive studies are much more significant than negative studies given that protective and nonprotective Abs exist and that the Ab response to *Mtb* is heterogeneous. In fact, the most straightforward interpretation of negative studies is that the particular serum or vaccine used in that study did not result in Ab-mediated protection. In contrast to negative studies, positive studies provide direct evidence for the ability of Ab-mediated immunity to contribute to the host defense against TB. Consequently, we interpret the available data to indicate that TB vaccines that induce Ab-mediated immunity as well as Ab-based therapy could result in enhanced protection. We note that the protective mechanisms against the tubercle bacillus are complex and highly interactive, rendering quantification of the relative contribution of B cells and Abs to the overall host resistance to *Mtb* difficult at this time. However, what is certain is that the TB field cannot go forward ignoring the contribution of Ab-mediated immunity if progress is going to be made in understanding the basis of host resistance and the design of future vaccines.

ACKNOWLEDGMENTS

This work was supported by funds from the National Institutes of Health (NIH)/National Institute of Allergy and Infectious Diseases (NIAID) (AI-067665 and AI-105684 to J.M.A., AI063537 and AI094745 to J.C., and AI-033774, AI-052733, and AI-033142 to A.C.), the National Heart, Lung, and Blood Institute (NHLBI) (HL-059842 to A.C.), the Center for AIDS Research (CFAR) at the Albert Einstein College of Medicine (AI-51519 to J.M.A.), the Aeras TB vaccine foundation (J.M.A. and A.C.), and the Food and Drug Administration (FDA) (1U18 FD004012/01 to J.M.A.). A.C. is also the recipient of a Bill & Melinda Gates Grand Challenge award and TB Vaccine Accelerator Program award. We thank Anke Ziegenbalg for her graphic assistance with the figures.

REFERENCES

Abel L, Casanova JL. 2000. Genetic predisposition to clinical tuberculosis: Bridging the gap between simple and complex inheritance. *Am J Hum Genet* **67:** 274–277.

Achkar JM, Jenny-Avital ER. 2011. Incipient and subclinical tuberculosis: Defining early disease states in the context of host immune response. *J Infect Dis* **204** (Suppl): S1179–S1186.

Achkar JM, Casadevall A. 2013. Antibody-mediated immunity against tuberculosis: Implications for vaccine development. *Cell Host Microbe* **13:** 250–262.

Ahmad Z, Fraig MM, Bisson GP, Nuermberger EL, Grosset JH, Karakousis PC. 2011. Dose-dependent activity of pyrazinamide in animal models of intracellular and extracellular tuberculosis infections. *Antimicrob Agents Chemother* **55:** 1527–1532.

Almeida LP, Trombone AP, Lorenzi JC, Rocha CD, Malardo T, Fontoura IC, Gembre AF, Silva RL, Silva CL, Castelo AP, et al. 2011. B cells can modulate the CD8 memory T cell after DNA vaccination against experimental tuberculosis. *Genet Vaccines Ther* **9:** 5.

Armstrong JA, Hart PD. 1971. Response of cultured macrophages to *Mycobacterium tuberculosis*, with observations on fusion of lysosomes with phagosomes. *J Exp Med* **134:** 713–740.

Armstrong JA, Hart PD. 1975. Phagosome-lysosome interactions in cultured macrophages infected with virulent tubercle bacilli. Reversal of the usual nonfusion pattern and observations on bacterial survival. *J Exp Med* **142:** 1–16.

Ballow M. 2011. The IgG molecule as a biological immune response modifier: Mechanisms of action of intravenous immune serum globulin in autoimmune and inflammatory disorders. *J Allergy Clin Immunol* **127:** 315–323; quiz 324-315.

Balu S, Reljic R, Lewis MJ, Pleass RJ, McIntosh R, van Kooten C, van Egmond M, Challacombe S, Woof JM, Ivanyi J. 2011. A novel human IgA monoclonal antibody protects against tuberculosis. *J Immunol* **186:** 3113–3119.

Beyazova U, Rota S, Cevheroglu C, Karsligil T. 1995. Humoral immune response in infants after BCG vaccination. *Tuber Lung Dis* **76:** 248–253.

Boggian K, Fierz W, Vernazza PL. 1996. Infrequent detection of lipoarabinomannan antibodies in human immunodeficiency virus–associated mycobacterial disease. Swiss HIV cohort study. *J Clin Microbiol* **34:** 1854–1855.

Bosio CM, Gardner D, Elkins KL. 2000. Infection of B cell-deficient mice with CDC 1551, a clinical isolate of *Mycobacterium tuberculosis*: Delay in dissemination and development of lung pathology. *J Immunol* **164:** 6417–6425.

Bruton OC. 1952. Agammaglobulinemia. *Pediatrics* **9:** 722–728.

Buccheri S, Reljic R, Caccamo N, Ivanyi J, Singh M, Salerno A, Dieli F. 2007. IL-4 depletion enhances host resistance and passive IgA protection against tuberculosis infection in BALB/c mice. *Eur J Immunol* **37:** 729–737.

Buccheri S, Reljic R, Caccamo N, Meraviglia S, Ivanyi J, Salerno A, Dieli F. 2009. Prevention of the post-chemotherapy relapse of tuberculous infection by combined immunotherapy. *Tuberculosis (Edinb)* **89:** 91–94.

Carroll MV, Lack N, Sim E, Krarup A, Sim RB. 2009. Multiple routes of complement activation by *Mycobacterium bovis* BCG. *Mol Immunol* **46:** 3367–3378.

Casadevall A. 1995. Antibody immunity and invasive fungal infections. *Infect Immun* **63:** 4211–4218.

Casadevall A. 1998. Antibody-mediated protection against intracellular pathogens. *Trends Microbiol* **6:** 102–107.

Casadevall A. 2003. Antibody-mediated immunity against intracellular pathogens: Two-dimensional thinking comes full circle. *Infect Immun* **71:** 4225–4228.

Casadevall A. 2004. The methodology for determining the efficacy of antibody-mediated immunity. *J Immunol Methods* **291:** 1–10.

Casadevall A, Pirofski LA. 2003. The damage–response framework of microbial pathogenesis. *Nat Rev Microbiol* **1:** 17–24.

Casadevall A, Pirofski LA. 2012a. Immunoglobulins in defense, pathogenesis, and therapy of fungal diseases. *Cell Host Microbe* **11:** 447–456.

Casadevall A, Pirofski LA. 2012b. A new synthesis for antibody-mediated immunity. *Nat Immunol* **13:** 21–28.

Casadevall A, Dadachova E, Pirofski LA. 2004. Passive antibody therapy for infectious diseases. *Nat Rev Microbiol* **2:** 695–703.

Casanova JL, Abel L. 2002. Genetic dissection of immunity to mycobacteria: The human model. *Annu Rev Immunol* **20:** 581–620.

Cassone A, Casadevall A. 2012. Recent progress in vaccines against fungal diseases. *Curr Opin Microbiol* **15:** 427–433.

Chambers MA, Gavier-Widen D, Hewinson RG. 2004. Antibody bound to the surface antigen MPB83 of *Mycobacterium bovis* enhances survival against high dose and low dose challenge. *FEMS Immunol Med Microbiol* **41:** 93–100.

Chan AC, Carter PJ. 2010. Therapeutic antibodies for autoimmunity and inflammation. *Nat Rev Immunol* **10:** 301–316.

Chang-hong S, Xiao-wu W, Hai Z, Ting-fen Z, Li-Mei W, Zhi-kai X. 2008. Immune responses and protective efficacy of the gene vaccine expressing Ag85B and ESAT6 fusion protein from *Mycobacterium tuberculosis*. *DNA Cell Biol* **27:** 199–207.

Chow SK, Smith C, MacCarthy T, Pohl MA, Bergman A, Casadevall A. 2013. Disease enhacing antibodies improve the efficacy of bacterial toxin-neutralizing antibodies. *Cell Host Microbe* **13:** 417–428.

Ciurana CL, Zwart B, van Mierlo G, Hack CE. 2004. Complement activation by necrotic cells in normal plasma environment compares to that by late apoptotic cells and involves predominantly IgM. *Eur J Immunol* **34:** 2609–2619.

Cliff JM, Lee JS, Constantinou N, Cho JE, Clark TG, Ronacher K, King EC, Lukey PT, Duncan K, Van Helden PD, et al. 2013. Distinct phases of blood gene expression pattern through tuberculosis treatment reflect modulation of the humoral immune response. *J Infect Dis* **207:** 18–29.

Clynes R. 2005. Immune complexes as therapy for autoimmunity. *J Clin Invest* **115:** 25–27.

Colditz GA, Brewer TF, Berkey CS, Wilson ME, Burdick E, Fineberg HV, Mosteller F. 1994. Efficacy of BCG vaccine in the prevention of tuberculosis. Meta-analysis of the published literature. *JAMA* **271:** 698–702.

Collins FM. 1974. Vaccines and cell-mediated immunity. *Bacteriol Rev* **38:** 371–402.

Conley ME, Dobbs AK, Farmer DM, Kilic S, Paris K, Grigoriadou S, Coustan-Smith E, Howard V, Campana D. 2009. Primary B cell immunodeficiencies: Comparisons and contrasts. *Annu Rev Immunol* **27:** 199–227.

Conti S, Fanti F, Magliani W, Gerloni M, Bertolotti D, Salati A, Cassone A, Polonelli L. 1998. Mycobactericidal activity of human natural, monoclonal, and recombinant yeast killer toxin-like antibodies. *J Infect Dis* **177:** 807–811.

Cooper AM. 2009. Cell-mediated immune responses in tuberculosis. *Annu Rev Immunol* **27:** 393–422.

Corominas M, Cardona V, Gonzalez L, Cayla JA, Rufi G, Mestre M, Buendia E. 2004. B-lymphocytes and co-stimulatory molecules in *Mycobacterium tuberculosis* infection. *Int J Tuberc Lung Dis* **8:** 98–105.

Costello AM, Kumar A, Narayan V, Akbar MS, Ahmed S, Abou-Zeid C, Rook GA, Stanford J, Moreno C. 1992. Does antibody to mycobacterial antigens, including lipoarabinomannan, limit dissemination in childhood tuberculosis? *Trans R Soc Trop Med Hyg* **86:** 686–692.

Cruz AT, Starke JR. 2007. Clinical manifestations of tuberculosis in children. *Paediatr Respir Rev* **8:** 107–117.

Cubas RA, Mudd JC, Savoye AL, Perreau M, van Grevenynghe J, Metcalf T, Connick E, Meditz A, Freeman GJ, Abesada-Terk G Jr., et al. 2013. Inadequate T follicular cell help impairs B cell immunity during HIV infection. *Nat Med* **19:** 494–499.

Czuczman MS, Gregory SA. 2010. The future of CD20 monoclonal antibody therapy in B-cell malignancies. *Leuk Lymphoma* **51:** 983–994.

Dayal R, Singh A, Katoch VM, Joshi B, Chauhan DS, Singh P, Kumar G, Sharma VD. 2008. Serological diagnosis of tuberculosis. *Indian J Pediatr* **75:** 1219–1221.

de Valliere S, Abate G, Blazevic A, Heuertz RM, Hoft DF. 2005. Enhancement of innate and cell-mediated immunity by antimycobacterial antibodies. *Infect Immun* **73:** 6711–6720.

Dhodapkar KM, Kaufman JL, Ehlers M, Banerjee DK, Bonvini E, Koenig S, Steinman RM, Ravetch JV, Dhodapkar

MV. 2005. Selective blockade of inhibitory Fcγ receptor enables human dendritic cell maturation with IL-12p70 production and immunity to antibody-coated tumor cells. *Proc Natl Acad Sci* **102:** 2910–2915.

Donald PR, Marais BJ, Barry CE, 3rd. 2010. Age and the epidemiology and pathogenesis of tuberculosis. *Lancet* **375:** 1852–1854.

Driver ER, Ryan GJ, Hoff DR, Irwin SM, Basaraba RJ, Kramnik I, Lenaerts AJ. 2012. Evaluation of a mouse model of necrotic granuloma formation using C3HeB/FeJ mice for testing of drugs against *Mycobacterium tuberculosis*. *Antimicrob Agents Chemother* **56:** 3181–3195.

Dromer F, Charreire J, Contrepois A, Carbon C, Yeni P. 1987. Protection of mice against experimental cryptococcosis by anti–*Cryptococcus neoformans* monoclonal antibody. *Infect Immun* **55:** 749–752.

Encinales L, Zuniga J, Granados-Montiel J, Yunis M, Granados J, Almeciga I, Clavijo O, Awad C, Collazos V, Vargas-Rojas MI, et al. 2010. Humoral immunity in tuberculin skin test anergy and its role in high-risk persons exposed to active tuberculosis. *Mol Immunol* **47:** 1066–1073.

Ernst JD. 2012. The immunological life cycle of tuberculosis. *Nat Rev Immunol* **12:** 581–591.

Fairchok MP, Rouse JH, Morris SL. 1995. Age-dependent humoral responses of children to mycobacterial antigens. *Clin Diagn Lab Immunol* **2:** 443–447.

Fletcher HA, Tanner R, Wallis RS, Meyer J, Manjaly ZR, Harris S, Satti I, Silver RF, Hoft D, Kampmann B, et al. 2013. Inhibition of mycobacterial growth in vitro following primary but not secondary vaccination with BCG. *Clin Vaccine Immunol* **20:** 1683–1689.

Flynn JL, Chan J. 2001. Immunology of tuberculosis. *Annu Rev Immunol* **19:** 93–129.

Flynn JL, Klein E. 2010. Pulmonary tuberculosis in monkeys. In *A color atlas of comparative pulmonary tuberculosis histopathology* (ed. Leong J). Taylor & Francis, Oxford.

Fortin A, Abel L, Casanova JL, Gros P. 2007. Host genetics of mycobacterial diseases in mice and men: Forward genetic studies of BCG-osis and tuberculosis. *Ann Rev Genomics Hum Genet* **8:** 163–192.

Giri PK, Verma I, Khuller GK. 2006. Enhanced immunoprotective potential of *Mycobacterium tuberculosis* Ag85 complex protein based vaccine against airway *Mycobacterium tuberculosis* challenge following intranasal administration. *FEMS Immunol Med Microbiol* **47:** 233–241.

Glatman-Freedman A. 2006. The role of antibody-mediated immunity in defense against *Mycobacterium tuberculosis*: Advances toward a novel vaccine strategy. *Tuberculosis (Edinb)* **86:** 191–197.

Glatman-Freedman A, Casadevall A. 1998. Serum therapy for tuberculosis revisited: Reappraisal of the role of antibody-mediated immunity against *Mycobacterium tuberculosis*. *Clin Microbiol Rev* **11:** 514–532.

Glatman-Freedman A, Mednick AJ, Lendvai N, Casadevall A. 2000. Clearance and organ distribution of *Mycobacterium tuberculosis* lipoarabinomannan (LAM) in the presence and absence of LAM-binding immunoglobulin M. *Infect Immun* **68:** 335–341.

Glatman-Freedman A, Casadevall A, Dai Z, Jacobs WR Jr., Li A, Morris SL, Navoa JA, Piperdi S, Robbins JB, Schneerson R, et al. 2004. Antigenic evidence of prevalence and diversity of *Mycobacterium tuberculosis* arabinomannan. *J Clin Microbiol* **42:** 3225–3231.

Gonzalez-Juarrero M, Turner OC, Turner J, Marietta P, Brooks JV, Orme IM. 2001. Temporal and spatial arrangement of lymphocytes within lung granulomas induced by aerosol infection with *Mycobacterium tuberculosis*. *Infect Immun* **69:** 1722–1728.

Good RA, Zak SJ. 1956. Disturbances in γ globulin synthesis as experiments of nature. *Pediatr Rev* **18:** 109–149.

Grosset J. 2003. *Mycobacterium tuberculosis* in the extracellular compartment: An underestimated adversary. *Antimicrob Agents Chemother* **47:** 833–836.

Grover A, Ahmed MF, Singh B, Verma I, Sharma P, Khuller GK. 2006. A multivalent combination of experimental antituberculosis DNA vaccines based on Ag85B and regions of difference antigens. *Microbes Infect* **8:** 2390–2399.

Guirado E, Amat I, Gil O, Diaz J, Arcos V, Caceres N, Ausina V, Cardona PJ. 2006. Passive serum therapy with polyclonal antibodies against *Mycobacterium tuberculosis* protects against post-chemotherapy relapse of tuberculosis infection in SCID mice. *Microbes Infect* **8:** 1252–1259.

Gupta S, Bhatia R, Datta KK. 1997. Serological diagnosis of childhood tuberculosis by estimation of mycobacterial antigen 60-specific immunoglobulins in the serum. *Tuber Lung Dis* **78:** 21–27.

Hamasur B, Haile M, Pawlowski A, Schroder U, Williams A, Hatch G, Hall G, Marsh P, Kallenius G, Svenson SB. 2003. *Mycobacterium tuberculosis* arabinomannan-protein conjugates protect against tuberculosis. *Vaccine* **21:** 4081–4093.

Hamasur B, Haile M, Pawlowski A, Schroder U, Kallenius G, Svenson SB. 2004. A mycobacterial lipoarabinomannan specific monoclonal antibody and its F(ab′) fragment prolong survival of mice infected with *Mycobacterium tuberculosis*. *Clin Exp Immunol* **138:** 30–38.

Hernandez J, Velazquez C, Valenzuela O, Robles-Zepeda R, Ruiz-Bustos E, Navarro M, Garibay-Escobar A. 2010. Low number of peripheral blood B lymphocytes in patients with pulmonary tuberculosis. *Immunol Invest* **39:** 197–205.

Hetland G, Wiker HG, Hogasen K, Hamasur B, Svenson SB, Harboe M. 1998. Involvement of antilipoarabinomannan antibodies in classical complement activation in tuberculosis. *Clin Diagn Lab Immunol* **5:** 211–218.

Hoff DR, Ryan GJ, Driver ER, Ssemakulu CC, De Groote MA, Basaraba RJ, Lenaerts AJ. 2011. Location of intra- and extracellular *M. tuberculosis* populations in lungs of mice and guinea pigs during disease progression and after drug treatment. *PLoS ONE* **6:** e17550.

Huygen K, Content J, Denis O, Montgomery DL, Yawman AM, Deck RR, DeWitt CM, Orme IM, Baldwin S, D'Souza C, et al. 1996. Immunogenicity and protective efficacy of a tuberculosis DNA vaccine. *Nat Med* **2:** 893–898.

Igietseme JU, Eko FO, He Q, Black CM. 2004. Antibody regulation of T-cell immunity: Implications for vaccine strategies against intracellular pathogens. *Expert Rev Vaccines* **3:** 23–34.

Ireton GC, Greenwald R, Liang H, Esfandiari J, Lyashchenko KP, Reed SG. 2010. Identification of *Mycobacterium tu-*

berculosis antigens of high serodiagnostic value. *Clin Vaccine Immunol* **17:** 1539–1547.

Isaacs D. 2013. Infectious risks associated with biologics. *Adv Exp Med Biol* **764:** 151–158.

Johnson CM, Cooper AM, Frank AA, Bonorino CB, Wysoki LJ, Orme IM. 1997. *Mycobacterium tuberculosis* aerogenic rechallenge infections in B cell-deficient mice. *Tuber Lung Dis* **78:** 257–261.

Kalergis AM, Ravetch JV. 2002. Inducing tumor immunity through the selective engagement of activating Fcγ receptors on dendritic cells. *J Exp Med* **195:** 1653–1659.

Karakousis PC, Yoshimatsu T, Lamichhane G, Woolwine SC, Nuermberger EL, Grosset J, Bishai WR. 2004. Dormancy phenotype displayed by extracellular *Mycobacterium tuberculosis* within artificial granulomas in mice. *J Exp Med* **200:** 647–657.

Keane J, Gershon S, Wise RP, Mirabile-Levens E, Kasznica J, Schwieterman WD, Siegel JN, Braun MM. 2001. Tuberculosis associated with infliximab, a tumor necrosis factor α-neutralizing agent. *N Engl J Med* **345:** 1098–1104.

Keyser A, Troudt JM, Taylor JL, Izzo AA. 2011. BCG substrains induce variable protection against virulent pulmonary *Mycobacterium tuberculosis* infection, with the capacity to drive Th2 immunity. *Vaccine* **29:** 9308–9315.

Kim MJ, Wainwright HC, Locketz M, Bekker LG, Walther GB, Dittrich C, Visser A, Wang W, Hsu FF, Wiehart U, et al. 2010. Caseation of human tuberculosis granulomas correlates with elevated host lipid metabolism. *EMBO Mol Med* **2:** 258–274.

Kohama H, Umemura M, Okamoto Y, Yahagi A, Goga H, Harakuni T, Matsuzaki G, Arakawa T. 2008. Mucosal immunization with recombinant heparin-binding haemagglutinin adhesin suppresses extrapulmonary dissemination of *Mycobacterium bovis* bacillus Calmette–Guérin (BCG) in infected mice. *Vaccine* **26:** 924–932.

Kondratieva TK, Rubakova EI, Linge IA, Evstifeev VV, Majorov KB, Apt AS. 2010. B cells delay neutrophil migration toward the site of stimulus: Tardiness critical for effective bacillus Calmette–Guérin vaccination against tuberculosis infection in mice. *J Immunol* **184:** 1227–1234.

Kozakiewicz L, Chen Y, Xu J, Wang Y, Dunussi-Joannopoulos K, Ou Q, Flynn JL, Porcelli SA, Jacobs WR Jr., Chan J. 2013a. B cells regulate neutrophilia during *Mycobacterium tuberculosis* infection and BCG vaccination by modulating the interleukin-17 response. *PLoS Pathog* **9:** e1003472.

Kozakiewicz L, Phuah J, Flynn J, Chan J. 2013b. The role of B cells and humoral immunity in *Mycobacterium tuberculosis* infection. *Adv Exp Med Biol* **783:** 225–250.

Kunnath-Velayudhan S, Salamon H, Wang HY, Davidow AL, Molina DM, Huynh VT, Cirillo DM, Michel G, Talbot EA, Perkins MD, et al. 2010. Dynamic antibody responses to the *Mycobacterium tuberculosis* proteome. *Proc Natl Acad Sci* **107:** 14703–14708.

Kunnath-Velayudhan S, Davidow AL, Wang HY, Molina DM, Huynh VT, Salamon H, Pine R, Michel G, Perkins MD, Xiaowu L, et al. 2012. Proteome-scale antibody responses and outcome of *Mycobacterium tuberculosis* infection in nonhuman primates and in tuberculosis patients. *J Infect Dis* **206:** 697–705.

Leemans JC, Juffermans NP, Florquin S, van Rooijen N, Vervoordeldonk MJ, Verbon A, van Deventer SJ, van der Poll T. 2001. Depletion of alveolar macrophages exerts protective effects in pulmonary tuberculosis in mice. *J Immunol* **166:** 4604–4611.

Leemans JC, Thepen T, Weijer S, Florquin S, van Rooijen N, van de Winkel JG, van der Poll T. 2005. Macrophages play a dual role during pulmonary tuberculosis in mice. *J Infect Dis* **191:** 65–74.

Lewinsohn DA, Gold MC, Lewinsohn DM. 2011. Views of immunology: Effector T cells. *Immunol Rev* **240:** 25–39.

Lin PL, Rodgers M, Smith L, Bigbee M, Myers A, Bigbee C, Chiosea I, Capuano SV, Fuhrman C, Klein E, et al. 2009. Quantitative comparison of active and latent tuberculosis in the cynomolgus macaque model. *Infect Immun* **77:** 4631–4642.

Locci M, Havenar-Daughton C, Landais E, Wu J, Kroenke MA, Arlehamn CL, Su LF, Cubas R, Davis MM, Sette A, et al. 2013. Human circulating $PD^{+}CXCR3^{-}CXCR5^{+}$ memory Tfh cells are highly functional and correlate with broadly neutralizing HIV antibody responses. *Immunity* **39:** 758–769.

Lopez Y, Yero D, Falero-Diaz G, Olivares N, Sarmiento ME, Sifontes S, Solis RL, Barrios JA, Aguilar D, Hernandez-Pando R, et al. 2009. Induction of a protective response with an IgA monoclonal antibody against *Mycobacterium tuberculosis* 16 kDa protein in a model of progressive pulmonary infection. *Int J Med Microbiol* **299:** 447–452.

Lux A, Aschermann S, Biburger M, Nimmerjahn F. 2010. The pro and anti-inflammatory activities of immunoglobulin G. *Ann Rheum Dis* **69** (Suppl 1)**:** i92–i96.

Lyashchenko K, Colangeli R, Houde M, Al Jahdali H, Menzies D, Gennaro ML. 1998. Heterogeneous antibody responses in tuberculosis. *Infect Immun* **66:** 3936–3940.

Lyashchenko KP, Greenwald R, Esfandiari J, Greenwald D, Nacy CA, Gibson S, Didier PJ, Washington M, Szczerba P, Motzel S, et al. 2007. PrimaTB STAT-PAK assay, a novel, rapid lateral-flow test for tuberculosis in nonhuman primates. *Clin Vaccine Immunol* **14:** 1158–1164.

Lyashchenko KP, Greenwald R, Esfandiari J, Chambers MA, Vicente J, Gortazar C, Santos N, Correia-Neves M, Buddle BM, Jackson R, et al. 2008. Animal-side serologic assay for rapid detection of *Mycobacterium bovis* infection in multiple species of free-ranging wildlife. *Vet Microbiol* **132:** 283–292.

Lyashchenko KP, Greenwald R, Esfandiari J, Mikota S, Miller M, Moller T, Vogelnest L, Gairhe KP, Robbe-Austerman S, Gai J, et al. 2012. Field application of serodiagnostics to identify elephants with tuberculosis prior to case confirmation by culture. *Clin Vaccine Immunol* **19:** 1269–1275.

Ma CS, Deenick EK, Batten M, Tangye SG. 2012. The origins, function, and regulation of T follicular helper cells. *J Exp Med* **209:** 1241–1253.

Maglione PJ, Chan J. 2009. How B cells shape the immune response against *Mycobacterium tuberculosis*. *Eur J Immunol* **39:** 676–686.

Maglione PJ, Xu J, Chan J. 2007. B cells moderate inflammatory progression and enhance bacterial containment upon pulmonary challenge with *Mycobacterium tuberculosis*. *J Immunol* **178:** 7222–7234.

Maglione PJ, Xu J, Casadevall A, Chan J. 2008. Fc γ receptors regulate immune activation and susceptibility during *Mycobacterium tuberculosis* infection. *J Immunol* **180:** 3329–3338.

Malik ZA, Denning GM, Kusner DJ. 2000. Inhibition of Ca^{2+} signaling by *Mycobacterium tuberculosis* is associated with reduced phagosome–lysosome fusion and increased survival within human macrophages. *J Exp Med* **191:** 287–302.

Manivannan S, Rao NV, Ramanathan VD. 2012. Role of complement activation and antibody in the interaction between *Mycobacterium tuberculosis* and human macrophages. *Indian J Exp Biol* **50:** 542–550.

McClelland EE, Nicola AM, Prados-Rosales R, Casadevall A. 2010. Ab binding alters gene expression in *Cryptococcus neoformans* and directly modulates fungal metabolism. *J Clin Invest* **120:** 1355–1361.

Moir S, Fauci AS. 2009. B cells in HIV infection and disease. *Nat Rev Immunol* **9:** 235–245.

Mossalayi MD, Vouldoukis I, Mamani-Matsuda M, Kauss T, Guillon J, Maugein J, Moynet D, Rambert J, Desplat V, Mazier D, et al. 2009. CD23 mediates antimycobacterial activity of human macrophages. *Infect Immun* **77:** 5537–5542.

Nimmerjahn F, Ravetch JV. 2008. Fcγ receptors as regulators of immune responses. *Nat Rev Immunol* **8:** 34–47.

Niu H, Hu L, Li Q, Da Z, Wang B, Tang K, Xin Q, Yu H, Zhang Y, Wang Y, et al. 2011. Construction and evaluation of a multistage *Mycobacterium tuberculosis* subunit vaccine candidate Mtb10.4-HspX. *Vaccine* **29:** 9451–9458.

North RJ, LaCourse R, Ryan L, Gros P. 1999. Consequence of Nramp1 deletion to *Mycobacterium tuberculosis* infection in mice. *Infect Immun* **67:** 5811–5814.

Nosanchuk JD, Steenbergen JN, Shi L, Deepe GS Jr., Casadevall A. 2003. Antibodies to a cell surface histone-like protein protect against Histoplasma capsulatum. *J Clin Invest* **112:** 1164–1175.

Nussbaum G, Yuan R, Casadevall A, Scharff MD. 1996. Immunoglobulin G3 blocking antibodies to the fungal pathogen *Cryptococcus neoformans*. *J Exp Med* **183:** 1905–1909.

Olivares N, Leon A, Lopez Y, Puig A, Cadiz A, Falero G, Martinez M, Sarmiento ME, Farinas M, Infante JF, et al. 2006. The effect of the administration of human γ globulins in a model of BCG infection in mice. *Tuberculosis (Edinb)* **86:** 268–272.

Ottenhoff TH. 2012. New pathways of protective and pathological host defense to mycobacteria. *Trends Microbiol* **20:** 419–428.

Ottenhoff TH, Kaufmann SH. 2012. Vaccines against tuberculosis: Where are we and where do we need to go? *PLoS Pathog* **8:** e1002607.

Palma C, Iona E, Giannoni F, Pardini M, Brunori L, Fattorini L, Del Giudice G, Cassone A. 2008. The LTK63 adjuvant improves protection conferred by Ag85B DNA-protein prime-boosting vaccination against *Mycobacterium tuberculosis* infection by dampening IFN-γ response. *Vaccine* **26:** 4237–4243.

Pethe K, Alonso S, Biet F, Delogu G, Brennan MJ, Locht C, Menozzi FD. 2001. The heparin-binding haemagglutinin of *M. tuberculosis* is required for extrapulmonary dissemination. *Nature* **412:** 190–194.

Pillai S. 2013. Love the one you're with: The HIV, B cell and TFH cell triangle. *Nat Med* **19:** 401–402.

Pohl MA, Rivera J, Nakouzi A, Chow SK, Casadevall A. 2013. Combinations of antibodies to anthrax toxin manifest emergent properties in neutralization assays. *Infect Immun* **81:** 1880–1888.

Rafiq K, Bergtold A, Clynes R. 2002. Immune complex-mediated antigen presentation induces tumor immunity. *J Clin Invest* **110:** 71–79.

Roca FJ, Ramakrishnan L. 2013. TNF dually mediates resistance and susceptibility to mycobacteria via mitochondrial reactive oxygen species. *Cell* **153:** 521–534.

Rodriguez A, Tjarnlund A, Ivanji J, Singh M, Garcia I, Williams A, Marsh PD, Troye-Blomberg M, Fernandez C. 2005. Role of IgA in the defense against respiratory infections IgA deficient mice exhibited increased susceptibility to intranasal infection with *Mycobacterium bovis* BCG. *Vaccine* **23:** 2565–2572.

Roy E, Stavropoulos E, Brennan J, Coade S, Grigorieva E, Walker B, Dagg B, Tascon RE, Lowrie DB, Colston MJ, et al. 2005. Therapeutic efficacy of high-dose intravenous immunoglobulin in *Mycobacterium tuberculosis* infection in mice. *Infect Immun* **73:** 6101–6109.

Rubbert-Roth A. 2012. Assessing the safety of biologic agents in patients with rheumatoid arthritis. *Rheumatology (Oxford)* **51** (Suppl 5): v38–v47.

Ruderman EM. 2012. Overview of safety of non-biologic and biologic DMARDs. *Rheumatology (Oxford)* **51** (Suppl 6): vi37–vi43.

Russo RT, Mariano M. 2010. B-1 cell protective role in murine primary *Mycobacterium bovis* bacillus Calmette–Guérin infection. *Immunobiology* **215:** 1005–1014.

Sada E, Ferguson LE, Daniel TM. 1990. An ELISA for the serodiagnosis of tuberculosis using a 30,000-Da native antigen of *Mycobacterium tuberculosis*. *J Infect Dis* **162:** 928–931.

Saylor C, Dadachova E, Casadevall A. 2009. Monoclonal antibody-based therapies for microbial diseases. *Vaccine* **27** (Suppl 6): G38–G46.

Schmitt N, Ueno H. 2013. Blood Tfh cells come with colors. *Immunity* **39:** 629–630.

Schoels M, Aletaha D, Smolen JS, Wong JB. 2012. Comparative effectiveness and safety of biological treatment options after tumour necrosis factor alpha inhibitor failure in rheumatoid arthritis: Systematic review and indirect pairwise meta-analysis. *Ann Rheum Dis* **71:** 1303–1308.

Schwebach JR. 2002. "The carbohydrate surface of *M. tuberculosis*: Antigenicity and antibody immunity." Thesis. Sue Golding Graduate Division of Medical Sciences. Albert Einstein College of Medicine, Bronx, NY.

Slight SR, Rangel-Moreno J, Gopal R, Lin Y, Fallert Junecko BA, Mehra S, Selman M, Becerril-Villanueva E, Baquera-Heredia J, Pavon L, et al. 2013. $CXCR5^+$ T helper cells mediate protective immunity against tuberculosis. *J Clin Invest* **123:** 712–726.

Smith MB, Boyars MC, Veasey S, Woods GL. 2000. Generalized tuberculosis in the acquired immune deficiency syndrome. *Arch Pathol Lab Med* **124:** 1267–1274.

Suga M, Tanaka F, Muranaka H, Nishikawa H, Ando M. 1996. Effect of antibacterial antibody on bactericidal activities of superoxide and lysosomal enzyme from alveolar macrophages in rabbits. *Respirology* **1:** 127–132.

Sutherland JS, Loxton AG, Haks MC, Kassa D, Ambrose L, Lee JS, Ran L, van Baarle D, Maertzdorf J, Howe R, et al. 2013. Differential gene expression of activating Fcγ receptor classifies active tuberculosis regardless of human immunodeficiency virus status or ethnicity. *Clin Microbiol Infect* **20:** O230–O238.

Tameris MD, Hatherill M, Landry BS, Scriba TJ, Snowden MA, Lockhart S, Shea JE, McClain JB, Hussey GD, Hanekom WA, et al. 2013. Safety and efficacy of MVA85A, a new tuberculosis vaccine, in infants previously vaccinated with BCG: A randomised, placebo-controlled phase 2b trial. *Lancet* **381:** 1021–1028

Teitelbaum R, Glatman-Freedman A, Chen B, Robbins JB, Unanue E, Casadevall A, Bloom BR. 1998. A mAb recognizing a surface antigen of *Mycobacterium tuberculosis* enhances host survival. *Proc Natl Acad Sci* **95:** 15688–15693.

Teixeira FM, Teixeira HC, Ferreira AP, Rodrigues MF, Azevedo V, Macedo GC, Oliveira SC. 2006. DNA vaccine using *Mycobacterium bovis* Ag85B antigen induces partial protection against experimental infection in BALB/c mice. *Clin Vaccine Immunol* **13:** 930–935.

Tjarnlund A, Rodriguez A, Cardona PJ, Guirado E, Ivanyi J, Singh M, Troye-Blomberg M, Fernandez C. 2006. Polymeric IgR knockout mice are more susceptible to mycobacterial infections in the respiratory tract than wild-type mice. *Int Immunol* **18:** 807–816.

Townsend MJ, Monroe JG, Chan AC. 2010. B-cell targeted therapies in human autoimmune diseases: An updated perspective. *Immunol Rev* **237:** 264–283.

Tsai MC, Chakravarty S, Zhu G, Xu J, Tanaka K, Koch C, Tufariello J, Flynn J, Chan J. 2006. Characterization of the tuberculous granuloma in murine and human lungs: Cellular composition and relative tissue oxygen tension. *Cell Microbiol* **8:** 218–232.

Ulrichs T, Kosmiadi GA, Trusov V, Jorg S, Pradl L, Titukhina M, Mishenko V, Gushina N, Kaufmann SH. 2004. Human tuberculous granulomas induce peripheral lymphoid follicle-like structures to orchestrate local host defence in the lung. *J Pathol* **204:** 217–228.

Vinuesa CG. 2012. HIV and T follicular helper cells: A dangerous relationship. *J Clin Invest* **122:** 3059–3062.

Vinuesa CG, Tangye SG, Moser B, Mackay CR. 2005. Follicular B helper T cells in antibody responses and autoimmunity. *Nat Rev Immunol* **5:** 853–865.

Vordermeier HM, Venkataprasad N, Harris DP, Ivanyi J. 1996. Increase of tuberculous infection in the organs of B cell-deficient mice. *Clin Exp Immunol* **106:** 312–316.

Vouldoukis I, Mazier D, Moynet D, Thiolat D, Malvy D, Mossalayi MD. 2011. IgE mediates killing of intracellular *Toxoplasma gondii* by human macrophages through CD23-dependent, interleukin-10 sensitive pathway. *PLoS ONE* **6:** e18289.

Weiner LM, Surana R, Wang S. 2010. Monoclonal antibodies: Versatile platforms for cancer immunotherapy. *Nat Rev Immunol* **10:** 317–327.

Williams A, Reljic R, Naylor I, Clark SO, Falero-Diaz G, Singh M, Challacombe S, Marsh PD, Ivanyi J. 2004. Passive protection with immunoglobulin A antibodies against tuberculous early infection of the lungs. *Immunology* **111:** 328–333.

Xue T, Stavropoulos E, Yang M, Ragno S, Vordermeier M, Chambers M, Hewinson G, Lowrie DB, Colston MJ, Tascon RE. 2004. RNA encoding the MPT83 antigen induces protective immune responses against *Mycobacterium tuberculosis* infection. *Infect Immun* **72:** 6324–6329.

Yano M, Gohil S, Coleman JR, Manix C, Pirofski LA. 2011. Antibodies to *Streptococcus pneumoniae* capsular polysaccharide enhance pneumococcal quorum sensing. *mBio* **2:** e0076-11.

Yao S, Huang D, Chen CY, Halliday L, Wang RC, Chen ZW. 2014. $CD4^+$ T cells contain early extrapulmonary tuberculosis (TB) dissemination and rapid TB progression and sustain multieffector functions of $CD8^+$ T and CD3-lymphocytes: Mechanisms of $CD4^+$ T cell immunity. *J Immunol* **192:** 2120–2132.

Yu X, Prados-Rosales R, Jenny-Avital ER, Sosa K, Casadevall A, Achkar JM. 2012. Comparative evaluation of profiles of antibodies to mycobacterial capsular polysaccharides in tuberculosis patients and controls stratified by HIV status. *Clin Vaccine Immunol* **19:** 198–208.

Zhang M, Zheng X, Zhang J, Zhu Y, Zhu X, Liu H, Zeng M, Graner MW, Zhou B, Chen X. 2012. $CD19^+CD1d^+CD5^+$ B cell frequencies are increased in patients with tuberculosis and suppress Th17 responses. *Cell Immunol* **274:** 89–97.

Ziegenbalg A, Prados-Rosales R, Jenny-Avital ER, Kim RS, Casadevall A, Achkar JM. 2013. Immunogenicity of mycobacterial vesicles in humans: Identification of a new tuberculosis antibody biomarker. *Tuberculosis (Edinb)* **93:** 448–455.

Immunity and Immunopathology in the Tuberculous Granuloma

Antonio J. Pagán[1] and Lalita Ramakrishnan[1,2,3]

[1]Department of Microbiology, University of Washington, Seattle, Washington 98195

[2]Department of Medicine, University of Washington, Seattle, Washington 98195

[3]Department of Immunology, University of Washington, Seattle, Washington 98195

Correspondence: lalitar@u.washington.edu; apagan@u.washington.edu

Granulomas, organized aggregates of immune cells, are a defining feature of tuberculosis (TB). Granuloma formation is implicated in the pathogenesis of a variety of inflammatory disorders. However, the tuberculous granuloma has been assigned the role of a host protective structure which "walls-off" mycobacteria. Work conducted over the past decade has provided a more nuanced view of its role in pathogenesis. On the one hand, pathogenic mycobacteria accelerate and exploit granuloma formation for their expansion and dissemination by manipulating host immune responses to turn leukocyte recruitment and cell death pathways in their favor. On the other hand, granuloma macrophages can preserve granuloma integrity by exerting a microbicidal immune response, thus preventing an even more rampant expansion of infection in the extracellular milieu. Even this host-beneficial immune response required to maintain the bacteria intracellular must be tempered, as an overly vigorous immune response can also cause granuloma breakdown, thereby directly supporting bacterial growth extracellularly. This review will discuss how mycobacteria manipulate inflammatory responses to drive granuloma formation and will consider the roles of the granuloma in pathogenesis and protective immunity, drawing from clinical studies of TB in humans and from animal models—rodents, zebrafish, and nonhuman primates. A deeper understanding of TB pathogenesis and immunity in the granuloma could suggest therapeutic approaches to abrogate the host-detrimental aspects of granuloma formation to convert it into the host-beneficial structure that it has been thought to be for nearly a century.

Pathogenic mycobacteria are exquisitely adapted to surviving in their hosts, and they have evolved a variety of virulence mechanisms to evade and co-opt immune responses, which allow them to infect the host, replicate within it, and transmit to new hosts. A major hurdle that mycobacteria must face is that for much of their life within the host, they reside within macrophages and dendritic cells (DCs), phagocytes that play pivotal roles in immunity to tuberculosis (TB) (Philips and Ernst 2012). For instance, to fulfill its life cycle, *Mycobacterium tuberculosis*, which causes human TB, must gain access to growth-permissive phagocytes, avoid microbicidal phagocytes, dampen productive innate and adaptive immune responses, and finally,

Cite this article as *Cold Spring Harb Perspect Med* doi: 10.1101/cshperspect.a018499

exit the intracellular environment so as to gain access to the lung airspace where it can become aerosolized and infect new hosts. How do mycobacteria achieve these remarkable feats? Most of these processes do not occur in isolated macrophages, but rather in the context of the granuloma, a cellular aggregate primarily consisting of several types of infected and uninfected phagocytes (macrophages, monocytes, DCs, and neutrophils) and T lymphocytes (Ramakrishnan 2012). A better understanding of TB pathogenesis then requires tackling its epicenter, the granuloma. This review will provide an overview of our current understanding of the granuloma, its formation, maturation, maintenance, and role in disease outcome, highlighting recent findings and new concepts emerging from studies in animal models (Table 1) and clinical studies of human TB.

LEADING UP TO THE GRANULOMA

Poor Microbicidal Macrophages Transport *M. tuberculosis* to Granuloma Initiation Sites in Deeper Tissues

Human epidemiological studies and animal studies have suggested that TB begins with the inhalation of as few as one to three *M. tuberculosis* bacilli and their deposition in the lower respiratory tract, where alveolar macrophages are thought to engulf the bacteria and transport them from the airspace across the lung epithelium into the parenchyma (Fig. 1) (Wells et al. 1948; Bates et al. 1965; Dannenberg 1993; Wolf et al. 2007). Experiments in zebrafish larvae modeling these early interactions show that macrophages recruited to the site of infection engulf the mycobacteria and transport them into deeper tissues (Clay et al. 2007). The observation that macrophage depletion prevents tissue dissemination underscores the role of macrophages in transporting the bacteria from their site of pathogen entry into distal tissues, a step that is required for development and transmission of TB.

Our laboratory recently identified a mechanism in mice and zebrafish by which *M. tuberculosis* and the closely related pathogen *Mycobacterium marinum* evade immune recognition via the Toll-like receptor (TLR)-MyD88 pathway to recruit and infect permissive macrophages that transport them across the epithelium (Cambier et al. 2014). These mycobacteria use the cell-wall-associated lipid phthiocerol dimycoceroserate (PDIM) to mask underlying PAMPs (pathogen-associated molecular patterns), thereby avoiding the recruitment of microbicidal macrophages through TLR-MyD88-dependent pathways (Cambier et al. 2014). The surface-associated phenolic glycolipid (PGL), a molecule that is structurally related to PDIMs (Onwueme et al. 2005), induces expression of the macrophage-monocyte chemokine CCL2 to recruit and infect mycobacterium-permissive CCR2-expressing macrophages. These newly infected macrophages then migrate into deeper tissues where they can incite granuloma formation.

Mycobacteria Induce Granuloma Formation in the Context of Innate Immunity

Real-time visualization of the events following *M. marinum* infection of zebrafish larvae shows that within 2–3 d of the infected macrophage reaching deeper tissues, granulomas can form around it, through a second wave of macrophage migration (Davis et al. 2002). These structures are not simple macrophage aggregates, but bona fide granulomas as evidenced by two features—first, the participating macrophages undergo the cardinal "epithelioid" transformation described for mature tuberculous granulomas in humans and mammalian animal models (Spector 1969; Adams 1976; Williams and Williams 1983; Bouley et al. 2001; Ramakrishnan 2012), and second, these structures induce the expression of mycobacterial granuloma-activated genes that are expressed in the mature granulomas of adult frogs but not in axenic cultures or in cultured macrophages (Ramakrishnan et al. 2000; Davis et al. 2002). Indeed, within the same larvae, these genes are not activated when the bacteria infect individual macrophages, but only when they participate in granuloma formation (Davis et al. 2002).

The finding that the tuberculous granuloma is an innate immune-cell-derived structure

Table 1. Animal models of tuberculous granuloma formation

	Advantages	Disadvantages	Reference(s)
Animal models of *M. tuberculosis*			
Rabbit	Forms lesions similar to humans, including necrotic mature granulomas	Few immunological reagents Few genetic tools	Flynn 2006; Helke et al. 2006
Guinea pig	Forms nonnecrotic mature granulomas	Few immunological reagents Few genetic tools Rarely forms necrotic granulomas	Flynn 2006; Helke et al. 2006
Mouse	Many immunological reagents Numerous genetic tools Well-characterized immune cell subsets and immunodominant *M. tuberculosis* epitopes Isogenic strains enable cell transfer studies Amenable to intravital microscopy	Most commonly used mouse strains form loose, nonnecrotic granulomas Persistent infection differs from human disease	Flynn 2006; Helke et al. 2006; Egen et al. 2008; Ernst 2012
Nonhuman primate (cynomolgus and rhesus macaques)	Similarity to humans Heterogeneous disease outcomes from active to latent disease Heterogeneous lesions, including necrotic mature granulomas Amenable to noninvasive imaging techniques	Few genetic tools Expensive	Flynn 2006; Helke et al. 2006; Lin et al. 2014
Animal models of *M. marinum*			
Zebrafish	Natural host of *M. marinum* Forms lesions similar to humans, including necrotic mature granulomas Genetically tractable Larvae are transparent, and thus well-suited for intravital microscopy Large clutch sizes enable high-throughput studies (e.g., genetic and pharmacological screens)	No lungs Poorly defined immune cell subsets Few immunological reagents	Swaim et al. 2006; Takaki et al. 2012; Ramakrishnan 2014
Leopard frog	Natural host of *M. marinum* Asymptomatic infection resembles latency in humans Forms nonnecrotic mature granulomas	Poorly defined immune cell subsets Few immunological reagents Few genetic tools	Ramakrishnan et al. 1997

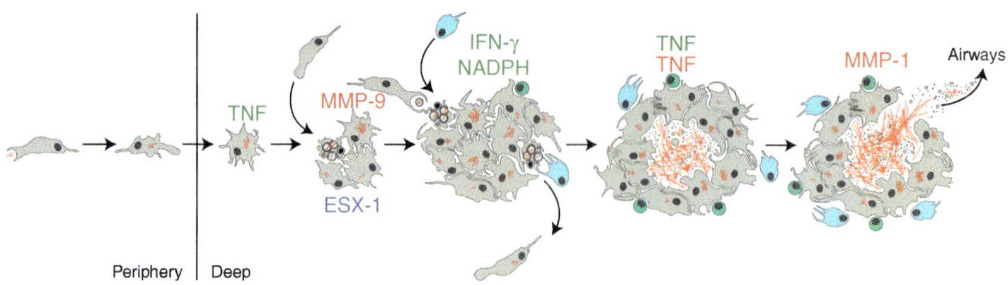

Figure 1. Overview of tuberculosis infection development. Host factors that are protective (green) or detrimental (red) are listed above the drawings. Note that the tumor necrosis factor (TNF) can have both beneficial and pathogenic roles. Macrophages (gray) engulf extracellular *M. tuberculosis* bacilli (red) in the alveolar space and transport them into deeper sites in the lung. Mycobacteria replicate within minimally microbicidal macrophages that antagonize bacterial growth via TNF-dependent mechanisms. Mycobacteria induce infected macrophage apoptosis and expression of host MMP9 in an ESX-1-dependent manner. Newly recruited macrophages engulf infected cell debris, contributing to granuloma expansion. Some of these newly infected macrophages can exit the primary granuloma and establish secondary granulomas in distal tissues. Neutrophils (light blue) can also scavenge dying infected cells and kill bacteria through an NADPH-dependent mechanism. *M. tuberculosis*-specific T cells (green) arrive at the granuloma and produce interferon-γ (IFN-γ) to enhance the microbicidal activity of macrophages. TNF excess and strong T-cell immunity can lead to macrophage necrosis and release of mycobacteria into the extracellular space, where they can grow relatively unchecked. Subsequent induction of MMP1 causes granuloma cavitation and release of mycobacteria into the airways.

was made possible mainly by the unprecedented temporal and spatial resolution afforded by real-time studies in the transparent zebrafish larva. It was the beginning of the new understanding that the granuloma, at least in its incipient stages, is a structure built by mycobacteria for their expansion and dissemination, thus challenging the long-held view that granulomas are strictly host-protective structures.

INSIDE THE GRANULOMA

Mycobacteria Use the Granuloma as a Vehicle for Expansion through Intercellular Spread Enhanced by the RD1/ESX-1 Virulence Locus

If mycobacterial interactions with innate immunity induce granulomas, is there a specific mycobacterial determinant involved? The answer to this came from a serendipitous observation on the pattern of infection with an ESX-1-deficient *M. marinum* strain (Volkman et al. 2004) and was recently confirmed in vitro in a human lung tissue model of *M. tuberculosis* granuloma formation (Parasa et al. 2014). ESX-1 is a type VII secretion system that is expressed by pathogenic mycobacteria, including *M. tuberculosis*, *Mycobacterium bovis*, and *M. marinum*, and is strongly implicated in *M. tuberculosis* virulence (Simeone et al. 2009). In fact, a molecular explanation for the reduced virulence of the Bacillus Calmette–Guérin (BCG) live attenuated vaccine strain of *M. bovis* came from genomic and genetic studies that linked BCG's attenuation to the loss of the region of difference 1 (RD1) locus that contains this secretion system (Behr et al. 1999; Pym et al. 2002; Hsu et al. 2003; Guinn et al. 2004). After ascertaining that the *M. marinum* ΔRD1 mutant was attenuated in adult leopard frogs and zebrafish, which are two of its natural hosts, an exploratory study comparing wild-type and ΔRD1 *M. marinum* infection in zebrafish larvae was conducted to try to identify the cellular basis of ΔRD1's attenuation in vivo (Volkman et al. 2004; Swaim et al. 2006). If granulomas were strictly host-protective, one would expect attenuated mycobacteria to show accelerated or at least unimpaired granuloma formation. Instead, ΔRD1 *M. marinum* infection resulted in more delayed and smaller granuloma formation than wild-type mycobacteria (Volkman et al. 2004). Importantly, the defective granuloma formation was in the face of grossly normal growth of the ΔRD1 *M. marinum* strain in the individual macrophages; despite becoming heavily infected with time, they simply did not aggregate (Volkman et al. 2004). The normal intracellular growth of ΔRD1 *M. marinum* was in contrast to a different *M. marinum* mutant in another secreted virulence protein, Erp, famous for being the first mycobacterial virulence determinant to be identified by molecular genetics (Berthet et al. 1998). Δ*erp M. marinum* displayed an intracellular growth defect in individual zebrafish larval macrophages, thus was compromised at an earlier step than ΔRD1 (Fig. 1) (Cosma et al. 2006). Despite having no intracellular growth defect, ΔRD1 was as attenuated as Δ*erp* for overall growth in the animals.

The finding that ΔRD1 infection had a primary defect at the step of granuloma formation and resulted in lower bacterial numbers suggested that the granuloma expands rather than restricts bacterial numbers (Volkman et al. 2004). Macrophage aggregation might impact bacterial numbers by facilitating the spread of bacteria to uninfected macrophages that are recruited to the aggregates. If so, then aggregate formation in wild-type infection should correlate with a dramatic increase in the number of infected macrophages and bacterial burdens, a hypothesis made eminently testable by the feasibility of direct and serial observation of granuloma formation combined with infected macrophage enumeration in the larvae. Indeed, the number of infected macrophages did not change significantly until aggregates formed and only on aggregation did the number of infected macrophages increase dramatically. Similarly, the number of viable bacteria also did not increase until after aggregation occurred 3–5 d postinfection. Collectively, these data suggested that granuloma formation driven by the ESX-1 system promotes intercellular bacterial spread, thereby providing the bacteria with a means to expand the infection niche.

In fact, the idea that the granuloma might benefit mycobacteria first came from earlier studies in chronically infected adult frogs and zebrafish with mature granulomas (Cosma et al. 2004). When these animals were superinfected with an isogenic virulent strain that was differentially marked, the new strain was found to preferentially migrate rapidly within host macrophages into the preexisting granulomas, including their necrotic centers. This trafficking phenomenon was pathogen-specific, as superinfecting *Salmonella* was largely excluded from granulomas. The superinfecting strain grew robustly within the preformed granulomas, suggesting that the granuloma is a microenvironment of impaired immunity that supports mycobacterial growth. A follow-up study in mice showed that superinfecting *M. tuberculosis* also migrates to mature lung granulomas (Cosma et al. 2008). These experiments also indicate that even mature granulomas are open structures that allow cellular influx, challenging the notion that they serve as physical barriers which "wall-off" mycobacteria.

Cellular Basis of the Granuloma's Role in Bacterial Expansion

The granuloma drives bacterial expansion by coordinately inducing infected macrophage apoptosis and uninfected macrophage recruitment to nascent granulomas (Fig. 1) (Davis and Ramakrishnan 2009). Time-lapse microscopy showed that newly recruited macrophages migrate within the growing granuloma and engulf the apoptotic debris of infected macrophages together with their bacterial contents. Quantitative analyses of infected cell death and phagocytosis by new recruits revealed that during wild-type *M. marinum* infection, ~80% of the infected granuloma macrophages die within 24 h and that on average, two or three new recruits become infected for every single dying macrophage. In contrast, ΔRD1 *M. marinum* induces the death of ~50% fewer infected macrophages as wild-type mycobacteria and recruits ~25% the number of uninfected macrophages, and only ~50% of these new recruits become infected. The rate of bacterial growth estimated by measuring fluorescence area was proportional to the increase in number of infected macrophages, suggesting that the process of infected cell death and rephagocytosis could explain most, if not all, of granuloma expansion. Because the kinetics of cell death and recruitment are slower during ΔRD1 *M. marinum* infection, these observations might also largely explain the cellular basis of attenuation of ΔRD1 mycobacteria in vivo. Rather than inhibiting macrophage responses that are generally protective against nonpathogenic mycobacteria (exemplified by case of the attenuated BCG/RD1 mutant) (Adams 1976; Dannenberg 2003), virulent mycobacteria have evolved mechanisms (i.e., their ESX-1 secretion system) for accelerating these responses, ultimately molding them into tools for infection development. Studies in adult mice and zebrafish suggest that the ESX-1 locus continues to play a role in mature granuloma formation/maintenance in the context of adaptive immunity, as the attenuated infection with RD1-mutant bacteria is associated with loose, poorly developed granulomas (Sherman et al. 2004; Volkman et al. 2004; Swaim et al. 2006).

Mechanistic Basis of Bacterial ESX-1 Induced Granuloma Formation: Co-Option of Host MMP9

An initial clue to the mechanism of RD1-induced granuloma formation came from the finding that the RD1 mutant's aggregation defect could be rescued by superinfecting the animals with wild-type bacteria marked with a different fluorescent protein; the superinfecting strain infected individual macrophages that were then able to cause the aggregation of the ΔRD1-infected macrophages that had remained isolated before (Volkman et al. 2004). Moreover, at least one wild-type-infected macrophage was required to serve as a nidus for each aggregate, suggesting that the presence of a macrophage infected with RD1-competent bacteria creates a chemotactic gradient that recruits macrophages (Volkman et al. 2004).

A better understanding of this chemotactic pathway came from a differential screen for host genes that are induced during wild-type but not ΔRD1 *M. marinum* infection in zebrafish larvae (Volkman et al. 2010). Transcriptional induction of matrix metalloproteinase-9 (MMP9) was greater with wild-type than the ΔRD1 bacteria, and this difference was further amplified when MMP9-dependent gelatinase activity was assayed in vivo; wild-type infection induced robust MMP9-dependent gelatinase activity whereas ΔRD1 infection had barely any activity. Genetic knockdown of *mmp9* in wild-type *M. marinum*-infected fish phenocopied the granuloma defect observed during ΔRD1 *M. marinum* infection and concomitantly reduced bacterial burdens and improved host survival (Volkman et al. 2010). The cellular pattern of ESX-1-dependent MMP9 induction was intriguing: It was more prominent in the epithelial cells surrounding the granuloma than in the granuloma macrophages themselves. Because ESX-1-dependent MMP9 induction occurred even in macrophage-depleted larvae, it appeared to be a consequence of the direct interaction between the bacterial secretion system and the epithelial cells rather than via signals from the infected macrophages. Furthermore, the ESX-1-dependent MMP9 induction could be attributed to ESAT-6, a small secreted protein substrate of the ESX-1 secretion system that has long been identified as one of the earliest proteins to be recognized by the T-cell response in humans (giving it its name early secretory antigenic target of T cells of 6 kDa size that abbreviates to ESAT-6) (Andersen et al. 1995; Ravn et al. 1999).

Compositely, the zebrafish findings suggested a model for granuloma formation in which ESAT-6 induces MMP9 in epithelial cells neighboring the nascent granuloma. The details of this mechanism and the relative importance of macrophage versus epithelial cell MMP9 in pathogenesis are yet to be worked out. ESX-1-dependent induction of MMP9 in the epithelium might benefit mycobacteria by providing a means of signal amplification. For example, a single infected macrophage might be sufficient to induce MMP9 in multiple epithelial cells and thus jumpstart the recruitment of uninfected macrophages. The mechanisms by which ESX-1 induces MMP9 and how epithelium-derived MMP9 promotes macrophage recruitment to nascent granulomas remain unknown and are under active study. As to how MMP9 induces macrophage chemotaxis, a potential mechanism of action might involve enhancing the activity of CCL7 or other chemokines via proteolysis of the amino terminus (Parks et al.

2004). CCL7 is an appealing candidate because it is a substrate of MMP9 in vivo (Greenlee et al. 2006), is produced by macrophages in response to mycobacterial infection (Scott and Flynn 2002), and can recruit monocytes from the bloodstream (Soehnlein and Lindbom 2010). Other nonmutually exclusive mechanisms could involve remodeling of the extracellular matrix at the site of infection through the release of a sequestered chemoattractant (e.g., glycan-bound chemokines) (Sarris et al. 2012) or degradation of a physical barrier (e.g., α-dystroglycan proteolysis along basement membranes) (Parks et al. 2004; Agrawal et al. 2006).

Again, the zebrafish findings all have parallels in humans. MMP9 levels are elevated in human TB (Price et al. 2003; Sheen et al. 2009), and in lung TB, it is expressed prominently in the epithelium surrounding the granulomas in addition to the macrophages themselves (Elkington et al. 2007). Among pleural TB patients, pleural fluid MMP9 concentrations are higher in those patients with granulomatous pleural disease than in those with nongranulomatous disease (Sheen et al. 2009). Among tuberculous meningitis patients, increased MMP9 levels in the cerebrospinal fluid are associated with worse outcomes (Price et al. 2003). In a mouse model of *M. tuberculosis* aerosol infection, MMP9 knockout mice recruited fewer macrophages to the lung and formed smaller granulomas, features that were associated with reduced lung bacterial loads as early as 2 wk postinfection and continuing through the 120-d assay period (Taylor et al. 2006). These data implicate MMP9 and granuloma formation in pathogenesis similar to the zebrafish and human data. It is perplexing then that the authors instead designated MMP9 as a host resistance factor that acts by promoting granuloma formation; this misinterpretation of the data at hand so as to align the conclusions with the protective granuloma model may attest to how entrenched the model is among TB researchers. Given the broad conservation of the MMP9-induced susceptibility, identifying the mycobacterial and host factors involved in macrophage recruitment to nascent granulomas would be a key step in designing targeted therapies to reduce the kinetics of granuloma formation just to the point where it is no longer host-detrimental.

Macrophage Apoptosis in the Granuloma: Protective or Pathogenic?

Studies of granuloma development in the zebrafish suggest that infected macrophage apoptosis plays a role in expanding infection (Davis and Ramakrishnan 2009). Detailed observations of the growing granuloma show that the uninfected macrophages recruited through RD1-MMP9 signaling remain motile within the granuloma as if moving in the context of a gradientless signal. A second signal emanating from dead or dying macrophages appears to draw these macrophages to them, and their encased bacteria are then phagocytosed to create new infected cells. Indeed, RD1-competent mycobacteria also induce more apoptotic death of infected macrophages in the granuloma (Volkman et al. 2004; Davis and Ramakrishnan 2009), consistent with studies showing that the RD1-encoded virulence determinant ESAT-6 can induce multiple programs associated with cell death in vitro (Guinn et al. 2004; Derrick and Morris 2007; van der Wel et al. 2007; Choi et al. 2010; Mishra et al. 2010; Aguilo et al. 2013). It would be predicted that the coordinated acceleration of new macrophage recruitment and infected macrophage apoptosis would be required to maximize bacterial expansion in the granuloma. However, because both processes are dependent on the same locus, RD1, the specific contribution of bacterially induced apoptosis in expanding infection has been difficult to tease out. Engineering host MMP9 deficiency dissociates the two processes; it reduces macrophage recruitment to the granuloma and virulence without affecting apoptosis of infected macrophages (Volkman et al. 2010). This finding suggests that RD1-mediated macrophage apoptosis is not sufficient for macrophage recruitment but does not tell us if its acceleration further expands infection.

Further confounding the role of apoptosis, pathogenic mycobacteria express virulence genes that inhibit apoptosis of cultured macrophages—*nuoG*, *secA2*, and *pknE*. *nuoG* encodes a subunit of the type I NADH dehydrogenase complex, *secA2* encodes a mycobacterial secretion system, and *pknE* encodes a serine/threonine kinase (Braunstein et al. 2003; Hinchey et al. 2007; Velmurugan et al. 2007; Briken and Miller 2008; Jayakumar et al. 2008). Pathogenic mycobacteria deficient in any of these genes show growth defects in cultured macrophages and in mice or zebrafish (Braunstein et al. 2003; Hinchey et al. 2007; Velmurugan et al. 2007; Jayakumar et al. 2008; Sullivan et al. 2012; Watkins et al. 2012; van der Woude et al. 2014). However, a direct link between their attenuation and impaired inhibition of macrophage apoptosis has not been made. It is not known if these bacterial mutants induce more apoptosis in vivo, much less if inhibition of apoptosis by targeting the corresponding host pathways restores their virulence. These experiments would be particularly important because NuoG, SecA2, and PknE participate broadly in cellular processes whose disruption might be responsible for their attenuation.

Based on in vitro studies, it has been proposed that apoptosis is a host strategy that is detrimental to the infecting mycobacteria, in contrast to necrosis, which favors bacterial growth (Fratazzi et al. 1997; Oddo et al. 1998; Keane et al. 2002; Gan et al. 2008; Behar et al. 2011). Some of these studies have caveats: the use of genetically undefined mutant strains and/or additional agents to induce specific apoptotic death pathways that might override mycobacterially induced pathways (Molloy et al. 1994; Fratazzi et al. 1997; Oddo et al. 1998; Keane et al. 2000; Gan et al. 2008). In terms of apoptotic pathways, apoptosis induced by Fas ligand or ATP have opposite effects on intracellular mycobacterial viability (Lammas et al. 1997). ESAT-6-induced apoptotic cell death per se may use bacterium-sparing pathways. Even if apoptosis is detrimental to mycobacteria, the rapid rephagocytosis of the dead macrophages in the context of the granuloma may nullify any bactericidal effects of apoptosis. In summary, it is possible that mycobacteria inhibit or induce macrophage apoptosis depending on the stage of infection. Mycobacteria might benefit from inhibiting macrophage apoptosis during the earliest stages of infection, when they rely on these cells to access deeper tissues, and then induce macrophage apoptosis to expand within the granuloma.

Neutrophils in the Granuloma: Protective or Pathogenic?

In early zebrafish granulomas, in contrast to arriving macrophages, neutrophils arriving at the granuloma may help control infection (Fig. 1) (Yang et al. 2012). Their recruitment to the granulomas is via signals from the dying macrophages, which they engulf to become infected just as the macrophages do. A subset of neutrophils kills the ingested mycobacteria in an NADPH oxidase-dependent manner. Experimentally preventing neutrophil entry into granulomas by sequestering neutrophils in hematopoietic tissues enhanced mycobacterial expansion and granuloma growth. In the context of the granuloma, neutrophil clearance of infected dying macrophages appears to be protective via two mechanisms: (1) directly lowering mycobacterial loads, and (2) simultaneously reducing the kinetics of intercellular spread into uninfected macrophages and their subsequent death. Work in other animal models and in humans has also identified a protective role of neutrophils in early TB. Neutrophil depletion in mice increased bacterial burdens. This effect could be mitigated by neutralization of interleukin-10 (IL-10) or administration of IL-12, interventions that likely enhanced the microbicidal activity of macrophages (Pedrosa et al. 2000). In rats, neutrophil depletion exacerbated TB infection, whereas transient neutrophilia enhanced control (Sugawara et al. 2004). Humans with chronic granulomatous disease (CGD), a genetic disorder caused by NADPH deficiency and characterized by severely impaired neutrophil oxidative burst (Amulic et al. 2012), are susceptible to mycobacterial infections, including TB (Lee et al. 2008; Dogru et al. 2010). Finally, work in mice suggests an indirect role for how neutrophils might be host-protective. DCs can engulf the apoptotic remnants of infected neutrophils and migrate to the draining lymph node, where they support *M. tuberculosis*–specific T-cell priming (Blomgran et al. 2012). However, the relative importance of this mode of antigen transfer on T-cell priming is unclear given that migratory DCs can also transfer unprocessed, soluble *M. tuberculosis* antigens to lymph node–resident DCs through a mechanism not involving apoptosis (Srivastava and Ernst 2014).

As with macrophages, the role of neutrophils in TB protection is confounded by studies showing they are pathological. In mouse TB infection, aggressive neutrophil responses to *M. tuberculosis* have been documented in genetically susceptible mice (Eruslanov et al. 2005); in cases of suboptimal macrophage immune responses, such as during CARD9 (Dorhoi et al. 2010) or miR-223 deficiency (Dorhoi et al. 2013); in the context of impaired IFN-γ-mediated immunoregulation (Desvignes and Ernst 2009; Nandi and Behar 2011), and as a consequence of pathogenic Th17 responses (Cruz et al. 2006, 2010). Together, these studies assign a pathological role to neutrophils.

So it is likely that neutrophils, similar to macrophages, play a nuanced role in TB pathogenesis; they may participate in protective immunity during early infection but may cause immunopathology in advanced stages of the disease. Both roles are potentially relevant in human TB where neutrophils are readily detected in the blood of patients with active TB by a signature IFN gene expression profile (Berry et al. 2010), in the cerebrospinal fluid of tuberculous meningitis (Thwaites et al. 2002; Lowe et al. 2012) an a in pulmonary TB, where they can be abundant in both early granulomas and late cavitary granulomas (Canetti 1955; Eum et al. 2010).

EXITING THE GRANULOMA

Egress of Infected Macrophages from the Primary Granuloma

At least in the innate stages of granuloma development, even as uninfected macrophages are being recruited to feed the granuloma, some newly infected macrophages exit the nascent granuloma and establish secondary granulomas, thus disseminating the infection within the host (Fig. 1) (Davis and Ramakrishnan 2009). Indeed, close temporal monitoring of the spread of infection from a primary granuloma focus tightly linked departing macrophages to the spread of infection. A similar phenomenon was recently documented in a transplantation model of TB in mice, where infected DCs were observed to exit the primary granuloma and spread the infection into distal tissues (Schreiber et al. 2011). Although the mechanism of infected macrophage egress remains unclear, it does appear to be the main mode of establishing multiple infection foci early in infection. It is conceivably a mycobacterial bet-hedging strategy because different granulomas within the same individual can expand or contract from the earliest stages of infection as shown by close monitoring of guinea pigs, zebrafish, and monkeys and surmised from detailed histopathological studies of the lungs of infected humans in the prechemotherapy era (Balasubramanian et al. 1994; Davis and Ramakrishnan 2009; Adams et al. 2011; Lin et al. 2014).

Exiting the Intracellular Environment through Macrophage Necrosis

Although mycobacteria exploit macrophages to infect and spread within a host, they enhance their transmission to a new host by becoming extracellular (Fig. 1). Mycobacteria are notoriously adapted to intracellular growth, so the vast majority of mycobacterial pathogenesis research has focused on mechanisms of intracellular survival. However, it has long been known that in humans, necrotic granulomas, called caseating granulomas for their cheesy appearance on macroscopic examination, thought to result from the necrotic breakdown of infected macrophages, are a major contributor to morbidity and transmission (Rich 1946; Canetti 1955; Grosset 2003; Ramakrishnan 2012). Detailed histological studies of tuberculous organs obtained from autopsies in the prechemotherapy era revealed that areas of caseation in early granulomas were associated with more numerous bacteria than noncaseating lesions (Canetti 1955). Corroborating these old human studies, work in *M. marinum*-infected adult zebrafish (Swaim et al. 2006), as well in *M. tuberculosis*-infected macaques (Lin et al. 2014), similarly find that caseation is associated from early on with high bacterial burdens. Virulent *M. tuberculosis* grown in culture acquires a corded appearance characterized by the formation of long, intertwined serpentine structures (Koch 1882). This in vitro phenotype correlates well with virulence (Middlebrook et al. 1947) and has been described to occur in vivo under conditions in which mycobacteria grow extracellularly (Clay et al. 2007, 2008). A recent study of *Mycobacterium abscessus* infection in zebrafish suggests that the cording morphology helps mycobacteria avoid macrophage-mediated immunity; uninfected macrophages that were recruited to sites of bacterial cording failed to rephagocytose the bacterial cords, perhaps because they were too large to be engulfed (Bernut et al. 2014). Finally, the bacterial RD1 virulence locus promotes necrosis of mature granulomas, either by postapoptotic necrosis or through yet-undefined independent mechanisms (Volkman et al. 2004; Swaim et al. 2006; Ramakrishnan 2012). These observations suggest that extracellular survival may be an important part of mycobacterium's ability to grow to high numbers in the compartment most conducive for transmission, a critical survival trait for a pathogen.

Previous studies could not discern whether high bacterial burdens promote necrosis, and the numerous bacteria released can simply survive in the necrotic debris, or whether the necrotic debris and/or extracellular milieu actually promote bacterial growth. Work in the zebrafish larvae has shed light on this issue and has provided evidence that although the early granuloma promotes growth, mycobacterial growth is further enhanced in the extracellular milieu when bacteria are released after macrophage necrosis, or if macrophages are absent altogether (Clay et al. 2007, 2008; Tobin et al. 2010, 2012; Ramakrishnan 2012; Roca and Ramakrishnan 2013). Several immune mechanisms have been implicated in necrosis.

Foamy Macrophages

Lipid-laden foamy macrophages are thought to contribute to caseum formation. In vitro granuloma models suggest that foamy macrophages form through a host transcription-dependent process involving peroxisome proliferator γ (PPARγ) and testicular receptor 4 (TR4) and induced by mycobacterial oxygenated mycolic acids, which leads to the accumulation of low-density lipoprotein-derived lipids (Peyron et al. 2008; Mahajan et al. 2012). ESX-1-competent mycobacteria induce the foamy phenotype by diverting glycolitic metabolism toward ketone body synthesis and inducing the expression of the antilipolytic G-protein-coupled receptor GPR109A (Singh et al. 2012). These macrophages are common in caseating granulomas, typically around the edges of the necrotic core, but rarely present in nonnecrotic lesions (Caceres et al. 2009). Foamy macrophages are poorly bactericidal compared with their nonfoamy counterparts, attributed in part to increased M2-type macrophage activation and IL-10 production (Mahajan et al. 2012) and impaired autophagy and lysosomal acidification (Singh et al. 2012). In fact, recent work indicates that M1-type macrophage polarization inhibits foamy macrophage development. Activation of the vitamin D pathway, which is induced on IFN-γ-mediated stimulation (Fabri et al. 2011), prevents lipid accumulation by reducing PPARγ expression (Salamon et al. 2014).

Bacteria can be found inside lipid bodies and contain lipid inclusions, suggesting that they can use host lipids as nutrient sources (Peyron et al. 2008; Russell et al. 2009). The lipid composition of the caseum reflects that of foamy macrophages, suggesting a link between foamy macrophages and caseum formation. It has been proposed that foamy macrophages contribute to caseum formation by undergoing necrosis, thereby spilling their intracellular contents (Russell et al. 2009). The lipids released into the extracellular space might serve as a nutrient source for enhanced mycobacterial growth in an environment of impaired cell-mediated immunity.

Tumor Necrosis Factor Deficiency as a Cause of Granuloma Macrophage Necrosis

In general, the failure of the infected macrophage to control bacterial replication caused

 Cite this article as *Cold Spring Harb Perspect Med* doi: 10.1101/cshperspect.a018499

by tumor necrosis factor (TNF) deficiency results in their accelerated necrotic death and release of bacteria (Fig. 1) (Clay et al. 2008; Tobin et al. 2010). Numerous lines of evidence have established the importance of the proinflammatory cytokine TNF in immunity to *M. tuberculosis*. Early studies in mice showed that TNF deficiency enhances mycobacterial growth and disease progression (Flynn et al. 1995), and they have been corroborated by studies in humans showing that therapeutic neutralization of TNF for the treatment of autoimmune diseases such as rheumatoid arthritis and noninfectious inflammatory disorders such as Crohn's disease increases TB susceptibility (Keane 2005). TNF signaling deficiency in mice produces disorganized tuberculous lesions teeming with extracellular mycobacteria (Flynn et al. 1995). The stark morphological differences between the organized granulomas of TNF-sufficient mice and the disorganized, necrotic structures of TNF-deficient mice helped establish the idea that TNF participates in granuloma formation and supported the notion that granulomas are host-protective structures formed by the immune system (Ramakrishnan 2012). However, the sequential monitoring of granuloma development that is possible in zebrafish larvae provides a more nuanced view of TNF involvement in immunity to TB and granuloma formation (Clay et al. 2008). Larvae rendered deficient in TNF-signaling via knockdown of TNF Receptor 1 showed increased intramacrophage mycobacterial loads and, unexpectedly, accelerated granuloma formation. The accelerated kinetics of granuloma formation are likely caused by an increased abundance of ESX-1 substrates in the extracellular space, which would induce MMP9 expression on the epithelial cells surrounding the infected macrophages. These heavily infected granuloma macrophages eventually became necrotic, releasing mycobacteria into the extracellular milieu. These observations suggest that TNF is not required for granuloma formation per se, but rather preserves granuloma integrity by inhibiting mycobacterial growth and preventing macrophage death. A live imaging study in mice showed that TNF blockade in established granulomas led to their disintegration (Egen et al. 2008), adding credence to the idea that TNF is critical for granuloma maintenance. Consistent with the zebrafish work, a study in cynomolgus macaques showed that TNF inhibition increased mycobacterial burdens and extrapulmonary dissemination of the infection without impeding granuloma formation (Lin et al. 2010). During active disease, granulomas in the treated group became more invasive, extending into adjacent vessels and airways. Strikingly, TNF inhibition did not appear to disrupt the architecture of established granulomas, but secondary granulomas in adjacent tissue and in distal organs nonetheless formed (Lin et al. 2010). These findings are in agreement with the observations in humans undergoing anti-TNF therapies who can develop organized caseating granulomas (Garcia Vidal et al. 2005; Iliopoulos et al. 2006). Because only some of the macrophages in established granulomas are infected, TNF deficiency would only cause the necrosis of these, thus forming a necrotic core within a cellular granuloma that would facilitate an exit strategy for the bacteria.

TNF Excess as a Cause of Granuloma Necrosis

Unexpectedly, excessive TNF in the granuloma is also host detrimental by inducing macrophage necrosis, but through a different mechanism from TNF deficiency (Fig. 1). Excess TNF caused excessive inflammation leading to Receptor-interacting serine/threonine kinase (RIPK) 1- and RIPK3-dependent necrosis of granuloma macrophages via production of mitochondrial reactive oxygen species (ROS) (Tobin et al. 2012; Roca and Ramakrishnan 2013). Accordingly, and in stark contrast to TNF-deficiency, macrophages experiencing an excess of TNF signaling initially have enhanced control of intracellular mycobacterial growth because of the ROS. But this ROS then causes cell necrosis through multiple mechanisms rendering the bacteria extracellular.

T Cells and Granuloma Necrosis

Like phagocytes, $CD4^+$ T cells can also play a dual role in TB protection and pathology, and have also been implicated in granuloma necrosis (Fig. 1). HIV-positive individuals with low $CD4^+$ T-cell counts in the blood are less likely to have cavitary TB lesions than individuals with normal $CD4^+$ T-cell frequencies and are less likely to transmit disease (Kwan and Ernst 2011). A recent study documented that human T-cell epitopes in the *M. tuberculosis* complex are highly conserved, suggesting that pathogenic mycobacteria benefit from T-cell recognition (Comas et al. 2010; Ernst 2012). The mechanism by which $CD4^+$ T cells contribute to necrosis is unclear, but it might involve an overly exuberant mycobacteria-specific response that induces the necrotic death of infected cells. It is plausible that the specific effector is TNF, and this might explain the widespread incidence of necrotic granulomas among patients with advanced TB. The effects of excessive TNF production might be present, albeit at a smaller scale, in the normal spectrum of TB lesions in nongenetically susceptible individuals and might contribute to caseum formation in established granulomas.

Cytotoxic T lymphocyte antigen-4 (CTLA-4) and program death-1 (PD-1), two members of the CD28 family of receptors (Greenwald et al. 2005), have been implicated in determining whether a T-cell response in TB is host-protective or host-detrimental. These receptors are induced during T-cell activation and recognize ligands decorating the surface of antigen-presenting cells (APCs). Engagement of these receptors dampens stimulatory signals transduced through the T-cell antigen receptor (TCR) signaling complex on TCR binding to cognate peptide:major histocompatibility complex (p:MHC) molecules displayed by the APCs (Greenwald et al. 2005). Although these receptors exert critical roles in preventing autoimmunity by restraining autoreactive T-cell responses, their engagement in the context of several infections and cancers is host-detrimental because it inhibits the development of robust pathogen- or tumor-specific T-cell immunity (Peggs et al. 2009; Fife and Pauken 2011; Odorizzi and Wherry 2012; Kamphorst and Ahmed 2013). A study of pulmonary TB in a West African cohort identified a single nucleotide polymorphism (SNP) in the 3′-untranslated region of *CTLA4* that correlated with increased disease severity (Thye et al. 2009). Patients bearing the +6230G allele had larger and more numerous lesions than those with an A/A genotype at the same position, and the +6230G individuals appeared to have more cavitary granulomas. Interestingly, this same SNP has been associated with several autoimmune diseases (Ueda et al. 2003), suggesting that the susceptibility in TB is due to a dysfunctional T-cell response. The effects of CTLA-4 inhibition on mouse models of TB remain largely unexplored. A study of BCG infection found that CTLA-4 blockade accelerated the kinetics of T-cell activation and enhanced IFN-γ production but did not alter bacterial burdens or tissue pathology (Kirman et al. 1999). It remains to be determined if CTLA-4 blockade during *M. tuberculosis* infection elicits a similar response. At the very least, this study shows that CTLA-4 exerts an inhibitory function during a mycobacterial infection. Nonetheless, studies of PD-1 in a mouse model of TB make a compelling case for the involvement of inhibitory receptors in preventing T-cell immunopathology in TB (Lazar-Molnar et al. 2010; Barber et al. 2011). PD-1 deficiency enhanced *M. tuberculosis*-specific $CD4^+$ T-cell expansion, increased the levels of proinflammatory cytokines in the lungs, including TNF, caused extensive tissue necrosis, and precipitated death (Lazar-Molnar et al. 2010; Barber et al. 2011). Again, TNF is a plausible culprit for widespread necrosis observed in the context of PD-1 deficiency. It will be interesting to determine if genetic polymorphisms in the TNF pathway, PD-1, and other inhibitory coreceptors or their ligands modulate susceptibility to TB in humans and, specifically, development of cavitary granulomas.

Cavitary Granulomas as Vehicles for TB Transmission

The formation of cavities that harbor very large numbers of bacteria greatly facilitates aerosol transmission in the advanced stages of human lung TB (Fig. 1). Patients harboring radiologically apparent cavitary lesions are more likely to have burdens of *M. tuberculosis* in their expectorated sputum and to transmit TB than those that do not have as advanced lesions (Palaci et al. 2007). Individual cavitary lesions may contain 10^7-10^9 bacilli (Canetti 1965). The high level of bacterial replication observed in cavitary granulomas may also contribute to the selection of genetic resistance to antitubercular drugs (Howard et al. 1949).

Recent work argues that the pathogenesis of cavitation is distinct from necrosis and that although necrosis is a prerequisite for cavitation, it is not sufficient. The collagenase matrix metalloproteinase-1 (MMP1) has been implicated in the final steps of granuloma cavitation through the degradation of the fibrous extracellular matrix surrounding the granuloma (Fig. 1) (Elkington et al. 2011c). SNPs in *MMP1* that increase protein abundance or enzymatic activity have been associated with TB hypersusceptibility (Ganachari et al. 2010; Wang et al. 2010). *M. tuberculosis* infection in humans induces MMP1 expression in epithelial cells surrounding the granuloma and in leukocytes (Elkington et al. 2005). Overexpression of human MMP1 in mice infected with *M. tuberculosis* induced granuloma breakdown (Elkington et al. 2011a). Although the specific mycobacterial signals that induce MMP1 (Ganachari et al. 2010) have not been identified, it has been noted that *M. bovis* BCG is a poor inducer compared with virulent *M. tuberculosis* (Elkington et al. 2005), suggesting that MMP1 induction might share similarities with that of MMP9. The factors that induce cavitation could be therapeutically intercepted to reduce tissue destruction and minimize transmission (Elkington et al. 2011b).

SUMMARY: A NEW ROLE FOR THE GRANULOMA FROM A HISTORICAL PERSPECTIVE

Work over the last decade has revised the role of the granuloma from host-protective structure to one that substantially benefits mycobacterial expansion. The protective granuloma model was based on several lines of circumstantial evidence from traditional animal models in which only single endpoint analyses of tissue histology and bacterial burdens were possible (Ramakrishnan 2012). In particular, the surmise that granuloma formation was dependent on adaptive immunity, the development of which is accompanied by a plateau in bacterial load contributed to this thinking (Andersen 1997; Saunders and Cooper 2000; North and Jung 2004; Urdahl et al. 2011). The idea has been that adaptive immunity is required for granuloma formation, which in turn restricts bacterial growth. In this model, mycobacterium-specific T cells migrate to the site of infection and interact with infected macrophages through the secretion of cytokines such as IFN-γ and TNF that induce granuloma formation while enhancing macrophage microbicidal functions. Whereas IFN-γ and TNF can be produced by innate immune cells, T cells are potent producers of these cytokines and have been shown to be critical for controlling mycobacterial infection in animal models and humans (Szabo et al. 2003; Al-Muhsen and Casanova 2008; Kwan and Ernst 2011; Philips and Ernst 2012; Tubo and Jenkins 2014). Mice deficient in $CD4^+$ T cells, IFN-γ signaling, or TNF signaling show disorganized macrophage aggregates that become necrotic (Kindler et al. 1989; Flynn et al. 1993, 1995; Bean et al. 1999; Caruso et al. 1999; Scanga et al. 2000; Flynn and Chan 2001; Roach et al. 2002; Algood et al. 2005; Stenger 2005; Chakravarty et al. 2008; Wallis and Schluger 2010). These observations associated granuloma formation with a protective immune response to TB.

The finding that granuloma formation can occur in the sole context of innate immunity was instrumental in starting to appreciate the granuloma's role in TB pathogenesis. Indeed, granuloma formation is accelerated by the very mycobacteria that it was said to "wall-off," turning a fundamentally host-beneficial process into a bacterium-beneficial one. Therefore, slowing the kinetics of granuloma formation may in fact benefit the host by allowing processes such as macrophage apoptosis to play out in the host's favor. Furthermore, maintaining macrophage cellularity by preventing their necrosis is also favorable to the host by keeping mycobacteria from the extracellular environment, which is even more growth-permissive than the intracellular milieu.

In summary then, the granuloma, as constructed and deconstructed by the pathogenic mycobacteria, is a pathological entity from its inception when it promotes intracellular bacterial spread to its advanced stages when it promotes extracellular bacterial growth and transmission. An understanding of which processes are pathogenic, and to what extent, may allow their modulation so as to render the tuberculous granuloma into a structure that promotes immunity without immunopathology.

ACKNOWLEDGMENTS

We thank C.J. Cambier for critical review. This work was funded by grants from the National Institutes of Health (NIH) (T32-AI055396 to A.J.P; A154503 and A136396 to L.R). L.R. is a recipient of the NIH Director's Pioneer Award.

REFERENCES

Adams DO. 1976. The granulomatous inflammatory response. A review. *Am J Pathol* **84:** 164–192.

Adams KN, Takaki K, Connolly LE, Wiedenhoft H, Winglee K, Humbert O, Edelstein PH, Cosma CL, Ramakrishnan L. 2011. Drug tolerance in replicating mycobacteria mediated by a macrophage-induced efflux mechanism. *Cell* **145:** 39–53.

Agrawal S, Anderson P, Durbeej M, van Rooijen N, Ivars F, Opdenakker G, Sorokin LM. 2006. Dystroglycan is selectively cleaved at the parenchymal basement membrane at sites of leukocyte extravasation in experimental autoimmune encephalomyelitis. *J Exp Med* **203:** 1007–1019.

Aguilo JI, Alonso H, Uranga S, Marinova D, Arbues A, de Martino A, Anel A, Monzon M, Badiola J, Pardo J, et al. 2013. ESX-1-induced apoptosis is involved in cell-to-cell spread of *Mycobacterium tuberculosis*. *Cell Microbiol* **15:** 1994–2005.

Al-Muhsen S, Casanova JL. 2008. The genetic heterogeneity of mendelian susceptibility to mycobacterial diseases. *J Allergy Clin Immunol* **122:** 1043–1051; quiz 1052–1043.

Algood HM, Lin PL, Flynn JL. 2005. Tumor necrosis factor and chemokine interactions in the formation and maintenance of granulomas in tuberculosis. *Clin Infect Dis* **41:** S189–S193.

Amulic B, Cazalet C, Hayes GL, Metzler KD, Zychlinsky A. 2012. Neutrophil function: From mechanisms to disease. *Annu Rev Immunol* **30:** 459–489.

Andersen P. 1997. Host responses and antigens involved in protective immunity to *Mycobacterium tuberculosis*. *Scand J Immunol* **45:** 115–131.

Andersen P, Andersen AB, Sorensen AL, Nagai S. 1995. Recall of long-lived immunity to *Mycobacterium tuberculosis* infection in mice. *J Immunol* **154:** 3359–3372.

Balasubramanian V, Wiegeshaus EH, Taylor BT, Smith DW. 1994. Pathogenesis of tuberculosis: Pathway to apical localization. *Tuber Lung Dis* **75:** 168–178.

Barber DL, Mayer-Barber KD, Feng CG, Sharpe AH, Sher A. 2011. CD4 T cells promote rather than control tuberculosis in the absence of PD-1-mediated inhibition. *J Immunol* **186:** 1598–1607.

Bates JH, Potts WE, Lewis M. 1965. Epidemiology of primary tuberculosis in an industrial school. *N Engl J Med* **272:** 714–717.

Bean AG, Roach DR, Briscoe H, France MP, Korner H, Sedgwick JD, Britton WJ. 1999. Structural deficiencies in granuloma formation in TNF gene-targeted mice underlie the heightened susceptibility to aerosol *Mycobacterium tuberculosis* infection, which is not compensated for by lymphotoxin. *J Immunol* **162:** 3504–3511.

Behar SM, Martin CJ, Booty MG, Nishimura T, Zhao X, Gan HX, Divangahi M, Remold HG. 2011. Apoptosis is an innate defense function of macrophages against *Mycobacterium tuberculosis*. *Mucosal Immunol* **4:** 279–287.

Behr MA, Wilson MA, Gill WP, Salamon H, Schoolnik GK, Rane S, Smal PM. 1999. Comparative genomics of BCG vaccines by whole-genome DNA microarray. *Science* **284:** 1520–1523.

Bernut A, Herrmann JL, Kissa K, Dubremetz JF, Gaillard JL, Lutfalla G, Kremer L. 2014. *Mycobacterium abscessus* cording prevents phagocytosis and promotes abscess formation. *Proc Natl Acad Sci* **111:** E943–E952.

Berry MP, Graham CM, McNab FW, Xu Z, Bloch SA, Oni T, Wilkinson KA, Banchereau R, Skinner J, Wilkinson RJ, et al. 2010. An interferon-inducible neutrophil-driven blood transcriptional signature in human tuberculosis. *Nature* **466:** 973–977.

Berthet FX, Lagranderie M, Gounon P, Laurent-Winter C, Ensergueix D, Chavarot P, Thouron F, Maranghi E, Pelicic V, Portnoi D, et al. 1998. Attenuation of virulence by disruption of the *Mycobacterium tuberculosis* erp gene. *Science* **282:** 759–762.

Blomgran R, Desvignes L, Briken V, Ernst JD. 2012. *Mycobacterium tuberculosis* inhibits neutrophil apoptosis, leading to delayed activation of naive CD4 T cells. *Cell Host Microbe* **11:** 81–90.

Bouley DM, Ghori N, Mercer KL, Falkow S, Ramakrishnan L. 2001. Dynamic nature of host-pathogen interactions in *Mycobacterium marinum* granulomas. *Infect Immun* **69:** 7820–7831.

Braunstein M, Espinosa BJ, Chan J, Belisle JT, Jacobs WR Jr. 2003. SecA2 functions in the secretion of superoxide dismutase A and in the virulence of *Mycobacterium tuberculosis*. *Mol Microbiol* **48:** 453–464.

Briken V, Miller JL. 2008. Living on the edge: Inhibition of host cell apoptosis by *Mycobacterium tuberculosis*. *Future Microbiol* **3:** 415–422.

Caceres N, Tapia G, Ojanguren I, Altare F, Gil O, Pinto S, Vilaplana C, Cardona PJ. 2009. Evolution of foamy macrophages in the pulmonary granulomas of experimental tuberculosis models. *Tuberculosis (Edinb)* **89:** 175–182.

Cambier CJ, Takaki KK, Larson RP, Hernandez RE, Tobin DM, Urdahl KB, Cosma CL, Ramakrishnan L. 2014. Mycobacteria manipulate macrophage recruitment through coordinated use of membrane lipids. *Nature* **505:** 218–222.

Canetti G. 1955. The tubercle bacillus in the pulmonary lesion of man; histobacteriology and its bearing on the therapy of pulmonary tuberculosis. Springer, New York.

Canetti G. 1965. Present aspects of bacterial resistance in tuberculosis. *Am Rev Respir Dis* **92:** 687–703.

Caruso AM, Serbina N, Klein E, Triebold K, Bloom BR, Flynn JL. 1999. Mice deficient in CD4 T cells have only transiently diminished levels of IFN-γ, yet succumb to tuberculosis. *J Immunol* **162:** 5407–5416.

Chakravarty SD, Zhu G, Tsai MC, Mohan VP, Marino S, Kirschner DE, Huang L, Flynn J, Chan J. 2008. Tumor necrosis factor blockade in chronic murine tuberculosis enhances granulomatous inflammation and disorganizes granulomas in the lungs. *Infect Immun* **76:** 916–926.

Choi HH, Shin DM, Kang G, Kim KH, Park JB, Hur GM, Lee HM, Lim YJ, Park JK, Jo EK, et al. 2010. Endoplasmic reticulum stress response is involved in *Mycobacterium tuberculosis* protein ESAT-6-mediated apoptosis. *FEBS Lett* **584:** 2445–2454.

Clay H, Davis JM, Beery D, Huttenlocher A, Lyons SE, Ramakrishnan L. 2007. Dichotomous role of the macrophage in early *Mycobacterium marinum* infection of the zebrafish. *Cell Host Microbe* **2:** 29–39.

Clay H, Volkman HE, Ramakrishnan L. 2008. Tumor necrosis factor signaling mediates resistance to mycobacteria by inhibiting bacterial growth and macrophage death. *Immunity* **29:** 283–294.

Comas I, Chakravartti J, Small PM, Galagan J, Niemann S, Kremer K, Ernst JD, Gagneux S. 2010. Human T cell epitopes of *Mycobacterium tuberculosis* are evolutionarily hyperconserved. *Nat Genet* **42:** 498–503.

Cosma CL, Humbert O, Ramakrishnan L. 2004. Superinfecting mycobacteria home to established tuberculous granulomas. *Nat Immunol* **5:** 828–835.

Cosma CL, Klein K, Kim R, Beery D, Ramakrishnan L. 2006. *Mycobacterium marinum* Erp is a virulence determinant required for cell wall integrity and intracellular survival. *Infect Immun* **74:** 3125–3133.

Cosma CL, Humbert O, Sherman DR, Ramakrishnan L. 2008. Trafficking of superinfecting mycobacterium organisms into established granulomas occurs in mammals and is independent of the Erp and ESX-1 mycobacterial virulence loci. *J Infect Dis* **198:** 1851–1855.

Cruz A, Khader SA, Torrado E, Fraga A, Pearl JE, Pedrosa J, Cooper AM, Castro AG. 2006. Cutting edge: IFN-γ regulates the induction and expansion of IL-17-producing CD4 T cells during mycobacterial infection. *J Immunol* **177:** 1416–1420.

Cruz A, Fraga Ag, Fountain JJ, Rangel-Moreno J, Torrado E, Saraiva M, Pereira DR, Randall TD, Pedrosa J, Cooper AM, et al. 2010. Pathological role of interleukin 17 in mice subjected to repeated BCG vaccination after infection with *Mycobacterium tuberculosis*. *J Exp Med* **207:** 1609–1616.

Dannenberg AM Jr. 1993. Immunopathogenesis of pulmonary tuberculosis. *Hosp Pract (Off Ed)* **28:** 51–58.

Dannenberg AM Jr. 2003. Macrophage turnover, division and activation within developing, peak and "healed" tuberculous lesions produced in rabbits by BCG. *Tuberculosis (Edinb)* **83:** 251–260.

Davis JM, Ramakrishnan L. 2009. The role of the granuloma in expansion and dissemination of early tuberculous infection. *Cell* **136:** 37–49.

Davis JM, Clay H, Lewis JL, Ghori N, Herbomel P, Ramakrishnan L. 2002. Real-time visualization of mycobacterium-macrophage interactions leading to initiation of granuloma formation in zebrafish embryos. *Immunity* **17:** 693–702.

Derrick SC, Morris SL. 2007. The ESAT6 protein of *Mycobacterium tuberculosis* induces apoptosis of macrophages by activating caspase expression. *Cell Microbiol* **9:** 1547–1555.

Desvignes L, Ernst JD. 2009. Interferon-γ-responsive nonhematopoietic cells regulate the immune response to *Mycobacterium tuberculosis*. *Immunity* **31:** 974–985.

Dogru D, Kiper N, Ozcelik U, Yalcin E, Tezcan I. 2010. Tuberculosis in children with congenital immunodeficiency syndromes. *Tuberk Toraks* **58:** 59–63.

Dorhoi A, Desel C, Yeremeev V, Pradl L, Brinkmann V, Mollenkopf HJ, Hanke K, Gross O, Ruland J, Kaufmann SH. 2010. The adaptor molecule CARD9 is essential for tuberculosis control. *J Exp Med* **207:** 777–792.

Dorhoi A, Iannaccone M, Farinacci M, Fae KC, Schreiber J, Moura-Alves P, Nouailles G, Mollenkopf HJ, Oberbeck-Muller D, Jorg S, et al. 2013. MicroRNA-223 controls susceptibility to tuberculosis by regulating lung neutrophil recruitment. *J Clin Invest* **123:** 4836–4848.

Egen JG, Rothfuchs AG, Feng CG, Winter N, Sher A, Germain RN. 2008. Macrophage and T cell dynamics during the development and disintegration of mycobacterial granulomas. *Immunity* **28:** 271–284.

Elkington PT, O'Kane CM, Friedland JS. 2005. The paradox of matrix metalloproteinases in infectious disease. *Clin Exp Immunol* **142:** 12–20.

Elkington PT, Green JA, Emerson JE, Lopez-Pascual LD, Boyle JJ, O'Kane CM, Friedland JS. 2007. Synergistic up-regulation of epithelial cell matrix metalloproteinase-9 secretion in tuberculosis. *Am J Respir Cell Mol Biol* **37:** 431–437.

Elkington P, Shiomi T, Breen R, Nuttall RK, Ugarte-Gil CA, Walker NF, Saraiva L, Pedersen B, Mauri F, Lipman M, et al. 2011a. MMP-1 drives immunopathology in human tuberculosis and transgenic mice. *J Clin Invest* **121:** 1827–1833.

Elkington PT, D'Armiento JM, Friedland JS. 2011b. Tuberculosis immunopathology: The neglected role of extracellular matrix destruction. *Sci Transl Med* **3:** 71–76.

Elkington PT, Ugarte-Gil CA, Friedland JS. 2011c. Matrix metalloproteinases in tuberculosis. *Eur Respir J* **38:** 456–464.

Ernst JD. 2012. The immunological life cycle of tuberculosis. *Nat Rev Immunol* **12:** 581–591.

Eruslanov EB, Lyadova IV, Kondratieva TK, Majorov KB, Scheglov IV, Orlova MO, Apt AS. 2005. Neutrophil responses to *Mycobacterium tuberculosis* infection in genetically susceptible and resistant mice. *Infect Immun* **73:** 1744–1753.

Eum SY, Kong JH, Hong MS, Lee YJ, Kim JH, Hwang SH, Cho SN, Via LE, Barry CE III. 2010. Neutrophils are the predominant infected phagocytic cells in the airways of patients with active pulmonary TB. *Chest* **137:** 122–128.

Fabri M, Stenger S, Shin DM, Yuk JM, Liu PT, Realegeno S, Lee HM, Krutzik SR, Schenk M, Sieling PA, et al. 2011. Vitamin D is required for IFN-γ-mediated antimicrobial activity of human macrophages. *Sci Transl Med* **3:** p104ra102.

Fife BT, Pauken KE. 2011. The role of the PD-1 pathway in autoimmunity and peripheral tolerance. *Ann N Y Acad Sci* **1217:** 45–59.

Flynn JL. 2006. Lessons from experimental *Mycobacterium tuberculosis* infections. *Microbes Infect* **8:** 1179–1188.

Flynn JL, Chan J. 2001. Immunology of tuberculosis. *Annu Rev Immunol* **19:** 93–129.

Flynn JL, Chan J, Triebold KJ, Dalton DK, Stewart TA, Bloom BR. 1993. An essential role for interferon γ in resistance to *Mycobacterium tuberculosis* infection. *J Exp Med* **178:** 2249–2254.

Flynn JL, Goldstein MM, Chan J, Triebold KJ, Pfeffer K, Lowenstein CJ, Schreiber R, Mak TW, Bloom BR. 1995. Tumor necrosis factor-α is required in the protective immune response against *Mycobacterium tuberculosis* in mice. *Immunity* **2:** 561–572.

Fratazzi C, Arbeit RD, Carini C, Remold HG. 1997. Programmed cell death of *Mycobacterium avium* serovar 4-infected human macrophages prevents the mycobacteria from spreading and induces mycobacterial growth inhibition by freshly added, uninfected macrophages. *J Immunol* **158:** 4320–4327.

Gan H, Lee J, Ren F, Chen M, Kornfeld H, Remold HG. 2008. *Mycobacterium tuberculosis* blocks crosslinking of annexin-1 and apoptotic envelope formation on infected macrophages to maintain virulence. *Nat Immunol* **9:** 1189–1197.

Ganachari M, Ruiz-Morales JA, Gomez de la Torre Pretell JC, Dinh J, Granados J, Flores-Villanueva PO. 2010. Joint effect of MCP-1 genotype GG and MMP-1 genotype 2G/2G increases the likelihood of developing pulmonary tuberculosis in BCG-vaccinated individuals. *PLoS ONE* **5:** e8881.

Garcia Vidal C, Rodriguez Fernandez S, Martinez Lacasa J, Salavert M, Vidal R, Rodriguez Carballeira M, Garau J. 2005. Paradoxical response to antituberculous therapy in infliximab-treated patients with disseminated tuberculosis. *Clin Infect Dis* **40:** 756–759.

Greenlee KJ, Corry DB, Engler DA, Matsunami RK, Tessier P, Cook RG, Werb Z, Kheradmand F. 2006. Proteomic identification of in vivo substrates for matrix metalloproteinases 2 and 9 reveals a mechanism for resolution of inflammation. *J Immunol* **177:** 7312–7321.

Greenwald RJ, Freeman GJ, Sharpe AH. 2005. The B7 family revisited. *Annu Rev Immunol* **23:** 515–548.

Grosset J. 2003. *Mycobacterium tuberculosis* in the extracellular compartment: An underestimated adversary. *Antimicrob Agents Chemother* **47:** 833–836.

Guinn KM, Hickey MJ, Mathur SK, Zakel KL, Grotzke JE, Lewinsohn DM, Smith S, Sherman DR. 2004. Individual RD1-region genes are required for export of ESAT-6/CFP-10 and for virulence of *Mycobacterium tuberculosis*. *Mol Microbiol* **51:** 359–370.

Helke KL, Mankowski JL, Manabe YC. 2006. Animal models of cavitation in pulmonary tuberculosis. *Tuberculosis (Edinb)* **86:** 337–348.

Hinchey J, Lee S, Jeon BY, Basaraba RJ, Venkataswamy MM, Chen B, Chan J, Braunstein M, Orme IM, Derrick SC, et al. 2007. Enhanced priming of adaptive immunity by a proapoptotic mutant of *Mycobacterium tuberculosis*. *J Clin Invest* **117:** 2279–2288.

Howard WL, Maresh F, Mueller EE, Yanitelli SA, Woodruff GF. 1949. The role of pulmonary cavitation in the development of bacterial resistance to streptomycin. *Am Rev Tuberc* **59:** 391–401.

Hsu T, Hingley-Wilson SM, Chen B, Chen M, Dai AZ, Morin PM, Marks CB, Padiyar J, Goulding C, Gingery M, et al. 2003. The primary mechanism of attenuation of bacillus Calmette-Guerin is a loss of secreted lytic function required for invasion of lung interstitial tissue. *Proc Natl Acad Sci* **100:** 12420–12425.

Iliopoulos A, Psathakis K, Aslanidis S, Skagias L, Sfikakis PP. 2006. Tuberculosis and granuloma formation in patients receiving anti-TNF therapy. *Int J Tuberc Lung Dis* **10:** 588–590.

Jayakumar D, Jacobs WR Jr, Narayanan S. 2008. Protein kinase E of *Mycobacterium tuberculosis* has a role in the nitric oxide stress response and apoptosis in a human macrophage model of infection. *Cell Microbiol* **10:** 365–374.

Kamphorst AO, Ahmed R. 2013. Manipulating the PD-1 pathway to improve immunity. *Curr Opin Immunol* **25:** 381–388.

Keane J. 2005. TNF-blocking agents and tuberculosis: New drugs illuminate an old topic. *Rheumatology (Oxford)* **44:** 714–720.

Keane J, Remold HG, Kornfeld H. 2000. Virulent *Mycobacterium tuberculosis* strains evade apoptosis of infected alveolar macrophages. *J Immunol* **164:** 2016–2020.

Keane J, Shurtleff B, Kornfeld H. 2002. TNF-dependent BALB/c murine macrophage apoptosis following *Mycobacterium tuberculosis* infection inhibits bacillary growth in an IFN-γ independent manner. *Tuberculosis (Edinb)* **82:** 55–61.

Kindler V, Sappino AP, Grau GE, Piguet PF, Vassalli P. 1989. The inducing role of tumor necrosis factor in the development of bactericidal granulomas during BCG infection. *Cell* **56:** 731–740.

Kirman J, McCoy K, Hook S, Prout M, Delahunt B, Orme I, Frank A, Le Gros G. 1999. CTLA-4 blockade enhances the immune response induced by mycobacterial infection but does not lead to increased protection. *Infect Immun* **67:** 3786–3792.

Koch R. 1882. The aetiology of tuberculosis. National Tuberculosis Association, New York.

Kwan CK, Ernst JD. 2011. HIV and tuberculosis: A deadly human syndemic. *Clin Microbiol Rev* **24:** 351–376.

Lammas DA, Stober C, Harvey CJ, Kendrick N, Panchalingam S, Kumararatne DS. 1997. ATP-induced killing of mycobacteria by human macrophages is mediated by purinergic P2Z(P2X7) receptors. *Immunity* **7:** 433–444.

Lazar-Molnar E, Chen B, Sweeney KA, Wang EJ, Liu W, Lin J, Porcelli SA, Almo SC, Nathenson SG, Jacobs WR Jr. 2010. Programmed death-1 (PD-1)-deficient mice are extraordinarily sensitive to tuberculosis. *Proc Natl Acad Sci* **107:** 13402–13407.

Lee PP, Chan KW, Jiang L, Chen T, Li C, Lee TL, Mak PH, Fok SF, Yang X, Lau YL. 2008. Susceptibility to mycobacterial infections in children with X-linked chronic granulomatous disease: A review of 17 patients living in a region endemic for tuberculosis. *Pediatr Infect Dis J* **27:** 224–230.

Lin PL, Myers A, Smith L, Bigbee C, Bigbee M, Fuhrman C, Grieser H, Chiosea I, Voitenek NN, Capuano SV, et al. 2010. Tumor necrosis factor neutralization results in disseminated disease in acute and latent *Mycobacterium tuberculosis* infection with normal granuloma structure in a cynomolgus macaque model. *Arthritis Rheum* **62:** 340–350.

Lin PL, Ford CB, Coleman MT, Myers AJ, Gawande R, Ioerger T, Sacchettini J, Fortune SM, Flynn JL. 2014. Sterilization of granulomas is common in active and latent tuberculosis despite within-host variability in bacterial killing. *Nat Med* **20:** 75–79.

Lowe DM, Redford PS, Wilkinson RJ, O'Garra A, Martineau AR. 2012. Neutrophils in tuberculosis: Friend or foe? *Trends Immunol* **33:** 14–25.

Mahajan S, Dkhar HK, Chandra V, Dave S, Nanduri R, Janmeja AK, Agrewala JN, Gupta P. 2012. *Mycobacterium tuberculosis* modulates macrophage lipid-sensing nuclear receptors PPARγ and TR4 for survival. *J Immunol* **188:** 5593–5603.

Middlebrook G, Dubos RJ, Pierce C. 1947. Virulence and morphological characteristics of mammalian tubercle bacilli. *J Exp Med* **86:** 175–184.

Mishra BB, Moura-Alves P, Sonawane A, Hacohen N, Griffiths G, Moita LF, Anes E. 2010. *Mycobacterium tuberculosis* protein ESAT-6 is a potent activator of the NLRP3/ASC inflammasome. *Cell Microbiol* **12:** 1046–1063.

Molloy A, Laochumroonvorapong P, Kaplan G. 1994. Apoptosis, but not necrosis, of infected monocytes is coupled with killing of intracellular bacillus Calmette-Guerin. *J Exp Med* **180:** 1499–1509.

Nandi B, Behar SM. 2011. Regulation of neutrophils by interferon-γ limits lung inflammation during tuberculosis infection. *J Exp Med* **208:** 2251–2262.

North RJ, Jung YJ. 2004. Immunity to tuberculosis. *Annu Rev Immunol* **22:** 599–623.

Oddo M, Renno T, Attinger A, Bakker T, MacDonald HR, Meylan PR. 1998. Fas ligand-induced apoptosis of infected human macrophages reduces the viability of intracellular *Mycobacterium tuberculosis*. *J Immunol* **160:** 5448–5454.

Odorizzi PM, Wherry EJ. 2012. Inhibitory receptors on lymphocytes: Insights from infections. *J Immunol* **188:** 2957–2965.

Onwueme KC, Vos CJ, Zurita J, Ferreras JA, Quadri LE. 2005. The dimycocerosate ester polyketide virulence factors of mycobacteria. *Prog Lipid Res* **44:** 259–302.

Palaci M, Dietze R, Hadad DJ, Ribeiro FK, Peres RL, Vinhas SA, Maciel EL, do Valle Dettoni V, Horter L, Boom WH, et al. 2007. Cavitary disease and quantitative sputum bacillary load in cases of pulmonary tuberculosis. *J Clin Microbiol* **45:** 4064–4066.

Parasa VR, Rahman MJ, Ngyuen Hoang AT, Svensson M, Brighenti S, Lerm M. 2014. Modeling *Mycobacterium tuberculosis* early granuloma formation in experimental human lung tissue. *Dis Model Mech* **7:** 281–288.

Parks WC, Wilson CL, Lopez-Boado YS. 2004. Matrix metalloproteinases as modulators of inflammation and innate immunity. *Nat Rev Immunol* **4:** 617–629.

Pedrosa J, Saunders BM, Appelberg R, Orme IM, Silva MT, Cooper AM. 2000. Neutrophils play a protective nonphagocytic role in systemic *Mycobacterium tuberculosis* infection of mice. *Infect Immun* **68:** 577–583.

Peggs KS, Quezada SA, Allison JP. 2009. Cancer immunotherapy: Co-stimulatory agonists and co-inhibitory antagonists. *Clin Exp Immunol* **157:** 9–19.

Peyron P, Vaubourgeix J, Poquet Y, Levillain F, Botanch C, Bardou F, Daffe M, Emile JF, Marchou B, Cardona PJ, et al. 2008. Foamy macrophages from tuberculous patients' granulomas constitute a nutrient-rich reservoir for *M. tuberculosis* persistence. *PLoS Pathog* **4:** e1000204.

Philips JA, Ernst JD. 2012. Tuberculosis pathogenesis and immunity. *Annu Rev Pathol* **7:** 353–384.

Price NM, Gilman RH, Uddin J, Recavarren S, Friedland JS. 2003. Unopposed matrix metalloproteinase-9 expression in human tuberculous granuloma and the role of TNF-α-dependent monocyte networks. *J Immunol* **171:** 5579–5586.

Pym AS, Brodin P, Brosch R, Huerre M, Cole ST. 2002. Loss of RD1 contributed to the attenuation of the live tuberculosis vaccines *Mycobacterium bovis* BCG and *Mycobacterium microti*. *Mol Microbiol* **46:** 709–717.

Ramakrishnan L. 2012. Revisiting the role of the granuloma in tuberculosis. *Nat Rev Immunol* **12:** 352–366.

Ramakrishnan L. 2013. The zebrafish guide to tuberculosis immunity and treatment. *Cold Spring Harb Symp Quant Biol* **78:** 179–192.

Ramakrishnan L, Valdivia RH, McKerrow JH, Falkow S. 1997. *Mycobacterium marinum* causes both long-term subclinical infection and acute disease in the leopard frog (*Rana pipiens*). *Infect Immun* **65:** 767–773.

Ramakrishnan L, Federspiel NA, Falkow S. 2000. Granuloma-specific expression of mycobacterium virulence proteins from the glycine-rich PE-PGRS family. *Science* **288:** 1436–1439.

Ravn P, Demissie A, Eguale T, Wondwosson H, Lein D, Amoudy HA, Mustafa AS, Jensen AK, Holm A, Rosenkrands I, et al. 1999. Human T cell responses to the ESAT-6 antigen from *Mycobacterium tuberculosis*. *J Infect Dis* **179:** 637–645.

Rich AR. 1946. *Pathogenesis of tuberculosis*. Charles C. Thomas, Springfield, IL.

Roach DR, Bean AG, Demangel C, France MP, Briscoe H, Britton WJ. 2002. TNF regulates chemokine induction essential for cell recruitment, granuloma formation, and clearance of mycobacterial infection. *J Immunol* **168:** 4620–4627.

Roca FJ, Ramakrishnan L. 2013. TNF dually mediates resistance and susceptibility to mycobacteria via mitochondrial reactive oxygen species. *Cell* **153:** 521–534.

Russell DG, Cardona PJ, Kim MJ, Allain S, Altare F. 2009. Foamy macrophages and the progression of the human tuberculosis granuloma. *Nat Immunol* **10:** 943–948.

Salamon H, Bruiners N, Lakehal K, Shi L, Ravi J, Yamaguchi KD, Pine R, Gennaro ML. 2014. Cutting edge: Vitamin D regulates lipid metabolism in *Mycobacterium tuberculosis* infection. *J Immunol* **193:** 30–34.

Sarris M, Masson JB, Maurin D, Van der Aa LM, Boudinot P, Lortat-Jacob H, Herbomel P. 2012. Inflammatory chemokines direct and restrict leukocyte migration within live tissues as glycan-bound gradients. *Curr Biol* **22:** 2375–2382.

Saunders BM, Cooper AM. 2000. Restraining mycobacteria: Role of granulomas in mycobacterial infections. *Immunol Cell Biol* **78:** 334–341.

Scanga CA, Mohan VP, Yu K, Joseph H, Tanaka K, Chan J, Flynn JL. 2000. Depletion of CD4(+) T cells causes reactivation of murine persistent tuberculosis despite continued expression of interferon γ and nitric oxide synthase 2. *J Exp Med* **192:** 347–358.

Schreiber HA, Harding JS, Hunt O, Altamirano CJ, Hulseberg PD, Stewart D, Fabry Z, Sandor M. 2011. Inflammatory dendritic cells migrate in and out of transplanted chronic mycobacterial granulomas in mice. *J Clin Invest* **121:** 3902–3913.

Scott HM, Flynn JL. 2002. *Mycobacterium tuberculosis* in chemokine receptor 2-deficient mice: Influence of dose on disease progression. *Infect Immun* **70:** 5946–5954.

Sheen P, O'Kane CM, Chaudhary K, Tovar M, Santillan C, Sosa J, Caviedes L, Gilman RH, Stamp G, Friedland JS. 2009. High MMP-9 activity characterises pleural tuberculosis correlating with granuloma formation. *Eur Respir J* **33:** 134–141.

Sherman DR, Guinn KM, Hickey MJ, Mathur SK, Zakel KL, Smith S. 2004. *Mycobacterium tuberculosis* H37Rv: ΔRD1 is more virulent than *M. bovis* bacille Calmette-Guerin in long-term murine infection. *J Infect Dis* **190:** 123–126.

Simeone R, Bottai D, Brosch R. 2009. ESX/type VII secretion systems and their role in host-pathogen interaction. *Curr Opin Microbiol* **12:** 4–10.

Singh V, Jamwal S, Jain R, Verma P, Gokhale R, Rao KV. 2012. *Mycobacterium tuberculosis*-driven targeted recalibration of macrophage lipid homeostasis promotes the foamy phenotype. *Cell Host Microbe* **12:** 669–681.

Soehnlein O, Lindbom L. 2010. Phagocyte partnership during the onset and resolution of inflammation. *Nat Rev Immunol* **10:** 427–439.

Spector WG. 1969. The granulomatous inflammatory exudate. *Int Rev Exp Pathol* **8:** 1–55.

Srivastava S, Ernst JD. 2014. Cell-to-cell transfer of *M. tuberculosis* antigens optimizes CD4 T cell priming. *Cell Host Microbe* **15:** 741–752.

Stenger S. 2005. Immunological control of tuberculosis: Role of tumour necrosis factor and more. *Ann Rheum Dis* **64:** iv24–iv28.

Sugawara I, Udagawa T, Yamada H. 2004. Rat neutrophils prevent the development of tuberculosis. *Infect Immun* **72:** 1804–1806.

Sullivan JT, Young EF, McCann JR, Braunstein M. 2012. The *Mycobacterium tuberculosis* SecA2 system subverts phagosome maturation to promote growth in macrophages. *Infect Immun* **80:** 996–1006.

Swaim LE, Connolly LE, Volkman HE, Humbert O, Born DE, Ramakrishnan L. 2006. *Mycobacterium marinum* infection of adult zebrafish causes caseating granulomatous tuberculosis and is moderated by adaptive immunity. *Infect Immun* **74:** 6108–6117.

Szabo SJ, Sullivan BM, Peng SL, Glimcher LH. 2003. Molecular mechanisms regulating Th1 immune responses. *Annu Rev Immunol* **21:** 713–758.

Takaki K, Cosma CL, Troll MA, Ramakrishnan L. 2012. An in vivo platform for rapid high-throughput antitubercular drug discovery. *Cell Rep* **2:** 175–184.

Taylor JL, Hattle JM, Dreitz SA, Troudt JM, Izzo LS, Basaraba RJ, Orme IM, Matrisian LM, Izzo AA. 2006. Role for matrix metalloproteinase 9 in granuloma formation during pulmonary *Mycobacterium tuberculosis* infection. *Infect Immun* **74:** 6135–6144.

Thwaites GE, Chau TT, Stepniewska K, Phu NH, Chuong LV, Sinh DX, White NJ, Parry CM, Farrar JJ. 2002. Diagnosis of adult tuberculous meningitis by use of clinical and laboratory features. *Lancet* **360:** 1287–1292.

Thye T, Scarisbrick G, Browne EN, Chinbuah MA, Gyapong J, Osei I, Owusu-Dabo E, Niemann S, Rusch-Gerdes S, Meyer CG, et al. 2009. CTLA4 autoimmunity-associated genotype contributes to severe pulmonary tuberculosis in an African population. *PLoS ONE* **4:** e6307.

Tobin DM, Vary JC Jr, Ray JP, Walsh GS, Dunstan SJ, Bang ND, Hagge DA, Khadge S, King MC, Hawn TR, et al. 2010. The lta4 h locus modulates susceptibility to mycobacterial infection in zebrafish and humans. *Cell* **140:** 717–730.

Tobin DM, Roca FJ, Oh SF, McFarland R, Vickery TW, Ray JP, Ko DC, Zou Y, Bang ND, Chau TT, et al. 2012. Host genotype-specific therapies can optimize the inflammatory response to mycobacterial infections. *Cell* **148:** 434–446.

Tubo NJ, Jenkins MK. 2014. $CD4^+$ T cells: Guardians of the phagosome. *Clin Microbiol Rev* **27:** 200–213.

Ueda H, Howson JM, Esposito L, Heward J, Snook H, Chamberlain G, Rainbow DB, Hunter KM, Smith AN, Di Genova G, et al. 2003. Association of the T-cell regulatory gene CTLA4 with susceptibility to autoimmune disease. *Nature* **423:** 506–511.

Urdahl KB, Shafiani S, Ernst JD. 2011. Initiation and regulation of T-cell responses in tuberculosis. *Mucosal Immunol* **4:** 288–293.

van der Wel N, Hava D, Houben D, Fluitsma D, van Zon M, Pierson J, Brenner M, Peters PJ. 2007. *M. tuberculosis* and *M. leprae* translocate from the phagolysosome to the cytosol in myeloid cells. *Cell* **129:** 1287–1298.

van der Woude AD, Stoop EJ, Stiess M, Wang S, Ummels R, van Stempvoort G, Piersma SR, Cascioferro A, Jimenez CR, Houben EN, et al. 2014. Analysis of SecA2-dependent substrates in *Mycobacterium marinum* identifies protein kinase G (PknG) as a virulence effector. *Cell Microbiol* **16:** 280–295.

Velmurugan K, Chen B, Miller JL, Azogue S, Gurses S, Hsu T, Glickman M, Jacobs WR Jr, Porcelli SA, Briken V. 2007. *Mycobacterium tuberculosis* nuoG is a virulence gene that inhibits apoptosis of infected host cells. *PLoS Pathog* **3:** e110.

Volkman HE, Clay H, Beery D, Chang JC, Sherman DR, Ramakrishnan L. 2004. Tuberculous granuloma formation is enhanced by a mycobacterium virulence determinant. *PLoS Biol* **2:** e367.

Volkman HE, Pozos TC, Zheng J, Davis JM, Rawls JF, Ramakrishnan L. 2010. Tuberculous granuloma induction via interaction of a bacterial secreted protein with host epithelium. *Science* **327:** 466–469.

Wallis RS, Schluger NW. 2010. Pulmonary infectious complications of tumor necrosis factor blockade. *Infect Dis Clin North Am* **24:** 681–692.

Wang CH, Lin HC, Lin SM, Huang CD, Liu CY, Huang KH, Hsieh LL, Chung KF, Kuo HP. 2010. MMP-1(-1607G) polymorphism as a risk factor for fibrosis after pulmonary tuberculosis in Taiwan. *Int J Tuberc Lung Dis* **14:** 627–634.

Watkins BY, Joshi SA, Ball DA, Leggett H, Park S, Kim J, Austin CD, Paler-Martinez A, Xu M, Downing KH, et al. 2012. *Mycobacterium marinum* SecA2 promotes stable granulomas and induces tumor necrosis factor α in vivo. *Infect Immun* **80:** 3512–3520.

Wells WF, Ratcliffe HL, Grumb C. 1948. On the mechanics of droplet nuclei infection; quantitative experimental airborne tuberculosis in rabbits. *Am J Hyg* **47:** 11–28.

Williams GT, Williams WJ. 1983. Granulomatous inflammation—A review. *J Clin Pathol* **36:** 723–733.

Wolf AJ, Linas B, Trevejo-Nunez GJ, Kincaid E, Tamura T, Takatsu K, Ernst JD. 2007. *Mycobacterium tuberculosis* infects dendritic cells with high frequency and impairs their function in vivo. *J Immunol* **179:** 2509–2519.

Yang CT, Cambier CJ, Davis JM, Hall CJ, Crosier PS, Ramakrishnan L. 2012. Neutrophils exert protection in the early tuberculous granuloma by oxidative killing of mycobacteria phagocytosed from infected macrophages. *Cell Host Microbe* **12:** 301–312.

Novel Vaccination Strategies against Tuberculosis

Peter Andersen[1] and Stefan H.E. Kaufmann[2]

[1]Statens Serum Institut, DK-2300 Copenhagen S, Denmark

[2]Max Planck Institute for Infection Biology, 10117 Berlin, Germany

Correspondence: pa@ssi.dk

The tuberculosis (TB) pandemic continues to rampage despite widespread use of the BCG (Bacillus Calmette–Guérin) vaccine. Novel vaccination strategies are urgently needed to arrest global transmission and prevent the uncontrolled development of multidrug-resistant forms of *Mycobacterium tuberculosis.* Over the last two decades, considerable progress has been made in the field of vaccine development with numerous innovative preclinical candidates and more than a dozen vaccines in clinical trials. These vaccines are developed either as boosters of the current BCG vaccine or as novel prime vaccines to replace BCG. Given the enormous prevalence of latent TB infection, vaccines that are protective on top of an already established infection remain a high priority and a significant scientific challenge. Here we discuss the current state of TB vaccine research and development, our understanding of the underlying immunology, and the requirements for an efficient TB vaccine.

Vaccination is one of the most successful medical measures to reduce morbidity and mortality (Kaufmann 2010). It has liberated us from the threat of numerous infectious diseases including polio, measles, hepatitis B, and smallpox. Increasing accessibility to vaccines of resource-poor regions by the Expanded Program on Immunization (EPI) has reduced child mortality from 20 million in 1960 to less than 10 million in 2005. In 1974, Bacille Calmette–Guérin (BCG) vaccination against tuberculosis (TB) was included in the EPI and now covers 80% of all infants on this globe. With more than 4 billion administrations, this vaccine has saved many infants' lives by protecting against serious forms of disseminated TB (Hatherill 2011; WHO 2013). Yet, the vaccine has had a minor impact on TB incidences because it fails to protect against the most prevalent form of this disease, pulmonary TB. The World Health Organization (WHO) has proposed to reduce prevalence by half in 2015, as compared to 1990—a goal that will be largely achieved by currently available intervention measures (Kaufmann et al. 2010; StopTBPartnership and WHO 2011). The more ambitious goal to eliminate TB by 2050, however, can only be accomplished if better diagnostics, drugs, and vaccines become available in due time (Kaufmann et al. 2010; StopTBPartnership and WHO 2011). In-

Cite this article as *Cold Spring Harb Perspect Med* doi: 10.1101/cshperspect.a018523

deed, the last decade has witnessed the development of novel vaccine candidates with more than a dozen undergoing clinical assessment (Kaufmann 2011, 2012). Here we describe general principles underlying TB vaccination, and the vaccine candidates that have entered the clinical trial pipeline. We will also discuss chances of success of current vaccine candidates and the need for further research and development to keep the vaccine pipeline viable. It cannot be excluded that vaccine candidates currently in the pipeline will fail, as was the case for the first vaccine candidate who completed a phase IIb efficacy trial without evidence of protection (Tameris et al. 2013) and another candidate who dropped out because of serious adverse events (Kupferschmidt 2011).

BCG, THE CURRENT VACCINE AGAINST TB

Mycobacterium bovis BCG is the only vaccine currently available against TB, and it has been in use for more than 80 years. The vaccine was developed at the Institute Pasteur, Lille, France, after more than 13 years of continuous in vitro passage of *M. bovis*, the pathogen responsible for TB in cattle (Calmette et al. 1927; Calmette and Plotz 1929). The genetic background for the attenuation of BCG was unknown until advances in molecular biology allowed direct comparisons between the genomes of *M. bovis* and the various strains of BCG. It became clear that the long-term in vitro propagation had resulted in the loss of several gene segments clustered in different regions of difference (RDs) (Behr et al. 1999). The RD1 is the original mutation resulting in attenuation of *M. bovis*, and this segment is lacking in all strains of BCG and encodes important virulence factors and T-cell antigens, such as early secretory antigenic 6 kDa (ESAT-6) and culture filtrate protein 10 (CFP10).

The efficacy of BCG was studied extensively in clinical trials during the 1930s and the vaccine was widely deployed after World War II. BCG is one of the most widely administered vaccines worldwide and has been part of the EPI since the early 1970s. BCG vaccination prevents disseminated disease (especially military and meningeal TB) in children, but despite inducing a strong T helper 1 (Th1) response, the efficacy of BCG is highly variable and the vaccine inadequately prevents pulmonary TB in all age groups, in particular in high-TB-endemic regions. Some of the hypotheses to explain the variable performance of BCG relates to the variation to technical factors of BCG itself (Tolderlund 1952; Janaszek 1991). However, the fact that BCG provides protection against extrapulmonary TB in childhood but not against pulmonary TB in adults suggests that the major problem with BCG is not only its efficacy per se but also waning or changed immune responses in adolescence. The simple explanation is that immunological memory after one vaccination does not last lifelong, and being a live vaccine, BCG is not considered for a secondary booster immunization later in life. The existence of abundant atypical mycobacteria in environmental samples in high-endemic regions adds to the complexity by providing their own level of anti-TB immunity to the population that may mask the effect of BCG or prevent the necessary vaccine replication (the so-called blocking hypothesis) (reviewed in Andersen and Doherty 2005). Although the millions of doses of BCG administered clearly emphasizes that this vaccine is generally safe, the WHO Global Advisory Committee on Vaccine Safety has changed its recommendations to advise against the use of BCG in HIV^+ children based on reported cases of disseminated BCG disease (Hesseling et al. 2004). This new policy obviously highlights the need for new and safe vaccines for both priming and boosting.

In their early studies on BCG vaccination, Calmette and Guérin already observed that BCG vaccination not only protected infants against death due to TB, but also reduced general mortality in infants who did not suffer from TB disease (Calmette et al. 1927). This topic was largely ignored for decades. More recently, epidemiologic evidence has been presented from several low-income countries that BCG vaccination is correlated with reduced general infant mortality (Roth et al. 2006; Benn et al. 2013). This is an intriguing observation that could influence decisions about continuation of BCG, even after licensure of novel vaccine candidates.

IMMUNE EFFECTOR CELLS AND MECHANISMS: WHAT SHOULD A TB VACCINE DO?

Immunity against TB is cell-mediated with T lymphocytes serving as mediators and mononuclear phagocytes as effectors of protection and pathology (Collins and Kaufmann 2001; Ernst 2012; O'Garra et al. 2013). Immunity against TB is a local event focused on granulomatous lesions with solid granulomas reflecting protection and caseous granulomas mirroring disease (Gengenbacher and Kaufmann 2012; Reece and Kaufmann 2012). Immune mechanisms involve CD4 T lymphocytes of Th1 type. These cells produce interferon γ (IFN-γ), which activates increased antimycobacterial activities in macrophages. Although, the central role of this axis in protective immunity against TB is beyond doubt, it has become increasingly clear that it is insufficient (Kaufmann 2013). Other T lymphocytes, notably CD8 T lymphocytes, and CD4 T cells producing interleukin (IL)-17 (Khader et al. 2007; Cruz et al. 2010), are likely involved in protective immunity (Woodworth and Behar 2006; Ottenhoff 2012). The Th17 cells seem to participate in the initiation of protective immunity. CD8 T cells can contribute to protection by secreting killer molecules (comprising perforin and granulysin, which directly attack macrophages and *M. tuberculosis* [*Mtb*], respectively) and by secreting IFN-γ (Stenger et al. 1998). Several unconventional T lymphocytes have been proposed to participate in immunity as well including γδ T cells and CD1-restricted T cells (Brigl and Brenner 2004; Bonneville and Scotet 2006). Aside from IFN-γ, other cytokines thought to participate in protection include tumor necrosis factor (TNF), granulocyte–monocyte colony-stimulating factor (GM-CSF), IL-1β, and the small molecule, vitamin D (Bermudez and Young 1990; Liu et al. 2006; Fabri et al. 2011). Even though the precise roles of different cells and mediators have not been fully elucidated, it is likely that the cross talk between the different elements has to be highly regulated, both with respect to timing and to location. Uncontrolled hyper- or hyporeactions of any participant of the cross talk can lead to disease reactivation of a previously well-controlled LTBI. Indeed protection and pathology are likely based on similar mechanisms—protection prevails as long as immunity is tightly controlled, whereas pathology develops once this control wanes (Ernst 2012).

Protection and pathology are focused to granulomatous lesions, which are primarily composed of T lymphocytes, mononuclear phagocytes, dendritic cells (DCs), and B lymphocytes (Gengenbacher and Kaufmann 2012; Reece and Kaufmann 2012). As long as the cellular components control each other, the lesion remains well-structured and contains *Mtb* successfully, even though the pathogen is not eradicated. Disturbances in the granuloma result in exaggerated cell death causing necrosis leading to liquefaction (Gengenbacher and Kaufmann 2012; Reece and Kaufmann 2012). These caseous granulomas not only fail to constrain *Mtb* but rather provide a fertile soil for *Mtb* growth and expansion. The different stages of granulomas need to be viewed within a continuum where the different forms coexist in TB patients (Barry et al. 2009; Gengenbacher and Kaufmann 2012). Thus, in one granuloma of a given patient, *Mtb* may still be contained, whereas in another, it may already have taken over.

Activated macrophages primarily inhibit *Mtb* growth and rarely eradicate the pathogen fully. Growth control is achieved by a combination of reactive oxygen and nitrogen intermediates supported by lysosomal enzyme attack (MacMicking et al. 1997). On the other hand, *Mtb* is capable of interfering with phagosome maturation (Rohde et al. 2007). It arrests the phagosome at an early stage, thus prohibiting fusion with lysosomes containing antibacterial enzymes. Aside from mononuclear phagocytes, neutrophils possess potent antibacterial effector functions (Amulic et al. 2012; Cooper and Torrado 2012). Yet, these short-lived phagocytes also have a high intrinsic risk of causing tissue damage (Kaufmann and Dorhoi 2013).

Mtb persisting in macrophages within solid granulomas enter a stage of dormancy in which they shut down their replicative and metabolic activity. These dormant *Mtb* express a different gene profile and therefore different antigens that may have a role in vaccines targeting LTBI (Leyten et al. 2006; Andersen 2007). Moreover, dormant *Mtb* are highly resistant to immune attack (Gengenbacher and Kaufmann 2012). The dormant *Mtb* does not harm the host but resists its elimination. Before TB disease reactivation, *Mtb* undergoes resuscitation, resulting in a highly replicative and metabolically active stage, which is characteristic for active TB disease.

Human TB is a spectral disease depending on the capacity of the immune system to contain *Mtb* in granulomas or not. In ca. 2 billion individuals, LTBI remains lifelong, whereas in almost 9 million individuals, disease develops every year (WHO 2013). It is clear that defined immunosuppressive mechanisms tip the balance in favor of the pathogen. Thus, HIV infection, affecting CD4 T lymphocytes, is the driving force for the current TB pandemic (UNAIDS and WHO 2013); treatment of patients with chronic inflammation such as rheumatoid arthritis with LTBI causes TB reactivation (Keane et al. 2001; Dixon et al. 2010), and individuals with genetic deficiency in the IFN-γ signaling pathways have a heightened risk of TB (Bustamante et al. 2011). Yet, in the majority of cases, the subtle changes, which lead to active disease, remain far from being understood. Better understanding of these mechanisms could provide a blueprint for future vaccine development (Kaufmann 2013). Current vaccine candidates try to mimic the immune response that prevails in LTBI (i.e., stimulation of IFN-γ-producing CD4 T cells) combined with some activation of Th17 cells, and of CD8 T cells. This strategy anticipates that vaccination can induce a protective immune response in susceptible individuals prone to risk of active TB in a similar way as natural *Mtb* infection does in individuals with lifelong LTBI. Ideally, next-generation vaccines should do better and not only induce containment of *Mtb* but also achieve its eradication (Kaufmann 2013). Prevention of *Mtb* infection by vaccination would be an alternative strategy (Kaufmann 2013).

LONG-LIVED IMMUNOLOGICAL MEMORY—A DESIRABLE QUALITY FOR A TB VACCINE

The purpose of vaccination is to establish a long-lived state of immunological memory, and for a chronic infection like LTBI, this is obviously a central goal. The most important obstacle with the current vaccine, BCG, is the lack of protection in adults, which may be related to insufficient immunological memory resulting in waning of immunity during childhood. What do we know about immunological memory against TB? The basic foundation was established in early animal studies that showed that a primary infection cleared by antibiotic treatment provided long-lived immunologic memory immunity, and various levels of increased resistance against secondary infection (Orme 1988; Andersen and Heron 1993; Mollenkopf et al. 2004). Protection was mediated by a CD4 T-cell population that was rapidly recruited to the site of infection, and if the CD4 T-cell subset was purified from memory immune animals, they could adoptively transfer protection against subsequent TB in recipient mice (Orme and Collins 1984; Andersen and Smedegaard 2000). CD4 T cells are not one homogenous population and can be subdivided based on their anatomical location, expression of various cell surface markers, and cytokine secretion into effector and memory T-cell subsets (Sallusto et al. 2004; Seder et al. 2008). Effector memory T cells (T_{em}) have low expression of CD62L and CCR7. They are found in peripheral tissues and produce effector cytokines like IFN-γ and TNF-α, often together with IL-2. In their final stage of differentiation, they lose their ability to proliferate and produce IL-2, and at this stage are referred to as terminal or short-lived effector T cells (T_{eff}). Recent data suggest that for both CD4 and CD8 T cells, the T_{eff} subset can be phenotypically defined by their expression of the killer cell lectin-like receptor G1 (KLGR1) (Joshi et al. 2007; Reiley et al. 2010; Lindenstrom et al. 2013). Central memory T cells (T_{cm}), are opposite to T_{eff} based on most of these fundamental parameters. They are characterized by a high expression of CD62L and CCR7 (which direct them through lymph nodes), and produce abundant IL-2 (Sallusto et al. 2004; Seder et al. 2008). The T_{cm} subset is of particular importance for the maintenance of immunologic memory after vaccination because of its continuous proliferation, and it was shown by adoptive transfer studies in the TB mouse model to mediate a highly efficient protection in the lung against an aerosol challenge with *Mtb* (Andersen and Smedegaard 2000).

In addition to phenotypic markers, the breakthrough in the definition of T-cell subsets based on their cytokine profile defined by intracellular (IC) flow cytometry (Seder et al. 2008) has resulted in the functional characterization of T cells based on the expression of different combinations of cytokines. Data from animal models as well as human clinical trials have led to the paradigm that the quality (i.e., protective potential) of T cells correlates with the number of cytokines coexpressed by the vaccine-promoted CD4 T cells. Moreover, if more than two cytokines are expressed, they are defined as high-quality multifunctional T cells (Darrah et al. 2007). Several independent reports of TB subunit vaccines have correlated enhancement of such multifunctional Th1 cells with growth reduction following aerosol *Mtb* infection of mice (Forbes et al. 2008; Derrick et al. 2011). However, for the discussion of these data in relation to immunological memory, the use of the term "multifunctional" can be misleading. For example, in an intracellular cytokine staining (ICS) assay where IFN-γ, TNFα, and IL-2 coexpression are compared, defining CD4 T cells with two functions as multifunctional would combine IFN-γ/TNFα, IFN-γ/IL-2, and TNFα/IL-2 producers. However, IFN-γ/TNFα cells are T_{eff}, whereas TNFα/IL-2 cells are T_{cm}, and these two subsets have markedly different roles in the maintenance of immunological memory. In comparative studies of an adjuvanted subunit vaccine and BCG, the subunit vaccine very efficiently maintained a population of IL-2^+ T_{cm} for up to 2 years postvaccination, whereas this population was only transiently expressed after BCG vaccination (Lindenstrom et al. 2009).

This pattern was also seen in chronically infected mice, where mice boosted with the subunit vaccine maintained a robust T_{cm} population in the infected organs in contrast to BCG-vaccinated animals that were characterized by terminally differentiated effector T cells and failure to control bacterial replication (Lindenstrom et al. 2013). A lack of long-lived T_{cm} may therefore represent one of BCG's major shortcomings (Orme 2010; Lindenstrom et al. 2013). In a recent study of BCG vaccination in humans it was observed that although the T-cell responses had phenotypic markers that resemble T_{cm}, their cytokine profiles (mostly IFN-γ) and their lack of proliferation had T_{eff} characteristics (Soares et al. 2013). That the IL-2^+ T_{cm} population is of importance for long-term containment of *Mtb* infection in humans is also suggested by a direct comparison of IFN-γ and IL-2 release in a modified QuantiFERON test, where IL-2 was characteristic for LTBI in contrast to active TB patients that produced IFN-γ only (Biselli et al. 2010). Of importance for the discussion of vaccine-promoted memory, the induction of T_{cm} is dependent on both vector/adjuvant delivery (Billeskov et al. 2013) and vaccine dose (Aagaard et al. 2009). Low doses of antigen in a slow-release vehicle seem to maintain T_{cm} and memory responses very efficiently.

HOW CAN WE TARGET TB WITH VACCINES (PRE/POST AND THERAPEUTIC)

Principally, TB vaccines can be administered at three different stages of infection/disease (Table 1; Fig. 1). Preexposure vaccines are administered prior to infection with *Mtb*. The current vaccine BCG, the recombinant (r) viable vaccine candidates, and most subunit vaccines that will be used to boost BCG have been designed as preexposure vaccines (Kaufmann 2012; Frick 2013). The target population is infants, vaccinated soon after birth. BCG is given during the first weeks of life, and whereas the viable vaccine candidates are supposed to replace BCG, the subunit vaccines are considered as boosters of priming with BCG or with a replacement vaccine. Postexposure vaccines target adolescents and adults with LTBI. More recent subunit vaccine candidates have been tailored for this strategy as so-called multistage vaccines by integrat-

Table 1. Overview of tuberculosis vaccines in clinical trial

Vaccine name	Target indication	Antigen name or Rv number	Antigen function	Delivery system	Descriptive notes	Phase	Reference(s)
MTBVAC	Preventive	NA	NA	Live mycobacteria	Attenuated MTB with two gene deletions	I	Arbues et al. 2013
VPM 1002	Preventive	NA	NA	Live rBCG strain expressing listeriolysin, urease-deleted	Improved antigenicity due to perforation of phagosome membrane	IIa	Grode et al. 2005, 2013
Ad5 Ag85A	Preventive	Ag85A	Mycolyltransferase	Adenovirus 5 vector	Replication-deficient viral delivery system	I	Smaill et al. 2013
Ad35/MVA85A	Preventive	Ag85A, Ag85B TB10.4	Mycolyltransferase Virulence factor	Adenovirus 35 and modified vaccinia Ankara vector	Prime boost combination of two viral delivery systems	I	Radosevic et al. 2007; Abel et al. 2010
Ad35/AERAS-402	Preventive	Ag85A, Ag85B TB10.4	Mycolyltransferase Virulence factor	Adenovirus 35 vector + modified vaccinia Ankara virus	Replication-deficient viral delivery system	IIa	Radosevic et al. 2007; Abel et al. 2010
H4/IC31	Preventive	Ag85B TB10.4	Mycolyltransferase Virulence factor	IC31	Formulation of cationic peptide and a synthetic TLR-9 agonist	IIa	Dietrich et al. 2005; Aagaard et al. 2009; Billeskov et al. 2012
MVA85A	Preventive	Ag85A	Mycolyltransferase	Modified vaccinia Ankara	Replication-deficient viral delivery system	IIb	McShane et al. 2004; Beveridge et al. 2007; Verreck et al. 2009; Tameris et al. 2013; White et al. 2013

M72	Preventive; postexposure	Rv1196 Rv0125	PPE family protein Peptidase	AS01E	Liposomes incorporating the TLR-4 agonist MPL	IIa	Reed et al. 2009; Day et al. 2013; Leroux-Roels et al. 2013
ID93	Preventive/ Postexposure/ Therapeutic	Rv2608 Rv3619, Rv3620 Rv1813	PPE family protein Virulence factor Latency-associated protein	GLA-SE	Synthetic TLR-4 agonist in oil-in-water emulsion	I	Bertholet et al. 2010; Coler et al. 2013
H1/H56/IC31	Preventive/ Postexposure/ Therapeutic	Ag85B ESAT-6 Rv2660c	Mycolyltransferase Virulence factor Latency-associated protein	IC31	Formulation of cationic peptide and a synthetic TLR-9 agonist	IIa	Weinrich Olsen et al. 2001; van Dissel et al. 2010; Aagaard et al. 2011
RUTI	Therapeutic	N/A	N/A	Whole fragmented *Mtb*		I	Cardona 2006
Mycobacterium vaccae	Therapeutic	N/A	N/A	Whole killed mycobacteria		III	deBruyn and Garner 2010; von Reyn et al. 2010; Yang et al. 2011
Mycobacterium indicus pranii	Therapeutic	N/A	N/A	Whole killed mycobacteria		III	Gupta et al. 2012a

NA, not applicable.

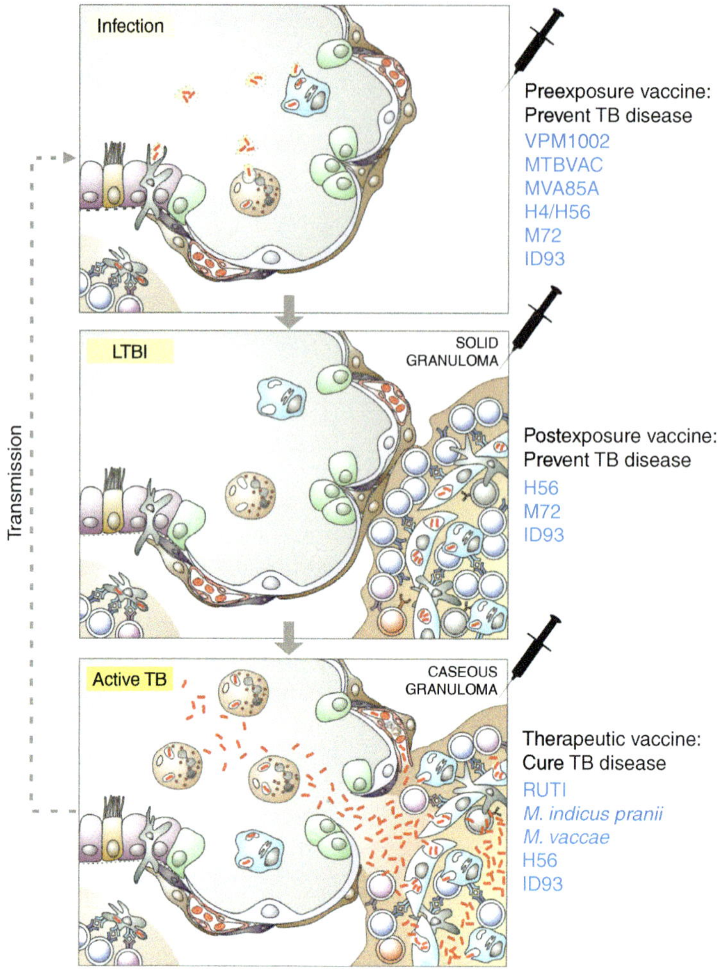

Figure 1. Novel vaccination strategies in the context of tuberculosis (TB) immunology and pathology. The three stages of TB are shown: infection, latent TB infection (LTBI), and active TB. Soon after *Mycobacterium tuberculosis* (*Mtb*) has entered a lung alveolus, it will be taken up by alveolar macrophages (blue) and neutrophils (orange) in the alveolar space and dendritic cells interspersed in the epithelial layer. These dendritic cells transport *Mtb* into draining lymph nodes where acquired immunity is stimulated. During LTBI solid granulomas contain *Mtb* inside mononuclear phagocytes. These solid granulomas are highly structured under the orchestration of T lymphocytes. During active TB, granulomas deteriorate and become caseous. As a consequence, *Mtb* multiplies in an unrestricted way and is spread through capillaries to other organs and through ruptures into the alveolar space, to the environment. Preexposure vaccines (*top*) to prevent TB disease are given before infection. VPM1002 and MTBVAC are live replacement vaccines given for prime instead of BCG and MVA85A; H4/H56, ID93, and M72 are booster vaccines on top of BCG. MVA85A is viral-vectored, whereas H4/H56, ID93 and M72 are protein adjuvant formulations; the target population is infants. Postexposure vaccines (*middle*) to prevent TB disease are given during LTBI as booster of a BCG prime. H56, M72, and ID93 are protein adjuvant formulations; the target population is adolescents and adults. Therapeutic vaccines (*bottom*) are given to patients with active TB in adjunct to or following chemotherapy, to cure TB or to prevent recurrence. RUTI is a semipurified preparation of *Mtb*, and *Mycobacterium indicus pranii* and *Mycobacterium vaccae* are killed preparations of atypical mycobacteria; the target population is TB patients, notably coinfected with HIV and/or suffering from multidrug or extensively drug-resistant TB.

ing latency antigens of *Mtb* (Andersen 2007) (see Table 1, Fig 1). Again, these vaccines are considered as booster vaccines of BCG (or BCG replacement) prime given at infancy. Therapeutic vaccines target patients with active TB in adjunct to (and to shorten) chemotherapy or patients suffering from extensively or totally drug-resistant (XDR and TDR, respectively) TB (Frick 2013; Prabowo et al. 2013). A candidate of this type is a killed *Mycobacterium vaccae* preparation that was used to treat patients with HIV coinfection suffering from miliary TB, with ambiguous outcome (von Reyn et al. 2010). Another *M. vaccae* vaccine has also failed to prove therapeutic benefit (deBruyn and Garner 2010; Yang et al. 2011; Frick 2013). RUTI, a semipurified preparation of killed *Mtb*, has completed phase II assessment in HIV-infected and -uninfected individuals with LTBI (Cardona 2006). Killed *Mycobacterium indicus pranii* was originally designed as vaccine against leprosy but found to have potential effects against TB. This vaccine has been licensed in India and is currently undergoing clinical phase III testing for TB treatment (Gupta et al. 2012a,b). In the following we will focus on preventive vaccines.

LIVE VACCINES

Currently, two types of live vaccines are under clinical assessment, an rBCG and an r*Mtb* deletion mutant (Grode et al. 2005; Arbues et al. 2013; Grode et al. 2013). The rBCG VPM1002 (rBCGΔUreC::hly) expresses listeriolysin (hly) from *Listeria monocytogenes*. Moreover, the urease C (ureC) gene was deleted in this construct. The absence of ureC allows stronger acidification of the phagosome in which VPM1002 resides. The more acidic pH in turn provides the optimum for biological activity of hly, a membrane-perforating molecule (Palmer 2001). Perforation allows egression of rBCG-derived antigens into the cytosol resulting in apoptosis of macrophages harboring the vaccine. These two alterations likely cause improved immunogenicity of the vaccine. Moreover, hly is only active at acidic pH and contains a PEST sequence comprised of proline (P), glutamate (E), serine (S), and threonine (T), which induces rapid aggregation and degradation of this molecule in the cytosol (Decatur and Portnoy 2000). These two features contribute to the safety of the vaccine candidate. VPM1002 has successfully passed two phase I trials and completed the direct observational stage of a phase IIa trial, in infants in South Africa (Grode et al. 2013; Kaufmann et al. 2014). The other live vaccine candidate MTBVAC is a double-deletion mutant of *Mtb* with deleted PhoP and FadD26 (Arbues et al. 2013). PhoP acts as a transcription factor in *Mtb*, which covers a broad range of some 80 genes, many of which are involved in virulence. Because of the request by WHO that *Mtb*-based live vaccine should comprise at least two mutations (Walker et al. 2010), FadD26, which encodes a critical enzymes in the biosynthesis of phthiocerol dimycocerosates, was deleted in addition. This vaccine is currently undergoing a phase I trial (Arbues et al. 2013).

SUBUNIT VACCINES

The first successful attempts to develop a nonviable subunit vaccine against TB were based on complex culture filtrate preparations, and these vaccines were found by several groups to impart considerable protection in various animal models (reviewed in Andersen 1994). Subunit vaccines for boosting BCG-induced responses can be divided into adjuvanted recombinant proteins or viral vector systems. Both strategies depend on the induction of immune responses to a single or a few antigens that are immunodominant during infection.

Viral Vectors

Viral vectors are replication-deficient variants of virus that, in their virulent form, are pathogens for humans or closely related nonhuman primates. Vaccinia and adenovirus are the most clinically advanced and both have proved immunogenic for boosting BCG responses in clinical trials (McShane et al. 2004; Abel et al. 2010). Both adenovirus and vaccinia virus are potent mucosal vaccines that give improved protection when administered through the mucosal route compared to conventional parenteral routes

(Goonetilleke et al. 2003; Wang et al. 2004; White et al. 2013).

The modified vaccinia virus Ankara expressing Ag85A (MVA85A) was the first novel BCG booster vaccine to reach the stage of clinical testing and evaluated to be safe and immunogenic in naïve healthy individuals and in volunteers vaccinated with BCG (McShane et al. 2004). In terms of immunogenicity, MVA85A markedly boosted the preexisting BCG-induced immune responses and promoted strong boosting of IFN-γ measured by ELISPOT and polyfunctional immune responses (Beveridge et al. 2007). Since these initial promising results, a very ambitious clinical program that culminated with the first efficacy trial of a novel vaccine since BCG was developed (Tameris et al. 2013). In this trial, 2797 BCG-vaccinated infants were enrolled, and although MVA85A was found to induce immune responses with a similar profile as in previous studies, the magnitude of responses in infants was more modest. Using a series of end points for TB disease and a QuantiFERON conversion as a measure of *Mtb*-infection, the efficacy of MVA85A against TB was 17.3% (−31.9 to 48.2) and against infection −3.8% (−28.1 to 15.9), showing no evidence of protection against TB disease or *Mtb* infection (Tameris et al. 2013). When discussing lessons learned from this trial, it is important to bear in mind that MVA85A may simply have been unable to improve on the protection provided by BCG in infants, where BCG provides its best protection (which is, however, still insufficient to eliminate the TB in children). In this regard the clinical data from the MVA85A trial are in agreement with the modest and nonsignificant added value when this vaccine was evaluated as a BCG booster in nonhuman primates (Verreck et al. 2009; Beverley 2013). The vaccine is currently under evaluation in a phase IIb clinical trial in HIV^{+} adults. Independent of the underlying reason for the failure, the trial can provide valuable insights when the immune data are scrutinized in greater detail and correlated with clinical outcome.

Replication-deficient adenoviral systems have either used Ad5 or Ad35 platforms. The replication-deficient Ad35 vector expressing Ag85A, Ag85B, and TB10.4 (AERAS-402) (Radosevic et al. 2007) was chosen to avoid preexisting and neutralizing antibody responses often found with Ad, but to which extent such antibodies represent a real problem for vaccine take is questioned by recent data that found no evidence that preexisting immunity significantly dampened the potency of an Ad5-based TB vaccine in a clinical phase I trial (at least over the duration of the trial) (Smaill et al. 2013). Adenovirus-based vaccines differ from the majority of the other vaccines by inducing an immune response biased toward the induction of CD8 T cells observed in both preclinical studies as well as in BCG-vaccinated adults in South Africa (Radosevic et al. 2007; Abel et al. 2010). However, the extent to which adenovirus promoted CD8 epitopes are available for recognition during natural *Mtb* infection and involved in protective immunity is the subject of ongoing debate (Bennekov et al. 2006; Elvang et al. 2009). The AERAS-402 vaccine is currently undergoing clinical phase IIa, but has in addition recently entered clinical trials in prime–boost combinations with MVA85A. The negative outcome of the STEP trial (where a recombinant adenovirus increased the risk of HIV/AIDS) (News in Brief 2007), however, makes it questionable if an adenovirus-based vaccine will ever be recommended for widespread use in the areas of the globe where *Mtb* and HIV coexist.

Adjuvanted Vaccines

When the first fusion proteins (H1 from SSI and M72 from GSK) were ready for clinical testing, only alum and MF59 were approved for human use, and both of these adjuvants are known to induce antibodies exclusively and have very limited protective potential in TB vaccines (Doherty and Andersen 2005). This has recently changed and today we have several novel adjuvant formulations in clinical trials (Table 1). Significant progress has been made in the construction and testing of recombinant proteins, mostly fusion proteins that combine two or more immunodominant antigens of *Mtb*. The first fusion protein-based vaccine was the Hybrid 1 (H1) fusion protein which consists of

Ag85B fused to ESAT-6 (Weinrich Olsen et al. 2001). This molecule has been tested with various adjuvants and has been taken into clinical trials formulated in the IC31 adjuvant, which activates human Toll-like receptor (TLR)9, facilitates antigen uptake by DCs and provides a slow release depot (Lingnau et al. 2007). IC31 stimulates robust IFN-γ production by CD4 Th1 cells in humans and its most striking feature is its ability to maintain long-lasting memory immune responses still detectable 2.5 yr after the last vaccination (van Dissel et al. 2010). The H1 fusion protein in IC31 adjuvant is currently in a phase IIa trial. A novel molecule, H56, based on the H1 backbone but incorporating the late-stage Rv2660c antigen (combined into a so-called multistage vaccine—see below) is currently in clinical phase I and may take over the role of H1 as the leading subunit vaccine for adolescent boost (Aagaard et al. 2011). Another polyprotein called H4 consists of Ag85B fused to the antigen TB10.4 (which in contrast to ESAT-6 is expressed also by BCG) (Dietrich et al. 2005; Billeskov et al. 2012) and is developed by Sanofi in a parallel clinical development program (Table 1). Both the H1/H56 and H4 fusion molecules have (in addition to the IC31 adjuvant) been extensively evaluated in preclinical animal models together with the CAF01 adjuvant (Weinrich Olsen et al. 2001; Lindenstrom et al. 2009). This liposome-based formulation combines the cationic surfactant dimethyldioctadecylammonium (DDC) with trehalose-dibehenate (TDB), a synthetic analog of the mycobacterial cord factor. This adjuvant signals through the innate immune receptor monocyte-inducible C-type lectin (Mincle) and has strong adjuvant properties comprising long-lived memory Th1 and Th17 responses (Lindenstrom et al. 2009, 2012; Desel et al. 2013) in adult as well as in neonatal mice (Kamath et al. 2009). The CAF01 adjuvant combined with the H1 molecule has recently successfully completed a clinical phase I trial.

The M72 fusion protein, consisting of *Mtb* antigens Rv1196 and Rv0125 originally developed as a collaboration between Corixa and GSK, has been successfully evaluated in various preclinical models including nonhuman primates (Reed et al. 2009). A phase I/II trial comparing the adjuvants AS01 (monophosphoryl lipid A [MPL] combined with the saponin derivative QS21 in liposomes) and AS02 (based on the same components in an oil-in-water emulsion) identified the liposomal formulation as the most immunogenic form in terms of inducing a CD4 T-cell response and led to the selection of AS01 for further clinical development in high endemic regions (Day et al. 2013; Leroux-Roels et al. 2013). Currently, a multicenter phase IIb trial involving vaccination of adults in the 18- to 50-yr age range is projected to start in early 2014.

The most recent TB vaccine entering clinical trial is ID93 from the Infectious Disease Research Institute (IDRI) (Bertholet et al. 2010). This vaccine combines a novel set of antigens (Rv2608, Rv3619, Rv3620, and Rv1813) not previously tested in humans and synthetic MPL formulated in a glucopyranosyl lipid stable emulsion (GLA-SE) and is designed to target both active and latent TB. In preclinical studies, this vaccine was protective almost at BCG levels in mice and the combination of BCG with an ID93 booster was able to reduce mortality in guinea pigs compared to BCG alone (Bertholet et al. 2010). In nonhuman primates the administration of ID93 on top of conventional anti-TB treatment reduced the lung pathology associated with disease (Coler et al. 2013). In an ongoing phase I trial, the safety and immunogenicity will be tested in healthy adults.

VACCINES AGAINST LATENT TB

An estimated 2 billion individuals are already infected with *Mtb*; they represent a huge reservoir for disease reactivation. With a reactivation rate of ~5%–10%, this is an incredible number of people who are at risk of developing TB disease and can infect other individuals. Thus, preventing latently infected individuals from reactivating disease is a high priority for any novel TB vaccination strategy. Mathematical modeling has shown that the most effective way to accelerate the global control of TB is a conventional preexposure vaccine combined with an efficient postexposure vaccine (Abu-Raddad et al. 2009). A late BCG booster (to be given to adolescents) will frequently be administered postexposure because of the high prevalence of latent TB in this age group. Over the years there has been much debate on safety of a post-exposure vaccine strategy, stimulated by the original failure (and death of several patients) of Koch's tuberculin as a therapeutic vaccine (Guttstadt 1891; Kaufmann and Winau 2005).

However, based on both animal data and recent clinical data there is so far no evidence to support this theoretical concern. Vaccination with 12 different vaccine preparations in a low-bacterial-burden mouse model developed to reflect LTBI did not induce any reactivation or worsening of pathology (Derrick et al. 2008), and by now several of the new experimental vaccines have been in clinical trials in individuals with LTBI with no apparent safety problem (Scriba et al. 2012; Day et al. 2013; Grode et al. 2013). Yet, there are still significant scientific challenges to overcome before an efficient post-exposure vaccine to prevent TB reactivation has become a reality. As *Mtb* adapts to the conditions in the immune host, the current data suggest that the bacteria transform from a growing metabolically active state to nonreplicating persistence with low metabolic activity (Andersen 2007; Barry et al. 2009; Gengenbacher and Kaufmann 2012; Reece and Kaufmann 2012). In this process the bacteria change their gene expression profile, which results in a different or modified antigenic repertoire where, for example, the genes encoding the Ag85 family are down-regulated to very low levels (Shi et al. 2004; Bold et al. 2011; Aagaard et al. 2011; Commandeur et al. 2013). The changed antigen repertoire has been confirmed in human studies showing that the antigens preferentially recognized by the immune system in latently infected healthy individuals differed from patients with active TB disease (Demissie et al. 2006; Leyten et al. 2006; Schuck et al. 2009). Mimicking conditions thought to reflect the environment inside the granuloma in vitro and evaluating the transcriptional response has thus been the subject of intensive research in recent years. The antigens under consideration are (i) DosR regulon and the enduring hypoxic response—both sets of overlapping genes are up-regulated in response to hypoxia (Park et al. 2003; Rustad et al. 2008); (ii) starvation antigens—up-regulated by *Mtb* upon depletion of nutrients (Betts et al. 2002); and (iii) resuscitation antigens that are produced as the bacteria resumes growth (Gupta et al. 2010; Commandeur et al. 2011). Addition of late-stage antigens to the well-established prophylactic vaccines may provide the basis for multistage TB vaccines with activity against all stages of infection (Andersen 2007). A multistage vaccine (H56) that combined the H1 (Ag85B ESAT-6) backbone and the *Mtb* starvation/latency antigen Rv2660c induced superior protection against late-stage infection in the mouse model of long-term persistent TB (Aagaard et al. 2011). The vaccine also prevented TB reactivation in a nonhuman primate model where animals received immunosuppressive anti-TNF treatment (Lin et al. 2012). The role of Rv2660 in the improved protection promoted by the H56 vaccine is the subject of ongoing evaluation. The antigen encoded by this gene is recognized in individuals with LTBI (Govender et al. 2010), and strong responses are found after TB challenge in nonhuman primates (Lin et al. 2012). The protein was identified in a high-resolution proteomic analysis of BCG (Zheng et al. 2012), but a recent strand-specific PCR analysis suggests that the gene is not translated into a protein in the *Mtb* strains analyzed (Houghton et al. 2013). It is therefore presently not clear if the Rv2660c gene product mediates its beneficial influence on the H56 molecule directly as an antigen or has an indirect influence of the overall immune profile of the H56 polyprotein fusion. A phase I clinical trial of H56 has just been completed and an ongoing phase IIa trial will optimize the dose of H56 in individuals with LTBI in South Africa.

The ID93 vaccine, which incorporates the latency-associated antigen encoded by Rv1813, was recently tested in TB-infected nonhuman primates in combination with conventional chemotherapy and this treatment was shown to reduce the duration of treatment compared with chemotherapy alone (Coler et al. 2013). Other recent studies have taken the same approach and combined different classes of antigens into fusion molecules or cocktails delivered in adjuvants. In a study by Jeon and colleagues, a vaccine based on the early antigen Ag85A was compared to the late antigen HspX (Jeon et al. 2011). Whereas the vaccine based on Ag85A protected best at day 30, the HspX-based vaccine gave the best protection at 90 d and the combination protected at both time points. Reece and Kaufmann (2012) expressed three different late antigens (Rv3407, Rv1733c, and Rv2659c) in rBCG (VPM1002 backbone). Also in this study, a characteristic feature was an improved late-stage protection with improved survival after 200 d.

A recent study evaluated the potential of ESAT-6 and the closely related antigen TB10.4 (EsxH) as components in preventive and postexposure TB vaccines (Hoang et al. 2013). In this study four different fusion-protein vaccines were constructed that only differed in these two components, and whereas all vaccines induced protection in a conventional prophylactic vaccination model, only the ESAT-6 containing vaccines had an effect when administered postexposure. The vaccine effect was influenced by the infectious load at the time point of vaccination and abolished in chronically infected animals with high bacterial loads at the onset of vaccination (Hoang et al. 2013). The findings are in agreement with a previous observation of postexposure activity of ESAT-6 containing vaccines in the guinea pig model measured both by growth and pathology (Henao-Tamayo et al. 2009). In this study the vaccines were administered once on top of early acute infection, which may explain that only a transient effect with no impact on long-term survival was seen. Therefore, although enhancing immunity to TB in animal models after exposure to *Mtb* infection has proved difficult, there are still grounds for optimism.

CONCLUDING REMARKS

With more than a dozen vaccine candidates moving forward in the clinical trial pipeline, comprising replacement vaccines for prime and subunit vaccines for boost, vaccines for pre- and postexposure with *Mtb*, as well as TB therapy, a broad TB portfolio has been developed. Yet, most of the current vaccine candidates induce immune responses qualitatively similar to those operative in healthy individuals with LTBI. The question remains whether this will suffice to achieve TB elimination by 2050 as claimed by the StopTB Partnership of the WHO (StopTBPartnership and WHO 2011). The most likely scenario is that this first generation of vaccines will be succeeded by a second generation of further improved vaccines. Design of these second-generation vaccines can benefit from information generated in ongoing clinical trials about mechanisms underlying protection. Biomarker studies, notably global gene expression profiling, therefore need to become an essential part of such vaccine trials (Maertzdorf et al. 2012; Weiner et al. 2013; Weiner and Kaufmann 2014). Longitudinal studies monitoring healthy contacts of patients with active TB, who do or do not develop active TB disease, can add valuable information. The disappointing outcome of the MVA85A phase IIb vaccine trial has stimulated new and innovative ideas on a number of aspects of TB vaccine development. First of all, there is now ongoing discussion and planning of future trials to enable the early monitoring of signs of vaccine efficacy. Some of the ideas that are currently being discussed build on either the conversion of the diagnostic IFN-γ release assay (the QuantiFERON test) as an indicator of ongoing infection (Andersen et al. 2007) or the prevention of recurrence of disease by vaccination of TB patients following completed chemotherapy. If successful, these designs may allow a very cost-effective and accelerated identification of promising vaccine candidates.

The need to go beyond the most popular antigens in TB vaccine, such as the Ag85 cognates, is also the subject of renewed interest, and recent discovery efforts have provided a number of very promising protective antigens selected to provide target molecules stably expressed also in LTBI (Bertholet et al. 2010; Aagaard et al. 2011; Knudsen et al. 2014), a phase where Ag85-based vaccines may have their limitations because gene expression is shut down (Shi et al. 2004; Bold et al. 2011; Aagaard et al. 2011; Commandeur et al. 2013).

Finally, the fact that the MVA85A throughout the preclinical and clinical development program was optimized to promote powerful Th1 responses has reemphasized that we need to look broader (and beyond IFN-γ), in our optimization of novel vaccines. Studies in both animal models and human clinical trials have shown that the IFN-γ response to BCG vaccination is not predictive of subsequent protection from TB (Elias et al. 2005; Mittrucker et al. 2007; Kagina et al. 2010), and recent data suggest that instead of boosting "more of the same" Th1 response it may be better to promote responses that are insufficiently promoted by BCG and mediated by T cells devoid of or low in IFN-γ expression (Goldsack and Kirman 2007; Lindenstrom et al. 2013).

As we gain access to the expanded data sets from the multiparametric analyses of ongoing and planned proof-of-concept phase IIb clinical trials of the candidate vaccines under evaluation, they will hopefully provide the conceptual basis for the optimal design of vaccines targeting a pathogen that has refined its survival strategy for at least 6000 years.

ACKNOWLEDGMENTS

We thank Mary Louise Grossman and Christina Gry Paulsen for help preparing the manuscript and Diane Schad for preparing the figure. S.H.E.K. and P.A. are supported by the European Union's Seventh Framework Programme (EU FP7), ADITEC (HEALTH-F4-2011-280873), and NEWTBVAC (HEALTH-F3-2009-241745); the Bill & Melinda Gates Foundation Grand Challenges in Global Health Program (BMGF GC6-74, #37772 and GC12, #37885; GC6-2013 #OPP 1055806, GC6-2013 #OPP 1065330); and the Innovative Medicines Initiative (IMI) Joint Undertaking "Biomarkers for Enhanced Vaccine Safety" BIOVACSAFE (IMI JU Grant No. 115308).

REFERENCES

Aagaard C, Hoang TT, Izzo A, Billeskov R, Troudt J, Arnett K, Keyser A, Elvang T, Andersen P, Dietrich J. 2009. Protection and polyfunctional T cells induced by Ag85B-TB10.4/IC31 against *Mycobacterium tuberculosis* is highly dependent on the antigen dose. *PLoS ONE* **4:** e5930.

Aagaard C, Hoang T, Dietrich J, Cardona PJ, Izzo A, Dolganov G, Schoolnik GK, Cassidy JP, Billeskov R, Andersen P. 2011. A multistage tuberculosis vaccine that confers efficient protection before and after exposure. *Nat Med* **17:** 189–194.

Abel B, Tameris M, Mansoor N, Gelderbloem S, Hughes J, Abrahams D, Makhethe L, Erasmus M, deKock M, vanderMerwe L, et al. 2010. The novel tuberculosis vaccine, AERAS-402, induces robust and polyfunctional $CD4^+$ and $CD8^+$ T cells in adults. *Am J Respir Crit Care Med* **181:** 1407–1417.

Abu-Raddad LJ, Sabatelli L, Achterberg JT, Sugimoto JD, Longini IM Jr, Dye C, Halloran ME. 2009. Epidemiological benefits of more-effective tuberculosis vaccines, drugs, and diagnostics. *Proc Natl Acad Sci* **106:** 13980–13985.

Amulic B, Cazalet C, Hayes GL, Metzler KD, Zychlinsky A. 2012. Neutrophil function: From mechanisms to disease. *Annu Rev Immunol* **30:** 459–489.

Andersen P. 1994. The T cell response to secreted antigens of *Mycobacterium tuberculosis*. *Immunobiology* **191:** 537–547.

Andersen P. 2007. Vaccine strategies against latent tuberculosis infection. *Trends Microbiol* **15:** 7–13.

Andersen P, Doherty TM. 2005. The success and failure of BCG—Implications for a novel tuberculosis vaccine. *Nat Rev Microbiol* **3:** 656–662.

Andersen P, Heron I. 1993. Specificity of a protective memory immune response against *Mycobacterium tuberculosis*. *Infect Immun* **61:** 844–851.

Andersen P, Smedegaard B. 2000. $CD4^+$ T-cell subsets that mediate immunological memory to *Mycobacterium tuberculosis* infection in mice. *Infect Immun* **68:** 621–629.

Andersen P, Doherty TM, Pai M, Weldingh K. 2007. The prognosis of latent tuberculosis: Can disease be predicted? *Trends Mol Med* **13:** 175–182.

Arbues A, Aguilo JI, Gonzalo-Asensio J, Marinova D, Uranga S, Puentes E, Fernandez C, Parra A, Cardona PJ, Vilaplana C, et al. 2013. Construction, characterization and preclinical evaluation of MTBVAC, the first live-attenuated *M. tuberculosis*–based vaccine to enter clinical trials. *Vaccine* **31:** 4867–4873.

Barry CE 3rd, Boshoff HI, Dartois V, Dick T, Ehrt S, Flynn J, Schnappinger D, Wilkinson RJ, Young D. 2009. The spectrum of latent tuberculosis: Rethinking the biology and intervention strategies. *Nat Rev Microbiol* **7:** 845–855.

Behr MA, Wilson MA, Gill WP, Salamon H, Schoolnik GK, Rane S, Small PM. 1999. Comparative genomics of BCG vaccines by whole-genome DNA microarray. *Science* **284:** 1520–1523.

Benn CS, Netea MG, Selin LK, Aaby P. 2013. A small jab—A big effect: Nonspecific immunomodulation by vaccines. *Trends Immunol* **34:** 431–439.

Bennekov T, Dietrich J, Rosenkrands I, Stryhn A, Doherty TM, Andersen P. 2006. Alteration of epitope recognition pattern in Ag85B and ESAT-6 has a profound influence on vaccine-induced protection against *Mycobacterium tuberculosis*. *Eur J Immunol* **36:** 3346–3355.

Bermudez LE, Young LS. 1990. Recombinant granulocyte—Macrophage colony-stimulating factor activates human macrophages to inhibit growth or kill *Mycobacterium avium* complex. *J Leukoc Biol* **48:** 67–73.

Bertholet S, Ireton GC, Ordway DJ, Windish HP, Pine SO, Kahn M, Phan T, Orme IM, Vedvick TS, Baldwin SL, et al. 2010. A defined tuberculosis vaccine candidate boosts BCG and protects against multidrug-resistant *Mycobacterium tuberculosis*. *Sci Transl Med* **2:** 53ra74.

Betts JC, Lukey PT, Robb LC, McAdam RA, Duncan K. 2002. Evaluation of a nutrient starvation model of *Mycobacterium tuberculosis* persistence by gene and protein expression profiling. *Mol Microbiol* **43:** 717–731.

Beveridge NE, Price DA, Casazza JP, Pathan AA, Sander CR, Asher TE, Ambrozak DR, Precopio ML, Scheinberg P, Alder NC, et al. 2007. Immunisation with BCG and recombinant MVA85A induces long-lasting, polyfunctional *Mycobacterium tuberculosis*-specific $CD4^+$ memory T lymphocyte populations. *Eur J Immunol* **37:** 3089–3100.

Beverley P. 2013. TB vaccine failure was predictable. *Nature* **503:** 469.

Billeskov R, Elvang TT, Andersen PL, Dietrich J. 2012. The HyVac4 subunit vaccine efficiently boosts BCG-primed anti-mycobacterial protective immunity. *PLoS ONE* **7:** e39909.

Billeskov R, Christensen JP, Aagaard C, Andersen P, Dietrich J. 2013. Comparing adjuvanted H28 and modified vaccinia virus ankara expressing H28 in a mouse and a non-human primate tuberculosis model. *PLoS ONE* **8:** e72185.

Biselli R, Mariotti S, Sargentini V, Sauzullo I, Lastilla M, Mengoni F, Vanini V, Girardi E, Goletti D, D'Amelio R, et al. 2010. Detection of interleukin-2 in addition to interferon-γ discriminates active tuberculosis patients, latently infected individuals, and controls. *Clin Microbiol Infect* **16:** 1282–1284.

Bold TD, Banaei N, Wolf AJ, Ernst JD. 2011. Suboptimal activation of antigen-specific $CD4^+$ effector cells enables persistence of *M. tuberculosis* in vivo. *PLoS Pathog* **7:** e1002063.

Bonneville M, Scotet E. 2006. Human Vγ9Vδ2 T cells: Promising new leads for immunotherapy of infections and tumors. *Curr Opin Immunol* **18:** 539–546.

Brigl M, Brenner MB. 2004. CD1: Antigen presentation and T cell function. *Annu Rev Immunol* **22:** 817–890.

Bustamante J, Picard C, Boisson-Dupuis S, Abel L, Casanova JL. 2011. Genetic lessons learned from X-linked Mendelian susceptibility to mycobacterial diseases. *Ann NY Acad Sci* **1246:** 92–101.

Calmette A, Plotz H. 1929. Protective inoculation against tuberculosis with BCG. *Am Rev Tuberc* **19:** 567–572.

Calmette A, Guérin C, Boquet A, Négre L. 1927. *La vaccination préventive contre la tuberculose par le "BCG"*. Masson, Paris.

Cardona PJ. 2006. RUTI: A new chance to shorten the treatment of latent tuberculosis infection. *Tuberculosis (Edinburgh)* **86:** 273–289.

Coler RN, Bertholet S, Pine SO, Orr MT, Reese V, Windish HP, Davis C, Kahn M, Baldwin SL, Reed SG. 2013. Therapeutic immunization against *Mycobacterium tuberculosis* is an effective adjunct to antibiotic treatment. *J Infect Dis* **207:** 1242–1252.

Collins HL, Kaufmann SH. 2001. Prospects for better tuberculosis vaccines. *Lancet Infect Dis* **1:** 21–28.

Commandeur S, vanMeijgaarden KE, Lin MY, Franken KL, Friggen AH, Drijfhout JW, Oftung F, Korsvold GE, Geluk A, Ottenhoff TH. 2011. Identification of human T-cell responses to *Mycobacterium tuberculosis* resuscitation-promoting factors in long-term latently infected individuals. *Clin Vaccine Immunol* **18:** 676–683.

Commandeur S, vanMeijgaarden KE, Prins C, Pichugin AV, Dijkman K, vandenEeden SJ, Friggen AH, Franken KL, Dolganov G, Kramnik I, Schoolnik GK, et al. 2013. An unbiased genome-wide *Mycobacterium tuberculosis* gene expression approach to discover antigens targeted by human T cells expressed during pulmonary infection. *J Immunol* **190:** 1659–1671.

Cooper AM, Torrado E. 2012. Protection versus pathology in tuberculosis: Recent insights. *Curr Opin Immunol* **24:** 431–437.

Cruz A, Fraga AG, Fountain JJ, Rangel-Moreno J, Torrado E, Saraiva M, Pereira DR, Randall TD, Pedrosa J, Cooper AM, et al. 2010. Pathological role of interleukin 17 in mice subjected to repeated BCG vaccination after infection with *Mycobacterium tuberculosis*. *J Exp Med* **207:** 1609–1616.

Darrah PA, Patel DT, DeLuca PM, Lindsay RW, Davey DF, Flynn BJ, Hoff ST, Andersen P, Reed SG, Morris SL, et al. 2007. Multifunctional T_H1 cells define a correlate of vaccine-mediated protection against *Leishmania major*. *Nat Med* **13:** 843–850.

Day CL, Tameris M, Mansoor N, vanRooyen M, deKock M, Geldenhuys H, Erasmus M, Makhethe L, Hughes EJ, Gelderbloem S, et al. 2013. Induction and regulation of T-cell immunity by the novel tuberculosis vaccine M72/AS01 in South African adults. *Am J Respir Crit Care Med* **188:** 492–502.

deBruyn G, Garner P. 2010. *Mycobacterium vaccae* immunotherapy for treating tuberculosis. *The Cochrane Library* **1:** 1–17.

Decatur AL, Portnoy DA. 2000. A PEST-like sequence in listeriolysin O essential for *Listeria monocytogenes* pathogenicity. *Science* **290:** 992–995.

Demissie A, Leyten EM, Abebe M, Wassie L, Aseffa A, Abate G, Fletcher H, Owiafe P, Hill PC, Brookes R, et al. 2006. Recognition of stage-specific mycobacterial antigens differentiates between acute and latent infections with *Mycobacterium tuberculosis*. *Clin Vaccine Immunol* **13:** 179–186.

Derrick SC, Perera LP, Dheenadhayalan V, Yang A, Kolibab K, Morris SL. 2008. The safety of post-exposure vaccination of mice infected with *Mycobacterium tuberculosis*. *Vaccine* **26:** 6092–6098.

Derrick SC, Yabe IM, Yang A, Morris SL. 2011. Vaccine-induced anti-tuberculosis protective immunity in mice correlates with the magnitude and quality of multifunctional CD4 T cells. *Vaccine* **29:** 2902–2909.

Desel C, Werninghaus K, Ritter M, Jozefowski K, Wenzel J, Russkamp N, Schleicher U, Christensen D, Wirtz S, Kirschning C, et al. 2013. The Mincle-activating adjuvant TDB induces MyD88-dependent Th1 and Th17 responses through IL-1R signaling. *PLoS ONE* **8:** e53531.

Dietrich J, Aagaard C, Leah R, Olsen AW, Stryhn A, Doherty TM, Andersen P. 2005. Exchanging ESAT6 with TB10.4 in an Ag85B fusion molecule-based tuberculosis subunit vaccine: Efficient protection and ESAT6-based sensitive monitoring of vaccine efficacy. *J Immunol* **174:** 6332–6339.

Dixon WG, Hyrich KL, Watson KD, Lunt M, Galloway J, Ustianowski A, Symmons DP. 2010. Drug-specific risk of tuberculosis in patients with rheumatoid arthritis treated with anti-TNF therapy: Results from the British Society for Rheumatology Biologics Register (BSRBR). *Ann Rheum Dis* **69:** 522–528.

Doherty TM, Andersen P. 2005. Vaccines for tuberculosis: Novel concepts and recent progress. *Clin Microbiol Rev* **18:** 687–702.

Elias D, Akuffo H, Britton S. 2005. PPD induced in vitro interferon γ production is not a reliable correlate of protection against *Mycobacterium tuberculosis*. *Trans R Soc Trop Med Hyg* **99:** 363–368.

Elvang T, Christensen JP, Billeskov R, Thi Kim Thanh Hoang T, Holst P, Thomsen AR, Andersen P, Dietrich J. 2009. CD4 and CD8 T cell responses to the *M. tuberculosis* Ag85B-TB10.4 promoted by adjuvanted subunit, adenovector or heterologous prime boost vaccination. *PLoS ONE* **4:** e5139.

Ernst JD. 2012. The immunological life cycle of tuberculosis. *Nat Rev Immunol* **12:** 581–591.

Fabri M, Stenger S, Shin DM, Yuk JM, Liu PT, Realegeno S, Lee HM, Krutzik SR, Schenk M, Sieling PA, et al. 2011. Vitamin D is required for IFN-γ-mediated antimicrobial activity of human macrophages. *Sci Transl Med* **3:** 104ra102.

Forbes EK, Sander C, Ronan EO, McShane H, Hill AV, Beverley PC, Tchilian EZ. 2008. Multifunctional, high-level cytokine-producing Th1 cells in the lung, but not spleen, correlate with protection against *Mycobacterium tuberculosis* aerosol challenge in mice. *J Immunol* **181:** 4955–4964.

Frick M. 2013. Where are we going, where have we been? In *The HIV, HCV, TB pipeline report*, pp. 263–283. http://www.pipelinereport.org.

Gengenbacher M, Kaufmann SH. 2012. *Mycobacterium tuberculosis*: Success through dormancy. *FEMS Microbiol Rev* **36:** 514–532.

Goldsack L, Kirman JR. 2007. Half-truths and selective memory: Interferon γ, CD4^{+} T cells and protective memory against tuberculosis. *Tuberculosis (Edinburgh)* **87:** 465–473.

Goonetilleke NP, McShane H, Hannan CM, Anderson RJ, Brookes RH, Hill AV. 2003. Enhanced immunogenicity and protective efficacy against *Mycobacterium tuberculosis* of bacille Calmette–Guérin vaccine using mucosal administration and boosting with a recombinant modified vaccinia virus Ankara. *J Immunol* **171:** 1602–1609.

Govender L, Abel B, Hughes EJ, Scriba TJ, Kagina BM, de-Kock M, Walzl G, Black G, Rosenkrands I, Hussey GD, et al. 2010. Higher human CD4 T cell response to novel *Mycobacterium tuberculosis* latency associated antigens Rv2660 and Rv2659 in latent infection compared with tuberculosis disease. *Vaccine* **29:** 51–57.

Grode L, Seiler P, Baumann S, Hess J, Brinkmann V, Nasser-Eddine A, Mann P, Goosmann C, Bandermann S, Smith D, et al. 2005. Increased vaccine efficacy against tuberculosis of recombinant *Mycobacterium bovis* bacille Calmette–Guérin mutants that secrete listeriolysin. *J Clin Invest* **115:** 2472–2479.

Grode L, Ganoza CA, Brohm C, Weiner J III, Eisele B, Kaufmann SH. 2013. Safety and immunogenicity of the recombinant BCG vaccine VPM1002 in a phase 1 open-label randomized clinical trial. *Vaccine* **31:** 1340–1348.

Gupta RK, Srivastava BS, Srivastava R. 2010. Comparative expression analysis of rpf-like genes of *Mycobacterium tuberculosis* H37Rv under different physiological stress and growth conditions. *Microbiology* **156:** 2714–2722.

Gupta A, Ahmad FJ, Ahmad F, Gupta UD, Natarajan M, Katoch V, Bhaskar S. 2012a. Efficacy of *Mycobacterium indicus pranii* immunotherapy as an adjunct to chemotherapy for tuberculosis and underlying immune responses in the lung. *PLoS ONE* **7:** e39215.

Gupta A, Ahmad FJ, Ahmad F, Gupta UD, Natarajan M, Katoch VM, Bhaskar S. 2012b. Protective efficacy of *Mycobacterium indicus pranii* against tuberculosis and underlying local lung immune responses in guinea pig model. *Vaccine* **30:** 6198–6209.

Guttstadt A. 1891. *Die Wirksamkeit des Koch'schen Heilmittels gegen Tuberculose*. Springer, Berlin (in German).

Hatherill M. 2011. Prospects for elimination of childhood tuberculosis: The role of new vaccines. *Arch Dis Child* **96:** 851–856.

Henao-Tamayo M, Palaniswamy GS, Smith EE, Shanley CA, Wang B, Orme IM, Basaraba RJ, DuTeau NM, Ordway D. 2009. Post-exposure vaccination against *Mycobacterium tuberculosis*. *Tuberculosis (Edinburgh)* **89:** 142–148.

Hesseling AC, Schaaf HS, Victor T, Beyers N, Marais BJ, Cotton MF, Wiid I, Gie RP, van Helden P, Warren RM. 2004. Resistant *Mycobacterium bovis* bacillus Calmette–Guérin disease: Implications for management of bacillus Calmette–Guérin disease in human immunodeficiency virus-infected children. *Pediatr Infect Dis J* **23:** 476–479.

Hoang T, Aagaard C, Dietrich J, Cassidy JP, Dolganov G, Schoolnik GK, Lundberg CV, Agger EM, Andersen P. 2013. ESAT-6 (EsxA) and TB10.4 (EsxH) based vaccines for pre- and post-exposure tuberculosis vaccination. *PLoS ONE* **8:** e80579.

Houghton J, Cortes T, Schubert O, Rose G, Rodgers A, De Ste Croix M, Aebersold R, Young DB, Arnvig KB. 2013. A small RNA encoded in the Rv2660c locus of *Mycobacterium tuberculosis* is induced during starvation and infection. *PLoS ONE* **8:** e80047.

Janaszek W. 1991. Evaluation of thermostability of lyophilized BCG vaccines by using an accelerated thermal degradation test. *Med Dosw Mikrobiol* **43:** 43–49.

Jeon BY, Kim SC, Eum SY, Cho SN. 2011. The immunity and protective effects of antigen 85A and heat-shock protein X against progressive tuberculosis. *Microbes Infect* **13:** 284–290.

Joshi NS, Cui W, Chandele A, Lee HK, Urso DR, Hagman J, Gapin L, Kaech SM. 2007. Inflammation directs memory precursor and short-lived effector CD8^{+} T cell fates via the graded expression of T-bet transcription factor. *Immunity* **27:** 281–295.

Kagina BM, Abel B, Scriba TJ, Hughes EJ, Keyser A, Soares A, Gamieldien H, Sidibana M, Hatherill M, Gelderbloem S, et al. 2010. Specific T cell frequency and cytokine expression profile do not correlate with protection against tuberculosis after bacillus Calmette–Guérin vaccination of newborns. *Am J Respir Crit Care Med* **182:** 1073–1079.

Kamath AT, Rochat AF, Christensen D, Agger EM, Andersen P, Lambert PH, Siegrist CA. 2009. A liposome-based mycobacterial vaccine induces potent adult and neonatal multifunctional T cells through the exquisite targeting of dendritic cells. *PLoS ONE* **4:** e5771.

Kaufmann SHE. 2010. *The new plagues—Pandemics and poverty in a globalized world.* Haus Publishing Limited, London.

Kaufmann SH. 2011. Fact and fiction in tuberculosis vaccine research: 10 years later. *Lancet Infect Dis* **11:** 633–640.

Kaufmann SH. 2012. Tuberculosis vaccine development: Strength lies in tenacity. *Trends Immunol* **33:** 373–379.

Kaufmann SH. 2013. Tuberculosis vaccines: Time to think about the next generation. *Semin Immunol* **25:** 172–181.

Kaufmann SH, Dorhoi A. 2013. Inflammation in tuberculosis: Interactions, imbalances and interventions. *Curr Opin Immunol* **25:** 441–449.

Kaufmann SH, Winau F. 2005. From bacteriology to immunology: The dualism of specificity. *Nat Immunol* **6:** 1063–1066.

Kaufmann SH, Hussey G, Lambert PH. 2010. New vaccines for tuberculosis. *Lancet* **375:** 2110–2119.

Kaufmann SH, Cotton MF, Eisele B, Gengenbacher M, Grode L, Hesseling AC, Waltzl G. 2014. The BCG replacement vaccine VPM1002: From drawing board to clinical trail. *Expert Rev Vaccines* **13:** 619–630.

Keane J, Gershon S, Wise RP, Mirabile-Levens E, Kasznica J, Schwieterman WD, Siegel JN, Braun MM. 2001. Tuberculosis associated with infliximab, a tumor necrosis factor α-neutralizing agent. *N Engl J Med* **345:** 1098–1104.

Khader SA, Bell GK, Pearl JE, Fountain JJ, Rangel-Moreno J, Cilley GE, Shen F, Eaton SM, Gaffen SL, Swain SL, et al. 2007. IL-23 and IL-17 in the establishment of protective pulmonary $CD4^+$ T cell responses after vaccination and during *Mycobacterium tuberculosis* challenge. *Nat Immunol* **8:** 369–377.

Knudsen NP, Norskov-Lauritsen S, Dolganov GM, Schoolnik GK, Lindenstrom T, Andersen P, Agger EM, Aagaard C. 2014. Tuberculosis vaccine with high predicted population coverage and compatibility with modern diagnostics. *Proc Natl Acad Sci* **111:** 1096–1101.

Kupferschmidt K. 2011. Infectious disease. Taking a new shot at a TB vaccine. *Science* **334:** 1488–1490.

Leroux-Roels I, Forgus S, DeBoever F, Clement F, Demoitie MA, Mettens P, Moris P, Ledent E, Leroux-Roels G, Ofori-Anyinam O, et al. 2013. Improved $CD4^+$ T cell responses to *Mycobacterium tuberculosis* in PPD-negative adults by M72/AS01 as compared to the M72/AS02 and Mtb72F/AS02 tuberculosis candidate vaccine formulations: A randomized trial. *Vaccine* **31:** 2196–2206.

Leyten EM, Lin MY, Franken KL, Friggen AH, Prins C, van Meijgaarden KE, Voskuil MI, Weldingh K, Andersen P, Schoolnik GK, et al. 2006. Human T-cell responses to 25 novel antigens encoded by genes of the dormancy regulon of *Mycobacterium tuberculosis. Microbes Infect* **8:** 2052–2060.

Lin PL, Dietrich J, Tan E, Abalos RM, Burgos J, Bigbee C, Bigbee M, Milk L, Gideon HP, Rodgers M, et al. 2012. The multistage vaccine H56 boosts the effects of BCG to protect cynomolgus macaques against active tuberculosis and reactivation of latent *Mycobacterium tuberculosis* infection. *J Clin Invest* **122:** 303–314.

Lindenstrom T, Agger EM, Korsholm KS, Darrah PA, Aagaard C, Seder RA, Rosenkrands I, Andersen P. 2009. Tuberculosis subunit vaccination provides long-term protective immunity characterized by multifunctional CD4 memory T cells. *J Immunol* **182:** 8047–8055.

Lindenstrom T, Woodworth J, Dietrich J, Aagaard C, Andersen P, Agger EM. 2012. Vaccine-induced Th17 cells are maintained long-term postvaccination as a distinct and phenotypically stable memory subset. *Infect Immun* **80:** 3533–3544.

Lindenstrom T, Knudsen NP, Agger EM, Andersen P. 2013. Control of chronic *mycobacterium tuberculosis* infection by CD4 $KLRG1^-$ IL-2-secreting central memory cells. *J Immunol* **190:** 6311–6319.

Lingnau K, Riedl K, von Gabain A. 2007. IC31 and IC30, novel types of vaccine adjuvant based on peptide delivery systems. *Expert Rev Vaccines* **6:** 741–746.

Liu PT, Stenger S, Li H, Wenzel L, Tan BH, Krutzik SR, Ochoa MT, Schauber J, Wu K, Meinken C, et al. 2006. Toll-like receptor triggering of a vitamin D-mediated human antimicrobial response. *Science* **311:** 1770–1773.

MacMicking J, Xie QW, Nathan C. 1997. Nitric oxide and macrophage function. *Annu Rev Immunol* **15:** 323–350.

Maertzdorf J, Weiner J III, Kaufmann SH. 2012. Enabling biomarkers for tuberculosis control. *Int J Tuberc Lung Dis* **16:** 1140–1148.

McShane H, Pathan AA, Sander CR, Keating SM, Gilbert SC, Huygen K, Fletcher HA, Hill AV. 2004. Recombinant modified vaccinia virus Ankara expressing antigen 85A boosts BCG-primed and naturally acquired antimycobacterial immunity in humans. *Nat Med* **10:** 1240–1244.

Mittrucker HW, Steinhoff U, Kohler A, Krause M, Lazar D, Mex P, Miekley D, Kaufmann SH. 2007. Poor correlation between BCG vaccination-induced T cell responses and protection against tuberculosis. *Proc Natl Acad Sci* **104:** 12434–12439.

Mollenkopf HJ, Kursar M, Kaufmann SH. 2004. Immune response to postprimary tuberculosis in mice: *Mycobacterium tuberculosis* and *Mycobacterium bovis* bacille Calmette–Guérin induce equal protection. *J Infect Dis* **190:** 588–597.

News in Brief. 2007. HIV vaccine failure prompts Merck to halt trial. *Nature* **449:** 390.

O'Garra A, Redford PS, McNab FW, Bloom CI, Wilkinson RJ, Berry MP. 2013. The immune response in tuberculosis. *Annu Rev Immunol* **31:** 475–527.

Orme IM. 1988. Characteristics and specificity of acquired immunologic memory to *Mycobacterium tuberculosis* infection. *J Immunol* **140:** 3589–3593.

Orme IM. 2010. The Achilles heel of BCG. *Tuberculosis (Edinburgh)* **90:** 329–332.

Orme IM, Collins FM. 1984. Adoptive protection of the *Mycobacterium tuberculosis*-infected lung. Dissociation between cells that passively transfer protective immunity and those that transfer delayed-type hypersensitivity to tuberculin. *Cell Immunol* **84:** 113–120.

Ottenhoff TH. 2012. New pathways of protective and pathological host defense to mycobacteria. *Trends Microbiol* **20:** 419–428.

Palmer M. 2001. The family of thiol-activated, cholesterol-binding cytolysins. *Toxicon* **39:** 1681–1689.

Park HD, Guinn KM, Harrell MI, Liao R, Voskuil MI, Tompa M, Schoolnik GK, Sherman DR. 2003. Rv3133c/dosR is a transcription factor that mediates the hypoxic response of *Mycobacterium tuberculosis*. *Mol Microbiol* **48:** 833–843.

Prabowo SA, Groschel MI, Schmidt ED, Skrahina A, Mihaescu T, Hasturk S, Mitrofanov R, Pimkina E, Visontai I, deJong B, et al. 2013. Targeting multidrug-resistant tuberculosis (MDR-TB) by therapeutic vaccines. *Med Microbiol Immunol* **202:** 95–104.

Radosevic K, Wieland CW, Rodriguez A, Weverling GJ, Mintardjo R, Gillissen G, Vogels R, Skeiky YA, Hone DM, Sadoff JC, et al. 2007. Protective immune responses to a recombinant adenovirus type 35 tuberculosis vaccine in two mouse strains: CD4 and CD8 T-cell epitope mapping and role of γ interferon. *Infect Immun* **75:** 4105–4115.

Reece ST, Kaufmann SH. 2012. Floating between the poles of pathology and protection: Can we pin down the granuloma in tuberculosis? *Curr Opin Microbiol* **15:** 63–70.

Reed SG, Coler RN, Dalemans W, Tan EV, DeLaCruz EC, Basaraba RJ, Orme IM, Skeiky YA, Alderson MR, Cowgill KD, et al. 2009. Defined tuberculosis vaccine, Mtb72F/AS02A, evidence of protection in cynomolgus monkeys. *Proc Natl Acad Sci* **106:** 2301–2306.

Reiley WW, Shafiani S, Wittmer ST, Tucker-Heard G, Moon JJ, Jenkins MK, Urdahl KB, Winslow GM, Woodland DL. 2010. Distinct functions of antigen-specific CD4 T cells during murine *Mycobacterium tuberculosis* infection. *Proc Natl Acad Sci* **107:** 19408–19413.

Rohde K, Yates RM, Purdy GE, Russell DG. 2007. *Mycobacterium tuberculosis* and the environment within the phagosome. *Immunol Rev* **219:** 37–54.

Roth A, Garly ML, Jensen H, Nielsen J, Aaby P. 2006. Bacillus Calmette–Guérin vaccination and infant mortality. *Expert Rev Vaccines* **5:** 277–293.

Rustad TR, Harrell MI, Liao R, Sherman DR. 2008. The enduring hypoxic response of *Mycobacterium tuberculosis*. *PLoS ONE* **3:** e1502.

Sallusto F, Geginat J, Lanzavecchia A. 2004. Central memory and effector memory T cell subsets: Function, generation, and maintenance. *Annu Rev Immunol* **22:** 745–763.

Schuck SD, Mueller H, Kunitz F, Neher A, Hoffmann H, Franken KL, Repsilber D, Ottenhoff TH, Kaufmann SH, Jacobsen M. 2009. Identification of T-cell antigens specific for latent *Mycobacterium tuberculosis* infection. *PLoS ONE* **4:** e5590.

Scriba TJ, Tameris M, Smit E, van der Merwe L, Hughes EJ, Kadira B, Mauff K, Brittain N, Lawrie A, Mulenga H, et al. 2012. A phase IIa trial of the new tuberculosis vaccine, MVA85A, in HIV- and/or *Mycobacterium tuberculosis*-infected adults. *Am J Respir Crit Care Med* **185:** 769–778.

Seder RA, Darrah PA, Roederer M. 2008. T-cell quality in memory and protection: Implications for vaccine design. *Nat Rev Immunol* **8:** 247–258.

Shi L, North R, Gennaro ML. 2004. Effect of growth state on transcription levels of genes encoding major secreted antigens of *Mycobacterium tuberculosis* in the mouse lung. *Infect Immun* **72:** 2420–2424.

Smaill F, Jeyanathan M, Smieja M, Medina MF, Thanthrige-Don N, Zganiacz A, Yin C, Heriazon A, Damjanovic D, Puri L, et al. 2013. A human type 5 adenovirus-based tuberculosis vaccine induces robust T cell responses in humans despite preexisting anti-adenovirus immunity. *Sci Transl Med* **5:** 205ra134.

Soares AP, KwongChung CK, Choice T, Hughes EJ, Jacobs G, van Rensburg EJ, Khomba G, deKock M, Lerumo L, Makhethe L, et al. 2013. Longitudinal changes in CD4$^+$ T-cell memory responses induced by BCG vaccination of newborns. *J Infect Dis* **207:** 1084–1094.

Stenger S, Hanson DA, Teitelbaum R, Dewan P, Niazi KR, Froelich CJ, Ganz T, Thoma-Uszynski S, Melian A, Bogdan C, et al. 1998. An antimicrobial activity of cytolytic T cells mediated by granulysin. *Science* **282:** 121–125.

StopTBPartnership, WHO. 2011. *The global plan to stop TB 2011–2015.*

Tameris MD, Hatherill M, Landry BS, Scriba TJ, Snowden MA, Lockhart S, Shea JE, McClain JB, Hussey GD, Hanekom WA, et al. 2013. Safety and efficacy of MVA85A, a new tuberculosis vaccine, in infants previously vaccinated with BCG: A randomised, placebo-controlled phase 2b trial. *Lancet* **381:** 1021–1028.

Tolderlund K. 1952. Preliminary report of laboratory investigations on the effect of light on BCG vaccine. *Acta Pathol Microbiol Scand Suppl* **93:** 299–307.

UNAIDS, WHO. 2013. *Global Report: UNAIDS report on the global AIDS epidemic 2013.* WHO, Geneva.

van Dissel JT, Arend SM, Prins C, Bang P, Tingskov PN, Lingnau K, Nouta J, Klein MR, Rosenkrands I, Ottenhoff TH, et al. 2010. Ag85B-ESAT-6 adjuvanted with IC31 promotes strong and long-lived *Mycobacterium tuberculosis* specific T cell responses in naive human volunteers. *Vaccine* **28:** 3571–3581.

Verreck FA, Vervenne RA, Kondova I, van Kralingen KW, Remarque EJ, Braskamp G, van der Werff NM, Kersbergen A, Ottenhoff TH, Heidt PJ, et al. 2009. MVA.85A boosting of BCG and an attenuated, phoP deficient *M. tuberculosis* vaccine both show protective efficacy against tuberculosis in rhesus macaques. *PLoS ONE* **4:** e5264.

von Reyn CF, Mtei L, Arbeit RD, Waddell R, Cole B, Mackenzie T, Matee M, Bakari M, Tvaroha S, Adams LV, et al. 2010. Prevention of tuberculosis in Bacille Calmette–Guérin–primed, HIV-infected adults boosted with an inactivated whole-cell mycobacterial vaccine. *AIDS* **24:** 675–685.

Walker KB, Brennan MJ, Ho MM, Eskola J, Thiry G, Sadoff J, Dobbelaer R, Grode L, Liu MA, Fruth U, et al. 2010. The second Geneva Consensus: Recommendations for novel live TB vaccines. *Vaccine* **28:** 2259–2270.

Wang J, Thorson L, Stokes RW, Santosuosso M, Huygen K, Zganiacz A, Hitt M, Xing Z. 2004. Single mucosal, but not parenteral, immunization with recombinant adenoviral-based vaccine provides potent protection from pulmonary tuberculosis. *J Immunol* **173:** 6357–6365.

Weiner J, Kaufmann SHE. 2014. Recent advances towards tuberculosis control: Vaccines and biomarkers. *J Intern Med* **275:** 467–480.

Weiner J, Maertzdorf J, Kaufmann SH. 2013. The dual role of biomarkers for understanding basic principles and devising novel intervention strategies in tuberculosis. *Ann NY Acad Sci* **1283:** 22–29.

Weinrich Olsen A, van Pinxteren LA, Meng Okkels L, Birk Rasmussen P, Andersen P. 2001. Protection of mice with a tuberculosis subunit vaccine based on a fusion protein of antigen 85B and ESAT-6. *Infect Immun* **69:** 2773–2778.

White AD, Sibley L, Dennis MJ, Gooch K, Betts G, Edwards N, Reyes-Sandoval A, Carroll MW, Williams A, Marsh PD, et al. 2013. Evaluation of the safety and immunogenicity of a candidate tuberculosis vaccine, MVA85A, delivered by aerosol to the lungs of macaques. *Clin Vaccine Immunol* **20:** 663–672.

WHO. 2013. *Global tuberculosis report 2013.* WHO, Geneva.

Woodworth JS, Behar SM. 2006. *Mycobacterium tuberculosis*-specific $CD8^+$ T cells and their role in immunity. *Crit Rev Immunol* **26:** 317–352.

Yang XY, Chen QF, Li YP, Wu SM. 2011. *Mycobacterium vaccae* as adjuvant therapy to anti-tuberculosis chemotherapy in never-treated tuberculosis patients: A meta-analysis. *PLoS ONE* **6:** e23826.

Zheng J, Liu L, Wei C, Leng W, Yang J, Li W, Wang J, Jin Q. 2012. A comprehensive proteomic analysis of *Mycobacterium bovis* bacillus Calmette–Guérin using high resolution Fourier transform mass spectrometry. *J Proteomics* **77:** 357–371.

Toward a Unified Biosignature for Tuberculosis

Jeroen Maertzdorf, Stefan H.E. Kaufmann, and January Weiner III

Max Planck Institute for Infection Biology, Department of Immunology, 10117 Berlin, Germany

Correspondence: maertzdorf@mpiib-berlin.mpg.de

Accurate and rapid diagnosis of active tuberculosis (TB) disease is still hampered by inadequate tools. Although current assays relying on single-marker readouts mostly display inadequate sensitivity and/or specificity, host-related multimarker signatures are especially poorly developed. As a consequence, research programs have been initiated to search for combinations of markers—so-called biosignatures with superior performance. Many such investigations harness high-throughput platforms to analyze the host response during infection and disease. A major challenge for these activities is the analysis of vast amounts of data produced. Specialized bioinformatic tools are being applied to identify the most robust biosignatures for classification of exposed and diseased individuals and prognosis of risk of disease in endemic areas. Validation of the most promising biosignatures in ongoing multicohort studies will bring us a step closer to the identification of an accurate unified signature.

Whereas most current diagnostic assays identify the presence of the pathogen in the host, host-related biomarkers hold promise for use in prognostic research and vaccine trials and for monitoring treatment responses. Over the last decade, host-related biomarker research in tuberculosis (TB) has witnessed a clear shift from investigations on single markers to high-throughput studies revealing signatures consisting of multiple integrated markers (Weiner et al. 2013). On the one hand, such high-throughput profiling has become feasible by advanced modern technologies. On the other hand, researchers in the field have realized that single markers usually lack the sensitivity and/or specificity of a true correlate that can successfully be implemented in a clinical setting. Biosignatures are believed to hold higher promise for clinical application in areas such as pathology and immunology and to be suitable to discriminate etiologically different diseases with similar clinical features in a single assay (Weiner et al. 2013). These apparent improvements of multimarker biosignatures, however, suffer from the drawback of complex readout and interpretation. Whereas single-marker assays can be easily interpreted and evaluated, studies relying on high-throughput platforms are faced with the challenge of highly dimensional data sets, thereby requiring more sophisticated bioinformatics tools and more in-depth interpretation skills.

HIGH-THROUGHPUT BIOMARKER PLATFORMS

High-throughput platforms currently used in TB biomarker research comprise (1) proteo-

Cite this article as *Cold Spring Harb Perspect Med* doi: 10.1101/cshperspect.a018531

mics, assessing the total composition of proteins and peptides in a given biological sample; (2) metabolomics, which measures small molecules involved in, or an end product of, basic metabolic processes taking place in biological systems; and (3) transcriptomics, which covers the expression of genes in relation to disease or in response to a pathogenic insult. Transcriptomics has become the most widely applied experimental readout in TB biomarker research. Microarray platforms have thus far been the method of choice to simultaneously quantify the transcriptional activity of all genes in host cells. This approach has revealed a multitude of potential biosignatures in TB, which can potentially be integrated into clinical settings to identify active TB disease in suspected cases (Maertzdorf et al. 2012a; Joosten et al. 2013). More recent studies also attempt to combine the transcriptional activity of both human cells and the pathogen to investigate host–pathogen interactions in more detail.

One drawback of microarray technologies is the lack of absolute and detailed evaluation of gene expression. Modern deep sequencing technologies provide quantitative and qualitative information on gene expression and genomic composition down to the single-nucleotide level (Normand and Yanai 2013). Because of the high cost and time-consuming process of such deep sequencing analyses, this technology is currently mostly restricted to small-scale exploratory studies, in which evaluation and validation of identified biomarkers are assessed by more standard methods.

Although high-throughput platforms currently in use have their own strengths and weaknesses, they share the inevitable need for complex analysis of the huge amount of data generated.

A prerequisite of successfully applying high-throughput platforms is the high quality of the biological samples. In the case of TB, most studies rely on peripheral blood as the source for transcriptional, metabolic, and proteomic profiling. Although the immunological battle against the invading pathogen is focused at the site of infection and pathogen persistence (i.e., the lung), this pathologic status is reflected in the peripheral blood by circulating immune cells (Weiner et al. 2013). For studies focused on proteomic and genomic analysis of blood cells, the complexity of such biological samples poses an additional challenge. The many different types of cells present in the blood and their varying composition between individuals add an additional level of complexity to the already staggering number of readout parameters being assessed (Jacobsen et al. 2006). This biological variation between individuals, and between different ethnic groups, renders validation studies in distinct cohorts an essential requirement to assess the potential clinical validity of biomarkers and biosignatures.

SINGLE BIOMARKERS IN TB DIAGNOSTICS—A MATTER OF SENSITIVITY AND SPECIFICITY

Among the major challenges in using single canonical biomarkers in TB diagnostics is the issue of sensitivity and specificity. Generally, current clinical diagnosis applies a combination of "old" and "new" biomarkers. One of the most broadly used assays is the sputum smear test, which detects the presence of acid-fast bacteria in sputum of (suspected) TB cases (Norbis et al. 2013). This sputum smear test has the benefits of being low cost and easy to handle and of the fact that a positive result provides certainty about the presence of mycobacteria. However, there are several important drawbacks to this assay. First and foremost of all, this test often results in false-negative results, thereby missing a substantial number of patients with active pulmonary TB (Harries et al. 1998). Second, the assay does not distinguish between live and dead bacteria, and thus it cannot detect active bacterial replication as a hallmark of active TB disease, which is of importance for monitoring treatment responses. Thus, although the sputum smear test has a high specificity, its overall sensitivity is low (Davies and Pai 2008).

A more sensitive and widely applied diagnostic test to detect the presence of live bacilli is culture from sputum. Although a positive culture result directly proves the presence of live and replicating mycobacteria in the lungs of a suspected TB patient, the slow growth characteristics of *Mycobaterium tuberculosis* (*Mtb*) make the culture assay a lengthy procedure lasting up to several weeks. Although new technologies such as liquid culture have brought this down to several days, it still is a long time for rapid patient management (Norbis et al. 2013).

The more recently developed GeneXpert assay is designed to detect mycobacteria in sputum of suspected cases. Instead of staining, this assay uses the much more sensitive (quantitative) polymerase chain reaction (PCR) to detect specific sequences in the bacterial genome. Although much more sensitive than the smear test, it too does not distinguish between live and dead bacteria. The GeneXpert assay has very high specificity and reasonably good sensitivity (Steingart et al. 2013) and has been endorsed by the World Health Organization. It is relatively costly (making routine screening in clinical settings unaffordable for countries with low financial resources) and requires special equipment operating on a constant and reliable power supply.

Often performed in combination with sputum smear or GeneXpert assays is the examination of chest X rays. Principally, lung lesions and inflammatory tissue are readily recognized in patients with active TB (Walzl et al. 2011). However, X ray does not detect active bacterial replication and may produce false-negative results, especially in early stages of TB disease development. The specificity of chest X rays is restricted by the inability to identify the causative agent or processes underlying pulmonary pathology and lung damage. Therefore, chest X ray is inconclusive for diagnosis of TB (Al-Zamel 2009).

Another group of clinical assays, targeted at host responses, rely on biomarkers of immune activation and memory to mycobacterial antigen(s). The widely used tuberculin skin test (TST) assesses local immunological responses elicited by mycobacterial antigens (Bekmurzayeva et al. 2013) and is primarily used to show prior sensitization and latent infection. Subcutaneous injection of an extract of heat-killed *Mtb* proteins evokes a delayed-type hypersensitivity (DTH) reaction, causing transient swelling and reddening of the skin. Although of low cost, the test has profound limitations for detecting latent infections both with respect to sensitivity and specificity, which range widely depending on the population tested and can be affected by HIV infection and Bacillus Calmette–Guérin (BCG) vaccination (Bekmurzayeva et al. 2013).

The more recent approach in this group of diagnostic tests, the interferon-γ release assays (IGRAs), such as the Quantiferon test, rely on ex vivo activation of T lymphocytes secreting interferon-γ (IFN-γ) on stimulation with defined *Mtb*-specific proteins (Bekmurzayeva et al. 2013). Although a positive test result indicates previous exposure of a person's cellular immune response to *Mtb*, it is not a measure of bacterial activity or even persistence of the bacillus. As such, failure to discriminate latent *Mtb* infection (LTBI) from active TB is a major drawback of IGRAs (Bekmurzayeva et al. 2013; Norbis et al. 2013). IGRAs have a sensitivity equal to the TST but are more specific. However, particularly in highly TB-endemic regions, IGRAs are unsuitable for diagnosing active TB disease (Walzl et al. 2011). Some individual cases under clinical suspicion of having TB can also present with negative results, which in turn increases the risk of false exclusion of TB (Mazurek et al. 2007). The test may also be impaired by T-cell anergy in HIV$^+$ individuals (Barth et al. 2008).

The lack of sensitivity and specificity of current diagnostic tools illustrate that a single marker is unlikely to fulfill the requirements for reliable discrimination between active TB and other pulmonary or related infections. As a consequence, researchers have started searching for combinations of biomarkers, often referred to as biosignatures, to tackle the issue of sensitivity and specificity in TB diagnosis.

GENETIC BIOSIGNATURES IN TB DISEASE

One of the most pronounced genetic biosignatures present in the blood of TB patients is the elevated expression of transcripts involved in IFN signaling. First described in detail by Berry et al. (2010), this signature, consisting of both IFN type I and type II, was shown to be mainly driven by neutrophils. Albeit a prominent signature in TB disease, an IFN gene expression profile has also been observed in other chronic inflammatory conditions like systemic lupus erythematosus (SLE) and sarcoidosis (Koth et al. 2011; Maertzdorf et al. 2012b; Bloom et al. 2013). As such, an IFN signature in itself is insufficient for a definitive identification of TB, but it may be implemented for the identification of a more generic underlying inflammatory condition. Likely, it will also be of value for the definition of predictive biomarkers (e.g., for progression of LTBI toward active TB disease before actual clinical signs are observed).

Another pronounced transcript signature, which has been described in several studies, is the increased activity of the Fc γ receptor signaling pathways. First described as an increased expression of CD64 (another alias for FCGR1A) in TB patients (Jacobsen et al. 2007) and later confirmed by others (Maertzdorf et al. 2011a; Joosten et al. 2012), its expression was shown to be strongly correlated with other inflammatory markers with a central role for the JAK-STAT pathway (Maertzdorf et al. 2011b). This feature is also illustrated by its connection to IFN-inducible genes and its association with Toll-like receptors (TLRs), guanylate-binding proteins (GBPs), and components of the complement system (Maertzdorf et al. 2011a). Key regulators within the JAK-STAT pathway are cognates of the suppressor of cytokine signaling (SOCS) family. Dysregulated expression of SOCS3 in T lymphocytes from TB patients has also been suggested to play a role in susceptibility to TB (Jacobsen et al. 2011).

Activation of the complement system, as indicated by increased gene expression of multiple factors herein, may, on the one hand, reflect an innate defense mechanism against *Mtb*. On the other hand, its chronic activation may significantly contribute to inflammation-mediated tissue damage (Welsh et al. 2012), contributing to the pathogenesis of the disease.

Involvement of the complement system is also observed in autoimmune diseases like SLE (Ballanti et al. 2013), in which the disease is not triggered by a pathogen, but rather by a dysregulated chronic activation of the complement system. Complement activation in TB and similarities with SLE are also illustrated by the high enrichment of TB-induced genes in signatures associated with SLE (Maertzdorf et al. 2011a).

A recent publication was the first to combine information of all genetic biosignatures in blood of TB patients described so far (Joosten et al. 2012). As the diverse platforms used in transcriptome analysis for TB biomarkers by various authors are not directly comparable with canonical analytical methods, the authors have analyzed a "superset" of transcripts, which have been found in the previous experimental studies. This resulted in improved sensitivity, allowing identification of significant enrichment in pathways and groups of genes which were until now not linked to a TB signature. While confirming the presence of most described signatures in multiple studies, their study identified a hitherto underappreciated role of the B-cell compartment. The results also point to an involvement of TREM1 signaling in active TB disease, something that had not been described in any of the previous studies separately (see also Walzl et al. 2014). Shortly after, Cliff et al. (2013) also identified significant changes in expression of a network of B-cell-related genes during disease resolution.

The major biological pathways active in TB can be clearly grouped into three dominant clusters—that is, (1) signaling and inflammation pathways, (2) IFN and immune pathways, and (3) T- and B-cell pathways—based on a set of 1446 differentially expressed transcripts, as recently shown by Bloom et al. (2013). First described by Maertzdorf et al. (2012b), this study revealed similarities, but also significant differences in blood gene expression signatures between TB and sarcoidosis. Moreover, Bloom et al. also included pneumonia and lung cancer in their study, indicating that, whereas TB and sarcoidosis share the dominant IFN signatures, the other two pulmonary diseases show distinct signatures dominated by inflammatory genes.

Although the above-described biological signatures reflecting TB pathology have been identified in multiple studies, their unique specificity for TB is low and many signatures are shared with other inflammatory diseases. These features provide important insights into the biology underlying TB pathology; yet they are of lesser value for clinical applications such as distinguishing TB patients from healthy individuals or from patients suffering from other diseases. Several studies have therefore tried to identify gene expression signatures that can specifically accomplish such distinctions, regardless of their biological relevance. The number of gene transcripts in such signatures range from three (Jacobsen et al. 2007) to hundreds (Berry et al. 2010; Bloom et al. 2013). Although the sensitivity and specificity of these signatures in distinguishing TB patients from healthy individuals are quite robust in most studies, they also seem to contain cohort-specific information at least to some degree. This is, for example, illustrated by the study by Bloom et al. (2013), applying signatures from two other studies (Koth et al. 2011; Maertzdorf et al. 2012b) onto their own data set led to a significant reduction in sensitivity in class predictions (Bloom et al. 2013). A global analysis combining genetic signatures in numerous cohorts of TB patients and controls from various TB-endemic areas around the world would allow the identification of a unified and general signature.

METABOLIC PROFILING BIOMARKERS IN TB

Although gene expression biomarkers from whole blood RNA have been widely applied to characterize differences between TB patients and control groups, other avenues have been taken as well. Assuming that RNA expression from whole blood predominantly reflects changes in peripheral blood cells, additional information can be gained by measuring molecules that are derived directly from the site of infection (Maertzdorf et al. 2012a). Weiner et al. (2012) analyzed metabolic profiles in serum samples of TB patients and healthy controls and showed that a biosignature based on metabolic profiles can achieve sensitivity and specificity, at least on par with transcription profiles (Weiner et al. 2012). Some of the predictive metabolites were directly derived from the site of infection. Kynurenine, which was found at significantly higher levels in the sera of TB patients than in controls, is synthesized from tryptophan by the enzyme IDO1, induced in macrophages and dendritic cells in contact with *Mtb*. It is likely that high kynurenine abundance in serum reflects release of this molecule from granulomas.

Among groups of metabolites that were found at different abundance in TB patients and healthy controls, distinct amino acids (e.g., histidine and cysteine), bile acids and uremic toxins (such as taurocholate and glycocholenate), *N*-acetylneuraminate, cortisol, fibrinopeptides, and lysophosphatidylcholines were most prevalent (Weiner et al. 2012). Intriguingly, several processes comprising changes in their metabolic components (including higher levels of kynurenine and cortisol and lower abundance of lysophosphatidilcholines, which may be caused by inhibition of phospholipase A2) can be linked to immunosuppressive mechanisms.

In a parallel approach, cytokines were determined in the same study groups. Distinct cytokines correlated with defined metabolites, showing the link between metabolite abundance in serum and the immune processes in response to TB disease. For example, the chemokine C-X-C motif chemokine 10 (CXCL10, IP-10), the cytokine interleukin 6, and the growth factor granulocyte colony-stimulating factor (GCSF) showed a negative correlation with abundances of several amino acids (for example, glutamine and tryptophan) and positive correlation with metabolic markers elevated in sera of TB patients, including *N*-acetylneuraminate and hypoxanthine.

VARIABILITY OF BIOMARKERS IN TB PATIENTS

Both transcriptomics and metabolomics revealed that the variance of the variables was higher in TB patients than in healthy subjects (J. Weiner, unpubl.). This becomes most apparent when visualization techniques such as Chernoff faces or spider plots are applied—the corresponding features are more profound in patients than in healthy individuals. A proximate explanation for this phenomenon is that the disease induces higher expression of several genes, and expression strength may correlate with variance of the measured expression signal. However, differential variability of gene expression (Ho et al. 2008) has been found in immune-modulated, stress-induced, and hormonally regulated genes in mice (Pritchard et al. 2001).

Some other chronic infectious diseases are characterized by a spectrum of clinical manifestations. Notably, in leprosy, a disease caused by *Mycobacterium leprae*, clinical manifestations range from tuberculoid leprosy to lepromatous leprosy. Furthermore, despite the fact that TB is often depicted as having two stages (latent and active TB), the reality is more complex (Barry et al. 2009), and the spectrum of clinical TB disease includes a diversity of manifestations and stages that falls between these two extremes and depends on a balance between pro- and anti-inflammatory responses (Lin and Flynn 2010). Moreover, even within an individual host, the granulomatous lesions show a remarkable diversity both in pathology and in response to treatment (Lin et al. 2014). Thus, the host response to TB is variable, and consequently individual variability is reflected by gene expression and metabolic profiles. This merits a more detailed analysis.

BIOSIGNATURES AND MACHINE LEARNING

Biosignatures are often presented as lists of genes that distinguish between groups of interest (e.g., between TB patients, patients with other diseases, and healthy controls). Generally, these genes are differentially expressed between groups. However, the reverse need not be true: Generating a biomarker set or a multivariate biosignature is not limited to selecting genes that differ most profoundly between conditions. A biosignature must be capable of distinguishing not only the samples it was derived from (the *training set*), but more importantly, any novel sample set that it will be confronted with. For example, if one has selected a number of genes that differentiate between the conditions in a given sample set, one needs to test whether these genes distinguish between conditions in another, independent set (the *validation set*). In essence, this is an application of supervised machine learning (ML).

An ML model is defined not only by a list of genes, metabolites, or other predictive variables, but also by the specific values of these variables and model parameters, such as weights which determine how each variable influences the model. Kaforou et al. (2013) analyzed a substantial number of samples from 12 different groups, from two cohorts (Malawi and South Africa, see Table 1), and three disease states (healthy control subjects, TB patients, and patients from a disease other than TB, which includes TB in differential diagnosis) (Kaforou et al. 2013). Furthermore, the study included HIV^- and HIV^+ individuals. The authors developed a simple, yet effective ML algorithm. Based on the training set, a list of less than 50 genes was compiled to differentiate between distinct disease states, and each gene was assigned a weight of $+1$ or -1 depending on whether it was more highly expressed in TB ($+1$) or in the control group (-1). The expression values from the selected list were multiplied by the weights and then summed and compared with a threshold calculated based on the levels of gene expression in the training set. Thus, the actual biosignature consisted of (1) a list of genes, (2) the assigned weights, and (3) a parameter (disease risk score [DRS] threshold) based on expression levels from the training set. In more complex ML algorithms the number of parameters required can be even higher. Notably, this same signature may not necessarily be successful if applied to another study based on an unrelated cohort and an independent readout platform.

MACHINE LEARNING ALGORITHMS

Several supervised ML algorithms exist, of which only a few have been exploited for TB data set analyses thus far (Table 1, see Method column).

k-*nearest neighbors* (KNN) (related to an unsupervised clustering method, k-means clustering) has been successfully applied by Berry et al. (2010). In KNN, the variates are treated as coordinates in an N-dimensional space,

Table 1. List of studies of human whole blood transcriptome in the context of active TB

Cohort	Study groups (sample size)	Classification error measures and error rates	Method	Study
United Kingdom (training set)	TB (13), LTBI (17), CTRL (12)	All results TB versus non-TB: sensitivity, 91.7%; specificity, 96.6%	*k*-nearest neighbor	Berry et al. 2010[a]
United Kingdom (test set)	TB (21), LTBI (21), CTRL (12)	Sensitivity, 61.7%; specificity, 93.8%; indeterminate, 1.9%	*k*-nearest neighbor	Berry et al. 2010
South Africa (validation set)	TB (20), LTBI (31)	Sensitivity, 94.1%; specificity, 96.7%; indeterminate, 7.8%	*k*-nearest neighbor	Berry et al. 2010
South Africa	TB (33), LTBI (34), CTRL (9)	TB versus LTBI using a four-gene signature: sensitivity, 94%; specificity, 97%	Random forest with LOO cross-validation	Maertzdorf et al. 2011b
Gambia	TB (46), LTBI (25), CTRL (37)	TB versus non-TB[e]: accuracy, 82%; sensitivity, 74%; specificity, 87%	Random forest with LOO cross-validation	Maertzdorf et al. 2011a
United States	CTRL (12)	Accuracy, 100%	PAM-R	Lesho et al. 2011
Brazil	LTBI (6), TB (5)	Accuracy, 100%	PAM-R	
Germany	TB(8), sarcoidosis (18), CTRL (18)	Three-way classification error rates: sarcoidosis, 5.6%; TB, 12.5%; CTRL, 0% (overall error rate, 4.55%)	Random forest with LOO cross-validation	Maertzdorf et al. 2012b
United Kingdom; France (training set)	TB (16), sarcoidosis (25), pneumonia (8), lung cancer (8), CTRL (38)	TB versus non-TB: sensitivity, 88%; specificity, 94%	Support vector machines	Bloom et al. 2013
United Kingdom; France (test set)	TB(11), sarcoidosis (25), pneumonia (6), lung cancer (8), CTRL (52)	Sensitivity, 82%; specificity, 91%	Support vector machines	Bloom et al. 2013
United Kingdom; France (validation set)	TB (8), sarcoidosis (11), CTRL (23)	Sensitivity, 88%; specificity, 92%	Support vector machines	Bloom et al. 2013
South Africa	TB/HIV⁺ (49), TB (47), LTBI HIV⁺ (48), LTBI/ (50), OD/HIV⁺ (68), OD/(49)	TB versus LTBI: sensitivity, 95%; specificity, 90%. TB versus OD: sensitivity, 93%; specificity, 88%	DRS	Kaforou et al. 2013
Northern Malawi	TB/HIV⁺ (60), TB/ (59), LTBI HIV⁺ (41), LTBI/ (36), OD/HIV⁺ (38), OD/(39)	TB versus LTBI: sensitivity, 95%; specificity, 90%. TB versus OD: sensitivity, 93%; specificity, 88%	DRS	Kaforou et al. 2013
South Africa	TB (10), cured (10)[c], recurrent(10)[c], LTBI (10)	Accuracy, 93.75%	Stepwise linear discriminant analysis	Mistry et al. 2007
Indonesia	TB (23)[d], CTRL (23)	Not used for classification task		Ottenhoff et al. 2012
South Africa	LTBI (38), TB (29)	Not used for classification task		Bloom et al. 2012
United Kingdom	TB (8)[b]	Not used for classification task		

Continued

Table 1. *Continued*

Cohort	Study groups (sample size)	Classification error measures and error rates	Method	Study
South Africa (training set)	TB (18) at time of diagnosis, and 1, 2, 4, and 26 weeks postdiagnosis	Overall accuracy, 92.6%	Neuronal network	Cliff et al. 2013
South Africa (test set)	TB (9)			

Donors were HIV$^-$ unless indicated otherwise.

CTRL, healthy controls; DRS, disease risk score; HIV$^+$, human immunodeficiency virus positive; LOO, leave one out; LTBI, latent tuberculosis infection; OD, other diseases; PAM-R, prediction analysis of microarrays with R; TB, tuberculosis.

[a] Data for the 393-transcript signature.

[b] Eight patients were followed up during TB treatment.

[c] Cured, cured patients who underwent one episode of TB; recurrent, cured patients who underwent two or three recurring episodes of TB; six individuals from each group were used as a training set, and the remaining four individuals were used as a test set.

[d] Samples from 23 patients were collected before, during, and after successful completion of the treatment.

[e] Data provided by the authors (J Maertzdorf, pers. comm.).

where N is the number of variables (e.g., genes, for which expression has been measured). For each group, its center is determined by averaging the position of all samples that belong to the group. Classification of new samples relies on determining the distance from each of the centers and choosing the center closest to the sample in question. A major advantage of this method is that decisions can be easily interpreted. The DSR algorithm described above and used by Kaforou et al. (2013) can be considered as a variant of this method, using Manhattan distances (in which the expression levels of single genes are summed) instead of Euclidean distances (in which the distance is measured as a square root of sum of squared differences in gene expression).

Random Forests (RF) ML algorithm is an ensemble-based algorithm closely related to another class of ML algorithms, decision trees. RF generates a large number of decision trees; when applied to a sample of the validation set, the decision how to classify this sample is based on the majority vote from the trees. RF has been successfully applied in several settings; in gene expression analysis, it compares favorably with other methods. A major advantage of RF is the fact that high accuracy can be obtained with only a few predictors (Diaz-Uriarte et al. 2006) and that accurate cross-validated error rates are provided "out of the box" (so-called OOB classification error rates).

Support vector machines (SVMs) are a type of generalized linear classifiers. Data points (samples) are mapped onto a multidimensional space in such a way that it is possible to calculate a hyperplane (a multidimensional plane), which separates the classes of samples. Whereas originally suitable only for two-class data, it can be extended to analyze also multiclass problems.

PERFORMANCE OF BIOSIGNATURES

Some 500 gene expression profiles have been collected from TB patients in different studies and the majority of these have been used in an ML context to generate biosignatures of TB (Table 1). Several groups have attempted to compare the signatures generated based on their data with the signatures based on lists of genes from other publications, with the overall outcome of achieving lower error rates when the signature was defined from the same data set than when a signature derived from another data set and a different algorithm were applied. Analyzing disease-specific biosignatures, Bloom et al. (2013) applied lists of genes corresponding to the biosignatures published by Maertzdorf et al. (2012b) and Koth et al. (2011). They found that the derived SVM models had a much lower performance when applied to their data set. Similarly, Kaforou et al. (2013) used the 393-gene list derived from Berry et al. (2010) and found that when applied to their method and their data, its performance was much lower than the models corresponding to the list of genes originally derived by Kaforou et al. (2013).

Some sets of genes can (and do) perform objectively better than others when used in a classification task *ceteris paribus*. Yet, lists of genes derived from a biosignature comprising specific parameters and applied to a specific data set generated with a specific microarray or RNAseq platform need not be compatible with other data sets and other algorithms. Gene lists produced by variable selection will differ even for the same data set when different algorithms are applied to the same data set. For a meaningful comparison, complete biosignatures, including the specific algorithms and parameters, such as weights or decision trees, should be directly applied to the same data set. Such a comparison has not yet been performed. Consequently, one of the major challenges awaiting the field of TB biomarkers is the unification of diverse platforms and data sets to achieve a platform-independent, global signature of TB.

A supervised ML algorithm is trained using a set of samples with known associations to groups (e.g., healthy controls and TB patients). Applied to a new set of samples, the algorithm should correctly classify these samples. In a simple setting with only two classifications (e.g., disease vs. healthy, or one selected class against all other classes), the errors of the algorithm correspond to type I and type II errors in a hypothesis-testing framework. Type I errors (false positives) arise when a "negative" sample (e.g., from a healthy patient) is classified as "positive" (e.g., TB disease). Type II errors (false negatives) arise in the opposite situation: A positive sample is classified as negative. Therefore, it is logical to describe the performance of an algorithm by its overall error rate (also termed accuracy) (Table 2).

For a single sample, the probabilities of type I and type II errors can be given. However, the actual number of false-positive and -negative predictions (e.g., in a clinical setting) also depends on the population demography. The actual numbers of incorrect predictions depend on the relative frequency of each group. An algorithm with sensitivity and specificity of 99% each will produce 10 times more false positives than false negatives if applied for detection of a disease with a 10% incidence in a population. This is known as the "accuracy paradox": If the prevalence of a group is sufficiently low, then an algorithm that uniformly predicts that a sample belongs to a majority group (e.g., healthy rather than TB disease) can have a higher accuracy (lower overall error rate).

More suitable measures of performance of an algorithm are available. Precision rate (also called positive predictive value, PPV) is the proportion of true positives among all samples that have been classified as positive. Another group of measures is derived from the receiver–operator characteristics (ROC) curves. If an ML algorithm is applied to a test set, the pre-

Table 2. Measures of machine learning algorithm performance

		Prediction		
		Negative	Positive	Accuracy measure
Reality	**Negative**	TN	FP, type I error	Specificity = TN/(TN + FP)
	Positive	FN, type II error	TP	Sensitivity = TP/(FN + TP)
	Accuracy measure	NPV = TN/(TN + FN)	PPV = TP/(FP + TP)	Accuracy = (TP + TN)/N =1 − overall error

FP, false positive; FN, false negative; NPV, negative predictive value; PPV, positive predictive value; TN, true negative; TP, true positive.

dictions of that algorithm are sorted by their confidence to derive an ROC curve. The area under the curve is a test statistic with known characteristics; a set of random predictions will form a diagonal, and the greater the area, the better the predictions.

Attempts to estimate the predictive power of a whole set of transcript biomarkers in TB have reported strikingly similar results (Fig. 1; Joosten et al. 2013). The accuracies, specificities, and sensitivities frequently range between 85% and 95% (Table 1). Although two studies obtained no misclassifications in some comparisons, this would be attributable to the small sample size used: Given an error rate of 5% and a total sample size of 20, one expects on average only one incorrect classification. Intriguingly, a study focusing on metabolic profiles rather than transcriptomes also revealed 3%–5% overall errors (Weiner et al. 2012). This could indicate an upper limit for the performance of biomarkers derived from blood samples.

Note that the performance of biomarkers can only be as good as the quality of the training set—in this case, the accuracy of clinical diagnosis of TB. If the training set includes misclassified individuals, then the performance of the biosignature will inadvertently suffer. This is particularly important when considering comparisons of TB patients with clinically healthy, but latently infected individuals. Most attempts to harness biomarkers for the segregation of healthy uninfected and individuals with LTBI have produced relatively large error rates (often $>30\%$), which could be the result of low sensitivity and low specificity of the tests used to determine the infection status. Considering that both groups are free of active disease, their blood signatures are more similar, resulting in a lower discriminative power to distinguish the two groups. Moreover, subclinical TB may already progress to clinical disease in some of these individuals and manifest as an apparent TB-like signature. However, if this were the case, it could in fact be harnessed for diagnosis TB in early stages using a biomarker-based diagnostic approach.

Another important issue has been raised by Kaforou et al. (2013). These authors compared the performance of biomarkers depending on whether the biosignature was based on a training set which included, in addition to samples from HIV^- donors, also HIV^+ TB patients and HIV^+ controls. They observed that performance substantially increased when HIV^+ TB patients were included; biomarkers derived from such a test set could be used to accurately classify HIV^- patients, but not vice versa: if the model construction was based on HIV^- TB patients only and controls only, then its performance in the HIV^+ population was poor.

PREDICTIVE BIOSIGNATURES FOR TB

A large body of evidence shows that diagnostic biosignatures of active TB disease can be defined. However, a high-throughput biosignature capable of predicting TB disease at a subclinical stage remains to be identified. This could be used for predicting (1) TB reactivation (progression from latent to active TB), (2) protective vaccine efficacy, and (3) treatment outcome.

It is tempting to assume that a host response signature can be defined at the molecular level, which precedes clinical diagnosis. This issue is being addressed by two ongoing efforts, a biomarker study based on an adolescent cohort (Mahomed et al. 2013) and GC6-74 (http://www.biomarkers-for-tb.net/consortium). In these studies, household contacts of active TB patients are being monitored over years to define signatures that can predict progression from infection to active TB disease. In the GC6 study, for example, ~3% of ~4500 household contacts developed active TB disease during the observation period of 2 years. Currently, metabolic and transcriptomic signatures are being defined that predict active TB disease at an early stage (i.e., before clinical TB diagnosis). It is hoped that it will be possible to capture early changes in gene expression and metabolic composition predictive of clinical TB onset thereafter.

The effect of drug treatment of TB on transcriptomic profiles has been investigated in independent studies by Bloom et al. (2012) and Cliff et al. (2013), who both detected rapid changes in IFN signaling and in innate immu-

 Cite this article as *Cold Spring Harb Perspect Med* doi: 10.1101/cshperspect.a018531

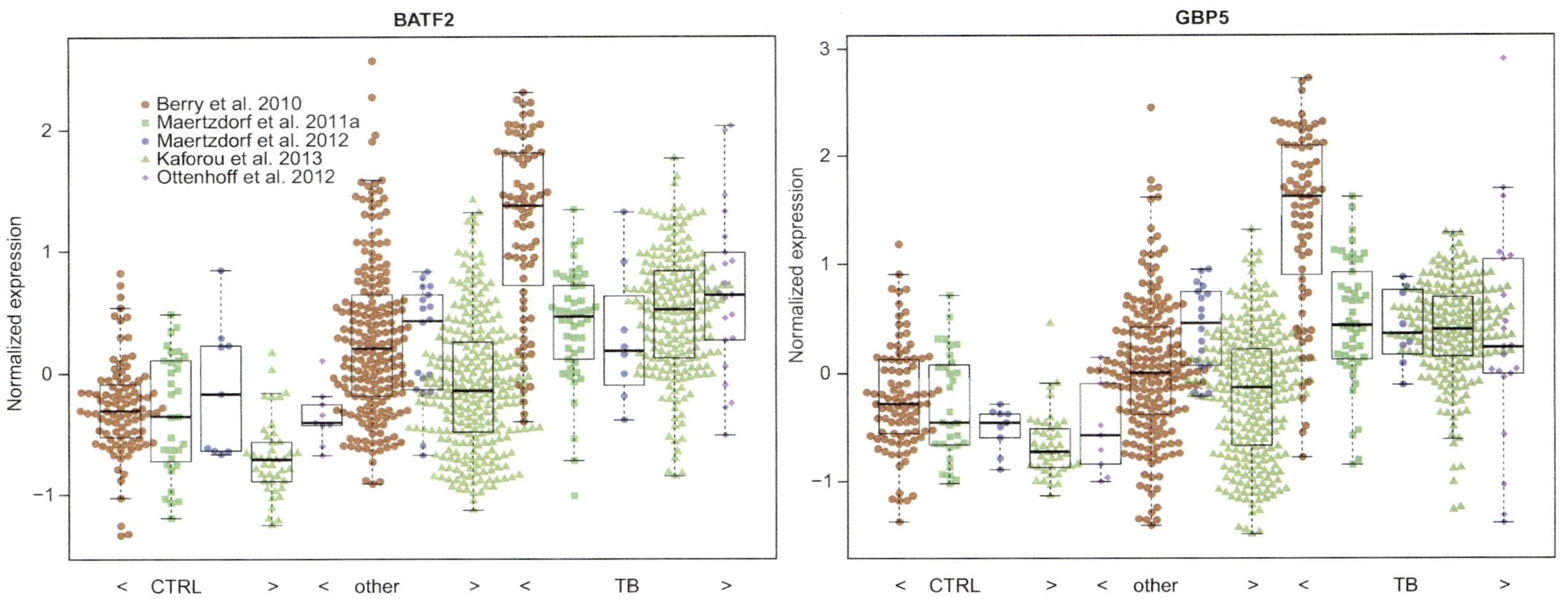

Figure 1. Normalized expression profiles of two selected genes (BATF2, basic leucine zipper transcription factor ATF-Like 2; GBP5, guanylate-binding protein 5) across different studies and study groups show a consistent landscape of TB responses on transcriptional level. CTRL, healthy donors (uninfected or with latent TB); other, other diseases; TB, clinical TB diagnosed.

nity, as early as 1 to 2 weeks after initiation of treatment. This finding suggests that it would be possible to quantitatively measure the response to TB treatment at an early stage of chemotherapy, although larger studies are needed for validation.

CONCLUSIONS

Most current diagnostic assays for TB have their own specific drawbacks and often rely on canonical single biomarkers with insufficient sensitivity and specificity. These limitations have prompted intensive search for multimarker host signatures with better predictive accuracy and improved diagnostic validity. High-throughput platforms, notably transcriptomics and metabolomics, have revealed numerous TB-related features, the majority of which have been confirmed in multiple studies. Focusing on the host response in TB, results are to a large extent compatible and reveal that the overall accuracy of a transcript biosignature can be as high as 95%. Bioinformatic analyses of the signatures identified are currently under validation in multicohort studies, bringing us a step closer to the identification of a unified signature of general applicability. Future efforts will be focused on validating the existing findings and, most importantly, on derivation of predictive signatures, useful for early diagnosis of risk of disease in infected healthy individuals.

ACKNOWLEDGMENTS

We thank Mary Louise Grossman for help preparing the manuscript. The authors are supported by the European Union's Seventh Framework Programme (EU FP7) ADITEC (HEALTH-F4-2011-280873) and NEWTBVAC (HEALTH-F3-2009-241745); the Bill and Melinda Gates Foundation Grand Challenges in Global Health Program (BMGF GC6-74, #37772 and GC12, #37885), and the EU/EFPIA Innovative Medicines Initiative Joint Undertaking (BioVacSafe) Grant No. 115308.

REFERENCES

*Reference is also in this subject collection.

Al-Zamel FA. 2009. Detection and diagnosis of *Mycobacterium tuberculosis*. *Expert Rev Anti Infect Ther* **7:** 1099–1108.

Ballanti E, Perricone C, Greco E, Ballanti M, Di MG, Chimenti MS, Perricone R. 2013. Complement and autoimmunity. *Immunol Res* **56:** 477–491.

Barry CE III, Boshoff HI, Dartois V, Dick T, Ehrt S, Flynn J, Schnappinger D, Wilkinson RJ, Young D. 2009. The spectrum of latent tuberculosis: Rethinking the biology and intervention strategies. *Nat Rev Microbiol* **7:** 845–855.

Barth RE, Mudrikova T, Hoepelman AI. 2008. Interferon-γ release assays (IGRAs) in high-endemic settings: Could they play a role in optimizing global TB diagnostics? Evaluating the possibilities of using IGRAs to diagnose active TB in a rural African setting. *Int J Infect Dis* **12:** e1–e6.

Bekmurzayeva A, Sypabekova M, Kanayeva D. 2013. Tuberculosis diagnosis using immunodominant, secreted antigens of *Mycobacterium tuberculosis*. *Tuberculosis (Edinb)* **93:** 381–388.

Berry MP, Graham CM, McNab FW, Xu Z, Bloch SA, Oni T, Wilkinson KA, Banchereau R, Skinner J, Wilkinson RJ, et al. 2010. An interferon-inducible neutrophil-driven blood transcriptional signature in human tuberculosis. *Nature* **466:** 973–977.

Bloom CI, Graham CM, Berry MP, Wilkinson KA, Oni T, Rozakeas F, Xu Z, Rossello-Urgell J, Chaussabel D, Banchereau J, et al. 2012. Detectable changes in the blood transcriptome are present after two weeks of antituberculosis therapy. *PLoS ONE* **7:** e46191.

Bloom CI, Graham CM, Berry MP, Rozakeas F, Redford PS, Wang Y, Xu Z, Wilkinson KA, Wilkinson RJ, Kendrick Y, et al. 2013. Transcriptional blood signatures distinguish pulmonary tuberculosis, pulmonary sarcoidosis, pneumonias and lung cancers. *PLoS ONE* **8:** e70630.

Cliff JM, Lee JS, Constantinou N, Cho JE, Clark TG, Ronacher K, King EC, Lukey PT, Duncan K, van Helden PD, et al. 2013. Distinct phases of blood gene expression pattern through tuberculosis treatment reflect modulation of the humoral immune response. *J Infect Dis* **207:** 18–29.

Davies PD, Pai M. 2008. The diagnosis and misdiagnosis of tuberculosis. *Int J Tuberc Lung Dis* **12:** 1226–1234.

Diaz-Uriarte R, Alvarez de AS. 2006. Gene selection and classification of microarray data using random forest. *BMC Bioinformatics* **7:** 3.

Harries AD, Maher D, Nunn P. 1998. An approach to the problems of diagnosing and treating adult smear-negative pulmonary tuberculosis in high-HIV-prevalence settings in sub-Saharan Africa. *Bull World Health Organ* **76:** 651–662.

Ho JW, Stefani M, dos Remedios CG, Charleston MA. 2008. Differential variability analysis of gene expression and its application to human diseases. *Bioinformatics* **24:** i390–i398.

Jacobsen M, Repsilber D, Gutschmidt A, Neher A, Feldmann K, Mollenkopf HJ, Kaufmann SH, Ziegler A. 2006. Deconfounding microarray analysis—Independent measurements of cell type proportions used in a regression model to resolve tissue heterogeneity bias. *Methods Inf Med* **45:** 557–563.

Jacobsen M, Repsilber D, Gutschmidt A, Neher A, Feldmann K, Mollenkopf HJ, Ziegler A, Kaufmann SH. 2007. Candidate biomarkers for discrimination between infection and disease caused by *Mycobacterium tuberculosis. J Mol Med (Berl)* **85:** 613–621.

Jacobsen M, Repsilber D, Kleinsteuber K, Gutschmidt A, Schommer-Leitner S, Black G, Walzl G, Kaufmann SH. 2011. Suppressor of cytokine signaling-3 is affected in T-cells from tuberculosis TB patients. *Clin Microbiol Infect* **17:** 1323–1331.

Joosten SA, Goeman JJ, Sutherland JS, Opmeer L, de Boer KG, Jacobsen M, Kaufmann SH, Finos L, Magis-Escurra C, Ota MO, et al. 2012. Identification of biomarkers for tuberculosis disease using a novel dual-color RT-MLPA assay. *Genes Immun* **13:** 71–82.

Joosten SA, Fletcher HA, Ottenhoff TH. 2013. A helicopter perspective on TB biomarkers: Pathway and process based analysis of gene expression data provides new insight into TB pathogenesis. *PLoS ONE* **8:** e73230.

Kaforou M, Wright VJ, Oni T, French N, Andersen ST, Bangani N, Banwell CM, Brent AJ, Crampin AC, Dockrell HM, et al. 2013. Detection of tuberculosis in HIV-infected and -uninfected African adults using whole blood RNA expression signatures: A case-control study. *PLoS Med* **10:** e1001538.

Koth LL, Solberg OD, Peng JC, Bhakta NR, Nguyen CP, Woodruff PG. 2011. Sarcoidosis blood transcriptome reflects lung inflammation and overlaps with tuberculosis. *Am J Respir Crit Care Med* **184:** 1153–1163.

Lesho E, Forestiero FJ, Hirata MH, Hirata RD, Cecon L, Melo FF, Paik SH, Murata Y, Ferguson EW, Wang Z, et al. 2011. Transcriptional responses of host peripheral blood cells to tuberculosis infection. *Tuberculosis (Edinb)* **91:** 390–399.

Lin PL, Flynn JL. 2010. Understanding latent tuberculosis: A moving target. *J Immunol* **185:** 15–22.

Lin PL, Ford CB, Coleman MT, Myers AJ, Gawande R, Ioerger T, Sacchettini J, Fortune SM, Flynn JL. 2014. Sterilization of granulomas is common in active and latent tuberculosis despite within-host variability in bacterial killing. *Nat Med* **20:** 75–79.

Maertzdorf J, Ota M, Repsilber D, Mollenkopf HJ, Weiner J, Hill PC, Kaufmann SH. 2011a. Functional correlations of pathogenesis-driven gene expression signatures in tuberculosis. *PLoS ONE* **6:** e26938.

Maertzdorf J, Repsilber D, Parida SK, Stanley K, Roberts T, Black G, Walzl G, Kaufmann SH. 2011b. Human gene expression profiles of susceptibility and resistance in tuberculosis. *Genes Immun* **12:** 15–22.

Maertzdorf J, Weiner J III, Kaufmann SH. 2012a. Enabling biomarkers for tuberculosis control. *Int J Tuberc Lung Dis* **16:** 1140–1148.

Maertzdorf J, Weiner J III, Mollenkopf HJ, Bauer T, Prasse A, Muller-Quernheim J, Kaufmann SH. 2012b. Common patterns and disease-related signatures in tuberculosis and sarcoidosis. *Proc Natl Acad Sci* **109:** 7853–7858.

Mahomed H, Ehrlich R, Hawkridge T, Hatherill M, Geiter L, Kafaar F, Abrahams DA, Mulenga H, Tameris M, Geldenhuys H, et al. 2013. TB incidence in an adolescent cohort in South Africa. *PLoS ONE* **8:** e59652.

Mazurek GH, Weis SE, Moonan PK, Daley CL, Bernardo J, Lardizabal AA, Reves RR, Toney SR, Daniels LJ, LoBue PA. 2007. Prospective comparison of the tuberculin skin test and 2 whole-blood interferon-γ release assays in persons with suspected tuberculosis. *Clin Infect Dis* **45:** 837–845.

Mistry R, Cliff JM, Clayton CL, Beyers N, Mohamed YS, Wilson PA, Dockrell HM, Wallace DM, van Helden PD, Duncan K, et al. 2007. Gene-expression patterns in whole blood identify subjects at risk for recurrent tuberculosis. *J Infect Dis* **195:** 357–365.

Norbis L, Miotto P, Alagna R, Cirillo DM. 2013. Tuberculosis: Lights and shadows in the current diagnostic landscape. *New Microbiol* **36:** 111–120.

Normand R, Yanai I. 2013. An introduction to high-throughput sequencing experiments: Design and bioinformatics analysis. *Methods Mol Biol* **1038:** 1–26.

Ottenhoff TH, Dass RH, Yang N, Zhang MM, Wong HE, Sahiratmadja E, Khor CC, Alisjahbana B, van CR, Marzuki S, et al. 2012. Genome-wide expression profiling identifies type 1 interferon response pathways in active tuberculosis. *PLoS ONE* **7:** e45839.

Pritchard CC, Hsu L, Delrow J, Nelson PS. 2001. Project normal: Defining normal variance in mouse gene expression. *Proc Natl Acad Sci* **98:** 13266–13271.

Steingart KR, Sohn H, Schiller I, Kloda LA, Boehme CC, Pai M, Dendukuri N. 2013. Xpert® MTB/RIF assay for pulmonary tuberculosis and rifampicin resistance in adults. *Cochrane Database Syst Rev* **1:** CD009593.

Walzl G, Ronacher K, Hanekom W, Scriba TJ, Zumla A. 2011. Immunological biomarkers of tuberculosis. *Nat Rev Immunol* **11:** 343–354.

* Walzl G, Haks MC, Joosten SA, Kleynhans L, Ronacher K, Ottenhoff THM. 2014. Clinical immunology and multiplex biomarkers of human tuberculosis. *Cold Spring Harb Perspect Med* doi: 10.1101/cshperspect.a018515.

Weiner J III, Parida SK, Maertzdorf J, Black GF, Repsilber D, Telaar A, Mohney RP, Arndt-Sullivan C, Ganoza CA, Fae KC, et al. 2012. Biomarkers of inflammation, immunosuppression and stress with active disease are revealed by metabolomic profiling of tuberculosis patients. *PLoS ONE* **7:** e40221.

Weiner J, Maertzdorf J, Kaufmann SH. 2013. The dual role of biomarkers for understanding basic principles and devising novel intervention strategies in tuberculosis. *Ann NY Acad Sci* **1283:** 22–29.

Welsh KJ, Lewis CT, Boyd S, Braun MC, Actor JK. 2012. Complement factor C7 contributes to lung immunopathology caused by *Mycobacterium tuberculosis. Clin Dev Immunol* **2012:** 429675.

Clinical Immunology and Multiplex Biomarkers of Human Tuberculosis

Gerhard Walzl[2], Mariëlle C. Haks[1,3], Simone A. Joosten[1,3], Léanie Kleynhans[2,3], Katharina Ronacher[2,3], and Tom H.M. Ottenhoff[1]

[1]Department of Infectious Diseases, Leiden University Medical Center, 2300 RC Leiden, The Netherlands

[2]DST/NRF Centre of Excellence for Biomedical TB Research/MRC Centre for Molecular and Cellular Biology, Division of Molecular Biology and Human Genetics, Faculty of Medicine and Health Sciences, Stellenbosch University, Tygerberg 7505, South Africa

Correspondence: gwalzl@sun.ac.za

The discovery of tuberculosis (TB) biomarkers is an important goal in current TB research, because the availability of such markers would have significant impact on TB prevention and treatment. Correlates of protection would greatly facilitate vaccine development and evaluation, whereas correlates of TB disease risk would facilitate early diagnosis and help installing early or preventive treatment. Currently, no such markers are available. This review describes several strategies that are currently being pursued to identify TB biomarkers and places these in a clinical context. The approaches discussed include both targeted and untargeted hypothesis-free strategies. Among the first are the measurements of specific biomarkers in antigen-stimulated peripheral blood, in serum or plasma, and detailed immune cell phenotyping. Among the latter are proteomic, genomic, and transcriptomic (mRNA, miRNA) approaches. Recent and promising developments are described.

KEY CLINICAL IMMUNOLOGICAL ASPECTS OF TUBERCULOSIS

Three to eight weeks after initial infection with *Mycobacterium tuberculosis* (*Mtb*), cell-mediated immunity develops. This is characterized by a delayed type hypersensitivity reaction, which forms the basis for a positive reaction to the tuberculin skin test. The majority of infected individuals contain the infection (latent tuberculosis), but in ~10% active tuberculosis (TB) disease develops. It is thought that latent and active tuberculosis are not two separate states, but rather a continuum of host and pathogen interactions with a spectrum of immune responses (Barry et al. 2009).

The underlying immunology of protection against TB is not fully understood and certainly involves both innate and adaptive responses; however, T helper 1 (Th1) cell-mediated immune responses appear to play a major role (Ottenhoff 2012a; Ottenhoff and Kaufmann 2012). The initial infection is dominated by a Th1-type immune response; however, if the infection is not contained, a gradual shift toward T helper 2 responses occurs (Fletcher

[3]Authorship in alphabetical order.

Cite this article as *Cold Spring Harb Perspect Med* doi: 10.1101/cshperspect.a018515

2007). Th1 cells are activated and proliferate in response to interleukin-12 (IL-12) produced by *Mtb*-infected macrophages, as well as other cytokines released by antigen-presenting cells such as IL-18 and IL-23 (Raja 2004). Activated Th1 cells are the major source of interferon-γ (IFN-γ), which is crucial for macrophage activation and containment of the infection. At this stage, elimination of *Mtb* before establishment of adaptive immunity is possible; however, *Mtb* has evolved immune evasion mechanisms that allow the bacteria to survive in the host for prolonged periods (Flynn and Chan 2003; Ottenhoff 2012b).

The importance of the IL-12/IL-23/IFN-γ axis for protective immunity against mycobacteria is discussed in the section Primary Immune Deficiency and Mendelian Susceptibility to Mycobacterial Diseases. However, despite the importance of IFN-γ, this cytokine alone is not sufficient for protection. Tumor necrosis factor-α (TNF-α), which induces chemokine secretion from macrophages, is equally important in controlling primary infection by supporting the formation of granulomas. Individuals treated with TNF-α receptor antagonists for rheumatologic diseases frequently suffer from reactivation TB, highlighting the importance of this cytokine in containment of mycobacteria (Dietrich and Doherty 2009). Although TNF-α is required for protection, high IL-4 levels together with TNF-α appear to promote immunopathology (Dietrich and Doherty 2009). In fact, IL-4 levels directly correlate with severity of disease. Similarly, IFN-γ and IL-2Rα are present at higher levels in bronchoalveolar lavages (BALs) from TB patients with severe disease than in those from moderate TB disease cases (Jo et al. 2003). Cytokines can give an indication not only to the severity of pathology, but also to the type of active TB. Patients with pleural TB generally have elevated levels of markers of systemic inflammation such as IL-6 and IL-8, whereas patients with classical pulmonary TB tend to have increased levels of cytokines associated with cell-mediated immunity (IL-12p40, sCD40L) (Djoba Siawaya et al. 2009b).

Other T-cell subsets playing an important role during *Mtb* infection are Th17 cells, which facilitate the recruitment of Th1 cells to the site of disease (Khader et al. 2007) and regulatory T cells (Tregs), which control excessive immunopathology (Joosten and Ottenhoff 2008; Green et al. 2010). Our understanding of immune responses against TB, however, remains incomplete, because, for example, the importance of B cells is not well-defined, despite their presence in granulomas. Apart from B and T cells, other cell subsets also play a role during *Mtb* infection including myeloid-derived cells. Myeloid-derived suppressor cells (MDSCs) suppress T-cell function in cancer biology (Gorgun et al. 2013) and infectious diseases (Qin et al. 2013), including TB (du Plessis et al. 2013). MDSCs are present in higher frequencies and suppress T-cell activation and trafficking in TB patients and in individuals recently infected with *Mtb* (du Plessis et al. 2013).

PRIMARY IMMUNE DEFICIENCY AND MENDELIAN SUSCEPTIBILITY TO MYCOBACTERIAL DISEASES

Although TB occurs most commonly in immunocompetent individuals in high-transmission settings and in acquired immunodeficient people due to HIV coinfection (or less commonly in people with diabetes mellitus or other systemic disorders), primary immune deficiency may present with disease because of less virulent mycobacteria or with unusual presentations of infection with *Mtb*. A group of inherited deficiencies in the immune system that are associated with increased susceptibility to mycobacterial diseases is collectively known as primary immune deficiency (PID) diseases. Among these, a high level of genetic heterogeneity exists in syndromes referred to as Mendelian susceptibility to mycobacterial diseases (MSMD) (Ottenhoff et al. 2002; reviewed in Al-Muhsen and Casanova 2008). MSMD is a rare mostly congenital syndrome, which confers a predisposition to mycobacterial infections caused by weakly virulent mycobacteria such as BCG (Bacillus Calmette–Guérin) vaccines and nontuberculous environmental mycobacteria (NTMs) as well as virulent mycobacterial species such as *Mtb*. Mutations in six MSMD-causing genes have been identified, and these genes include an X-linked gene (nuclear factor-κB-essential modulator [*NEMO*]) and five autosomal genes (IFN-γ receptor 1 and 2 [*IFNGR1, IFNGR2*], signal transducer and activator of transcription 1 [*STAT1*], IL-12p40 subunit [*IL12B*], and IL-12 receptor β-subunit [*IL12RB1*]) (reviewed in Al-Muhsen and Casanova 2008). Mutations in these genes either prevent or result in the dysfunctional expression of the encoded proteins. Patients with these mutations often present with a severe clinical phenotype, causing early and often fatal mycobacterial infections. IFNγR1 deficiency results histologically in lepromatous-type granulomas, which are poorly differentiated. These granulomas contain relatively few giant cells and lymphocytes, but they do contain abundant macrophages with high bacillary loads. Affected patients with partial IFNγR1 deficiency display less severe clinical disease phenotypes than patients completely deficient for IFNγR1 (Ottenhoff et al. 2002; reviewed in Al-Muhsen and Casanova 2008). NEMO and STAT1 mutations are associated with several infectious diseases, with a spectrum extending beyond mycobacteria, including fungal, bacterial, and viral infections (reviewed in Al-Muhsen and Casanova 2008; Lee et al. 2011). Monocytes from patients with X-linked recessive NEMO deficiency have an intrinsic defect in T-cell-dependent IL-12 production, which leads to impaired IFN-γ production by T cells. In the X-linked MSMD syndrome chronic granulomatous disease (CGD) mutations in the CYBB gene result in a diminished respiratory burst (release of reactive oxygen species mediated by NADPH oxidase) in monocyte-derived macrophages, but not in monocytes or granulocytes (Bustamante et al. 2011). Other PID diseases enhancing susceptibility to severe mycobacterial infections can be caused by autosomal dominant mutations in the interferon regulatory factor 8 (IRF8) as well as the excessive production of neutralizing autoantibodies to IFN-γ. These disorders result in the depletion of circulating monocytes and dendritic cells and block downstream mediators of IFN-γ, respectively, highlighting the importance of these cells and mediators in antimycobacterial immunity (Lee et al. 2011).

Mycobacterium bovis BCG can cause life-threatening diseases in children with PIDs like MSMD and severe combined immunodeficiencies (SCID). The most common initial presentation is the development of persistent ulcerations at the BCG inoculation site followed by systemic dissemination that can present as osteomyelitis, pneumonia, bone marrow involvement, and hepatosplenic abscesses (Ottenhoff et al. 2002; reviewed in Lee and Lau 2013). BCG-related complications soon after birth might therefore provide early warning of possible underlying immunodeficiencies before more serious infections take root.

Two steps are important for the successful treatment of MSMD. First, the underlying gene mutations responsible for the impaired immunity need to be ascertained and, second, the causative microorganism needs to be identified. Cytokine neutralization assays may point to the presence of anticytokine autoantibodies, and flow cytometry and gene sequencing (polymerase chain reaction [PCR]) can detect defects in candidate markers or receptors (van de Vosse et al. 2004; Wang et al. 2012). Oligonucleotide arrays could serve as rapid and useful alternative methods to identify mycobacteria because characterization can be completed within hours, in contrast to mycobacterial culture which could take up to several weeks (Wang et al. 2012).

IMPORTANCE OF DEVELOPING IMMUNOLOGIC TB BIOMARKERS FOR EARLY (DEVELOPING) DISEASE

Up to now, sputum smear and culture, and more recently the GeneXpert MTB/RIF (mycobacterium TB/rifampicin) tests, are the most frequently used sputum-based diagnostic tests to detect active TB disease. Sputum smear requires 10,000 bacteria/mL and has a relatively low sensitivity of 24% (Davies and Pai 2008). Although sputum culture is more sensitive, with a sensitivity of 40%, and can detect as little as 150 bacteria/mL, it can take up to 2 mo to obtain culture results (Horne et al. 2010). The PCR-based GeneXpert MTB/RIF test can be performed within 2 h with a sensitivity of >98% in smear-positive pulmonary TB and 68% in smear-negative TB, and at the same time, it detects rifampicin resistance (Boehme et al. 2010; Steingart et al. 2013). However, all of these diagnostic tests require an *Mtb*-positive sputum, and many active TB patients, including but not exclusively HIV-positive individuals, diabetes patients, and children, often do not present with *Mtb*-positive sputum (Bacakoglu et al. 2001; Walzl et al. 2011). Similarly, extrapulmonary disease is characterized by *Mtb*-negative sputum.

In addition to diagnosing TB through the detection of mycobacteria or their products in body fluids, immune responses of the host to mycobacterial antigens have been exploited for diagnostic tests. The tuberculin skin test (TST) measures a delayed-type hypersensitivity reaction at the injection site and IFN-γ release assays (IGRAs) measure IFN-γ secretion of peripheral blood cells to mycobacterial antigens. However, detection of immune reactivity against *Mtb* may also be the result of vaccination, latent infection with TB, or infection with nontuberculous mycobacteria and does not prove TB disease.

For this reason, identification of biomarkers that can reliably distinguish between latent TB infection and active TB disease (as well as vaccination or NTM infection) is of utmost importance, particularly because early detection of active TB is crucial to stop transmission of *Mtb* and thus reduce TB incidence rates. Therefore, there is currently an actively ongoing search for other types of TB biomarkers. Biomarkers of disease progression would provide insights in which latently infected individuals are likely to progress to active TB. Once identified, these individuals can be closely monitored or offered prophylactic therapy. In addition, there is a search for biomarkers of treatment response, which would allow stratification of patients into different treatment options, including shortened, standard, or prolonged courses of antibiotic therapy. Biomarkers of treatment response would thus contribute to reducing drug resistance due to nonadherence and also improve the validation of novel TB drugs and shorten clinical trials. Markers of treatment failure and relapse would accelerate recognition of poor outcomes, regardless of whether this is due to poor adherence, drug resistance, ineffective drugs in a clinical trial, or host factors that increase susceptibility. Therefore, not only diagnostic markers but also biomarkers of disease progression, infection status, treatment response, and treatment outcome would provide critical tools in the global fight against TB. Finally, biomarkers of protection against TB disease would be very useful in distinguishing protected from potential disease susceptible individuals, as well as be of tremendous value in TB vaccine trials, because such correlates of protection could predict in an early stage whether or not the administered vaccine would be protective. This could dramatically, shorten TB vaccine trials. Ideally, such correlates should work also in the immunocompromised (HIV-coinfected individuals) or in comorbidities such as type 2 diabetes.

Below, we discuss various strategies that are currently followed in the global TB research community to discover and refine TB biomarkers for the key phenotypes discussed above.

PROTEIN-BASED APPROACHES TO TB BIOMARKER DISCOVERY

Targeted Approaches

Biomarkers in Antigen-Stimulated Peripheral Blood

IGRAs determine the release of IFN-γ after stimulation of peripheral whole blood or peripheral blood mononuclear cells (PBMCs) in response to *Mtb*-specific antigens (ESAT6, CFP10, TB7.7) (Lalvani et al. 2001; Mori et al. 2004). These assays have become the gold standard for assessing infection with *Mtb* rather than the less specific TST (tuberculin skin test) (Janssens 2007). IGRAs are not able to distinguish between latent and active TB; however, although interestingly, a substantial increase of IFN-γ production has been reported in latently infected individuals shortly before diagnosis of TB (Diel et al. 2008; Higuchi et al. 2008). Antigen-stimulated multicytokine signatures, however, can differentiate between latent and active TB in adults. In *Mtb* infection phase-dependent antigen-stimulated whole-blood cultures, multiple cytokines other than IFN-γ showed diagnostic potential (Chegou et al. 2012). Similarly in

QuantiFERON tube supernatants, levels of epidermal growth factor (EGF), soluble CD40 ligand (sCD40L), macrophage inflammatory protein-1β (MIP-1β), vascular endothelial growth factor (VEGF), transforming growth factor-α (TGF-α), and IL-1α could differentiate between latent and active TB (Chegou et al. 2009). Even in HIV-positive and -negative children, a diagnostically challenging population group, the levels of IFN-α2, IL-1Ra, sCD40L, IP-10 (interferon-induced protein-10), and VEGF in QuantiFERON supernatant proved useful in differentiating active and latent TB (Chegou et al. 2013).

Biomarkers in Serum and Plasma

Biomarkers measured directly in serum or plasma without additional antigen stimulation would reduce the time to test results and thus offers a distinct advantage. Multicytokine signatures in serum have indeed been found to be useful for the differentiation between latent and active TB. Plasma concentrations of EGF, fractalkine, IFN-γ, IL-4, MCP-3 (monocyte chemoattractant protein-3), and IP-10 were found to be significantly different between TB patients and healthy household contacts (Mihret et al. 2013). An earlier study showed that serum levels of proinflammatory cytokines IL-6 and IP-10 were significantly lower in latently infected individuals than in TB patients, whereas MCP-1 levels were higher (Djoba Siawaya et al. 2009a). Cytokine profiles during early TB treatment were also able to predict month-2 culture conversion and hold promise in predicting treatment outcome and future relapse (Walzl et al. 2011; K Ronacher, unpubl.). Plasma granulysin levels also correlate with treatment response (plasma granulysin levels and cellular IFN-γ production correlate with curative host responses in TB, whereas plasma IFN-γ levels correlate with TB disease activity in adults) (Sahiratmadja et al. 2007).

Plasma levels of markers involved in the Toll-like receptor 4 pathway, like soluble CD14 (sCD14) and myeloid differentiation-2 (MD-2), have furthermore been shown to differentiate between latently infected individuals and TB patients (Feruglio et al. 2013).

Immune Cell Phenotyping

Polychromatic flow cytometry is often used to measure different cell surface markers and intracellular cytokine production, allowing for the characterization of different types of immune cells. Phenotyping of immune cells using this approach has shown that different T-cell subsets can differentiate between latent and active TB. *Mtb*-specific $CD4^+$ and $CD8^+$ T-cell subsets secreting TNF-α only, IFN-γ only, and dual TNF-α/IFN-γ appear in higher frequencies in TB patients compared with latently infected individuals (Pollock et al. 2013). $CD4^+$ T cells from individuals latently infected are polyfunctional and express TNF-α, IFN-γ, and IL-2 compared with the dominant TNF-α-only response of TB patients (Harari et al. 2011). During active disease, *Mtb*-specific $CD4^+$ T cells also switch from central to effector memory T cells, which are accompanied by a decrease in IL-7 receptor α expression (Pollock et al. 2013). PPD-specific TNF-α-only secreting $CD4^+$ T cells with an effector memory phenotype might therefore discriminate active disease and latent TB infection (LTBI) with promising accuracy.

Untargeted Approaches and New Technologies

Untargeted approaches can include transcriptomic, proteomic, or metabolomic approaches. Transcriptomic approaches will be discussed in detail in the section Transcriptomic Approaches to TB Biomarker Discovery, whereas the current section will focus on protein-based untargeted approaches. Proteomic profiling by mass spectrometry or protein chip technology allows for nontargeted screening of large numbers of peptides between TB patients and controls. Proteomic fingerprinting of serum for host markers identified three markers (transthyretin, C-reactive protein [CRP], and neopterin) that could discriminate with high accuracy between TB patients and controls with other infectious and inflammatory conditions (Agranoff et al. 2006). Similarly, serum proteomic profiles could differentiate sputum smear-negative and smear-positive TB patients from controls with reasonable accuracy (Liu et al. 2010). High-throughput screening was also applied to detect antibodies in sera against antigens from culture filtrate (Sartain et al. 2006) and later to the entire *Mtb* proteome (Kunnath-Velayudhan et al. 2010) and identified a small pool of antibodies with diagnostic potential.

A novel highly multiplexed proteomic technique has recently been applied in the search for TB treatment response markers. De Groote et al. (2013) used an unbiased proteomic analysis approach using *SOMA*mers (slow off-rate modified aptamers) to identify protein markers associated with active TB and to determine alterations in their expression levels in response to TB treatment. Serum concentrations of serum amyloid A (SAA) and CRP were shown to decrease from baseline to week 8 of anti-TB treatment, whereas serum albumin levels increased. Some serum markers—CRP, SAA, and NPS-PLA2—were able to distinguish TB patients based on their disease severity before or shortly after initiation of treatment.

Nontargeted metabolomic approaches have led to the discovery of metabolic profiles that correlate with different TB disease states and anti-TB treatment outcome. Although metabolomic approaches will be discussed in detail in a separate article, it is nevertheless important to note that biosignatures of small-molecule molecular features (MFs) have been identified in urine sample of TB patients using mass spectrometry (Mahapatra et al. 2014). In these samples, levels of 45 MFs changed significantly by month 1 of anti-TB treatment, with levels of 23 MFs consistently changing in abundance until the end of treatment (Mahapatra et al. 2014). This approach of identifying urine-based anti-TB treatment response biosignatures serves as proof of concept for further metabolomics investigations.

TRANSCRIPTOMIC APPROACHES TO TB BIOMARKER DISCOVERY

A Meta-Like Analysis of Genome-Wide Approaches Used to Identify TB Biomarkers of Disease and Early Disease Progression

Early detection of active TB infection is key toward better control of the TB pandemic, because it would allow initiation of curative treatment before TB transmission can occur. However, the early identification of "asymptomatic" TB progressors remains a major challenge. Current diagnostic tools rely on detecting live *Mtb* (bacterial cultures, *Mtb* DNA) in samples from individuals that present with already active disease, which in all likelihood have already transmitted infection. Approaches are needed to identify biomarkers that predict, or detect at a very early stage, the risk of developing active TB disease.

A number of recent studies have attempted to identify biomarkers of TB disease by performing unbiased genome-wide human gene expression studies. These studies mostly relied on peripheral blood samples from patients with active (pulmonary) TB disease directly after diagnosis and contrasted gene expression profiles to those of healthy (infected) controls or patients with other inflammatory/pulmonary disorders (Jacobsen et al. 2007; Mistry et al. 2007; Berry et al. 2010; Maertzdorf et al. 2011a,b, 2012; Ottenhoff et al. 2012; Bloom et al. 2013; Cliff et al. 2013; Kaforou et al. 2013). Each individual study performed extensive data analysis to identify key signatures that could discriminate TB disease from the respective control group(s). The studies used either unseparated peripheral blood or isolated leucocytes thereof to study TB disease–related gene expression profiles, although the blood is not the primary site of TB disease. Despite the rather limited sample sizes of most individual studies, the studies were able to identify active TB disease–associated signatures and could link these to known biological pathways and processes. IFN-α/β signaling was found to be a key process in TB disease; it was first identified by Berry et al. (2010) and subsequently confirmed in several other studies. IFN-α/β signaling had been known mostly for its association with intracellular viral infections. The activation of similar signaling pathways by *Mtb* and viruses reveals the activation of overlapping intracellular response pathways triggered by quite diverse microbial danger signals. The upstream events triggering IFN-α/β signaling in TB are incompletely defined as yet.

 Cite this article as *Cold Spring Harb Perspect Med* doi: 10.1101/cshperspect.a018515

We recently performed a combined analysis of all human genes identified by the above-cited published genome-wide gene expression studies (except the studies by Kaforou et al. 2013 and Anderson et al. 2014, which were not available at the time of our analysis), aiming to assess potentially novel pathways involved in TB pathogenesis (Joosten et al. 2013). The combination of all genes identified to be associated with TB disease by the individual studies resulted in a gene set of 409 genes. Subsequent combined modular analysis (Chaussabel et al. 2008), ingenuity-based pathway analysis, and gene set enrichment analysis (GSEA) resulted in the identification of several novel pathways associated with TB pathogenesis. Somewhat surprisingly, analysis of the combined data did not yield IFN-α/β signaling as the strongest process in TB disease. Instead, a strong myeloid-derived inflammatory signature was found to be of particular importance. Myeloid-related processes that were strongly represented in the data set included signaling through pattern recognition receptors, FcR activation, and enhanced communication between innate and adaptive immune cells. In addition, we identified the TREM-1 (triggering receptor expressed on myeloid cells) signaling pathway as a potential new target pathway involved in TB. Increased secretion of TREM-1 has been described in the lungs of patients with TB, although this was not unique for infection with *Mtb* (Richeldi et al. 2004; Chan et al. 2007; Tintinger et al. 2012). In addition, B-cell activation was identified to be important for TB disease pathogenesis, and indeed B cells have been identified in human TB lesions but their function in TB pathogenesis and protective immunity remains largely unknown (Ulrichs et al. 2004). As a next step, in-depth studies are needed to unravel the potential role of TREM-1 signaling, FcR signaling, and B cells in TB. Functional and gene/protein expression studies will help in determining the role of these cells and molecules in infection and decipher new pathways involved in TB disease pathogenesis. These insights should provide a more rational basis for identifying biomarkers of TB disease risk and early progression.

MicroRNA-Based Profiling as a New Nontargeted Approach

Nontargeted approaches such as RNA sequencing, including the identification of host microRNA (miRNA) signatures, can contribute to the discovery of biomarkers for pulmonary tuberculosis. An miRNA signature in serum, consisting of 15 miRNAs, could potentially discriminate patients with pulmonary TB from individuals with latent TB and was able to categorize them with a diagnostic accuracy of 82% (Miotto et al. 2013). Zhang et al. (2013) furthermore identified six serum miRNAs that had a sensitivity and specificity of 95% and 92%, respectively, to diagnose TB. miRNAs shown to contribute to biomarker signatures in TB patients include, among others, let-7e, miR-29c, miR-146a, miR-148a, miR-178, miR-192, miR-193a-5p, miR-365, miR-378, and miR-483 (Miotto et al. 2013; Zhang et al. 2013).

Focused Transcriptomic Approaches to Identify TB Biomarkers of Disease and Early Disease Progression

Quantitative changes in RNA expression levels to identify TB biomarkers are currently primarily being analyzed using hypothesis-free genome-wide (microarray/RNA-Seq) screening methods at the transcriptomic level (see subsection A Meta-Like Analysis of Genome-Wide Approaches Used to Identify TB Biomarkers of Disease and Early Disease Progression). However, because TB biomarker signatures identifying those infected individuals that are at risk of progressing to active TB (vs. those whose immune system will effectively contain the infection) will most likely encompass a limited set of multiple gene transcripts, neither genome-wide (microarray/RNA-Seq) nor single-gene (real-time PCR) approaches are ideally suited to develop practically useful TB biomarker assays. Furthermore, microarray analysis, RNA-Seq, and real-time PCR are technically challenging and too costly to be applied on a routine basis in resource-poor settings.

To identify and monitor multicomponent host biomarker signatures in large human cohort studies, techniques have been developed that combine sets of markers at the transcriptomic level. Fluidigm, for example, provides high-throughput real-time quantitative PCR based on proprietary microfluidic chips (Rahimov et al. 2012). These gene expression assays are commercially available, but they are still costly and require specialized equipment not routinely available in laboratories in most TB-endemic areas. In contrast, dual-color reverse-transcriptase multiplex ligation-dependent probe amplification (dcRT-MLPA) is an inexpensive and robust technique permitting rapid and accurate RNA expression profiling of as many as 90 transcripts in a single reaction. As the assay is high-throughput, it is exceptionally suited to determine biomarker signatures on a population scale. We have used dcRT-MLPA to characterize the human immune response in the peripheral blood during TB infection as well as in the response to curative treatment in several cohort studies in genetically and geographically diverse populations (Sutherland et al. 2011, 2013; Joosten et al. 2012). Biomarker signatures were identified and validated with excellent classifying values between TB cases versus healthy infected or uninfected controls. Biomarkers within the signatures included apoptosis-related genes and T-cell/B-cell markers, suggesting important contributions of adaptive immunity to TB pathogenesis (Joosten et al. 2012). In a follow-up study with 523 participants across four sub-Saharan countries (Ethiopia, Malawi, South Africa, and The Gambia), differing also in TB and HIV status, we found a number of genes to be expressed at lower levels in active diseased compared with latently infected individuals, which normalized during treatment. A remarkably consistent classifier of active disease appeared to be the high-affinity IgG Fc receptor 1 FCGR1A (CD64), which was expressed at significantly higher levels in active TB regardless of HIV status or genetic background (Sutherland et al. 2013).

The classifying value of the identified biomarker signatures may be further enhanced in future studies by including markers derived from recent microarray studies highlighting a potential role for type I IFN-αβ signaling pathways (Berry et al. 2010) and/or myeloid-derived inflammatory pathways (Joosten et al. 2013). Moreover, probing immunological differences between TB progressors and nonprogressors at early time points after contact with a TB case identified several markers that may predict the onset of active TB at a very early stage after infection (Sutherland et al. 2011). Once these markers have been validated in larger studies, they will provide an initial platform to prospectively identify people at risk of developing TB.

BRIDGING FOCUSED ("BIASED") AND GENOME-WIDE ("UNBIASED") APPROACHES: TOWARD TB DISEASE–SPECIFIC BIOMARKER SIGNATURES

From the genome-wide host gene expression studies discussed above and in Maertzdorf et al. (2014), it is evident that a predominantly inflammatory signature is detectable during active TB disease. This signature is detectable systemically, probably reflecting dynamic leukocyte trafficking through the inflamed lung tissue. Indeed, TB granulomas are highly dynamic structures with significant cellular influx and efflux. Although the robust inflammatory signature in TB is rather unsurprising, an important issue is that this signature is shared with many other inflammatory disorders, including sarcoidosis (which poses a differential diagnostic dilemma for TB and nontuberculous mycobacteria [NTM] pulmonary disease) as well as melioidosis, which is caused by the intracellular bacterial pathogen *Burkholderia pseudomallei* (Koh et al. 2013). The 86-gene signature, which was initially believed to be specific for TB because it was absent from individuals with *Staphylococcus aureus* or *Streptococcus pyogenes* infections or those affected by autoimmune disease (SLE [systemic lupus erythematosus] and Still's disease) (Berry et al. 2010), was later found to be present also in melioidosis and sarcoidosis patients (Maertzdorf et al. 2012; Koh et al. 2013). Thus, the IFN-α/β signaling signature in itself is unlikely to be of clinical diagnostic relevance in TB, although it might be of value as part of a diagnostic signature identifying individuals as early TB progressors. Kaforou et al. (2013) identified a diagnostic, active TB disease-specific signature based on a limited number of host genes, mostly distinct from the IFN-α/β signaling cascade (see below).

The different nature of the diseases with a prominent IFN-α/β signaling signature (viral and bacterial vs. infection; bacterial infection vs. autoimmune/inflammatory disease) would suggest that more discriminatory signatures should be identifiable. Such more specific signatures might be obscured by the overwhelmingly present inflammatory phenotype. One way to uncover these more specific signatures is through antigen-specific stimulation approaches, such as discussed in the sections Importance of Developing Immunologic TB Biomarkers for Early (Developing) Disease and Protein-Based Approaches to TB Biomarker Discovery. The stimulation of blood cells by *Mtb* lysates, BCG, recombinant protein or lipid antigens, or peptides could strongly enrich for antigen-specific disease-related immune reactivity. These responses can be profiled at the level of the expression of genes, proteins, or metabolic products or changes in cell phenotype and function. Sources could encompass unseparated blood cells, offering the advantage that all cell types are represented, including those with less-defined but possibly important roles in anti-TB immunity. These include, besides T cells, also B cells, natural killer (NK) cells, natural killer T (NKT) cells, mucosal-associated invariant T (MAIT) cells, innate lymphoid cells (ILCs), different myeloid cell subsets (monocytes, dendritic cells, neutrophils), and other less conventional circulating cells. Alternatively, but not mutually exclusive, isolated purified cell subsets can be analyzed to dissect more precisely *Mtb*-stimulation- or infection-induced events in key cell types. When biomarkers are identified through such approaches, new algorithms can be developed to mine data from genome-wide whole-blood transcriptomic data sets to analyze selectively immunity-related specific key genes or pathways.

Another, complementary focused strategy to identify TB biomarkers is to select markers involved in specific pathways known to play important roles in TB control. These encompass both adaptive immunity–related markers, including Th1, Th2, Th17, and Treg subsets (e.g., transcriptional regulators, hallmark effector cytokines), as well as innate signaling and autophagy pathway markers (see, e.g., the subsections Targeted Approaches and Biomarkers in Serum and Plasma). Although not studied directly in an antigen-specific setting, the fact that these cells and pathways play important roles in TB infection and pathogenesis enhances their plausibility of delivering new biomarkers and significant signatures.

CONCLUDING REMARKS AND PERSPECTIVE

New approaches to TB biomarker discovery seem to start yielding promising results. A major and challenging next step now is to translate basic biomarker discovery into clinically useful algorithms that can be applied in the field, using relatively simple tests. Second, such algorithms should be able to distinguish between (early) TB, latent TB, and other diseases that pose a diagnostic dilemma because they present as entities with TB in the differential diagnosis. A third and major challenge is that these algorithms should also work in the immunocompromised, as many TB cases are HIV-coinfected. In a recent study, which was conducted in South Africa and Malawi, important progress was made in each of these areas (Kaforou et al. 2013). Blood transcriptional signatures were identified that were able to distinguish TB from other diseases prevalent in both HIV-uninfected and HIV-infected African adults. These other diseases included patients with other (mostly pulmonary infectious) disorders in which TB was considered in the differential diagnosis but then excluded. The diagnostic signatures were robust and were validated in other data sets, including those of Berry et al. (2010). Subsequently, minimal sets of genes were selected that could robustly differentiate between TB, LTBI, and other diseases in both HIV-infected and HIV-uninfected individuals. Using a set of 27 genes, it was possible to accurately identify

TB versus LTBI, and a set of 44 genes was able to differentiate TB from other diseases. A disease risk score was developed that can now be developed into a simple test format suitable for use in HIV-infected TB populations. A more recent study extended this work also to TB-infected infants, with similar results in terms of the identification of useful diagnostic TB disease mRNA biosignature (Anderson et al. 2014). Prospective studies using such tests are now needed to validate their actual performance. Nevertheless, these transcriptomic signatures in any case are highly promising and have the potential to translate new TB biomarkers to clinically relevant settings where these tests (e.g., Joosten et al. 2012) are urgently needed.

ACKNOWLEDGMENTS

We gratefully acknowledge the support of the following organizations: The Netherlands Organization of Scientific Research (NWO); the European Commission (grants to IDEA, ADITEC, NEWTBVAC, EURIPRED, TANDEM); The Bill & Melinda Gates Foundation Grand Challenges in Global Health (grants GC6#74 and GC12#82); the European & Developing Countries Clinical Trials Partnership (EDCTP) (grant to AE-TBC, EDCTP IP. 09.32040.011); The South African Medical Research Council (MRC), and National Research Foundation (NRF), as well as the DST/NRF Centre of Excellence for Biomedical Tuberculosis Research. The funders had no role in study design, data collection and analysis, decision to publish, or preparation of the manuscript. We thank all members of our laboratories for their support.

REFERENCES

Reference is also in this subject collection.

Agranoff D, Fernandez-Reyes D, Papadopoulos MC, Rojas SA, Herbster M, Loosemore A, Tarelli E, Sheldon J, Schwenk A, Pollok R, et al. 2006. Identification of diagnostic markers for tuberculosis by proteomic fingerprinting of serum. *Lancet* **368:** 1012–1021.

Al-Muhsen S, Casanova JL. 2008. The genetic heterogeneity of Mendelian susceptibility to mycobacterial diseases. *J Allergy Clin Immunol* **122:** 1043–1051; quiz 1052–1053.

Anderson ST, Kaforou M, Brent AJ, Wright VJ, Banwell CM, Chagaluka G, Crampin AC, Dockrell HM, French N, Hamilton MS, et al. 2014. Diagnosis of childhood TB in African countries by host RNA expression. *N Engl J Med* **370:** 1712–1723.

Bacakoglu F, Basoglu OK, Cok G, Sayiner A, Ates M. 2001. Pulmonary tuberculosis in patients with diabetes mellitus. *Respiration* **68:** 595–600.

Barry CE, 3rd, Boshoff HI, Dartois V, Dick T, Ehrt S, Flynn J, Schnappinger D, Wilkinson RJ, Young D. 2009. The spectrum of latent tuberculosis: Rethinking the biology and intervention strategies. *Nat Rev Microbiol* **7:** 845–855.

Berry MP, Graham CM, McNab FW, Xu Z, Bloch SA, Oni T, Wilkinson KA, Banchereau R, Skinner J, Wilkinson RJ, et al. 2010. An interferon-inducible neutrophil-driven blood transcriptional signature in human tuberculosis. *Nature* **466:** 973–977.

Bloom CI, Graham CM, Berry MP, Rozakeas F, Redford PS, Wang Y, Xu Z, Wilkinson KA, Wilkinson RJ, Kendrick Y, et al. 2013. Transcriptional blood signatures distinguish pulmonary tuberculosis, pulmonary sarcoidosis, pneumonias and lung cancers. *PLoS ONE* **8:** e70630.

Boehme CC, Nabeta P, Hillemann D, Nicol MP, Shenai S, Krapp F, Allen J, Tahirli R, Blakemore R, Rustomjee R, et al. 2010. Rapid molecular detection of tuberculosis and rifampin resistance. *N Engl J Med* **363:** 1005–1015.

Bustamante J, Arias AA, Vogt G, Picard C, Galicia LB, Prando C, Grant AV, Marchal CC, Hubeau M, Chapgier A, et al. 2011. Germline CYBB mutations that selectively affect macrophages in kindreds with X-linked predisposition to tuberculous mycobacterial disease. *Nat Immunol* **12:** 213–221.

Chan MC, Chang KM, Chao WC, Lin LY, Kuo BI, Hsu JY, Wu CL. 2007. Evaluation of a new inflammatory molecule (triggering receptor expressed on myeloid cells-1) in the diagnosis of pleural effusion. *Respirology* **12:** 333–338.

Chaussabel D, Quinn C, Shen J, Patel P, Glaser C, Baldwin N, Stichweh D, Blankenship D, Li L, Munagala I, et al. 2008. A modular analysis framework for blood genomics studies: Application to systemic lupus erythematosus. *Immunity* **29:** 150–164.

Chegou NN, Black GF, Kidd M, van Helden PD, Walzl G. 2009. Host markers in QuantiFERON supernatants differentiate active TB from latent TB infection: Preliminary report. *BMC Pulm Med* **9:** 21.

Chegou NN, Essone PN, Loxton AG, Stanley K, Black GF, van der Spuy GD, van Helden PD, Franken KL, Parida SK, Klein MR, et al. 2012. Potential of host markers produced by infection phase-dependent antigen-stimulated cells for the diagnosis of tuberculosis in a highly endemic area. *PLoS ONE* **7:** e38501.

Chegou NN, Detjen AK, Thiart L, Walters E, Mandalakas AM, Hesseling AC, Walzl G. 2013. Utility of host markers detected in Quantiferon supernatants for the diagnosis of tuberculosis in children in a high-burden setting. *PLoS ONE* **8:** e64226.

Cliff JM, Lee JS, Constantinou N, Cho JE, Clark TG, Ronacher K, King EC, Lukey PT, Duncan K, Van Helden PD, et al. 2013. Distinct phases of blood gene expression pattern through tuberculosis treatment reflect modulation of the humoral immune response. *J Infect Dis* **207:** 18–29.

Davies PD, Pai M. 2008. The diagnosis and misdiagnosis of tuberculosis. *Int J Tuberc Lung Dis* **12:** 1226–1234.

De Groote MA, Nahid P, Jarlsberg L, Johnson JL, Weiner M, Muzanyi G, Janjic N, Sterling DG, Ochsner UA. 2013. Elucidating novel serum biomarkers associated with pulmonary tuberculosis treatment. *PLoS ONE* **8:** e61002.

Diel R, Loddenkemper R, Meywald-Walter K, Niemann S, Nienhaus A. 2008. Predictive value of a whole blood IFN-γ assay for the development of active tuberculosis disease after recent infection with *Mycobacterium tuberculosis*. *Am J Respir Crit Care Med* **177:** 1164–1170.

Dietrich J, Doherty TM. 2009. Interaction of *Mycobacterium tuberculosis* with the host: Consequences for vaccine development. *APMIS* **117:** 440–457.

Djoba Siawaya JF, Beyers N, van Helden P, Walzl G. 2009a. Differential cytokine secretion and early treatment response in patients with pulmonary tuberculosis. *Clin Exp Immunol* **156:** 69–77.

Djoba Siawaya JF, Chegou NN, van den Heuvel MM, Diacon AH, Beyers N, van Helden P, Walzl G. 2009b. Differential cytokine/chemokines and KL-6 profiles in patients with different forms of tuberculosis. *Cytokine* **47:** 132–136.

du Plessis N, Loebenberg L, Kriel M, von Groote-Bidlingmaier F, Ribechini E, Loxton AG, van Helden PD, Lutz MB, Walzl G. 2013. Increased frequency of myeloid-derived suppressor cells during active tuberculosis and after recent *Mycobacterium tuberculosis* infection suppresses T-cell function. *Am J Respir Crit Care Med* **188:** 724–732.

Feruglio SL, Troseid M, Damas JK, Kvale D, Dyrhol-Riise AM. 2013. Soluble markers of the Toll-like receptor 4 pathway differentiate between active and latent tuberculosis and are associated with treatment responses. *PLoS ONE* **8:** e69896.

Fletcher HA. 2007. Correlates of immune protection from tuberculosis. *Curr Mol Med* **7:** 319–325.

Flynn JL, Chan J. 2003. Immune evasion by *Mycobacterium tuberculosis*: Living with the enemy. *Curr Opin Immunol* **15:** 450–455.

Gorgun GT, Whitehill G, Anderson JL, Hideshima T, Maguire C, Laubach J, Raje N, Munshi NC, Richardson PG, Anderson KC. 2013. Tumor-promoting immune-suppressive myeloid-derived suppressor cells in the multiple myeloma microenvironment in humans. *Blood* **121:** 2975–2987.

Green AM, Mattila JT, Bigbee CL, Bongers KS, Lin PL, Flynn JL. 2010. CD4(+) regulatory T cells in a cynomolgus macaque model of *Mycobacterium tuberculosis* infection. *J Infect Dis* **202:** 533–541.

Harari A, Rozot V, Enders FB, Perreau M, Stalder JM, Nicod LP, Cavassini M, Calandra T, Blanchet CL, Jaton K, et al. 2011. Dominant TNF-α^+ *Mycobacterium tuberculosis*-specific $CD4^+$ T cell responses discriminate between latent infection and active disease. *Nat Med* **17:** 372–376.

Higuchi K, Harada N, Fukazawa K, Mori T. 2008. Relationship between whole-blood interferon-γ responses and the risk of active tuberculosis. *Tuberculosis (Edinb)* **88:** 244–248.

Horne DJ, Royce SE, Gooze L, Narita M, Hopewell PC, Nahid P, Steingart KR. 2010. Sputum monitoring during tuberculosis treatment for predicting outcome: Systematic review and meta-analysis. *Lancet Infect Dis* **10:** 387–394.

Jacobsen M, Repsilber D, Gutschmidt A, Neher A, Feldmann K, Mollenkopf HJ, Ziegler A, Kaufmann SH. 2007. Candidate biomarkers for discrimination between infection and disease caused by *Mycobacterium tuberculosis*. *J Mol Med (Berl)* **85:** 613–621.

Janssens JP. 2007. Interferon-γ release assay tests to rule out active tuberculosis. *Eur Respir J* **30:** 183–184; author reply 184–185.

Jo EK, Park JK, Dockrell HM. 2003. Dynamics of cytokine generation in patients with active pulmonary tuberculosis. *Curr Opin Infect Dis* **16:** 205–210.

Joosten SA, Ottenhoff TH. 2008. Human CD4 and CD8 regulatory T cells in infectious diseases and vaccination. *Hum Immunol* **69:** 760–770.

Joosten SA, Goeman JJ, Sutherland JS, Opmeer L, de Boer KG, Jacobsen M, Kaufmann SH, Finos L, Magis-Escurra C, Ota MO, et al. 2012. Identification of biomarkers for tuberculosis disease using a novel dual-color RT-MLPA assay. *Genes Immun* **13:** 71–82.

Joosten SA, Fletcher HA, Ottenhoff TH. 2013. A helicopter perspective on TB biomarkers: Pathway and process based analysis of gene expression data provides new insight into TB pathogenesis. *PLoS ONE* **8:** e73230.

Kaforou M, Wright VJ, Oni T, French N, Anderson ST, Bangani N, Banwell CM, Brent AJ, Crampin AC, Dockrell HM, et al. 2013. Detection of tuberculosis in HIV-infected and -uninfected African adults using whole blood RNA expression signatures: A case-control study. *PLoS Med* **10:** e1001538.

Khader SA, Bell GK, Pearl JE, Fountain JJ, Rangel-Moreno J, Cilley GE, Shen F, Eaton SM, Gaffen SL, Swain SL, et al. 2007. IL-23 and IL-17 in the establishment of protective pulmonary $CD4^+$ T cell responses after vaccination and during *Mycobacterium tuberculosis* challenge. *Nat Immunol* **8:** 369–377.

Koh GC, Schreiber MF, Bautista R, Maude RR, Dunachie S, Limmathurotsakul D, Day NP, Dougan G, Peacock SJ. 2013. Host responses to melioidosis and tuberculosis are both dominated by interferon-mediated signaling. *PLoS ONE* **8:** e54961.

Kunnath-Velayudhan S, Salamon H, Wang HY, Davidow AL, Molina DM, Huynh VT, Cirillo DM, Michel G, Talbot EA, Perkins MD, et al. 2010. Dynamic antibody responses to the *Mycobacterium tuberculosis* proteome. *Proc Natl Acad Sci* **107:** 14703–14708.

Lalvani A, Pathan AA, Durkan H, Wilkinson KA, Whelan A, Deeks JJ, Reece WH, Latif M, Pasvol G, Hill AV. 2001. Enhanced contact tracing and spatial tracking of *Mycobacterium tuberculosis* infection by enumeration of antigen-specific T cells. *Lancet* **357:** 2017–2021.

Lee PP, Lau YL. 2013. Endemic infections in Southeast Asia provide new insights to the phenotypic spectrum of primary immunodeficiency disorders. *Asian Pac J Allergy Immunol* **31:** 217–226.

Lee WI, Huang JL, Yeh KW, Jaing TH, Lin TY, Huang YC, Chiu CH. 2011. Immune defects in active mycobacterial diseases in patients with primary immunodeficiency diseases (PIDs). *J Formos Med Assoc* **110:** 750–758.

Liu Q, Chen X, Hu C, Zhang R, Yue J, Wu G, Li X, Wu Y, Wen F. 2010. Serum protein profiling of smear-positive and smear-negative pulmonary tuberculosis using SELDI-TOF mass spectrometry. *Lung* **188:** 15–23.

Maertzdorf J, Ota M, Repsilber D, Mollenkopf HJ, Weiner J, Hill PC, Kaufmann SH. 2011a. Functional correlations of pathogenesis-driven gene expression signatures in tuberculosis. *PLoS ONE* **6:** e26938.

Maertzdorf J, Repsilber D, Parida SK, Stanley K, Roberts T, Black G, Walzl G, Kaufmann SH. 2011b. Human gene expression profiles of susceptibility and resistance in tuberculosis. *Genes Immun* **12:** 15–22.

Maertzdorf J, Weiner J, 3rd, Mollenkopf HJ, Bauer T, Prasse A, Muller-Quernheim J, Kaufmann SH. 2012. Common patterns and disease-related signatures in tuberculosis and sarcoidosis. *Proc Natl Acad Sci* **109:** 7853–7858.

* Maertzdorf J, Kaufmann SHE, Weiner J III. 2014. Toward a unified biosignature for tuberculosis. *Cold Spring Harb Perspect Med* doi: 10.1101/cshperspect.a018531.

Mahapatra S, Hess AM, Johnson JL, Eisenach KD, Degroote MA, Gitta P, Joloba ML, Kaplan G, Walzl G, Boom WH, et al. 2014. A metabolic biosignature of early response to anti-tuberculosis treatment. *BMC Infect Dis* **14:** 53.

Mihret A, Bekele Y, Bobosha K, Kidd M, Aseffa A, Howe R, Walzl G. 2013. Plasma cytokines and chemokines differentiate between active disease and non-active tuberculosis infection. *J Infect* **66:** 357–365.

Miotto P, Mwangoka G, Valente IC, Norbis L, Sotgiu G, Bosu R, Ambrosi A, Codecasa LR, Goletti D, Matteelli A, et al. 2013. miRNA signatures in sera of patients with active pulmonary tuberculosis. *PLoS ONE* **8:** e80149.

Mistry R, Cliff JM, Clayton CL, Beyers N, Mohamed YS, Wilson PA, Dockrell HM, Wallace DM, van Helden PD, Duncan K, et al. 2007. Gene-expression patterns in whole blood identify subjects at risk for recurrent tuberculosis. *J Infect Dis* **195:** 357–365.

Mori T, Sakatani M, Yamagishi F, Takashima T, Kawabe Y, Nagao K, Shigeto E, Harada N, Mitarai S, Okada M, et al. 2004. Specific detection of tuberculosis infection: An interferon-γ-based assay using new antigens. *Am J Respir Crit Care Med* **170:** 59–64.

Ottenhoff TH. 2012a. The knowns and unknowns of the immunopathogenesis of tuberculosis. *Int J Tuberc Lung Dis* **16:** 1424–1432.

Ottenhoff TH. 2012b. New pathways of protective and pathological host defense to mycobacteria. *Trends Microbiol* **20:** 419–428.

Ottenhoff TH, Kaufmann SH. 2012. Vaccines against tuberculosis: Where are we and where do we need to go? *PLoS Pathog* **8:** e1002607.

Ottenhoff TH, Verreck FA, Lichtenauer-Kaligis EG, Hoeve MA, Sanal O, van Dissel JT. 2002. Genetics, cytokines and human infectious disease: Lessons from weakly pathogenic mycobacteria and salmonellae. *Nat Genet* **32:** 97–105.

Ottenhoff TH, Dass RH, Yang N, Zhang MM, Wong HE, Sahiratmadja E, Khor CC, Alisjahbana B, van Crevel R, Marzuki S, et al. 2012. Genome-wide expression profiling identifies type 1 interferon response pathways in active tuberculosis. *PLoS ONE* **7:** e45839.

Pollock KM, Whitworth HS, Montamat-Sicotte DJ, Grass L, Cooke GS, Kapembwa MS, Kon OM, Sampson RD, Taylor GP, Lalvani A. 2013. T-cell immunophenotyping distinguishes active from latent tuberculosis. *J Infect Dis* **208:** 952–968.

Qin A, Cai W, Pan T, Wu K, Yang Q, Wang N, Liu Y, Yan D, Hu F, Guo P, et al. 2013. Expansion of monocytic myeloid-derived suppressor cells dampens T cell function in HIV-1-seropositive individuals. *J Virol* **87:** 1477–1490.

Rahimov F, King OD, Leung DG, Bibat GM, Emerson CP Jr, Kunkel LM, Wagner KR. 2012. Transcriptional profiling in facioscapulohumeral muscular dystrophy to identify candidate biomarkers. *Proc Natl Acad Sci* **109:** 16234–16239.

Raja A. 2004. Immunology of tuberculosis. *Indian J Med Res* **120:** 213–232.

Richeldi L, Mariani M, Losi M, Maselli F, Corbetta L, Buonsanti C, Colonna M, Sinigaglia F, Panina-Bordignon P, Fabbri LM. 2004. Triggering receptor expressed on myeloid cells: Role in the diagnosis of lung infections. *Eur Respir J* **24:** 247–250.

Sahiratmadja E, Alisjahbana B, Buccheri S, Di Liberto D, de Boer T, Adnan I, van Crevel R, Klein MR, van Meijgaarden KE, Nelwan RH, et al. 2007. Plasma granulysin levels and cellular interferon-γ production correlate with curative host responses in tuberculosis, while plasma interferon-γ levels correlate with tuberculosis disease activity in adults. *Tuberculosis (Edinb)* **87:** 312–321.

Sartain MJ, Slayden RA, Singh KK, Laal S, Belisle JT. 2006. Disease state differentiation and identification of tuberculosis biomarkers via native antigen array profiling. *Mol Cell Proteomics* **5:** 2102–2113.

Steingart KR, Sohn H, Schiller I, Kloda LA, Boehme CC, Pai M, Dendukuri N. 2013. Xpert(R) MTB/RIF assay for pulmonary tuberculosis and rifampicin resistance in adults. *Cochrane Database Syst Rev* **1:** CD009593.

Sutherland JS, Hill PC, Adetifa IM, de Jong BC, Donkor S, Joosten SA, Opmeer L, Haks MC, Ottenhoff TH, Adegbola RA, et al. 2011. Identification of probable early-onset biomarkers for tuberculosis disease progression. *PLoS ONE* **6:** e25230.

Sutherland JS, Loxton AG, Haks MC, Kassa D, Ambrose L, Lee JS, Ran L, van Baarle D, Maertzdorf J, Howe R, et al. 2013. Differential gene expression of activating Fcγ receptor classifies active tuberculosis regardless of human immunodeficiency virus status or ethnicity. *Clin Microbiol Infect* **20:** O230–O238.

Tintinger GR, van der Merwe JJ, Fickl H, Rheeder P, Feldman C, Anderson R. 2012. Soluble triggering receptor expressed on myeloid cells in sputum of patients with community-acquired pneumonia or pulmonary tuberculosis: A pilot study. *Eur J Clin Microbiol Infect Dis* **31:** 73–76.

Ulrichs T, Kosmiadi GA, Trusov V, Jorg S, Pradl L, Titukhina M, Mishenko V, Gushina N, Kaufmann SH. 2004. Human tuberculous granulomas induce peripheral lymphoid follicle-like structures to orchestrate local host defence in the lung. *J Pathol* **204:** 217–228.

van de Vosse E, Hoeve MA, Ottenhoff TH. 2004. Human genetics of intracellular infectious diseases: Molecular and cellular immunity against mycobacteria and salmonellae. *Lancet Infect Dis* **4:** 739–749.

Walzl G, Ronacher K, Hanekom W, Scriba TJ, Zumla A. 2011. Immunological biomarkers of tuberculosis. *Nat Rev Immunol* **11:** 343–354.

Wang LH, Yen CL, Chang TC, Liu CC, Shieh CC. 2012. Impact of molecular diagnosis on treating Mendelian susceptibility to mycobacterial diseases. *J Microbiol Immunol Infect* **45:** 411–417.

Zhang X, Guo J, Fan S, Li Y, Wei L, Yang X, Jiang T, Chen Z, Wang C, Liu J, et al. 2013. Screening and identification of six serum microRNAs as novel potential combination biomarkers for pulmonary tuberculosis diagnosis. *PLoS ONE* **8:** e81076.

Mouse Model of Tuberculosis

Andrea M. Cooper

Trudeau Institute, Inc., Saranac Lake, New York 12983

Correspondence: acooper@trudeauinstitute.org

The mouse provides a tool with which to probe the complex interaction between the mammalian immune system and the slow-growing, inflammatory, and persistent bacterium, *Mycobacterium tuberculosis* (*Mtb*). Simple mouse models using genetic deletion or antibody inhibition have identified causal connections between specific components of the immune response and survival upon challenge with *Mtb*, and these studies have corresponded with observations made in humans. To improve on current intervention strategies, it is essential that the complex interactions between the components of the immune response that mediate and regulate the protective response to *Mtb* infection be dissected; furthermore, the pathways by which specific molecules and cells act must be delineated. The mouse model provides a tool with which to achieve this goal; however, experimental design and data interpretation must be made in the context of data sets generated from the entire tuberculosis field.

Organisms have increasing levels of complexity and when they interact, the level of complexity increases dramatically. Vertebrates have developed the ability to respond to exposure to lower-order organisms in the form of a targeted and highly regulated immune response. The immune response has simple elements at its base including recognition of "danger," recognition of nonself, the ability to adapt to novel antigens, the ability to remember previous antigens, and active regulation of the above responses. When these simple elements act in concert, the host response is immensely adaptable and capable of dealing with a vast array of potential pathogens. Of course, this ability can also lead to inappropriate responses, which contribute to damage and disease. Animal models have been used to identify definitive causal relationships between specific components of this complex immune response and the survival of the host following exposure to a variety of pathogens. Although these studies remain valid, the complexities of the pathways by which specific components of the immune response interact both to control the pathogen and to limit immunopathology are just now being fully realized. Defining the role of specific factors within complex pathways now requires highly refined and manipulatable tools, and recent developments within the mouse model provide these tools.

Within the context of mycobacterial disease, and tuberculosis in particular, the complexity arising from the persistence of this pathogen and the need for balance between protection and pathogenesis is at the core of our difficulty in controlling this pathogen. The cell types that contribute to the immunity to TB include my-

Cite this article as *Cold Spring Harb Perspect Med* doi: 10.1101/cshperspect.a018556

eloid and lymphoid cells but within these broad groupings are a wide range of cell phenotypes, the importance of which depend on location of the challenge, the nature of challenge, and the constituents of the microbiome, which play a large part in regulating the tonic state of the immune system (Erturk-Hasdemir et al. 2013). To deconvolute the complexity of the immune system and to drill down through the mechanisms that mediate its initiation, expansion, and regulation, it is critical to use a model wherein many of the variables can be controlled. The mouse does not provide a direct mimic of the human response to mycobacterial infection. It does, however, provide a living, breathing vertebrate lung on a small scale with the capacity to perform a large number of experiments with definitive outcomes. It also provides a manipulatable tool that represents the complexity of the vertebrate immune response to *Mycobacterium tuberculosis* (*Mtb*) while allowing definitive experimentation to isolate the critical components involved in both protection and pathogenesis. The recent increase in tools for the mouse model has allowed us to better define the interaction between the pathogen and the different components of the immune response, and the outcomes have been surprising.

GENETIC APPROACHES

A powerful tool provided by the mouse is the ability to investigate complex genetic traits in a mammalian model. Mutant mouse strains can be used for "reverse" genetic approaches to query the role of a specific gene in the development of mycobacterial disease in the vertebrate host; this is almost entirely performed with murine models at the current time. "Forward" genetics use random mutation as well as the comparison of inbred strains of mice, which differ in their susceptibility to mycobacterial disease to probe for novel genes in an unbiased manner (Fortin et al. 2007). The variety of susceptibility within inbred mouse strains is highlighted by the fact that CBA, C3HeB/FeJ, DBA/2, and 129SvJ are susceptible to *Mtb*, whereas C57BL/6 J and BALB/c are resistant (Medina et al. 1998). By crossing the inbred strains and generating congenic lines, loci associated with the susceptible phenotype have been identified. The use of this tool has resulted in the determination of several independent loci responsible for susceptibility such as *sst1*, which contains the *Ipr1* gene (Pan et al. 2005); loci on chromosomes 9 and 3, which mediate interstrain differences between susceptible I/St and resistant A/Sn strains (Sánchez et al. 2003); and the *Trl1-4* loci, which contribute to susceptibility of the DBA/2 J strain (Marquis et al. 2009). Importantly these susceptibility loci are associated with different arms of the protective response and highlight the importance of the balanced integration of the lymphoid, myeloid, and subsequent inflammatory response in maintaining control of *Mtb* in vivo.

TARGETED CELLULAR APPROACHES

Early events occurring during infection are difficult to model and analyze even in the mouse model. It is thought that aerosol delivery of a suspension of bacteria at a low concentration mimics natural infection, and indeed most of the animal models use this or a variation of this delivery system. Whether this is a true mimic is not clear, as the nature of infectious bacteria arriving from the transmitting individual to the exposed individual is not yet defined. Using this low-dose model, however, results in very few early events and renders investigation of these events difficult. Indirect measures have therefore been used within the mouse model to investigate the importance of specific cell types in the early initiation of the acquired cellular response, which is critical for control of *Mtb*. One such model includes genetically modified mice that allow for the timed depletion of specific cells, which express the diphtheria toxin receptor (DTR) (Saito et al. 2001). Recently the use of this model to deplete cells positive for C-C chemokine receptor 2 (CCR2) resulted in the surprising observation that inflammatory monocytes (which express CCR2) are required to deliver invading bacteria to the draining lymph node (Samstein et al. 2013). Dendritic cells had been thought to be responsible for this transport, and indeed they appear to act in this capacity once infection is established (Wolf et al.

2007); however, the inflammatory monocytes, although responsible for delivery, were not responsible for driving T-cell activation (Samstein et al. 2013). Using the $CD11c^+$ DTR model (Jung et al. 2002), it was found that T cells were compromised in their ability to be activated if $CD11c^+$ cells lacked the IL-12Rβ1 (Robinson et al. 2010). There are other genetic systems available that can be used for timed depletion of specific cell types or of specific molecules within specific cell types such as the cre/loxP system (Kühn et al. 2002). Concerns with these models that must be considered when using them in the context of *Mtb* infection include the ability of the depleting agent to penetrate the macrophage-dominated lesion and the impact of significant cell death on the integrity of the granulomatous lesion. Despite these concerns, the use of these targeting systems to deplete molecules and cells within a defined time frame and within specific cell types have increased the power of the initial genetic-deletion techniques that were used to confirm the roles of specific components of the immune response such as IFN-γ, TNF, and IL-12 in controlling *Mtb* infection (Cooper et al. 1993, 1997; Flynn et al. 1993, 1995).

EXAMINING T-CELL RESPONSES WITHIN THE *Mtb*-INFECTED MOUSE

Understanding how the body recognizes invasion by *Mtb* and initiates the expansion of antigen-specific T cells is important in understanding pathogenesis and in vaccine design. Because of the low frequency of initiating events following low-dose aerosol infection, it is necessary to have indirect measures of antigen presentation. In recent studies with the mouse model, one aspect of early infection was highlighted when it became clear that the acquired immune response largely ignores the arrival of the bacterium in the lung following aerosol infection (Chackerian et al. 2002; Reiley et al. 2008; Wolf et al. 2008). In these papers, analyses of antigen-specific cellular responses were made using specific antigens and/or T-cell receptor transgenic (TCRTg) T cells. The importance of the TCRTg T cells is that they provide a highly sensitive tool with which to indicate the kinetics and location of appropriately presented antigen when delivered exogenously and examined at specific times posttransfer (Kearney et al. 1994). In three separate laboratories the timing of initial naïve T-cell activation was found to be delayed relative to challenge (~7–9 d) and was found to occur within the lung-draining lymph node and not to any great extent with the lung (Gallegos et al. 2008; Reiley et al. 2008; Wolf et al. 2008). The use of TCRTg cells was critical to this insight as the very low frequency of the endogenous response meant that the earliest events could not be detected directly. Although TCRTg cells represent a powerful tool, they should be used with care as they are an artificial T cell and do not develop identically to endogenous T cells. It is also critical to keep the transferred precursor level low as it is known that the precursor frequency of naïve T cells impacts the outcome of the immune response (Kearney et al. 1994; Jenkins et al. 2012; Sprent 2013).

The function of T cells within the inflamed site induced by *Mtb* infection is also a subject that has been investigated using the mouse model. In this respect, use of immunohistochemistry and live imaging has been crucial. Early intravital studies supported the key role of TNF in development of the macrophage matrix of the *Mtb*-induced granuloma (Egen et al. 2008) and also showed that T cells within the macrophage-dominated lesion fail to undergo migration arrest and only occasionally secreted cytokine in a targeted manner (Egen et al. 2011). In a different study, using flow-cytometric examination of T-cell function immediately ex vivo, a low level of antigen availability within the granuloma was associated with poor cytokine production in vivo (Bold et al. 2011). These studies, along with those implicating the importance of correct chemokine receptor expression in T-cell function (Slight et al. 2013), support the importance of T-cell location relative to the *Mtb*-infected macrophage in mediating the control of bacterial growth. A recent mouse study addressed the importance of direct T-cell interaction with infected macrophages using a bone marrow chimera model. In these chimeras, bone marrow is transferred into an irradiated host and repopulates the radiosensitive portions of the hematopoietic system (Shizuru et al. 1996). Using donors that differ in the ability to express specific molecules and that can be differentiated by the expression of a congenic marker, the response of these cells can be compared in vivo with the same stimuli and within the same context. Using this tool it was found that within the same host, only those infected macrophages expressing MHC class II showed CD4 T-cell-dependent reduction of bacterial numbers (Srivastava et al. 2013); thus addressing a long-term question of whether direct T-cell macrophage interaction was required for antibacterial activity by the macrophage. This type of bone marrow chimera model is very useful for a range of immunological investigations of the chronic inflammation induced by *Mtb*. Key points are that intact and deficient cells are within the same environment and will not undergo rejection over the long term (which transferred cells would undergo). Concerns include the fact that long-lived, nondividing hematopoietic cells (memory T cells, tissue macrophages, etc.) will not be fully removed by irradiation, and this should be considered and controlled for wherever possible.

Full investigation of the function and phenotype of T cells during mycobacterial disease has been greatly impacted recently by the use of tetramer staining (Altman et al. 1996) and cell sorting. The tetramer stains used to identify a subset of the antigen-specific cells within an endogenous population of responding cells have proven particularly useful in identifying T-cell trends that were not apparent when studying the bulk population of activated T cells. By focusing on T cells of one antigen specificity, it has been possible to define several subsets of responding cells, such as those expressing markers associated with antigen exposure (e.g., PD-1 and KLRG-1 [Reiley et al. 2010]). Importantly, the addition of cell sorting to the study of T cells from infected mice has allowed the functional capacity of T-cell subsets to be assessed. Thus, when T cells were subsetted based on their expression of PD-1 or KLRG-1, they were found to have different abilities to produce cytokine and to proliferate and persist with an infected host (Reiley et al. 2010). The increased use of tetramer stains in human studies to identify and characterize antigen-specific T cells (Lindestam Arlehamn et al. 2013) will allow the work in the mice to undergo even more refinement and allow for observations made in the mouse to be fully translated to the antigen-specific population in humans. This very powerful set of tools is set to transform our understanding of T-cell function within the human.

PATHOLOGIC CONSEQUENCES OF *Mtb* INFECTION IN THE MOUSE

Using histological techniques, many studies have been made of the pathologic consequences of infection in the mouse lung, and inclusion of this parameter in any mouse model provides important information regarding the health of the lung tissue. Importantly, although increased bacterial burden and decreased granuloma integrity are usually seen together, it is also the case that the granulomatous response develops over time despite little change in bacterial number (Rhoades et al. 1997). A recent development in our understanding of the role of B-cell follicles in immunity was prompted by the repeated observation of these follicles associated with *Mtb*-induced inflammation in the mouse. Using mouse models of gene deletion, bone marrow chimeras, and antibody/serum treatment, the role of B cells in *Mtb* infection has been examined. Recently, it has been shown that B cells serve to regulate the IL-17 response and thereby reduce neutrophil recruitment to the infection site (Kondratieva et al. 2010; Kozakiewicz et al. 2013). Using genetically depleted mice it was also found that loss of the activating receptor FcγR compromises control of *Mtb* growth, whereas loss of the inhibitory receptor FcγRIIB improves control (Maglione et al. 2008). In contrast, in models where B cells are present but are unable to generate circulating immunoglobulin, they act to inhibit immunity in association with excess IL-10 production (Torrado et al. 2013). Recent work has indicated an association between B-cell follicles in migration of T cells from the blood vessels throughout the inflamed area of the lungs in mice (Khader et al. 2009, 2011), and this work was extended to nonhuman primates (NHPs) and humans. It was found that B-cell follicles were in a minority of lesions from active TB patients, and that B-cell follicles were dominant in latently infected relative to actively infected NHPs (Slight et al. 2013). The mouse model was then used to investigate the causative connection between the B-cell follicles and bacterial control (Slight et al. 2013). It was found that although B-cell follicles are associated with control, they are not required for it and that they are a consequence of the appearance of C-X-C chemokine receptor 5 (CXCR5)-expressing CD4 T cells, which respond to CXCL13 and which act as follicular helper T cells. The expression of CXCR5 on the T cells is required to mediate appropriate migration of the activated T cell from the blood vessel to colocalize with infected phagocytes and thereby mediate macrophage activation (Slight et al. 2013). This work is a fine example of how the use of multiple models allows for the identification of a phenomenon followed by the definition of the pathways by which the phenomenon occurs.

Although activation of infected macrophages requires colocalization with antigen-specific T cells, these T cells are also actively regulated by the environment which they create. Although the ability of T cells to undergo migration arrest and mediate antibacterial function is low (see above), they are very able to activate the accumulated macrophages within the *Mtb*-induced lesion to generate a highly inflamed site. How T cells function within this site and how the site is regulated have been extensively addressed using mouse models. Original observations using gene-deleted mice indicated that IFN-γ and IL-12p40 were essential for control of *Mtb* infection in the mouse model (Cooper et al. 1993, 1997, 2002b), and these studies were complementary to the observation in humans that absence of these genes resulted in Mendelian susceptibility to mycobacterial disease (MSMD) (Filipe-Santos et al. 2006). However, the role of IFN-γ has been questioned because of the observation that the simple number of IFN-γ-producing T cells in the peripheral blood of humans does not strongly correlate with ability to control mycobacterial disease. Recent studies with mice, using gene-deleted and bone marrow chimera models, have shown that IFN-γ expression by T cells acts to limit the accumulation of neutrophils (Pearl et al. 2001; Nandi et al. 2011), and that it also regulates IL-17 activity (Desvignes et al. 2009; Nandi et al. 2011) within the inflamed site. IFN-γ also acts directly to limit the accumulation of activated T cells within the mycobacterial lesion (Gomes et al. 1999; Cooper et al. 2002a; Nandi et al. 2011), and this may contribute to the inability of the vertebrate host to eliminate the infection. One consequence of IFN-γ production is the generation of nitric oxide by macrophages within the granuloma. Although nitric oxide is critical to limit growth of *Mtb*, it is also known to regulate the pathologic response to mycobacterial infection (Cooper et al. 2002a). In this regard an antibiotic-dependent *Mtb* was recently used to specifically probe the anti-inflammatory activity of nitric oxide. It was found that lymphocyte-derived IFN-γ limited the production of IL-1 and subsequent immunopathology via the induction of nitric oxide–mediated inhibition of the NLRP3 inflammasome (Mishra et al. 2013). Nitric oxide also acts to limit the accumulation of activated T-cell subsets within mycobacterially infected tissue (Pearl et al. 2012).

Although the pathologic response to *Mtb* infection in the mouse lung does not recapitulate the complete set of outcomes seen in diseased human tissue, manipulation of the mouse model can be used to determine the factors involved in initiating and regulating inflammation. Comparative pathology can then be used to identify factors that, when dysregulated, allow for the type of pathology seen in humans.

USE OF THE MOUSE MODEL TO DEVELOP DRUGS AND VACCINES

Although the real power of the mouse model lies in the delineation of in vivo immunological and pathological pathways, it can also be used as a small animal model to study drugs and vaccines. It is in these studies where overinterpretation can cause problems. It is essential that the investigator ensures that the tool being used will answer the question being asked and also that the scientific community interprets the observations made in light of the constraints of the model. Within drug development it is necessary to understand the context of the bacteria within the mouse; thus, if one wants to screen a drug for its ability to target bacteria in a macrophage-dominated lesion in the lung within an immunocompetent host, then a B6 mouse infected with *Mtb* via the aerosol route is potentially suitable. If, however, one needs to target bacteria growing within a neutrophil-dominated or necrotic lesion, then one can use a mouse lacking IFN-γ production or signaling (Desvignes et al. 2009; Nandi et al. 2011) or an inbred strain such as I/St (Eruslanov et al. 2005) or mice with the sst1-susceptible locus (Pichugin et al. 2009). The above also applies when considering vaccination; it has been shown that the susceptibility profiles of different mouse strains are maintained after vaccination with BCG (Bacillus Calmette–Guérin) (Medina et al. 1999). Thus if one wants to test a vaccine in a model wherein expression of immunity is compromised, then a susceptible mouse strain is the correct one to use. In terms of vaccine development, however, the mouse most effectively represents the capacity to investigate potential mechanisms of protection rather than a tool to decide which vaccines move forward.

CONCLUSION

The mouse model allows for both definitive and unbiased approaches with which to probe the interaction between *Mtb* and a vertebrate host. It also provides a manipulatable environment that can reflect aspects of the human infection and disease progression. Overinterpretation and inappropriate translation to human disease can lead to issues, but judicious interpretation within the context of the field as a whole can lead to much greater understanding of the pathways mediating pathogenesis in tuberculosis.

ACKNOWLEDGMENTS

A.M.C. is supported by Trudeau Institute, Inc., National Institutes of Health grants AI69121, AI46530, and AI73564, and the Bill and Melinda Gates Foundation.

REFERENCES

Altman J, Moss P, Goulder P, Barouch D, McHeyzer-Williams M, Bell J, McMichael A, Davis M. 1996. Phenotypic analysis of antigen-specific T lymphocytes. *Science* **274:** 94–96.

Bold TD, Banaei N, Wolf AJ, Ernst JD. 2011. Suboptimal activation of antigen-specific $CD4^+$ effector cells enables persistence of *M. tuberculosis* in vivo. *PLoS Pathog* **7:** e1002063.

Chackerian A, Alt J, Perera T, Dascher C, SM B. 2002. Dissemination of *Mycobacterium tuberculosis* is influenced by host factors and precedes the initiation of T-cell immunity. *Infect Immun* **70:** 4501–4509.

Cooper AM, Dalton DK, Stewart TA, Griffin JP, Russell DG, Orme IM. 1993. Disseminated tuberculosis in interferon γ gene-disrupted mice. *J Exp Med* **178:** 2243–2247.

Cooper AM, Magram J, Ferrante J, Orme IM. 1997. IL-12 is crucial to the development of protective immunity in mice intravenously infected with *Mycobacterium tuberculosis*. *J Exp Med* **186:** 39–46.

Cooper AM, Adams LB, Dalton DK, Appelberg R, Ehlers S. 2002a. IFN-γ and NO in mycobacterial disease: New jobs for old hands. *Trends Microbiol* **10:** 221–226.

Cooper AM, Kipnis A, Turner J, Magram J, Ferrante J, Orme IM. 2002b. Mice lacking bioactive IL-12 can generate protective, antigen-specific cellular responses to mycobacterial infection only if the IL-12 p40 subunit is present. *J Immunol* **168:** 1322–1327.

Desvignes L, Ernst JD. 2009. Interferon-γ-responsive nonhematopoietic cells regulate the immune response to *Mycobacterium tuberculosis*. *Immunity* **31:** 974–985.

Egen J, Rothfuchs A, Feng C, Winter N, Sher A, Germain R. 2008. Macrophage and T cell dynamics during the development and disintegration of mycobacterial granulomas. *Immunity* **28:** 271–284.

Egen JG, Rothfuchs AG, Feng CG, Horwitz MA, Sher A, Germain RN. 2011. Intravital imaging reveals limited antigen presentation and T cell effector function in mycobacterial granulomas. *Immunity* **34:** 807–819.

Erturk-Hasdemir D, Kasper DL. 2013. Resident commensals shaping immunity. *Curr Opin Immunol* **25:** 450–455.

Eruslanov E, Lyadova I, Kondratieva T, Majorov K, Scheglov I, Orlova M, Apt A. 2005. Neutrophil responses to *Mycobacterium tuberculosis* infection in genetically susceptible and resistant mice. *Infect Immun* **73:** 1744–1753.

Filipe-Santos O, Bustamante J, Chapgier A, Vogt G, de Beaucoudrey L, Feinberg J, Jouanguy E, Boisson-Dupuis S, Fieschi C, Picard C, et al. 2006. Inborn errors of IL-12/23- and IFN-γ-mediated immunity: Molecular, cellular, and clinical features. *Semin Immunol* **18:** 347–361.

Flynn JL, Chan J, Triebold KJ, Dalton DK, Stewart TA, Bloom BR. 1993. An essential role for interferon γ in resistance to *Mycobacterium tuberculosis* infection. *J Exp Med* **178:** 2249–2254.

Flynn JL, Goldstein MM, Chan J, Triebold KJ, Pfeffer K, Lowenstein CJ, Schreiber R, Mak TW, Bloom BR. 1995.

Tumor necrosis factor-α is required in the protective immune response against *Mycobacterium tuberculosis* in mice. *Immunity* **2:** 561–572.

Fortin A, Abel L, Casanova JL, Gros P. 2007. Host genetics of mycobacterial diseases in mice and men: Forward genetic studies of BCG-osis and tuberculosis. *Ann Rev Genom Hum Genet* **8:** 163–192.

Gallegos A, Pamer E, Glickman M. 2008. Delayed protection by ESAT-6-specific effector CD4$^+$ T cells after airborne *M. tuberculosis* infection. *J Exp Med* **205:** 2359–2368.

Gomes MS, Florido M, Pais TF, Appelberg R. 1999. Improved clearance of *Mycobacterium avium* upon disruption of the inducible nitric oxide synthase gene. *J Immunol* **162:** 6734–6739.

Jenkins MK, Moon JJ. 2012. The role of naive T cell precursor frequency and recruitment in dictating immune response magnitude. *J Immunol* **188:** 4135–4140.

Jung S, Unutmaz D, Wong P, Sano G, De los Santos K, Sparwasser T, Wu S, Vuthoori S, Ko K, Zavala F, et al. 2002. In vivo depletion of CD11c$^+$ dendritic cells abrogates priming of CD8$^+$ T cells by exogenous cell-associated antigens. *Immunity* **17:** 211–220.

Kearney ER, Pape KA, Loh DY, Jenkins MK. 1994. Visualization of peptide-specific T cell immunity and peripheral tolerance induction in vivo. *Immunity* **1:** 327–339.

Khader S, Rangel-Moreno J, Fountain J, Martino C, Reiley W, Pearl J, Winslow G, Woodland D, Randall T, Cooper A. 2009. In a murine tuberculosis model, the absence of homeostatic chemokines delays granuloma formation and protective immunity. *J Immunol* **183:** 8004–8014.

Khader SA, Guglani L, Rangel-Moreno J, Gopal R, Fallert Junecko BA, Fountain JJ, Martino C, Pearl JE, Tighe M, Lin YY, et al. 2011. IL-23 is required for long-term control of *Mycobacterium tuberculosis* and B cell follicle formation in the infected lung. *J Immunol* **187:** 5402–5407.

Kondratieva T, Rubakova E, Linge I, Evstifeev V, Majorov K, Apt A. 2010. B cells delay neutrophil migration toward the site of stimulus: Tardiness critical for effective bacillus Calmette-Guérin vaccination against tuberculosis infection in mice. *J Immunol* **184:** 1227–1234.

Kozakiewicz L, Chen Y, Xu J, Wang Y, Dunussi-Joannopoulos K, Ou Q, Flynn JL, Porcelli SA, Jacobs WR Jr, Chan J. 2013. B cells regulate neutrophilia during *Mycobacterium tuberculosis* infection and BCG vaccination by modulating the interleukin-17 response. *PLoS Pathog* **9:** e1003472.

Kühn R, Torres RM. 2002. Cre/loxP recombination system and gene targeting. In *Transgenesis techniques* (ed. Clarke A), Vol. 180, pp. 175–204. Springer, New York.

Lindestam Arlehamn CS, Gerasimova A, Mele F, Henderson R, Swann J, Greenbaum JA, Kim Y, Sidney J, James EA, Taplitz R, et al. 2013. Memory T cells in latent *Mycobacterium tuberculosis* infection are directed against three antigenic islands and largely contained in a CXCR$^+$ CCR$^+$ Th1 subset. *PLoS Pathog* **9:** e1003130.

Maglione P, Xu J, Casadevall A, Chan J. 2008. Fcγ receptors regulate immune activation and susceptibility during *Mycobacterium tuberculosis* infection. *J Immunol* **180:** 3329–3338.

Marquis J, Lacourse R, Ryan L, North R, Gros P. 2009. Genetic and functional characterization of the mouse Trl3 locus in defense against tuberculosis. *J Immunol* **182:** 3757–3767.

Medina E, North RJ. 1998. Resistance ranking of some common inbreb mouse strains to *Mycobacterium tuberculosis* and realtionship to major histocompatibiltiy complex haplotype and *Nramp1* genotype. *Immunology* **93:** 270–274.

Medina E, North R. 1999. Genetically susceptible mice remain proportionally more susceptible to tuberculosis after vaccination. *Immunology* **96:** 16–21.

Mishra BB, Rathinam VAK, Martens GW, Martinot AJ, Kornfeld H, Fitzgerald KA, Sassetti CM. 2013. Nitric oxide controls the immunopathology of tuberculosis by inhibiting NLRP3 inflammasome-dependent processing of IL-1β. *Nat Immunol* **14:** 52–60.

Nandi B, Behar SM. 2011. Regulation of neutrophils by interferon-γ limits lung inflammation during tuberculosis infection. *J Exp Med* **208:** 2251–2262.

Pan H, Yan B, Rojas M, Shebzukhov Y, Zhou H, Kobzik L, Higgins D, Daly M, Bloom B, Kramnik I. 2005. *Ipr1* gene mediates innate immunity to tuberculosis. *Nature* **434:** 767–772.

Pearl JE, Saunders BM, Ehlers S, Orme IM, Cooper AM. 2001. Inflammation and lymphocyte activation during mycobacterial infection in the interferon-γ-deficient mouse. *Cell Immunol* **211:** 43–50.

Pearl JE, Torrado E, Tighe M, Fountain JJ, Solache A, Strutt T, Swain S, Appelberg R, Cooper AM. 2012. Nitric oxide inhibits the accumulation of CD4$^+$CD44^{hi}Tbet$^+$CD69^{lo} T cells in mycobacterial infection. *Eur J Immunol* **42:** 3267–3279.

Pichugin AV, Yan B-S, Sloutsky A, Kobzik L, Kramnik I. 2009. Dominant role of the *sst1* locus in pathogenesis of necrotizing lung granulomas during chronic tuberculosis infection and reactivation in genetically resistant hosts. *Am J Pathol* **174:** 2190–2201.

Reiley W, Calayag M, Wittmer S, Huntington J, Pearl J, Fountain J, Martino C, Roberts A, Cooper A, Winslow G, et al. 2008. ESAT-6-specific CD4 T cell responses to aerosol *Mycobacterium tuberculosis* infection are initiated in mediastinal lymph nodes. *Proc Natl Acad Sci* **105:** 10961–10966.

Reiley WW, Shafiani S, Wittmer ST, Tucker-Heard G, Moon JJ, Jenkins MK, Urdahl KB, Winslow GM, Woodland DL. 2010. Distinct functions of antigen-specific CD4 T cells during murine *Mycobacterium tuberculosis* infection. *Proc Natl Acad Sci* **107:** 19408–19413.

Rhoades ER, Frank AA, Orme IM. 1997. Progression of chronic pulmonary tuberculosis in mice aerogenically infected with virulent *Mycobacterium tuberculosis*. *Tuber Lung Dis* **78:** 57–66.

Robinson R, Khader S, Martino C, Fountain J, Teixeira-Coelho M, Pearl J, Smiley S, Winslow G, Woodland D, Walter M, et al. 2010. *Mycobacterium tuberculosis* infection induces il12rb1 splicing to generate a novel IL-12Rβ1 isoform that enhances DC migration. *J Exp Med* **207:** 591–605.

Saito M, Iwawaki T, Taya C, Yonekawa H, Noda M, Inui Y, Mekada E, Kimata Y, Tsuru A, Kohno K. 2001. Diphtheria toxin receptor-mediated conditional and targeted cell ablation in transgenic mice. *Nat Biotechnol* **19:** 746–750.

Samstein M, Schreiber HA, Leiner IM, Sušac B, Glickman MS, Pamer EG, Lanzavecchia A. 2013. Essential yet limited role for CCR2$^+$ inflammatory monocytes during *Mycobacterium tuberculosis*–specific T cell priming. *eLife* **2:** e01086.

Sánchez F, Radaeva TV, Nikonenko BV, Persson A-S, Sengul S, Schalling M, Schurr E, Apt AS, Lavebratt C. 2003. Multigenic control of disease severity after virulent *Mycobacterium tuberculosis* infection in mice. *Infect Immun* **71:** 126–131.

Shizuru J, Jerabek L, Edwards C, Weissman I. 1996. Transplantation of purified hematopoietic stem cells: Requirements for overcoming the barriers of allogeneic engraftment. *Biol Blood Marrow Transplant* **2:** 3–14.

Slight SR, Rangel-Moreno J, Gopal R, Lin Y, Fallert Junecko BA, Mehra S, Selman M, Becerril-Villanueva E, Baquera-Heredia J, Pavon L, et al. 2013. CXCR5$^+$ T helper cells mediate protective immunity against tuberculosis. *J Clin Invest* **123:** 712–726.

Sprent J. 2013. The power of dilution: Using adoptive transfer to study TCR transgenic T cells. *J Immunol* **191:** 5325–5326.

Srivastava S, Ernst JD. 2013. Cutting edge: Direct recognition of infected cells by CD4 T cells is required for control of intracellular *Mycobacterium tuberculosis* in vivo. *J Immunol* **191:** 1016–1020.

Torrado E, Fountain JJ, Robinson RT, Martino CA, Pearl JE, Rangel-Moreno J, Tighe M, Dunn R, Cooper AM. 2013. Differential and site specific impact of B cells in the protective immune response to *Mycobacterium tuberculosis* in the mouse. *PLoS ONE* **8:** e61681.

Wolf AJ, Linas B, Trevejo-Nunez GJ, Kincaid E, Tamura T, Takatsu K, Ernst JD. 2007. *Mycobacterium tuberculosis* infects dendritic cells with high frequency and impairs their function in vivo. *J Immunol* **179:** 2509–2519.

Wolf A, Desvignes L, Linas B, Banaiee N, Tamura T, Takatsu K, Ernst J. 2008. Initiation of the adaptive immune response to *Mycobacterium tuberculosis* depends on antigen production in the local lymph node, not the lungs. *J Exp Med* **205:** 105–115.

Animal Models of Tuberculosis: Guinea Pigs

Simon Clark, Yper Hall, and Ann Williams

Microbiology Services, Public Health England, Porton Down, Salisbury SP4 0JG, United Kingdom

Correspondence: ann.rawkins@phe.gov.uk

The progression of the disease that follows infection of guinea pigs with *Mycobacterium tuberculosis* displays many features of human tuberculosis (TB), and the guinea pig model of TB has been used for more than 100 years as a research tool to understand and describe disease mechanisms. Changes in the bacterial burden and pathology following infection can be readily monitored and used to evaluate the impact of TB interventions. Demonstration of the protective efficacy of vaccines in the low-dose aerosol guinea pig model is an important component of the preclinical data package for novel vaccines in development, and there is a continual need to improve the model to facilitate progression of vaccines to the clinic. Development of better tools with which to dissect the immune responses of guinea pigs is a focus of current research.

Guinea pigs are synonymous with experimentation and this animal has been used to model several diseases of man (Padilla-Carlin et al. 2008). From the studies performed by Robert Koch to identify the causative agent of tuberculosis (TB) to the present day, the guinea pig has played its part to understand disease processes, to define important components of *Mycobacterium tuberculosis*, and to test the potency of vaccines and therapies. In general, researchers have favored the outbred Dunkin–Hartley strain of guinea pig, although inbred strains are available. It is possible to induce disease with very low doses of *M. tuberculosis*, particularly when delivered by the aerosol route (Smith and Harding 1977). Guinea pigs are therefore more susceptible to TB than other model species and this has both advantages and disadvantages. Infection with *M. tuberculosis* can be established following injection into various body compartments or instillation to the lungs via the trachea or intranasally but the most relevant and well-characterized guinea pig model of TB uses the aerosol route of challenge. There have been many excellent reviews written about the aerosol infection guinea pig model of TB and these are referenced frequently to provide the reader with further details. The aim of this article is to give an overview of the main features of the model, highlighting what has been learned through using the guinea pig to study TB, and to suggest areas for refinement and development in the future.

WHAT IS THE MODEL?

Clinical Picture

Although guinea pigs are susceptible to TB, outwardly the signs of infection are only apparent

Cite this article as *Cold Spring Harb Perspect Med* doi: 10.1101/cshperspect.a018572

in the latter stages of disease. Weight loss is a sensitive indicator of progressive infection, and it is usually the most significant component of clinical scoring systems that are used to monitor animal welfare and trigger a humane end point, whereby the animal is killed prior to suffering. General behavior, condition of the coat, and changes to normal feeding and drinking patterns are other components of the humane end point, which is sometimes referred to as a modified Karnofsky score (Williams et al. 2009). Temperature changes have been suggested as an early indicator of disease outcome (Grover et al. 2009), but temperature monitoring is not adopted widely.

Infection invariably leads to death of the animal, but the time taken to reach the humane end point varies according to the initial dose and virulence of the strain of *M. tuberculosis*. Initial studies performed to establish and characterize the guinea pig model of TB infection were based on very low-dose aerosol inoculation. This "rational animal model of TB" was developed by Smith and colleagues and is expertly described by McMurray (1994). Unsensitized animals infected with less than five bacilli succumbed to disease from week 14 postchallenge, but even after 40 wk, 20% of the animals had survived (Wiegeshaus et al. 1970). In contrast, studies performed more recently generally use aerosol doses of 20–50 bacilli and, even though this is still regarded as low-dose, the progression to severe disease is more rapid and 100% of animals have met humane end points by week 30 (Brandt et al. 2004; Williams et al. 2009; Grover et al. 2012). Even higher aerosol doses (~500–1000) have been used, which result in accelerated times to humane end points of between 8 and 20 wk. This very high-dose challenge model has been used in vaccine evaluation studies to show improved efficacy over BCG (Bacillus Calmette–Guérin) (Williams et al. 2005a), but, because of the very acute nature of the disease that develops, high-dose challenge is less clinically relevant.

M. tuberculosis Replication

The pattern or profile of multiplication of *M. tuberculosis* in the lungs and spleens of guinea pigs following aerosol infection has been comprehensively described by Alsaadi and Smith (1973). In the lung, as illustrated in Figure 1, an initial period of logarithmic growth up to ~16 d postchallenge, is followed by an extended period of many weeks during which the bacterial load is stable, neither increasing nor decreasing. This profile of bacterial load is similar in animals infected with different doses, but dose affects the maximum concentration attained in the lung and this is proportional—a 10-fold increase in the dose results in a 10-fold increase in the num-

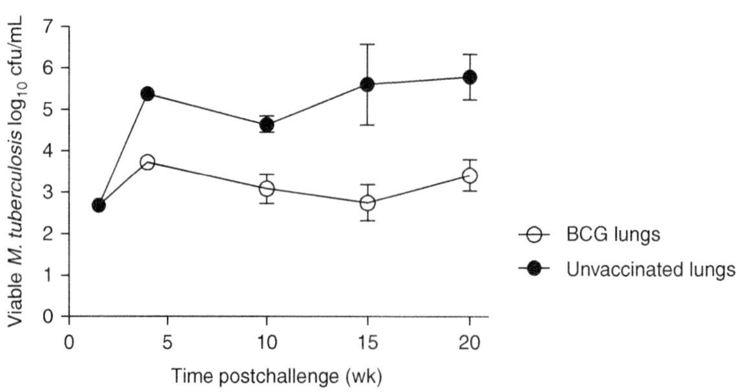

Figure 1. Bacterial load (mean $\log_{10}$ colony forming units per mL of tissue) in the lungs of guinea pigs following low-dose (10- to 20-CFU) aerosol infection with *M. tuberculosis* H37Rv. Solid circles show unvaccinated animals; open circles are animals vaccinated with Bacillus Calmette–Guérin (BCG) (5×10^4 CFU, 12 wk before aerosol infection). Error bars are standard error of the mean.

 Cite this article as *Cold Spring Harb Perspect Med* doi: 10.1101/cshperspect.a018572

ber of bacteria at ~16 d postchallenge. Ultimately, the control of bacterial replication is lost and a further increase in bacterial load is synonymous with the humane end point (Williams et al. 2009).

In the spleen, there is an initial period in which no bacteria are detected by culturing spleen samples on agar and this is ~14 d postchallenge (Alsaadi and Smith 1973). It is entirely possible that viable bacteria are present before this but they are below the threshold of detection. Dissemination to the spleen has been used as a sensitive way to compare the virulence or fitness of mycobacterial strains, with an increased rate of dissemination being associated with higher virulence (Balasubramanian et al. 1992; Williams et al. 2005b). Similar to the profile in the lungs, a stable control of replication occurs from ~4–6 wk postchallenge, and this is maintained until animals meet humane end points.

Enumeration of bacterial load in lungs and spleens is frequently used to define the burden of disease, and this is usually measured by culturing homogenized tissue on appropriate agar plates. The colonies that arise are counted and the bacterial load is commonly expressed as colony forming units (CFU) per mL or gram of tissue. Culture on solid agar has limitations, and there is a consensus that a subpopulation of bacteria may be viable even if not culturable. Alternative techniques to measure viability have been described, which include using fluorescently tagged bacteria or viability stains, but these currently lack the reproducibility and sensitivity of culture on agar. Broth culture using automated detection systems to identify metabolic activity offer an alternative to CFU that might be more sensitive and reliable.

Pathology

Pathological changes that occur in the lungs and extrapulmonary sites of guinea pigs following aerosol infection have been described extensively in the context of previously naïve animals, and these observations have been fundamental to the understanding of experimental TB in guinea pigs (Smith and Harding 1977; Turner et al. 2003; Basaraba et al. 2006; Basaraba 2008; Palanisamy et al. 2008). Key features of the pathology include human-like granulomas with central necrosis enclosed by lymphocytes, macrophages, and multinucleate giant cells and a fibrotic capsule. Cavitation is observed only rarely—for example, with certain strains of *M. tuberculosis* (Kato-Maeda et al. 2012).

Comparative assessments of pathology have become an accepted means of defining the pathogenicity of strains or evaluating the efficacy of treatments, such as vaccines or drugs (Dascher et al. 2003; Basaraba 2008; Ordway et al. 2008). There is an increasing trend to introduce more quantitative assessments of pathology using a scoring system that is used by a certified pathologist to record the key changes in terms of their severity or quantity (Williams et al. 2005b; Palanisamy et al. 2008). An illustration of the type of data generated when comparing vaccines using such scoring system is shown in Figure 2C.

Immune Response

The guinea pig was frequently used in early studies to determine the effect on the immune system of tuberculosis infection or inoculation with mycobacterial components. Lymphocyte proliferation assays and dermal reactivity were used to characterize and compare the delayed-type hypersensitivity reactions induced, and guinea pigs have continued to be useful for evaluating reagents which are used for diagnostic skin tests (Haslov et al. 1984, 1995; Malaghini et al. 2011). However, compared with other laboratory animal species, there has been limited development of immunological reagents specific for the guinea pig. Despite this, key features of the guinea pig response to *M. tuberculosis* and BCG have been studied by using methodologies such as antibody blocking, bioassays, and relative gene expression, including a boutique microarray covering key cytokines, chemokines, and their receptors/ligands (Tree et al. 2006). These studies have shown the importance of both the innate and adaptive arms of the immune system as summarized by Padilla-Carlin et al. (2008) and the role of CD1-restricted T cells (Hiromatsu et al. 2002) in the interaction

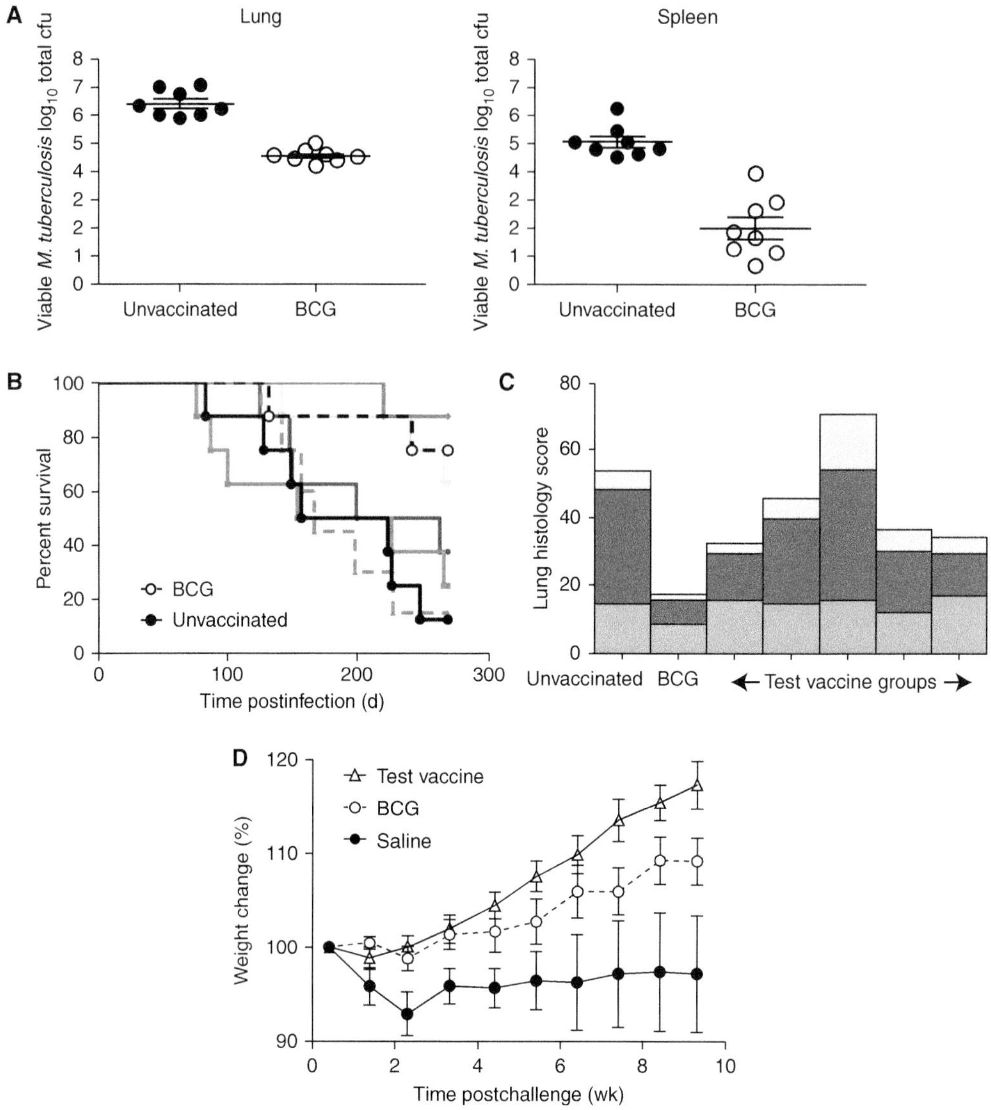

Figure 2. Examples of measurements of disease used to evaluate the efficacy of vaccines. (*A*) Bacterial load measured at week 4 postinfection, data from unvaccinated (solid circles) and BCG-vaccinated (open circles) animals are shown; each circle is an individual animal. (*B*) Kaplan–Meier survival plot showing unvaccinated (solid circles, solid line) and BCG-vaccinated (open circles, dashed line) animals and various test vaccines. (*C*) Semiquantitative scoring system showing extent of consolidation (mid-gray), caseation/necrosis (dark gray), and calcification (light gray), for unvaccinated animals, BCG-vaccinated animals, and animals vaccinated with test vaccines. (*D*) Changes in body weight measured over time postchallenge relative to the weight at challenge. Mean percentage weight change (±S.E.M.) is shown for each group of animals, which were either unvaccinated (solid circles), BCG-vaccinated (open circles), or given a test vaccine (open triangles).

of *M. tuberculosis* with the host. Ordway et al. (2007) have pioneered flow cytometry techniques for characterizing the changes in the cellular response to *M. tuberculosis* in relevant tissues such as lungs, spleen, and lymph nodes. Using this technique in combination with quantitative polymerase chain reaction (qPCR), Ordway and her colleagues have been able to track changes in lymphocyte populations and have revealed important differences in the response to clinical isolates of *M. tuberculosis* in comparison to laboratory strains, notably the induction of regulatory T cells by highly virulent strains belonging to the W-Beijing genotype (Shang et al. 2011). However, the lack of well-defined, commercially available assays with which to monitor immune responses to vaccines has largely restricted the guinea pig model to efficacy testing, with immunogenicity data derived from mouse studies. This is less than ideal because the differences between mouse and guinea pig immune systems do not enable protection to be correlated with immune response.

WHAT DID WE LEARN FROM THIS MODEL?

Analysis of the subject matter of 550 publications (from 1980s to present) involving tuberculosis and guinea pigs reveals that this animal model has contributed widely to our knowledge of the disease, across several disciplines. The distribution of subject categories is shown in Figure 3.

Vaccine Research

A large proportion of the publications describe vaccine evaluations in the guinea pig, because guinea pigs are the preferred small animal model to show the protective efficacy of vaccines. Advantages of guinea pigs over mice include their greater size, enabling more analyses to be performed in the same animal, and the wider range of vaccine types that can be tested compared with mice, which lack some immunological features (e.g., CD1b that are needed to respond to glycolipid antigens). In the absence of positive clinical efficacy data, the predictive value for humans of data obtained in guinea pigs remains unknown but demonstration of efficacy in this model is currently the main "gatekeeper" to progression of a vaccine toward clinical development. Efficacy of the vaccine is measured either by a reduction in the bacterial load in lungs and spleens at 4–5 wk postinfection or by the mean survival time over a prolonged follow-up period, compared with positive (BCG) and negative (unvaccinated)

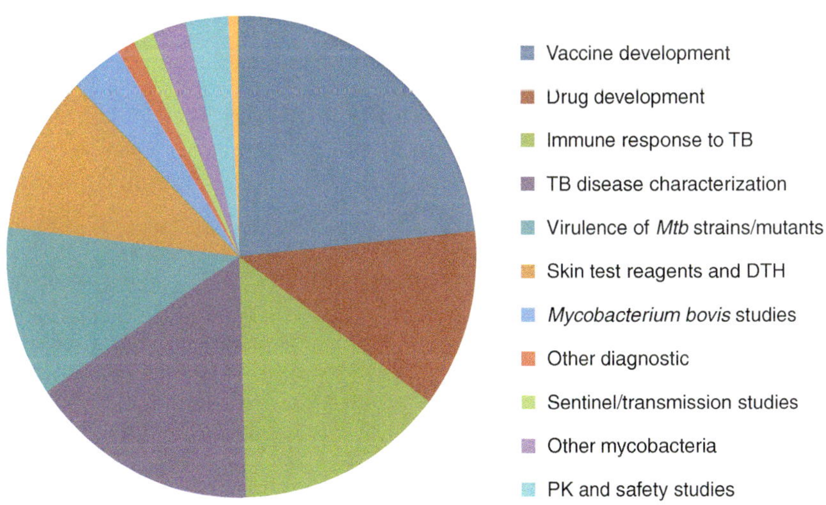

Figure 3. Pie chart showing distribution of the subject matter of 550 publications from 1982 to the present. The source of the publications was an NCBI (National Center for Biotechnology Information) PubMed search using the term "guinea pig tuberculosis."

controls. Evaluations based on bacterial load have increased statistical power to discriminate vaccines and are more rapid and less costly than survival studies, but the latter may be preferred to test the long-term impact of vaccination to prevent severe disease. Subjective or semiquantitative assessment of the pathology at the time of necropsy is also made and, in some studies, improved weight gain over the course of the postchallenge period has been used to define protection (Horwitz et al. 2000). Figure 2 shows examples of these efficacy readouts. Several reviews are recommended for further information, all of which conclude that the guinea pig model has provided essential preclinical efficacy and safety information on vaccine candidates (Orme et al. 2001; McMurray 2003; Orme 2005, 2006; Gupta et al. 2007; Williams et al. 2009).

In addition to its use as a means of proving/confirming efficacy, the guinea pig model has played a key role in identifying antigenic targets for incorporation into vaccines. This was particularly evident in the early days of antigen discovery as described in the previous section of this review. More recently, the key measure of immunogenicity has been the ability to elicit a Th1 response, characterized by the production of interferon γ, which is more readily tested in mice than guinea pigs, and, therefore, mice now tend to be used to test for putative antigenicity.

A less prominent but very important role of the guinea pig in vaccine research has been in preclinical product development. Guinea pigs are used among the battery of tests to show the safety of live attenuated vaccines according to EU regulations and guidelines, and as illustrated in the development of novel live vaccine candidates (Walker et al. 2010; Arbues et al. 2013; Grode et al. 2013). In the future, it would be preferable for such tests to be replaced by in vitro alternatives that would allow, for example, batch-release assays to be conducted without the need for animal testing.

Host–Pathogen Interactions—Identification of Key Pathogenic Mechanisms

Around one-quarter of the publications were related to the use of guinea pigs in understanding host–pathogen interactions, either through the careful study of the disease progression or via screening gene knockout *M. tuberculosis* mutants for their ability to cause disease. This has led to the identification of key pathogenic mechanisms of *M. tuberculosis*. The model has also revealed a number of important, host-related factors that have an impact on the susceptibility of individuals to TB. The effect of malnutrition has been extensively studied and is reviewed by Cegielski and McMurray (2004), who describe the detrimental impact of restricting dietary zinc, vitamin D, and particularly protein on the resistance to *M. tuberculosis* infection. The importance of regulation of iron by both the host and pathogen has been clearly shown in guinea pig studies (Basaraba et al. 2008; Thom et al. 2012). Similarly, studies in the guinea pig showed the strong association of hyperglycemia with exacerbation of disease, which may explain the link between TB disease and diabetes (Podell et al. 2012).

Drug Development

Although mice are commonly used to screen compounds for their potency to kill *M. tuberculosis* in vivo, testing of drug efficacy in guinea pigs is considered important because a wider range of pathological lesions develop and these are not only more reflective of human pathology but also represent a more stringent target for chemotherapy (Basaraba 2008). The necrotic granulomas that are a feature of guinea pig lung pathology are proposed to harbor bacteria that are refractory to standard chemotherapy regimens. Lenaerts et al. (2007) clearly showed the presence of extracellular, biofilm-like clusters of acid-fast bacilli in granulomas of guinea pigs, and this was associated with the failure of standard chemotherapy to sterilize the lungs. Therefore, guinea pigs are a highly relevant species to test novel drugs or regimens to show activity against persisting bacilli.

Studies of *Mycobacterium bovis* Infection

Despite the opportunities to study infection caused by *Mycobacterium bovis* in the natural hosts (e.g., cattle and deer), guinea pigs have proven useful as an experimental tool to develop diagnostic skin test reagents (van Pinxteren et al. 2000), screen mutants (Collins 2001), or perform early-stage down-selection of vaccines intended for use in cattle or wildlife (De Lisle et al. 1999; Chambers et al. 2002; Clark et al. 2008).

FUTURE PERSPECTIVES FOR THE MODEL

Vaccine Evaluation and Natural Transmission Studies

It is likely that the guinea pig model will remain an important in vivo system to test the potency of interventions to reduce disease burden, at least until a reliable marker of protective immunity is defined. Researchers with expertise in the model are continually seeking ways to improve the model and advances in methods to quantify disease burden, such as advanced imaging and the use of bacterial reporter strains, are on the horizon. Developments that allow disease progression to be monitored in real time in the same animal will help to clarify which are the optimal readouts to define protective efficacy. There is a renewed interest in understanding natural transmission of TB with a view to improving control measures. In the original natural transmission studies performed by Riley in the 1950s (Riley 1961), guinea pigs were used to sensitively "capture" tubercle bacilli, which were shed from patients with TB disease, and similar experimental systems are being developed (Dharmadhikari et al. 2011) with funding initiatives such as the Bill and Melinda Gates Foundation, TB Vaccine Accelerator grants. The reliance on the guinea pig model has sparked several new initiatives to develop immunological reagents and assays to monitor responses to exposure/infection. These new tools will substantially improve vaccine evaluation studies by allowing vaccination schedules to be optimized before performing lengthy and costly challenge studies and will additionally enable correlates of protection and immune markers of disease progression to be identified.

Postexposure Vaccination and Clinically Relevant Scenarios

Although mice are the more commonly used species to test therapeutic or postexposure vaccines, guinea pigs might be considered to measure both efficacy (to prevent reactivation of persisting organisms) and the safety of vaccines or immunotherapies because the characteristic necrotic granulomas, which develop in guinea pigs, are an environment that has been associated with persistence of bacteria and the expression of antigens believed to be important in latent *M. tuberculosis* infection.

Guinea pigs have been shown to be useful to study TB in the context of other underlying factors such as diabetes and malnutrition. The development of immunological tools should make possible the manipulation of host factors to determine their specific interactions with *M. tuberculosis*.

CONCLUDING REMARKS

The guinea pig has been the faithful servant of the TB researcher for more than 200 years, providing information to understand disease processes and identify virulence determinants of *M. tuberculosis*. It has enabled preclinical safety and efficacy screening of new drugs and vaccines, which are urgently needed. Although overshadowed for many years by mouse models, which have allowed identification and study of the immune responses to *M. tuberculosis*, guinea pigs have generally been regarded as the more relevant species to replicate human disease. New immunological tools are being developed, sparked by the use of guinea pigs as recipients of naturally transmitted *M. tuberculosis*; such tools will further increase the usefulness of the guinea pig in the future.

REFERENCES

Alsaadi AI, Smith DW. 1973. The fate of virulent and attenuated mycobacteria in guinea pigs infected by the respiratory route. *Am Rev Respir Dis* **107:** 1041–1046.

Arbues A, Aguilo JI, Gonzalo-Asensio J, Marinova D, Uranga S, Puentes E, Fernandez C, Parra A, Cardona PJ, Vilaplana C, et al. 2013. Construction, characterization and preclinical evaluation of MTBVAC, the first live-attenuated *M. tuberculosis*-based vaccine to enter clinical trials. *Vaccine* **31:** 4867–4873.

Balasubramanian V, Guo-Zhi W, Wiegeshaus E, Smith D. 1992. Virulence of *Mycobacterium tuberculosis* for guinea pigs: A quantitative modification of the assay developed by Mitchison. *Tuber Lung Dis* **73:** 268–272.

Basaraba RJ. 2008. Experimental tuberculosis: The role of comparative pathology in the discovery of improved tuberculosis treatment strategies. *Tuberculosis* **88:** S35–47.

Basaraba RJ, Dailey DD, McFarland CT, Shanley CA, Smith EE, McMurray DN, Orme IM. 2006. Lymphadenitis as a major element of disease in the guinea pig model of tuberculosis. *Tuberculosis* **86:** 386–394.

Basaraba RJ, Bielefeldt-Ohmann H, Eschelbach EK, Reisenhauer C, Tolnay AE, Taraba LC, Shanley CA, Smith EA, Bedwell CL, Chlipala EA, et al. 2008. Increased expression of host iron-binding proteins precedes iron accumulation and calcification of primary lung lesions in experimental tuberculosis in the guinea pig. *Tuberculosis* **88:** 69–79.

Brandt L, Skeiky YA, Alderson MR, Lobet Y, Dalemans W, Turner OC, Basaraba RJ, Izzo AA, Lasco TM, Chapman PL, et al. 2004. The protective effect of the *Mycobacterium bovis* BCG vaccine is increased by coadministration with the *Mycobacterium tuberculosis* 72-kilodalton fusion polyprotein Mtb72F in *M. tuberculosis*-infected guinea pigs. *Infect Immun* **72:** 6622–6632.

Cegielski JP, McMurray DN. 2004. The relationship between malnutrition and tuberculosis: Evidence from studies in humans and experimental animals. *Int J Tuberc Lung Dis* **8:** 286–298.

Chambers MA, Williams A, Hatch G, Gavier-Widen D, Hall G, Huygen K, Lowrie D, Marsh PD, Hewinson RG. 2002. Vaccination of guinea pigs with DNA encoding the mycobacterial antigen MPB83 influences pulmonary pathology but not hematogenous spread following aerogenic infection with *Mycobacterium bovis*. *Infect Immun* **70:** 2159–2165.

Clark S, Cross ML, Nadian A, Vipond J, Court P, Williams A, Hewinson RG, Aldwell FE, Chambers MA. 2008. Oral vaccination of guinea pigs with a *Mycobacterium bovis* bacillus Calmette-Guerin vaccine in a lipid matrix protects against aerosol infection with virulent *M. bovis*. *Infect Immun* **76:** 3771–3776.

Collins DM. 2001. Virulence factors of *Mycobacterium bovis*. *Tuberculosis* **81:** 97–102.

Dascher CC, Hiromatsu K, Xiong X, Morehouse C, Watts G, Liu G, McMurray DN, LeClair KP, Porcelli SA, Brenner MB. 2003. Immunization with a mycobacterial lipid vaccine improves pulmonary pathology in the guinea pig model of tuberculosis. *Int Immunol* **15:** 915–925.

De Lisle GW, Wilson T, Collins DM, Buddle BM. 1999. Vaccination of guinea pigs with nutritionally impaired avirulent mutants of *Mycobacterium bovis* protects against tuberculosis. *Infect Immun* **67:** 2624–2626.

Dharmadhikari AS, Basaraba RJ, Van Der Walt ML, Weyer K, Mphahlele M, Venter K, Jensen PA, First MW, Parsons S, McMurray DN, et al. 2011. Natural infection of guinea pigs exposed to patients with highly drug-resistant tuberculosis. *Tuberculosis* **91:** 329–338.

Grode L, Ganoza CA, Brohm C, Weiner J 3rd, Eisele B, Kaufmann SH. 2013. Safety and immunogenicity of the recombinant BCG vaccine VPM1002 in a phase 1 open-label randomized clinical trial. *Vaccine* **31:** 1340–1348.

Grover A, Taylor J, Troudt J, Keyser A, Arnett K, Izzo L, Rholl D, Izzo A. 2009. Kinetics of the immune response profile in guinea pigs after vaccination with *Mycobacterium bovis* BCG and infection with *Mycobacterium tuberculosis*. *Infect Immun* **77:** 4837–4846.

Grover A, Troudt J, Arnett K, Izzo L, Lucas M, Strain K, McFarland C, Hall Y, McMurray D, Williams A, et al. 2012. Assessment of vaccine testing at three laboratories using the guinea pig model of tuberculosis. *Tuberculosis* **92:** 105–111.

Gupta UD, Katoch VM, McMurray DN. 2007. Current status of TB vaccines. *Vaccine* **25:** 3742–3751.

Haslov K, Closs O, Moller S, Bentzon MW. 1984. Studies on the development of tuberculin sensitivity in immunized guinea pigs with demonstration of a close relationship between results of skin tests and the lymphocyte transformation technique. *Int Arch Allergy Appl Immunol* **73:** 114–122.

Haslov K, Andersen A, Nagai S, Gottschau A, Sorensen T, Andersen P. 1995. Guinea pig cellular immune responses to proteins secreted by *Mycobacterium tuberculosis*. *Infect Immun* **63:** 804–810.

Hiromatsu K, Dascher CC, LeClair KP, Sugita M, Furlong ST, Brenner MB, Porcelli SA. 2002. Induction of CD1-restricted immune responses in guinea pigs by immunization with mycobacterial lipid antigens. *J Immunol* **169:** 330–339.

Horwitz MA, Harth G, Dillon BJ, Maslesa-Galic S. 2000. Recombinant bacillus Calmette–Guérin (BCG) vaccines expressing the *Mycobacterium tuberculosis* 30-kDa major secretory protein induce greater protective immunity against tuberculosis than conventional BCG vaccines in a highly susceptible animal model. *Proc Natl Acad Sci* **97:** 13853–13858.

Kato-Maeda M, Shanley CA, Ackart D, Jarlsberg LG, Shang S, Obregon-Henao A, Harton M, Basaraba RJ, Henao-Tamayo M, Barrozo JC, et al. 2012. Beijing sublineages of *Mycobacterium tuberculosis* differ in pathogenicity in the guinea pig. *Clin Vaccine Immunol* **19:** 1227–1237.

Lenaerts AJ, Hoff D, Aly S, Ehlers S, Andries K, Cantarero L, Orme IM, Basaraba RJ. 2007. Location of persisting mycobacteria in a guinea pig model of tuberculosis revealed by r207910. *Antimicrob Agents Chemother* **51:** 3338–3345.

Malaghini M, Thomaz-Soccol V, Probst CM, Krieger MA, Preti H, Kritski A, Soccol CR. 2011. Recombinant antigen production for assays of intradermoreaction for diagnosis and surveillance of tuberculosis. *J Biotechnol* **156:** 56–58.

McMurray DN. 1994. Guinea pig model of tuberculosis. In *Tuberculosis: Pathogenesis, protection and control* (ed. Bloom BR), pp. 135–147. American Society for Microbiology, Washington, DC.

McMurray DN. 2003. Recent progress in the development and testing of vaccines against human tuberculosis. *Int J Parasitol* **33:** 547–554.

Ordway D, Palanisamy G, Henao-Tamayo M, Smith EE, Shanley C, Orme IM, Basaraba RJ. 2007. The cellular immune response to *Mycobacterium tuberculosis* infection in the guinea pig. *J Immunol* **179:** 2532–2541.

Ordway D, Henao-Tamayo M, Shanley C, Smith EE, Palanisamy G, Wang B, Basaraba RJ, Orme IM. 2008. Influence of *Mycobacterium bovis* BCG vaccination on cellular immune response of guinea pigs challenged with *Mycobacterium tuberculosis*. *Clin Vaccine Immunol* **15:** 1248–1258.

Orme IM. 2005. Tuberculosis vaccines: Current progress. *Drugs* **65:** 2437–2444.

Orme IM. 2006. Preclinical testing of new vaccines for tuberculosis: A comprehensive review. *Vaccine* **24:** 2–19.

Orme IM, McMurray DN, Belisle JT. 2001. Tuberculosis vaccine development: Recent progress. *Trends Microbiol* **9:** 115–118.

Padilla-Carlin DJ, McMurray DN, Hickey AJ. 2008. The guinea pig as a model of infectious diseases. *Comp Med* **58:** 324–340.

Palanisamy GS, Smith EE, Shanley CA, Ordway DJ, Orme IM, Basaraba RJ. 2008. Disseminated disease severity as a measure of virulence of *Mycobacterium tuberculosis* in the guinea pig model. *Tuberculosis* **88:** 295–306.

Podell BK, Ackart DF, Kirk NM, Eck SP, Bell C, Basaraba RJ. 2012. Non-diabetic hyperglycemia exacerbates disease severity in *Mycobacterium tuberculosis* infected guinea pigs. *PloS ONE* **7:** e46824.

Riley RL. 1961. Airborne pulmonary tuberculosis. *Bacteriol Rev* **25:** 243–248.

Shang S, Harton M, Tamayo MH, Shanley C, Palanisamy GS, Caraway M, Chan ED, Basaraba RJ, Orme IM, Ordway DJ. 2011. Increased Foxp3 expression in guinea pigs infected with W-Beijing strains of *M. tuberculosis*. *Tuberculosis* **91:** 378–385.

Smith DW, Harding GE. 1977. Animal model of human disease. Pulmonary tuberculosis. Animal model: Experimental airborne tuberculosis in the guinea pig. *Am J Pathol* **89:** 273–276.

Thom RE, Elmore MJ, Williams A, Andrews SC, Drobniewski F, Marsh PD, Tree JA. 2012. The expression of ferritin, lactoferrin, transferrin receptor and solute carrier family 11A1 in the host response to BCG-vaccination and *Mycobacterium tuberculosis* challenge. *Vaccine* **30:** 3159–3168.

Tree JA, Elmore MJ, Javed S, Williams A, Marsh PD. 2006. Development of a guinea pig immune response-related microarray and its use to define the host response following *Mycobacterium bovis* BCG vaccination. *Infect Immun* **74:** 1436–1441.

Turner OC, Basaraba RJ, Orme IM. 2003. Immunopathogenesis of pulmonary granulomas in the guinea pig after infection with *Mycobacterium tuberculosis*. *Infect Immun* **71:** 864–871.

van Pinxteren LA, Ravn P, Agger EM, Pollock J, Andersen P. 2000. Diagnosis of tuberculosis based on the two specific antigens ESAT-6 and CFP10. *Clin Diagn Lab Immunol* **7:** 155–160.

Walker KB, Brennan MJ, Ho MM, Eskola J, Thiry G, Sadoff J, Dobbelaer R, Grode L, Liu MA, Fruth U, et al. 2010. The second Geneva Consensus: Recommendations for novel live TB vaccines. *Vaccine* **28:** 2259–2270.

Wiegeshaus EH, McMurray DN, Grover AA, Harding GE, Smith DW. 1970. Host-parasite relationships in experimental airborne tuberculosis. 3. Relevance of microbial enumeration to acquired resistance in guinea pigs. *Am Rev Respir Dis* **102:** 422–429.

Williams A, Hall Y, Orme IM. 2009. Evaluation of new vaccines for tuberculosis in the guinea pig model. *Tuberculosis* **89:** 389–397.

Williams A, Hatch GJ, Clark SO, Gooch KE, Hatch KA, Hall GA, Huygen K, Ottenhoff TH, Franken KL, Andersen P, et al. 2005a. Evaluation of vaccines in the EU TB Vaccine Cluster using a guinea pig aerosol infection model of tuberculosis. *Tuberculosis* **85:** 29–38.

Williams A, James BW, Bacon J, Hatch KA, Hatch GJ, Hall GA, Marsh PD. 2005b. An assay to compare the infectivity of *Mycobacterium tuberculosis* isolates based on aerosol infection of guinea pigs and assessment of bacteriology. *Tuberculosis* **85:** 177–184.

Animal Models of Tuberculosis: Zebrafish

Lisanne M. van Leeuwen[1,2], Astrid M. van der Sar[1], and Wilbert Bitter[1,3]

[1]Department of Pediatric Infectious Diseases and Immunology, VU University Medical Center, 1081 HV Amsterdam, The Netherlands

[2]Department of Medical Microbiology and Infection control, VU University Medical Center, 1081 BT Amsterdam, The Netherlands

[3]Department of Molecular Microbiology, VU University, 1081 HV Amsterdam, The Netherlands

Correspondence: a.vandersar@vumc.nl

Over the past decade the zebrafish (*Danio rerio*) has become an attractive new vertebrate model organism for studying mycobacterial pathogenesis. The combination of medium-throughput screening and real-time in vivo visualization has allowed new ways to dissect host pathogenic interaction in a vertebrate host. Furthermore, genetic screens on the host and bacterial sides have elucidated new mechanisms involved in the initiation of granuloma formation and the importance of a balanced immune response for control of mycobacterial pathogens. This article will highlight the unique features of the zebrafish–*Mycobacterium marinum* infection model and its added value for tuberculosis research.

Why would one use zebrafish (*Danio rerio*) to study tuberculosis (TB)? Although zebrafish are vertebrates, they do not have lungs, an obvious caveat for studying a pulmonary disease. Furthermore, at present it is unclear whether *Mycobacterium tuberculosis* can give rise to successful infections in cold-blooded animals. Robert Koch tried to infect cold-blooded animals, including a turtle, a goldfish, three eels, and five frogs. After two months, none of them showed any sign of disease, whereas most mammals were either clearly ill or showed tubercles upon autopsy (Koch 1884). Despite these drawbacks, zebrafish have emerged as a valuable organism to study infectious diseases and especially TB (Grunwald and Eisen 2002; Meeker and Trede 2008; Ramakrishnan 2013). The power of the model, real-time imaging of biological processes, was first exploited for TB by the group of Ramakrishnan (Davis et al. 2002), leading the way to study mycobacterial virulence factors and host characteristics in real time in a living vertebrate animal. In recent years, the strength of the zebrafish model has been greatly extended with the increasing availability of transgenic zebrafish lines, improved imaging techniques, and a growing list of genetic tools and large-scale mutant analysis. This article will highlight the unique features of the zebrafish–*Mycobacterium marinum* infection model and its added value for TB research.

WHAT IS THE ZEBRAFISH–*M. marinum* MODEL OF TUBERCULOSIS?

To appreciate the zebrafish—*M. marinum* model of TB, it is important to discuss the basic traits and tools of both the zebrafish and its natural pathogen *M. marinum*.

Cite this article as *Cold Spring Harb Perspect Med* doi: 10.1101/cshperspect.a018580

General Properties of Zebrafish

Advantageous features of the zebrafish include their small size (adults are 3- to 5-cm long), the possibility of keeping them at high population density (5 fish/L), and their ease of breeding—a single female can lay up to 300 eggs a week (Meijer and Spaink 2011). Zebrafish embryos develop externally and are transparent during embryo and larval stages, making it possible to follow host–pathogen interaction in real time. In contrast to other animal models, the zebrafish can be studied during the first weeks of development. In this period, the embryo solely relies on the innate immune system (Fig. 1) (van der Sar et al. 2004b; Meeker and Trede 2008; Novoa and Figueras 2012; van der Vaart et al. 2012), which provides the opportunity to study the contribution of innate immunity to disease in an isolated fashion. Furthermore, it allows for distinguishing between this arm of immunity and a combined innate and adaptive immune response in the context of infection, like in adult fish, which have a complex adaptive immune system akin to that of mammals (Fig. 1) (Traver et al. 2003; Meeker and Trede 2008; Renshaw and Trede 2012; van der Vaart et al. 2012). The finalized whole-genome sequence of zebrafish (Howe et al. 2013) reveals that ~70% of human genes have at least one obvious zebrafish ortholog.

Because of the genetic possibilities (Amsterdam and Hopkins 2006; Lesley and Ramakrishnan 2008; Meijer and Spaink 2011; Blackburn et al. 2013) and the specimen availability and size (and therefore screening options), zebrafish are often seen as a bridge between cell culture systems and mammals (Brittijn et al. 2009).

General Properties of *M. marinum*

Because *M. tuberculosis* does not seem to cause disease in cold-blooded animals, an alternative pathogen is used. Zebrafish are susceptible to a number of mycobacterial pathogens, of which *M. marinum* is the most interesting candidate (Watral and Kent 2007). *M. marinum* naturally inhabits aquatic environments and is the causative agent of a tuberculosis-like disease in cold-blooded animals (Tobin and Ramakrishnan 2008). Furthermore, this species is a close genetic relative of *M. tuberculosis*. At 6.6 Mb, the genome of *M. marinum* is ~1.5 times the size of that of *M. tuberculosis*, which likely reflects its expanded host range and capabilities to survive in the environment. Orthologous coding sequences share an average amino acid identity of 85% (Stinear et al. 2008). Furthermore, the two species share different mechanisms for intracellular growth and host survival. *M. tuberculosis* genes can usually complement mutations in *M. marinum* orthologs and vice versa (Gao et al. 2003; Stinear et al. 2008; Tobin and Ramakrishnan 2008; Stoop et al. 2011). Similar

Figure 1. Development of zebrafish immunity in comparison with the human immune system. Zebrafish possess a complex immune system, similar to that of humans. Development of zebrafish larvae is shown in *A* and a time line is shown in *B*. The appearance of components of the immune system is shown in *C*, and comparison is made with human immune components. Components of the innate immune system are detectable and active in the first days postfertilization (dpf) (e.g., macrophages, neutrophils, eosinophils, and mast cells). Adaptive immunity takes longer to develop and starts with thymus development at 60 hours postfertilization (hpf) and the appearance of the first lymphocytic markers at ~4 dpf. At 21 dpf, the thymus is fully matured, and the first mature T cells and B cells are detected; humoral immunity is functional at 28 dpf. wpf, weeks postfertilization; TCR, T-cell receptor; NK, natural killer; MHC, major histocompatibility complex; DC, dendritic cell; APC, antigen-presenting cell; TLR, Toll-like receptor; NITR, novel immune-type receptor; TNF-α, tumor necrosis factor-α; IFN, interferon. References cited in figure as follows: a, Herbomel et al. 1999; b, Herbomel et al. 2001; c, Traver et al. 2003; d, Meijer and Spaink 2011; e, Novoa and Figueras 2012; f, Renshaw et al. 2006; g, Le Guyader et al. 2008; h, Renshaw and Trede 2012; i, Bertrand et al. 2007; j, Balla et al. 2010; k, Meeker and Trede 2008; l, Dobson et al. 2008; m, Lam et al. 2002; n, Trede et al. 2004; o, Danilova et al. 2004; p, Schorpp et al. 2006; q, Meeker et al. 2010; r, Laing and Hansen 2011; s, Lam et al. 2004; t, Danilova et al. 2005; u, Page et al. 2013; v, Yoder 2009; w, Yoder et al. 2010; x, van der Sar et al. 2004b; y, van der Vaart et al. 2012; z, Palha et al. 2013; aa, de Jong et al. 2011; bb, de Jong and Zon 2012; cc, Lugo-Villarino et al. 2010.

A B

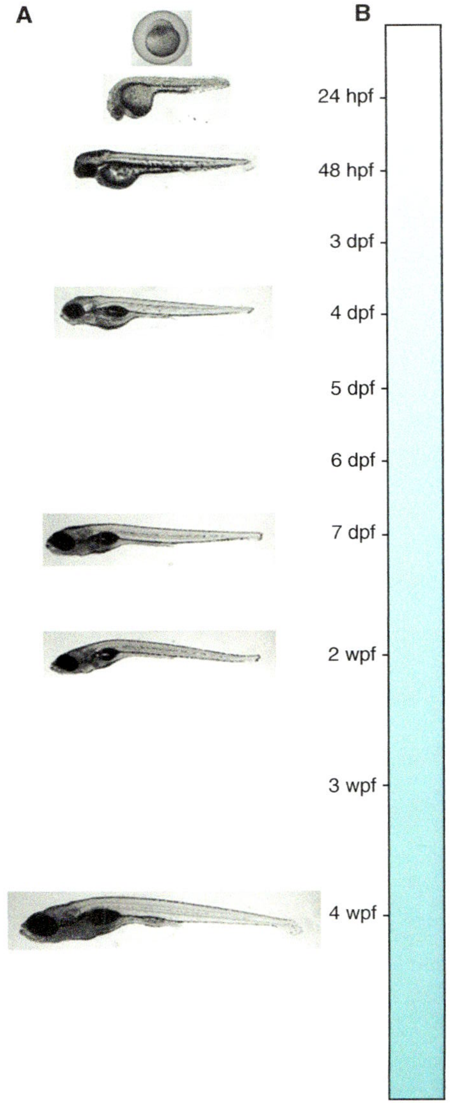

C

	Zebrafish	Human	Development	Ref
Myeloid				
Monocytes/macrophages			24 hpf (1)	a, b, c, d, e
Motility	+	+		
Phagocytic activity	+	+		
Ability to activate T/B cells	+	+		c
Different marker subsets	+	+		
Neutrophils			48 hpf (2)	d, e, f, g, h
Motility	+	+		
Phagocytic activity	+	+		
Myeloperoxidase	+	+		
Eosinophils			36 hpf (3)	h, i, j
Motility	+	+		
Degranulation	Only shown in response to *Heligmosomoides polygyrus* in zebrafish			
Basophils	Currently not characterized in zebrafish			k
Mast cells	Share structural and functional characteristics		24–28 hpf (4)	h, l
Degranulation	+	+		
Lymphoid				
T cells			Thymus 60 hpf-21dpf (5)	c, d, h, m, n,
Educated in thymus	+	+	First lymphocytic markers 4 dpf (6)	o, p, k, q, r,
TCR	Zebrafish TCR-α,β,γ,δ identified			
Gene expression	Similarities in *ikaros*, *lck*, *GATA-3*, *rag*		Mature T cells 21 dpf (7)	
CD4⁺ helper/cytotoxic CD8⁺/ CD4⁺CD25⁺ regulatory T cells	Genetic evidence for existence in zebrafish, functional assays are lacking			
B cells			First B cells: 20–21 dpf (8)	s, t, u
Ig subtypes	D,M,Z	A,D,E,G,M	Onset humoral immunity: 28 dpf (9)	
Antibody response to immunization	+	+		
NK cells				e, h, v, w
Receptor	NITR	classical NK receptors		
	NITRs probably functional orthologs of mammalian NK receptors			
General				
Complement system	Highly developed complement system in zebrafish, with shared human elements			c, e, x
Identified components	C3, C4, Factor B & H, MBL			
Inflammatory proteins	Homology in human and zebrafish in: IL1β, IL10, TNFα, IL8,			y
	CXCR1&2			z
	IFNø1, IFNø2	Structural homology with IFN type I resp. III		
MHC	Type I & II identified, share functional characteristics			c, aa, bb,
DC & other APCs	Share morphological and functional characteristics			h, cc
TLR	TLR2, TLR3, TLR5 specificity conserved in mammals			y
	TLR4 identified in zebrafish, differs in specificity			
TLR-signaling pathway	Myd88, Mal/Tirap, Trif/Ticam1, Sarm, Traf6 identified in zebrafish, share homology with mammals			y

Figure 1. *See facing page for legend.*

to *M. tuberculosis*, specific genotypic lineages of *M. marinum* are associated with variability in virulence (van der Sar et al. 2004a; Ostland et al. 2008; Hernandez-Pando et al. 2012). Apart from the free-living stage, another clear difference for *M. marinum* is its restricted growth temperature, which lies between 28°C and 30°C. Growth is normally halted at 37°C, which is considered as one of the main factors that limits *M. marinum* infections to cooler surface of the skin (Kent et al. 2006). *M. marinum* is primarily associated with human skin lesions called fish tank granulomas. Interestingly, these local granulomas are often histopathologically indistinguishable from *M. tuberculosis* dermal granulomas (Travis et al. 1985; MacGregor 1995) (Fig. 2). *M. marinum* has several other advantages over working with *M. tuberculosis*, including fewer biosafety restrictions (BSL2 instead of BSL3) and a relatively short replication time (4 h) (Tobin and Ramakrishnan 2008).

ROUTES OF INFECTION

The natural infection route for *M. marinum* has not been fully elucidated, but the available evidence strongly indicates that the gastrointestinal tract is the port of entry (Harriff et al. 2007). Furthermore, transmission was significantly enhanced when the bacteria were supplied within free-living unicellular eukaryotes, including amoeba and paramecium (Harriff et al. 2007; Peterson et al. 2013). However, these more natural routes of transmission are not really applicable for infection experiments, as the infection dose and timing cannot be easily controlled. Therefore, to study mycobacterial pathogenesis in vivo, zebrafish are infected with *M. marinum* via different inoculation routes (Fig. 3). Adult zebrafish are usually infected by intraperitoneal or intramuscular injection, whereas the most commonly used infection route in embryos is injection into the caudal vein at 28 hpf (Meijer and Spaink 2011; Benard et al. 2012). Local in-

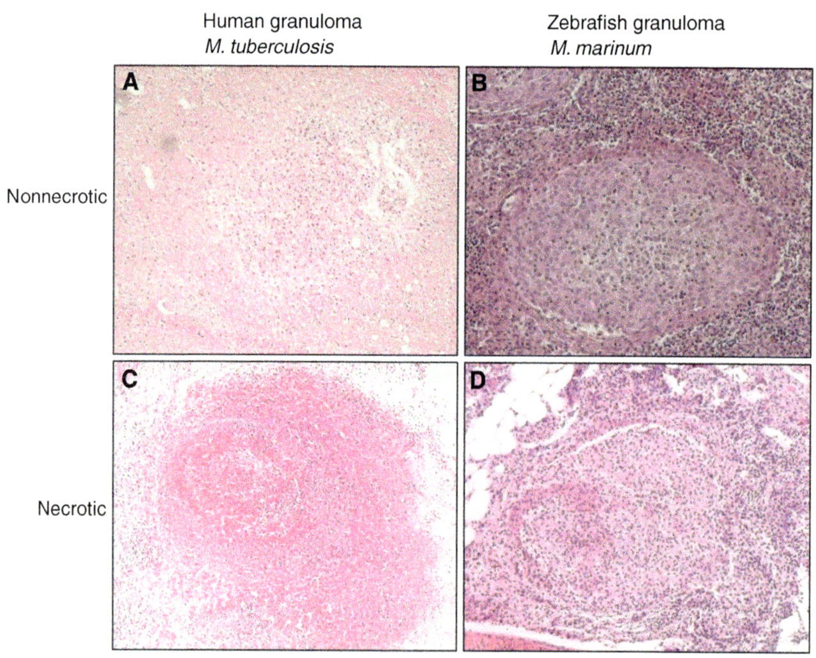

Figure 2. Pathology in adult fish compared with human granulomas. Zebrafish granulomas caused by *M. marinum* show great similarities with human granulomas formed after infection with *M. tuberculosis*. Panels represent nonnecrotic early granuloma in human (*A*) and zebrafish (*B*) and granulomas with a necrotic center in human (*C*) and zebrafish (*D*). Human granulomas obtained from a neuropathology study in our Department of Pediatric Infectious Diseases and Immunology (D Zaharie, S Roest, M van der Kulp, AM van Furth, pers. comm.).

 Cite this article as *Cold Spring Harb Perspect Med* doi: 10.1101/cshperspect.a018580

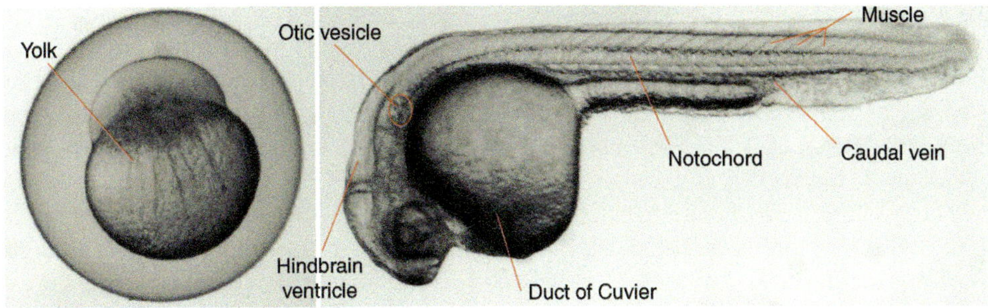

Figure 3. Routes of infection. Zebrafish are infected with *M. marinum* at different time points and via different inoculation routes. Systemic infection is achieved by injection into the caudal vein at 28 hpf or inoculation via the duct of Cuvier in embryos at 2–3 dpf (Benard et al. 2012). Local injection routes are the hindbrain ventricle, muscle, notochord (Alibaud et al. 2011), or otic vesicle. In addition to intravenous injection at 24–28 hpf, yolk injection can be applied at the one- to four-cell stage in a high-throughput setting (Benard et al. 2012).

oculation routes (e.g., via the hindbrain ventricle, muscle, notochord, or otic vesicle [Fig. 3]) can be used to study macrophage and neutrophil chemotaxis. Alternatively, yolk injection at the one- to four-cell stage can be applied for early infections in a high-throughput setting (Meijer and Spaink 2011).

KEY FEATURES OF *M. marinum* INFECTION IN ZEBRAFISH

Actually two zebrafish infection models exist, the adult and the embryonic-larval model. Each has its own characteristics and benefits and both will be discussed.

Pathology in Adult Fish

Adult zebrafish develop on intraperitoneal injection with *M. marinum*, a chronic infection with necrotic (caseating) granulomas, a key feature of human TB (Pozos and Ramakrishnan 2004; van der Sar et al. 2004a; Berg and Ramakrishnan 2012). These granulomas are preferentially formed in fatty tissue and are most commonly found in the pancreas, adipose tissue, liver, spleen, and gonads (Swaim et al. 2006; Parikka et al. 2012; Oksanen et al. 2013; Stoop et al. 2013). The first granulomas can already be found in the first weeks postinfection (Swaim et al. 2006; Parikka et al. 2012). Even the first signs of necrosis, consisting of cytoplasmic and nuclear debris, are present at this time. The induction of a latent, chronic, or active mycobacterial disease depends on the infection dose and the *M. marinum* strain used (van der Sar et al. 2004a; Swaim et al. 2006; Parikka et al. 2012). A low infection dose results in a latent disease with stable numbers of granulomas over time, whereas a high-dose infection leads to a more progressive and active disease (Parikka et al. 2012). During a chronic disease course in zebrafish, bacterial growth seems to mimic growth curves of various other animal models of TB—growth for the first 3–4 wk and reaching a plateau when adaptive immunity develops (North and Jung 2004; van der Sar et al. 2004a; Swaim et al. 2006; Parikka et al. 2012; Ramakrishnan 2012). At 16–20 wk postinfection, most granulomas contain a necrotic center, which is also the location where the bacteria are predominantly present. Most granulomas form a fibrotic and/or cellular cuff, which separates them from the surrounding tissue at this time point (Swaim et al. 2006; Parikka et al. 2012; Ramakrishnan 2012).

As in human TB, maximal control of *M. marinum* infection in zebrafish is dependent on an intact adaptive immune system (Swaim et al. 2006; Parikka et al. 2012; Ramakrishnan 2012). Because of the lack of immune markers, characterization of the immune response of zebrafish during mycobacterial infection is mainly based on transcriptome and deep sequencing studies (Meijer et al. 2005; Hegedus et al. 2009; Meijer and Spaink 2011; van der Vaart et al. 2012). These studies show a modest but complex host response in the early stages of infection (Meijer et al. 2005; Hegedus et al. 2009). Detailed analysis of immune factors involved in mycobacterial disease depends on the generation of more knockout zebrafish and development of specific antibodies directed against immune cells and chemokines/cytokines.

Pathology in Embryos

Pathology in zebrafish embryos is, because of practical/ethical reasons, usually only studied for 5–6 d. Within this short time frame early granuloma formation can be studied by real-time imaging (Fig. 4). This allows visualization of early steps in mycobacterial pathogenesis in the context of innate immunity. On infection, *M. marinum* is readily phagocytosed by macrophages (Lesley and Ramakrishnan 2008; Yang et al. 2012; Ramakrishnan 2013), which traverse endothelial and epithelial barriers and form infectious clusters in deeper tissue within 4 d (Davis et al. 2002; Lesley and Ramakrishnan 2008; Tobin and Ramakrishnan 2008). Once early granulomas form, macrophages adopt a distinctive epithelioid morphology. Within these clusters mycobacteria activate genes that are known to be specifically activated within mature granulomas in adults, confirming that these infectious clusters actually resemble granulomas (Tobin and Ramakrishnan 2008). This means that innate immune determinants are sufficient to drive *M. marinum* granuloma formation/initiation (Tobin and Ramakrishnan 2008; Meijer and Spaink 2011; Ramakrishnan 2013).

LESSONS LEARNED FROM THE ZEBRAFISH INFECTION MODEL

We will discuss a number of bacterial features and host characteristics important during the early steps of mycobacterial infection that

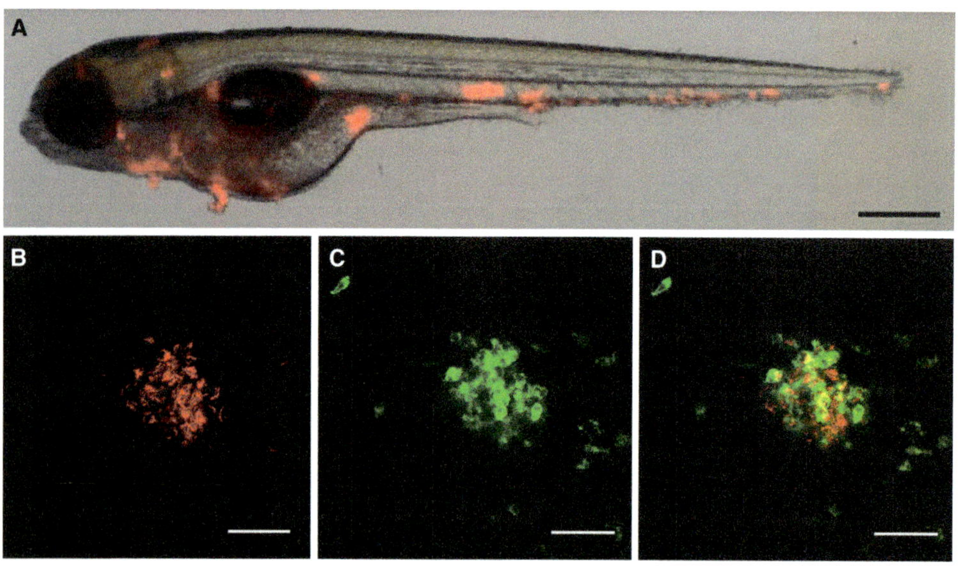

Figure 4. Pathology in embryos. (*A*) Merged bright-field and fluorescent image of a zebrafish embryo infected with red fluorescent *M. marinum* and photographed at 5 dpi. (Adapted with permission from Stoop et al. 2011.) Clustering of mycobacteria and early granuloma formation is shown as red spots. (*B–D*) Higher magnification of an early granuloma at 5 dpi formed after bloodstream infection, derived from analysis using confocal imaging by our research group. (*B*) *M. marinum* E11 (in red), (*C*) phagocytes stained with anti-L-Plastin (in green), (*D*) merge of *B* and *C* confirming the colocalization of these cells in early granulomas in zebrafish embryos. Scale bar, 35 μm.

have been discovered using the zebrafish model (Fig. 5).

Dynamic Granulomas

Classically the granuloma is regarded as a static structure "walling off" bacteria from the rest of the body and therefore critical for host protection (Ulrichs and Kaufmann 2006; Rubin 2009; Schaaf and Zumla 2009). This idea was changed upon observation of the early stages of granuloma formation in zebrafish embryos, which revealed the dynamics of this process (Ramakrishnan 2012). Elegant studies with photobleaching of distinctive clusters in zebrafish embryos and reinfection experiments showed that infected macrophages can detach from the established granuloma and wander off to new locations to form secondary granulomas, thereby disseminating *M. marinum* (Lesley and Ramakrishnan 2008; Ramakrishnan 2013). Furthermore, macrophages attracted to existing granulomas consume damaged/apoptotic infected cells and their bacterial content in the center of the granuloma, leading to expansion of the early aggregate. These experiments revealed two things: (1) Granuloma formation might actually aid bacterial proliferation, because accelerated bacterial proliferation coincides with granuloma formation (Lesley and Ramakrishnan 2008); and (2) early granulomas are not fixed in size and location. Subsequently, TB studies in mice and nonhuman primates further supported the notion that granulomas are actually highly dynamic structures (Egen et al. 2008; Lin et al. 2013; Ramakrishnan 2013).

Genetic Susceptibility to TB

A broad variation in TB susceptibility and differences between individuals is a long-understood concept.

In the search for candidates for host susceptibility, the zebrafish model has contributed by using forward genetic screens. Tobin et al. (2010) used this method to identify mutant zebrafish with increased susceptibility to *M. marinum*. Genetic analysis of one such mutant showed that the *lta4h* locus was affected. This locus controls the balance between pro- and anti-inflammatory eicosanoids. Also in humans LTA4H polymorphisms seem to play a role in the control of infection and inflammation during TB (Tobin et al. 2010). This characterization led to the conclusion that inflammation must be balanced, and misbalance can result in either an inadequate inflammatory or tissue-destructive hyperinflammatory state. Additional research (Tobin et al. 2012) showed that therapies directed to a specific profile could favor disease outcome (Berg and Ramakrishnan 2012), highlighting how well the zebrafish model resembles aspects of human TB and how useful this model can be to study features of this disease.

In addition to the *lta4h* locus, other genes seem to be required to maintain the balance of mycobacterial infection. For instance, *ptpn6* morphant embryos, in which the gene is temporarily knocked down, show a hyperinflammation phenotype (Kanwal et al. 2013). The *ptpn6* gene is associated with chronic inflammatory disease in human and plays an important role as a negative regulator of the innate immune system, probably by regulating the induction levels of several kinases in TLR signaling (Kanwal et al. 2013).

Complementary Features of the Embryo and Adult Systems

An illustrative example in which virulence patterns showed large differences in the embryo model compared with the adult model is described by Stoop et al. (2013). In this study they examined the effect of a knockout in the mycobacterial *mptC* gene, which is required for mannan core branching of lipomannan and lipoarabinomannan. This modification has been linked to TLR-2 activation (Nigou et al. 2008). Interestingly, although this mutant is clearly attenuated in embryos, the effect is only minor in the context of the adaptive immune system. The reverse is also possible, as was shown by Weerdenburg et al. (2012). An *M. marinum* mutant disrupted in ESX-5 secretion was slightly attenuated in embryos, but showed increased virulence in adult zebrafish, characterized by highly increased bacterial loads and early onset of granuloma formation. The molecular basis for

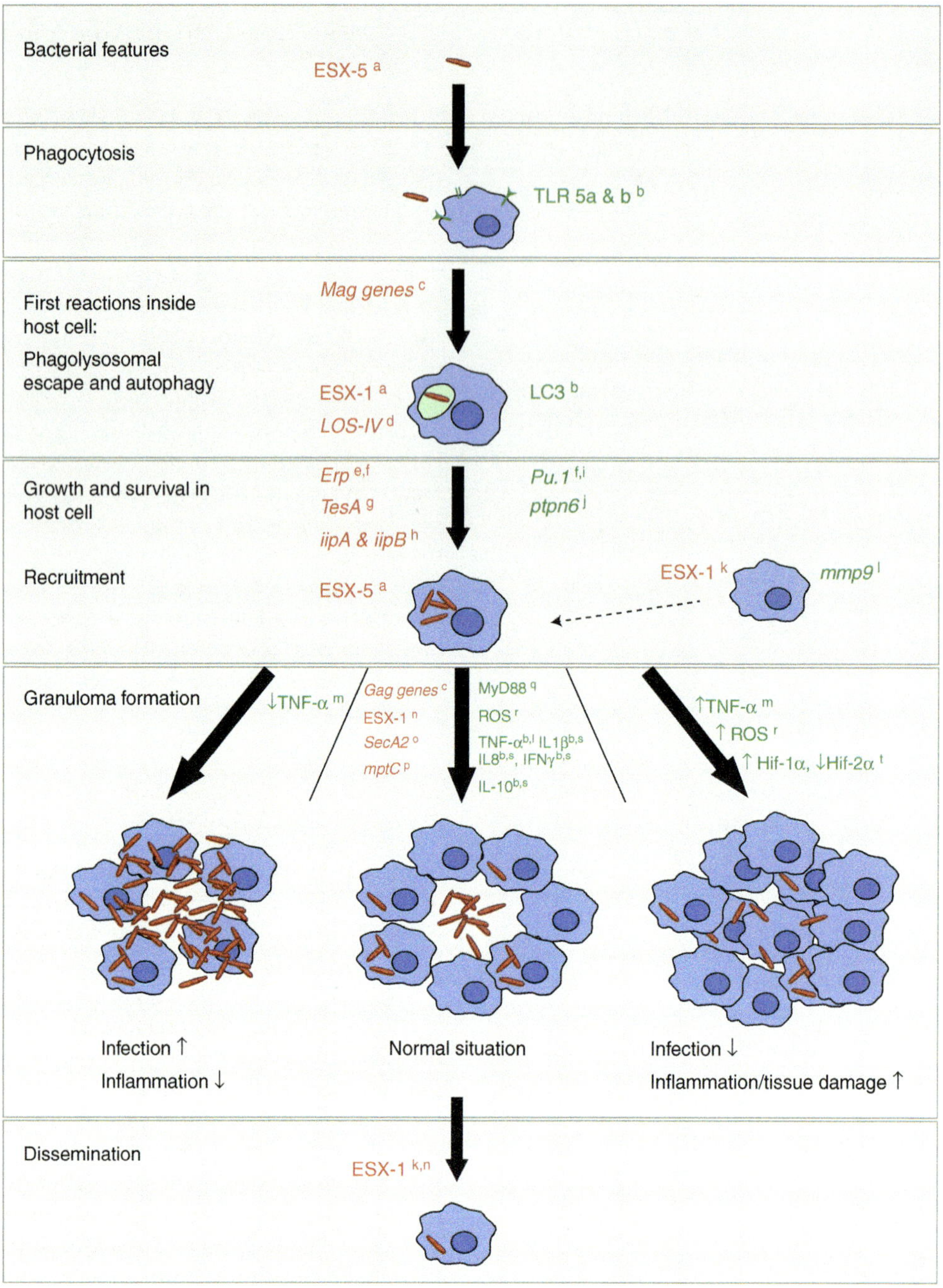

Figure 5. Graphical summary. This summary shows bacterial and host characteristics important in mycobacterial pathogenesis derived from and validated in the zebrafish infection model. The different hallmarks of pathogenesis are shown. For each step, red shows identified mycobacterial factors important for the pathogen to survive and cope with the immune system of the host, and green shows host factors required for an appropriate immune response. Three types of granuloma are described and schematically depicted in this summary. The granuloma in the *middle* is the normal granuloma with a balance between inflammation and infection; at the *left* and *right*, granulomas without the right balance are depicted with high infection and high inflammation, respectively. Labels in the figure refer to the following references: a, Stoop et al. 2012; b, van der Vaart et al. 2012; c, Davis et al. 2002; d, van der Woude et al. 2012; e, Cosma et al. 2006; f, Meijer and Spaink 2011; g Alibaud et al. 2011; h, Gao et al. 2006; I, Clay et al. 2007; j, Kanwal et al. 2013; k, Davis and Ramakrishnan 2009; l, Volkman et al. 2010; m, Tobin et al. 2010; n, Volkman et al. 2004; o, van der Woude et al. 2013; p, Stoop et al. 2013; q, van der Vaart et al. 2013; r, Roca and Ramakrishnan 2013; s, van der Sar et al. 2009; t, Elks et al. 2013.

this difference has not been identified yet, but seems to be independent of the adaptive immune response, as the hypervirulence phenotype was also observed in zebrafish *rag* mutants. These studies highlight the importance of studying both the embryo and adult systems.

Mycobacterial Virulence Factors

The zebrafish embryo is an excellent model to study the importance of different mycobacterial virulence factors in different steps of infection. The *erp* (*pirG*) gene, coding for a cell wall–associated protein with unknown function, was first identified as required for virulence in *M. tuberculosis* (Berthet et al. 1998; Cosma et al. 2006). Using microscopic examination of infected zebrafish embryos it could be shown that *M. marinum* lacking Erp failed to grow and survive upon phagocytosis, an event very early in granuloma pathogenesis (Cosma et al. 2006; Meijer and Spaink 2011). Subsequently, macrophages were eliminated in zebrafish embryos by injection of pu.1 morpholino, thereby knocking down the pu.1 transcription factor, which is required for myeloid development (Meijer and Spaink 2011). Now, growth of the *erp* mutant was restored, indicating that in vivo attenuation was specifically linked to defective growth inside macrophages (Lesley and Ramakrishnan 2008).

A number of studies have used different setups to identify *M. marinum* virulence factors, most of which seem to underscore the similarities between *M. marinum* and *M. tuberculosis*. The most elaborate screen was performed by Stoop et al. (Stoop et al. 2011, 2013; van der Woude et al. 2013), who screened in total 1000 random transposon mutants for early granuloma formation and virulence. With nearly half of the highly attenuated mutants, the most prominent virulence locus identified in these experiments was *esx-1*. This is not entirely surprising, as the *esx-1* locus is probably the most extensively studied virulence locus in pathogenic mycobacteria. The *esx-1* locus is coding for components of a protein secretion system and its substrates, and although the actual mechanism is still not completely resolved, the most compelling data suggests that ESX-1 effector proteins are required for phagolysosomal escape (Stamm et al. 2003; Houben et al. 2012). In addition to the phagosome escape phenotype, macrophage recruitment and dissemination of disease (Volkman et al. 2004; Davis and Ramakrishnan 2009; Stoop et al. 2011) have also been attributed to the ESX-1 system, although these effects could be indirect because *esx-1*-deficient *M. marinum* does not reach its normal location within the phagocytosing cell. Importantly, phagosomal escape of pathogenic mycobacteria was first convincingly shown for *M. marinum* (Stamm et al. 2003) and only later for *M. tuberculosis*, underscoring the importance of this model.

In conclusion, the combination of real-time imaging and high-throughput settings seem ideally suited to screen for bacterial factors involved in the establishment of a successful infection.

Using Zebrafish to Identify New Antimycobacterial Compounds

The search for new antimicrobial compounds or therapies can be accelerated using the zebrafish model. Activity and dosage of antimycobacterial compounds in zebrafish closely resemble characteristics in humans (Adams et al. 2011). In addition, the zebrafish model has helped to challenge the model that persistence is linked to arrested growth (Adams et al. 2011; Philips and Ernst 2011). Using the zebrafish model, it was shown, by spatial monitoring of the behavior of fluorescent bacteria after treatment with antibiotics, that both macrophages and granulomas play a role in the induction and dissemination of drug-tolerant bacteria. The intramacrophage-mediated oxidative stress induces the expression of bacterial efflux pumps in actively replicating bacteria. It was also shown that bacterial efflux pump inhibitors (e.g., verapamil) can be added to the standard antibiotic treatment to reduce macrophage-induced drug tolerance and possibly shorten treatment (Adams et al. 2011; Philips and Ernst 2011; Berg and Ramakrishnan 2012; Zumla et al. 2013).

Another example of using zebrafish embryos in the identification of new antimycobacterial drugs is a recent study by Makarov, who produced and analyzed a new generation of benzathiozinones (Makarov et al. 2014). These compounds bind DprE1 and thereby selectively inhibit the biosynthesis of crucial cell wall components. The most effective second-generation compound (i.e., PBTZ169) was compared with the first-generation lead compound in a zebrafish embryo infection model. Although both compounds reduced bacterial load in zebrafish embryos, this model showed an important difference in toxicity, whereas the original compound led to developmental abnormalities, like deposits in the notochord and subsequent shortening of the anteroposterior axes, and PBTZ169 did not. These examples show that effectiveness and toxicity of antimycobacterial compounds can be assessed accurately using zebrafish embryos.

CONCLUDING REMARKS

The use of zebrafish larvae for studying microbial infection has led to important new insights in host defense mechanisms, which often appear to be common for higher vertebrates (Table 1). However, we still need to extend our comparison of zebrafish model with the mammalian systems to show the translational value for biomedical applications. The rapid increase of available high-throughput technologies in the zebrafish toolbox, such as advances in robotic injection and automated readouts of zebrafish embryos (Spaink et al. 2013), will lead to new approaches for TB research. In addition, new reporter lines of zebrafish that provide readouts for activation of the immune system are highly useful tools for even better in vivo visualization of mycobacterial infections (Kanther and Rawls 2010; Palha et al. 2013). What we still need are specific antibodies for distinguishing immune cell types and technologies for generating cell-specific and conditional knockout mutants.

Zebrafish provide an excellent opportunity to address questions that are difficult to solve in mammalian systems. In return, discoveries in zebrafish must be confirmed in mammalian systems to maximize their translational impact.

Table 1. Top five advantages of the zebrafish model in mycobacterial research

1	Fast model, small animal, ease of breeding, ease of genetic manipulation
2	Transparency and availability of transgenic zebrafish lines make real-time imaging possible
3	Innate and adaptive immunity can be studied separately
4	*Mycobacterium marinum* is strongly related to *Mycobacterium tuberculosis* and causes granulomatous disease in zebrafish with shared characteristics to human granulomatous disease
5	Screens possible for (i) mycobacterial virulence factors; (ii) host factors; (iii) therapeutic compounds, like antibiotics

REFERENCES

Adams KN, Takaki K, Connolly LE, Wiedenhoft H, Winglee K, Humbert O, Edelstein PH, Cosma CL, Ramakrishnan L. 2011. Drug tolerance in replicating mycobacteria mediated by a macrophage-induced efflux mechanism. *Cell* **145:** 39–53.

Alibaud L, Rombouts Y, Trivelli X, Burguiere A, Cirillo SL, Cirillo JD, Dubremetz JF, Guerardel Y, Lutfalla G, Kremer L. 2011. A *Mycobacterium marinum* TesA mutant defective for major cell wall-associated lipids is highly attenuated in *Dictyostelium discoideum* and zebrafish embryos. *Mol Microbiol* **80:** 919–934.

Amsterdam A, Hopkins N. 2006. Mutagenesis strategies in zebrafish for identifying genes involved in development and disease. *Trends Genet* **22:** 473–478.

Balla KM, Lugo-Villarino G, Spitsbergen JM, Stachura DL, Hu Y, Banuelos K, Romo-Fewell O, Aroian RV, Traver D. 2010. Eosinophils in the zebrafish: Prospective isolation, characterization, and eosinophilia induction by helminth determinants. *Blood* **116:** 3944–3954.

Benard EL, van der Sar AM, Ellett F, Lieschke GJ, Spaink HP, Meijer AH. 2012. Infection of zebrafish embryos with intracellular bacterial pathogens. *J Vis Exp* **61:** e3781.

Berg RD, Ramakrishnan L. 2012. Insights into tuberculosis from the zebrafish model. *Trends Mol Med* **18:** 689–690.

Berthet FX, Lagranderie M, Gounon P, Laurent-Winter C, Ensergueix D, Chavarot P, Thouron F, Maranghi E, Pelicic V, Portnoi D, et al. 1998. Attenuation of virulence by disruption of the *Mycobacterium tuberculosis erp* gene. *Science* **282:** 759–762.

Bertrand JY, Kim AD, Violette EP, Stachura DL, Cisson JL, Traver D. 2007. Definitive hematopoiesis initiates through a committed erythromyeloid progenitor in the zebrafish embryo. *Development* **134:** 4147–4156.

Blackburn PR, Campbell JM, Clark KJ, Ekker SC. 2013. The CRISPR system—Keeping zebrafish gene targeting fresh. *Zebrafish* **10:** 116–118.

Brittijn SA, Duivesteijn SJ, Belmamoune M, Bertens LF, Bitter W, de Bruijn JD, Champagne DL, Cuppen E, Flik G, Vandenbroucke-Grauls CM, et al. 2009. Zebrafish development and regeneration: New tools for biomedical research. *Int J Dev Biol* **53:** 835–850.

Clay H, Davis JM, Beery D, Huttenlocher A, Lyons SE, Ramakrishnan L. 2007. Dichotomous role of the macrophage in early *Mycobacterium marinum* infection of the zebrafish. *Cell Host Microbe* **2:** 29–39.

Cosma CL, Klein K, Kim R, Beery D, Ramakrishnan L. 2006. *Mycobacterium marinum* Erp is a virulence determinant required for cell wall integrity and intracellular survival. *Infect Immun* **74:** 3125–3133.

Danilova N, Hohman VS, Sacher F, Ota T, Willett CE, Steiner LA. 2004. T cells and the thymus in developing zebrafish. *Dev Comp Immunol* **28:** 755–767.

Danilova N, Bussmann J, Jekosch K, Steiner LA. 2005. The immunoglobulin heavy-chain locus in zebrafish: Identification and expression of a previously unknown isotype, immunoglobulin Z. *Nat Immunol* **6:** 295–302.

Davis JM, Ramakrishnan L. 2009. The role of the granuloma in expansion and dissemination of early tuberculous infection. *Cell* **136:** 37–49.

Davis JM, Clay H, Lewis JL, Ghori N, Herbomel P, Ramakrishnan L. 2002. Real-time visualization of mycobacterium-macrophage interactions leading to initiation of granuloma formation in zebrafish embryos. *Immunity* **17:** 693–702.

de Jong JL, Zon LI. 2012. Histocompatibility and hematopoietic transplantation in the zebrafish. *Adv Hematol* **2012:** 282318.

de Jong JL, Burns CE, Chen AT, Pugach E, Mayhall EA, Smith AC, Feldman HA, Zhou Y, Zon LI. 2011. Characterization of immune-matched hematopoietic transplantation in zebrafish. *Blood* **117:** 4234–4242.

Dobson JT, Seibert J, Teh EM, Da'as S, Fraser RB, Paw BH, Lin TJ, Berman JN. 2008. Carboxypeptidase A5 identifies a novel mast cell lineage in the zebrafish providing new insight into mast cell fate determination. *Blood* **112:** 2969–2972.

Egen JG, Rothfuchs AG, Feng CG, Winter N, Sher A, Germain RN. 2008. Macrophage and T cell dynamics during the development and disintegration of mycobacterial granulomas. *Immunity* **28:** 271–284.

Elks PM, Brizee S, van der Vaart M, Walmsley SR, van Eeden FJ, Renshaw SA, Meijer AH. 2013. Hypoxia inducible factor signaling modulates susceptibility to mycobacterial infection via a nitric oxide dependent mechanism. *PLoS Pathog* **9:** e1003789.

Gao LY, Groger R, Cox JS, Beverley SM, Lawson EH, Brown EJ. 2003. Transposon mutagenesis of *Mycobacterium marinum* identifies a locus linking pigmentation and intracellular survival. *Infect Immun* **71:** 922–929.

Gao LY, Pak M, Kish R, Kajihara K, Brown EJ. 2006. A mycobacterial operon essential for virulence in vivo and invasion and intracellular persistence in macrophages. *Infect Immun* **74:** 1757–1767.

Grunwald DJ, Eisen JS. 2002. Headwaters of the zebrafish—Emergence of a new model vertebrate. *Nat Rev Genet* **3:** 717–724.

Harriff MJ, Bermudez LE, Kent ML. 2007. Experimental exposure of zebrafish, *Danio rerio* (Hamilton), to *Mycobacterium marinum* and *Mycobacterium peregrinum* reveals the gastrointestinal tract as the primary route of infection: A potential model for environmental mycobacterial infection. *J Fish Dis* **30:** 587–600.

Hegedus Z, Zakrzewska A, Agoston VC, Ordas A, Racz P, Mink M, Spaink HP, Meijer AH. 2009. Deep sequencing of the zebrafish transcriptome response to mycobacterium infection. *Mol Immunol* **46:** 2918–2930.

Herbomel P, Thisse B, Thisse C. 1999. Ontogeny and behaviour of early macrophages in the zebrafish embryo. *Development* **126:** 3735–3745.

Herbomel P, Thisse B, Thisse C. 2001. Zebrafish early macrophages colonize cephalic mesenchyme and developing brain, retina, and epidermis through a M-CSF receptor-dependent invasive process. *Dev Biol* **238:** 274–288.

Hernandez-Pando R, Marquina-Castillo B, Barrios-Payan J, Mata-Espinosa D. 2012. Use of mouse models to study the variability in virulence associated with specific genotypic lineages of *Mycobacterium tuberculosis*. *Infect Genet Evol* **12:** 725–731.

Houben D, Demangel C, van Ingen J, Perez J, Baldeon L, Abdallah AM, Caleechurn L, Bottai D, van Zon M, de Punder K, et al. 2012. ESX-1-mediated translocation to the cytosol controls virulence of mycobacteria. *Cell Microbiol* **14:** 1287–1298.

Howe K, Clark MD, Torroja CF, Torrance J, Berthelot C, Muffato M, Collins JE, Humphray S, McLaren K, Matthews L, et al. 2013. The zebrafish reference genome sequence and its relationship to the human genome. *Nature* **496:** 498–503.

Kanther M, Rawls JF. 2010. Host-microbe interactions in the developing zebrafish. *Curr Opin Immunol* **22:** 10–19.

Kanwal Z, Zakrzewska A, den Hertog J, Spaink HP, Schaaf MJ, Meijer AH. 2013. Deficiency in hematopoietic phosphatase ptpn6/Shp1 hyperactivates the innate immune system and impairs control of bacterial infections in zebrafish embryos. *J Immunol* **190:** 1631–1645.

Kent ML, Watral V, Wu M, Bermudez LE. 2006. In vivo and in vitro growth of *Mycobacterium marinum* at homoeothermic temperatures. *FEMS Microbiol Lett* **257:** 69–75.

Koch R. 1884. Die Ätiologie der Tuberkulose, Mitteilungen aus dem Kaiserl. *Gesundheitsamte* **2:** 1–88.

Laing KJ, Hansen JD. 2011. Fish T cells: Recent advances through genomics. *Dev Comp Immunol* **35:** 1282–1295.

Lam SH, Chua HL, Gong Z, Wen Z, Lam TJ, Sin YM. 2002. Morphologic transformation of the thymus in developing zebrafish. *Dev Dyn* **225:** 87–94.

Lam SH, Chua HL, Gong Z, Lam TJ, Sin YM. 2004. Development and maturation of the immune system in zebrafish, *Danio rerio*: A gene expression profiling, in situ hybridization and immunological study. *Dev Comp Immunol* **28:** 9–28.

Le Guyader D, Redd MJ, Colucci-Guyon E, Murayama E, Kissa K, Briolat V, Mordelet E, Zapata A, Shinomiya H, Herbomel P. 2008. Origins and unconventional behavior of neutrophils in developing zebrafish. *Blood* **111:** 132–141.

Lesley R, Ramakrishnan L. 2008. Insights into early mycobacterial pathogenesis from the zebrafish. *Curr Opin Microbiol* **11:** 277–283.

Lin PL, Coleman T, Carney JP, Lopresti BJ, Tomko J, Fillmore D, Dartois V, Scanga C, Frye LJ, Janssen C, et al. 2013. Radiologic responses in cynomolgous macaques for assessing tuberculosis chemotherapy regimens. *Antimicrob Agents Chemother* doi: 10.1128/AAC.00277-13.

Lugo-Villarino G, Balla KM, Stachura DL, Banuelos K, Werneck MB, Traver D. 2010. Identification of dendritic antigen-presenting cells in the zebrafish. *Proc Natl Acad Sci* **107:** 15850–15855.

MacGregor RR. 1995. Cutaneous tuberculosis. *Clin Dermatol* **13:** 245–255.

Makarov V, Lechartier B, Zhang M, Neres J, van der Sar AM, Raadsen SA, Hartkoorn RC, Ryabova OB, Vocat A, Decosterd LA, et al. 2014. Towards a new combination therapy for tuberculosis with next generation benzothiazinones. *EMBO Mol Med* **6:** 372–383.

Meeker ND, Trede NS. 2008. Immunology and zebrafish: Spawning new models of human disease. *Dev Comp Immunol* **32:** 745–757.

Meeker ND, Smith AC, Frazer JK, Bradley DF, Rudner LA, Love C, Trede NS. 2010. Characterization of the zebrafish T cell receptor β locus. *Immunogenetics* **62:** 23–29.

Meijer AH, Spaink HP. 2011. Host-pathogen interactions made transparent with the zebrafish model. *Curr Drug Targets* **12:** 1000–1017.

Meijer AH, Verbeek FJ, Salas-Vidal E, Corredor-Adamez M, Bussman J, van der Sar AM, Otto GW, Geisler R, Spaink HP. 2005. Transcriptome profiling of adult zebrafish at the late stage of chronic tuberculosis due to *Mycobacterium marinum* infection. *Mol Immunology* **42:** 1185–1203.

Nigou J, Vasselon T, Ray A, Constant P, Gilleron M, Besra GS, Sutcliffe I, Tiraby G, Puzo G. 2008. Mannan chain length controls lipoglycans signaling via and binding to TLR2. *J Immunol* **180:** 6696–6702.

North RJ, Jung YJ. 2004. Immunity to tuberculosis. *Annu Rev Immunol* **22:** 599–623.

Novoa B, Figueras A. 2012. Zebrafish: Model for the study of inflammation and the innate immune response to infectious diseases. *Adv Exp Med Biol* **946:** 253–275.

Oksanen KE, Halfpenny NJ, Sherwood E, Harjula SK, Hammaren MM, Ahava MJ, Pajula ET, Lahtinen MJ, Parikka M, Ramet M. 2013. An adult zebrafish model for preclinical tuberculosis vaccine development. *Vaccine* **31:** 5202–5209.

Ostland VE, Watral V, Whipps CM, Austin FW, St-Hilaire S, Westerman ME, Kent ML. 2008. Biochemical, molecular, and virulence characteristics of select *Mycobacterium marinum* isolates in hybrid striped bass *Morone chrysops* × *M. saxatilis* and zebrafish *Danio rerio*. *Dis Aquat Organ* **79:** 107–118.

Page DM, Wittamer V, Bertrand JY, Lewis KL, Pratt DN, Delgado N, Schale SE, McGue C, Jacobsen BH, Doty A, et al. 2013. An evolutionarily conserved program of B-cell development and activation in zebrafish. *Blood* **122:** e1–e11.

Palha N, Guivel-Benhassine F, Briolat V, Lutfalla G, Sourisseau M, Ellett F, Wang CH, Lieschke GJ, Herbomel P, Schwartz O, et al. 2013. Real-time whole-body visualization of Chikungunya Virus infection and host interferon response in zebrafish. *PLoS Pathog* **9:** e1003619.

Parikka M, Hammaren MM, Harjula SK, Halfpenny NJ, Oksanen KE, Lahtinen MJ, Pajula ET, Iivanainen A, Pesu M, Ramet M. 2012. *Mycobacterium marinum* causes a latent infection that can be reactivated by γ irradiation in adult zebrafish. *PLoS Pathog* **8:** e1002944.

Peterson TS, Ferguson JA, Watral VG, Mutoji KN, Ennis DG, Kent ML. 2013. Paramecium caudatum enhances transmission and infectivity of *Mycobacterium marinum* and *M. chelonae* in zebrafish *Danio rerio*. *Dis Aquat Organ* **106:** 229–239.

Philips JA, Ernst JD. 2011. Directly observing therapy: A new view of drug tolerance in tuberculosis. *Cell* **145:** 13–14.

Pozos TC, Ramakrishnan L. 2004. New models for the study of mycobacterium-host interactions. *Curr Opin Immunol* **16:** 499–505.

Ramakrishnan L. 2012. Revisiting the role of the granuloma in tuberculosis. *Nat Rev Immunol* **12:** 352–366.

Ramakrishnan L. 2013. Looking within the zebrafish to understand the tuberculous granuloma. *Adv Exp Med Biol* **783:** 251–266.

Renshaw SA, Trede NS. 2012. A model 450 million years in the making: Zebrafish and vertebrate immunity. *Dis Model Mech* **5:** 38–47.

Renshaw SA, Loynes CA, Trushell DM, Elworthy S, Ingham PW, Whyte MK. 2006. A transgenic zebrafish model of neutrophilic inflammation. *Blood* **108:** 3976–3978.

Roca FJ, Ramakrishnan L. 2013. TNF dually mediates resistance and susceptibility to mycobacteria via mitochondrial reactive oxygen species. *Cell* **153:** 521–534.

Rubin EJ. 2009. The granuloma in tuberculosis—Friend or foe? *N Engl J Med* **360:** 2471–2473.

Schaaf HS, Zumla A. 2009. *Tuberculosis: A comprehensive clinical reference*. Saunders, Edinburgh.

Schorpp M, Bialecki M, Diekhoff D, Walderich B, Odenthal J, Maischein HM, Zapata AG, Boehm T. 2006. Conserved functions of Ikaros in vertebrate lymphocyte development: Genetic evidence for distinct larval and adult phases of T cell development and two lineages of B cells in zebrafish. *J Immunol* **177:** 2463–2476.

Spaink HP, Cui C, Wiweger MI, Jansen HJ, Veneman WJ, Marin-Juez R, de Sonneville J, Ordas A, Torraca V, van der Ent W, et al. 2013. Robotic injection of zebrafish embryos for high-throughput screening in disease models. *Methods* **62:** 246–254.

Stamm LM, Morisaki JH, Gao LY, Jeng RL, McDonald KL, Roth R, Takeshita S, Heuser J, Welch MD, Brown EJ. 2003. *Mycobacterium marinum* escapes from phagosomes and is propelled by actin-based motility. *J Exp Med* **198:** 1361–1368.

Stinear TP, Seemann T, Harrison PF, Jenkin GA, Davies JK, Johnson PD, Abdellah Z, Arrowsmith C, Chillingworth T, Churcher C, et al. 2008. Insights from the complete genome sequence of *Mycobacterium marinum* on the evolution of *Mycobacterium tuberculosis*. *Genome Res* **18:** 729–741.

Stoop EJ, Schipper T, Huber SK, Nezhinsky AE, Verbeek FJ, Gurcha SS, Besra GS, Vandenbroucke-Grauls CM, Bitter W, van der Sar AM. 2011. Zebrafish embryo screen for mycobacterial genes involved in the initiation of granuloma formation reveals a newly identified ESX-1 component. *Dis Model Mech* **4:** 526–536.

Stoop EJ, Bitter W, van der Sar AM. 2012. Tubercle bacilli rely on a type VII army for pathogenicity. *Trend Microbiol* **20:** 477–484.

Stoop EJ, Mishra AK, Driessen NN, van Stempvoort G, Bouchier P, Verboom T, van Leeuwen LM, Sparrius M, Raadsen SA, van Zon M, et al. 2013. Mannan core branching of lipo(arabino)mannan is required for mycobacterial virulence in the context of innate immunity. *Cell Microbiol* **15:** 2093–2108.

Swaim LE, Connolly LE, Volkman HE, Humbert O, Born DE, Ramakrishnan L. 2006. *Mycobacterium marinum* infection of adult zebrafish causes caseating granulomatous tuberculosis and is moderated by adaptive immunity. *Infect Immun* **74:** 6108–6117.

Tobin DM, Ramakrishnan L. 2008. Comparative pathogenesis of *Mycobacterium marinum* and *Mycobacterium tuberculosis*. *Cell Microbiol* **10:** 1027–1039.

Tobin DM, Vary JC Jr., Ray JP, Walsh GS, Dunstan SJ, Bang ND, Hagge DA, Khadge S, King MC, Hawn TR, et al. 2010. The lta4 h locus modulates susceptibility to mycobacterial infection in zebrafish and humans. *Cell* **140:** 717–730.

Tobin DM, Roca FJ, Oh SF, McFarland R, Vickery TW, Ray JP, Ko DC, Zou Y, Bang ND, Chau TT, et al. 2012. Host genotype-specific therapies can optimize the inflammatory response to mycobacterial infections. *Cell* **148:** 434–446.

Traver D, Herbomel P, Patton EE, Murphey RD, Yoder JA, Litman GW, Catic A, Amemiya CT, Zon LI, Trede NS. 2003. The zebrafish as a model organism to study development of the immune system. *Adv Immunol* **81:** 253–330.

Travis WD, Travis LB, Roberts GD, Su DW, Weiland LW. 1985. The histopathologic spectrum in *Mycobacterium marinum* infection. *Arch Pathol Lab Med* **109:** 1109–1113.

Trede NS, Langenau DM, Traver D, Look AT, Zon LI. 2004. The use of zebrafish to understand immunity. *Immunity* **20:** 367–379.

Ulrichs T, Kaufmann SH. 2006. New insights into the function of granulomas in human tuberculosis. *J Pathol* **208:** 261–269.

van der Sar AM, Abdallah AM, Sparrius M, Reinders E, Vandenbroucke-Grauls CM, Bitter W. 2004a. *Mycobacterium marinum* strains can be divided into two distinct types based on genetic diversity and virulence. *Infect Immun* **72:** 6306–6312.

van der Sar AM, Appelmelk BJ, Vandenbroucke-Grauls CM, Bitter W. 2004b. A star with stripes: Zebrafish as an infection model. *Trends Microbiol* **12:** 451–457.

van der Sar AM, Spaink HP, Zakrzewska A, Bitter W, Meijer AH. 2009. Specificity of the zebrafish host transcriptome response to acute and chronic mycobacterial infection and the role of innate and adaptive immune components. *Mol Immunol* **46:** 2317–2332.

van der Vaart M, Spaink HP, Meijer AH. 2012. Pathogen recognition and activation of the innate immune response in zebrafish. *Adv Hematol* **2012:** 159807.

van der Vaart M, van Soest JJ, Spaink HP, Meijer AH. 2013. Functional analysis of a zebrafish myd88 mutant identifies key transcriptional components of the innate immune system. *Dis Model Mech* **6:** 841–854.

van der Woude AD, Sarkar D, Bhatt A, Sparrius M, Raadsen SA, Boon L, Geurtsen J, van der Sar AM, Luirink EN, et al. 2012. Unexpected link between lipooligosaccharide biosynthesis and surface protein release in *Mycobacterium marinum*. *J Biol Chem* **287:** 20417–20429.

van der Woude AD, Stoop EJ, Stiess M, Wang S, Ummels R, van Stempvoort G, Piersma SR, Cascioferro A, Jimenez CR, Houben EN, et al. 2013. Analysis of SecA2-dependent substrates in *Mycobacterium marinum* identifies protein kinase G (PknG) as a virulence effector. *Cell Microbiol* **16:** 280–295.

Volkman HE, Clay H, Beery D, Chang JC, Sherman DR, Ramakrishnan L. 2004. Tuberculous granuloma formation is enhanced by a mycobacterium virulence determinant. *PLoS Biol* **2:** e367.

Volkman HE, Pozos TC, Zheng J, Davis JM, Rawls JF, Ramakrishnan L. 2010. Tuberculous granuloma induction via interaction of a bacterial secreted protein with host epithelium. *Science* **327:** 466–469.

Watral V, Kent ML. 2007. Pathogenesis of mycobacterium spp. in zebrafish (*Danio rerio*) from research facilities. *Comp Biochem Physiol C Toxicol Pharmacol* **145:** 55–60.

Weerdenburg EM, Abdallah AM, Mitra S, de Punder K, van der Wel NN, Bird S, Appelmelk BJ, Bitter W, van der Sar AM. 2012. ESX-5-deficient *Mycobacterium marinum* is hypervirulent in adult zebrafish. *Cell Microbiol* **14:** 728–739.

Yang CT, Cambier CJ, Davis JM, Hall CJ, Crosier PS, Ramakrishnan L. 2012. Neutrophils exert protection in the early tuberculous granuloma by oxidative killing of mycobacteria phagocytosed from infected macrophages. *Cell Host Microbe* **12:** 301–312.

Yoder JA. 2009. Form, function and phylogenetics of NITRs in bony fish. *Dev Comp Immunol* **33:** 135–144.

Yoder JA, Turner PM, Wright PD, Wittamer V, Bertrand JY, Traver D, Litman GW. 2010. Developmental and tissue-specific expression of NITRs. *Immunogenetics* **62:** 117–122.

Zumla A, Nahid P, Cole ST. 2013. Advances in the development of new tuberculosis drugs and treatment regimens. *Nat Rev Drug Discov* **12:** 388–404.

Modeling Tuberculosis in Nonhuman Primates

Charles A. Scanga and JoAnne L. Flynn

Department of Microbiology and Molecular Genetics, University of Pittsburgh School of Medicine, Pittsburgh, Pennsylvania 15261

Correspondence: joanne@pitt.edu

Nonhuman primates have emerged as an excellent model of human tuberculosis, in large part because they recapitulate the full spectrum of infection outcome and pathology seen in humans. Several variables inherent to the nonhuman primate models of tuberculosis are discussed in this review, including the monkey species, *Mycobacterium tuberculosis* strains, and routes of infection, all of which can influence the model to be chosen for various studies. New technologies for studying the microbiology, immunology, and pathogenesis of tuberculosis in nonhuman primates have greatly expanded the capabilities of this model for basic and translational studies, including the development and testing of new treatment and prevention strategies for tuberculosis.

Exposure to *Mycobacterium tuberculosis* results in a wide range of outcomes, from clearance of the pathogen without establishment of infection, to active tuberculosis (TB), to asymptomatic, latent infection. Latent TB is a complex infection state (Barry et al. 2009; Lin and Flynn 2010) that can reactivate and cause active TB. TB has diverse clinical presentations and can arise in practically any organ system, although the lungs are most commonly involved. Granulomas are the pathologic hallmark of TB and primarily responsible for the immunopathology of TB. They are classically described as organized inflammatory structures consisting of a necrotic core containing both infected and uninfected macrophages as well as multinucleated giant cells (Langerhans cells), surrounded by B and T lymphocytes, encased by a rim of fibroblasts. In reality, lesions in active TB can vary widely, even within the same patient, and can be necrotic (caseous), nonnecrotizing, or suppurative (Flynn and Klein 2011). Tuberculous pneumonia, consolidations, and cavities may also be present. Similarly, lesions associated with latent TB may be caseous, fibrocalcific, sclerotic, or mineralized.

Existing antituberculous drugs require 6- to 9-month regimens and drug resistance increasingly limits their effectiveness. The vaccine against TB, *Mycobacterium bovis* Bacillus Calmette Guérin (BCG), was developed nearly 100 years ago and has only limited efficacy (Andersen and Doherty 2005). New antibiotics, vaccines, and novel therapeutics are needed urgently. Developing these requires a model system that recapitulates the complexity of human TB. The ideal animal model would include (1) susceptibility to the same *M. tuberculosis* strains that cause human disease; (2) similar disease presentations and complex lesional histopathology; (3) recapitulation of the entire spectrum of possible infection outcomes; (4) latent TB states

Cite this article as *Cold Spring Harb Perspect Med* doi: 10.1101/cshperspect.a018564

that can be reactivated by the same triggers as in humans; (5) immunologic similarity to humans, allowing for cross-reactive immunologic tools and vaccine responses predictive of those in humans; (6) outbred animals reflecting human genetic diversity; and, last, (6) physiologic and metabolic similarity to humans, facilitating translational drug development. Numerous animal models of TB exist, each possessing unique advantages and disadvantages. However, only the nonhuman primate (NHP) model shows all of the features listed above (Flynn et al. 2008). NHPs have been used in TB research for decades and have become a unique and powerful research tool that recapitulates all important aspects of human disease.

HISTORICAL USE OF NHPs IN TB RESEARCH

NHPs are susceptible to natural *M. tuberculosis* infection. Outbreaks in both feral (Keet et al. 2000; Michel et al. 2013) and captive (Schroeder 1938; Benson et al. 1955; Mayhall et al. 1981; Fourie and Odendaal 1983; Shin et al. 1995; Panarella and Bimes 2010; Payne et al. 2011) colonies have been reported. All NHP species are considered potentially susceptible to *M. tuberculosis* infection (Good 1984), with a general susceptibility hierarchy of Old World species (most susceptible), followed by apes, and New World monkeys (least susceptible) (Montali et al. 2001).

NHPs were first used for TB research in pioneering work by Leon Schmidt who used rhesus macaques (*Macaca mulatta*) to study antituberclous drugs (Schmidt 1956, 1966; Schmidt et al. 1959). After intratracheal instillation of $10^2 - 10^3$ colony-forming units (CFU) *M. tuberculosis* 5159, all macaques succumbed to active TB with caseous granulomas and cavitary disease in the lungs. This work established the rhesus macaque as susceptible to even moderately low doses of *M. tuberculosis*. Robert Good extended the use of this rhesus model to show that BCG conferred marked protection from *M. tuberculosis* challenge (Good 1968). Barclay et al. (1970) further refined the use of rhesus for vaccine research by introducing the aerosol infection route and by using the virulent H37Rv *M. tuberculosis* strain still commonly used in TB research laboratories. Unlike the extensive and confluent pulmonary disease resulting from direct intratracheal instillation of *M. tuberculosis* reported by both Schmidt and Good (Schmidt 1956; Good 1968), aerogenic infection of rhesus macaques with a low-dose inoculum (<50 CFU) resulted in discrete granulomas, the initial number of which approximated the calculated infectious dose (Barclay et al. 1970). Aerogenic infection still resulted in progressive TB that was proportional in rate to the infective dose and BCG vaccination afforded striking protection from this challenge. Notably, tuberculous hilar lymphadenopathy was a much more prominent feature of disease initiated by aerosol than by intratracheal instillation. Over the next few years, low-dose, aerogenic challenge of rhesus macaques with virulent *M. tuberculosis* remained the NHP model of choice for vaccine studies (Baram et al. 1971; Ribi et al. 1971; Barclay et al. 1973; Janicki et al. 1973; Chaparas et al. 1975). Perhaps because of reduced availability of rhesus macaques for experimentation and waning interest in TB research, no TB studies using monkeys appeared in the literature from 1975 until 1996. The emergence of the human immunodeficiency virus (HIV) pandemic reinvigorated interest in modeling infectious diseases in NHPs, especially the use of macaques experimentally infected with simian immunodeficiency virus (SIV). The increasing prevalence of AIDS resulted in a resurgence of TB in many countries (Corbett et al. 2003) and renewed interest in TB research. In 1996, Walsh et al. established a novel NHP model of TB using cynomolgus macaques (*Macaca fasicularis*) (Walsh et al. 1996), heralding the beginning of a new era that has witnessed a tremendous increase in the use of NHPs to model TB.

NHP SPECIES

From Schmidt's initial study in 1956 (Schmidt 1956) until the 1990s, rhesus macaques exclusively were used for TB research. Seeking to take advantage of the ready supply of captive-bred cynomolgus macaques in the Philippines, Marcus Horwitz initiated a study to evaluate this species as a model of human TB (Walsh et al. 1996). Animals were infected intratracheally with a wide dose range of Erdman strain *M. tuberculosis* (10^1-10^5 CFU) and monitored for up to 7 months. The outcome was clearly dose-dependent. Macaques receiving high infectious doses (10^5 and 10^4 CFU) succumbed to TB after 7–13 wk with extensive bilateral tuberculous pneumonia with abundant necrosis and extrapulmonary manifestations such as ocular TB, meningitis, and spondylitis (Pott's disease). Animals receiving a moderate infectious dose (10^3 CFU) developed more slowly progressive disease that caused mortality by 14–24 wk. Pulmonary pathology was still widespread but showed less necrosis and more cellular infiltration, but there was less extrapulmonary disease. The disease in macaques infected with low doses of *M. tuberculosis* ($<10^2$ CFU) progressed even more slowly and these animals survived $\geq$19 wk postinfection. Granulomas arising in these animals were much smaller and densely cellular, resembling lesions typical of human TB. Most strikingly, three of the eight macaques receiving $<10^2$ CFU did not show any clinical or radiographic signs of disease after 7 mo, despite immunologically confirmed infection. Necropsy revealed disease mostly confined to the lungs. This report (Walsh et al. 1996) of subclinical disease in three NHPs infected with a low dose of *M. tuberculosis* revealed the potential of NHPs to model both latent and active TB. This concept was further developed in a seminal study in which 17 cynomolgus macaques were infected with ~25 CFU *M. tuberculosis* Erdman by bronchoscopic instillation (Capuano et al. 2003). Despite being infected with the same dose, the animals showed a range of outcomes from rapidly progressive TB to latent TB that, in some animals, was stably maintained for >20 mo. A wide spectrum of granuloma morphologies was noted from caseous, to solid cellular, to fibrocalcific that recapitulated the range of histopathology in human TB (Fig. 1). These studies further established that cynomolgus macaques could manifest the various TB disease states seen in humans, with ~40% of animals developing active TB and 60% developing latent infection. Lin et al. (2009) identified clinical parameters indicative of active disease, such as weight loss, abnormal chest X-ray (CXR), culture-positive gastric aspirates, and elevated erythrocyte sedimentation rate (ESR). Monkeys with latent TB therefore could be identified as those animals that presented none of these clinical signs within 6 mo postinfection (Lin et al. 2009). These clinical classifications were confirmed by gross pathology and bacterial load scoring at necropsy. This "low-dose inoculum" cynomolgus model of TB was used by our group to study both acute (up to 6 wk postinfection) and chronic (>1 yr postinfection) *M. tuberculosis* infection (Lin et al. 2006, 2009). Cynomolgus macaques therefore can model all manifestations of the entire spectrum of infection outcomes in humans (Table 1).

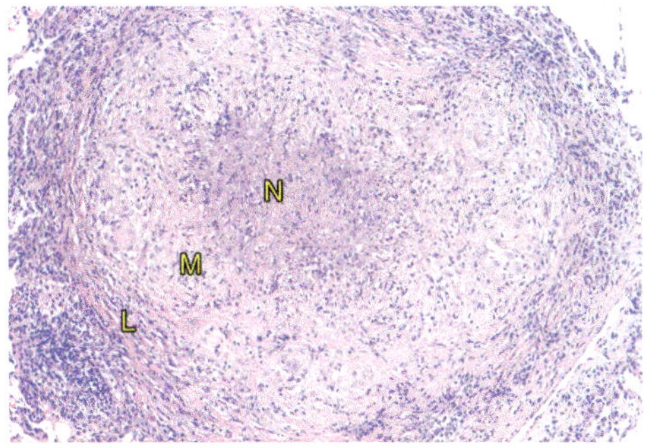

Figure 1. Pulmonary granuloma from a cynomolgus macaque 20 wk after *Mycobacterium tuberculosis* infection showing striking similarity to classical TB histopathology in humans. A macrophage-enriched zone (M) surrounds a central area of necrosis (N) with an outer lymphocytic/fibrocytic cuff (L). Original magnification 10×. (Courtesy of Dr. Edwin Klein, University of Pittsburgh.)

Cynomolgus macaques used for research typically come from large colonies in Asia or Indonesia and show substantial genetic diversity. Cynomolgus macaques from the isolated island of Mauritius, on the other hand, have much less genetic diversity (Krebs et al. 2005), and their MHC alleles are limited and well-defined. This makes Mauritian cynomolgus macaques ideal for developing MHC:peptide tetramers that can be used to identify, track, and isolate antigen-specific T cells, a feature that has been exploited in SIV research (Burwitz et al.

Table 1. Summary of nonhuman primate species used to model tuberculosis

Monkey species	Advantages	Disadvantages
Cynomolgus macaque (*Macaca fascicularis*)	Best represents the entire spectrum of human TB Can develop either latent or active TB Well-developed immunologic reagents Relatively resistant to *Mtb* Readily available	Expensive to purchase and to maintain Large size: limits housing capacity, requires more product for drug studies
Rhesus macaque (*Macaca mulatta*)	Recapitulates many aspects of human TB Relatively susceptible to *Mtb* Well-developed immunologic reagents	Expensive and large More limited availability
Common marmoset (*Callithrix jacchus*)	Recapitulates many aspects of human TB Much smaller than macaques, increasing housing capacity and decreasing amount of test substance needed for drug studies Easily group-housed Frequent dizygotic twinning	Limited number of suppliers More limited immunologic reagents Smaller size limits biological sampling frequency/amount

2009; Budde et al. 2012). Although there are no published reports yet of experimental TB in Mauritian cynomolgus macaques, these animals have the potential to expand our repertoire of tetrameric immunologic probes targeting mycobacteria-specific T cells from the single tetramer reported so far (Wei et al. 2009).

Although several studies (Walsh et al. 1996; Capuano et al. 2003; Lin et al. 2009) firmly establish that cynomolgus macaques are relatively resistant to *M. tuberculosis* and can model the entire spectrum of human TB including latent disease, rhesus macaques appear more susceptible. Early studies showed that even relatively low doses of *M. tuberculosis* caused progressive, fatal TB in rhesus monkeys (Good 1968; Ribi et al. 1971). In a dose–response study in which rhesus macaques were infected intratracheally with 50, 200, 500, or 3000 CFU *M. tuberculosis* H37Rv, all doses resulted in active TB with disease progression rate correlated with inoculum size (Zhang et al. 2011). Three studies have directly compared the susceptibility to TB in rhesus and cynomolgus macaques. Motzel et al. infected cynomolgus macaques ($n = 6$), rhesus macaques ($n = 6$), and vervets (*Chlorocebus pygerythrus*) ($n = 5$) using 100 CFU of *M. tuberculosis* Erdman injected intrathecally. Based on survival times, vervets were by far most susceptible, with rhesus and, especially, cynomolgus macaques showing more resistance (Motzel et al. 2003). In another direct comparison study, both rhesus and cynomolgus macaques were intratracheally infected with 3000 CFU *M. tuberculosis* (Erdman strain) and the rhesus showed more extensive lung disease and extrapulmonary spread (Langermans et al. 2001). More recently, Sharpe et al. (2009) showed greater susceptibility in rhesus macaques compared with cynomolgus macaques following low-dose (30–75-CFU) aerosol infection with *M. tuberculosis* Erdman. In contrast, several studies show resistance in rhesus macaques. Gormus et al. (2004) reported subclinical TB in rhesus monkeys infected with the H37Rv strain of *M. tuberculosis*, whereas animals infected with strain Erdman developed progressive TB. Latent TB was reported in rhesus macaques infected with the less virulent *M. tuberculosis* strain CDC1551 (Mehra et al. 2011). Rhesus macaques used for research are of either Chinese or Indian origin and substantial genetic differences exist between the two subspecies (Yan et al. 2011). Interestingly, the studies reporting latent TB in rhesus macaques used animals of Indian origin (Safi et al. 2003; Gormus et al. 2004; Mehra et al. 2011), whereas the study showing susceptibility of rhesus macaques to low-dose inocula used animals from China (Zhang et al. 2011), suggesting distinct resistance patterns between Chinese and Indian rhesus, although a direct comparison has not been reported. Overall, experimental TB in rhesus macaques resembles many key aspects of human disease, but it is widely considered to reflect TB in susceptible individuals because of the overwhelming tendency of this species to develop active TB regardless of the inoculating dose (Table 1).

Recently, a new NHP model of TB using the common marmoset (*Callithrix jacchus*) was described (Via et al. 2013). Marmosets are New World monkeys that are much smaller (300–500 g) than Old World primates such as macaques (2 to more than 10 kg). Via et al. tested the susceptibility of marmosets to mycobacteria of differing virulence: the virulent K04 clinical isolate and Erdman strain, the less virulent *M. tuberculosis* strain CDC1551, and the *M. tuberculosis* complex member *M. africanum*. Low-dose aerogenic infection with all mycobacterial strains resulted in fulminant TB that progressed at a rate proportional to the virulence of the strain used (Via et al. 2013). Intratracheal infection with strain Erdman also resulted in extensive disease. Marmosets thus display a striking susceptibility to mycobacteria and, like larger NHP species, recapitulate some of the clinicopathologic manifestations of human TB. An advantage of marmosets, in addition to their small size, is that they have a high incidence of dizygotic twinning. Because a number of cross-reactive immunologic reagents are also available (Brok et al. 2001), elegant immunologic studies are possible in this novel small NHP model of TB.

EFFECT OF INOCULUM STRAIN, DOSE, AND ROUTE

The mycobacterial strain, inoculum dose, and infection route can greatly affect the outcome of NHP infection. Different *M. tuberculosis* strains can show distinct virulence characteristics in mice (Caceres et al. 2012), guinea pigs (Palanisamy et al. 2008), and rabbits (Tsenova et al. 2005). Head-to-head comparisons of bacterial strain virulence have not been performed in NHPs. Thus, inferences must be made by comparing outcomes reported in separate NHP studies, which frequently are performed by different researchers, at different times, using different strain isolates, doses, and infection routes. Nonetheless, some conclusions may be drawn from the literature.

Different strains of *M. tuberculosis* can display distinct virulence patterns in NHPs, as in other animal species (Tsenova et al. 2005; Palanisamy et al. 2008; Caceres et al. 2012). CDC1551, a clinical isolate of *M. tuberculosis* that is highly immunogenic (Manca et al. 1999), appears to be less virulent than other *M. tuberculosis* strains in some animal models (Tsenova et al. 2005) but not others (Palanisamy et al. 2008). When used to infect 12 rhesus macaques, CDC1551 (500 CFU, aerosol) resulted in early, active TB in only one animal, whereas the other 11 developed subclinical infection (Mehra et al. 2011). Conversely, marmosets appear quite susceptible to low dose (<25 CFU) aerosolized CDC1551, succumbing to the infection within 70 days (Via et al. 2013).

The majority of TB studies in NHPs were performed using the Erdman strain (Walsh et al. 1996; Langermans et al. 2001; Capuano et al. 2003; Chen et al. 2009; Lin et al. 2009; Sharpe et al. 2009, 2010; Lin et al. 2012c, 2014), although several used H37Rv (Shen et al. 2002b; Gormus et al. 2004; Zhang et al. 2011; Rayner et al. 2013). Although Erdman is generally thought to be more virulent in NHPs, this might not be so clear-cut. The most powerful piece of evidence for this belief is the report by Gormus et al., in which rhesus macaques infected intrabronchially with ≥10 CFU of *M. tuberculosis* Erdman all developed active TB, whereas infection with ≤200 CFU of *M. tuberculosis* H37Rv resulted in subclinical disease in all animals (Gormus et al. 2004). In another study, six rhesus macaques chronically infected with SIV were challenged with *M. tuberculosis* H37Rv (200 CFU) and half the animals developed latent TB, despite their presumed immunodeficiency (Safi et al. 2003). The H37Rv strain can be quite virulent for NHPs as well. Not surprisingly, high-dose (≥1000 CFU) H37Rv uniformly results in active TB in rhesus macaques (Lewinsohn et al. 2006; Sugawara et al. 2009). When delivered by aerosol to rhesus macaques, 400–500 CFU of the H37Rv strain caused fatal TB in 4–6 wk (Shen et al. 2002b). However, in contrast to Gormus et al. (2004) and Safi et al. (2003), two reports showed that rhesus macaques infected with as few as 50 CFU of *M. tuberculosis* H37Rv all developed active disease (Zhang et al. 2011; Min et al. 2013). The reports of latent or subclinical TB in rhesus macaques infected with H37Rv may be related more to the geographic source of the animals and less to the virulence of the infecting strain because both reports of limited disease following *M. tuberculosis* H37Rv infection used rhesus of Indian, rather than Chinese, origin (Safi et al. 2003; Gormus et al. 2004). It is also possible that different isolates or preparations of the same strain have varying levels of virulence.

Although the Erdman strain of *M. tuberculosis* appears more virulent in NHPs because of its ability to cause progressive TB in both rhesus (Langermans et al. 2001; Gormus et al. 2004; Sharpe et al. 2009, 2010) and cynomolgus (Walsh et al. 1996; Langermans et al. 2001; Capuano et al. 2003; Sharpe et al. 2009; Lin et al. 2010, 2012b) macaques, low doses (25 CFU) of Erdman in cynomolgus macaques lead to latent TB in half the monkeys (Lin et al. 2009, 2010, 2012b,c; Diedrich et al. 2010; Mattila et al. 2011). When larger inocula (250–500 CFU) of the same Erdman strain were similarly delivered to cynomolgus macaques, all progressed to active TB (Lin et al. 2012b; Chen et al. 2013). Thus, the outcome of infection with *M. tuberculosis* Erdman in cynomolgus monkeys is dose-dependent, as first shown by Walsh et al. (1996). A similar relationship between inoculum size and disease progression following *M. tuberculosis* H37Rv infection in rhesus macaques also exists (Zhang et al. 2011).

The method used to infect NHPs also plays a role in determining disease progression and outcome. The two most commonly used routes of infection for NHP studies of TB are intra-airway instillation and inhalation of aerosolized bacilli. The earliest reports of experimental *M. tuberculosis* infection of NHPs used intratracheal instillation (Schmidt 1956, 1966; Schmidt et al. 1959), as did several more recent studies (Walsh et al. 1996; Langermans et al. 2001). This protocol was improved on by introducing a flexible fiber-optic bronchoscope (Capuano et al. 2003), and bronchoscopic instillation has become the standard method for intra-airway inoculation of *M. tuberculosis*. The bronchoscope facilitates precise delivery of inocula directly into targeted lung segments using direct fiber-optic visualization. The inoculum volume and concentration can be measured to accurately calculate the infecting dose. Following low-dose bronchoscopic infection, granulomas appear first in the lungs 3–4 wk postinfection and then in the draining hilar lymph nodes by ~5 wk (Lin et al. 2006). Although initially uniformly caseous (Lin et al. 2006), these granulomas eventually develop into a wide spectrum of lesion types (Lin et al. 2009). However, even though monkeys infected intrabronchially can show the entire spectrum of TB seen in humans (Capuano et al. 2003; Lin et al. 2009), this route does not reflect the natural transmission of TB and bypasses host defenses of the upper respiratory tract.

Because infectious aerosols transmit TB, experimental infection by aerosolized bacteria is thought to best reflect the natural route of *M. tuberculosis* transmission. Early vaccine studies used aerogenic infection (Barclay et al. 1970, 1973; Baram et al. 1971; Ribi et al. 1971; Janicki et al. 1973; Chaparas et al. 1975; Shen et al. 2002b). Following aerosol infection of rhesus macaques with *M. tuberculosis* H37Rv, lesions appear in the lungs and hilar lymph nodes within 3 wk postinfection and show varied histopathologic appearance (Rayner et al. 2013). Sharpe et al. recently sought to further refine the aerosol infection route (Sharpe et al. 2010). Rhesus macaques of Indian origin were exposed to ~50 CFU *M. tuberculosis* Erdman, and clinical (body weight, ESR, CXR) and postmortem parameters (gross pathology, lung pathology, bacterial load) were assessed. All animals progressed to active TB despite substantial animal-to-animal variation, especially in terms of survival times that ranged from 6 to 48 wk. Much of the variability is likely due to genetic differences between animals, but at least some can be attributed to the many variables involved in preparing and delivering aerogenic inocula to individual animals (Clark et al. 2011). Coupling aerosol infection with real-time plethysmography may reduce variation (Sharpe et al. 2009). This infection route also requires larger, more specialized equipment than intrabronchial instillation. Although bronchoscopic instillation does bypass innate defenses of the upper respiratory tract, aerosol infection typically delivers monodispersed bacteria in uniform droplets ~2 μM in diameter. Although this approximates the droplet size considered most infectious in the aerosol cloud emanating from coughing TB patients (Fennelly et al. 2012), the infectious nuclei generated by a laboratory nebulizer differ physiochemically from the complex aerosols generated by the cough of a tuberculous person and may interact differently with the innate immune system within the airway. Although a direct comparison between aerosol and bronchoscopic infection has not been performed, some evidence suggests that the aerosol route is more virulent. Aerosol infection of cynomolgus macaques with 30–40-CFU *M. tuberculosis* Erdman resulted in varied disease progression rates but without evidence of true latent TB within the 12-wk follow-up period (Sharpe et al. 2009). In a more limited study, aerogenic infection of cynomolgus macaques with <20 CFU strain Erdman resulted in progressive disease in all four animals (J Flynn, C Scanga, and P Lin, unpubl.).

Thus, the choice of *M. tuberculosis* strain, size of the inoculating dose, and route of infection can all affect the outcome of experimental TB in NHPs. All these parameters must be carefully considered when planning studies or evaluating results.

IN VIVO IMAGING OF NHPs INFECTED WITH *M. tuberculosis*

Small animal models of TB that show minimal animal-to-animal variability (e.g., mice, guinea pigs, rabbits) provide the opportunity to kill small numbers of animals at various time points following infection to understand dynamic processes. This approach is less feasible with NHPs, which are much more variable and resource-intensive. A distinct advantage of low-dose infection of cynomolgus macaques is that different disease states (e.g., active or latent TB) can develop. When animals are killed at early time points, there is no way to know a priori if that animal was destined to develop active or latent TB. In vivo imaging offers a way to monitor disease progression over time within the same animal. Beginning with some of the earliest studies (Schmidt 1966), CXR is often used to monitor TB progression (Verreck et al. 2009). However, the resolution of conventional CXR is poor and cannot detect subtle changes in pulmonary lesions. A large step forward was made in 2006 when computed tomography (CT) was used to serially assess disease development in rhesus macaques following high-dose *M. tuberculosis* infection (Lewinsohn et al. 2006). CT offers both a 10-fold increase in spatial resolution and the ability to assess extrapulmonary organs. Magnetic resonance imaging (MRI), which is especially good at producing high-resolution images of soft tissue, has also been used to visualize lung lesion distribution (Sharpe et al. 2009, 2010; Rayner et al. 2013) and can be combined with stereology to quantitatively measure lung disease volume (Sharpe et al. 2009). Although MRI has the potential to serially follow disease development, it has so far been applied only ex vivo to excised and fixed lungs. The most recent imaging advance for TB studies combined high-resolution CT with positron emission tomography (PET) in living animals (Davis et al. 2009; Via et al. 2012). In PET imaging, ^{18}F-fluorodeoxyglucose (FDG) injected intravenously is taken up and trapped within metabolically active cells (e.g., inflammatory cells within a granuloma). PET/CT imaging therefore conveys both the anatomic detail of CT as well as functional information (i.e., metabolic activity). PET/CT imaging has been used to follow TB progression in both marmosets (Via et al. 2013) and macaques (Lin et al. 2013, 2014). PET/CT imaging allows one to follow the appearance and distribution of individual granulomas; track changes in their size, shape, and metabolic activity over time; and then identify and analyze those individual lesions at necropsy. This allows one to correlate the in vivo evolution of lesions with ex vivo pathologic, immunologic, and bacteriologic parameters—all at the level of the individual granuloma.

APPLICATIONS OF THE NHP MODEL

New Insights into TB Pathogenesis

Infection of cynomolgus macaques using low-dose (~25-CFU) *M. tuberculosis* results in varied outcomes that closely mimic all forms of TB in humans (Capuano et al. 2003; Lin et al. 2009). This model system facilitates investigations of basic concepts of TB pathogenesis. Infection is initiated when bacilli enter the lungs, get taken up by phagocytes such as alveolar macrophages and dendritic cells, and begin to replicate. Bacilli spread to lung-draining lymph nodes, presumably via migrating dendritic cells. Recent work using bar-coded *M. tuberculosis* isolates shows that each granuloma in the lung arises from a single bacterium (Lin et al. 2014). Using PET/CT imaging and/or necropsy, these lesions can be detected within 2–4 wk of infection in both lungs and lymph nodes, coincident with the developing adaptive immune response to the pathogen and influx of inflammatory cells (Lin et al. 2006, 2014; Rayner et al. 2013). Early lesions show some central necrosis (Lin et al. 2006) and are likely hypoxic (Via et al. 2008).

Studies in NHPs have expanded our understanding of the granuloma itself. Tuberculous granulomas are not uniform structures and, instead, display a wide variety of gross and histopathological appearances. Multiple lesion types can coexist even within the same individual. These same features can be seen in experimentally infected NHPs (Lin et al. 2009; Flynn and Klein 2011). Recently, developing lesions in infected cynomolgus macaques were tracked using FDG PET/CT imaging, and bacterial killing was assessed within each individual granuloma at necropsy (Lin et al. 2014). The physical and metabolic characteristics of individual lesions *within the same animal* were dynamic, followed independent trajectories, and showed a 10,000-fold range of bacterial burden. Early (4 wk) postinfection, all granulomas had culturable bacteria, but by 11 wk, ~10% of lesions had been sterilized, and increased to >30% by 6 mo. Strikingly, the degree of mycobacterial killing varied within lesions from the same animal regardless of whether the disease was active or latent, although there were more sterile lesions in latent animals (Lin et al. 2014). This study highlights the lesional heterogeneity within the same animal and suggests strongly that the ultimate outcome of infection is predicated on responses at a lesional, rather than a global level. The NHP model of TB uniquely recapitulates the spectrum of disease outcomes and granuloma characteristics observed in humans and provides an ideal platform with which to study TB pathogenesis.

INVESTIGATING LATENT AND REACTIVATION TB

In the traditional binary view of TB pathogenesis, the host can either control bacterial replication to establish a latent TB infection, or bacteria may continue to replicate and spread, resulting in active TB and progressive immunopathology. We now understand that TB exists as a continuous spectrum of disease states, from dormant to fulminant infection (Barry et al. 2009; Lin et al. 2009; Lin and Flynn 2010; Gideon and Flynn 2011). Where a TB patient falls along this spectrum has important implications for diagnosis, prognosis, and treatment, highlighting the importance of macaques as the only animal model that recapitulates these variable outcomes. Persons latently infected with *M. tuberculosis* are at risk for reactivation and represent a huge reservoir of potential cases of active, infectious TB. More research is needed to help better predict those most at risk for reactivation and to develop targeted therapies that may eliminate either the infection itself or the potential for reactivation. The well-characterized cynomolgus model of latent TB (Lin et al. 2009; Lin and Flynn 2010; Gideon and Flynn 2011) provides a unique opportunity to investigate important gaps in knowledge about latent *M. tuberculosis* infection.

The metabolic state of the bacilli during clinical latency is unknown. However, genetic mutations accumulate at the same rate in macaques with latent or active TB (Ford et al. 2011), suggesting that host bactericidal activity determines latency rather than bacterial replication rate—a hypothesis further supported by recent studies (Lin et al. 2014). PET/CT imaging of latently infected animals typically reveals lesions in lung-draining lymph nodes and a small number of discrete, heterogeneously FDG-avid granulomas within the lungs (J Flynn, unpubl.). As in humans, latent TB in cynomolgus macaques can be stably maintained, can spontaneously reactivate, or can reactivate in response to some immune suppression (Lin et al. 2009; Lin and Flynn 2010). TNF (tumor necrosis factor) is a key cytokine in antituberculous immunity (reviewed in O'Garra et al. 2013), and TNF neutralization in humans is associated with reactivation of latent TB (Keane 2004). Likewise, TNF blockade induces reactivation in ~70% of latently infected macaques (Lin et al. 2010). This NHP model creates opportunities to investigate interventions that may reduce the reactivation risk. In one such study of prophylactic chemotherapy, a 2-mo course of metronidazole, a drug effective only in low oxygen microenvironments, was found to be as efficacious as 6 mo of isoniazid or 2 mo of isoniazid and rifampin in preventing anti-TNF-induced reactivation (Lin et al. 2012a). In another, vaccination of macaques with a BCG/H56 heterologous prime-boost regimen before low-dose infection greatly reduced the risk of reactivation following TNF neutralization (Lin et al. 2012b).

MODELING HIV-TB COINFECTIONS

The World Health Organization estimates 14 million people are coinfected with HIV and *M. tuberculosis*, and TB accounts for ~26% of all AIDS-related deaths (WHO 2013). The magnitude of this public health problem demands urgent research into the synergy between these two pathogens and new approaches to treating coinfected individuals. Macaques are the only species besides humans susceptible to infection with both immunodeficiency virus and *M. tuberculosis*, making them ideal to model coinfection. Because HIV infects only humans, NHP studies use the closely related SIV or chimeric SIV-HIV (SHIV). Early investigations of mycobacterial coinfection showed that immunodeficient monkeys were susceptible to *M. tuberculosis* or even to the attenuated mycobacterial vaccine BCG (Zhou et al. 1999; Croix et al. 2000; Shen et al. 2002a; Safi et al. 2003). In fact, the susceptibility of SIV-infected macaques to mycobacterial coinfection has been used to show the safety of novel vaccines based on highly attenuated *M. tuberculosis* strains (Sampson et al. 2011; Jensen et al. 2012). Continued work with this model should provide insights into the mechanisms by which *M. tuberculosis* can accelerate HIV replication and hasten progression of both TB and SIV disease.

In humans, coinfection with HIV is the most powerful risk factor for reactivating latent TB, increasing the risk of reactivation ~20-fold (Pawlowski et al. 2012). Diedrich et al. (2010) modeled this clinical scenario by using SIV to coinfect cynomolgus macaques with established latent TB, resulting in reactivation in all macaques. Interestingly, although animals with the biggest decline in $CD4^+$ T cell counts reactivated first, those with near-normal $CD4^+$ T cell counts also reactivated, albeit at later times (7–11 mo), analogous to humans coinfected with HIV/*M. tuberculosis* in which reactivation TB can occur before $CD4^+$ T cells decline (Lawn and Churchyard 2009). The role of $CD4^+$ T cells in maintaining latent TB was explored further in another NHP study in which $CD4^+$ T cells were depleted from latently infected cynomolgus macaques and reactivation occurred in only half the animals, suggesting that exacerbation of TB following HIV coinfection is not simply caused by the loss of $CD4^+$ T cells (Lin et al. 2012c). Additional studies of macaques with latent TB suggest that SIV coinfection affects $CD8^+$ T cell and monocyte function, which may be, at least in part, responsible for the TB reactivation (Mattila et al. 2011; Diedrich et al. 2013).

EVALUATING NEW DRUGS AND VACCINES

Current antimycobacterial drug regimens are lengthy—at least 6 mo—and drug resistance continues to emerge in *M. tuberculosis*. New drugs that can circumvent resistance mechanisms or shorten chemotherapy courses are critically needed. Because of their relatively high throughput, small animal models of TB (e.g., mice) are often used to screen drug candidates.

However, results in mice do not always predict drug efficacy in humans (Cynamon et al. 1999; Mitchison and Chang 2009; Williams et al. 2009; Lee et al. 2012). Furthermore, the tuberculous pathology in mice differs dramatically from that in humans. Mice do not show diverse granuloma types and do not develop cavitary disease—all common features in human TB. Testing the most promising new chemotherapeutic agents in NHPs before advancing them into clinical trials has distinct advantages. First, drugs in NHPs display pharmacokinetics similar to those observed in humans (Lin et al. 2012a), enabling simple allometric-based dose calculations (McLeay et al. 2012). Second, cynomolgus macaques infected with *M. tuberculosis* often show a wide spectrum of lesion types including cavities (Lin et al. 2009), an important feature because it is reasonable to assume disparate drug efficacies on bacilli residing in distinct granuloma morphologies. Third, unlike humans, single-drug regimens can be tested in macaques to determine efficacy. Although NHPs are expensive to purchase and house, new advances in PET/CT imaging facilitate serial assessment of tuberculous disease before, during, and after a treatment regimen in the same animals (Lin et al. 2013). This reduces the number of animals needed. Furthermore, individual lesions can be followed by PET/CT and can be independently analyzed and considered, further enhancing the statistical power of studies with limited animals (Lin et al. 2013). A drawback to testing novel chemical compounds in large monkeys is the amount of drug that must be synthesized, often at great expense. Recently, marmosets experimentally infected with *M. tuberculosis* were shown to offer many of the same advantages of larger NHPs yet weigh ~10-fold less, making them an attractive option for testing new antimycobacterial drugs (Via et al. 2013).

An increasing number of TB vaccine candidates are available and must be down-selected to advance the most promising into clinical trials (Brennan et al. 2012; Ottenhoff and Kaufmann 2012). NHPs have long been used to test TB vaccines (Good 1968) and offer distinct advantages over other animal models. Their phylogenetic closeness to humans means they have very similar immune systems and a wealth of immunologic tools exists for studying immune responses in monkeys. Serial samples of blood and BAL (bronchoalveolar lavage) fluid can be obtained and used for immunologic assays enabling dynamic and quantitative measurements of vaccine immunogenicity. After vaccination, monkeys can be challenged with *M. tuberculosis* to assess vaccine efficacy. Because macaques can be used to model both active and latent TB, therapeutic (i.e., postinfection) vaccine regimens targeted to either disease state can be evaluated, in addition to the more conventional prophylactic (i.e., preinfection) vaccines.

Evaluating published TB vaccine studies in NHPs is confounded by multiple variables including monkey species, timing of vaccinations and challenge, route of challenge, and inoculum size. Rhesus macaques are the most commonly used species for testing TB vaccines, both historically (Barclay et al. 1970; Ribi et al. 1971; Janicki et al. 1973) and recently (Langermans et al. 2001; Sugawara et al. 2009; Verreck et al. 2009; Sharpe et al. 2010; Rahman et al. 2012), but cynomolgus macaques increasingly are being used (Langermans et al. 2001; Okada et al. 2009; Reed et al. 2009; Kita et al. 2011; Lin et al. 2012b). In the sole direct comparison study, BCG vaccination provided better protection against high-dose *M. tuberculosis* challenge in cynomolgus compared with rhesus macaques (Langermans et al. 2001), suggesting that rhesus were the preferred species in which to test whether a live vaccine candidate conferred better protection than BCG. However, this is contradicted by both earlier (Barclay et al. 1970; Ribi et al. 1971; Janicki et al. 1973) and more recent studies, which showed significant protection by BCG alone in rhesus (Shen et al. 2002b; Verreck et al. 2009; Sharpe et al. 2010). A wide range of challenge dose has been reported, from 3000 CFU (Sugawara et al. 2009) to as few as 25 CFU (Lin et al. 2012b). Too large an inoculum will overwhelm any protective effect, whereas too low a dose, especially in cynomolgus macaques, will result in latent TB in some control animals. In most vaccine studies, *M. tuberculosis* is delivered intratracheally or intrabronchially. However, aerosol challenge of vaccinated animals may more closely replicate natural transmission (Shen et al. 2002b; Sharpe et al. 2010). As discussed above, however, aerogenic infection may be more virulent than intrabronchial delivery and may mask subtle protective effects. The *M. tuberculosis* strain used to challenge vaccinated animals may affect the outcome because of differential virulence. The most commonly used challenge strains for TB vaccine studies are H37Rv and Erdman, which do show distinct virulence profiles (see above). Clearly, a harmonized protocol for testing vaccine candidates in NHPs would be hugely beneficial, but, as yet, no consensus exists regarding these model components.

The outcome measures of protection are important considerations in NHP studies of TB vaccines or therapeutic agents. Clinical assessment (body weight, hematological parameters, and CXR) has been used during the in-life challenge phase (Verreck et al. 2009; Lin et al. 2012b), but their predictive value has not been established. Postchallenge survival times of animals subjected to different vaccine regimens can be compared (Reed et al. 2009; Sharpe et al. 2010; Kita et al. 2011; Lin et al. 2012b). However, this poses both ethical concerns and statistical challenges, because genetic variability often results in large differences in survival times within experimental groups (Sharpe et al. 2010). Animals can be necropsied at fixed end points to compare pathology and bacterial loads between groups (Langermans et al. 2001; Okada et al. 2009; Rahman et al. 2012), but such analyses are complicated. First, the time point(s) chosen is a variable that may influence a study's conclusions. Second, the extent of pathology is difficult to quantitatively assess. Although a number of scoring systems have been developed (Lin et al. 2009; Verreck et al. 2009), there is inherent subjectivity in such analyses. Last, determining bacterial load in monkeys is technically challenging. Some researchers homogenize whole lungs for plating (Langermans et al. 2001; Verreck et al. 2009), some use a stereologic approach to guide the selection of random tissue sections for plating (Luciw et al. 2011), and some use a combination of lesion collection and random sampling (Lin et al. 2009). Many researchers report bacterial burden as CFU/gram of tissue (Langermans et al. 2001; Reed et al. 2009; Verreck et al. 2009) or CFU/lung (Kita et al. 2011). Lin et al. devised a methodology to generate both a "CFU score" for quantitative analysis of bacterial burden and a calculable measure of bacterial dissemination (Lin et al. 2009, 2012a). However, given that the number of live bacteria within individual granulomas can vary by more than several orders of magnitude even within the same animal (Lin et al. 2014), perhaps the most accurate method to comprehensively assess bacterial burden is to use pre-necropsy imaging (e.g., PET/CTor MRI) as a road map to identify and harvest individual lesions. These can be homogenized and plated to determine CFU/granuloma. Regions of generalized pathology (i.e., TB pneumonia or large consolidations) and the remaining grossly normal tissue can be randomly sampled (Lin et al. 2013, 2014). This methodology is less susceptible to skewing by a few granulomas that have extraordinarily high CFU. The power of this approach is increased if a portion of each lesion is subjected to quantitative PCR to enumerate *M. tuberculosis* genomes (chromosomal equivalents, or CEQ). Because mycobacterial genomes remain long after bacilli are killed (Munoz-Elias et al. 2005), CEQ reflects the cumulative number of bacteria (alive or dead) that ever existed in a particular lesion and so the CFU/CEQ ratio reflects bacterial killing within each granuloma (Lin et al. 2014). This comprehensive approach assesses both bacterial replication and bactericidal activity for each lesion and is especially powerful in assessing vaccines or drugs, which may affect heterogenously each nidus of infection (Fig. 2).

CONCLUDING REMARKS

There is still much to learn about TB pathogenesis, and improved diagnostics, prophylactics, and therapeutics need to be developed. To take full advantage of recent advances in immunology, genomics, proteomics, metabolomics, and mathematical modeling (Marino et al. 2011), tractable animal models of TB that recapitulate as much as possible the features of human dis-

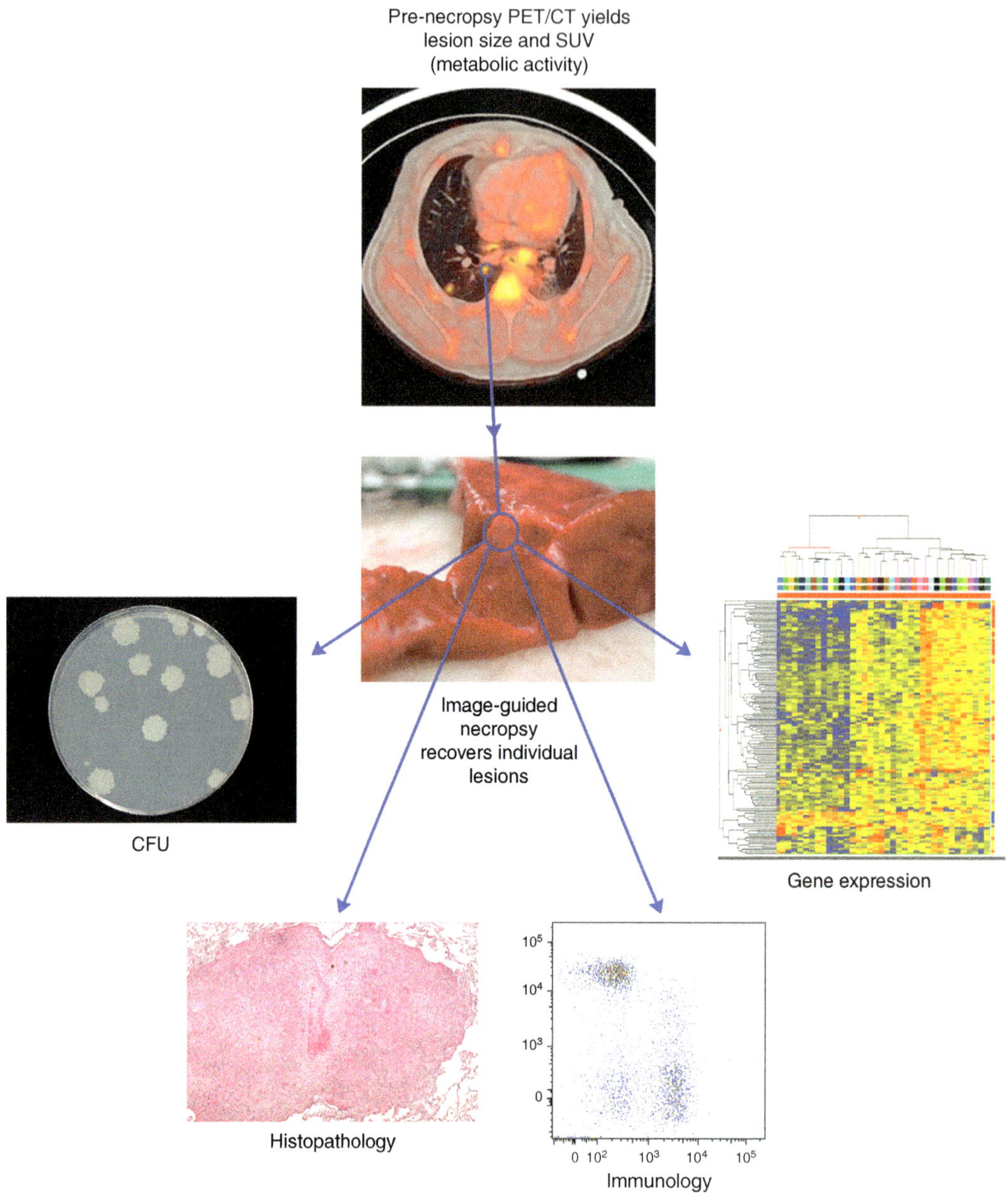

Figure 2. Modeling TB in NHPs facilitates studies based on local responses within individual lesions. Disease can be monitored over time with imaging technologies. Here, serial PET/CT imaging provides the history of a lesion, in terms of size and metabolic activity, over the course of the study. A pre-necropsy scan guides the harvesting of these individual lesions as small as 1 mm that can be portioned out to obtain data on bacterial load, histopathology, immunology, and gene expression. These data are distinct from global immunologic and transcriptional responses (i.e., from PBMC) and can differ from lesion-to-lesion within the same animal. SUV, standardized uptake value; CFU, colony-forming unit. (Figure credit: Chelsea L. Chedrick and Dr. Hannah P. Gideon, University of Pittsburgh.)

ease are needed. Their phylogenetic closeness to humans, their ability to model active, latent, and reactivation TB, and their suitability for serial sampling and imaging make NHPs an ideal experimental platform. Because of the high costs associated with purchasing and housing NHPs, particularly under ABSL-3 containment, small animal models of TB will continue to play important roles in TB research. However, NHP studies are critically important, particularly where alternative models are lacking (e.g., studies of latent TB) and to assist in selecting novel therapies or vaccines to advance into clinical trials.

ACKNOWLEDGMENTS

We gratefully acknowledge the contributions of all Flynn laboratory members, past and present; Drs. Edwin Klein and Hannah P. Gideon for supplying data for the figures; and Chelsea L. Chedrick for assistance with the figures. Our work is supported by the National Institutes of Health (grants AI50732, HL106804, EB012579, AI094745, HL110811, and AI105422), the Bill and Melinda Gates Foundation, and the Aeras Global Fund.

REFERENCES

Andersen P, Doherty TM. 2005. The success and failure of BCG—Implications for a novel tuberculosis vaccine. *Nat Rev Microbiol* **3:** 656–662.

Baram P, Soltysik L, Condoulis W. 1971. The in vitro assay of tuberculin hypersensitivity in *Macaca mulatta* sensitized with bacille Calmette Guérin cell wall vaccine and-or infected with virulent *Mycobacterium tuberculosis*. *Lab Anim Sci* **21:** 727–733.

Barclay WR, Anacker RL, Brehmer W, Leif W, Ribi E. 1970. Aerosol-induced tuberculosis in subhuman primates and the course of the disease after intravenous BCG vaccination. *Infect Immun* **2:** 574–582.

Barclay WR, Busey WM, Dalgard DW, Good RC, Janicki BW, Kasik JE, Ribi E, Ulrich CE, Wolinsky E. 1973. Protection of monkeys against airborne tuberculosis by aerosol vaccination with bacillus Calmette–Guérin. *Am Rev Resp Dis* **107:** 351–358.

Barry CE 3rd, Boshoff HI, Dartois V, Dick T, Ehrt S, Flynn J, Schnappinger D, Wilkinson RJ, Young D. 2009. The spectrum of latent tuberculosis: Rethinking the biology and intervention strategies. *Nat Rev Microbiol* **7:** 845–855.

Benson RE, Fremming BD, Young RJ. 1955. A tuberculosis outbreak in a *Macaca mulatta* colony. *Am Rev Tuberc* **72:** 204–209.

Brennan MJ, Stone MR, Evans T. 2012. A rational vaccine pipeline for tuberculosis. *Int J Tuberc Lung Dis* **16:** 1566–1573.

Brok HP, Hornby RJ, Griffiths GD, Scott LA, Hart BA. 2001. An extensive monoclonal antibody panel for the phenotyping of leukocyte subsets in the common marmoset and the cotton-top tamarin. *Cytometry* **45:** 294–303.

Budde ML, Greene JM, Chin EN, Ericsen AJ, Scarlotta M, Cain BT, Pham NH, Becker EA, Harris M, Weinfurter JT, et al. 2012. Specific $CD8^+$ T cell responses correlate with control of simian immunodeficiency virus replication in Mauritian cynomolgus macaques. *J Virol* **86:** 7596–7604.

Burwitz BJ, Pendley CJ, Greene JM, Detmer AM, Lhost JJ, Karl JA, Piaskowski SM, Rudersdorf RA, Wallace LT, Bimber BN, et al. 2009. Mauritian cynomolgus macaques share two exceptionally common major histocompatibility complex class I alleles that restrict simian immunodeficiency virus–specific $CD8^+$ T cells. *J Virol* **83:** 6011–6019.

Caceres N, Llopis I, Marzo E, Prats C, Vilaplana C, de Viedma DG, Samper S, Lopez D, Cardona PJ. 2012. Low dose aerosol fitness at the innate phase of murine infection better predicts virulence amongst clinical strains of *Mycobacterium tuberculosis*. *PloS ONE* **7:** e29010.

Capuano SV 3rd, Croix DA, Pawar S, Zinovik A, Myers A, Lin PL, Bissel S, Fuhrman C, Klein E, Flynn JL. 2003. Experimental *Mycobacterium tuberculosis* infection of cynomolgus macaques closely resembles the various manifestations of human *M. tuberculosis* infection. *Infect Immun* **71:** 5831–5844.

Chaparas SD, Good RC, Janicki BW. 1975. Tuberculin-induced lymphocyte transformation and skin reactivity in monkeys vaccinated or not vaccinated with Bacille Calmette–Guérin, then challenged with virulent *Mycobacterium tuberculosis*. *Am Rev Respir Dis* **112:** 43–47.

Chen CY, Huang D, Wang RC, Shen L, Zeng G, Yao S, Shen Y, Halliday L, Fortman J, McAllister M, et al. 2009. A critical role for CD8 T cells in a nonhuman primate model of tuberculosis. *PLoS Pathog* **5:** e1000392.

Chen CY, Yao S, Huang D, Wei H, Sicard H, Zeng G, Jomaa H, Larsen MH, Jacobs WR Jr, Wang R, et al. 2013. Phosphoantigen/IL2 expansion and differentiation of Vγ2Vδ2 T cells increase resistance to tuberculosis in nonhuman primates. *PLoS Pathog* **9:** e1003501.

Clark SO, Hall Y, Kelly DL, Hatch GJ, Williams A. 2011. Survival of *Mycobacterium tuberculosis* during experimental aerosolization and implications for aerosol challenge models. *J Appl Microbiol* **111:** 350–359.

Corbett EL, Watt CJ, Walker N, Maher D, Williams BG, Raviglione MC, Dye C. 2003. The growing burden of tuberculosis: Global trends and interactions with the HIV epidemic. *Arch Intern Med* **163:** 1009–1021.

Croix DA, Capuano S 3rd, Simpson L, Fallert BA, Fuller CL, Klein EC, Reinhart TA, Murphey-Corb M, Flynn JL. 2000. Effect of mycobacterial infection on virus loads and disease progression in simian immunodeficiency virus-infected rhesus monkeys. *AIDS Res Hum Retrovir* **16:** 1895–1908.

Cynamon MH, Klemens SP, Sharpe CA, Chase S. 1999. Activities of several novel oxazolidinones against *Mycobacterium tuberculosis* in a murine model. *Antimicrob Agents Chemother* **43:** 1189–1191.

Davis SL, Nuermberger EL, Um PK, Vidal C, Jedynak B, Pomper MG, Bishai WR, Jain SK. 2009. Noninvasive pulmonary [^{18}F]-2-fluoro-deoxy-D-glucose positron emission tomography correlates with bactericidal activity of tuberculosis drug treatment. *Antimicrob Agents Chemother* **53:** 4879–4884.

Diedrich CR, Mattila JT, Klein E, Janssen C, Phuah J, Sturgeon TJ, Montelaro RC, Lin PL, Flynn JL. 2010. Reactivation of latent tuberculosis in cynomolgus macaques infected with SIV is associated with early peripheral T cell depletion and not virus load. *PloS ONE* **5:** e9611.

Diedrich CR, Mattila JT, Flynn JL. 2013. Monocyte-derived IL-5 reduces TNF production by *Mycobacterium tuberculosis*-specific CD4 T cells during SIV/M. tuberculosis coinfection. *J Immunol* **190:** 6320–6328.

Fennelly KP, Jones-Lopez EC, Ayakaka I, Kim S, Menyha H, Kirenga B, Muchwa C, Joloba M, Dryden-Peterson S, Reilly N, et al. 2012. Variability of infectious aerosols produced during coughing by patients with pulmonary tuberculosis. *Am J Respir Crit Care Med* **186:** 450–457.

Flynn JL, Klein E. 2011. Pulmonary tuberculosis in monkeys. In *A color atlas of comparative pulmonary tuberculosis histopathology* (ed. Leong VDJ, Dick T), pp. 83–106. CRC, Boca Raton, FL.

Flynn JL, Tsenova L, Izzo A, Kaplan G. 2008. Experimental animal models of tuberculosis. In *Handbook of tuberculosis: Immunology and cell biology* (ed. Kaufmann SHE, Britton WJ), pp. 389–417. Wiley-VCH, Weinheim, Germany.

Ford CB, Lin PL, Chase MR, Shah RR, Iartchouk O, Galagan J, Mohaideen N, Ioerger TR, Sacchettini JC, Lipsitch M, et al. 2011. Use of whole genome sequencing to estimate the mutation rate of *Mycobacterium tuberculosis* during latent infection. *Nat Genet* **43:** 482–486.

Fourie PB, Odendaal MW. 1983. *Mycobacterium tuberculosis* in a closed colony of baboons (*Papio ursinus*). *Lab Anim* **17:** 125–128.

Gideon HP, Flynn JL. 2011. Latent tuberculosis: What the host "sees"? *Immunol Res* **50:** 202–212.

Good RC. 1968. Biology of the mycobacterioses. Simian tuberculosis: Immunologic aspects. *Ann NY Acad Sci* **154:** 200–213.

Good RC. 1984. Diseases in nonhuman primates. In *The mycobacteria: A sourcebook* (ed. Kubica GP, Wayne LG), pp. 903–921. Dekker, New York.

Gormus BJ, Blanchard JL, Alvarez XH, Didier PJ. 2004. Evidence for a rhesus monkey model of asymptomatic tuberculosis. *J Med Primatol* **33:** 134–145.

Janicki BW, Good RC, Minden P, Affronti LF, Hymes WF. 1973. Immune responses in rhesus monkeys after bacillus Calmette–Guérin vaccination and aerosol challenge with *Mycobacterium tuberculosis*. *Am Rev Respir Dis* **107:** 359–366.

Jensen K, Ranganathan UD, Van Rompay KK, Canfield DR, Khan I, Ravindran R, Luciw PA, Jacobs WR Jr, Fennelly G, Larsen MH, et al. 2012. A recombinant attenuated *Mycobacterium tuberculosis* vaccine strain is safe in immunosuppressed simian immunodeficiency virus-infected infant macaques. *Clin Vac Immunol* **19:** 1170–1181.

Keane J. 2004. Tumor necrosis factor blockers and reactivation of latent tuberculosis. *Clin Infect Dis* **39:** 300–302.

Keet DF, Kriek NP, Bengis RG, Grobler DG, Michel A. 2000. The rise and fall of tuberculosis in a free-ranging chacma baboon troop in the Kruger National Park. *Onderstepoort J Vet Res* **67:** 115–122.

Kita Y, Okada M, Nakajima T, Kanamaru N, Hashimoto S, Nagasawa T, Kaneda Y, Yoshida S, Nishida Y, Nakatani H, et al. 2011. Development of therapeutic and prophylactic vaccine against tuberculosis using monkey and transgenic mice models. *Hum Vaccin* **7:** 108–114.

Krebs KC, Jin Z, Rudersdorf R, Hughes AL, O'Connor DH. 2005. Unusually high frequency MHC class I alleles in Mauritian origin cynomolgus macaques. *J Immunol* **175:** 5230–5239.

Langermans JA, Andersen P, van Soolingen D, Vervenne RA, Frost PA, van der Laan T, van Pinxteren LA, van den Hombergh J, Kroon S, Peekel I, et al. 2001. Divergent effect of bacillus Calmette–Guérin (BCG) vaccination on *Mycobacterium tuberculosis* infection in highly related macaque species: Implications for primate models in tuberculosis vaccine research. *Proc Natl Acad Sci* **98:** 11497–11502.

Lawn SD, Churchyard G. 2009. Epidemiology of HIV-associated tuberculosis. *Curr Opin HIVAIDS* **4:** 325–333.

Lee M, Lee J, Carroll MW, Choi H, Min S, Song T, Via LE, Goldfeder LC, Kang E, Jin B, et al. 2012. Linezolid for treatment of chronic extensively drug-resistant tuberculosis. *New Engl J Med* **367:** 1508–1518.

Lewinsohn DM, Tydeman IS, Frieder M, Grotzke JE, Lines RA, Ahmed S, Prongay KD, Primack SL, Colgin LM, Lewis AD, et al. 2006. High resolution radiographic and fine immunologic definition of TB disease progression in the rhesus macaque. *Microbes Infect* **8:** 2587–2598.

Lin PL, Flynn JL. 2010. Understanding latent tuberculosis: A moving target. *J Immunol* **185:** 15–22.

Lin PL, Pawar S, Myers A, Pegu A, Fuhrman C, Reinhart TA, Capuano SV, Klein E, Flynn JL. 2006. Early events in *Mycobacterium tuberculosis* infection in cynomolgus macaques. *Infect Immun* **74:** 3790–3803.

Lin PL, Rodgers M, Smith L, Bigbee M, Myers A, Bigbee C, Chiosea I, Capuano SV, Fuhrman C, Klein E, et al. 2009. Quantitative comparison of active and latent tuberculosis in the cynomolgus macaque model. *Infect Immun* **77:** 4631–4642.

Lin PL, Myers A, Smith L, Bigbee C, Bigbee M, Fuhrman C, Grieser H, Chiosea I, Voitenek NN, Capuano SV, et al. 2010. Tumor necrosis factor neutralization results in disseminated disease in acute and latent *Mycobacterium tuberculosis* infection with normal granuloma structure in a cynomolgus macaque model. *Arthritis Rheum* **62:** 340–350.

Lin PL, Dartois V, Johnston PJ, Janssen C, Via L, Goodwin MB, Klein E, Barry CE III, Flynn JL. 2012a. Metronidazole prevents reactivation of latent *Mycobacterium tuberculosis* infection in macaques. *Proc Natl Acad Sci* **109:** 14188–14193.

Lin PL, Dietrich J, Tan E, Abalos RM, Burgos J, Bigbee C, Bigbee M, Milk L, Gideon HP, Rodgers M, et al. 2012b. The multistage vaccine H56 boosts the effects of BCG to protect cynomolgus macaques against active tuberculosis and reactivation of latent *Mycobacterium tuberculosis* infection. *J Clin Invest* **122:** 303–314.

Lin PL, Rutledge T, Green AM, Bigbee M, Fuhrman C, Klein E, Flynn JL. 2012c. CD4 T cell depletion exacerbates acute *Mycobacterium tuberculosis* while reactivation of latent infection is dependent on severity of tissue depletion in cynomolgus macaques. *AIDS Res Hum Retrovir* **28:** 1693–1702.

Lin PL, Coleman T, Carney JP, Lopresti BJ, Tomko J, Fillmore D, Dartois V, Scanga C, Frye LJ, Janssen C, et al. 2013. Radiologic responses in cynomolgous macaques for assessing tuberculosis chemotherapy regimens. *Antimicrob Agents Chemother* **57:** 4237–4244.

Lin PL, Ford CB, Coleman MT, Myers AJ, Gawande R, Ioerger T, Sacchettini J, Fortune SM, Flynn JL. 2014. Sterilization of granulomas is common in active and latent tuberculosis despite within-host variability in bacterial killing. *Nat Med* **20:** 75–79.

Luciw PA, Oslund KL, Yang XW, Adamson L, Ravindran R, Canfield DR, Tarara R, Hirst L, Christensen M, Lerche NW, et al. 2011. Stereological analysis of bacterial load and lung lesions in nonhuman primates (rhesus macaques) experimentally infected with *Mycobacterium tuberculosis*. *Am J Physiol Lung Cell Mol Physiol* **301:** L731–L738.

Manca C, Tsenova L, Barry CE III, Bergtold A, Freeman S, Haslett PA, Musser JM, Freedman VH, Kaplan G. 1999. *Mycobacterium tuberculosis* CDC1551 induces a more vigorous host response in vivo and in vitro, but is not more virulent than other clinical isolates. *J Immunol* **162:** 6740–6746.

Marino S, Linderman JJ, Kirschner DE. 2011. A multifaceted approach to modeling the immune response in tuberculosis. *Wiley Interdiscip Rev Syst Biol Med* **3:** 479–489.

Mattila JT, Diedrich CR, Lin PL, Phuah J, Flynn JL. 2011. Simian immunodeficiency virus-induced changes in T cell cytokine responses in cynomolgus macaques with latent *Mycobacterium tuberculosis* infection are associated with timing of reactivation. *J Immunol* **186:** 3527–3537.

Mayhall CG, Lamb VA, Coleman PH. 1981. Infection in rhesus (*Macaca mulatta*) and squirrel (*Saimiri sciureus*) monkeys due to *Mycobacterium tuberculosis* phage type B. Outbreak in a primate colony. *J Med Primatol* **10:** 302–311.

McLeay SC, Morrish GA, Kirkpatrick CM, Green B. 2012. The relationship between drug clearance and body size: Systematic review and meta-analysis of the literature published from 2000 to 2007. *Clin Pharmacokinet* **51:** 319–330.

Mehra S, Golden NA, Dutta NK, Midkiff CC, Alvarez X, Doyle LA, Asher M, Russell-Lodrigue K, Monjure C, Roy CJ, et al. 2011. Reactivation of latent tuberculosis in rhesus macaques by coinfection with simian immunodeficiency virus. *J Med Primatol* **40:** 233–243.

Michel AL, Hlokwe TM, Espie IW, van Zijll Langhout M, Koeppel K, Lane E. 2013. *Mycobacterium tuberculosis* at the human/wildlife interface in a high TB burden country. *Transbound Emerg Dis* **60:** 46–52.

Min F, Zhang Y, Pan J, Wang J, Yuan W. 2013. *Mycobacterium tuberculosis* infection in rhesus monkeys (*Macaca mulatta*) and evaluation of ESAT-6 and CFP10 as immunodiagnostic antigens. *Exp Anim* **62:** 281–293.

Mitchison DA, Chang KC. 2009. Experimental models of tuberculosis: Can we trust the mouse? *Am J Respir Crit Care Med* **180:** 201–202.

Montali RJ, Mikota SK, Cheng LI. 2001. *Mycobacterium tuberculosis* in zoo and wildlife species. *Rev Sci Tech* **20:** 291–303.

Motzel SL, Schachner RD, Kornegay RW, Fletcher MA, Kanaya B, Gomez JA, Ngai DT-W, Pouch WJ, Washington MV, Handt LA, et al. 2003. Diagnosis of tuberculosis in nonhuman primates. In *International perspectives: The future of nonhuman primate resources*, pp. 156–159. National Academies Press, Washington, DC.

Munoz-Elias EJ, Timm J, Botha T, Chan WT, Gomez JE, McKinney JD. 2005. Replication dynamics of *Mycobacterium tuberculosis* in chronically infected mice. *Infect Immun* **73:** 546–551.

O'Garra A, Redford PS, McNab FW, Bloom CI, Wilkinson RJ, Berry MP. 2013. The immune response in tuberculosis. *Ann Rev Immunol* **31:** 475–527.

Okada M, Kita Y, Nakajima T, Kanamaru N, Hashimoto S, Nagasawa T, Kaneda Y, Yoshida S, Nishida Y, Nakatani H, et al. 2009. Novel prophylactic and therapeutic vaccine against tuberculosis. *Vaccine* **27:** 3267–3270.

Ottenhoff TH, Kaufmann SH. 2012. Vaccines against tuberculosis: Where are we and where do we need to go? *PLoS Pathog* **8:** e1002607.

Palanisamy GS, Smith EE, Shanley CA, Ordway DJ, Orme IM, Basaraba RJ. 2008. Disseminated disease severity as a measure of virulence of *Mycobacterium tuberculosis* in the guinea pig model. *Tuberculosis* **88:** 295–306.

Panarella ML, Bimes RS. 2010. A naturally occurring outbreak of tuberculosis in a group of imported cynomolgus monkeys (*Macaca fascicularis*). *J Am Assoc Lab Anim Sci* **49:** 221–225.

Pawlowski A, Jansson M, Skold M, Rottenberg ME, Kallenius G. 2012. Tuberculosis and HIV co-infection. *PLoS Pathog* **8:** e1002464.

Payne KS, Novak JJ, Jongsakul K, Imerbsin R, Apisitsaowapa Y, Pavlin JA, Hinds SB. 2011. *Mycobacterium tuberculosis* infection in a closed colony of rhesus macaques (*Macaca mulatta*). *J Am Assoc Lab Anim Sci* **50:** 105–108.

Rahman S, Magalhaes I, Rahman J, Ahmed RK, Sizemore DR, Scanga CA, Weichold F, Verreck F, Kondova I, Sadoff J, et al. 2012. Prime-boost vaccination with rBCG/rAd35 enhances $CD8^+$ cytolytic T-cell responses in lesions from *Mycobacterium tuberculosis*-infected primates. *Mol Med* **18:** 647–658.

Rayner EL, Pearson GR, Hall GA, Basaraba RJ, Gleeson F, McIntyre A, Clark S, Williams A, Dennis MJ, Sharpe SA. 2013. Early lesions following aerosol infection of rhesus macaques (*Macaca mulatta*) with *Mycobacterium tuberculosis* strain H37RV. *J Comp Pathol* **149:** 475–485.

Reed SG, Coler RN, Dalemans W, Tan EV, DeLa Cruz EC, Basaraba RJ, Orme IM, Skeiky YA, Alderson MR, Cowgill KD, et al. 2009. Defined tuberculosis vaccine, Mtb72F/AS02A, evidence of protection in cynomolgus monkeys. *Proc Natl Acad Sci* **106:** 2301–2306.

Ribi E, Anacker RL, Barclay WR, Brehmer W, Harris SC, Leif WR, Simmons J. 1971. Efficacy of mycobacterial cell walls as a vaccine against airborne tuberculosis in the Rheusus monkey. *J Infect Dis* **123:** 527–538.

Safi H, Gormus BJ, Didier PJ, Blanchard JL, Lakey DL, Martin LN, Murphey-Corb M, Vankayalapati R, Barnes PF. 2003. Spectrum of manifestations of *Mycobacterium tuberculosis* infection in primates infected with SIV. *AIDS Res Hum Retroviruses* **19:** 585–595.

Sampson SL, Mansfield KG, Carville A, Magee DM, Quitugua T, Howerth EW, Bloom BR, Hondalus MK. 2011. Extended safety and efficacy studies of a live attenuated double leucine and pantothenate auxotroph of *Mycobacterium tuberculosis* as a vaccine candidate. *Vaccine* **29:** 4839–4847.

Schmidt LH. 1956. Some observations on the utility of simian pulmonary tuberculosis in defining the therapeutic potentialities of isoniazid. *Am Rev Tuberc* **74:** 138–153; discussion, 153–159.

Schmidt LH. 1966. Studies on the antituberculous activity of ethambutol in monkeys. *Ann NY Acad Sci* **135:** 747–758.

Schmidt L, Grover A, Hoffmann R. 1959. The comparative therapeutic activities of thiocarbanidin and para-aminosalicylic acid administered alone and in combination with isoniazid. *Trans 18th VA-Armed Forces Conf Chemother Tuberculosis* 312–317.

Schroeder CR. 1938. Acquired tuberculosis in the primate in laboratories and zoological collections. *Am J Pub Health Nations Health* **28:** 469–475.

Sharpe SA, Eschelbach E, Basaraba RJ, Gleeson F, Hall GA, McIntyre A, Williams A, Kraft SL, Clark S, Gooch K, et al. 2009. Determination of lesion volume by MRI and stereology in a macaque model of tuberculosis. *Tuberculosis* **89:** 405–416.

Sharpe SA, McShane H, Dennis MJ, Basaraba RJ, Gleeson F, Hall G, McIntyre A, Gooch K, Clark S, Beveridge NE, et al. 2010. Establishment of an aerosol challenge model of tuberculosis in rhesus macaques and an evaluation of endpoints for vaccine testing. *Clin Vaccine Immunol* **17:** 1170–1182.

Shen Y, Zhou D, Chalifoux L, Shen L, Simon M, Zeng X, Lai X, Li Y, Sehgal P, Letvin NL, et al. 2002a. Induction of an AIDS virus-related tuberculosis-like disease in macaques: A model of simian immunodeficiency virus–mycobacterium coinfection. *Infect Immun* **70:** 869–877.

Shen Y, Zhou D, Qiu L, Lai X, Simon M, Shen L, Kou Z, Wang Q, Jiang L, Estep J, et al. 2002b. Adaptive immune response of $V\gamma2V\delta2^{+}$ T cells during mycobacterial infections. *Science* **295:** 2255–2258.

Shin NS, Kwon SW, Han DH, Bai GH, Yoon J, Cheon DS, Son YS, Ahn K, Chae C, Lee YS. 1995. *Mycobacterium tuberculosis* infection in an orangutan (*Pongo pygmaeus*). *The J Vet Med Sci* **57:** 951–953.

Sugawara I, Sun L, Mizuno S, Taniyama T. 2009. Protective efficacy of recombinant BCG Tokyo (Ag85A) in rhesus monkeys (*Macaca mulatta*) infected intratracheally with H37Rv *Mycobacterium tuberculosis*. *Tuberculosis* **89:** 62–67.

Tsenova L, Ellison E, Harbacheuski R, Moreira AL, Kurepina N, Reed MB, Mathema B, Barry CE 3rd, Kaplan G. 2005. Virulence of selected *Mycobacterium tuberculosis* clinical isolates in the rabbit model of meningitis is dependent on phenolic glycolipid produced by the bacilli. *J Infect Dis* **192:** 98–106.

Verreck FA, Vervenne RA, Kondova I, van Kralingen KW, Remarque EJ, Braskamp G, van der Werff NM, Kersbergen A, Ottenhoff TH, Heidt PJ, et al. 2009. MVA.85A boosting of BCG and an attenuated, phoP deficient *M. tuberculosis* vaccine both show protective efficacy against tuberculosis in rhesus macaques. *PloS ONE* **4:** e5264.

Via LE, Lin PL, Ray SM, Carrillo J, Allen SS, Eum SY, Taylor K, Klein E, Manjunatha U, Gonzales J, et al. 2008. Tuberculous granulomas are hypoxic in guinea pigs, rabbits, and nonhuman primates. *Infect Immun* **76:** 2333–2340.

Via LE, Schimel D, Weiner DM, Dartois V, Dayao E, Cai Y, Yoon YS, Dreher MR, Kastenmayer RJ, Laymon CM, et al. 2012. Infection dynamics and response to chemotherapy in a rabbit model of tuberculosis using [^{18}F]2-fluoro-deoxy-D-glucose positron emission tomography and computed tomography. *Antimicrob Agents Chemother* **56:** 4391–4402.

Via LE, Weiner DM, Schimel D, Lin PL, Dayao E, Tankersley SL, Cai Y, Coleman MT, Tomko J, Paripati P, et al. 2013. Differential virulence and disease progression following *Mycobacterium tuberculosis* complex infection of the common marmoset (*Callithrix jacchus*). *Infect Immun* **81:** 2909–2919.

Walsh GP, Tan EV, dela Cruz EC, Abalos RM, Villahermosa LG, Young LJ, Cellona RV, Nazareno JB, Horwitz MA. 1996. The Philippine cynomolgus monkey (*Macaca fasicularis*) provides a new nonhuman primate model of tuberculosis that resembles human disease. *Nat Med* **2:** 430–436.

Wei H, Wang R, Yuan Z, Chen CY, Huang D, Halliday L, Zhong W, Zeng G, Shen Y, Shen L, et al. 2009. DR*W201/P65 tetramer visualization of epitope-specific CD4 T-cell during *M. tuberculosis* infection and its resting memory pool after BCG vaccination. *PloS ONE* **4:** e6905.

WHO. 2013. *Global tuberculosis report 2013*. World Health Organization, http://www.who.int/tb/publications/global_report/en/.

Williams KN, Stover CK, Zhu T, Tasneen R, Tyagi S, Grosset JH, Nuermberger E. 2009. Promising antituberculosis activity of the oxazolidinone PNU-100480 relative to that of linezolid in a murine model. *Antimicrob Agents Chemother* **53:** 1314–1319.

Yan G, Zhang G, Fang X, Zhang Y, Li C, Ling F, Cooper DN, Li Q, Li Y, van Gool AJ, et al. 2011. Genome sequencing and comparison of two nonhuman primate animal models, the cynomolgus and Chinese rhesus macaques. *Nat Biotechnol* **29:** 1019–1023.

Zhang J, Ye YQ, Wang Y, Mo PZ, Xian QY, Rao Y, Bao R, Dai M, Liu JY, Guo M, et al. 2011. *M. tuberculosis* H37Rv infection of Chinese rhesus macaques. *J Neuroimmune Pharmacol* **6:** 362–370.

Zhou D, Shen Y, Chalifoux L, Lee-Parritz D, Simon M, Sehgal PK, Zheng L, Halloran M, Chen ZW. 1999. *Mycobacterium bovis* bacille Calmette–Guérin enhances pathogenicity of simian immunodeficiency virus infection and accelerates progression to AIDS in macaques: A role of persistent T cell activation in AIDS pathogenesis. *J Immunol* **162:** 2204–2216.

Mycobacterial Growth

Iria Uhía[1], Kerstin J. Williams[1], Vahid Shahrezaei[2], and Brian D. Robertson[1]

[1]Department of Medicine, MRC Centre for Molecular Bacteriology and Infection, Imperial College London, London, SW7 2AZ, United Kingdom

[2]Department of Mathematics, Imperial College London, London, SW7 2AZ, United Kingdom

Correspondence: b.robertson@imperial.ac.uk

In this work, we review progress made in understanding the molecular underpinnings of growth and division in mycobacteria, concentrating on work published since the last comprehensive review (Hett and Rubin 2008). We have focused on exciting work making use of new time-lapse imaging technologies coupled with reporter-gene fusions and antimicrobial treatment to generate insights into how mycobacteria grow and divide in a heterogeneous manner. We try to reconcile the different observations reported, providing a model of how they might fit together. We also review the topic of mycobacterial spores, which has generated considerable discussion during the last few years. Resuscitation promoting factors, and regulation of growth and division, have also been actively researched, and we summarize progress in these areas.

The answers to many biological questions are facilitated by technological advances that allow us to observe and interrogate objects easier, faster, and more accurately than before. Time-lapse observations of bacteria have been around for many years, even for more difficult to grow prokaryotes, such as mycobacteria. Elegant studies by Brieger and Glauert more than 60 yr ago show what can be performed with ingenuity and patience (Brieger and Glauert 1952, 1956; Brieger et al. 1953, and references therein). We now have autofocus microscopes with motorized stages, digital cameras with more and more pixels, and software to control it all. Historically, the basics of growing bacteria for imaging used bacterial agar; recently, however, microfluidics arrived on the microscope stage, which allowed us to grow bacteria in suspension and to control growth conditions with relative ease. These systems make it possible to change growth medium in a controlled manner, introduce antimicrobials, and image what happens, as frequently as the bacteria will tolerate exposure to the high-intensity light needed to excite the fluorophores they express. The availability of commercial systems means that investigations of bacterial growth and division and the response to environmental changes are once again only constrained by our ingenuity.

MYCOBACTERIAL IMAGING

Technological advances in micro- and nanotechnology permit the study of microorganisms at the single-cell level. Electron microscopy provided insights into mycobacterial cell division (Dahl 2004), showing *Mycobacterium tuberculosis* forming branching structures with

Cite this article as *Cold Spring Harb Perspect Med* doi: 10.1101/cshperspect.a021097

V-shaped cells undergoing a "snapping" mechanism of cell division common to actinomycetes. Electron micrographs allow high cellular detail to be visualized, but tell nothing about the dynamics of cell division and chromosome segregation; this requires time-resolved images that represent separate growth stages to visualize the process in its entirety. Live-cell time-lapse imaging allows single cells to be imaged periodically, so that the movement of a protein during cell growth and division can be observed directly and quantified to assess cell-to-cell variability (Locke and Elowitz 2009). Advances in microscopy, fluorescent proteins, and dye technologies have allowed multiple protein and cellular structures to be viewed simultaneously, which, coupled with time-lapse imaging, is emerging as a powerful tool to investigate mycobacterial cell division.

Live-Cell Time-Lapse Imaging

To date, only a few studies of cell division in mycobacteria have been reported using this technology (Joyce et al. 2011, 2012; Aldridge et al. 2012; Golchin et al. 2012; Santi et al. 2013; Wakamoto et al. 2013). The method is not without challenges; mycobacteria grow slowly and tend to divide to form disorganized microcolonies, which impacts on the imaging protocol to ensure the microscopy conditions remain permissive for growth and capture in-focus images. Fluorescence microscopy requires an excitation source (laser, xenon, or helium lamp) to produce a detectable emission from the fluorophore, but prolonged high-intensity light causes phototoxicity, affecting cell viability. Two methods of growing mycobacteria on thin agar pads or in microfluidic devices, both housed in temperature controlled chambers and imaged by bright-field or confocal microscopy, have been reported. Growth on thin agar pads on a microscope slide has been used to study fundamental processes such as bacterial growth patterns, protein localization dynamics, antibiotic action, and bacterial persistence (Fiebig et al. 2006; Thanbichler and Shapiro 2006; Letek et al. 2008). However, the environmental conditions are difficult to manipulate, and it is challenging to prevent desiccation of the agar pad and maintain levels of oxygen and nutrients for the longer experiments needed for slow-growing mycobacteria. A modified agar pad method for mycobacteria was developed (Joyce et al. 2011) using glass-bottomed dishes and an agar pad, with the bacteria sandwiched between coverslip and agar, and imaged with an inverted microscope. This method allowed imaging over longer times (>65 h); can be used with fluorescence microscopy and permits some manipulation of environmental conditions, by diffusion through the thin agar pad during imaging (Joyce et al. 2012). The availability of multiwell glass-bottomed plates and automated microscope stages means that this method could be used for higher-throughput analyses. However, more complex alterations of environmental conditions, such as changing the medium composition or removal of antibiotics, are impractical.

Microfluidic devices are more sophisticated and expensive, but they are a rapidly advancing technology, with commercial platforms now available as an alternative to in-house devices. This technology has been used to study mycobacterial cell division (Aldridge et al. 2012; Golchin et al. 2012; Santi et al. 2013; Wakamoto et al. 2013). Typical custom-built microfluidic devices use photolithographic methods to create a positive template of microchannels which is used to cast negative-aspect replicas in polydimethylsiloxane (PDMS). The PDMS structures are bonded to glass slides, and holes are added to make input and output channels for the addition and removal of growth medium using syringe pumps (Aldridge et al. 2012; Golchin et al. 2012; Santi et al. 2013; Wakamoto et al. 2013). Continuous perfusion of the cells ensures a suitable growth environment for long-term experiments and permits manipulation of environmental conditions, such as the addition or removal of antibiotics. Such devices have the advantage that they can restrict movement of the cells in the Z-plane, keeping them in focus, although it is unclear as yet whether this is detrimental to mycobacterial growth. To date, only imaging of the fast-growing *Mycobacterium smegmatis* has been reported using microfluidics. Recent advances include the development of microfluidic plates and automated perfusion systems (e.g., the CellASIC ONIX Microfluidic Perfusion Platform [Lee et al. 2009]) permitting higher-throughput and automated methods of single-cell tracking. Although not without drawbacks, live-cell imaging using microfluidics is arguably now the method of choice, and it will be interesting to see if super-resolution microscopy can be incorporated into such systems.

ASYMMETRIC GROWTH

Several groups have studied cell elongation and septum placement in mycobacteria, reaching different conclusions about the asymmetry or symmetry of these processes. However, some of the disagreements may be attributed to the use of different experimental conditions and analysis methods (Table 1 and Fig. 1), as will be discussed below.

Unipolar/Bipolar Growth

The absence from actinomycete genomes of the actin homolog MreB, which directs lateral wall biogenesis (Carballido-López 2006), together with the localization of nascent peptidoglycan synthesis to the cell tips of mycobacterial and corynebacterial cells, supports polar growth in these bacteria (Daniel and Errington, 2003; Thanky et al. 2007; Hett and Rubin 2008). Additional work showed a role for Wag31—homolog of the Gram-positive cell-division protein DivIVA—in the maintenance of cell morphology (Kang et al. 2008).

Polar growth has been the topic of several recent studies. Aldridge et al. (2012) proposed that mycobacterial growth is unipolar and mainly from the old cell pole. However, exclusively unipolar growth was not observed by other authors, although some did notice a different growth rate between poles without reference to pole age (Joyce et al. 2012; Singh et al. 2013). Another study showed the same rate of mycobacterial growth from both poles (Santi et al. 2013). According to the Aldridge model, after division, one daughter cell inherits the growing (old) pole, whereas its sibling creates a new growth pole, leading to a slower elongation rate. As the growth pole matures, cells elongate faster and birth length increases, assuming that cell cycle is dependent on time, not cell size (Aldridge et al. 2012). The results and conclusions reached by Santi et al. (2013) are nonetheless quite different. In their model, old and new poles elongate at the same rate. However, they quantified exponential growth rate, considering elongation velocity to be size-dependent (larger cells growing faster), and their data show that the cells inheriting the old pole tend to be larger at division and so grow faster than the new pole cells (Santi et al. 2013). The elongation rate remains nevertheless the same in sibling cells, as described by Wakamoto et al. (2013). Thus, this model supports the exponential growth of single cells, as suggested for other bacteria (Godin et al. 2010; Mir et al. 2011), and is in agreement with a size-control mechanism that would prevent cells from dividing before reaching a minimum size; once achieved, the division would proceed in a random fashion (Santi et al. 2013).

Antibiotic Susceptibility/Persistence

Supporters of unipolar growth suggested related consequences for antibiotic susceptibility (Aldridge et al. 2012). The cells inheriting the growing pole were more sensitive to several peptidoglycan synthesis inhibitors, as expected, and also to isoniazid, targeting mycolic acid synthesis, but more resistant to the RNA polymerase inhibitor, rifampicin (Aldridge et al. 2012). Thus, variability in the susceptibility of these two populations of cells to antibiotics was proposed (Aldridge et al. 2012). The association between growth rates and sensitivity to isoniazid was later challenged, as other investigators did not find a correlation (Wakamoto et al. 2013). In contrast, a weak positive association was described between survival in the presence of isoniazid and the inheritance of the old pole (Wakamoto et al. 2013). Santi et al. (2013) also did not find any difference between old pole and new pole cells regarding sensitivity to the antibiotics tested by Aldridge et al. (2012), although the possibility that the different techniques used

Table 1. Summary of reported live cell time-lapse imaging studies of mycobacterial cell division

Study	Growth conditions	Size-dependent cell division	Septum marker	Septum placement	Asymmetric growth	Asymmetric division	Growth rate estimation method
Joyce et al. 2011, 2012	Agar pad	No	PBP1a-mCherry (mid)	Toward midcell (87% within central 20th percentile)	Yes Bipolar, but unequal velocities	Yes	Exponential
Aldridge et al. 2012	Microfluidics	No (time-dependent)	None	n.d.	Yes Unipolar	Yes	Linear
Singh et al. 2013	Agar pad	No	FtsZ-mCherry (early)	Random	Yes Bipolar, but unequal and unipolar	Yes	n.d.
Santi et al. 2013	Microfluidics	No (or time-dependent)	Wag31-GFP (late)	Toward midcell but slight bias toward new cell pole	Yes Bipolar, but equal velocities	Yes	Exponential

Summary of results reported for the recently published studies, highlighting the marker used and results obtained.
n.d., not determined.

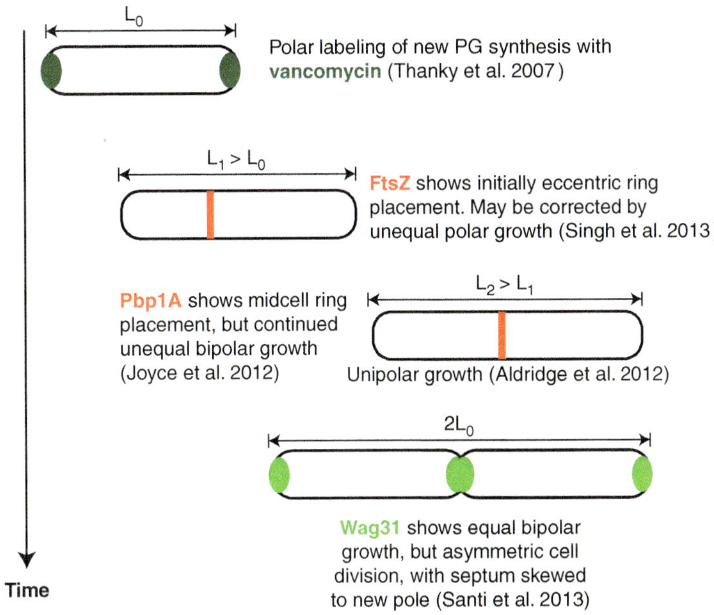

Figure 1. Cartoon summarizing the results published to date on mycobacterial cell division using time-lapse imaging. A timeline has been constructed to try to reconcile the different results reported for polar and asymmetric growth. PG, peptidoglycan.

could affect the results cannot be discarded (Santi et al. 2013). Survival in the presence of isoniazid was attributed to single-cell dynamics of KatG, the isoniazid-activating enzyme; cells expressing KatG in stochastic pulses would be more sensitive to the drug (Wakamoto et al. 2013). As the survival of sibling cells was positively correlated, it was suggested that epigenetics contribute to this phenomenon. This result supports the opinion that persistent cells may continue to grow in the presence of antibiotics and that the stochastic expression of any factor which promotes or inhibits the activity of the antibiotic could be key in the survival of single cells (Wakamoto et al. 2013). That the persistent state of *M. tuberculosis* in chronic infection may be attributable to on-going bacterial replication is in opposition to models that defend a nonreplicating state (Gill et al. 2009). Other work on *M. smegmatis* showed that some cells exit dormancy stochastically and independently of time or environmental factors, perhaps through the stochastic expression or repression of a master regulatory gene (Buerger et al. 2012). These results suggest that slowing of growth may not be the only common strategy for microorganisms to achieve persistence (Buerger et al. 2012).

Septum Positioning

The apparently asymmetric septum placement observed could be a consequence of the asymmetric polar growth reported (Aldridge et al. 2012; Joyce et al. 2012; Singh et al. 2013). Indeed, this is the conclusion of Joyce et al. (2012), using penicillin-binding protein 1a (PBP1a) and Van-BODIPY as markers of poles and septum, respectively. They found that septum placement is less accurate in mycobacteria than in corynebacteria, but a mid-cell position was favored. However, this was altered by subsequent unequal polar growth, leading to asymmetric division. Septum placement was independent of cell length (Joyce et al. 2012); other investigators state that cells need to reach a critical size before division (Santi et al. 2013; Singh et al. 2013). Singh et al. (2013) showed that FtsZ ring positioning was nearly random, but when using membrane (FM4-64) or cell wall (FL-Vanco) markers, the septum position was found to be more symmetric. Finally, when using the late-division protein Wag31 as a septum marker, it was biased toward the new pole (Santi et al. 2013). These discrepancies might be because of the use of different markers; FtsZ is probably the earliest component in septum formation, with membranes, PBP1a, and cell wall components recruited at later stages. Alternative explanations taking this into account may bring these apparently disparate observations together. If the FtsZ ring is placed nonsymmetrically, then subsequent unequal polar growth may lead to an apparent mid-cell positioning of later septum components. As growth continues, the septum is again found in an asymmetric position before cell division, when Wag31 is located there (Joyce et al. 2012; Santi et al. 2013; Singh et al. 2013). Asymmetric division sites have been reported over the nucleoids, requiring a DNA translocase to transfer the DNA through the septum before it closes (Singh et al. 2013); however, this has not been reported by others. More observations are required to account for the heterogeneity reported in mycobacterial growth and division, and investigations using consensus cell division markers in the different experimental systems would further help clarify the situation.

Asymmetric growth and division is widespread in bacteria and may have evolved multiple times (Kysela et al. 2013), because it influences population aging and produces phenotypic heterogeneity. This could provide fitness advantages for the population through a bet-hedging strategy (Kussell and Leibler 2005). The recent work in mycobacteria suggests that phenotypic heterogeneity could arise at multiple levels through asymmetric polar growth and inaccurate cell division. The ultimate importance of the specific forms of growth asymmetries in host–pathogen interactions is a key area for further investigations.

Drug-Resistant Strains: Growth and Division

It is interesting to note the characteristic morphology observed in resistant *M. tuberculosis* strains (Velayati et al. 2009a,b; Farnia et al. 2010). During exponential growth, multidrug-resistant (MDR) and susceptible isolates are mainly rod-shaped, whereas oval, rounded, or branching cells are seen in extensively drug-resistant (XDR) isolates (Farnia et al. 2010). XDR subpopulations also displayed an extremely thick wall (Velayati et al. 2009b). Symmetrical, asymmetrical, and branching division were observed in all isolates, but XDR isolates displayed a novel division type in which a rod-shaped mother cell produced a small round bacillus (Farnia et al. 2010). These changes in morphology may help these strains escape immune responses and adapt to the host environment (Champion and Mitragotri 2006; Farnia et al. 2010).

CHROMOSOME SEGREGATION

Before cell division, the replicated chromosomes must be partitioned into the daughter cells. The presence of chromosomal homologs of the genes needed to segregate low-copy-number plasmids during cell division raises the possibility that chromosomes are segregated in a similar way. Both plasmid and chromosome encoded *par* loci consist of an ATPase (ParA), a site-specific DNA-binding protein (ParB) that interacts with ParA, and a DNA sequence motif (*parS*) to which ParB binds. The type I plasmid-encoded *par* loci encode a Walker A Cytoskeletal ATPase and are the ones also found on bacterial chromosomes (Ebersbach and Gerdes 2005).

The chromosomal ParAB system has been studied in several bacteria including *Mycobacterium spp.* (Jakimowicz et al. 2007; Casart et al. 2008; Maloney et al. 2009; Nisa et al. 2010; Chaudhuri and Dean 2011; Ginda et al. 2013). In *Caulobacter crescentus* (Ptacin and Shapiro 2010), the only species in which *parA* and *parB* are essential, a model was proposed in which ParA dimerizes when bound to ATP and forms linear polymers. These polymers are dissociated from the ends, stimulated by the binding of the ParB-*parS* partition complex. As ParA depolymerizes, the partition complex moves toward the new pole during chromosome segregation.

Chromosomal *par* loci are located proximal to and upstream of *oriC* (Lin and Grossman 1998). Genes homologous to *parA* and *parB* have been identified in all mycobacteria se-

 Cite this article as *Cold Spring Harb Perspect Med* doi: 10.1101/cshperspect.a021097

quenced so far (Jakimowicz et al. 2007). Two *parS* copies, identical to those in *Streptomyces coelicolor* (Jakimowicz et al. 2002), have been identified in *M. smegmatis*, *Mycobacterium bovis* BCG (Bacillus Calmette–Guérin) and *M. tuberculosis* (Jakimowicz et al. 2007; Casart et al. 2008), and a third *parS* copy with one mismatch to the consensus is also located close to *oriC*. These *parS* sequences interact with ParB in *M. smegmatis* (Jakimowicz et al. 2007). The *par* genes are arranged in an operon, where they cluster with another six conserved genes (including *gidB*), upstream and divergent to the *dnaA* gene (Casart et al. 2008). One *parS* sequence is located in the *gidB* promoter, and the other is in the coding region of *parA*, suggesting that *parB* could regulate both *gidB* and *parA* expression and control the levels of Par proteins (Casart et al. 2008). Indeed, the amino-terminal domain of ParB does interact with *parS* (Chaudhuri and Dean 2011). The mycobacterial ParB–*parS* partition complex involves ParB–ParB interactions (Ginda et al. 2013). On binding to *parS* sequences, it has been proposed that in *M. tuberculosis*, ParB dimers undergo a drastic compaction, which primes ParB spreading on the *parS*-adjacent DNA scaffold to form the type of higher-order partition assembly (Chaudhuri and Dean 2011) described for other bacteria (Murray et al. 2006; Breier and Grossman 2007).

The *parA* and *parB* genes are annotated as essential in *M. tuberculosis* based on transposon mutagenesis (Sassetti et al. 2003; Zhang et al. 2012). However, they are nonessential in *M. smegmatis* (Jakimowicz et al. 2007; Ginda et al. 2013), in which both locate to the poles of the cell (Maloney et al. 2009; Ginda et al. 2013). However, this localization pattern was only studied with static microscopy, and it may be dynamic in live cells, as seen in *C. crescentus* (Ptacin and Shapiro 2010). In fact, a gradient of ParA from one pole toward the other has been observed in *M. smegmatis* using in vivo time-lapse microscopy (G Joyce, KJ Williams, and BD Robertson, unpubl.). In contrast in *Corynebacterium glutamicum*, ParB remains stably attached to the cell poles during time-lapse experiments (Donovan et al. 2010). The bipolar localization of ParB observed in static microscopy is altered when *parA* is deleted; however, the deletion of *parB* does not seem to alter ParA localization, suggesting that mislocalized partition complexes have a more negative influence on chromosome segregation than their complete absence (Ginda et al. 2013).

Overproduction or deletion of ParA or ParB causes growth inhibition and severe chromosome segregation defects (Jakimowicz et al. 2007; Maloney et al. 2009; Ginda et al. 2013). Deletion of either *parA* or *parB* leads to a high percentage of anuclear cells, three times higher in the *parA* deletion strain (Ginda et al. 2013). Surprisingly, the *parAB* mutants have milder growth defects and fewer anucleate cells, suggesting that a specific ParA:ParB ratio is crucial for correct operation. ParA colocalizes and interacts with Wag31, and aberrations in cell length (elongated or shortened cells) were observed in all three mutants (Ginda et al. 2013). Thus, the ParAB system could coordinate chromosome segregation with other cell cycle processes through interaction with a polar determinant, as has been proposed in *C. crescentus* and *C. glutamicum* (Ptacin and Shapiro 2010; Donovan et al. 2012).

To achieve a mechanistic understanding of chromosome segregation, septum placement, asymmetric growth, and their interdependence, mathematical modeling of the spatiotemporal dynamics of the key players will be essential. Similar modeling approaches have provided insight into the Min system in *Escherichia coli* (Kruse et al. 2007) and ParAB-mediated plasmid partitioning (Ringgaard et al. 2009). Quantitative data can be used to test the validity of different mechanisms, for example, theory sets physical limits to the positional information and accuracy provided by protein gradients (Tostevin et al. 2007). Modeling can also shed light on fitness advantages of observed asymmetries and heterogeneities in growth and division (Kussell and Leibler 2005).

Regulation of Growth and Cell Division

Bacterial eukaryotic-type serine/threonine protein kinases (STPKs) transmit signals from the extracellular environment via the reversible phosphorylation of proteins, permitting bacteria to adapt to external changes. In mycobacteria, these kinases are thought to be involved in several processes, including cell shape, growth, and cell division. *M. tuberculosis* possesses 11 STPKs (PknA-PknL, except C), whose biochemical activity and substrates have been widely studied and reviewed (Hett and Rubin 2008; Molle and Kremer 2010). More recently, PknA and PknB have been implicated in the phosphorylation of the lone Ser/Thr phosphatase (PstP) in *M. tuberculosis*, suggesting a signaling regulation of STPKs/PstP through mutually dependent mechanisms (Sajid et al. 2011). PknB—which localizes at mid-cell and poles (Mir et al. 2011)—phosphorylates the peptidoglycan biosynthetic protein MviNP, leading to the recruitment of FhaA, which modulates peptidoglycan synthesis at the cell poles and septum (Gee et al. 2012; Warner and Mizrahi 2012). Osmotic stress stimulates a signaling pathway in *M. tuberculosis* regulated by PknD (Hatzios et al. 2013). PknE kinase has been implicated in the suppression of apoptosis during nitrate stress and an adaptive response regulating cellular integrity and survival (Kumar and Narayanan 2012; Kumar et al. 2013). PknI and PknK are thought to be involved in slowing the growth of *M. tuberculosis* during infection (Gopalaswamy et al. 2009; Malhotra et al. 2010), whereas PknJ phosphorylation of pyruvate kinase A (mtPykA) affects central metabolism (Arora et al. 2012) and PknL may modulate apoptosis (Lakshminarayan et al. 2008).

Two-component systems (TCSs) are formed by a sensor kinase that autophosphorylates when receiving signals from the environment, transferring a phosphoryl group to a response regulator, which then activates specific regulons for adaptation to the signal sensed. *M. tuberculosis* encodes 11 TCSs, and the MtrAB system has been implicated in the maintenance of cell wall integrity (Moker et al. 2004; Cangelosi et al. 2006; Nguyen et al. 2010; Plocinska et al. 2012). Expression of the MtrA regulon is necessary for regulated cell division, and one of these genes encodes the essential cell wall hydrolase RipA (Plocinska et al. 2012). MtrB localizes at the cell poles, membranes, and septa in an FtsZ-dependent manner, and MtrA regulon expression is compromised under conditions that interfere with MtrB septal localization, suggesting that MtrB sensor kinase activation takes place at the septum (Plocinska et al. 2012).

Rpfs

The first resuscitation promoting factor protein (Rpf) was described in *Micrococcus luteus* (Mukamolova et al. 2002). Its name indicates its capacity to promote the resuscitation of dormant bacteria. This secreted protein has homologs among other high G + C Gram-positive bacteria, including *Mycobacterium* spp. *M. tuberculosis* contains five Rpf homologs, RpfA-E, scattered throughout the genome, that can resuscitate dormant BCG or *M. tuberculosis* (for review, see Kana and Mizrahi 2010). All of them contain putative signal sequences at the amino terminus, suggesting that they are active extracellularly (Kana and Mizrahi 2010). Rpfs share a conserved 70-amino-acid region, the Rpf domain, responsible for biological activity (Mukamolova et al. 2002). This domain is similar to C-type lysozyme and the *E. coli*–soluble lytic transglycosylase 70 (Cohen-Gonsaud et al. 2005), both involved in the degradation of peptidoglycan; the muralytic activity of this family of proteins has been shown (Mukamolova et al. 2006; Telkov et al. 2006). Peptidoglycan hydrolysis could produce muropeptides that might modulate innate immune responses or activate the cell resuscitation pathway (Jo 2008; Kana and Mizrahi 2010; Nikitushkin et al. 2013). Recently, a novel class of 2-nitrophenylthiocyanates has been found to inhibit the muralytic activity of Rpfs and prevent the resuscitation of dormant *M. smegmatis* and *M. tuberculosis*, which makes them interesting candidate compounds against nonreplicating mycobacteria (Demina et al. 2009). The crystal structure of RpfB catalytic domain in complex with the lysozyme inhibitor NAG3 suggests that Glu-292 is the sole residue essential for catalysis in this protein (Squeglia et al. 2013). The use of the structure of RpfB to model the catalytic domains of the other four Rpfs

 Cite this article as *Cold Spring Harb Perspect Med* doi: 10.1101/cshperspect.a021097

shows a high degree of similarity but also differences among these five proteins (Squeglia et al. 2013). The expression of all five *rpfs* varies in the function of the growth phase and under different stress conditions, but all of them are expressed in the early exponential phase, and the relative expression of all five is enhanced in resuscitation phase (Gupta et al. 2010). Differential expression of the five *rpf* genes in *M. tuberculosis* appears to be related to differential regulation. *rpfA* has been shown to be regulated by the cAMP receptor protein, and *rpfC* by the alternative σ factor SigD and the site two protease homolog, Rv2869c (Raman et al. 2004; Makinoshima and Glickman 2005; Rickman et al. 2005).

The five *M. tuberculosis rpf* genes are not essential for growth in vitro and in vivo, individually or collectively (Downing et al. 2004; Tufariello et al. 2004; Kana et al. 2008), but triple, quadruple, and quintuple mutants show impaired spontaneous resuscitation in vitro and are attenuated in vivo (Downing et al. 2005; Kana et al. 2008). The quintuple mutants show increased sensitivity to inhibitors of late peptidoglycan biosynthesis steps, probably owing to increased cell envelope permeability (Kana et al. 2010; Wivagg and Hung 2012). The in vivo attenuation of the multiple mutants led to their consideration as novel vaccine candidates. Both quadruple *rpf* deletion mutants, ΔACBD and ΔACDE, induced protection in the mouse model of tuberculosis infection (Kondratieva et al. 2011). RpfB and RpfE are sufficient for normal growth, suggesting a functional hierarchy (Kana et al. 2008), and both interact with the cell wall hydrolase RipA, whereas RpfB and RipA colocalize in the septum of dividing cells, suggesting that the RpfB–RipA interactions could be involved in the separation of daughter cells during reactivation (Hett et al. 2007, 2008). RipA also interacts with the PBP1, a peptidoglycan-synthesizing enzyme, and a model was proposed in which PBP1 competes with RpfB for binding to RipA, thus limiting RipA-RpfB peptidoglycan hydrolyzing activity (Hett et al. 2010). RpfB is considered a promising candidate for inclusion in novel tuberculosis vaccines (Romano et al. 2012).

THE CONTROVERSY OF MYCOBACTERIAL SPORULATION

The ability of *M. tuberculosis* to cause long-term subclinical infections that later develop into clinically active disease is one of the main obstacles to tuberculosis control. The production of spores by mycobacteria could be a bacterial strategy to survive during this long subclinical phase, but this possibility has not been widely accepted. Studies from the 1950s suggested the existence of spores in old mycobacterial cultures (e.g., see Brieger and Glauert 1956), but they were not reproducible and often declared to be caused by contamination or artifacts (for references, see Traag et al. 2010 and Singh et al. 2010).

More recently, Ghosh et al. (2009) reported the existence of endospores in old cultures of *M. marinum* on solid agar medium and suggested their existence in *M. bovis* BCG. To ensure the absence of contaminants, the germination of individual endospores was tracked, as was the return to sporulation in late stationary phase. An endospore-like structure was visualized using transmission electron microscopy, and the *M. marinum* endospores tested positive for spore-specific stains, resistance to heat and chemical stress, and the presence of dipicolinic acid (Ghosh et al. 2009). These investigators also suggested that the asymmetric placement of the septum during cell division observed in mycobacteria could be in agreement with their ability to form spores (Singh et al. 2010).

These results (Ghosh et al. 2009) were disputed by Traag et al. (2010), who failed to detect the presence of spores in *M. marinum* cultures after reproducing the experimental procedures of Gosh and colleagues. They were also unable to recover spores from frogs chronically infected by *M. marinum*. The observation that the endospores found were strikingly similar to those of *Bacillus subtilis* (Ghosh et al. 2009) suggested a possible contamination of the samples. In a follow-up paper from the Kirsebom laboratory, differences in the appearance between these two kinds of spores were reported (Singh et al. 2010). Traag et al. (2010) showed that mycobacteria lack orthologs of key genes involved in endospore formation in low G + C Gram-positive bacteria, perhaps unsurprising for high G + C mycobacterium species. It has also been noted that although rare, some species of *Streptomyces* can form endospores under specific conditions (Stastná et al. 1992) and that the absence of homologous sporulation genes does not prove the absence of proteins with similar function (Singh et al. 2010).

Although it remains possible that spores might be produced by *M. marinum* under certain conditions, Traag et al. (2010) were unable to reproduce this. More recently, spore-like structures were reported in a 1-yr-old liquid culture of *Mycobacterium avium* subsp. *paratuberculosis* (MAP) (Lamont et al. 2012). These spores were resistant to heat and chemical stresses and positive for MAP 16sRNA and dipicolinate, but not for gene elements of well-known endospore-forming strains. Although these resemble endospores, the authors note that they are also reminiscent of *Streptomyces spp.* aerial hyphae spores. The fact that MAP has been found as a contaminant in pasteurized food supports the existence of spores in this species (Lamont et al. 2012). The existence of spores in mycobacterium species is still controversial, and the exact conditions leading to their formation need to be more widely studied to produce sufficient data to clarify the situation.

CONCLUSIONS

This is an exciting time for research on bacteria at the single-cell level, and we now have the tools to address questions about phenotypic variation within genetically clonal populations, and how this impacts on cell survival in the face of environmental stress.

ACKNOWLEDGMENTS

I.U. is funded by a fellowship from the Fundación Alfonso Martin Escudero.

REFERENCES

Aldridge BB, Fernandez-Suarez M, Heller D, Ambravaneswaran V, Irimia D, Toner M, Fortune SM. 2012. Asymmetry and aging of mycobacterial cells lead to variable growth and antibiotic susceptibility. *Science* **335:** 100–104.

Arora G, Sajid A, Arulanandh MD, Singhal A, Mattoo AR, Pomerantsev AP, Leppla SH, Maiti S, Singh Y. 2012. Unveiling the novel dual specificity protein kinases in *Bacillus anthracis*: Identification of the first prokaryotic dual specificity tyrosine phosphorylation-regulated kinase (*dyrk*)-like kinase. *J Biol Chem* **287:** 26749–26763.

Breier AM, Grossman AD. 2007. Whole-genome analysis of the chromosome partitioning and sporulation protein Spo0J (ParB) reveals spreading and origin-distal sites on the *Bacillus subtilis* chromosome. *Mol Microbiol* **64:** 703–718.

Brieger EM, Glauert AM. 1952. A phase-contrast study of reproduction in mycelial strains of avian tubercle bacilli. *J Gen Microbiol* **7:** 287–294.

Brieger EM, Glauert AM. 1956. Sporelike structures in the tubercle bacillus. *Nature* **178:** 544.

Brieger EM, Cosslet VE, Glauert AM. 1953. Action of antibiotics on avian tubercle bacilli studied with the electron microscope. *Nature* **171:** 211–212.

Buerger S, Spoering A, Gavrish E, Leslin C, Ling L, Epstein SS. 2012. Microbial scout hypothesis, stochastic exit from dormancy, and the nature of slow growers. *Appl Environ Microbiol* **78:** 3221–3228.

Cangelosi GA, Do JS, Freeman R, Bennett JG, Semret M, Behr MA. 2006. The two-component regulatory system *mtrAB* is required for morphotypic multidrug resistance in *Mycobacterium avium*. *Antimicrob Agents Chemother* **50:** 461–468.

Carballido-López R. 2006. The bacterial actin-like cytoskeleton. *Microbiol Mol Biol Rev* **70:** 888–909.

Casart Y, Gamero E, Rivera-Gutierrez S, González-Y-Merchand JA, Salazar L. 2008. *par* genes in *Mycobacterium bovis* and *Mycobacterium smegmatis* are arranged in an operon transcribed from “SigGC” promoters. *BMC Microbiol* **8:** 51.

Champion JA, Mitragotri S. 2006. Role of target geometry in phagocytosis. *Proc Natl Acad Sci* **103:** 4930–4934.

Chaudhuri BN, Dean R. 2011. The evidence of large-scale DNA-induced compaction in the mycobacterial chromosomal ParB. *J Mol Biol* **413:** 901–907.

Cohen-Gonsaud M, Barthe P, Bagnéris C, Henderson B, Ward J, Roumestand C, Keep NH. 2005. The structure of a resuscitation-promoting factor domain from *Mycobacterium tuberculosis* shows homology to lysozymes. *Nat Struct Mol Biol* **12:** 270–273.

Dahl JL. 2004. Electron microscopy analysis of *Mycobacterium tuberculosis* cell division. *FEMS Microbiol Lett* **240:** 15–20.

Daniel RA, Errington J. 2003. Control of cell morphogenesis in bacteria: Two distinct ways to make a rod-shaped cell. *Cell* **113:** 767–776.

Demina GR, Makarov VA, Nikitushkin VD, Ryabova OB, Vostroknutova GN, Salina EG, Shleeva MO, Goncharenko AV, Kaprelyants AS. 2009. Finding of the low molecular weight inhibitors of resuscitation promoting factor enzymatic and resuscitation activity. *PLoS ONE* **4:** e8174.

Donovan C, Schwaiger A, Krämer R, Bramkamp M. 2010. Subcellular localization and characterization of the ParAB system from *Corynebacterium glutamicum*. *J Bacteriol* **192:** 3441–3451.

Donovan C, Sieger B, Krämer R, Bramkamp M. 2012. A synthetic *Escherichia coli* system identifies a conserved origin tethering factor in *Actinobacteria*. *Mol Microbiol* **84:** 105–116.

Downing KJ, Betts JC, Young DI, McAdam RA, Kelly F, Young M, Mizrahi V. 2004. Global expression profiling of strains harbouring null mutations reveals that the five *rpf*-like genes of *Mycobacterium tuberculosis* show functional redundancy. *Tuberculosis* **84:** 167–179.

Downing KJ, Mischenko VV, Shleeva MO, Young DI, Young M, Kaprelyants AS, Apt AS, Mizrahi V. 2005. Mutants of *Mycobacterium tuberculosis* lacking three of the five *rpf*-like genes are defective for growth in vivo and for resuscitation in vitro. *Infect Immun* **73:** 3038–3043.

Ebersbach G, Gerdes K. 2005. Plasmid segregation mechanisms. *Annu Rev Genet* **39:** 453–479.

Farnia P, Mohammad RM, Merza MA, Tabarsi P, Zhavnerko GK, Ibrahim TA, Kuan HO, Ghanavei J, Farnia P, Ranjbar R, et al. 2010. Growth and cell-division in extensive (XDR) and extremely drug resistant (XXDR) tuberculosis strains: Transmission and atomic force observation. *Int J Clin Exp Med* **3:** 308–314.

Fiebig A, Keren K, Theriot JA. 2006. Fine-scale time-lapse analysis of the biphasic, dynamic behaviour of the two *Vibrio cholerae* chromosomes. *Mol Microbiol* **60:** 1164–1178.

Gee CL, Papavinasasundaram KG, Blair SR, Baer CE, Falick AM, King DS, Griffin JE, Venghatakrishnan H, Zukauskas A, Wei J-R, et al. 2012. A phosphorylated pseudokinase complex controls cell wall synthesis in mycobacteria. *Sci Signal* **5:** ra7.

Ghosh J, Larsson P, Singh B, Pettersson BMF, Islam NM, Sarkar SN, Dasgupta S, Kirsebom LA. 2009. Sporulation in mycobacteria. *Proc Natl Acad Sci* **106:** 10781–10786.

Gill WP, Harik NS, Whiddon MR, Liao RP, Mittler JE, Sherman DR. 2009. A replication clock for *Mycobacterium tuberculosis*. *Nat Med* **15:** 211–214.

Ginda K, Bezulska M, Ziółkiewicz M, Dziadek J, Zakrzewska-Czerwińska J, Jakimowicz D. 2013. ParA of *Mycobacterium smegmatis* co-ordinates chromosome segregation with the cell cycle and interacts with the polar growth determinant DivIVA. *Mol Microbiol.* **87:** 998–1012.

Godin M, Delgado FF, Son S, Grover WH, Bryan AK, Tzur A, Jorgensen P, Payer K, Grossman AD, Kirschner MW, et al. 2010. Using buoyant mass to measure the growth of single cells. *Nat Methods* **7:** 387–390.

Golchin SA, Stratford J, Curry RJ, McFadden J. 2012. A microfluidic system for long-term time-lapse microscopy studies of mycobacteria. *Tuberculosis* **92:** 489–496.

Gopalaswamy R, Narayanan S, Chen B, Jacobs WR, Av-Gay Y. 2009. The serine/threonine protein kinase PknI controls the growth of *Mycobacterium tuberculosis* upon infection. *FEMS Microbiol Lett* **295:** 23–29.

Gupta RK, Srivastava BS, Srivastava R. 2010. Comparative expression analysis of *rpf*-like genes of *Mycobacterium tuberculosis* H37Rv under different physiological stress and growth conditions. *Microbiology* **156:** 2714–2722.

Hatzios SK, Baer CE, Rustad TR, Siegrist MS, Pang JM, Ortega C, Alber T, Grundner C, Sherman DR, Bertozzi CR. 2013. Osmosensory signaling in *Mycobacterium tuberculosis* mediated by a eukaryotic-like Ser/Thr protein kinase. *Proc Natl Acad Sci* **110:** E5069–E5077.

Hett EC, Rubin EJ. 2008. Bacterial growth and cell division: A mycobacterial perspective. *Microbiol Mol Biol Rev* **72:** 126–156, table of contents.

Hett EC, Chao MC, Steyn AJ, Fortune SM, Deng LL, Rubin EJ. 2007. A partner for the resuscitation-promoting factors of *Mycobacterium tuberculosis*. *Mol Microbiol* **66:** 658–668.

Hett EC, Chao MC, Deng LL, Rubin EJ. 2008. A mycobacterial enzyme essential for cell division synergizes with resuscitation-promoting factor. *PLoS Pathog* **4:** e1000001.

Hett EC, Chao MC, Rubin EJ. 2010. Interaction and modulation of two antagonistic cell wall enzymes of mycobacteria. *PLoS Pathog* **6:** e1001020.

Jakimowicz D, Chater K, Zakrzewska-Czerwínska J. 2002. The ParB protein of *Streptomyces coelicolor* A3(2) recognizes a cluster of *parS* sequences within the origin-proximal region of the linear chromosome. *Mol Microbiol* **45:** 1365–1377.

Jakimowicz D, Brzostek A, Rumijowska-Galewicz A, Zydek P, Dołzbłasz A, Smulczyk-Krawczyszyn A, Zimniak T, Wojtasz L, Zawilak-Pawlik A, Kois A, et al. 2007. Characterization of the mycobacterial chromosome segregation protein ParB and identification of its target in *Mycobacterium smegmatis*. *Microbiology* **153:** 4050–4060.

Jo E-K. 2008. Mycobacterial interaction with innate receptors: TLRs, C-type lectins, and NLRs. *Curr Opin Infect Dis* **21:** 279–286.

Joyce G, Robertson BD, Williams KJ. 2011. A modified agar pad method for mycobacterial live-cell imaging. *BMC Res Notes* **4:** 73.

Joyce G, Williams KJ, Robb M, Noens E, Tizzano B, Shahrezaei V, Robertson BD. 2012. Cell division site placement and asymmetric growth in mycobacteria. *PLoS ONE* **7:** e44582.

Kana BD, Mizrahi V. 2010. Resuscitation-promoting factors as lytic enzymes for bacterial growth and signaling. *FEMS Immunol Med Microbiol* **58:** 39–50.

Kana BD, Gordhan BG, Downing KJ, Sung N, Vostroktunova G, Machowski EE, Tsenova L, Young M, Kaprelyants A, Kaplan G, et al. 2008. The resuscitation-promoting factors of *Mycobacterium tuberculosis* are required for virulence and resuscitation from dormancy but are collectively dispensable for growth in vitro. *Mol Microbiol* **67:** 672–684.

Kana BD, Mizrahi V, Gordhan BG. 2010. Depletion of resuscitation-promoting factors has limited impact on the drug susceptibility of *Mycobacterium tuberculosis*. *J Antimicrob Chemother* **65:** 1583–1585.

Kang C-M, Nyayapathy S, Lee J-Y, Suh J-W, Husson RN. 2008. Wag31, a homologue of the cell division protein DivIVA, regulates growth, morphology and polar cell wall synthesis in mycobacteria. *Microbiology* **154:** 725–735.

Kondratieva T, Rubakova E, Kana BD, Biketov S, Potapov V, Kaprelyants A, Apt A. 2011. *Mycobacterium tuberculosis* attenuated by multiple deletions of rpf genes effectively protects mice against TB infection. *Tuberculosis* **91:** 219–223.

Kruse K, Howard M, Margolin W. 2007. An experimentalist's guide to computational modelling of the Min system. *Mol Microbiol* **63:** 1279–1284.

Kumar D, Narayanan S. 2012. *pknE*, a serine/threonine kinase of *Mycobacterium tuberculosis* modulates multiple apoptotic paradigms. *Infect Genet Evol* **12:** 737–747.

Kumar D, Palaniyandi K, Challu VK, Kumar P, Narayanan S. 2013. PknE, a serine/threonine protein kinase from *Mycobacterium tuberculosis* has a role in adaptive responses. *Arch Microbiol* **195:** 75–80.

Kussell E, Leibler S. 2005. Phenotypic diversity, population growth, and information in fluctuating environments. *Science* **309:** 2075–2078.

Kysela DT, Brown PJB, Huang KC, Brun YV. 2013. Biological consequences and advantages of asymmetric bacterial growth. *Annu Rev Microbiol* **67:** 417–435.

Lakshminarayan H, Narayanan S, Bach H, Sundaram KGP, Av-Gay Y. 2008. Molecular cloning and biochemical characterization of a serine threonine protein kinase, PknL, from *Mycobacterium tuberculosis*. *Protein Expr Purif* **58:** 309–317.

Lamont EA, Bannantine JP, Armién A, Ariyakumar DS, Sreevatsan S. 2012. Identification and characterization of a spore-like morphotype in chronically starved *Mycobacterium avium* subsp. *paratuberculosis* cultures. *PLoS ONE* **7:** e30648.

Lee PJ, Gaige TA, Hung PJ. 2009. Dynamic cell culture: A microfluidic function generator for live cell microscopy. *Lab Chip* **9:** 164–166.

Letek M, Fiuza M, Ordóñez E, Villadangos AF, Ramos A, Mateos LM, Gil JA. 2008. Cell growth and cell division in the rod-shaped actinomycete *Corynebacterium glutamicum*. *Antonie Van Leeuwenhoek* **94:** 99–109.

Lin DC, Grossman AD. 1998. Identification and characterization of a bacterial chromosome partitioning site. *Cell* **92:** 675–685.

Locke JCW, Elowitz MB. 2009. Using movies to analyse gene circuit dynamics in single cells. *Nat Rev Microbiol* **7:** 383–392.

Makinoshima H, Glickman MS. 2005. Regulation of *Mycobacterium tuberculosis* cell envelope composition and virulence by intramembrane proteolysis. *Nature* **436:** 406–409.

Malhotra V, Arteaga-Cortés LT, Clay G, Clark-Curtiss JE. 2010. *Mycobacterium tuberculosis* protein kinase K confers survival advantage during early infection in mice and regulates growth in culture and during persistent infection: Implications for immune modulation. *Microbiology* **156:** 2829–2841.

Maloney E, Madiraju M, Rajagopalan M. 2009. Overproduction and localization of *Mycobacterium tuberculosis* ParA and ParB proteins. *Tuberculosis* **89:** S65–S69.

Mir M, Wang Z, Shen Z, Bednarz M, Bashir R, Golding I, Prasanth SG, Popescu G. 2011. Optical measurement of cycle-dependent cell growth. *Proc Natl Acad Sci* **108:** 13124–13129.

Moker N, Brocker M, Schaffer S, Kramer R, Morbach S, Bott M. 2004. Deletion of the genes encoding the MtrA-MtrB two-component system of *Corynebacterium glutamicum* has a strong influence on cell morphology, antibiotics susceptibility and expression of genes involved in osmoprotection. *Mol Microbiol* **54:** 420–438.

Molle V, Kremer L. 2010. Division and cell envelope regulation by Ser/Thr phosphorylation: *Mycobacterium* shows the way. *Mol Microbiol* **75:** 1064–1077.

Mukamolova GV, Turapov OA, Kazarian K, Telkov M, Kaprelyants AS, Kell DB, Young M. 2002. The *rpf* gene of *Micrococcus luteus* encodes an essential secreted growth factor. *Mol Microbiol* **46:** 611–621.

Mukamolova GV, Murzin AG, Salina EG, Demina GR, Kell DB, Kaprelyants AS, Young M. 2006. Muralytic activity of *Micrococcus luteus* Rpf and its relationship to physiological activity in promoting bacterial growth and resuscitation. *Mol Microbiol* **59:** 84–98.

Murray H, Ferreira H, Errington J. 2006. The bacterial chromosome segregation protein Spo0J spreads along DNA from parS nucleation sites. *Mol Microbiol* **61:** 1352–1361.

Nguyen HT, Wolff KA, Cartabuke RH, Ogwang S, Nguyen L. 2010. A lipoprotein modulates activity of the MtrAB two-component system to provide intrinsic multidrug resistance, cytokinetic control and cell wall homeostasis in *Mycobacterium*. *Mol Microbiol* **76:** 348–364.

Nikitushkin VD, Demina GR, Shleeva MO, Kaprelyants AS. 2013. Peptidoglycan fragments stimulate resuscitation of "non-culturable" mycobacteria. *Antonie Van Leeuwenhoek* **103:** 37–46.

Nisa S, Blokpoel MCJ, Robertson BD, Tyndall JDA, Lun S, Bishai WR, O'Toole R. 2010. Targeting the chromosome partitioning protein ParA in tuberculosis drug discovery. *J Antimicrob Chemother* **65:** 2347–2358.

Plocinska R, Purushotham G, Sarva K, Vadrevu IS, Pandeeti EVP, Arora N, Plocinski P, Madiraju MV, Rajagopalan M. 2012. Septal localization of the *Mycobacterium tuberculosis* MtrB sensor kinase promotes MtrA regulon expression. *J Biol Chem* **287:** 23887–23899.

Ptacin JL, Shapiro L. 2010. Initiating bacterial mitosis: Understanding the mechanism of ParA-mediated chromosome segregation. *Cell Cycle* **9:** 4033–4034.

Raman S, Hazra R, Dascher CC, Husson RN. 2004. Transcription regulation by the *Mycobacterium tuberculosis* alternative sigma factor SigD and its role in virulence. *J Bacteriol* **186:** 6605–6616.

Rickman L, Scott C, Hunt DM, Hutchinson T, Menéndez MC, Whalan R, Hinds J, Colston MJ, Green J, Buxton RS. 2005. A member of the cAMP receptor protein family of transcription regulators in *Mycobacterium tuberculosis* is required for virulence in mice and controls transcription of the *rpfA* gene coding for a resuscitation promoting factor. *Mol Microbiol* **56:** 1274–1286.

Ringgaard S, van Zon J, Howard M, Gerdes K. 2009. Movement and equipositioning of plasmids by ParA filament disassembly. *Proc Natl Acad Sci* **106:** 19369–19374.

Romano M, Aryan E, Korf H, Bruffaerts N, Franken CLMC, Ottenhoff THM, Huygen K. 2012. Potential of *Mycobacterium tuberculosis* resuscitation-promoting factors as antigens in novel tuberculosis sub-unit vaccines. *Microbes Infect* **14:** 86–95.

Sajid A, Arora G, Gupta M, Upadhyay S, Nandicoori VK, Singh Y. 2011. Phosphorylation of *Mycobacterium tuberculosis* Ser/Thr phosphatase by PknA and PknB. *PLoS ONE* **6:** e17871.

Santi I, Dhar N, Bousbaine D, Wakamoto Y, McKinney JD. 2013. Single-cell dynamics of the chromosome replication and cell division cycles in mycobacteria. *Nat Commun* **4:** 2470.

Sassetti CM, Boyd DH, Rubin EJ. 2003. Genes required for mycobacterial growth defined by high density mutagenesis. *Mol Microbiol* **48:** 77–84.

Singh B, Ghosh J, Islam NM, Dasgupta S, Kirsebom LA. 2010. Growth, cell division and sporulation in mycobacteria. *Antonie Van Leeuwenhoek* **98:** 165–177.

Singh B, Nitharwal RG, Ramesh M, Pettersson BMF, Kirsebom LA, Dasgupta S. 2013. Asymmetric growth and division in *Mycobacterium* spp.: Compensatory mechanisms for non-medial septa. *Mol Microbiol* **88:** 64–76.

Squeglia F, Romano M, Ruggiero A, Vitagliano L, De Simone A, Berisio R. 2013. Carbohydrate recognition by RpfB from *Mycobacterium tuberculosis* unveiled by crystallographic and molecular dynamics analyses. *Biophys J* **104:** 2530–2539.

Stastná J, Goodfellow M, Kristůfek V, Novotná J, Jizba J, Cáslavská J, Kofronová O, Blumauerová M. 1992. Characteristics of *Streptomyces globisporus* strain 0234A forming endospores in submerged cultures. *Folia Microbiol (Praha)* **37:** 111–116.

Telkov MV, Demina GR, Voloshin SA, Salina EG, Dudik TV, Stekhanova TN, Mukamolova GV, Kazaryan KA, Goncharenko AV, Young M, et al. 2006. Proteins of the Rpf (resuscitation promoting factor) family are peptidoglycan hydrolases. *Biochemistry (Mosc)* **71:** 414–422.

Thanbichler M, Shapiro L. 2006. MipZ, a spatial regulator coordinating chromosome segregation with cell division in *Caulobacter*. *Cell* **126:** 147–162.

Thanky NR, Young DB, Robertson BD. 2007. Unusual features of the cell cycle in mycobacteria: Polar-restricted growth and the snapping-model of cell division. *Tuberculosis* **87:** 231–236.

Tostevin F, Wolde ten PR, Howard M. 2007. Fundamental limits to position determination by concentration gradients. *PLoS Comp Biol* **3:** e78.

Traag BA, Driks A, Stragier P, Bitter W, Broussard G, Hatfull G, Chu F, Adams KN, Ramakrishnan L, Losick R. 2010. Do mycobacteria produce endospores? *Proc Natl Acad Sci* **107:** 878–881.

Tufariello JM, Jacobs WR, Chan J. 2004. Individual *Mycobacterium tuberculosis* resuscitation-promoting factor homologues are dispensable for growth in vitro and in vivo. *Infect Immun* **72:** 515–526.

Velayati AA, Farnia P, Ibrahim TA, Haroun RZ, Kuan HO, Ghanavi J, Farnia P, Kabarei AN, Tabarsi P, Omar AR, et al. 2009a. Differences in cell wall thickness between resistant and nonresistant strains of *Mycobacterium tuberculosis*: Using transmission electron microscopy. *Chemotherapy* **55:** 303–307.

Velayati AA, Farnia P, Masjedi MR, Ibrahim TA, Tabarsi P, Haroun RZ, Kuan HO, Ghanavi J, Varahram M. 2009b. Totally drug-resistant tuberculosis strains: Evidence of adaptation at the cellular level. *Eur Respir J* **34:** 1202–1203.

Wakamoto Y, Dhar N, Chait R, Schneider K, Signorino-Gelo F, Leibler S, McKinney JD. 2013. Dynamic persistence of antibiotic-stressed mycobacteria. *Science* **339:** 91–95.

Warner DF, Mizrahi V. 2012. A pseudokinase debut at the mycobacterial cell wall. *Sci Signal* **5:** pe3.

Wivagg CN, Hung DT. 2012. Resuscitation-promoting factors are required for β-lactam tolerance and the permeability barrier in *Mycobacterium tuberculosis*. *Antimicrob Agents Chemother* **56:** 1591–1594.

Zhang YJ, Ioerger TR, Huttenhower C, Long JE, Sassetti CM, Sacchettini JC, Rubin EJ. 2012. Global assessment of genomic regions required for growth in *Mycobacterium tuberculosis*. *PLoS Pathog* **8:** e1002946.

The Mycobacterial Cell Envelope—Lipids

Mary Jackson

Mycobacteria Research Laboratories, Department of Microbiology, Immunology and Pathology, Colorado State University, Colorado 80523-1682

Correspondence: mary.jackson@colostate.edu

Mycobacterium tuberculosis (*Mtb*) lipids are indelibly imprinted in just about every key aspect of tuberculosis (TB) basic and translational research. Although the interest in these compounds originally stemmed from their abundance, structural diversity, and antigenicity, continued research in this field has been driven by their important contribution to TB pathogenesis and their interest from the perspective of drug, vaccine, diagnostic, and biomarker development. This article summarizes what is known of the roles of lipids in the physiology and pathogenicity of *Mtb* and the exciting developments that have occurred in recent years in identifying new lead compounds targeting their biogenesis.

The mycobacterial cell envelope is the dominant feature of the biology of *Mycobacterium tuberculosis* (*Mtb*) and other mycobacteria, based on sugars and lipids of exceptional structure. Cell envelope lipids constitute ~40% of the cell dry mass, although this percentage may vary depending on species/isolate and growth conditions (Goren and Brennan 1979; Minnikin et al. 1982). The particular chemical structures and organization of these lipids between the inner and outer membrane of the mycobacterial cell envelope account for much of its impermeability to biocides and for the unique staining properties of mycobacteria that aid in the diagnosis of infected specimens (Goren and Brennan 1979; Jarlier and Nikaido 1994; Brennan and Nikaido 1995). Being located at the interface between the bacterium and the host, the outer membrane and capsular lipids of *Mtb* also play important roles in directing host–pathogen interactions. Several lipid components of *Mtb* (e.g., isoprenoid lipids, glycerophospholipids, phosphatidylinositol mannosides, lipoarabinomannan, mycolic acids, and trehalose mycolates) are produced by all mycobacterial species, consistent with their requirement for growth. The biosynthesis of some of these lipids is the site of action of anti-TB drugs such as isoniazid (INH) and ethionamide (ETH), as well as multiple other lead compounds under development. Other lipids (e.g., long-chain polymethyl-branched fatty acid–containing acyltrehaloses and long-chain diols) are not essential for growth but are unique to pathogenic mycobacteria and have been involved in pathogenesis.

Studies initiated in 1927 by R.J. Anderson and colleagues mark the beginning of the pio-

Cite this article as *Cold Spring Harb Perspect Med* doi: 10.1101/cshperspect.a021105

neering work that has led to the discovery and early structural definition of some of the most biologically relevant lipids of *Mtb*, including phosphatidylinositol mannosides, mycolic acids, and branched fatty acids and polyols (Goren and Brennan 1979). Studies conducted for decades to follow by generations of outstanding biochemists in France, the United Kingdom, and the United States, in particular, have resulted in a thorough understanding of the chemical structures of these lipids. Their detailed descriptions have been compiled in several recent books and reviews and the reader is referred to these for further reading on this topic (Brennan 1988; Barry et al. 1998; Kaur et al. 2009; Daffé et al. 2014). Developments in the genetic manipulation of mycobacteria in the 1990s and the release of the first complete genome sequence of *Mtb* in 1998 have provided a major impetus to the study of the biosynthesis of these compounds with the result that many of the enzymes and transporters involved in their biogenesis have now been identified. Following the classification of *Mtb* into six major genetic lineages associated with specific geographical regions (Gagneux and Small 2007), recent years have also seen a return of interest in comparative analyses of the lipid content of clinical isolates from different regions of the world in the hope of identifying correlates of pathogenicity. Interestingly, not only are these studies providing new insights into the biochemical diversity of *Mtb* and the putative roles of some lipids in host–pathogen interactions (Daffé et al. 1991; Constant et al. 2002; Reed et al. 2004, 2007; Tsenova et al. 2005; Sinsimer et al. 2008; Huet et al. 2009; Krishnan et al. 2011), they are also shedding light on the genetic basis of observations made some 20 to 40 years ago by early investigators in the field (Goren et al. 1974a; Daffé et al. 1991; Krishnan et al. 2011; Supply et al. 2013). What is known of the biosynthesis of *Mtb* lipids has been reviewed recently (Daffé et al. 2014). This review focuses on our current understanding of the roles of cell wall lipids in the physiology and pathogenicity of *Mtb* and describes ongoing drug discovery efforts aimed at targeting their biosynthesis, export, and regulation.

PHYSICAL ORGANIZATION AND PHYSIOLOGICAL ROLES OF *Mtb* CELL ENVELOPE LIPIDS

Architecture of the *Mtb* Cell Envelope

A schematic representation of the cell envelope's architecture of *Mtb* is presented in Figure 1. The innermost layer is the plasma membrane that seems typical of bacterial membranes. Outside the plasma membrane is a massive cell wall "core" comprised of peptidoglycan (PG) covalently attached to the heteropolysaccharide arabinogalactan (AG), in turn esterified at its nonreducing ends to α-alkyl, β-hydroxy long-chain (C_{60}-C_{90}) mycolic acids. Intercalated within this lipid environment are the "free" (noncovalently linked) lipids and lipoglycans that have intrigued researchers for more than eight decades: the phosphatidylinositol mannosides (PIMs), the phthiocerol dimycocerosates (PDIMs), the phenolic glycolipids (PGLs), a variety of acyltrehaloses, mannose-capped lipoarabinomannan (ManLAM), etc. (Figs. 2 and 3). The covalently bound mycolic acids of the cell wall core and the free lipids form the inner and outer leaflets, respectively, of a highly impermeable asymmetrical bilayer (known as the "mycomembrane" or outer membrane) that confers to mycobacteria their characteristic resistance to many therapeutic agents (Minnikin et al. 1982; Jarlier and Nikaido 1994; Hoffmann et al. 2008; Zuber et al. 2008) (Fig. 1). Finally, a loosely attached capsular-like structure outside the outer membrane of *Mtb* was shown to mainly consist of polysaccharides and proteins with only minor amounts of lipids (2%–3% of the material) (Lemassu and Daffé 1994; Ortalo-Magné et al. 1995; Sani et al. 2010) (Fig. 1). Thus, in spite of being Gram-positive bacteria, mycobacteria possess a cell envelope characterized by the presence of an outer membrane and a periplasmic space.

Mycolic Acids

The interest in drugs targeting the biosynthesis of mycolic acids is clearly illustrated by the therapeutic efficacy of INH and ETH (Table 1). This essentially owes to their role as key structural elements of the outer membrane. The mycolic

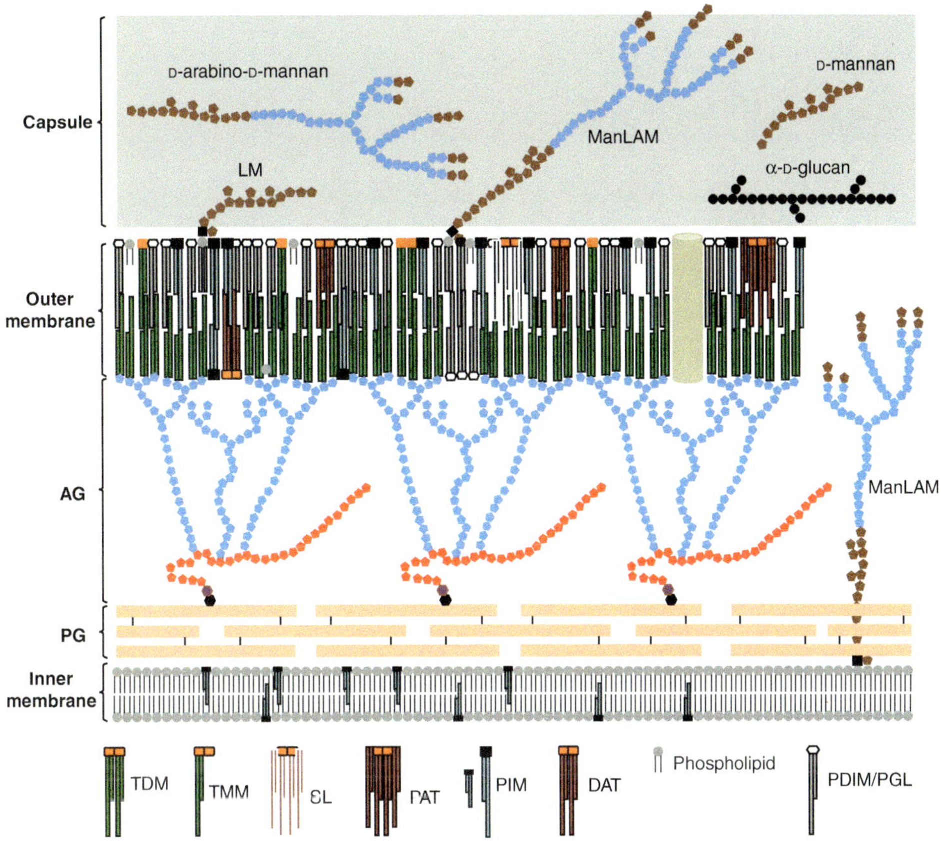

Figure 1. Schematic representation of the *Mtb* cell envelope. Many of the classes of (glyco)lipids discussed in the text are represented schematically and are shown in probable locations in the cell envelope. Light blue symbols represent arabinose residues, red symbols represent galactose residues, brown symbols represent mannose residues, and black circles represent glucose residues. D-arabino-D-mannan, D-glucan, and D-mannan are capsular polysaccharides. Mycolic acid chains are shown in dark green. LM, lipomannan; ManLAM, mannose-capped lipoarabinomannan; AG, arabinogalactan; PG, peptidoglycan.

acids covalently linked to AG represent about half of the weight of the cell wall core (Draper 1998). Mycolic acids also occur as acyl substituents esterifying a variety of outer membrane (glyco)lipids including trehalose mono- and dimycolates (Fig. 2), glycerol monomycolate, and glucose monomycolate. They play key roles in the permeability of the cell envelope, the ability of *Mtb* to form biofilms (Ojha et al. 2005, 2010; Sambandan et al. 2013), and the pathogenicity of the bacterium during the actively replicating and persistent stages of the infection (Barry et al. 1998; Daffé and Draper 1998; Yuan et al. 1998; Dubnau et al. 2000; Glickman et al. 2000; Sugawara et al. 2002; Vander Beken et al. 2011).

Inner and Outer Membrane Extractable Lipids

Glycerophospholipids, PIM, LM, and ManLAM. Glycerophospholipids (phosphatidylinositol [PI], phosphatidylglycerol, phosphatidylserine [PS], phosphatidylethanolamine [PE], cardiolipin [CL]), and mannosylated forms of PI known collectively as PIMs (Fig. 2) are the major lipid constituents of the plasma membrane of *Mtb*. In addition, the plasma membrane of *Mtb* contains major lipoglycans known as lipomannan (LM) and ManLAM (Fig. 3) (Pitarque et al. 2008), and a number of isoprenoids that play various critical functions in the cell. Among them, decaprenyl phosphate (Dec-P)

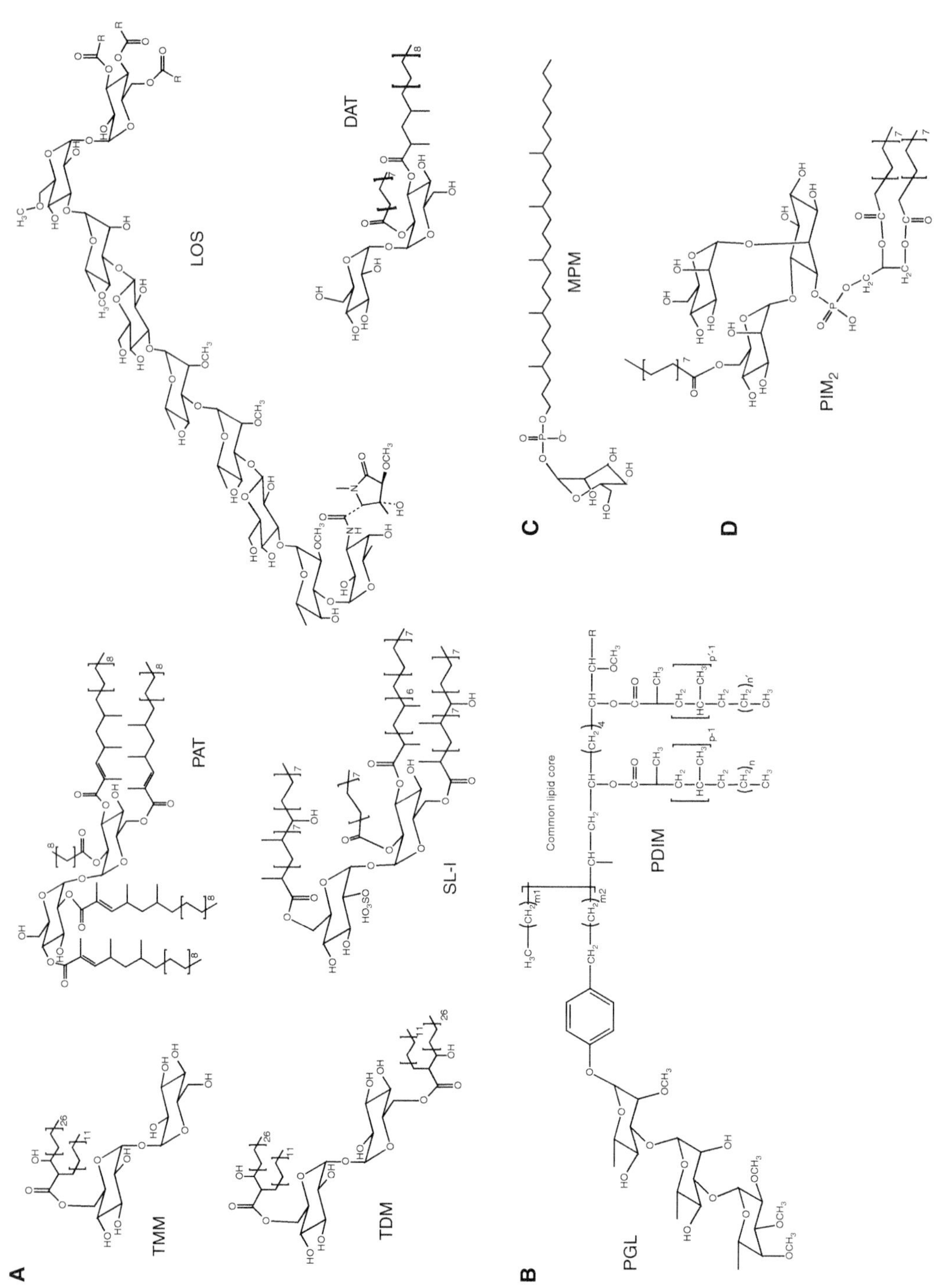

Figure 2. Structures of *Mtb* lipids. (*Legend continues on following page.*)

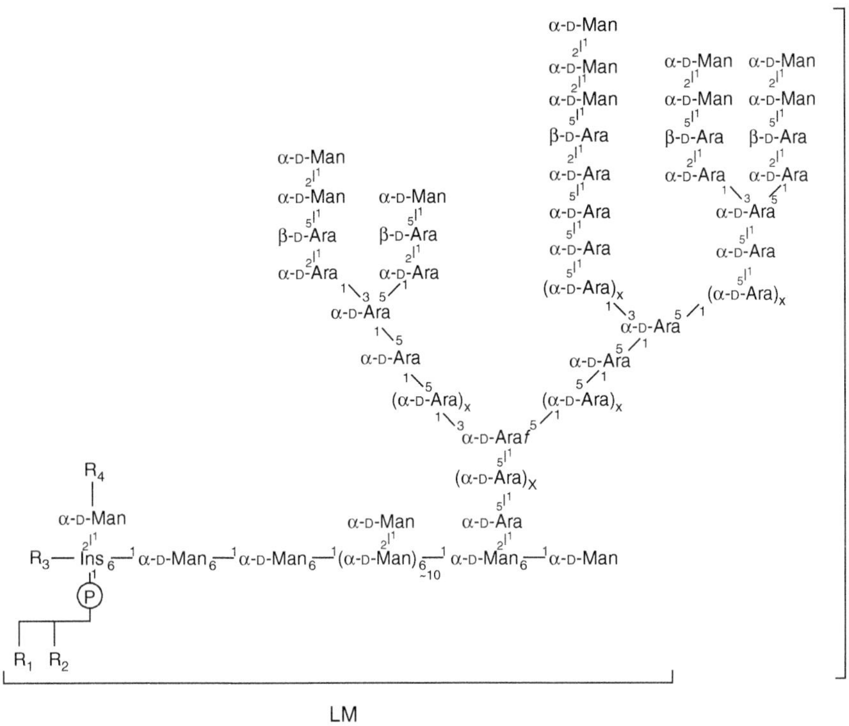

Figure 3. Structures of *Mtb* lipoglycans. Mannose-capped lipoarabinomannan (ManLAM); the mannan moiety of ManLAM consists of ~20–30 Man*p* residues and the arabinan polymers of ~60 Ara*f* units; the precise number of arabinan chain(s) attached to mannan is still uncertain. Lipomannan (LM) is devoid of the arabinan chains of ManLAM. R_1, R_2, R_3, R_4 are tuberculostearic acid, oleic acid, or palmitic acid.

serves as a carrier of activated sugars in the syn thesis of essential cell envelope polymers including PG, AG, LM, and ManLAM (Kaur et al. 2009), and menaquinones are essential components of the respiratory chain (Weinstein et al. 2005; Dhiman et al. 2009). Thus, as in other bacteria, plasma membrane lipids play a vital role in *Mtb*, providing a selective permeability barrier around the cell and participating in a number of critical physiological processes, including electron transport, ATP formation, DNA replication, and the biosynthesis of a variety of cell envelope components.

Glycerophospholipids (particularly PE), PIM, LM, and ManLAM are also found in the outermost layers of the cell envelope of *Mtb* and other *Mycobacterium* species where they may interact with the host (Ortalo-Magné et al.

Figure 2. (*Continued*) (*A*) Structures of acyltrehaloses: trehalose monomycolate (TMM); trehalose dimycolate (TDM); sulfolipid (SL-I); diacyltrehalose (DAT); polyacyltrehalose (PAT); and the lipooligosaccharide (LOS) of *Mtb* Canettii (R=Ac). The major sulfolipid SL-I (2,3,6,6′-tetraacyl α-α′-trehalose-2′-sulfate) is represented. In SL-I, trehalose is sulfated at the 2′ position and esterified with palmitic acid and the multimethyl-branched phthioceranic and hydroxyphthioceranic acids. In DAT (2,3-di-*O*-acyltrehalose), trehalose is esterified with palmitic acid and the multimethyl-branched mycosanoic acid. In PAT, trehalose is esterified with palmitic acid and the multimethyl-branched mycolipenic acids. (*B*) Structures of the phthiocerol dimycocerosate (PDIM) and phenolic glycolipid (PGL) of *Mtb*. p, p′ = 3–5; n, n′ = 16–18; m1 = 20–22; m2 = 15–17; R = CH_2-CH_3 or CH_3. (*C*) Structure of the predominant mannosyl-β-1-phosphomycoketide (MPM) from *Mtb* H37Rv. (*D*) Structure of a triacylated phosphatidylinositol dimannoside (PIM_2), one of the major forms of PIMs produced by *Mtb*.

Table 1. TB drug discovery pipeline showing the inhibitors targeting lipid biosynthesis

Pathway targeted	(Proposed) target protein	Inhibitor: Discovery	Inhibitor: Preclinical development	Inhibitor: Clinical development
Mycolic acids				
	InhA	CD117 (Vilchèze et al. 2011) Pyridomycin (Hartkoorn et al. 2012) Triclosan derivatives (Pan and Tonge 2012; North et al. 2013) Novel structural classes (GlaxoSmithKline)		
	HadABC	ISO and TAC analogs (Phetsuksiri et al. 1999; Bhowruth et al. 2006; Alahari et al. 2007; Shahab et al. 2010; Coxon et al. 2013) NAS-21, NAS-91 and analogs (Bhowruth et al. 2008; Gratraud et al. 2008)		
	KasA/KasB	Thiolactomycin and analogs (Pan and Tonge 2012; North et al. 2013)		
	Pks13	Thiophene compounds; Compound 3′ (Ioerger et al. 2013; Wilson et al. 2013)		
	FadD32	4,6-diaryl-5,7-dimethyl coumarins (Stanley et al. 2013)		
	Antigen 85 A, B, and C	Ebselen (Favrot et al. 2013) I3-AG85 (Warrier et al. 2012)		
	MmpL3	Adamantyl ureas (Grzegorzewicz et al. 2012a) BM212 and analogs (La Rosa et al. 2012; Poce et al. 2013) C215 (Stanley et al. 2012) SPIRO2 and THPP1 (Remuinan et al. 2013) Compound 2 (Ioerger et al. 2013)		SQ109 (Tahlan et al. 2012) (Sequella)
	Unknown (Inhibition of oxygenated mycolic acid biosynthesis)			PA-824 (Stover et al. 2000) OPC-67683 (Matsumoto et al. 2006)

Continued

Table 1. *Continued*

Pathway targeted	(Proposed) target protein	Inhibitor: Discovery	Inhibitor: Preclinical development	Inhibitor: Clinical development
	EthR	ETH "boosters": BDM 31343 and analogs (Willand et al. 2009; Villemagne et al. 2012)		
Decaprenyl phosphate				
	IspC	Fosfomidomycin analogs (Obiol-Pardo et al. 2011; Uh et al. 2011)		
Isoprenoid-based biosynthetic precursors				
PG biosynthesis	MraY	Capuramycin analogs (Sequella)	SQ641 (lead capuramycin analog) (Sequella)	
PG biosynthesis	WecA	Caprazamycin derivatives (CPZEN-45) (Ishizaki et al. 2013)		
LAM (and AG) biosynthesis	DprE1	DNB1 (Christophe et al. 2009) VI-9376 (Magnet et al. 2010) 377790 (Stanley et al. 2012) TCA-1 (Wang et al. 2013) Several synthetic compounds (TB Alliance, Scripps)	Benzothiazinones (BTZ043) (Makarov et al. 2009)	
Menaquinones				
	MenA	Aurachin RE, Ro 48-8071 and analogs (Dhiman et al. 2009; Debnath et al. 2012)		
	MenB	1,4-benzoxazines; 4-oxo-4-phenylbut-2-enoates (Li et al. 2010; 2011)		
	MenE	Sulfonyladenosine analogs (Lu et al. 2008; 2012)		
PGL				
	FadD22	5′-O-[*N*-(4-hydroxybenzoyl)sulfamoyl]-adenosine (Ferreras et al. 2008)		
Ser/Thr kinases				
	PknA PknB PknG	Several chemical scaffolds (Vertex Pharmaceuticals Inc.) (Magnet et al. 2010; Danilenko et al. 2011; Lougheed et al. 2011; Chapman et al. 2012)		

See text and the Working Group for New Drugs, Stop TB Partnership (http://www.newtbdrugs.org) for details.

1996; Pitarque et al. 2008; Dhiman et al. 2011). Whether *Mtb* requires phosphatidylglycerol, CL, PS, and PE for growth is at present not known. PI, PIM, LM, and ManLAM, in contrast, are all required for the viability of *Mtb* in vitro (Kaur et al. 2009; Guerin et al. 2010). Emerging data indicate that PIM play important roles in the permeability of the cell envelope, inner membrane integrity, and regulation of cell septation and division (Parish et al. 1997; Korduláková et al. 2002; Patterson et al. 2003; Morita et al. 2005, 2006). Likewise, structural defects in LM and ManLAM were shown to affect the β-lactam susceptibility and acid-fast staining properties of mycobacterial cells, indicating an equally important role of these molecules in cell envelope integrity (Fukuda et al. 2013).

Trehalose esters, PDIM, and PGL. Other outer membrane/surface-exposed lipids include trehalose monomycolates (TMM) and trehalose dimycolates (TDM), PDIM, sulfolipids (SL), diacyltrehaloses (DAT), polyacyltrehaloses (PAT), phenolic glycolipids (PGL), and lipooligosaccharides (LOS) (Fig. 2). In addition to serving as a mycolic acid donor in the formation of TDM and the cell wall core, TMM was recently identified as the likely form under which mycolic acids, which are synthesized in the cytoplasm, translocate to the periplasm or outer membrane (Grzegorzewicz et al. 2012a). Consistently, compounds that prevent TMM translocation are potent inhibitors of *Mtb* (Grzegorzewicz et al. 2012a; Tahlan et al. 2012; Stanley et al. 2012; La Rosa et al. 2012; Remuinan et al. 2013). In contrast to TDM and TMM, which are considered essential lipid components of the cell envelope of all mycobacteria, SL, DAT, PAT, and PDIM are more restricted in their distribution and are not essential for the growth of *Mtb* in vitro, although they have been involved in pathogenicity (see the section Roles of *Mtb* Lipids in Pathogenicity). PDIM and closely related phthiocerol diphthioceranates are essentially confined to pathogenic *Mycobacterium* species (Daffé and Lanéelle 1988). Consistent with their important roles in the permeability of the cell envelope (Camacho et al. 2001) and pathogenicity, PDIMs are apparently produced by all virulent clinical isolates of *Mtb*. DAT and PAT are confined to virulent isolates of the *Mycobacterium tuberculosis* complex (Goren and Brennan 1979; Jackson et al. 2007), and SL are exclusively found in the human pathogen *Mtb* (Goren 1990). Structural similarities between SL, DAT, and PAT and, to some extent PDIM, particularly the fact that they all are esterified with long-chain polymethyl-branched fatty acids, is suggestive of at least partially redundant functions in the cells. One of them is to alleviate the propionate-mediated stress undergone by *Mtb* when the bacterium switches to host cholesterol and fatty acids as major carbon sources (Singh et al. 2009; Lee et al. 2013). The propionyl-CoA generated upon β-oxidation of cholesterol is converted to methylmalonyl-CoA by the propionyl-CoA carboxylase and then used by dedicated polyketide synthases in the elongation of the polymethyl-branched fatty acids esterifying PDIM, SL, DAT, and PAT. Independent from this metabolic function and suggestive of their collective role in the permeability of the cell envelope, *Mtb* mutants deficient in the synthesis of more than one polymethyl-branched fatty acid–containing lipid (either PDIM and SL or DAT, PAT, and SL) but not mutants lacking only one lipid species, lose the ability to stain with neutral red (Cardona et al. 2006). Finally, DAT and PAT have been involved in the retention of the capsular material at the surface of *Mtb* (Rousseau et al. 2003a).

PGL and LOS are other lipids acylated by polymethyl-branched fatty acids produced by *Mtb* and related tubercle bacilli, albeit not all lineages (Fig. 2). LOS have thus far only been found in *Mycobacterium canettii* (Daffé et al. 1991), a representative of smooth tubercle bacilli that seem to have originated from the same pool of ancestors as *Mtb* but rarely causes human disease (Supply et al. 2013). Based on studies performed in *Mycobacterium marinum* (Ren et al. 2007), the presence of LOS in the cell envelope of *M. canettii* may account for the particular smooth colonial morphotype of this strain. The ability to synthesize PGL, on the other hand, has only been retained by *M. canettii* and some *Mtb* isolates of the East Asian/Beijing lineage (Daffé et al. 1987; Constant et al. 2002; Reed et al. 2004; Huet et al. 2009). PGL have been involved in pathogenicity (see the section Roles of *Mtb* Lipids in Pathogenicity). In an attempt to correlate the lipid content with the virulence of *Mtb* isolates, Goren et al. characterized a methoxylated phenolphthiocerol (a nonglycosylated variant of PGL), the so-called "attenuation indicator lipid" (Goren et al. 1974a). This lipid and its unmethylated form were detected in East Asian/Beijing isolates and found to accumulate in all Indo-Oceanic *Mtb* strains examined (Krishnan et al. 2011). Similarly, Beijing strains were reported to accumulate variants of PDIM and eventually PGL, known as phthiotriol and glycosylated phenolphthiotriol dimycocerosates (Huet et al. 2009). The correlation between the occurrence of these lipids and variations in virulence remains, however, unclear (Huet et al. 2009; Krishnan et al. 2011). PGL and LOS are clearly not essential for growth but they are potent B-cell antigens making them potentially useful, albeit lineage-specific, serodiagnostics (Brennan 1988; He et al. 1991; Vera-Cabrera et al. 1994; Simonney et al. 1995, 1996; Constant et al. 2002; Julian et al. 2002).

Other Lipids

Another family of lipids known as the mannosyl-β-1-phosphomycoketides (MPM) are produced by slow growing mycobacteria including *Mtb*, *Mycobacterium avium*, and *M. marinum* (Fig. 2). They are found inside the cells and released in the culture medium. They are not essential for the growth of *Mtb* but are thought to be involved in pathogenicity (Matsunaga and Sugita 2012).

Triglycerides (TAG) are considered intracellular lipids of *Mtb*. They represent the main apolar lipid when glycerol serves as the major carbon source in the medium (Brennan 1988). TAGs are thought to serve as an energy reserve for the long-term survival of *Mtb* during the persistence phase of infection (Brennan 1988; Daniel et al. 2004), as well as a means by which free fatty acids are detoxified. *Mtb* Beijing family isolates accumulate large quantities of TAG, possibly as a result of the up-regulation of the TAG synthase, Rv3130c (Reed et al. 2007).

Regulation of Lipid Synthesis

The physiological status of mycobacterial bacilli (i.e., age of the culture, actively replicating vs. persistent) and a number of environmental factors including temperature, oxygen tension, and nitrogen and carbon sources are known to impact their lipid composition, particularly phospholipids, TAG, PIM, LM, ManLAM, mycolic acid–based glycolipids, and polymethyl-branched fatty acid–containing lipids (Brennan 1988; Barry et al. 1998; Daffé and Draper 1998; Singh et al. 2009; Dhiman et al. 2011; Lee et al. 2013; Yang et al. 2013). Less is known of the regulation of lipid synthesis during host infection. PDIM and mycolic acids are apparently produced in abundant quantities by in vivo–grown tubercle bacilli (Kanai et al. 1970; Bhamidi et al. 2012). Yet, variations in the acid-fast characteristics of *Mtb* during mouse and guinea pig infection suggest that the bacterium undergoes drastic adaptative changes of its lipid composition in vivo (Ryan et al. 2010). Increased production of SL and DAT during host infection is supported by the up-regulation of biosynthetic genes on phagocytosis of *Mtb* by human primary macrophages or during progressive pulmonary TB infection in mice (Graham and Clark-Curtiss 1999; Rodriguez et al. 2013). The virulence-associated two-component regulator PhoP-PhoR may be involved in this up-regulation as it has been found to coordinately and positively regulate the synthesis of SL, DAT, and PAT in *Mtb* (Gonzalo-Asencio et al. 2006; Walters et al. 2006). The metabolic switching of *Mtb* to host lipids as carbon sources during infection and the associated increase in the production of PDIM, SL, DAT, and PAT were shown to be facilitated by the regulatory protein WhiB3 (Singh et al. 2009). In recent years, PknA, PknB, and other members of the Ser/Thr kinase family were found to regulate the activity of multiple enzymes and transporters involved in the biosynthesis of mycolic acids, ManLAMs, and PDIMs (Molle and Kremer 2010). It is thus apparent that lipid synthesis in *Mtb* is tightly controlled and that regulation occurs both at the transcriptional and post-translational levels.

ROLES OF *Mtb* LIPIDS IN PATHOGENICITY

Several excellent reviews have been published about the biological activities of *Mtb* lipids, including very recently (Daffé and Draper 1998; Russell et al. 2002; Karakousis et al. 2004; Bertozzi and Schelle 2008; Britton and Triccas 2008; Gilleron et al. 2008; Glickman 2008; Guilhot et al. 2008; Guenin-Macé et al. 2009; Neyrolles and Guilhot 2011; Russell 2011; Daffé et al. 2014). Thus, only a brief overview of what is known and remains to be investigated about the involvement of lipids in the pathogenesis of TB will be presented here.

The existence of a possible correlation between the lipid content of *Mtb* clinical isolates and their pathogenicity was noted early on by Middlebrook and Goren among others. These studies led to the identification of SL, TDM, and PDIM and derivatives as lipids of potential relevance to TB immunopathogenesis (Bloch 1950; Goren et al. 1974a,b; Daffé and Draper 1998). Further work on the biological activities of purified lipids in vitro and in vivo followed, in the postgenomic era, by an examination of the virulence phenotype and immune responses induced by *Mtb* mutants deficient in various aspects of their biosynthesis lent further support to the involvement of lipids in host–pathogen interactions. Their contribution to the infection process accompanies every step of the life cycle of the bacterium. The entry of *Mtb* inside host macrophages and dendritic cells is essentially mediated by specialized phagocytic receptors including complement receptors, scavenger receptors, and C-type lectins, such as the mannose receptor, DC-SIGN, and Mincle. PIM, TDM, and ManLAM are among the predominant glycolipids mediating *Mtb*'s interactions with these receptors (Villeneuve et al. 2005; Schlesinger et al. 2008; Ishikawa et al. 2009; Neyrolles and Guilhot 2011). Once inside phagocytic cells, *Mtb* resides in a phagosome that fails to fuse with lysozymes. The isoprenoid-derived compounds, isotuberculosinol and tuberculosinol, ManLAM, TDM, PDIM, SL, and DAT all have been implicated in the impairment of phagosome maturation, although the mechanisms involved and amount of supporting data varies for each compound (Daffé and Draper 1998; Brodin et al. 2010; Neyrolles and Guilhot 2011; Russell 2011; Mann and Peters 2012). Inside the cells, *Mtb* releases significant amounts of proteins and lipids, among them TMM, TDM, PIM, PGL, PE, phosphatidylglycerol, CL, and ManLAM, that traffic within the cell and may be released through exocytosis (Russell et al. 2002; Russell 2011). These molecules are not only taken up by bystander antigen-presenting cells, they also act as modulators of the function of the host cell and surrounding tissue, impacting the secretion of pro- and anti-inflammatory cytokines (e.g., PGL, TDM, mycolic acids, SL, PIM, LM, ManLAM, and lipoproteins), apoptosis (lipoproteins, PIM, ManLAM, and TDM), T-cell functions (ManLAM, DAT, and PAT), the induction of foamy macrophages (oxygenated mycolates and TDM), and granuloma formation (TMM, TDM, and ManLAM) (Daffé and Draper 1998; Jackson et al. 2007; Gilleron et al. 2008; Peyron et al. 2008; Guenin-Macé et al. 2009; Neyrolles and Guilhot 2011; Rajni et al. 2011; Russell 2011; Vander Beken et al. 2011; Li et al. 2012; Sakamoto et al. 2013; Vir et al. 2013). Importantly, several *Mtb* lipids, including diacylated forms of SL, PIM, ManLAM, MPM, and mycolyl lipids, represent themselves as antigens for immune recognition and are presented to T lymphocytes by MHC-I-like molecules of the CD1 family (Matsunaga and Sugita 2012; Arora et al. 2013; Ly et al. 2013; Van Rhijn et al. 2013). Some of these lipids may show potential as subunit vaccines (Guiard et al. 2009; Arora et al. 2013). Finally, ManLAM, SL, TDM, PGL, LOS, DAT, and lipoproteins are also potent inducers of humoral immune responses.

Although the critical involvement of PDIM and TDM in TB pathogenesis is now supported by a wealth of in vitro and in vivo data (Guilhot et al. 2008; Neyrolles and Guilhot 2011; Rajni et al. 2011; Li et al. 2012), the role(s) played by other prominent (glyco)lipids including (iso)-tuberculosinol, SL, DAT, PAT, PGL, some PDIM variants, and ManLAM during host infection are far from being as clear. Their roles in pathogenicity typically come into question when their demonstrated biological activities in vitro or in vivo (e.g., inhibition of phagosome maturation and immunomodulatory activities), usually as purified molecules, fail to translate into a clear "virulence" phenotype in *Mtb* strains genetically engineered to produce or, on the contrary, lose the ability to produce them. Classical examples of this include, for instance, SL, whose plethora of biological activities (Goren and Brennan 1979; Goren 1990; Daffé and Draper 1998; Bertozzi and Schelle 2008) fail to translate into a clear replication or persistence advantage in infected mice or guinea pigs (Rousseau et al. 2003b); DAT and PAT, whose absence from *Mtb* H37Rv does not hamper the ability of this strain to grow in mice (Rousseau et al. 2003a); or ManLAM, the suppression of the bioactive mannose caps of which fails to translate into any detectable phenotype in macrophages and animal models of infection (Afonso-Barroso et al. 2012). A combination of factors may account for this. First, no pathogenic trait of *Mtb* is attributable to a single virulence factor and so compensatory mechanisms within certain lipid families (e.g., polymethyl-branched fatty acid–containing lipids) or cell ligands (e.g., ManLAMs and mannosylated glycoproteins) are known to exist (Pitarque et al. 2005; Passemar et al. 2014). Second, an inherent flaw associated with studies that use purified molecules is that they may not accurately mimic qualitatively and/or quantitatively the way these molecules are presented to the host when carried by whole bacilli. Furthermore, the genetic background of the *Mtb* strain in which they are produced is likely to affect the way they interact with the host and their subsequent contribution to pathogenicity (e.g., PGL) (Sinsimer et al. 2008). Third, lipids such as SL and (iso)tuberculosinol are restricted to the human pathogen, *Mtb*, and may only show a clear phenotype in this specific host. The facts that the ability of *Mtb* to produce some PDIM variants and that PGL is relatively restricted to East-Asian isolates (Constant et al. 2002; Reed et al. 2004; Huet et al. 2009) suggest that the different *Mtb* lineages may even have evolved regionally to tailor their lipid composition to the genetic background of their human host (Neyrolles and Guilhot 2011). From a mechanistic standpoint, concluding to the direct effect of a lipid on a specific host function can be challenging. This owes to the roles that lipids often play in the structure and permeability of the cell envelope in addition to potentially interacting with the host. Thus, a deficiency in their production may not only cause *Mtb* to become more susceptible (i.e., more permeable) to host defense mechanisms (e.g., PDIMs and their impact on the resistance of *Mtb* to oxidative stress) (Rousseau et al. 2004), it may also profoundly alter the way other immunomodulatory antigens are presented at the cell surface and interact with host functions.

Mtb LIPIDS IN THE CONTEXT OF DRUG DISCOVERY

General Considerations

The previous sections have highlighted the diversity, unique structures, and essential roles played by cell envelope lipids in the physiology and pathogenicity of *Mtb*. These features account for the specificity and therapeutic efficacy of first- and second-line TB drugs such as INH and ETH, which inhibit the biosynthesis of mycolic acids (Banerjee et al. 1994; Vilchèze and Jacobs 2007; Grzegorzewicz et al. 2012b) (Fig. 4), and those of ethambutol (EMB), which inhibits the formation of the arabinan domains of ManLAM (Fig. 3) and AG (Mikušova et al. 1995). In addition, pyrazinamide was reported to be an inhibitor of the fatty acid synthase I (FAS-I) (Zimhony et al. 2000). With multidrug resistance on the increase, recent years have seen a marked intensification of TB drug discovery efforts with the result that many new lead compounds are now at various stages of the drug discovery and preclinical development pipeline. Interestingly, these efforts keep pointing at cell envelope lipids as one of the Achille's heels of *Mtb* (Table 1) (Jackson et al. 2013). As importantly, they are leading the TB field to revisit earlier impressions that drug targeting the biogenesis of the cell envelope lipids may not be synergistic with other drugs, useful against MRD-*Mtb* isolates, or active against persistent bacilli. This section summarizes recent developments that have occurred in the discovery of drugs targeting lipid synthesis in *Mtb*.

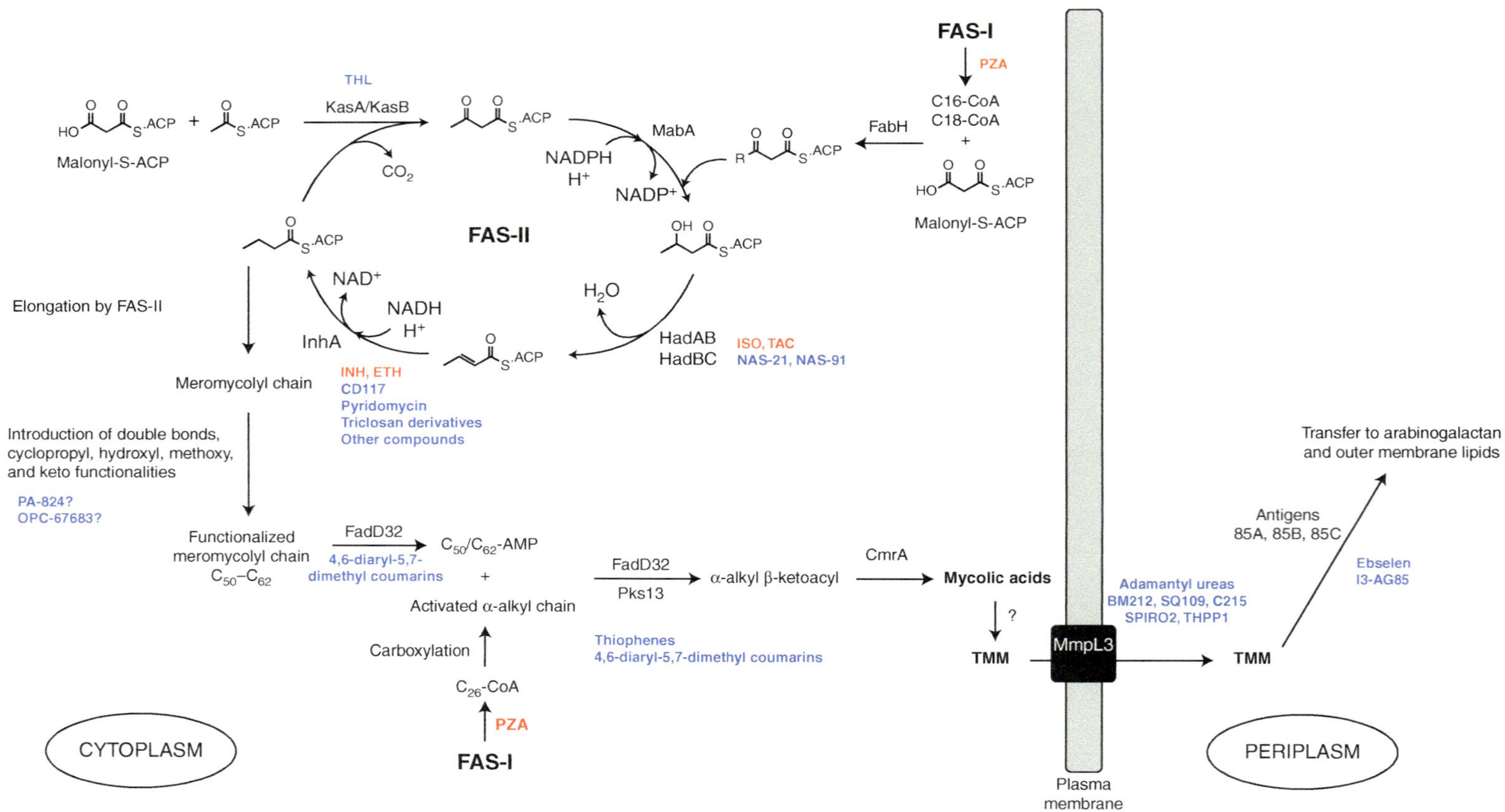

Figure 4. Biosynthetic pathway of mycolic acids in *Mtb* and site of action of anti-TB drugs. The saturated α-alkyl chain (C_{24} or C_{26} in *Mtb*) and the meromycoloyl chain (C_{50}–C_{62}) are synthesized by fatty-acid synthase-I (FAS-I) and fatty-acid synthase-II (FAS-II), respectively. The initial substrates of FAS-II are medium length keto-acyl-ACP resulting from the condensation by the *Mtb* FabH protein of the acyl-CoA products of FAS-I with malonyl-ACP. (*Legend continues on following page.*)

Drugs Targeting Mycolic Acid Biosynthesis and Export

The biosynthesis of mycolic acids is shown schematically in Figure 4. In the past 10 years, both target-based and whole cell–based approaches have been used toward the identification and development of inhibitors acting on virtually all portions of this biosynthetic pathway (Fig. 4 and Table 1). A comprehensive review of these efforts was recently published by North et al. (2013), and we will here only briefly describe some of the most exciting developments that have occurred in the last few years. Target-based screening uses biochemical and structural approaches to design, screen, and further evaluate a compound's activity against a specific molecular target. This type of approach has been used extensively to rationally optimize inhibitors of the FAS-II elongation cycle—in particular, analogs of thiolactomycin as inhibitors of KasA/KasB and triclosan derivatives as inhibitors of InhA (Pan and Tonge 2012). The screening of inhibitors showing activity against the *Plasmodium falciparum* enoyl reductase and β-hydroxyacyl-ACP dehydratase, FabZ, identified compounds that appear to target the corresponding FAS-II enzymes in *Mtb* and display an MIC against whole mycobacterial cells (Bhowruth et al. 2008; Gratraud et al. 2008; Vilchèze et al. 2011). Pyridomycin, a cyclic depsipeptide isolated from *Streptomyces* with an MIC value of 0.4 μg/mL against *Mtb*, is now known to also target InhA (Haatkoorn et al. 2012), as are novel structural classes of inhibitors in the lead-optimization phase reported by the Working Group on New TB Drugs (Table 1). Incidentally, the recent elucidation of the mode of action of isoxyl (ISO) and thiacetazone (TAC), two prodrugs formerly used in the clinical treatment of *Mtb*, revealed that they both inhibit the dehydration step of the FAS-II cycle catalyzed by HadAB and HadBC (Grzegorzewicz et al. 2012b). The finding that relatively simple structural modifications of the parent ISO and TAC compounds can increase the potency of analogs more than 20-fold is encouraging in that it suggests that it may be possible to identify compounds that could be administered at a lower dose, thereby reducing side effects (Phetsuksiri et al. 1999; Bhowruth et al. 2006; Alahari et al. 2007; Shahab et al. 2010; Coxon et al. 2013).

Because of their pivotal roles in the final assembly of mycolic acids and their transfer to cell envelope acceptors, Pks13, FadD32, and the mycoloyltransferases of the antigen 85 complex are also receiving a lot of attention from the perspective of drug development (Fig. 4). High-throughput screening assays were reported for FadD32 (Galandrin et al. 2013) and the antigens 85 (Boucau et al. 2009; Flamin et al. 2009; Sanki et al. 2009; Favrot et al. 2013). The latter assays led to the identification of a number of inhibitors of antigens 85, one of them, known as ebselen, also shows activity against *Mtb* in culture (MIC of 20 μg/mL). The molecular mechanism of inhibition of antigens 85 by ebselen was elucidated and found to be particularly interesting in the sense that it is unlikely to lead to the selection of drug-resistant isolates (Favrot et al. 2013). Small molecule binders of antigen 85C identified by magnetic resonance spectroscopy also showed activity against *Mtb* in

Figure 4. (*Continued*) After reduction by the β-keto-acyl-ACP reductase MabA, dehydration by the (*3R*)-hydroxyl-dehydratases HadAB and HadBC and reduction by the enoyl-CoA reductase InhA, either the β-ketoacyl-ACP synthase KasA or KasB catalyzes the condensation of the resulting product with malonyl-ACP units, thereby initiating the next round of elongation. Methyltransferases and other as yet unknown enzymes modify the meromycolyl chain introducing double bonds, cyclopropyl, hydroxy, methoxy, and keto functionalities. These two chains are coupled together via Claisen condensation by the acyl-AMP ligase FadD32 and the polyketide synthase Pks13. Upon release from Pks13, reduction by CmrA yields mycolic acids, which are then translocated to the periplasm under the form of TMM by partially elucidated translocation machinery involving the essential integral membrane transporter, MmpL3, and attached to AG or another molecule of TMM to form TDM, by the antigen 85 complex. The sites of action of *Mtb* inhibitors are indicated. Drugs presently or formerly used in the clinical treatment of TB are in red; inhibitors under development are in blue (see Table 1). THL, thiolactomycin; PZA, pyrazinamide.

vitro and inside macrophages in the 100-µM range (Warrier et al. 2012). The return of interest in whole cell–based screening that the TB field has witnessed in recent years has led to the identification of thiophenes and other compounds active against Pks13 (Ioerger et al. 2013; Wilson et al. 2013), diaryl coumarin–based compounds active against FadD32 (Stanley et al. 2013), and diverse chemotypes active against the TMM transporter, MmpL3 (Grzegorzewicz et al. 2012a; Stanley et al. 2012; Ioerger et al. 2013; Remuinan et al. 2013). BM212 and derivatives (La Rosa et al. 2012; Poce et al. 2013) and SQ109, a drug candidate originally designed to be an EMB analog and currently undergoing phase II clinical trials (Sacksteder et al. 2012; Tahlan et al. 2012), were also shown to kill *Mtb* through the inhibition of MmpL3. The reason why so many different chemical scaffolds apparently inhibit the MmpL3-mediated translocation of TMM is unclear. Establishing a validated assay for the direct measurement of MmpL3 inhibition is a high priority, because it would greatly facilitate the further development of these inhibitors and could potentially reveal new scaffolds for development.

In summary, recent drug discovery efforts have yielded a number of chemotypes inhibiting various aspects of the synthesis of mycolic acid, some of which are promising candidates for further development. Inhibiting the FAS-II system and MmpL3 currently appear to be the most attractive/druggable targets for TB drug discovery in this pathway.

Isoprenoids and Related Lipids

Inhibitors of the MEP pathway. As a lipid carrier of activated saccharide subunits, polyisoprenyl phosphate (Dec-P) is involved in the biosynthesis of the arabinan portion of AG, the mannan and arabinan domains of arabinomannan, LM, and ManLAM, the lipid I and lipid II precursors of PG, and the biosynthesis of the "linker unit" between AG and PG (Kaur et al. 2009; Daffé et al. 2014) (Fig. 1). The discovery that Dec-P synthesis in *Mtb* proceeds through the methylerythritol phosphate pathway, which has no homolog in humans, has provided stimulus for the characterization and identification of inhibitors of the relevant enzymes. Fosmidomycin, which is currently in clinical studies for the treatment of malaria, is a competitive inhibitor of the second enzyme of the pathway, 1-deoxy-D-xylulose-5-phosphate reductoisomerase (IspC). Several derivatives of this antibiotic have been synthesized, some of which have shown promising results against *Mtb* (Jackson et al. 2013) (Table 1).

Inhibitors of lipid-linked biosynthetic precursors. The phospho-*N*-acetylmuramyl pentapeptide translocase (MraY) catalyzes the exchange of UDP-N-acetylmuramic acid pentapeptide from UDP to Dec-P thereby generating lipid I in PG biosynthesis. The synthesis of capuramycin analogs as inhibitors of this enzyme has led to the identification of several compounds with 2- to 4-µg/mL MICs against drug-susceptible and MDR *Mtb* isolates (Jackson et al. 2013). Although its mode of action has yet to be confirmed in whole *Mtb* cells, one of them, SQ641, is at the stage of preclinical development (Table 1).

Very recently, the caprazamycin derivative CPZEN-45 was shown to be an inhibitor of *Mtb*'s decaprenyl-phosphate-GlcNAc-1-phosphate transferase, WecA, in the biosynthesis of AG (Ishizaki et al. 2013).

Decaprenylphosphoryl arabinose (DPA) is the only known arabinose donor in the building of the arabinan domains of the two essential cell envelope (lipo)polysaccharides, AG, and ManLAM. In the last 4 years, whole cell–based screening of compounds against *Mtb* has produced several inhibitors of the essential epimerase DprE1 required for the formation of DPA (Table 1). The molecular mechanism of action of some of these compounds has been thoroughly investigated and several DPA inhibitors are now reported to be in the hit-to-lead or preclinical development phases (Table 1) (Jackson et al. 2013).

Menaquinones. The lipoquinones involved in the respiratory chains of mycobacteria consist of menaquinones (2-methyl-3-polyprenyl-1,4-naphthoquinones) (Daffé et al. 2014). Evidence based on transcriptomics profiling and the inhibitory activity of menaquinone inhibitors against *Mtb* in culture has highlighted the requirement of this bacterium for electron transport and, therefore, menaquinone synthesis both during active replication and microaerophilic persistence (Dhiman et al. 2009). Accordingly, three key enzymes of the menaquinone biosynthetic pathway of *Mtb*, MenB (1,4-dihydroxy-2-napthoic acid synthase), MenE (O-succinylbenzoyl-CoA synthase), and MenA (1,4-dihydroxy-2-napthoic acid octaprenyl transferase) have been studied as potential drug targets and a number of promising inhibitors synthesized (Table 1).

Inhibition of PIM, LM, and ManLAM Biosynthesis

The essential character of PIM, LM, and ManLAM, their restricted distribution to mycobacteria and closely related Actinomycetes, and their demonstrated impact on the structure and permeability of the cell envelope of *Mtb* make the biosynthetic enzymes of these molecules attractive candidates for the development of specific *Mtb* inhibitors with the potential to synergize with or potentiate the activity of other drugs used in combination. Accordingly, target-to-drug approaches are pursuing various essential enzymes acting both at early (e.g., PimA, PimB') and late (e.g., Emb proteins and other lipid-linked sugar-utilizing glycosyltransferases) stages of the pathway. Innovative high-throughput screening assays have been developed for some of these enzymes (Zhang et al. 2010, 2011). The most advanced ManLAM inhibitors to date are those targeting DPA synthesis, as described in the previous section.

Targeting Lipids Involved in the Replication and Persistence of *Mtb* In Vivo

Targeting TAG synthesis through inhibition of the primary TAG synthase of *Mtb*, Rv3130c (Daniel et al. 2004; Sirakova et al. 2006), may represent a viable approach to the eradication of persistent bacilli for the key role TAG is likely to play as an energy reserve for the long-term survival of *Mtb* during the persistence phase of infection.

As detailed in the previous section, PDIMs are critical components of the permeability barrier surrounding *Mtb* and contribute to a significant extent to the survival and ability of the bacterium to replicate in vivo. To the best of our knowledge, no specific PDIM inhibitors have yet been reported but promising compounds targeting the Ser/Thr kinases of *Mtb* that regulate their biosynthesis (among other physiological processes) are under development (Jackson et al. 2013) (Table 1). Another regulatory system of interest in the context of drug development is the two-component transcriptional regulator PhoP-PhoR, which regulates multiple virulence-associated processes in *Mtb*, including the biosynthesis of SL, DAT, and PAT (Gonzalo-Asencio et al. 2006). Finally, a compound inhibiting the production of PGL in whole *Mtb* cells has been reported (Ferreras et al. 2008).

CONCLUDING REMARKS

Mtb lipids have been for the last eight decades and still remain today the object of much research activity. One of the highlights of this research in the last five years is undoubtedly the discovery of a variety of novel chemical scaffolds inhibiting various aspects of lipid synthesis, particularly mycolic acids, ManLAM, and AG. Beyond their therapeutic applications, lipids involved in the immunopathogenesis of TB may also represent useful targets for future preventive interventions, as illustrated by current studies aimed at investigating the vaccine potential of CD1-restricted lipid antigens (G Puzo, pers. comm.) and that of an attenuated *phoP*-based *Mtb* knockout mutant (Nambiar et al. 2012). Although the interest in developing TB serodiagnostics based on *Mtb* lipids seems to have somewhat waned in the last decade, important efforts are currently focusing on their potential as biomarkers to monitor TB reactivation, as well as the efficacy of treatment and vaccination (Shui et al. 2012; Wallis et al. 2013; Chan et al. 2013).

ACKNOWLEDGMENTS

Vicki Jones is gratefully acknowledged for her help with the preparation of the figures. The author's research on cell envelope lipids and inhibitors is supported through the National Institutes of Health/National Institute of Allergy and Infectious Diseases grants AI064798 and AI063054.

REFERENCES

Afonso-Barroso A, Clark SO, Williams A, Rosa GT, Nobrega C, Silva-Gomes S, Vale-Costa S, Ummels R, Stoker N, Movahedzadeh F, et al. 2012. Lipoarabinomannan mannose caps do not affect mycobacterial virulence or the induction of protective immunity in experimental animal models of infection and have minimal impact on in vitro inflammatory responses. *Cell Microbiol* **15:** 660–674.

Alahari A, Trivelli X, Guerardel Y, Dover LG, Besra GS, Sacchettini JC, Reynolds RC, Coxon GD, Kremer L. 2007. Thiacetazone, an antitubercular drug that inhibits cyclopropanation of cell wall mycolic acids in mycobacteria. *PLoS ONE* **2:** e1343.

Arora P, Foster EL, Porcelli SA. 2013. CD1d and natural killer T cells in immunity to *Mycobacterium tuberculosis*. *Adv Exp Med Biol* **783:** 199–223.

Banerjee A, Dubnau E, Quémard A, Balasubramanian V, Um KS, Wilson T, Collins D, Lisle G, Jacobs WR Jr. 1994. *inhA*, a gene encoding a target for isoniazid and ethionamide in *Mycobacterium tuberculosis*. *Science* **263:** 227–230.

Barry CE III, Lee RE, Mdluli K, Sampson AE, Schroeder BG, Slayden RA, Yuan Y. 1998. Mycolic acids: Structure, biosynthesis and physiological functions. *Prog Lipid Res* **37:** 143–179.

Bertozzi CR, Schelle MW. 2008. Sulfated metabolites from *Mycobacterium tuberculosis*: Sulfolipid-1 and beyond. In *The mycobacterial cell envelope* (ed. Daffé M, Reyrat J-M), pp. 291–304. ASM, Washington, DC.

Bhamidi S, Shi L, Chatterjee D, Belisle JT, Crick DC, McNeil MR. 2012. A bioanalytical method to determine the cell wall composition of *Mycobacterium tuberculosis* grown *in vivo*. *Anal Biochem* **421:** 240–249.

Bhowruth V, Brown AK, Reynolds RC, Coxon GD, Mackay SP, Minnikin DE, Besra GS. 2006. Symmetrical and unsymmetrical analogues of isoxyl; active agents against *Mycobacterium tuberculosis*. *Bioorg Med Chem Lett* **16:** 4743–4747.

Bhowruth V, Brown AK, Besra GS. 2008. Synthesis and biological evaluation of NAS-21 and NAS-91 analogues as potential inhibitors of the mycobacterial FAS-II dehydratase enzyme Rv0636. *Microbiology* **154:** 1866–1875.

Bloch H. 1950. Studies on the virulence of tubercle bacilli; isolation and biological properties of a constituent of virulent organisms. *J Exp Med* **91:** 197–218, pl.

Boucau J, Sanki AK, Voss BJ, Sucheck SJ, Ronning DR. 2009. A coupled enzymatic assay measuring *Mycobacterium tuberculosis* antigen 85C enzymatic activity. *Anal Biochem* **385:** 120–127.

Brennan PJ. 1988. *Mycobacterium* and other actinomycetes. In *Microbial lipids* (ed. Ratledge C, Wilkinson SG), pp. 203–298. Academic, London.

Brennan PJ, Nikaido H. 1995. The envelope of mycobacteria. *Annu Rev Biochem* **64:** 29–63.

Britton WJ, Triccas JA. 2008. The constituents of the cell envelope and their impact on the host immune system. In *The mycobacterial cell envelope* (ed. Daffé M, Reyrat J-M), pp. 249–270. ASM, Washington, DC.

Brodin P, Poquet Y, Levillain F, Peguillet I, Larrouy-Maumus G, Gilleron M, Ewann F, Christophe T, Fenistein D, Jang J, et al. 2010. High content phenotypic cell-based visual screen identifies *Mycobacterium tuberculosis* acyltrehalose-containing glycolipids involved in phagosome remodeling. *PLoS Pathog* **6:** e1001100.

Camacho LR, Constant P, Raynaud C, Lanéelle MA, Triccas JA, Gicquel B, Daffé M, Guilhot C. 2001. Analysis of the phthiocerol dimycocerosate locus of *Mycobacterium tuberculosis*. Evidence that this lipid is involved in the cell wall permeability barrier. *J Biol Chem* **276:** 19845–19854.

Cardona P-J, Soto CY, Martin C, Gicquel B, Agusti G, Guirado E, Sirakova TD, Kolattukudy PE, Julian E, Luquin M. 2006. Neutral red reaction is related to virulence and cell wall methyl-branched lipids in *Mycobacterium tuberculosis*. *Microbes Infect* **8:** 183–190.

Chan CE, Zhao BZ, Cazenave-Gassiot A, Pang SW, Bendt AK, Wenk MR, Macary PA, Hanson BJ. 2013. Novel phage display–derived mycolic acid–specific antibodies with potential for tuberculosis diagnosis. *J Lipid Res* **54:** 2924–2932.

Chapman TM, Bouloc N, Buxton RS, Chugh J, Lougheed KE, Osborne SA, Saxty B, Smerdon SJ, Taylor DL, Whalley D. 2012. Substituted aminopyrimidine protein kinase B (PknB) inhibitors show activity against *Mycobacterium tuberculosis*. *Bioorg Med Chem Lett* **22:** 3349–3353.

Christophe T, Jackson M, Jeon HK, Fenistein D, Contreras-Dominguez M, Kim J, Genovesio A, Carralot JP, Ewann F, Kim EH, et al. 2009. High content screening identifies decaprenyl-phosphoribose 2′ epimerase as a target for intracellular antimycobacterial inhibitors. *PLoS Pathog* **5:** e1000645.

Constant P, Perez E, Malaga W, Lanéelle MA, Saurel O, Daffé M, Guilhot C. 2002. Role of the *pks15/1* gene in the biosynthesis of phenolglycolipids in the *Mycobacterium tuberculosis* complex. Evidence that all strains synthesize glycosylated *p*-hydroxybenzoic methyl esters and that strains devoid of phenolglycolipids harbor a frameshift mutation in the *pks15/1* gene. *J Biol Chem* **277:** 38148–38158.

Coxon GD, Craig D, Corrales RM, Vialla E, Gannoun-Zaki L, Kremer L. 2013. Synthesis, antitubercular activity and mechanism of resistance of highly effective thiacetazone analogues. *PloS ONE* **8:** e53162.

Daffé M, Lanéelle M-A. 1988. Distribution of phthiocerol diester, phenolic mycosides and related compounds in mycobacteria. *J Gen Microbiol* **134:** 2049–2055.

Daffé M, Draper P. 1998. The envelope layers of mycobacteria with reference to their pathogenicity. *Adv Microb Physiol* **39:** 131–203.

Daffé M, Lacave C, Lanéelle MA, Lanéelle G. 1987. Structure of the major triglycosyl phenol-phthiocerol of *Mycobacterium tuberculosis* (strain Canetti). *Eur J Biochem* **167:** 155–160.

Daffé M, McNeil MR, Brennan PJ. 1991. Novel type-specific lipooligosaccharides from *Mycobacterium tuberculosis*. *Biochemistry* **30:** 378–388.

Daffé M, Crick DC, Jackson M. 2014. Genetics of capsular polysaccharides and cell envelope (glyco)lipids. *Microbiol Spectrum* **2:** MGM2-0021-2013.

Daniel J, Deb C, Dubey VS, Sirakova TD, Abomoelak B, Morbidoni HR, Kolattukudy PE. 2004. Induction of a novel class of diacylglycerol acyltransferases and triacylglycerol accumulation in *Mycobacterium tuberculosis* as it goes into a dormancy-like state in culture. *J Bacteriol* **186:** 5017–5030.

Danilenko VN, Osolodkin DI, Lakatosh SA, Preobrazhenskaya MN, Shtil AA. 2011. Bacterial eukaryotic type serine-threonine protein kinases: From structural biology to targeted anti-infective drug design. *Curr Top Med Chem* **11:** 1352–1369.

Debnath J, Siricilla S, Wan B, Crick DC, Lenaerts AJ, Franzblau SG, Kurosu M. 2012. Discovery of selective menaquinone biosynthesis inhibitors against *Mycobacterium tuberculosis*. *J Med Chem* **55:** 3739–3755.

Dhiman RK, Mahapatra S, Slayden RA, Boyne ME, Lenaerts A, Hinshaw JC, Angala SK, Chatterjee D, Biswas K, Narayanasamy P, et al. 2009. Menaquinone synthesis is critical for maintaining mycobacterial viability during exponential growth and recovery from non-replicating persistence. *Mol Microbiol* **72:** 85–97.

Dhiman RK, Dinadayala P, Ryan GJ, Lenaerts AJ, Schenkel AR, Crick DC. 2011. Lipoarabinomannan localization and abundance during growth of *Mycobacterium smegmatis*. *J Bacteriol* **193:** 5802–5809.

Draper P. 1998. The outer parts of the mycobacterial envelope as permeability barriers. *Frontiers Biosci* **3:** D1253–D1261.

Dubnau E, Chan J, Raynaud C, Mohan VP, Lanéelle M-A, Yu K, Quémard A, Smith I, Daffé M. 2000. Oxygenated mycolic acids are necessary for virulence of *Mycobacterium tuberculosis* in mice. *Mol Microbiol* **36:** 630–637.

Elamin AA, Stehr M, Oehlmann W, Singh M. 2009. The mycolyltransferase 85A, a putative drug target of *Mycobacterium tuberculosis*: Development of a novel assay and quantification of glycolipid-status of the mycobacterial cell wall. *J Microbiol Method* **79:** 358–363.

Favrot L, Grzegorzewicz AE, Lajiness DH, Marvin RK, Boucau J, Isailovic D, Jackson M, Ronning DR. 2013. Mechanism of inhibition of *Mycobacterium tuberculosis* antigen 85 by ebselen. *Nat Commun* **4:** 2748.

Ferreras JA, Stirrett KL, Lu X, Ryu JS, Soll CE, Tan DS, Quadri LE. 2008. Mycobacterial phenolic glycolipid virulence factor biosynthesis: Mechanism and small-molecule inhibition of polyketide chain initiation. *Chem Biol* **15:** 51–61.

Fukuda T, Matsumura T, Ato M, Hamasaki M, Nishiuchi Y, Murakami Y, Maeda Y, Yoshimori T, Matsumoto S, Kobayashi K, et al. 2013. Critical roles for lipomannan and lipoarabinomannan in cell wall integrity of mycobacteria and pathogenesis of tuberculosis. *mBio* **4:** e00472-12.

Gagneux S, Small PM. 2007. Global phylogeography of *Mycobacterium tuberculosis* and implications for tuberculosis product development. *Lancet Infect Dis* **7:** 328–337.

Galandrin S, Guillet V, Rane RS, Leger M, Radha N, Eynard N, Das K, Balganesh TS, Mourey L, Daffé M, et al. 2013. Assay development for identifying inhibitors of the mycobacterial FadD32 activity. *J Biomol Screen.* **18:** 576–587.

Gilleron M, Jackson M, Nigou J, Puzo G. 2008. Structure, activities and biosynthesis of the phosphatidyl-*myo*-inositol-based lipoglycans. In *The mycobacterial cell envelope* (ed. Daffé M, Reyrat J-M), pp. 75–105. ASM, Washington, DC.

Glickman MS. 2008. Cording, cord factors and trehalose dimycolate. In *The mycobacterial cell envelope* (ed. Daffé M, Reyrat J-M), pp. 63–73. ASM, Washington DC.

Glickman MS, Cox JS, Jacobs WR Jr, 2000. A novel mycolic acid cyclopropane synthetase is required for cording, persistence, and virulence of *Mycobacterium tuberculosis*. *Mol Cell* **5:** 717–727.

Gonzalo Asensio J, Maia C, Ferrer NL, Barilone N, Laval F, Soto CY, Winter N, Daffe M, Gicquel B, Martin C, et al. 2006. The virulence-associated two-component PhoP-PhoR system controls the biosynthesis of polyketide-derived lipids in *Mycobacterium tuberculosis*. *J Biol Chem* **281:** 1313–1316.

Goren MB. 1990. Mycobacterial fatty acid esters of sugars and sulfosugars. In *handbook of lipid research glycolipids, phosphoglycolipids and sulfoglycolipids* (ed. Kates M), pp. 363–461. Plenum, New York.

Goren MB, Brennan PJ. 1979. Mycobacterial lipids: Chemistry and biologic activities. In *Tuberculosis* (ed. Youmans GP), pp. 63–193. W.B. Saunders, Philadelphia.

Goren MB, Brokl O, Schaefer WB. 1974a. Lipids of putative relevance to virulence in *Mycobacterium tuberculosis*: Phthiocerol dimycocerosate and the attenuation indicator lipid. *Infect Immun* **9:** 150–158.

Goren MB, Brokl O, Schaefer WB. 1974b. Lipids of putative relevance to virulence in *Mycobacterium tuberculosis*: Correlation of virulence with elaboration of sulfatides and strongly acidic lipids. *Infect Immun* **9:** 142–149.

Graham JE, Clark-Curtiss JE. 1999. Identification of *Mycobacterium tuberculosis* RNAs synthesized in response to phagocytosis by human macrophages by selective capture of transcribed sequences (SCOTS). *Proc Natl Acad Sci* **96:** 11554–11559.

Gratraud P, Surolia N, Besra GS, Surolia A, Kremer L. 2008. Antimycobacterial activity and mechanism of action of NAS-91. *Antimicrob Agents Chemother* **52:** 1162–1166.

Grzegorzewicz AE, Pham H, Gundi VAKB, Scherman MS, North EJ, Hess T, Jones V, Gruppo V, Born SEM, Korduláková J, et al. 2012a. Inhibition of mycolic acid transport across the *Mycobacterium tuberculosis* plasma membrane. *Nat Chem Biol* **8:** 334–341.

Grzegorzewicz AE, Korduláková J, Jones V, Born SE, Belardinelli JM, Vaquié A, Gundi VA, Madacki J, Slama N, Laval F, et al. 2012b. A common mechanism of inhibition of the *Mycobacterium tuberculosis* mycolic acid biosynthetic pathway by isoxyl and thiacetazone. *J Biol Chem* **287:** 38434–38441.

Guenin-Macé L, Simeone R, Demangel C. 2009. Lipids of pathogenic Mycobacteria: Contributions to virulence and host immune suppression. *Transbound Emerg Dis* **56:** 255–268.

Guerin ME, Kordulákova J, Alzari PM, Brennan PJ, Jackson M. 2010. Molecular basis of phosphatidyl-myo-inositol mannoside biosynthesis and regulation in mycobacteria. *J Biol Chem* **285:** 33577–33583.

Guiard J, Collmann A, Garcia-Alles LF, Mourey L, Brando T, Mori L, Gilleron M, Prandi J, De Libero G, Puzo G. 2009. Fatty acyl structures of *Mycobacterium tuberculosis* sulfoglycolipid govern T cell response. *J Immunol* **182:** 7030–7037.

Guilhot C, Chalut C, Daffé M. 2008. Biosynthesis and roles of phenolic glycolipids and related molecules in *Mycobacterium tuberculosis*. In *The mycobacterial cell envelope* (ed. Daffé M, Reyrat J-M), pp. 273–289. ASM, Washington, DC.

Hartkoorn RC, Sala C, Neres J, Pojer F, Magnet S, Mukherjee R, Uplekar S, Boy-Rottger S, Altmann KH, Cole ST. 2012. Towards a new tuberculosis drug: Pyridomycin—Nature's isoniazid. *EMBO Mol Med* **4:** 1032–1042.

He H, Oka S, Han YK, Yamamura Y, Kusunose E, Kusunose M, Yano I. 1991. Rapid serodiagnosis of human mycobacteriosis by ELISA using cord factor (trehalose-6,6′-dimycolate) purified from *Mycobacterium tuberculosis* as antigen. *FEMS Microbiol Immunol* **3:** 201–204.

Hoffmann C, Leis A, Niederweis M, Plitzko JM, Engelhardt H. 2008. Disclosure of the mycobacterial outer membrane: Cryo-electron tomography and vitreous sections reveal the lipid bilayer structure. *Proc Natl Acad Sci* **105:** 3963–3967.

Huet G, Constant P, Malaga W, Lanéelle MA, Kremer K, van Soolingen D, Daffé M, Guilhot C. 2009. A lipid profile typifies the Beijing strains of *Mycobacterium tuberculosis*: Identification of a mutation responsible for a modification of the structures of phthiocerol dimycocerosates and phenolic glycolipids. *J Biol Chem* **284:** 27101–27113.

Ioerger TR, O'Malley T, Liao R, Guinn KM, Hickey MJ, Mohaideen N, Murphy KC, Boshoff HI, Mizrahi V, Rubin EJ, et al. 2013. Identification of new drug targets and resistance mechanisms in *Mycobacterium tuberculosis*. *PloS ONE* **8:** e75245.

Ishikawa E, Ishikawa T, Morita YS, Toyonaga K, Yamada H, Takeuchi O, Kinoshita T, Akira S, Yoshikai Y, Yamasaki S. 2009. Direct recognition of the mycobacterial glycolipid, trehalose dimycolate, by C-type lectin Mincle. *J Exp Med* **206:** 2879–2888.

Ishizaki Y, Hayashi C, Inoue K, Igarashi M, Takahashi Y, Pujari V, Crick DC, Brennan PJ, Nomoto A. 2013. Inhibition of the first step in synthesis of the mycobacterial cell wall core, catalyzed by the GlcNAc-1-phosphate transferase WecA, by the novel caprazamycin derivative CPZEN-45. *J Biol Chem* **288:** 30309–30319.

Jackson M, Stadthagen G, Gicquel B. 2007. Long-chain multiple methyl-branched fatty acid-containing lipids of *Mycobacterium tuberculosis*: Biosynthesis, transport, regulation and biological activities. *Tuberculosis* **87:** 78–86.

Jackson M, McNeil MR, Brennan PJ. 2013. Progress in targeting cell envelope biogenesis in *Mycobacterium tuberculosis*. *Future Microbiol* **8:** 855–875.

Jarlier V, Nikaido H. 1994. Mycobacterial cell wall: Structure and role in natural resistance to antibiotics. *FEMS Microbiol Lett* **123:** 11–18.

Julian E, Matas L, Perez A, Alcaide J, Laneelle MA, Luquin M. 2002. Serodiagnosis of tuberculosis: Comparison of immunoglobulin A (IgA) response to sulfolipid I with IgG and IgM responses to 2,3-diacyltrehalose, 2,3,6-triacyltrehalose, and cord factor antigens. *J Clin Microbiol* **40:** 3782–3788.

Kanai K, Wiegeshaus E, Smith DW. 1970. Demonstration of mycolic acid and phthiocerol dimycocerosate in "in vivo grown tubercle bacilli". *Jpn J Med Sci Biol* **23:** 327–333.

Karakousis PC, Bishai WR, Dorman SE. 2004. *Mycobacterium tuberculosis* cell envelope lipids and the host immune response. *Cell Microbiol* **6:** 105–116.

Kaur D, Guerin ME, Skovierova H, Brennan PJ, Jackson M. 2009. Chapter 2. Biogenesis of the cell wall and other glycoconjugates of *Mycobacterium tuberculosis*. *Adv Appl Microbiol* **69:** 23–78.

Kordulákova J, Gilleron M, Mikušová K, Puzo G, Brennan PJ, Gicquel B, Jackson M. 2002. Definition of the first mannosylation step in phosphatidylinositol synthesis: PimA is essential for growth of mycobacteria. *J Biol Chem* **277:** 31335–31344.

Krishnan N, Malaga W, Constant P, Caws M, Tran TH, Salmons J, Nguyen TN, Nguyen DB, Daffé M, Young DB, et al. 2011. *Mycobacterium tuberculosis* lineage influences innate immune response and virulence and is associated with distinct cell envelope lipid profiles. *PloS ONE* **6:** e23870.

La Rosa V, Poce G, Canseco JO, Buroni S, Pasca MR, Biava M, Raju RM, Porretta GC, Alfonso S, Battilocchio C, et al. 2012. MmpL3 is the cellular target of the antitubercular pyrrole derivative BM212. *Antimicrob Agents Chemother* **56:** 324–331.

Lee W, Vanderven BC, Fahey RJ, Russell DG. 2013. Intracellular *Mycobacterium tuberculosis* exploits host-derived fatty acids to limit metabolic stress. *J Biol Chem* **288:** 6788–6800.

Lemassu A, Daffé M. 1994. Structural features of the exocellular polysaccharides of *Mycobacterium tuberculosis*. *Biochem J* **297:** 351–357.

Li X, Liu N, Zhang H, Knudson SE, Slayden RA, Tonge PJ. 2010. Synthesis and SAR studies of 1,4-benzoxazine MenB inhibitors: Novel antibacterial agents against *Mycobacterium tuberculosis*. *Bioorg Med Chem Lett* **20:** 6306–6309.

Li X, Liu N, Zhang H, Knudson SE, Li HJ, Lai CT, Simmerling C, Slayden RA, Tonge PJ. 2011. CoA adducts of 4-oxo-4-phenylbut-2-enoates: Inhibitors of MenB from the *M. tuberculosis* menaquinone biosynthesis pathway. *ACS Med Chem Lett* **2:** 818–823.

Li C, Du Q, Deng W, Xie J. 2012. The biology of mycobacterium cord factor and roles in pathogen–host interaction. *Crit Rev Eukaryot Gene Expr* **22:** 289–297.

Lougheed KE, Osborne SA, Saxty B, Whalley D, Chapman T, Bouloc N, Chugh J, Nott TJ, Patel D, Spivey VL, et al. 2011. Effective inhibitors of the essential kinase PknB and their potential as anti-mycobacterial agents. *Tuberculosis (Edinb)* **91:** 277–286.

Lu X, Zhang H, Tonge PJ, Tan DS. 2008. Mechanism-based inhibitors of MenE, an acyl-CoA synthetase involved in bacterial menaquinone biosynthesis. *Bioorg Med Chem Lett* **18:** 5963–5966.

Lu X, Zhou R, Sharma I, Li X, Kumar G, Swaminathan S, Tonge PJ, Tan DS. 2012. Stable analogues of OSB-AMP: Potent inhibitors of MenE, the o-succinylbenzoate-CoA synthetase from bacterial menaquinone biosynthesis. *Chem Biochem* **13:** 129–136.

Ly D, Kasmar AG, Cheng TY, de Jong A, Huang S, Roy S, Bhatt A, van Summeren RP, Altman JD, Jacobs WR Jr, et al. 2013. CD1c tetramers detect ex vivo T cell responses to processed phosphomycoketide antigens. *J Exp Med* **210:** 729–741.

Magnet S, Hartkoorn RC, Szekely R, Pato J, Triccas JA, Schneider P, Szantai-Kis C, Orfi L, Chambon M, Banfi D, et al. 2010. Leads for antitubercular compounds from kinase inhibitor library screens. *Tuberculosis (Edinb)* **90:** 354–360.

Makarov V, Manina G, Mikušová K, Mollmann U, Ryabova O, Saint-Joanis B, Dhar N, Pasca MR, Buroni S, Lucarelli AP, et al. 2009. Benzothiazinones kill *Mycobacterium tuberculosis* by blocking arabinan synthesis. *Science* **324:** 801–804.

Mann FM, Peters RJ. 2012. Isotuberculosinol: The unusual case of an immunomodulatory diterpenoid from *Mycobacterium tuberculosis. Med Chem Comm* **3:** 899–904.

Matsumoto M, Hashizume H, Tomishige T, Kawasaki M, Tsubouchi H, Sasaki H, Shimokawa Y, Komatsu M. 2006. OPC-67683, a nitro-dihydro-imidazooxazole derivative with promising action against tuberculosis in vitro and in mice. *PLoS Med* **3:** e466.

Matsunaga I, Sugita M. 2012. Mycoketide: A CD1c-presented antigen with important implications in mycobacterial infection. *Clin Dev Immunol* **2012:** 981821.

Mikušová K, Slayden RA, Besra GS, Brennan PJ. 1995. Biogenesis of the mycobacterial cell wall and the site of action of ethambutol. *Antimicrob Agents Chemother* **39:** 2484–2489.

Minnikin DE. 1982. Lipids: Complex lipids, their chemistry, biosynthesis and roles. In *The biology of mycobacteria* (ed. Ratledge C, Stanford J), pp. 95–184. Academic, London.

Molle V, Kremer L. 2010. Division and cell envelope regulation by Ser/Thr phosphorylation: Mycobacterium shows the way. *Mol Microbiol* **75:** 1064–1077.

Morita YS, Velasquez R, Taig E, Waller RF, Patterson JH, Tull D, Williams SJ, Billman-Jacobe H, McConville MJ. 2005. Compartmentalization of lipid biosynthesis in mycobacteria. *J Biol Chem* **280:** 21645–21652.

Morita YS, Sena CCB, Waller RF, Kurokawa K, Sernee MF, Nakatani F, Haites RE, Billman-Jacobe H, McConville MJ, Maeda Y, et al. 2006. PimE is a polyprenol-phosphate-mannose-dependent mannosyltransferase that transfers the fifth mannose of phosphatidylinositol mannoside in mycobacteria. *J Biol Chem* **281:** 25143–25155.

Nambiar JK, Pinto R, Aguilo JI, Takatsu K, Martin C, Britton WJ, Triccas JA. 2012. Protective immunity afforded by attenuated, PhoP-deficient *Mycobacterium tuberculosis* is associated with sustained generation of $CD4^+$ T-cell memory. *Eur J Immunol* **42:** 385–392.

Neyrolles O, Guilhot C. 2011. Recent advances in deciphering the contribution of *Mycobacterium tuberculosis* lipids to pathogenesis. *Tuberculosis (Edinb)* **91:** 187–195.

North EJ, Jackson M, Lee RE. 2013. New approaches to target the mycolic acid biosynthesis pathway for the development of tuberculosis therapeutics. *Curr Pharm Des* (in press).

Obiol-Pardo C, Rubio-Martinez J, Imperial S. 2011. The methylerythritol phosphate (MEP) pathway for isoprenoid biosynthesis as a target for the development of new drugs against tuberculosis. *Curr Med Chem* **18:** 1325–1338.

Ojha A, Anand M, Bhatt A, Kremer L, Jacobs WR Jr, Hatfull GF. 2005. GroEL1: A dedicated chaperone involved in mycolic acid biosynthesis during biofilm formation in mycobacteria. *Cell* **123:** 861–873.

Ojha AK, Trivelli X, Guerardel Y, Kremer L, Hatfull GF. 2010. Enzymatic hydrolysis of trehalose dimycolate releases free mycolic acids during mycobacterial growth in biofilms. *J Biol Chem* **285:** 17380–17389.

Ortalo-Magné A, Dupont MA, Lemassu A, Andersen AB, Gounon P, Daffé M. 1995. Molecular composition of the outermost capsular material of the tubercle bacillus. *Microbiol* **141:** 1609–1620.

Ortalo-Magné A, Lemassu A, Lanéelle MA, Bardou F, Silve G, Gounon P, Marchal G, Daffé M. 1996. Identification of the surface-exposed lipids on the cell envelopes of *Mycobacterium tuberculosis* and other mycobacterial species. *J Bacteriol* **178:** 456–461.

Pan P, Tonge PJ. 2012. Targeting InhA, the FASII enoyl-ACP reductase: SAR studies on novel inhibitor scaffolds. *Curr Top Med Chem* **12:** 672–693.

Parish T, Liu J, Nikaido H, Stoker NG. 1997. A *Mycobacterium smegmatis* mutant with a defective inositol monophosphate phosphatase gene homolog has altered cell envelope permeability. *J Bacteriol* **179:** 7827–7833.

Passemar C, Arbues A, Malaga W, Mercier I, Moreau F, Lepourry L, Neyrolles O, Guilhot C, Astarie-Dequeker C. 2014. Multiple deletions in the polyketide synthase gene repertoire of *Mycobacterium tuberculosis* reveal functional overlap of cell envelope lipids in host-pathogen interactions. *Cell Microbiol* **16:** 195–213.

Patterson JH, Waller RF, Jeevarajah D, Billman-Jacobe H, McConville MJ. 2003. Mannose metabolism is required for mycobacterial growth. *Biochem J* **372:** 77–86.

Peyron P, Vaubourgeix J, Poquet Y, Levillain F, Botanch C, Bardou F, Daffé M, Emile JF, Marchou B, Cardona PJ, et al. 2008. Foamy macrophages from tuberculous patients' granulomas constitute a nutrient-rich reservoir for *M. tuberculosis* persistence. *PLoS Pathog* **4:** e1000204.

Phetsuksiri B, Baulard AR, Cooper A, Minnikin DE, Douglas JD, Besra GS, Brennan PJ. 1999. Antimycobacterial activities of isoxyl and new derivatives through the inhibition of mycolic acid synthesis. *Antimicrob Agents Chemother* **43:** 1042–1051.

Pitarque S, Herrmann JL, Duteyrat JL, Jackson M, Stewart GR, Lecointe F, Payre B, Schwartz O, Young DB, Marchal G, et al. 2005. Deciphering the molecular bases of *Mycobacterium tuberculosis* binding to the lectin DC-SIGN reveals an underestimated complexity. *Biochem J* **392:** 615–624.

Pitarque S, Larrouy-Maumus G, Payré B, Jackson M, Puzo G, Nigou J. 2008. The immunomodulatory lipoglycans, lipoarabinomannan and lipomannan, are exposed at the mycobacterial cell surface. *Tuberculosis* **88:** 560–565.

Poce G, Bates RH, Alfonso S, Cocozza M, Porretta GC, Ballell L, Rullas J, Ortega F, De Logu A, Agus E, et al. 2013.

Improved BM212 MmpL3 inhibitor analogue shows efficacy in acute murine model of tuberculosis infection. *PloS ONE* **8:** e56980.

Rajni, Rao N, Meena LS. 2011. Biosynthesis and virulent behavior of lipids produced by *Mycobacterium tuberculosis*: LAM and Cord Factor: An overview. *Biotechnol Res Int* **2011:** 274693.

Reed MB, Domenech P, Manca C, Su H, Barczak AK, Kreiswirth BN, Kaplan G, Barry CE III. 2004. A glycolipid of hypervirulent tuberculosis strains that inhibits the innate immune response. *Nature* **431:** 84–87.

Reed MB, Gagneux S, Deriemer K, Small PM, Barry CE 3rd. 2007. The W-Beijing lineage of *Mycobacterium tuberculosis* overproduces triglycerides and has the DosR dormancy regulon constitutively upregulated. *J Bacteriol* **189:** 2583–2589.

Remuinan MJ, Perez-Herran E, Rullas J, Alemparte C, Martinez-Hoyos M, Dow DJ, Afari J, Mehta N, Esquivias J, Jimenez E, et al. 2013. Tetrahydropyrazolo[1,5-*a*]pyrimidine-3-carboxamide and *N*-benzyl-6′,7′-dihydrospiro [piperidine-4,4′-thieno[3,2-c]pyran] analogues with bactericidal efficacy against *Mycobacterium tuberculosis* targeting MmpL3. *PloS ONE* **8:** e60933.

Ren H, Dover LG, Islam ST, Alexander DC, Chen JM, Besra GS, Liu J. 2007. Identification of the lipooligosaccharide biosynthetic gene cluster from *Mycobacterium marinum*. *Mol Microbiol* **63:** 1345–1359.

Rodriguez JE, Ramirez AS, Salas LP, Helguera-Repetto C, Gonzalez-y-Merchand J, Soto CY, Hernandez-Pando R. 2013. Transcription of genes involved in sulfolipid and polyacyltrehalose biosynthesis of *Mycobacterium tuberculosis* in experimental latent tuberculosis infection. *PloS ONE* **8:** e58378.

Rousseau C, Neyrolles O, Bordat Y, Giroux S, Sirakova TD, Prevost M-C, Kolattukudy PE, Gicquel B, Jackson M. 2003a. Deficiency in mycolipenate- and mycosanoate-derived acyltrehaloses enhances early interactions of *Mycobacterium tuberculosis* with host cells. *Cell Microbiol* **5:** 405–415.

Rousseau C, Turner OC, Rush E, Bordat Y, Sirakova TD, Kolattukudy PE, Ritter S, Orme IM, Gicquel B, Jackson M. 2003b. Sulfolipid deficiency does not affect the virulence of *Mycobacterium tuberculosis* H37Rv in mice and guinea pigs. *Infect Immun* **71:** 4684–4690.

Rousseau C, Winter N, Pivert E, Bordat Y, Neyrolles O, Ave P, Huerre M, Gicquel B, Jackson M. 2004. Production of phthiocerol dimycocerosates protects *Mycobacterium tuberculosis* from the cidal activity of reactive nitrogen intermediates produced by macrophages and modulates the early immune response to infection. *Cell Microbiol* **6:** 277–287.

Russell DG. 2011. *Mycobacterium tuberculosis* and the intimate discourse of a chronic infection. *Immunol Rev* **240:** 252–268.

Russell DG, Mwandumba HC, Rhoades EE. 2002. *Mycobacterium* and the coat of many lipids. *J Cell Biol* **158:** 421–426.

Ryan GJ, Hoff DR, Driver ER, Voskuil ML, Gonzalez-Juarrero M, Basaraba RJ, Crick DC, Spencer JS, Lenaerts AJ. 2010. Multiple *M. tuberculosis* phenotypes in mouse and guinea pig lung tissue revealed by a dual-staining approach. *PloS ONE* **5:** e11108.

Sacksteder KA, Protopopova M, Barry CE III, Andries K, Nacy CA. 2012. Discovery and development of SQ109: A new antitubercular drug with a novel mechanism of action. *Future Microbiol* **7:** 823–837.

Sakamoto K, Kim MJ, Rhoades ER, Allavena RE, Ehrt S, Wainwright HC, Russell DG, Rohde KH. 2013. Mycobacterial trehalose dimycolate reprograms macrophage global gene expression and activates matrix metalloproteinases. *Infect Immun* **81:** 764–776.

Sambandan D, Dao DN, Weinrick BC, Vilchèze C, Gurcha SS, Ojha A, Kremer L, Besra GS, Hatfull GF, Jacobs WR Jr. 2013. Keto-mycolic acid-dependent pellicle formation confers tolerance to drug-sensitive *Mycobacterium tuberculosis*. *mBio* **4:** e00222–00213.

Sani M, Houben ENG, Geurtsen J, Pierson J, de Punder K, van Zon M, Wever B, Piersma SR, Jimenez CR, Daffé M, et al. 2010. Direct visualization by cryo-EM of the mycobacterial capsular layer: A labile structure containing ESX-1-secreted proteins. *PLoS Pathog* **6:** e1000794.

Sanki AK, Boucau J, Ronning DR, Sucheck SJ. 2009. Antigen 85C-mediated acyl-transfer between synthetic acyl donors and fragments of the arabinan. *Glycoconj J* **26:** 589–596.

Schlesinger LS, Azad AK, Torrelles JB, Roberts E, Vergne I, Deretic V. 2008. Determinants of phagocytosis, phagosome biogenesis and autophagy for *Mycobacterium tuberculosis*. In *Handbook of tuberculosis: Immunology and cell biology* (ed. Kaufmann SHE, Britton WJ), pp. 1–22. Wiley-VCH, Darmstadt, Germany.

Shahab FM, Kobarfard F, Shafaghi B, Dadashzadeh S. 2010. Preclinical pharmacokinetics of KBF611, a new antituberculosis agent in mice and rabbits, and comparison with thiacetazone. *Xenobiotica* **40:** 225–234.

Shui G, Bendt AK, Jappar IA, Lim HM, Laneelle M, Herve M, Via LE, Chua GH, Bratschi MW, Zainul Rahim SZ, et al. 2012. Mycolic acids as diagnostic markers for tuberculosis case detection in humans and drug efficacy in mice. *EMBO Mol Med* **4:** 27–37.

Simonney N, Molina JM, Molimard M, Oksenhendler E, Perronne C, Lagrange PH. 1995. Analysis of the immunological humoral response to *Mycobacterium tuberculosis* glycolipid antigens (DAT, PGLTb1) for diagnosis of tuberculosis in HIV-seropositive and -seronegative patients. *Eur J Clin Microbiol Infect Dis* **14:** 883–891.

Simonney N, Molina JM, Molimard M, Oksenhendler E, Lagrange PH. 1996. Comparison of A60 and three glycolipid antigens in an ELISA test for tuberculosis. *Clin Microbiol Infect* **2:** 214–222.

Singh A, Crossman DK, Mai D, Guidry L, Voskuil MI, Renfrow MB, Steyn AJ. 2009. *Mycobacterium tuberculosis* WhiB3 maintains redox homeostasis by regulating virulence lipid anabolism to modulate macrophage response. *PLoS Pathog* **5:** e1000545.

Sinsimer D, Huet G, Manca C, Tsenova L, Koo MS, Kurepina N, Kana B, Mathema B, Marras SA, Kreiswirth BN, et al. 2008. The phenolic glycolipid of *Mycobacterium tuberculosis* differentially modulates the early host cytokine response but does not in itself confer hypervirulence. *Infect Immun* **76:** 3027–3036.

Sirakova TD, Dubey VS, Deb C, Daniel J, Korotkova TA, Abomoelak B, Kolattukudy PE. 2006. Identification of a diacylglycerol acyltransferase gene involved in accumulation of triacylglycerol in *Mycobacterium tuberculosis* under stress. *Microbiology* **152:** 2717–2725.

Stanley SA, Grant SS, Kawate T, Iwase N, Shimizu M, Wivagg C, Silvis M, Kazyanskaya E, Aquadro J, Golas A, et al. 2012. Identification of novel inhibitors of *M. tuberculosis* growth using whole cell based high-throughput screening. *ACS Chem Biol* **7:** 1377–1384.

Stanley SA, Kawate T, Iwase N, Shimizu M, Clatworthy AE, Kazyanskaya E, Sacchettini JC, Ioerger TR, Siddiqi NA, Minami S, et al. 2013. Diarylcoumarins inhibit mycolic acid biosynthesis and kill *Mycobacterium tuberculosis* by targeting FadD32. *Proc Natl Acad Sci* **110:** 11565–11570.

Stover KC, Warrener P, VanDevanter DR, Sherman DR, Arain TM, Langhorne MH, Anderson SW, Towell JA, Yuan Y, McMurray DN, et al. 2000. A small-molecule nitroimidazopyran drug candidate for the treatment of tuberculosis. *Nature* **405:** 962–966.

Sugawara I, Udagawa T, Hua SC, Reza-Gholizadeh M, Otomo K, Saito Y, Yamada H. 2002. Pulmonary granulomas of guinea pigs induced by inhalation exposure of heat-treated BCG Pasteur, purified trehalose dimycolate and methyl ketomycolate. *J Med Microbiol* **51:** 131–137.

Supply P, Marceau M, Mangenot S, Roche D, Rouanet C, Khanna V, Majlessi L, Criscuolo A, Tap J, Pawlik A, et al. 2013. Genomic analysis of smooth tubercle bacilli provides insights into ancestry and pathoadaptation of *Mycobacterium tuberculosis*. *Nat Genet* **45:** 172–179.

Tahlan K, Wilson R, Kastrinsky DB, Arora K, Nair V, Fischer E, Barnes SW, Walker JR, Alland D, Barry CE 3rd, et al. 2012. SQ109 targets MmpL3, a membrane transporter of trehalose monomycolate involved in mycolic acid donation to the cell wall core of *Mycobacterium tuberculosis*. *Antimicrob Agents Chemother* **56:** 1797–1809.

Tsenova L, Ellison E, Harbacheuski R, Moreira AL, Kurepina N, Reed MB, Mathema B, Barry CE III, Kaplan G. 2005. Virulence of selected *Mycobacterium tuberculosis* clinical isolates in the rabbit model of meningitis is dependent on phenolic glycolipid produced by the bacilli. *J Infect Dis* **192:** 98–106.

Uh E, Jackson ER, San Jose G, Maddox M, Lee RE, Lee RE, Boshoff HI, Dowd CS. 2011. Antibacterial and antitubercular activity of fosmidomycin, FR900098, and their lipophilic analogs. *Bioorg Med Chem Lett* **21:** 6973–6976.

Van Rhijn I, Ly D, Moody DB. 2013. CD1a, CD1b, and CD1c in immunity against mycobacteria. *Adv Exp Med Biol* **783:** 181–197.

Vander Beken S, Al Dulayymi JR, Naessens T, Koza G, Maza-Iglesias M, Rowles R, Theunissen C, De Medts J, Lanckacker E, Baird MS, et al. 2011. Molecular structure of the *Mycobacterium tuberculosis* virulence factor, mycolic acid, determines the elicited inflammatory pattern. *Eur J Immunol* **41:** 450–460.

Vera-Cabrera L, Handzel V, Laszlo A. 1994. Development of an enzyme-linked immunosorbent assay (ELISA) combined with a streptavidin-biotin and enzyme amplification method to detect anti-2,3-di-o-acyltrehalose (DAT) antibodies in patients with tuberculosis. *J Immunol Methods* **177:** 69–77.

Vilchèze C, Jacobs WR Jr, 2007. The mechanism of isoniazid killing: Clarity through the scope of genetics. *Annu Rev Microbiol* **61:** 35–50.

Vilchèze C, Baughn AD, Tufariello J, Leung LW, Kuo M, Basler CF, Alland D, Sacchettini JC, Freundlich JS, Jacobs WR Jr. 2011. Novel inhibitors of InhA efficiently kill *Mycobacterium tuberculosis* under aerobic and anaerobic conditions. *Antimicrob Agents Chemother* **55:** 3889–3898.

Villemagne B, Crauste C, Flipo M, Baulard AR, Deprez B, Willand N. 2012. Tuberculosis: The drug development pipeline at a glance. *Eur J Med Chem* **51:** 1–16.

Villeneuve C, Gilleron M, Maridonneau-Parini I, Daffé M, Astarie-Dequeker C, Etienne G. 2005. Mycobacteria use their surface-exposed glycolipids to infect human macrophages through a receptor-dependent process. *J Lipid Res* **46:** 475–483.

Vir P, Gupta D, Agarwal R, Verma I. 2013. Immunomodulation of alveolar epithelial cells by *Mycobacterium tuberculosis* phosphatidylinositol mannosides results in apoptosis. *APMIS* **122:** 268–282.

Wallis RS, Kim P, Cole S, Hanna D, Andrade BB, Maeurer M, Schito M, Zumla A. 2013. Tuberculosis biomarkers discovery: Developments, needs, and challenges. *Lancet Infect Dis* **13:** 362–372.

Walters SB, Dubnau E, Kolesnikova I, Laval F, Daffé M, Smith I. 2006. The *Mycobacterium tuberculosis* PhoPR two-component system regulates genes essential for virulence and complex lipid biosynthesis. *Mol Microbiol* **60:** 312–330.

Wang F, Sambandan D, Halder R, Wang J, Batt SM, Weinrick B, Ahmad I, Yang P, Zhang Y, Kim J, et al. 2013. Identification of a small molecule with activity against drug-resistant and persistent tuberculosis. *Proc Natl Acad Sci* **110:** E2510–E2517.

Warrier T, Tropis M, Werngren J, Diehl A, Gengenbacher M, Schlegel B, Schade M, Oschkinat H, Daffé M, Hoffner S, et al. 2012. Antigen 85C inhibition restricts *Mycobacterium tuberculosis* growth through disruption of cord factor biosynthesis. *Antimicrob Agents Chemother* **56:** 1735–1743.

Weinstein EA, Yano T, Li LS, Avarbock D, Avarbock A, Helm D, McColm AA, Duncan K, Lonsdale JT, Rubin H. 2005. Inhibitors of type II NADH:menaquinone oxidoreductase represent a class of antitubercular drugs. *Proc Natl Acad Sci* **102:** 4548–4553.

Willand N, Dirie B, Carette X, Bifani P, Singhal A, Desroses M, Leroux F, Willery E, Mathys V, Deprez-Poulain R, et al. 2009. Synthetic EthR inhibitors boost antituberculous activity of ethionamide. *Nat Med* **15:** 537–544.

Wilson R, Kumar P, Parashar V, Vilchèze C, Veyron-Churlet R, Freundlich JS, Barnes SW, Walker JR, Szymonifka MJ, Marchiano E, et al. 2013. Antituberculosis thiophenes define a requirement for Pks13 in mycolic acid biosynthesis. *Nat Chem Biol* **9:** 499–506.

Yang L, Sinha T, Carlson TK, Keiser TL, Torrelles JB, Schlesinger LS. 2013. Changes in the major cell envelope components of *Mycobacterium tuberculosis* during in vitro growth. *Glycobiology* **23:** 926–934.

Yuan Y, Zhu Y, Crane DD, Barry CE III. 1998. The effect of oxygenated mycolic acid composition on cell wall function and macrophage growth in *Mycobacterium tuberculosis. Mol Microbiol* **29:** 1449–1458.

Zhang J, Amin AG, Holemann A, Seeberger PH, Chatterjee D. 2010. Development of a plate-based scintillation proximity assay for the mycobacterial AftB enzyme involved in cell wall arabinan biosynthesis. *Bioorg Med Chem* **18:** 7121–7131.

Zhang J, Angala SK, Pramanik PK, Li K, Crick DC, Liav A, Jozwiak A, Swiezewska E, Jackson M, Chatterjee D. 2011. Reconstitution of functional mycobacterial arabinosyltransferase aftc proteoliposome and assessment of decaprenylphosphorylarabinose analogues as arabinofuranosyl donors. *ACS Chem Biol* **6:** 819–828.

Zimhony O, Cox JS, Welch JT, Vilchèze C, Jacobs WR Jr. 2000. Pyrazinamide inhibits the eukaryotic-like fatty acid synthetase I (FASI) of *Mycobacterium tuberculosis. Nat Med* **6:** 1043–1047.

Zuber B, Chami M, Houssin C, Dubochet J, Griffiths G, Daffé M. 2008. Direct visualization of the outer membrane of mycobacteria and corynebacteria in their native state. *J Bact* **190:** 5672–5680.

The Mycobacterial Cell Wall—Peptidoglycan and Arabinogalactan

Luke J. Alderwick, James Harrison, Georgina S. Lloyd, and Helen L. Birch

Institute of Microbiology and Infection, School of Biosciences, University of Birmingham, Birmingham B15 2TT, United Kingdom

Correspondence: l.alderwick@bham.ac.uk

The mycobacterial bacillus is encompassed by a remarkably elaborate cell wall structure. The mycolyl-arabinogalactan-peptidoglycan (mAGP) complex is essential for the viability of *Mycobacterium tuberculosis* and maintains a robust basal structure supporting the upper "myco-membrane." *M. tuberculosis* peptidoglycan, although appearing to be unexceptional at first glance, contains a number of unique molecular subtleties that become particularly important as the TB-bacilli enters into nonreplicative growth during dormancy. Arabinogalactan, a highly branched polysaccharide, serves to connect peptidoglycan with the outer mycolic acid layer, and a variety of unique glycolsyltransferases are used for its assembly. In this review, we shall explore the microbial chemistry of this unique heteropolysacchride, examine the molecular genetics that underpins its fabrication, and discuss how the essential biosynthetic process might be exploited for the development of future anti-TB chemotherapies.

THE MYCOBACTERIAL CELL WALL—PEPTIDOGLYCAN AND ARABINOGALACTAN

The remarkable molecular complexity of the mycobacterial cell wall is a particularly distinguishing feature that set *Mycobacterium* species apart from the majority of other prokaryotes. Although classified as gram-positive organisms, their envelopes do in fact share notable features with Gram-negative cell walls, such as an outer permeability barrier acting as a pseudo-outer membrane (Minnikin 1982; Brennan and Nikaido 1995). Much of the early structural definition of the cell wall was conducted in the 1960s and 1970s (Adam et al. 1969; Petit et al. 1969; Lederer et al. 1975) and later continued by Minnikin, who in 1982 proposed the currently accepted structural model for the cell wall architecture (Minnikin 1982). The mycolyl-arabinogalactan-peptidoglycan (mAGP) complex, as it is commonly termed, represents the cell wall core structure that encompasses the mycobacterial bacilli.

Structural Features of Mycobacterial Peptidoglycan

Peptidoglycan (PG) is a complex macromolecular structure situated on the outside of the plasma membrane of almost all eubacteria (Schleifer and Kandler 1972; van Heijenoort

Cite this article as *Cold Spring Harb Perspect Med* doi: 10.1101/cshperspect.a021113

2001). Its mesh-like arrangement confers rigidity to the cell, allowing it to withstand osmotic pressure maintaining cell integrity and cellular shape. Relatively little is known about *Mycobacterium tuberculosis* PG synthesis, although it is generally assumed to be analogous to that of *Escherichia coli* (van Heijenoort 2001), also being classified as A1γ according to the classification system of Schleifer and Kandler (1972). Mycobacterial PG forms the basal layer of the mAGP complex and is composed of alternating *N*-acetylglucosamine (GlcNAc) and modified muramic acid (Mur) residues, linked in a β(1 → 4) configuration (Lederer et al. 1975). Unlike *E. coli* PG, the muramic acid residues in both *M. tuberculosis* and *Mycobacterium smegmatis* contain a mixture of *N*-acetyl and *N*-glycolyl derivatives, whereby the *N*-acetyl function has been oxidized to a *N*-glycolyl function to form MurNGly (Mahapatra et al. 2000, 2005; Raymond et al. 2005). Although the precise function of the *N*-glycolyl modifications is yet to be elucidated, it has been hypothesized that these additional glycolyl-containing residues might have the potential for additional hydrogen bonding interactions, strengthening the mesh-like structure of the PG layer (Brennan and Nikaido 1995), as well as possibly protecting the organism from degradation via lysozyme (Chatterjee et al. 1991). Tetrapeptide side chains consisting of L-alaninyl-D-*iso*glutaminyl-*meso*-diaminopimelyl-D-alanine are cross-linked with identical short peptides of neighboring glycan chains (Petit et al. 1969). These cross-links include the expected 3 → 4 *meso*-diaminopimelic acid (DAP) and D-alanine bond that is common to most prokaryotes, but also a high degree of 3 → 3 bonds between two residues of DAP (Ghuysen 1968; Wietzerbin-Falszpan et al. 1970). The proportion of cross-linking in *Mycobacterium* species is 70%–80% (Matsuhashi 1966), significantly more so than *E. coli*, with only 50% (Vollmer and Holtje 2004). An additional deviation from *E. coli* PG is the use of the muramic acid residues as attachment sites for the galactan domain of the arabinogalactan, whereby 6-OH of some of the muramic acid residues form a phosphodiester bond and are linked to the α-L-rhamnopyranose-(1 → 3)-α-D-GlcNAc (1 → P) linker unit of AG (McNeil et al. 1990).

One model proposed for the three-dimensional topology of the mAGP complex, consistent with the traditional models of PG architecture (Ghuysen 1968; Brennan and Nikaido 1995), suggests that the PG and the galactan moiety run parallel to the plasma membrane. However, an opposing model put forward by other modeling studies predicts that the PG and the AG polymers may in fact be coiled and are thus orientated perpendicular to the plane of the plasma membrane (Dmitriev et al. 2000, 2003). Minnikin et al. (2002) proposed that both AG and LAM polymers form coiled strands and integrate with the basal PG layer. Interestingly, a study by Meroueh et al. (2006) presented compelling evidence in the form of nuclear magnetic resonance (NMR) data that suggests that the PG glycan strand is orthogonal to the plane of the membrane; thus, the overall three-dimensional structure and topology remain open to debate.

Biosynthesis of Mycobacterial Peptidoglycan

Cytoplasmic Steps of Peptidoglycan Intermediate Metabolism

The biosynthesis of PG begins within the cytoplasm of all bacteria that contain a murein sacculus, and the activated sugar nucleotide UDP-GlcNAc is usually considered to be the "start point" of PG anabolism. UDP-GlcNAc is synthesized from D-fructose-6-phosphate in four steps and requires three enzymes. GlmS is an aminotransferase that converts D-fructose-6-phosphate to D-glucosamine-1-phosphate, and although a clear ortholog is present in *M. tuberculosis*, there has been no investigation of this gene or protein to date (Durand et al. 2008). GlmM is a mutase enzyme that converts D-glucosamine-1-phosphate to D-glucosamine-6-phosphate and has been shown to be an essential gene in *M. smegmatis* (Li et al. 2012). Indeed, the conversion of D-glucosamine-6-phosphate to D-glucosamine-1-phosphate is unique to prokaryotes and is considered a potential drug target (Li et al. 2011). GlmU is a bifunctional enzyme that carries out both acetylation and uridylation reactions, ultimately forming UDP-GlcNAc (Jagtap et al. 2012, 2013). The carboxy-terminal domain of GluU is responsible for catalyzing acylation of D-glucosamine-6-phosphate whereas the amino-terminal domain catalyzes uridylation of *N*-acetylglucosamine-1-phosphate. GlmU has been shown to be an essential gene in *M. smegmatis* (Zhang et al. 2008). Interestingly, a single threonine residue within the carboxy-terminal domain of GlmU is phosphorylated by the serine/threonine protein kinase PknB, resulting in a modulation of GlmU acetyltransferase activity (Parikh et al. 2009).

UDP-MurNAc is formed from UDP-GlcNAc in a two-step process involving the catalytic activities of two enzymes, MurA and MurB. MurA is a UDP-GlcNAc enolpyruvyl transferase that catalyzes the transfer of enolpyruvate from phosphoenoylpyruvate to the 3-position of the *N*-acetylglucosamine moiety of UDP-GlcNAc, liberating inorganic phosphate in the process. Fosfomycin is an analog of phosphoenoylpyruvate and it inhibits MurA by alkylating an active site cysteine residue (Kim et al. 1996). However, although fosfomycin is considered to be a broad-spectrum antibiotic, it has no ready utility as an antitubercular drug. *M. tuberculosis* is inherently resistant to fosfomycin because of the presence of an aspartic acid in place of the aforementioned cysteine, which usually confers sensitivity to the drug (De Smet et al. 1999). MurB is a reductase that uses NADPH as an electron donor to convert the enolpyruvate moiety to D-lactoyl, thus delivering UDP-MurNAc as a final product. To date, the investigation of MurB from mycobacteria has been limited to in silico homology modeling and molecular dynamics simulations (Kumar et al. 2011).

The intracellular ATP-dependent muramic acid ligase enzymes, MurC–MurF, work consecutively to synthesize UDP-*N*-acetylmuramyl pentapeptide and UDP-*N*-glycolylmuramyl pentapeptide from either UDP-MurNAc or UDP-MurNGlyc, respectively. *M. tuberculosis* UDP-MurNGlyc is initially generated by hydroxylation of the methyl group of the MurNAc moiety of UDP-MurNAc (Gateau et al. 1976; Essers and Schoop 1978). Conversion of UDP-MurNAc to UDP-MurNGlyc involves a monooxygenase encoded by the *namH* gene (Raymond et al. 2005). Chemical analysis of the nucleotide-linked PG intermediates from *M. tuberculosis* strongly suggests that this pool of metabolites is composed of a mixture of both MurNAc and MurNGlyc subtypes, in which the proportion of MurNAc precursors is heavily suppressed by the presence of D-cycloserine but not vancomycin (Mahapatra et al. 2005). The UDP-MurNGlyc and UDP-MurNAc intermediates are then perpetuated throughout the PG pathway by the successive additions of L-alanine (MurC), D-glutamate (MurD), *meso*-DAP (MurE), and D-alanyl-D-alanine (MurF), a unique prokaryotic pathway, which has been extensively reviewed by other investigators (Barreteau et al. 2008). The Mur ligases C–F share a common mechanism whereby the carboxyl group appended to the UDP substrate is activated by phosphorylation with ATP, generating ADP. The UDP-substrate phospho-intermediate is then attacked by an amino acid or dipeptide specific to the ligase catalyzing the reaction, resulting in extension by aminoacylation of the UDP precursor and the expulsion of inorganic phosphate (Falk et al. 1996; Bouhss et al. 1999). Both *M. tuberculosis* and *Mycobacterium leprae* MurC orthologs have been shown to be capable of ligating both L-alanine and L-glycine to UDP-MurNAc (Mahapatra et al. 2000). Apart from MurC, the only other ATP-dependent Mur ligase that has been biochemically characterized is MurE (Basavannacharya et al. 2010a,b).

Several other enzymes play vital roles in the cytoplasmic assembly of PG, two of which are the Alr and Ddl proteins that provide L-alanine racemase activity and D-alanine:D-alanine ligase activity, respectively (Feng and Barletta 2003). Several recent biochemical studies have provided comprehensive molecular insight into how D-cycloserine (currently used as a second-line anti-TB agent) inhibits the Ddl enzyme (Prosser and de Carvalho 2013a,b). In this regard, a number of high-throughput screening studies have identified Alr as being an equally interesting drug target (Anthony et al. 2011; Lee et al. 2013).

Polyprenyl phosphates play a crucial role in prokaryotic cell wall biosynthesis, providing a hydrophobic lipid anchor that enables cell envelope biosynthesis to occur while being tethered to the cytoplasmic membrane. In mycobacteria, MurX (usually termed MraY in other prokaryotes) is an integral membrane protein that transfers the phospho-MurNAc-pentapeptide to a decaprenol phosphate lipid. The result is the displacement of the UDP nucleotide moiety with a decaprenyl lipid carrier, thus forming lipid I from Park's nucleotide. Although the molecular genetics or biochemistry of MurX has not been studied in detail, it appears that MurX from *M. smegmatis* is capable of incorporating the muramyl-pentapeptide from both UDP-*N*-acetylmuramyl pentapeptide and UDP-*N*-glycolylmuramyl pentapeptide precursors with equal efficiency (Chen et al. 2013). MurG is a GT-B glycosyltransferase that uses UDP-GlcNAc as a substrate to form a $\beta(1 \rightarrow 4)$ glycosidic bond between GlcNAc and either the MurNAc or MurNGlyc sugar of lipid I. MurG from *M. tuberculosis* has been shown to be able to complement a *murG*-deficient strain of *E. coli* (Jha et al. 2012), and because of the essential nature of MurG, it is a target for the development of new antibacterial agents (Trunkfield et al. 2010). MurG marks the final "step" in the cytoplasmic pathway of PG biosynthesis, and its product is a cell wall intermediate termed lipid II.

The Latter Stages of Peptidoglycan Assembly

The cytoplasmic membrane presents a physical barrier that separates the cytoplasm from the outer periplasmic space of the mycobacterial cell, as well as a thermodynamic hurdle that must be overcome by numerous cell wall intermediates that are destined for deposition in the mycobacterial envelope. Lipid II separates the cytoplasm from the outer periplasmic space of the mycobacterial cell. Several biochemical and molecular genetic investigations in other nonmycobacterial prokaryotes have identified both MurJ and FtsW proteins as being candidate proteins that translocate lipid II across the bacterial cytoplasmic membrane (Ruiz 2008; Mohammadi et al. 2011; Butler et al. 2013; Mohamed and Valvano 2014). FtsW belongs to the shape, elongation, division, and sporulation (SEDS) family of proteins, all of which are integral membrane proteins involved in translocation of molecules across the cytoplasmic membrane. Interestingly, RodA is also a member of the SEDS family, and a recent study has shown that this protein also contributes lipid II flippase activity as well as having a direct interaction with the polar growth organizing protein, DivIVA (Sieger et al. 2013).

Two proteins, PonA1 and PonA2, encoded by *Rv0050* and *Rv3682*, respectively, are bifunctional penicillin-binding proteins that carry out both transglycoylase and transpeptidase enzymatic reactions, both of which use lipid II as a substrate. Studies on PonA1 from *M. smegmatis* have shown that apart from it being necessary for maintaining cell shape, viability, and integrity, this enzyme is also required for synergistic regulation of PG hydrolysis by interacting with the RipA-RpfB complex, a lytic transglycosylase and endopeptidase, respectively (Hett et al. 2010). PonA2 has also been attributed to having an important role in maintaining cell shape, integrity, and adaptation of *M. tuberculosis* into dormancy (Patru and Pavelka 2010). However, a recent biochemical and structural study of the PASTA domain from PonA2 has shown that this protein is unable to bind classical cognate ligands, such as muropeptides, β-lactams, or nascent PG (Calvanese et al. 2014).

PBPa and PBPb are two variants of the high-molecular-mass penicillin-binding proteins found in *M. tuberculosis*. PBPa is a class A penicillin-binding protein that plays an important role in the cell division process and maintenance of cell shape (Dasgupta et al. 2006). PknB, a serine/threonine-specific protein kinase, has been shown to phosphorylate PBPa on two key threonine residues T362 and T437, the latter of which is crucial to enable full signal transduction–mediated control of this important cell wall process (Dasgupta et al. 2006). Interestingly, both PBPa and PBPb have been shown to directly interact with the cell division complex and septal formation machinery FtsZ, FtsQ, and CrgA (Plocinski et al. 2011).

Although the PG of actively replicating *M. tuberculosis* contains a network of classical 3 → 4 transpeptide bonds, PG from nonreplicating *M. tuberculosis* contains significantly more nonclassical 3 → 3 linkages. Thus, a significant molecular rearrangement must occur in the PG of *M. tuberculosis* as its shifts its mode of growth from one of propagation into one of dormancy. The *M. tuberculosis* genome encodes at least five nonclassical L,D-transpeptidases (Ldt), which are the enzymes responsible for generating 3 → 3 linkages between opposing stem peptides in mycobacterial PG. *M. tuberculosis* deficient in both LdtMt1 and LdtMt2 activities shows an altered cell surface morphology and severely attenuates the growth and virulence of *M. tuberculosis* (Schoonmaker et al. 2014). Other biochemical studies have identified LdtM2 as being important for resistance to β-lactam antibiotics such as amoxicillin (Gupta et al. 2010) as well as carbapenems, and the structural basis for the inhibition of LdtMt2 by meropenem has been elucidated (Kim et al. 2013; Li et al. 2013). The X-ray crystal structure of LdtMt1 has also been solved in the apo and meropenem-bound form, highlighting some subtle differences between these two variants of L,D-transpeptidases (Correale et al. 2013).

ARABINOGALACTAN

Structural Features of Arabinogalactan

Arabinogalactan (AG) is a heteropolysaccharide that is covalently tethered to ~10%–12% of the muramic acid residues of PG via a phosphodiester bond (Amar and Vilkas 1973). Collectively, PG and AG form a huge macro polymer positioned between the cytoplasmic membrane and the outer mycolic acid layer of the TB bacilli. Early work showed that AG was composed predominantly of arabinose and galactose and constitutes ~35% of the total mass of the cell envelope (Misaki and Yukawa 1966; Azuma et al. 1968; Kanetsuna 1968; Kanetsuna et al. 1969). Both arabinose and galactose sugars are present in the furanoid ring form, D-galactofuranosyl (Gal*f*) and D-arabinofuranosyl (Ara*f*), which appear infrequently in nature (McNeil et al. 1987). A comprehensive characterization of oligomers generated from partial depolymerization of per-*O*-alkylated AG using gas chromatography–mass spectrometry (GC-MS), fast-atom bombardment–mass spectrometry (FAB-MS), and NMR spectroscopy resolved the detailed structure of the AG complex (McNeil et al. 1987; Daffé et al. 1990; McNeil et al. 1994; Besra et al. 1995). The molecular structure of AG can be segmented into three separate constituents: the linker unit (LU), galactan, and arabinan. Amar and Vilkas (1973) initially reported that AG is tethered to PG at intervals by a phosphodiester bond, supported by the presence of muramyl-6-phosphate in cell wall preparations from several mycobacterial species (Liu and Gotschlich 1967; Kanetsuna 1968). The chemical nature of this link was not answered until 20 years later when oligosaccharides containing Gal*f* from the galactan domain were isolated along with rhamnose (Rha) residues (McNeil et al. 1990). The further discovery of the disaccharide L-Rha*p*-(1 → 3)-D-GlcNAc led to the conclusion that these constituents make up the linkage unit and the inference that the GlcNAc is directly attached to the 6-position of a proportion of the muramyl residues of PG (McNeil et al. 1990). The D-galactan component of AG is composed of approximately 30 linear alternating β(1 → 5) and β(1 → 6) Gal*f* residues (Amar and Vilkas et al. 1973; McNeil et al. 1987) and is attached to the rhamnosyl residue of the LU. Three tricosamer domains of D-arabinan, each composed of approximately 23 Ara*f* residues, are affixed to the C-5 hydroxyl of β(1 → 6)-linked Gal*f* units (Besra et al. 1995) specifically to the 8th, 10th, and 12th Gal*f* residues of the galactan domain (Alderwick et al. 2005). The arabinan domain is a highly branched polysaccharide built on a backbone of α(1 → 5)-linked sugars with a number of α(1 → 3)-linked residues forming 3,5-Ara*f* branchpoints (Daffé et al. 1990). Further α(1 → 5)-linked Ara*f* sugars are attached subsequent to this branchpoint with the nonreducing ends terminated by β(1 → 2) Ara*f* residues. The final structural motif (Ara*f*-β(1 → 2)-Ara*f*-α(1-)$_2$

$\rightarrow$ 3,5-Ara*f*-α(1 $\rightarrow$ 5)-Ara*f*-α(1$\rightarrow$)) is a distinctive hexa-arabinoside (Ara_6) of which approximately two-thirds are esterified with mycolic acids (McNeil et al. 1991). AG from *M. tuberculosis* is also further decorated with succinyl residues and galactosamine (GalN) located on the 2-position of an inner 3,5-α-D-Ara*f* bifurcation point of approximately one-third of the arabinan tricosamers (Draper et al. 1997; Lee et al. 2006; Bhamidi et al. 2008; Peng et al. 2012). The last two decades has witnessed a dramatic increase in our understanding of how this complex polymer is assembled. Much emphasis has been placed on investigating the molecular genetics of how this complex structure is assembled in mycobacteria. The complete sequencing of several genomes from mycobacteria and other closely related species has provided major impetus in the identification and the study of the enzymes involved in the biosynthesis of this exceptional structure, with the hope of uncovering new drug targets.

Biosynthesis of Arabinogalactan

Biosynthesis of the Linker Unit

The crucial structural role of the LU in the attachment of AG to PG, as well as the presence of L-rhamnose, a sugar absent in humans, makes the biosynthetic pathway leading to the formation of this disaccharide an attractive drug target (Ma et al. 2001). In *M. tuberculosis*, LU biosynthesis is initiated on the isoprenoid lipid carrier decaprenyl-phosphate (C_{50}-P), whereby GlcNAc-phosphate is transferred from the activated sugar donor UDP-GlcNAc, thus forming C_{50}-P-P-GlcNAc, referred to as glycolipid 1 (GL-1) (Mikusova et al. 1996). Rv1302 shows a high degree of homology with the WecA protein from *E. coli* (Amer and Valvano 2002; Lehrer et al. 2007). Recent biochemical characterization of this enzyme shows that Rv1302 is indeed a decaprenyl-phosphate α-*N*-acetylglucosaminyltransferase responsible for the formation of GL-1 (Ishizaki et al. 2013), and the gene encoding WecA is essential for growth in *M. smegmatis* (Jin et al. 2010). The LU is completed by the subsequent action of the rhamnosyltransferase WbbL, which adds an L-Rha*p* to the 3-position of the GlcNAc of GL-1, this forming glycolipid 2 (GL-2) (Mills et al. 2004). WbbL uses the high-energy nucleotide sugar donor dTDP-rhamnose as a substrate for the formation of GL-2. Because formation of GL-2 is an essential biosynthetic step (Mills et al. 2004), the biosynthetic pathway leading to the formation dTDP-rhamnose has been heavily investigated, and a number of inhibitors of this process have been reported (Ma et al. 2001, 2002; Babaoglu et al. 2003; Kantardjieff et al. 2004). Synthesis of dTDP-Rha occurs via a linear 4-stage pathway using the gene products of *rmlABCD*. RmlA (Rv0334) sets in motion the sequence of reactions, converting dTTP + α-D-glucose 1-phosphate to dTDP-glucose + PP_i (Ma et al. 1997). The enzyme was cloned from *M. tuberculosis* and transformed into an *E. coli* strain devoid of four dTDP-Rha biosynthetic genes. Cellular extract analysis revealed an abundance of α-D-Glc-P thymidylyltransferase activity confirming its proposed function (Ma et al. 1997). The product of RmlA activity is then shuttled through three sequential reactions catalyzed by dTDP-D-glucose 4,6-dehydratase (Rv3464, RmlB), dTDP-4-keto-6-deoxy-D-glucose 3,5 epimerase (Rv3465, RmlC) and dTDP-Rha synthase (Rv3266, RmlD) (Hoang et al. 1999; Stern et al. 1999; Ma et al. 2001). Both *rmlB* and *rmlC* genes have also been shown as being essential for mycobacterial growth (Li et al. 2006).

Galactan Precursor Synthesis

The Gal*f* residues of the galactan domain are incorporated from the high-energy sugar nucleotide donor UDP-Gal*f*, which is formed via two reactions. In *E. coli*, galactosyl residues in the pyranose ring form (UDP-Gal*p*) are synthesized by the action of GalE, a UDP-glucose 4-epimerase, which uses UDP-glucopyranose (UDP-Glc*p*) as its substrate (Lemaire and Muller-Hill 1986). A study using cell-free extracts of *M. smegmatis* and radiolabeled UDP-Gal*p* showed the presence of UDP-glucose 4-epimerase activity, and the amino-terminal sequence of the isolated protein was shown to be similar to that of *M. tuberculosis* Rv3634 (Weston et al.

 Cite this article as *Cold Spring Harb Perspect Med* doi: 10.1101/cshperspect.a021113

1997). Conversion of UDP-Gal*p* to the furanose form occurs via ring contraction catalyzed by the flavoenzyme UDP-galactopyranose mutase (Glf) that was first recognized in *E. coli* (Nassau et al. 1996) and subsequently in *M. smegmatis* and *M. tuberculosis* (Rv3809c) (Weston et al. 1997). Allelic exchange experiments of *glf* in *M. smegmatis* highlighted the essentiality of this gene (Pan et al. 2001).

Arabinan Precursor Synthesis

As we shall see in the following section, mycobacterial D-arabinan assembly follows a linear biosynthetic pathway that involves an assortment of membrane-bound glycosyltransferases. Although D-arabinan contains a complex mixture of glycosidic linkages, decaprenylphosphoryl-β-D-arabinofuranose (DPA) is used exclusively by all of the enzymes involved in this pathway as a lipid-linked, activated Ara*f* substrate (Wolucka et al. 1994; Xin et al. 1997; Alderwick et al. 2005). Synthetically derived DP[^{14}C]A and an array of synthetic acceptors have determined that DPA provides Ara*f* units in the in vitro formation of 2-linked, 3-linked, and 5-linked arabinofuranosyl linkages present in the arabinans of AG and LAM (Belanger et al. 1996; Lee et al. 1997; Xin et al. 1997).

Because DPA is such an indispensable molecule required for mycobacterial cell wall biosynthesis, the elucidation of the biosynthetic pathway leading to its formation has received much attention. Classical biosynthesis of such polyprenylphosphate sugars chiefly involves the donation of a glycosyl residue from an activated sugar nucleotide donor to a polyprenylphosphate substrate. Interestingly sugar nucleotides of arabinose (UDP-Ara or GDP-Ara) have not been identified in mycobacteria. Instead, the carbon skeleton of the arabinosyl residues are derived from 5-phosphoribosyl-1-pyrophosphate (pRpp), a metabolite that emerges from the nonoxidative pentose shunt pathway (Scherman et al. 1995). *M. tuberculosis* has a single pRpp synthetase, which is responsible for the formation of pRpp and uses both ribose 5-phosphate and ATP as its substrates (Alderwick et al. 2011). The 5-phospho-α-D-ribose-1-pyrophosphate:decaprenyl phosphate 5-phosphoribosyl transferase (Rv3806c), also annotated as UbiA, transfers the ribose-5-phosphate moiety from pRpp to decaprenylphosphate, ultimately forming decaprenylphosphoryl-5-β-D-phosphoribofuranose (DPPR) (Huang et al. 2005, 2008). The essentiality of UbiA was highlighted in a study that used *Corynebacterium glutamicum* as a model organism to investigate the molecular genetics of mycobacterial D-arabinan biosynthesis. A *ubiA*-deficient strain of *C. glutamicum* resulted in a cell wall phenotype that was completely devoid of arabinose, giving incontrovertible evidence that DPA is indeed the only Ara*f* donor for D-arabinan biosynthesis (Alderwick et al. 2005, 2006a). DPPR is dephosphorylated to decaprenylphosphoryl-β-D-ribofuranose (DPR) by a phosphatase enzyme encoded by Rv3807c. Genetic deletion and subsequent phenotypic studies of the *M. smegmatis* homolog (MSMEG6402) suggest that although this gene is not essential, its enzymatic function is required to enable cell wall biosynthesis to continue unabated (Jiang et al. 2011). At this point, DPR is epimerized to DPA in a two-step epimerization process that involves two enzymes, DprE1 and DprE2. DprE1, encoded by *rv3790*, is an oxidoreductase that serves to oxidize the C-2 hydroxyl of the ribose moiety of DPR to form decaprenylphosphoryl-2-keto-β-D-erythro-pentofuranose (DPK), which is an intermediate metabolite of this essential pathway (Mikusova et al. 2005). DprE2, encoded by *rv3791*, then reduces the C2-keto of DPK, resulting in the complete synthesis of the sole Ara*f* donor, DPA (Mikusova et al. 2005).

At this point, it is worth giving special attention to DprE1, primarily because several recent chemical biology studies have shown that this enzyme is particularly susceptible to inhibition by a variety of small-molecule inhibitors that also show potent antimycobacterial activity. Benzothiazinones (BTZs) are a new class of sulfur-containing heterocyclic compounds that kill *M. tuberculosis* with nanomolar potency by targeting DprE1 (Makarov et al. 2009). Several biochemical and structural biology studies have shown that BTZs are suicide inhibitors, whereby BTZ is activated by DprE1, a FAD-dependent enzyme, forming a covalent semimercaptal bond with a key active-site cystine residue (Trefzer et al. 2010, 2012; Batt et al. 2012). Subsequent high-throughput screening and high-content screening experiments have revealed that DprE1 is an extremely "druggable" enzyme, with molecules such as the dinitrobenzamides (DNBs), nitrotriazoles, pyrazolopyridones, azaindoles, and a benzothiazoles (TCA1) (Christophe et al. 2009; Stanley et al. 2012; Shirude et al. 2013; Wang et al. 2013; Panda et al. 2014).

Because of the apparent vulnerability of DprE1 as a key enzyme in cell wall biosynthesis, it has been lauded by many within the mycobacterial research community as a "magic drug target." Targeting D-arabinan biosynthesis ultimately results in the removal of covalent linkage between peptidoglycan and the outer mycolate layers and is a salutary approach to the development of new antimycobacterial agents. However, this is insufficient evidence to explain the vulnerable nature of DprE1 as a "magic drug target." A recent investigation into the vulnerability of DprE1 as a drug target showed that the primary consequence of DprE1 inhibition is not simply the loss of DPA formation, rather it is the accumulation of DPR in the cytoplasmic membrane that induces synthetic lethality, depleting the TB bacilli of the limited supply of decaprenylphosphate that is required for both AG and PG biosynthesis to proceed unhindered (Grover et al. 2014). As we shall see, a variety of membrane-bound arabinofuranosyltransferases are required to assemble D-arabinan on the periplasmic face of the cytoplasmic membrane. Because DPA is synthesized on the inner leaflet of the cytoplasmic membrane, it is necessary for DPA to be translocated to position this Ara*f* donor in the correct orientation. Rv3789 has been identified as a DPA flippase responsible for this activity (Larrouy-Maumus et al. 2012).

Galactan Biosynthesis

The assortment of glycosyl linkages within the galactan moiety leads to the supposition that at least two Gal*f* transferases (GalTs) are required for its complete biosynthesis. GlfT1 (Rv3782) is classified as an inverting glycosyltransferase-2 (GT-2) of the GT-A superfamily, and it is recognized as the GalT responsible for the initial transfer of two Gal*f* residues, using UDP-Gal*f* as a substrate, to form both C_{50}-P-P-GlcNAc-Rha-Gal*f* (GL-3) and C_{50}-P-P-GlcNAc-Rha-Gal*f*-Gal*f* (GL-4) (Mikusova et al. 2006; Alderwick et al. 2008). Using a novel neoglycolipid acceptor assay that contained isolated *E. coli* membranes expressing GlfT2 (Rv3808c), it was shown that this enzyme has dual functionality, acting both as a UDP-Gal*f*:β-D-(1 → 5) GalT and UDP-Gal*f*:β-D-(1 → 6) GalT, responsible for the polymerization of approximately 30 Gal*f* residues with alternating β(1 → 5) and β(1 → 6) linkages (Kremer et al. 2001; Mikusova et al. 2006). Apart from being a bifunctional GalT, GlfT2 displays additional interesting features: By using a substrate tethering mechanism, it is able to have intrinsic control of the chain length of the galactan product (May et al. 2009). Further structural analysis of GlfT2 using X-ray crystallography and NMR has shed further light on how this unique enzyme is tetrameric and is able to control chain length processivity and bifunctionality using a single active site (Szczepina et al. 2009; Wheatley et al. 2012).

Arabinan Biosynthesis

A Brief Digression on Ethambutol. As discussed earlier, D-arabinan is a pivotal scaffold structure, which serves to covalently connect PG to the outer mycolic acid layer. Its biosynthesis is also targeted by the frontline drug ethambutol (EMB). EMB is a synthetic compound that was first recognized as an antimycobacterial agent in 1961 (Thomas et al. 1961). Early work by Kilburn and Greenberg observed an unanticipated increase in viable cells during the initial 4 h after addition of EMB to *M. smegmatis* cultures (Kilburn and Takayama 1981). It was postulated that large bacillary clusters disaggregated because of a possible reduction in lipid content, which would lead to the apparent increase in colony-forming units (CFUs) (Kilburn and Takayama 1981). This theory was supported by Takayama and coworkers who conducted a series of early studies into the effects of the EMB on *M. smegmatis*, reporting that inhibition of mycolic acid transfer into the cell wall and the simultaneous accumulation of trehalose-monomycolate (TMM), trehalose-dimycolate (TDM), and free mycolic acids occurred within 15 min of drug administration, suggesting that the target may be a mycolytransferase responsible for the transfer of mycolic acids onto the arabinan polymer (Takayama et al. 1979; Kilburn and Takayama 1981). However, it was later discovered, from observing the incorporation of [^{14}C]glucose into the cell wall D-arabinose monomers, that EMB inhibits the formation of D-arabinan (Takayama and Kilburn 1989), whereas synthesis of D-galactan of AG remained unaffected (Mikusova et al. 1995). A major breakthrough in the discovery of the precise EMB cellular target arose through exploitation of a moderately resistant strain from the related *Mycobacterium avium* species. A genomic library from the aforementioned strain was screened and overexpressed in an otherwise susceptible *M. smegmatis* host, leading to the identification of a resistance-conferring region encompassing three complete open reading frames (ORFs), *embR*, *embA*, and *embB* (Belanger et al. 1996). Moreover, use of an EMB-sensitive cell-free arabinan biosynthetic assay showed that arabinosyltransferase activity was restored with *embAB* overexpression. Interestingly, neither *embA* or *embB* alone was sufficient to confer multicopy resistance, thus supporting the supposition that they are translationally coupled, possibly forming a multienzyme complex (Belanger et al. 1996). EMB resistance was also used to identify the *embCAB* gene cluster from *M. smegmatis*, which was subsequently characterized in *M. tuberculosis* and *M. leprae*, all of which possess the same syntenic organization and encode homologs of the *embA* and *embB* genes from *M. avium* (Lety et al. 1997; Telenti et al. 1997). Escuyer et al. (2001) created individual genetic knockouts in *M. smegmatis*, *embC*, *embA*, and *embB*, all of which were viable, with the most profound effects observed in the *embB* mutant. Individual inactivation of *embA* and *embB* resulted in the diminished incorporation of arabinose into AG, specifically, the terminal disaccharide β-D-Ara*f* –(1 → 2)-α-D-Ara*f*, normally situated on the 3-OH of the 3,5-linked Ara*f* residue.

Identification of Novel Arabinofuranosyltransferases and the Use of C. glutamicum *and* M. smegmatis *as Model Organisms*

The Emb proteins, although novel, possess membrane topologies consistent with other glycosyltransferases (GTs) that use lipid-linked precursors, and do not resemble the more typical nucleotide-diphosphate (NDP) sugar donor requiring GTs. To date, the carbohydrate-active enzymes (CAZy) database has classified GTs into approximately 95 families with three large structural superfamilies, GT-A, GT-B, and GT-C (Liu and Mushegian 2003). GT-A and GT-B enzymes use NDP-sugar donors and are either globular or peripheral membrane proteins. The GT-C superfamily are large integral membrane proteins, all of which contain eight to 13 predicted transmembrane (TM) domains, with typically low sequence similarity but a conserved amino acid motif, called the DxD motif, generally positioned in the first or second predicted extracytoplasmic loop, and is thought to be required for binding the polyprenylphosphosugar substrate (Berg et al. 2007). The Emb proteins have been classified as GT-Cs, comprising approximately 1100 amino acids and 12–13 TM-spanning regions (Berg et al. 2005; Seidel et al. 2007b). Efforts to generate viable *embA*/*embB* mutants in *M. tuberculosis* and an *embAB* double mutant in *M. smegmatis* have so far proven unfruitful, highlighting their essentiality in mycobacteria. The Corynebacterianeae taxon encompasses *Mycobacterium* species as well as *Corynebacterium* species, such as *Corynebacterium diphtheriae* and *C. glutamicum*. *Corynebacterium* are deemed the archetype of Corynebacterianeae, and because they maintain a low frequency of gene duplications and modifications, they also possess a cell wall core remarkably similar to *M. tuberculosis* and have served as a useful tool and model organism to study otherwise essential orthologous *M. tuberculosis* genes. Alderwick et al.

(2005) successfully constructed a *C. glutamicum* mutant with its singular *emb* gene disrupted (Cg-*emb*), and subsequent phenotypic analyses of this mutant revealed an almost total loss of cell wall arabinan, except for terminal *t*-Ara*f* residues decorating the galactan backbone. Moreover, EMB treatment of wild-type *C. glutamicum* produced a profile identical to that of the mutant, illustrating that Cg-*emb* is indeed the target of EMB and furthermore that another AraT responsible for "priming" the galactan backbone must exist. As described earlier, disruption of the 5-phospho-α-D-ribose-1-pyrophosphate: decaprenyl phosphate 5-phosphoribosyl transferase ortholog (Cg-*ubiA*), resulted in total ablation of Ara*f* residues, indicating that the unidentified AraTwas also DPA-dependent (Alderwick et al. 2005). This pioneering study paved the way for the discovery of several novel GT-C arabinofuransyltransferases, each of which plays key roles in D-arabinan biosynthesis. AftA was identified as the enzyme responsible for priming the 8th, 10th, and 12th Gal*f* residues of the galactan backbone, which are elongated by the Emb proteins in an α(1 → 5)-linked fashion (Alderwick et al. 2006b). The *M. smegmatis* AftA homolog (MSMEG_6386) could only be chromosomally deleted in a merodiploid strain, highlighting its essentiality in mycobacteria (Shi et al. 2008). Both *C. glutamicum* and *M. smegmatis* model systems were used in combination to identify AftC as the enzyme responsible for introducing α(1 → 3) Ara*f* linkages into D-arabinan of AG and lipoarabinomannan (LAM) (Birch et al. 2008, 2010). Standing at 1400 amino acids in length and with a molecular mass of ~150 kDa, AftD represents the largest of the GT-C AraTs present in *M. tuberculosis.* It has been shown that AftD shows α(1 → 3) Ara*f* transferase activity, but because of its disproportionally large size, is speculated to have additional functions, such as being a scaffold protein for the recruitment of additional cell wall biosynthetic enzymes (Skovierova et al. 2009). Again, *C. glutamicum* was used to identify AftB as the enzyme that transfers terminal β(1 → 2) Ara*f* residues into the nonreducing Ara_6 motif of AG, thus bringing AG biosynthesis to a halt (Seidel et al. 2007a).

REFERENCES

Adam A, Petit JF, Wietzerbin-Falszpan J, Sinay P, Thomas DW, Lederer E. 1969. L'acide *N*-glycolylmuramique, constituant des parois de *Mycobacterium smegmatis*: Identification par spectrometrie de masse. *FEBS Lett* **4:** 87–92.

Alderwick LJ, Radmacher E, Seidel M, Gande R, Hitchen PG, Morris HR, Dell A, Sahm H, Eggeling L, Besra GS. 2005. Deletion of Cg-emb in Corynebacterianeae leads to a novel truncated cell wall arabinogalactan, whereas inactivation of Cg-ubiA results in an arabinan-deficient mutant with a cell wall galactan core. *J Biol Chem* **280:** 32362–32371.

Alderwick LJ, Dover LG, Seidel M, Gande R, Sahm H, Eggeling L, Besra GS. 2006a. Arabinan-deficient mutants of *Corynebacterium glutamicum* and the consequent flux in decaprenylmonophosphoryl-D-arabinose metabolism. *Glycobiology* **16:** 1073–1081.

Alderwick LJ, Seidel M, Sahm H, Besra GS, Eggeling L. 2006b. Identification of a novel arabinofuranosyltransferase (AftA) involved in cell wall arabinan biosynthesis in *Mycobacterium tuberculosis. J Biol Chem* **281:** 15653–15661.

Alderwick LJ, Dover LG, Veerapen N, Gurcha SS, Kremer L, Roper DL, Pathak AK, Reynolds RC, Besra GS. 2008. Expression, purification and characterisation of soluble GlfT and the identification of a novel galactofuranosyltransferase Rv3782 involved in priming GlfT-mediated galactan polymerisation in *Mycobacterium tuberculosis. Protein Expr Purif* **58:** 332–341.

Alderwick LJ, Lloyd GS, Lloyd AJ, Lovering AL, Eggeling L, Besra GS. 2011. Biochemical characterization of the *Mycobacterium tuberculosis* phosphoribosyl-1-pyrophosphate synthetase. *Glycobiology* **21:** 410–425.

Amar C, Vilkas E. 1973. [Isolation of arabinose phosphate from the walls of *Mycobacterium tuberculosis* H 37 Ra]. *C R Acad Sci Hebd Seances Acad Sci D* **277:** 1949–1951.

Amer AO, Valvano MA. 2002. Conserved aspartic acids are essential for the enzymic activity of the WecA protein initiating the biosynthesis of *O*-specific lipopolysaccharide and enterobacterial common antigen in *Escherichia coli. Microbiology* **148:** 571–582.

Anthony KG, Strych U, Yeung KR, Shoen CS, Perez O, Krause KL, Cynamon MH, Aristoff PA, Koski RA. 2011. New classes of alanine racemase inhibitors identified by high-throughput screening show antimicrobial activity against *Mycobacterium tuberculosis. PLoS ONE* **6:** e20374.

Azuma I, Kimura H, Niinaka T, Aoki T, Yamamura Y. 1968. Chemical and immunological studies on mycobacterial polysaccharides. 1. Purification and properties of polysaccharides from human tubercle bacilli. *J Bacteriol* **95:** 263–271.

Babaoglu K, Page MA, Jones VC, McNeil MR, Dong C, Naismith JH, Lee RE. 2003. Novel inhibitors of an emerging target in *Mycobacterium tuberculosis*; substituted thiazolidinones as inhibitors of dTDP-rhamnose synthesis. *Bioorg Med Chem Lett* **13:** 3227–3230.

Barreteau H, Kovac A, Boniface A, Sova M, Gobec S, Blanot D. 2008. Cytoplasmic steps of peptidoglycan biosynthesis. *FEMS Microbiol Rev* **32:** 168–207.

Basavannacharya C, Moody PR, Munshi T, Cronin N, Keep NH, Bhakta S. 2010a. Essential residues for the enzyme activity of ATP-dependent MurE ligase from *Mycobacterium tuberculosis*. *Protein Cell* **1:** 1011–1022.

Basavannacharya C, Robertson G, Munshi T, Keep NH, Bhakta S. 2010b. ATP-dependent MurE ligase in *Mycobacterium tuberculosis*: Biochemical and structural characterisation. *Tuberculosis (Edinb)* **90:** 16–24.

Batt SM, Jabeen T, Bhowruth V, Quill L, Lund PA, Eggeling L, Alderwick LJ, Futterer K, Besra GS. 2012. Structural basis of inhibition of *Mycobacterium tuberculosis* DprE1 by benzothiazinone inhibitors. *Proc Natl Acad Sci* **109:** 11354–11359.

Belanger AE, Besra GS, Ford ME, Mikusova K, Belisle JT, Brennan PJ, Inamine JM. 1996. The embAB genes of *Mycobacterium avium* encode an arabinosyl transferase involved in cell wall arabinan biosynthesis that is the target for the antimycobacterial drug ethambutol. *Proc Natl Acad Sci* **93:** 11919–11924.

Berg S, Starbuck J, Torrelles JB, Vissa VD, Crick DC, Chatterjee D, Brennan PJ. 2005. Roles of conserved proline and glycosyltransferase motifs of EmbC in biosynthesis of lipoarabinomannan. *J Biol Chem* **280:** 5651–5663.

Berg S, Kaur D, Jackson M, Brennan PJ. 2007. The glycosyltransferases of *Mycobacterium tuberculosis*—Roles in the synthesis of arabinogalactan, lipoarabinomannan, and other glycoconjugates. *Glycobiology* **17:** 35–56R.

Besra GS, Khoo KH, McNeil MR, Dell A, Morris HR, Brennan PJ. 1995. A new interpretation of the structure of the mycolyl-arabinogalactan complex of *Mycobacterium tuberculosis* as revealed through characterization of oligoglycosylalditol fragments by fast-atom bombardment mass spectrometry and 1H nuclear magnetic resonance spectroscopy. *Biochemistry* **34:** 4257–4266.

Bhamidi S, Scherman MS, Rithner CD, Prenni JE, Chatterjee D, Khoo KH, McNeil MR. 2008. The identification and location of succinyl residues and the characterization of the interior arabinan region allow for a model of the complete primary structure of *Mycobacterium tuberculosis* mycolyl arabinogalactan. *J Biol Chem* **283:** 12992–13000.

Birch HL, Alderwick LJ, Bhatt A, Rittmann D, Krumbach K, Singh A, Bai Y, Lowary TL, Eggeling L, Besra GS. 2008. Biosynthesis of mycobacterial arabinogalactan: Identification of a novel $\alpha(1\rightarrow3)$ arabinofuranosyltransferase. *Mol Microbiol* **69:** 1191–1206.

Birch HL, Alderwick LJ, Appelmelk BJ, Maaskant J, Bhatt A, Singh A, Nigou J, Eggeling L, Geurtsen J, Besra GS. 2010. A truncated lipoglycan from mycobacteria with altered immunological properties. *Proc Natl Acad Sci* **107:** 2634–2639.

Bouhss A, Dementin S, van Heijenoort J, Parquet C, Blanot D. 1999. Formation of adenosine 5′-tetraphosphate from the acyl phosphate intermediate: A difference between the MurC and MurD synthetases of *Escherichia coli*. *FEBS Lett* **453:** 15–19.

Brennan PJ, Nikaido H. 1995. The envelope of mycobacteria. *Annu Rev Biochem* **64:** 29–63.

Butler EK, Davis RM, Bari V, Nicholson PA, Ruiz N. 2013. Structure-function analysis of MurJ reveals a solvent-exposed cavity containing residues essential for peptidoglycan biogenesis in *Escherichia coli*. *J Bacteriol* **195:** 4639–4649.

Calvanese L, Falcigno L, Maglione C, Marasco D, Ruggiero A, Squeglia F, Berisio R, D'Auria G. 2014. Structural and binding properties of the PASTA domain of PonA2, a key penicillin binding protein from *Mycobacterium tuberculosis*. *Biopolymers* **101:** 712–719.

Chatterjee D, Bozic CM, McNeil M, Brennan PJ. 1991. Structural features of the arabinan component of the lipoarabinomannan of *Mycobacterium tuberculosis*. *J Biol Chem* **266:** 9652–9660.

Chen KT, Kuan YC, Fu WC, Liang PH, Cheng TJ, Wong CH, Cheng WC. 2013. Rapid preparation of mycobacterium *N*-glycolyl Lipid I and Lipid II derivatives: A biocatalytic approach. *Chemistry* **19:** 834–838.

Christophe T, Jackson M, Jeon HK, Fenistein D, Contreras-Dominguez M, Kim J, Genovesio A, Carralot JP, Ewann F, Kim EH, et al. 2009. High content screening identifies decaprenyl-phosphoribose 2′ epimerase as a target for intracellular antimycobacterial inhibitors. *PLoS Pathog* **5:** e1000645.

Correale S, Ruggiero A, Capparelli R, Pedone E, Berisio R. 2013. Structures of free and inhibited forms of the L,D-transpeptidase LdtMt1 from *Mycobacterium tuberculosis*. *Acta Crystallogr D Biol Crystallogr* **69:** 1697–1706.

Daffé M, Brennan PJ, McNeil M. 1990. Predominant structural features of the cell wall arabinogalactan of *Mycobacterium tuberculosis* as revealed through characterization of oligoglycosyl alditol fragments by gas chromatography/mass spectrometry and by ^{1}H and ^{13}C NMR analyses. *J Biol Chem* **265:** 6734–6743.

Dasgupta A, Datta P, Kundu M, Basu J. 2006. The serine/threonine kinase PknB of *Mycobacterium tuberculosis* phosphorylates PBPA, a penicillin-binding protein required for cell division. *Microbiology* **152:** 493–504.

De Smet KA, Kempsell KE, Gallagher A, Duncan K, Young DB. 1999. Alteration of a single amino acid residue reverses fosfomycin resistance of recombinant MurA from *Mycobacterium tuberculosis*. *Microbiology* **145:** 3177–3184.

Dmitriev BA, Ehlers S, Rietschel ET, Brennan PJ. 2000. Molecular mechanics of the mycobacterial cell wall: From horizontal layers to vertical scaffolds. *Int J Med Microbiol* **290:** 251–258.

Dmitriev BA, Toukach FV, Schaper KJ, Holst O, Rietschel ET, Ehlers S. 2003. Tertiary structure of bacterial murein: The scaffold model. *J Bacteriol* **185:** 3458–3468.

Draper P, Khoo KH, Chatterjee D, Dell A, Morris HR. 1997. Galactosamine in walls of slow-growing mycobacteria. *Biochem J* **327:** 519–525.

Durand P, Golinelli-Pimpaneau B, Mouilleron S, Badet B, Badet-Denisot MA. 2008. Highlights of glucosamine-6P synthase catalysis. *Arch Biochem Biophys* **474:** 302–317.

Escuyer VE, Lety MA, Torrelles JB, Khoo KH, Tang JB, Rithner CD, Frehel C, McNeil MR, Brennan PJ, Chatterjee D. 2001. The role of the *embA* and *embB* gene products in the biosynthesis of the terminal hexaarabinofuranosyl motif of *Mycobacterium smegmatis* arabinogalactan. *J Biol Chem* **276:** 48854–48862.

Essers L, Schoop HJ. 1978. Evidence for the incorporation of molecular oxygen, a pathway in biosynthesis of N-glycolylmuramic acid in *Mycobacterium phlei*. *Biochim Biophys Acta* **544:** 180–184.

Falk PJ, Ervin KM, Volk KS, Ho HT. 1996. Biochemical evidence for the formation of a covalent acyl-phosphate linkage between UDP-*N*-acetylmuramate and ATP in the *Escherichia coli* UDP-*N*-acetylmuramate:L-alanine ligase-catalyzed reaction. *Biochemistry* **35:** 1417–1422.

Feng Z, Barletta RG. 2003. Roles of *Mycobacterium smegmatis* D-alanine:D-alanine ligase and D-alanine racemase in the mechanisms of action of and resistance to the peptidoglycan inhibitor D-cycloserine. *Antimicrob Agents Chemother* **47:** 283–291.

Gateau O, Bordet C, Michel G. 1976. [Study of the formation of *N*-glycolylmuramic acid from *Nocardia asteroides* (author's transl)]. *Biochim Biophys Acta* **421:** 395–405.

Ghuysen JM. 1968. Use of bacteriolytic enzymes in determination of wall structure and their role in cell metabolism. *Bacteriol Rev* **32:** 425–464.

Grover S, Alderwick LJ, Mishra AK, Krumbach K, Marienhagen J, Eggeling L, Bhatt A, Besra GS. 2014. Benzothiazinones mediate killing of Corynebacterineae by blocking decaprenyl phosphate recycling involved in cell wall biosynthesis. *J Biol Chem* **289:** 6177–6187.

Gupta R, Lavollay M, Mainardi JL, Arthur M, Bishai WR, Lamichhane G. 2010. The *Mycobacterium tuberculosis* protein LdtMt2 is a nonclassical transpeptidase required for virulence and resistance to amoxicillin. *Nat Med* **16:** 466–469.

Hett EC, Chao MC, Rubin EJ. 2010. Interaction and modulation of two antagonistic cell wall enzymes of mycobacteria. *PLoS Pathog* **6:** e1001020.

Hoang TT, Ma Y, Stern RJ, McNeil MR, Schweizer HP. 1999. Construction and use of low-copy number T7 expression vectors for purification of problem proteins: Purification of *Mycobacterium tuberculosis* RmlD and pseudomonas aeruginosa LasI and RhlI proteins, and functional analysis of purified RhlI. *Gene* **237:** 361–371.

Huang H, Scherman MS, D'Haeze W, Vereecke D, Holsters M, Crick DC, McNeil MR. 2005. Identification and active expression of the *Mycobacterium tuberculosis* gene encoding 5-phospho-{α}-D-ribose-1-diphosphate: decaprenyl-phosphate 5-phosphoribosyltransferase, the first enzyme committed to decaprenylphosphoryl-d-arabinose synthesis. *J Biol Chem* **280:** 24539–24543.

Huang H, Berg S, Spencer JS, Vereecke D, D'Haeze W, Holsters M, McNeil MR. 2008. Identification of amino acids and domains required for catalytic activity of DPPR synthase, a cell wall biosynthetic enzyme of *Mycobacterium tuberculosis*. *Microbiology* **154:** 736–743.

Ishizaki Y, Hayashi C, Inoue K, Igarashi M, Takahashi Y, Pujari V, Crick DC, Brennan PJ, Nomoto A. 2013. Inhibition of the first step in synthesis of the mycobacterial cell wall core, catalyzed by the GlcNAc-1-phosphate transferase WecA, by the novel caprazamycin derivative CPZEN-45. *J Biol Chem* **288:** 30309–30319.

Jagtap PK, Soni V, Vithani N, Jhingan GD, Bais VS, Nandicoori VK, Prakash B. 2012. Substrate-bound crystal structures reveal features unique to *Mycobacterium tuberculosis* *N*-acetyl-glucosamine 1-phosphate uridyltransferase and a catalytic mechanism for acetyl transfer. *J Biol Chem* **287:** 39524–39537.

Jagtap PK, Verma SK, Vithani N, Bais VS, Prakash B. 2013. Crystal structures identify an atypical two-metal-ion mechanism for uridyltransfer in GlmU: Its significance to sugar nucleotidyl transferases. *J Mol Biol* **425:** 1745–1759.

Jha RK, Katagihallimath N, Hota SK, Das KS, de Sousa SM. 2012. An assay for exogenous sources of purified MurG, enabled by the complementation of *Escherichia coli* murG(Ts) by the *Mycobacterium tuberculosis* homologue. *FEMS Microbiol Lett* **326:** 161–167.

Jiang T, He L, Zhan Y, Zang S, Ma Y, Zhao X, Zhang C, Xin Y. 2011. The effect of MSMEG_6402 gene disruption on the cell wall structure of *Mycobacterium smegmatis*. *Microb Pathog* **51:** 156–160.

Jin Y, Xin Y, Zhang W, Ma Y. 2010. *Mycobacterium tuberculosis* Rv1302 and *Mycobacterium smegmatis* MSMEG_4947 have WecA function and MSMEG_4947 is required for the growth of *M. smegmatis*. *FEMS Microbiol Lett* **310:** 54–61.

Kanetsuna F. 1968. Chemical analyses of mycobacterial cell walls. *Biochim Biophys Acta* **158:** 130–143.

Kanetsuna F, Imaeda T, Cunto G. 1969. On the linkage between mycolic acid and arabinogalactan in phenol-treated myobacterial cell walls. *Biochim Biophys Acta* **173:** 341–344.

Kantardjieff KA, Kim CY, Naranjo C, Waldo GS, Lekin T, Segelke BW, Zemla A, Park MS, Terwilliger TC, Rupp B. 2004. *Mycobacterium tuberculosis* RmlC epimerase (Rv3465): A promising drug-target structure in the rhamnose pathway. *Acta Crystallogr D Biol Crystallogr* **60:** 895–902.

Kilburn JO, Takayama K. 1981. Effects of ethambutol on accumulation and secretion of trehalose mycolates and free mycolic acid in *Mycobacterium smegmatis*. *Antimicrob Agents Chemother* **20:** 401–404.

Kim DH, Lees WJ, Kempsell KE, Lane WS, Duncan K, Walsh CT. 1996. Characterization of a Cys115 to Asp substitution in the *Escherichia coli* cell wall biosynthetic enzyme UDP-GlcNAc enolpyruvyl transferase (MurA) that confers resistance to inactivation by the antibiotic fosfomycin. *Biochemistry* **35:** 4923–4928.

Kim HS, Kim J, Im HN, Yoon JY, An DR, Yoon HJ, Kim JY, Min HK, Kim SJ, Lee JY, et al. 2013. Structural basis for the inhibition of *Mycobacterium tuberculosis* L,D-transpeptidase by meropenem, a drug effective against extensively drug-resistant strains. *Acta Crystallogr D Biol Crystallogr* **69:** 420–431.

Kremer L, Dover LG, Morehouse C, Hitchin P, Everett M, Morris HR, Dell A, Brennan PJ, McNeil MR, Flaherty C, et al. 2001. Galactan biosynthesis in *Mycobacterium tuberculosis*. Identification of a bifunctional UDP-galactofuranosyltransferase. *J Biol Chem* **276:** 26430–26440.

Kumar V, Saravanan P, Arvind A, Mohan CG. 2011. Identification of hotspot regions of MurB oxidoreductase enzyme using homology modeling, molecular dynamics and molecular docking techniques. *J Mol Model* **17:** 939–953.

Larrouy-Maumus G, Skovierova H, Dhouib R, Angala SK, Zuberogoitia S, Pham H, Villela AD, Mikusova K, Noguera A, Gilleron M, et al. 2012. A small multidrug resistance-like transporter involved in the arabinosylation of arabinogalactan and lipoarabinomannan in mycobacteria. *J Biol Chem* **287:** 39933–39941.

Lederer E, Adam A, Ciorbaru R, Petit JF, Wietzerbin J. 1975. Cell walls of mycobacteria and related organisms; chemistry and immunostimulant properties. *Mol Cell Biochem* **7:** 87–104.

Lee RE, Brennan PJ, Besra GS. 1997. *Mycobacterial arabinan* biosynthesis: The use of synthetic arabinoside acceptors in the development of an arabinosyl transfer assay. *Glycobiology* **7:** 1121–1128.

Lee A, Wu SW, Scherman MS, Torrelles JB, Chatterjee D, McNeil MR, Khoo KH. 2006. Sequencing of oligoarabinosyl units released from mycobacterial arabinogalactan by endogenous arabinanase: Identification of distinctive and novel structural motifs. *Biochemistry* **45:** 15817–15828.

Lee Y, Mootien S, Shoen C, Destefano M, Cirillo P, Asojo OA, Yeung KR, Ledizet M, Cynamon MH, Aristoff PA, et al. 2013. Inhibition of mycobacterial alanine racemase activity and growth by thiadiazolidinones. *Biochem Pharmacol* **86:** 222–230.

Lehrer J, Vigeant KA, Tatar LD, Valvano MA. 2007. Functional characterization and membrane topology of *Escherichia coli* WecA, a sugar-phosphate transferase initiating the biosynthesis of enterobacterial common antigen and *O*-antigen lipopolysaccharide. *J Bacteriol* **189:** 2618–2628.

Lemaire HG, Muller-Hill B. 1986. Nucleotide sequences of the *gal E* gene and the *gal T* gene of *E. coli*. *Nucleic Acids Res* **14:** 7705–7711.

Lety MA, Nair S, Berche P, Escuyer V. 1997. A single point mutation in the embB gene is responsible for resistance to ethambutol in *Mycobacterium smegmatis*. *Antimicrob Agents Chemother* **41:** 2629–2633.

Li W, Xin Y, McNeil MR, Ma Y. 2006. rmlB and rmlC genes are essential for growth of mycobacteria. *Biochem Biophys Res Commun* **342:** 170–178.

Li Y, Zhou Y, Ma Y, Li X. 2011. Design and synthesis of novel cell wall inhibitors of *Mycobacterium tuberculosis* GlmM and GlmU. *Carbohydr Res* **346:** 1714–1720.

Li S, Kang J, Yu W, Zhou Y, Zhang W, Xin Y, Ma Y. 2012. Identification of *M. tuberculosis* Rv3441c and *M. smegmatis* MSMEG_1556 and essentiality of *M. smegmatis* MSMEG_1556. *PLoS ONE* **7:** e42769.

Li WJ, Li DF, Hu YL, Zhang XE, Bi LJ, Wang DC. 2013. Crystal structure of L,D-transpeptidase LdtMt2 in complex with meropenem reveals the mechanism of carbapenem against *Mycobacterium tuberculosis*. *Cell Res* **23:** 728–731.

Liu TY, Gotschlich EC. 1967. Muramic acid phosphate as a component of the mucopeptide of Gram-positive bacteria. *J Biol Chem* **242:** 471–476.

Liu J, Mushegian A. 2003. Three monophyletic superfamilies account for the majority of the known glycosyltransferases. *Protein Sci* **12:** 1418–1431.

Ma Y, Mills JA, Belisle JT, Vissa V, Howell M, Bowlin K, Scherman MS, McNeil M. 1997. Determination of the pathway for rhamnose biosynthesis in mycobacteria: Cloning, sequencing and expression of the *Mycobacterium tuberculosis* gene encoding α-D-glucose-1-phosphate thymidylyltransferase. *Microbiology* **143:** 937–945.

Ma Y, Stern RJ, Scherman MS, Vissa VD, Yan W, Jones VC, Zhang F, Franzblau SG, Lewis WH, McNeil MR. 2001. Drug targeting *Mycobacterium tuberculosis* cell wall synthesis: Genetics of dTDP-rhamnose synthetic enzymes and development of a microtiter plate-based screen for inhibitors of conversion of dTDP-glucose to dTDP-rhamnose. *Antimicrob Agents Chemother* **45:** 1407–1416.

Ma Y, Pan F, McNeil M. 2002. Formation of dTDP-rhamnose is essential for growth of mycobacteria. *J Bacteriol* **184:** 3392–3395.

Mahapatra S, Crick DC, Brennan PJ. 2000. Comparison of the UDP-*N*-acetylmuramate:L-alanine ligase enzymes from *Mycobacterium tuberculosis* and *Mycobacterium leprae*. *J Bacteriol* **182:** 6827–6830.

Mahapatra S, Scherman H, Brennan PJ, Crick DC. 2005. N Glycolylation of the nucleotide precursors of peptidoglycan biosynthesis of *Mycobacterium spp.* is altered by drug treatment. *J Bacteriol* **187:** 2341–2347.

Makarov V, Manina G, Mikusova K, Mollmann U, Ryabova O, Saint-Joanis B, Dhar N, Pasca MR, Buroni S, Lucarelli AP, et al. 2009. Benzothiazinones kill *Mycobacterium tuberculosis* by blocking arabinan synthesis. *Science* **324:** 801–804.

Matsuhashi M. 1966. [Biosynthesis in the bacterial cell wall]. *Tanpakushitsu Kakusan Koso* **11:** 875–886.

May JF, Splain RA, Brotschi C, Kiessling LL. 2009. A tethering mechanism for length control in a processive carbohydrate polymerization. *Proc Natl Acad Sci* **106:** 11851–11856.

McNeil M, Wallner SJ, Hunter SW, Brennan PJ. 1987. Demonstration that the galactosyl and arabinosyl residues in the cell-wall arabinogalactan of *Mycobacterium leprae* and *Mycobacterium tuberculosis* are furanoid. *Carbohydr Res* **166:** 299–308.

McNeil M, Daffe M, Brennan PJ. 1990. Evidence for the nature of the link between the arabinogalactan and peptidoglycan of mycobacterial cell walls. *J Biol Chem* **265:** 18200–18206.

McNeil M, Daffe M, Brennan PJ. 1991. Location of the mycolyl ester substituents in the cell walls of mycobacteria. *J Biol Chem* **266:** 13217–13223.

McNeil MR, Robuck KG, Harter M, Brennan PJ. 1994. Enzymatic evidence for the presence of a critical terminal hexa-arabinoside in the cell walls of *Mycobacterium tuberculosis*. *Glycobiology* **4:** 165–173.

Meroueh SO, Bencze KZ, Hesek D, Lee M, Fisher JF, Stemmler TL, Mobashery S. 2006. Three-dimensional structure of the bacterial cell wall peptidoglycan. *Proc Natl Acad Sci* **103:** 4404–4409.

Mikusova K, Slayden RA, Besra GS, Brennan PJ. 1995. Biogenesis of the mycobacterial cell wall and the site of action of ethambutol. *Antimicrob Agents Chemother* **39:** 2484–2489.

Mikusova K, Mikus M, Besra GS, Hancock I, Brennan PJ. 1996. Biosynthesis of the linkage region of the mycobacterial cell wall. *J Biol Chem* **271:** 7820–7828.

Mikusova K, Huang H, Yagi T, Holsters M, Vereecke D, D'Haeze W, Scherman MS, Brennan PJ, McNeil MR, Crick DC. 2005. Decaprenylphosphoryl arabinofuranose, the donor of the D-arabinofuranosyl residues of mycobacterial arabinan, is formed via a two-step epimerization of decaprenylphosphoryl ribose. *J Bacteriol* **187:** 8020–8025.

Mikusova K, Belanova M, Kordulakova J, Honda K, McNeil MR, Mahapatra S, Crick DC, Brennan PJ. 2006. Identification of a novel galactosyl transferase involved in biosynthesis of the mycobacterial cell wall. *J Bacteriol* **188:** 6592–6598.

Mills JA, Motichka K, Jucker M, Wu HP, Uhlik BC, Stern RJ, Scherman MS, Vissa VD, Pan F, Kundu M, et al. 2004. Inactivation of the mycobacterial rhamnosyltransferase, which is needed for the formation of the arabinogalactan-peptidoglycan linker, leads to irreversible loss of viability. *J Biol Chem* **279:** 43540–43546.

Minnikin DE. 1982. Lipids: Complex lipids, their chemistry, biosynthesis and roles. In *The biology of the mycobacteria* (eds. Ratledge C, Stanford J), pp. 95–184. Academic Press, London.

Minnikin DE, Kremer L, Dover LG, Besra GS. 2002. The methyl-branched fortifications of *Mycobacterium tuberculosis. Chem Biol* **9:** 545–553.

Misaki A, Yukawa S. 1966. Studies on cell walls of mycobacteria. II. Constitution of polysaccharides from BCG cell walls. *J Biochem (Tokyo)* **59:** 511–520.

Mohamed YF, Valvano MA. 2014. A *Burkholderia cenocepacia* MurJ (MviN) homolog is essential for cell wall peptidoglycan synthesis and bacterial viability. *Glycobiology* **24:** 564–576.

Mohammadi T, van Dam V, Sijbrandi R, Vernet T, Zapun A, Bouhss A, Diepeveen-de Bruin M, Nguyen-Disteche M, de Kruijff B, Breukink E. 2011. Identification of FtsW as a transporter of lipid-linked cell wall precursors across the membrane. *EMBO J* **30:** 1425–1432.

Nassau PM, Martin SL, Brown RE, Weston A, Monsey D, McNeil MR, Duncan K. 1996. Galactofuranose biosynthesis in *Escherichia coli* K-12: Identification and cloning of UDP-galactopyranose mutase. *J Bacteriol* **178:** 1047–1052.

Pan F, Jackson M, Ma Y, McNeil M. 2001. Cell wall core galactofuran synthesis is essential for growth of mycobacteria. *J Bacteriol* **183:** 3991–3998.

Panda M, Ramachandran S, Ramachandran V, Shirude PS, Humnabadkar V, Nagalapur K, Sharma S, Kaur P, Guptha S, Narayan A, et al. 2014. Discovery of pyrazolopyridones as a novel class of non-covalent DprE1 inhibitor with potent anti-mycobacterial activity. *J Med Chem.* **57:** 4761–4771.

Parikh A, Verma SK, Khan S, Prakash B, Nandicoori VK. 2009. PknB-mediated phosphorylation of a novel substrate, *N*-acetylglucosamine-1-phosphate uridyltransferase, modulates its acetyltransferase activity. *J Mol Biol* **386:** 451–464.

Patru MM, Pavelka MS Jr. 2010. A role for the class A penicillin-binding protein PonA2 in the survival of *Mycobacterium smegmatis* under conditions of nonreplication. *J Bacteriol* **192:** 3043–3054.

Peng W, Zou L, Bhamidi S, McNeil MR, Lowary TL. 2012. The galactosamine residue in mycobacterial arabinogalactan is α-linked. *J Org Chem* **77:** 9826–9832.

Petit JF, Adam A, Wietzerbin-Falszpan J, Lederer E, Ghuysen JM. 1969. Chemical structure of the cell wall of *Mycobacterium smegmatis*. I. Isolation and partial characterization of the peptidoglycan. *Biochem Biophys Res Commun* **35:** 478–485.

Plocinski P, Ziolkiewicz M, Kiran M, Vadrevu SI, Nguyen HB, Hugonnet J, Veckerle C, Arthur M, Dziadek J, Cross TA, et al. 2011. Characterization of CrgA, a new partner of the *Mycobacterium tuberculosis* peptidoglycan polymerization complexes. *J Bacteriol* **193:** 3246–3256.

Prosser GA, de Carvalho LP. 2013a. Kinetic mechanism and inhibition of *Mycobacterium tuberculosis* D-alanine:D-alanine ligase by the antibiotic D-cycloserine. *FEBS J* **280:** 1150–1166.

Prosser GA, de Carvalho LP. 2013b. Metabolomics reveal D-alanine:D-alanine ligase as the target of D-cycloserine. *ACS Med Chem Lett* **4:** 1233–1237.

Raymond JB, Mahapatra S, Crick DC, Pavelka MS Jr. 2005. Identification of the *namH* gene, encoding the hydroxylase responsible for the *N*-glycolylation of the mycobacterial peptidoglycan. *J Biol Chem* **280:** 326–333.

Ruiz N. 2008. Bioinformatics identification of MurJ (MviN) as the peptidoglycan lipid II flippase in *Escherichia coli. Proc Natl Acad Sci* **105:** 15553–15557.

Scherman M, Weston A, Duncan K, Whittington A, Upton R, Deng L, Comber R, Friedrich JD, McNeil M. 1995. Biosynthetic origin of mycobacterial cell wall arabinosyl residues. *J Bacteriol* **177:** 7125–7130.

Schleifer KH, Kandler O. 1972. Peptidoglycan types of bacterial cell walls and their taxonomic implications. *Bacteriol Rev* **36:** 407–477.

Schoonmaker MK, Bishai WR, Lamichhane G. 2014. Nonclassical transpeptidases of *Mycobacterium tuberculosis* alter cell size, morphology, the cytosolic matrix, protein localization, virulence, and resistance to β-lactams. *J Bacteriol* **196:** 1394–1402.

Seidel M, Alderwick LJ, Birch HL, Sahm H, Eggeling L, Besra GS. 2007a. Identification of a novel arabinofuranosyltransferase AftB involved in a terminal step of cell wall arabinan biosynthesis in Corynebacterianeae, such as *Corynebacterium glutamicum* and *Mycobacterium tuberculosis. J Biol Chem* **282:** 14729–14740.

Seidel M, Alderwick LJ, Sahm H, Besra GS, Eggeling L. 2007b. Topology and mutational analysis of the single Emb arabinofuranosyltransferase of *Corynebacterium glutamicum* as a model of Emb proteins of *Mycobacterium tuberculosis. Glycobiology* **17:** 210–219.

Shi L, Zhou R, Liu Z, Lowary TL, Seeberger PH, Stocker BL, Crick DC, Khoo KH, Chatterjee D. 2008. Transfer of the first arabinofuranose residue to galactan is essential for *Mycobacterium smegmatis* viability. *J Bacteriol* **190:** 5248–5255.

Shirude PS, Shandil R, Sadler C, Naik M, Hosagrahara V, Hameed S, Shinde V, Bathula C, Humnabadkar V, Kumar N, et al. 2013. Azaindoles: Noncovalent DprE1 inhibitors from scaffold morphing efforts, kill *Mycobacterium tuberculosis* and are efficacious in vivo. *J Med Chem* **56:** 9701–9708.

Sieger B, Schubert K, Donovan C, Bramkamp M. 2013. The lipid II flippase RodA determines morphology and growth in *Corynebacterium glutamicum. Mol Microbiol* **90:** 966–982.

Skovierova H, Larrouy-Maumus G, Zhang J, Kaur D, Barilone N, Kordulakova J, Gilleron M, Guadagnini S, Belanova M, Prevost MC, et al. 2009. AftD, a novel essential arabinofuranosyltransferase from mycobacteria. *Glycobiology* **19:** 1235–1247.

Stanley SA, Grant SS, Kawate T, Iwase N, Shimizu M, Wivagg C, Silvis M, Kazyanskaya E, Aquadro J, Golas A, et al. 2012. Identification of novel inhibitors of *M. tuberculosis* growth using whole cell based high-throughput screening. *ACS Chem Biol* **7:** 1377–1384.

Stern RJ, Lee TY, Lee TJ, Yan W, Scherman MS, Vissa VD, Kim SK, Wanner BL, McNeil MR. 1999. Conversion of dTDP-4-keto-6-deoxyglucose to free dTDP-4-ketorhamnose by the *rmlC* gene products of *Escherichia coli* and *Mycobacterium tuberculosis*. *Microbiology* **145:** 663–671.

Szczepina MG, Zheng RB, Completo GC, Lowary TL, Pinto BM. 2009. STD-NMR studies suggest that two acceptor substrates for GlfT2, a bifunctional galactofuranosyltransferase required for the biosynthesis of *Mycobacterium tuberculosis* arabinogalactan, compete for the same binding site. *Chembiochem* **10:** 2052–2059.

Takayama K, Armstrong EL, Kunugi KA, Kilburn JO. 1979. Inhibition by ethambutol of mycolic acid transfer into the cell wall of *Mycobacterium smegmatis*. *Antimicrob Agents Chemother* **16:** 240–242.

Takayama K, Kilburn JO. 1989. Inhibition of synthesis of arabinogalactan by ethambutol in *Mycobacterium smegmatis*. *Antimicrob Agents Chemother* **33:** 1493–1499.

Telenti A, Philipp WJ, Sreevatsan S, Bernasconi C, Stockbauer KE, Wieles B, Musser JM, Jacobs WR Jr. 1997. The emb operon, a gene cluster of *Mycobacterium tuberculosis* involved in resistance to ethambutol. *Nat Med* **3:** 567–570.

Thomas JP, Baughn CO, Wilkinson RG, Shepherd RG. 1961. A new synthetic compound with antituberculous activity in mice: Ethambutol (dextro-2,2′-(ethylenediimino)-di-l-butanol). *Am Rev Respir Dis* **83:** 891–893.

Trefzer C, Rengifo-Gonzalez M, Hinner MJ, Schneider P, Makarov V, Cole ST, Johnsson K. 2010. Benzothiazinones: Prodrugs that covalently modify the decaprenylphosphoryl-β-D-ribose 2′-epimerase DprE1 of *Mycobacterium tuberculosis*. *J Am Chem Soc* **132:** 13663–13665.

Trefzer C, Skovierova H, Buroni S, Bobovska A, Nenci S, Molteni E, Pojer F, Pasca MR, Makarov V, Cole ST, et al. 2012. Benzothiazinones are suicide inhibitors of mycobacterial decaprenylphosphoryl-β-D-ribofuranose 2′-oxidase DprE1. *J Am Chem Soc* **134:** 912–915.

Trunkfield AE, Gurcha SS, Besra GS, Bugg TD. 2010. Inhibition of *Escherichia coli* glycosyltransferase MurG and *Mycobacterium tuberculosis* Gal transferase by uridine-linked transition state mimics. *Bioorg Med Chem* **18:** 2651–2663.

van Heijenoort J. 2001. Formation of the glycan chains in the synthesis of bacterial peptidoglycan. *Glycobiology* **11:** 25R–36R.

Vollmer W, Holtje JV. 2004. The architecture of the murein (peptidoglycan) in gram-negative bacteria: Vertical scaffold or horizontal layer(s)? *J Bacteriol* **186:** 5978–5987.

Wang F, Sambandan D, Halder R, Wang J, Batt SM, Weinrick B, Ahmad I, Yang P, Zhang Y, Kim J, et al. 2013. Identification of a small molecule with activity against drug-resistant and persistent tuberculosis. *Proc Natl Acad Sci* **110:** E2510–E2517.

Weston A, Stern RJ, Lee RE, Nassau PM, Monsey D, Martin SL, Scherman MS, Besra GS, Duncan K, McNeil MR. 1997. Biosynthetic origin of mycobacterial cell wall galactofuranosyl residues. *Tuber Lung Dis* **78:** 123–131.

Wheatley RW, Zheng RB, Richards MR, Lowary TL, Ng KK. 2012. Tetrameric structure of the GlfT2 galactofuranosyltransferase reveals a scaffold for the assembly of mycobacterial arabinogalactan. *J Biol Chem* **287:** 28132–28143.

Wietzerbin-Falszpan J, Das BC, Azuma I, Adam A, Petit JF, Lederer E. 1970. Isolation and mass spectrometric identification of the peptide subunits of mycobacterial cell walls. *Biochem Biophys Res Commun* **40:** 57–63.

Wolucka BA, McNeil MR, de Hoffmann E, Chojnacki T, Brennan PJ. 1994. Recognition of the lipid intermediate for arabinogalactan/arabinomannan biosynthesis and its relation to the mode of action of ethambutol on mycobacteria. *J Biol Chem* **269:** 23328–23335.

Xin Y, Lee RE, Scherman MS, Khoo KH, Besra GS, Brennan PJ, McNeil M. 1997. Characterization of the in vitro synthesized arabinan of mycobacterial cell walls. *Biochim Biophys Acta* **1335:** 231–234.

Zhang W, Jones VC, Scherman MS, Mahapatra S, Crick D, Bhamidi S, Xin Y, McNeil MR, Ma Y. 2008. Expression, essentiality, and a microtiter plate assay for mycobacterial GlmU, the bifunctional glucosamine-1-phosphate acetyltransferase and *N*-acetylglucosamine-1-phosphate uridyltransferase. *Int J Biochem Cell Biol* **40:** 2560–2571.

Mycobacterium tuberculosis Metabolism

Digby F. Warner

Medical Research Council/National Health Laboratory Services/University of Cape Town Molecular Mycobacteriology Research Unit and Department of Science and Technology/National Research Foundation Centre of Excellence for Biomedical TB Research, Institute of Infectious Disease and Molecular Medicine and Division of Medical Microbiology, University of Cape Town, Rondebosch 7700, South Africa

Correspondence: digby.warner@uct.ac.za

Metabolism underpins the physiology and pathogenesis of *Mycobacterium tuberculosis*. However, although experimental mycobacteriology has provided key insights into the metabolic pathways that are essential for survival and pathogenesis, determining the metabolic status of bacilli during different stages of infection and in different cellular compartments remains challenging. Recent advances—in particular, the development of systems biology tools such as metabolomics—have enabled key insights into the biochemical state of *M. tuberculosis* in experimental models of infection. In addition, their use to elucidate mechanisms of action of new and existing antituberculosis drugs is critical for the development of improved interventions to counter tuberculosis. This review provides a broad summary of mycobacterial metabolism, highlighting the adaptation of *M. tuberculosis* as specialist human pathogen, and discusses recent insights into the strategies used by the host and infecting bacillus to influence the outcomes of the host–pathogen interaction through modulation of metabolic functions.

Ultimately, the process of pathogenicity itself will be describable in terms of the chemistry of the mycobacterial cell.

—Wheeler and Ratledge (1994)

The term "metabolism" has a very wide purview. For bacteria, it is commonly used to describe the full set of complex and interconnected chemical transformations that enable individual cells to survive and replicate. In turn, these might be broadly divided into the anabolic pathways that consume energy in generating biomass and the energy-releasing catabolic reactions that channel organic building blocks into diverse cellular structures and pathways. Metabolism also includes pathways that are essential to the ability of bacteria to respond to dynamic environments and to maintain structural integrity in the face of fluctuating nutrient availability. Therefore, in an obligate pathogen such as *Mycobacterium tuberculosis* whose entire life cycle is driven in the context of human infection, metabolism necessarily underpins both physiology and pathogenesis (Rhee 2013).

Owing to this dual role, the metabolism of *M. tuberculosis* has been the subject of intense research (Munoz-Elias and McKinney 2006; Beste and McFadden 2010). However, although experimental mycobacteriology—in particular, the use of genetic tools to disrupt enzymatic and regulatory functions—has provided critical insights into the metabolic pathways that are es-

Cite this article as *Cold Spring Harb Perspect Med* doi: 10.1101/cshperspect.a021121

sential for mycobacterial survival and pathogenesis, it remains extremely challenging to determine the precise metabolic status of bacilli during different stages of the infection cycle in vivo and, moreover, to elucidate the extent of heterogeneity in infecting populations located in discrete cellular (micro)environments in a single infected host. For the most part, investigations of mycobacterial metabolism have concentrated primarily on elucidating the metabolic *capacity* of the bacillus in vitro in defined growth media and under specific environmental conditions—or in experimental models of infection—rather than investigating metabolic function directly, and at the level of the complete biological system, during tuberculosis (TB) disease (Beste and McFadden 2010; Rhee et al. 2011). This is a subtle distinction, but it has significant ramifications for any attempts to catalog bacillary metabolic status and function during different disease stages (Barry et al. 2009) and, consequently, for downstream efforts to develop improved interventions to counter this pathogen, whether through novel antimycobacterial drugs (Lechartier et al. 2014), host-directed therapies (Schwegmann and Brombacher 2008; Hawn et al. 2013), or vaccines (Ernst 2012) (Fig. 1). Fortunately, recent developments—particularly the application of systems biology tools such as analysis of labeled metabolic intermediates (Marrero et al. 2010; Beste et al. 2011, 2013; Watanabe et al. 2011; Lee et al. 2013) in combination with major advances in mass spectrometery–based technologies (du Preez and Loots 2013; Rhee 2013; Loots 2014)—promise unprecedented access to the biochemical state of *M. tuberculosis* in experimental models of infection, as well as in determining the mechanisms of action of new and existing anti-TB drugs.

Different aspects of mycobacterial metabolism have been extensively reviewed in a number of excellent articles, and the interested reader is referred to these for detailed analyses (see Box 1).

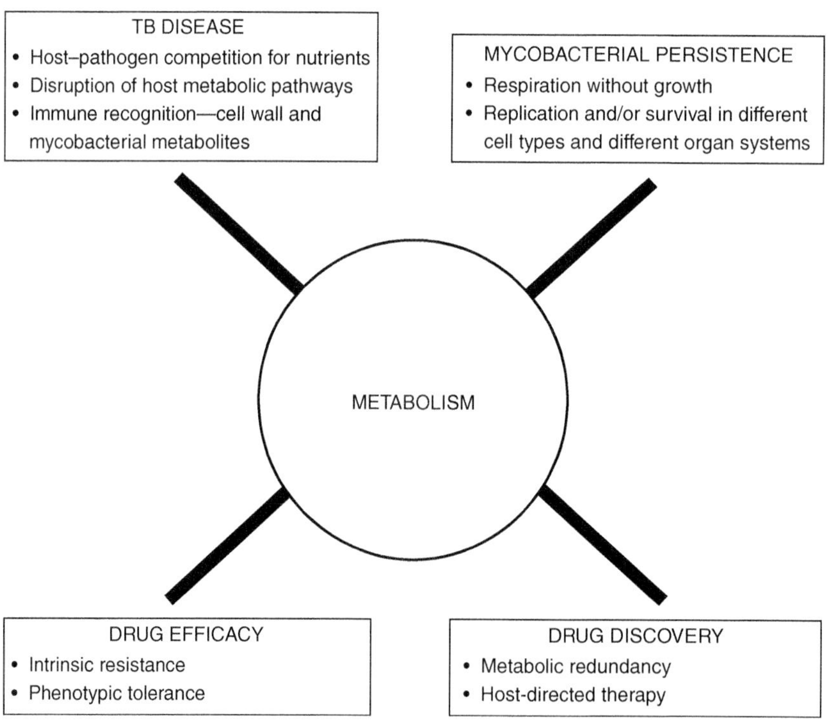

Figure 1. Metabolism impacts key features of *Mycobacterium tuberculosis* pathogenesis and tuberculosis (TB) disease, as well as drug efficacy and new TB drug development.

BOX 1. RECOMMENDED RESOURCES

Physiology of *Mycobacterium tuberculosis*

- Cook GM, Berney M, Gebhard S, Heinemann M, Cox RA, Danilchanka O, Niederweis M. 2009. Physiology of mycobacteria. *Adv Microb Physiol* **55:** 81–319.
- Russell DG. 2013. The evolutionary pressures that have molded *Mycobacterium tuberculosis* into an infectious adjuvant. *Curr Opin Microbiol* **16:** 78–84.

Central Carbon Metabolism

- Ehrt S, Rhee K. 2013. *Mycobacterium tuberculosis* metabolism and host interaction: Mysteries and paradoxes. *Curr Top Microbiol Immunol* **374:** 163–188.

Cofactor Metabolism

- Bi J, Wang H, Xie J. 2011. Comparative genomics of NAD(P) biosynthesis and novel antibiotic drug targets. *J Cell Physiol* **226:** 331–334.
- Salaemae W, Azhar A, Booker GW, Polyak SW. 2011. Biotin biosynthesis in *Mycobacterium tuberculosis*: Physiology, biochemistry and molecular intervention. *Protein Cell* **2:** 691–695.

Redox Homeostasis and Signal Transduction

- Kumar A, Farhana A, Guidry L, Saini V, Hondalus M, Steyn AJ. 2011. Redox homeostasis in mycobacteria: The key to tuberculosis control? *Expert Rev Mol Med* **13:** e39.
- Bretl DJ, Demetriadou C, Zahrt TC. 2011. Adaptation to environmental stimuli within the host: Two-component signal transduction systems of *Mycobacterium tuberculosis. Microbiol Mol Biol Rev* **75:** 566–582.

Sulfur, Nitrogen, and Phosphorus Metabolism

- Hatzios SK, Bertozzi CR. 2011. The regulation of sulfur metabolism in *Mycobacterium tuberculosis. PLoS Pathog* **7:** el002036.
- Amon J, Titgemeyer F, Burkovski A. 2009. A genomic view on nitrogen metabolism and nitrogen control in mycobacteria. *J Mol Microbiol Biotechnol* **17:** 20–29.
- Niederweis M. 2008. Nutrient acquisition by mycobacteria. *Microbiology* **154:** 679–692.

Metallobiology

- Rowland JL, Niederweis M. 2012. Resistance mechanisms of *Mycobacterium tuberculosis* against phagosomal copper overload. *Tuberculosis (Edinb)* **92:** 202–210.
- Riccardi G, Milano A, Pasca MR, Nies DH. 2008. Genomic analysis of zinc homeostasis in *Mycobacterium tuberculosis. FEMS Microbiol Lett* **287:** 1–7.

Enzymology

- Hudson SA, McLean KJ, Munro AW, Abell C. 2012. *Mycobacterium tuberculosis* cytochrome P450 enzymes: A cohort of novel TB drug targets. *Biochem Soc Trans* **40:** 573–579.
- Selengut JD, Haft DH. 2010. Unexpected abundance of coenzyme F420-dependent enzymes in *Mycobacterium tuberculosis* and other actinobacteria. *J Bacteriol* **192:** 5788–5798.

In addition, literature in this subject collection focused on specific areas of *M. tuberculosis* physiology and metabolism, including the factors influencing mycobacterial growth (Uhía et al. 2014) and cell wall composition and homeostasis (Alderwick et al. 2014; Jackson 2014). Therefore, this review will provide a broad overview of metabolism in *M. tuberculosis*, focusing primarily on the pathways involved in central carbon metabolism and highlighting recent findings implicating specific metabolic functions in mycobacterial pathogenesis. It will also consider the increasing impact of "omics" technologies in elucidating the metabolic state of bacilli in different models of infection, with special reference to the influence of mycobacterial metabolism on the host–pathogen interaction. As noted previously (Warner and Mizrahi 2008), investigations of core metabolic processes in *M. tuberculosis* are generally aimed (explicitly or implicitly) at identifying essential functions and potential vulnerabilities that might be targeted in novel intervention strategies; therefore, the discussion throughout will be framed within the context of new TB drug discovery, with an emphasis on recent insights into the influence of bacillary metabolic status on antibiotic efficacy, as well as in the application of advanced analytic tools to determine antibiotic mechanisms of action.

MYCOBACTERIAL METABOLISM AND HUMAN TB DISEASE

M. tuberculosis is transmitted in infectious aerosols, which are inhaled deep into the lung alveoli where the bacilli lodge in terminal air spaces and are engulfed by resident alveolar macrophages and recruited neutrophils (O'Garra et al. 2013). A hallmark of pathogenic mycobacteria is the ability to block normal acidification of phagosomes by preventing phagolysosomal fusion, enabling infecting bacilli to establish an intracellular niche that is conducive for replication in inactivated macrophages that offer limited antimicrobial defense (Russell 2011). There, the bacilli undergo several rounds of replication; however, following recruitment of innate immune components, host effectors such as reactive oxygen and nitrogen intermediates are released and mycobacterial replication slows. Immune activation results in the recruitment of lymphocytes and additional macrophages that assemble into a granuloma, a multicellular structure that sequesters the infecting bacteria from the surrounding tissue, and further inhibits the bacillary replication rate. Ultimately, the interior of the granuloma becomes necrotic (or "caseous") and hypoxic (Via et al. 2008), and bacilli are thought to enter a quiescent state characterized by limited or no replication and phenotypic resistance to drugs targeting processes such as cell wall biosynthesis (Karakousis et al. 2008). Evidence from various experimental systems, including macrophage (Rohde et al. 2012), mouse (Gill et al. 2009), and nonhuman primate (Lin et al. 2013) models, is consistent with the idea that, following infection, bacilli undergo several rounds of rapid replication, after which the increase in total bacterial number slows dramatically as a consequence of host-mediated killing and ultimately declines. Moreover, by applying a "clock plasmid" through both acute and chronic phases, it has been shown that replication continues throughout infection in the mouse model (Gill et al. 2009), an observation which appears to be supported in nonhuman primates as well in the emergence of chromosomal mutations during latent infection (Ford et al. 2011). In turn, this suggests that bacillary numbers are maintained at suppressed levels during long-term infection owing to active immune surveillance and killing.

M. tuberculosis is not restricted to specific host cellular compartments during infection (Dartois and Barry 2013; Dartois 2014). In cellular granulomas, bacilli are located predominantly within macrophages as well as in some extracellular niches; in caseous centers of necrotic granulomas, they are extracellular and considered metabolically quiescent (O'Garra et al. 2013). Bacilli are also found on the inner surface of open cavities within multiple cell types and even extracellular (Eum et al. 2010; Lowe et al. 2012), where they are protected from the immune system and able to replicate freely (Kaplan et al. 2003). In addition, there is molecular evidence that bacilli are located in a variety of cells in distal loci of the lung—despite the absence of any clear histological evidence of infection (Hernandez-Pando et al. 2000)—as well as in other organs (Barrios-Payan et al. 2012). The occupation of discrete tissues and cell types implies that individual bacteria from a clonal infecting population might be characterized by different physiological (and, in turn, metabolic) states, even where located within the same microenvironment—perhaps by analogy with the significant heterogeneity in host cell type and function within organized granulomas (Mattila et al. 2013).

From the perspective of mycobacterial metabolism, the bacilli are predicted to access glucose and triacylglycerides as primary carbon sources during early replication under aerobic conditions; thereafter the glucose-deficient macrophage environment forces a shift to the utilization of lipids (Boshoff and Barry 2005). As the infection proceeds, and there is increased immune activation and host-imposed stress, normal aerobic respiration becomes increasingly limited and the bacterium switches metabolism to ensure maintenance of an energized membrane in the absence of growth (Watanabe et al. 2011; Eoh and Rhee 2013). It is simplistic, therefore, to assume that mycobacterial metabolism has been selected to generate maximal bacillary numbers within a given microenvironment. The identification of immunopathology (*imp/pat*) mutants impaired in their ability to cause characteristic disease pathology despite showing no growth defect reinforces the important disconnect between bacillary number and disease outcome (Hingley-Wilson et al. 2003). Similarly, the idea that metabolic activity is designed to maximize mycobacterial biomass and energy production from limited nutrient sources is problematic (Rhee et al. 2011). *M. tuberculosis* does not have to outcompete other organisms within the same niche. Moreover, the pathology characteristic of TB disease is not mediated by bacterial toxins but instead reflects the host immune response to mycobacterial antigens (Ernst 2012).

Recent evidence from the nonhuman primate model indicates that the bacterial population within individual pulmonary lesions achieves a maximum size that is fairly consistent, numbering approximately 2×10^5 bacilli per lesion just before the onset of the adaptive immune response and stabilizing at a median of approximately 10^2 bacilli during active disease (Lin et al. 2013). It is only those permissive lesions that exceed the characteristic "carrying capacity" that spread locally or result in TB pneumonia (Lin et al. 2009). It seems likely, therefore, that maximal growth might be detrimental to the immediate fate of the infecting bacillus (individual host outcome) or to its long-term survival (evolutionary persistence within the human population). The phenotypes of hypervirulent mutants, for example, often result from mutations in structural and regulatory genes (Parish et al. 2003; Shimono et al. 2003; Hu et al. 2006), perhaps indicating that *M. tuberculosis* virulence is tightly controlled. As discussed below, however, the extent to which metabolic activity varies in different host tissues and within specific cell types remains unresolved, as does the manner in which host cell activation impacts bacillary metabolic state.

Cataloging Mycobacterial Metabolic Capacity

If the genetic repertoire of a pathogen can be used to infer key characteristics of its lifestyle, the *M. tuberculosis* genome suggested an organism equipped with metabolic flexibility and autonomy, as well as the inherent capacity to resist nutrient stress (Cole et al. 1998). *M. tuberculosis* is a prototroph, possessing the biosynthetic capacity for amino acids, vitamins, and cofactors. In addition to a massively expanded complement of genes involved in fatty acid metabolism, the mycobacterial genome encodes a functional tricarboxylic acid cycle, pentose phosphate and Embden–Meyerhof–Parnas pathways, as well as enzymes offering a metabolic link between glycolytic and tricarboxylic acid pathways, suggesting the ability to switch between sugars, host-derived fatty acids, glucose, tricarboxylic acids, amino acids, and cholesterol as sources of nitrogen, carbon, and energy during host infection. Consistent with early predictions, phenotypic and transcriptional analyses of bacilli grown under defined conditions in vitro, or harvested from clinical infections, reinforced the inferred dependence of *M. tuberculosis* on fatty acids as primary carbon source (Schnappinger et al. 2003; Timm et al. 2003; Rohde et al. 2012). These observations have been reinforced and refined in a large number of studies (McKinney et al. 2000; Pandey and Sassetti 2008; de Carvalho et al. 2010a; Marrero et al. 2010; Rhee et al. 2011; Lee et al. 2013), which have applied targeted gene-deletion and knockdown mutants, in some cases in combination with metabolomic approaches, in a variety of experimental models in vitro and in vivo to arrive at a common conclusion: *M. tuberculosis* uses fatty acids as its predominant source of carbon and energy during host infection (discussed below).

Central carbon metabolism intersects with pathways involved in maintaining nitrogen homeostasis at α-ketoglutarate, a substrate of the key tricarboxylic acid cycle enzyme, α-ketoglutarate dehydrogenase, as well as glutamate synthase. Competition for α-ketoglutarate is therefore subject to complex regulation to ensure efficient partitioning between energy generation and anabolism. Recent evidence in *M. tuberculosis* implicates GarA, a forkhead-associated (FHA) domain-containing protein, of controlling the activities of three enzymes that use α-ketoglutarate—inhibiting α-ketoglutarate dehydrogenase, activating glutamate synthase, and inhibiting glutamate dehydrogenase (Ventura et al. 2013). Because GarA is itself subject to phosphorylation and binds multiple kinases (Molle and Kremer 2010), this observation points to the critical, but largely unexplored, role of posttranslational modifications in regulating core metabolic processes in *M. tuberculosis*.

Recent Insights into Carbon Metabolism

The observed attenuation of mutants defective in gluconeogenesis, the glyoxylate cycle, and the methylcitrate cycle (McKinney et al. 2000; Munoz-Elias and McKinney 2005; Munoz-Elias et al. 2006; Marrero et al. 2013) supports the inferred importance of carbon metabolism for mycobacterial pathogenesis. Moreover, a series of studies have elucidated the functional plasticity inherent in the mycobacterial tricarboxlic acid cycle, in turn implying the ability to use a variety of substrates under different oxygen tensions and in nutritionally diverse host environments (Tian et al. 2005a,b; Baughn et al. 2009; Wagner et al. 2011; Watanabe et al. 2011). Recent analyses using ^{13}C-metabolic flux analysis suggest an additional, anabolic role for isocitrate lyase in a so-called "GAS pathway," in which pyruvate dissimilation is achieved at slow growth rates and in glycerol-limited conditions via the glyoxylate shunt and carboxylating anaplerotic reactions (involving phosphoenolpyruvate carboxykinase, pyruvate carboxylase, and malic enzyme), which enable fixation of exogenous CO_2 and generation of biomass via succinyl CoA (Beste et al. 2011). The ability to derive carbon from CO_2 was confirmed in follow-up studies from the same group in an experimental model that also suggested the ability of *M. tuberculosis* to assimilate amino acids including alanine, glutamate/glutamine, and asparagine/aspartate from the host macrophage (Beste et al. 2013). Importantly, these observations are consistent with prior in vitro results that established the ability of *M. tuberculosis* to cocatabolize multiple carbon sources simultaneously via compartmentalization of discrete metabolic processes (de Carvalho et al. 2010a). The capacity for differential catabolism through glycolytic, pentose phosphate, and/or tricarboxylic acid pathways suggests that in vitro growth media should be adjusted to ensure physiologically relevant metabolic activity, particularly in drug screens (discussed below). However, further research is required to determine the relative contribution of different metabolic functions to *M. tuberculosis* during different growth stages and in different cellular locations. In addition, recent evidence implicating the LpqY-SugA-SugB-SugC ATP-binding cassette transporter in the critical recycling of trehalose (Kalscheuer et al. 2010) raises questions about the potential role of carbohydrates in mycobacterial metabolism in vivo (Rhee et al. 2011).

The consumption of alternative carbon sources including odd- and branched-chain fatty acids, branched-chain amino acids, and cholesterol generates propionyl CoA as a three-carbon terminal product. This poses a problem for *M. tuberculosis* in terms of its ability to balance the relative intracellular levels of two- and three-carbon intermediates—propionate is a high-energy metabolite but is toxic to *M. tuberculosis* if accumulated in elevated concentrations. *M. tuberculosis* possesses two major pathways for propionate catabolism—the methylcitrate cycle, which depends on the function of isocitrate lyase (Munoz-Elias et al. 2006), and the methylmalonyl pathway, which uses a vitamin B_{12}-dependent methylmalonyl CoA mutase (Savvi et al. 2008). Consistent with the inferred importance of propionate metabolism for *M. tuberculosis* pathogenesis, previous evidence suggested that, during in vivo infection in a mouse model, bacilli synthesized high-mass phthiocerol dimycocerosate (PDIM) forms via methylmalonyl-CoA derived from the β-oxidation of host lipids (Jain et al. 2007). More recently, however, it has been shown that, in addition to these two pathways, *M. tuberculosis* is able to limit propionyl-CoA accumulation by shunting excess subunits into the methyl-branched virulence lipids, sulfolipid-1 and PDIM, which act as a "sink" (Lee et al. 2013). Moreover, by labeling macrophage lipid droplets with ^{14}C-propionate, ^{14}C-oleate, and ^{14}C-stearate before infection, the investigators showed that *M. tuberculosis* incorporates host-derived lipids into PDIM, thereby confirming the ability of intracellular bacilli to access host fatty acid stores. In addition to reinforcing the close metabolic interaction between infecting pathogen and its cellular environment, these observations suggest that fluctuations in the amount of propionate routed into cell wall lipids will affect the host–pathogen interaction. Furthermore, because the methylmalonyl pathway depends on vitamin B_{12} for activity, the availability of this cofactor is likely to determine relative flux through the different routes (Griffin et al. 2012). In turn, this observation reinforces the potential impact of metabolic activity on disease progression and pathology and highlights the importance of determining the levels of key metabolites and cofactors in different host compartments.

Metabolism in the Absence of Growth

A seminal review (Boshoff and Barry 2005) pointed out that even nonreplicating bacilli must retain sufficient basal metabolic activity to ensure maintenance of an energized cell membrane as well as core cellular processes. Of particular importance is the need to sustain low-level ATP production and the continual regeneration of reducing equivalents in the form of NAD^+ to maintain the proton motive force. The first of two key studies investigating this notion used metabolomics and isotopomer analyses to investigate the shift in central metabolism in *M. tuberculosis* during replication arrest under diminishing oxygen conditions (Watanabe et al. 2011). The results confirmed a significant decrease in intracellular ATP levels in oxygen-starved bacilli relative to active aerobic growth and a large increase in the ratio of NADH to NAD^+. To alleviate this effect, bacilli grown on glucose initiate a reversed TCA cycle, which results in the net incorporation of CO_2 and the active secretion of succinate in a fermentative respiratory strategy. The critical role of succinate in hypoxic adaptation in *M. tuberculosis* was reinforced in separate work that also measured intermediates of the mycobacterial TCA cycle during the shift to anoxia, although in this case acetate was supplied as primary carbon source so as to mimic the inferred importance of fatty acid metabolism for mycobacterial pathogenesis (Eoh and Rhee 2013). The results implicated the glyoxylate shunt in the generation of succinate and glycine, specifically identifying functional isocitrate lyase as critical to this process, and thereby establishing an additional role for the enzyme independent from its established contribution to fatty acid catabolism (Munoz-Elias and McKinney 2005). Based on these observations, the investigators proposed that succinate functions as a "metabolic battery" in *M. tuberculosis*, ensuring sustained membrane potential, ATP synthesis, and supply of TCA cycle intermediates. Although this suggests key components of the fermentative process as potential drug targets for latent TB, it also prompts an important question about the impact of secreted succinate on the local inflammatory response. Recent evidence implicating macrophage-derived succinate in innate immune signaling (Tannahill et al. 2013) raises the possibility that mycobacterial metabolic shutdown might be coupled with decreased host immune activity.

MYCOBACTERIAL METABOLISM AND THE HOST IMMUNE RESPONSE

M. tuberculosis has adapted to human infection over 70,000 years of coevolution (Comas et al. 2013). Any analysis of metabolic function in this bacterium must, therefore, consider the influence of metabolism on the host–pathogen interaction. Because infecting bacilli are wholly dependent on their human host for increased biomass, access to nutrients represents a critical point of conflict. For this reason, mechanisms directly regulating nutrient and trace metal availability are key to an effective host immune response and involve both starving (Wagner et al. 2005; Zhang et al. 2013b) or poisoning (Botella et al. 2011) the infecting bacilli, which themselves use countermeasures such as the mobilization of specific small molecule effectors including cAMP to modulate host immune function (Agarwal et al. 2009). Infection with *M. tuberculosis* can also impact cellular metabolism; for example, by diverting glycolysis toward ketone body biosynthesis, *M. tuberculosis* actively disrupts macrophage metabolic homeostasis to promote the accumulation of lipid bodies (Singh et al. 2012). This process, which is mediated by mycobacterial mycolic acids and ensures the incorporation of phagosomal bacilli into intracellular lipid bodies, induces a nonreplicating state in *M. tuberculosis*, suggesting that the resultant foamy macrophages constitute an important reservoir of persistent organisms (Peyron et al. 2008). Similarly, transcriptional and biochemical analyses are consistent with the idea that *M. tuberculosis* infection dysregulates host lipid metabolism so that the caseating granulomas characteristic of active TB disease comprise the preferred carbon sources of the bacillus—cholesterol, triacylglycerides, and glycosphingolipids (Kim et al. 2010).

It has been proposed, too, that *M. tuberculosis* causes a nutritional imbalance that triggers autophagy in infected macrophages (Kumar and Rao 2011). In support of these observations, pioneering RNAi screens to elucidate host factors that are critical to controlling intracellular infection identified genes involved in metabolic regulation and function (Jayaswal et al. 2010; Kumar et al. 2010). More recently, immunoresponsive gene 1 (*Irg1*) has been implicated in the inhibition of *M. tuberculosis* through the production of itaconic acid (Michelucci et al. 2013), a succinate analog that inhibits isocitrate lyase and is induced in activated macrophages (Strelko et al. 2011). Itaconate has been usefully applied in vitro to show the existence of a functional citramalate cycle in some bacteria (Berg et al. 2002); therefore, the detection of elevated citramalate concentrations in sputum samples from patients with active TB disease (du Preez and Loots 2013) is intriguing, particularly given the inferred importance of succinate in host immune function (Tannahill et al. 2013).

Emerging evidence from different bacterial systems, as well as *M. tuberculosis*, reinforces the notion that metabolism is fundamental to host–pathogen dynamics. For example, Group A *Streptococcus* directly modulates asparagine production by host cells, in turn triggering expression of an asparagine-responsive gene regulon that stimulates bacterial proliferation (Baruch et al. 2014). Critically, this study showed that degradation of asparagine through the administration of asparaginase resulted in bacterial growth arrest, thereby suggesting a novel antibacterial intervention targeting host amino acid homeostasis. Recent work by Eric Rubin and colleagues has similarly situated tryptophan homeostasis at the nexus of the mycobacterium–host interaction (Zhang et al. 2013b). Using a transposon insertion site-mapping method pioneered in the same laboratory (Sassetti and Rubin 2003), the investigators identified the set of mycobacterial genes that is essential to the ability of the bacillus to survive in an immune-competent host (Zhang et al. 2013b).

Consistent with previous observations, these included genes required for gluconeogenesis, reinforcing the inferred role of fatty acid catabolism in *M. tuberculosis* pathogenesis (Marrero et al. 2010). In addition, the analysis of underrepresented genes revealed a specific requirement for a functional tryptophan biosynthetic pathway. Immune activation triggers up-regulation of host indoleamine 2,3-dioxygenase, an enzyme involved in tryptophan catabolism, as part of an established antimicrobial response that effectively starves invading pathogens of the essential amino acid. Like some other bacteria, *M. tuberculosis* counters this mechanism by synthesizing tryptophan de novo, thereby identifying the tryptophan biosynthetic machinery as a potential therapeutic target. Using fluorinated anthranilate derivatives, the investigators showed that inhibition of the essential anthranilate synthase, TrpE, was bactericidal in vitro and limited growth in the mouse model (Zhang et al. 2013b).

Microbial metabolites are antigens for host immune detection; for example, vitamin B_2 and vitamin B_9 derivatives are natural ligands for the MHC class I–like related molecule (MR1) on mucosal-associated invariant T (MAIT) cells (Kjer-Nielsen et al. 2012), and they can also modulate host immune function (Smith et al. 2013). In turn, this implies that tight spatial and temporal control of metabolism is likely to be critical to an obligate pathogen whose entire life cycle occurs within the context of host infection and, therefore, immune surveillance. Indirect support of this idea is provided by the observation that metabolic enzymes are among the confirmed T-cell epitopes that appear to be hyperconserved (Comas et al. 2010), suggesting that the gene products as well as their metabolic functions are under direct negative selection—for example, glutamine synthetase, a secreted enzyme which is thought to be involved in bacillary regulation of host intracellular pH through disrupted ammonia metabolism (Kumar and Rao 2011). In contrast, comparative genomics suggests that various metabolic functions have been gained or lost during the evolution of modern *M. tuberculosis* strains from the ancestral smooth tubercle bacillus (Stinear et al. 2008; McGuire et al. 2012; Supply et al. 2013), including those required for the biosynthesis of cofactors such as molybdopterin (Williams et al. 2014) and vitamin B_{12} (Gopinath et al. 2013a). Similarly, inactivating polymorphisms and large deletions affecting genes involved in intermediary metabolism are overrepresented in comparative genomic analyses of circulating clinical isolates, suggesting strong selection pressure on specific metabolic functions (Tsolaki et al. 2004; Warner et al. 2007). The extent to which the loss of these genes impacts the short-term competitive survival and, on a longer timescale, the persistence of the evolved mutant within the human population is unclear and requires further investigation.

INVESTIGATING MYCOBACTERIAL METABOLISM IN VIVO

Auxotrophs as Bioprobes of Host Environments

There has been considerable activity around the construction of amino acid auxotrophs (Hinshelwood and Stoker 1992; McAdam et al. 1995; Gordhan et al. 2002; Parish 2003), mainly for their possible development as live-attenuated vaccines (Chambers et al. 2000; Smith et al. 2001; Pavelka et al. 2003; Sampson et al. 2004, 2011). In different mouse models, arginine (Gordhan et al. 2002), lysine (Pavelka et al. 2003), leucine (McAdam et al. 1995; Chambers et al. 2000), methionine, proline, and tryptophan auxotrophs (Smith et al. 2001) are severely attenuated, suggesting the inability of the infecting mycobacteria to scavenge adequate sources of the respective essential amino acids from the host. Double-auxotrophic mutants of *Mtb* have also been constructed carrying inactivating deletions in pantothenate (vitamin B_5) and either lysine (Sambandamurthy et al. 2005; Larsen et al. 2009) or leucine (Sampson et al. 2004, 2011) biosynthetic pathways and fail to cause disease in multiple animal models. These attenuated strains have also found practical use under biological safety II conditions—for example, in a complex high-throughput drug screen to identify compounds that are active against nonreplicating bacilli (Gold et al. 2012).

Notwithstanding the potential prophylactic applications, auxotrophic mutants can prove extremely useful as probes of the host environment. For example, the profound in vivo attenuation of the arginine auxotroph (Gordhan et al. 2002) is unexpected given the critical role of arginine as substrate for nitric oxide (NO) production in *M. tuberculosis*–infected macrophages (Qualls et al. 2012), implying the inability of the bacillus to transport specific amino acids in vivo. Alternatively, it might indicate the capacity of infected host cells to sequester specific amino acids, as described for tryptophan (Zhang et al. 2013b). As noted above, amino acids such as asparagine, glutamate, and aspartate serve as organic sources of nitrogen, which implicates amino acid transport and assimilatory mechanisms in pathogenesis independent of the corresponding biosynthetic pathways. For example, recent work has established that *M. tuberculosis* requires host-derived aspartate (Gouzy et al. 2013). Deletion of the aspartate transporter, AnsP1, resulted in severe growth attenuation during infection of both wild-type and immunodeficient mice and was associated with reduced pathology. In addition to identifying the aspartate transporter, this study is notable for two reasons. First, the observation that in vitro models do not necessarily reproduce key aspects of the host environment—the *ansP1* mutant showed no growth defect in macrophages, in contrast to the profound phenotype observed in vivo. Second, the involvement of AnsP1 in aspartate assimilation—the MTB genome encodes paralogous AnsP1 and AnsP2 proteins that show significant identity to asparagine transporters, yet although AnsP1 is essential for aspartate uptake, follow-up work from the same group has implicated AnsP2 in a asparagine transport and catabolism in combination with the secreted asparaginase, AnsA (Gouzy et al. 2014). Deletion of AnsP2 does not eliminate nitrogen assimilation from asparagine, suggesting that another protein(s) compensates for loss of function. By analogy with the recent identification of the mycobacterial corrinoid (Gopinath et al. 2013b) and heme (Tullius et al. 2011; Owens et al. 2013) transporters, this observation reinforces the need to identify the mechanisms that mediate uptake of essential nutrients, cofactors, and trace elements in *M. tuberculosis* and simultaneously highlights the unique adaptation of conserved proteins to specialist functions in an obligate pathogen (discussed below). In addition, the dual role of the *ansA*-encoded asparaginase in mycobacterial nitrogen homeostasis and the defense against host-mediated acid stress reinforces the intersection of physiology and virulence in core metabolic functions.

Advances in the Postgenomic Era

Knockout mutants, whether containing targeted or random disruptions of metabolic enzymes, are limited in their ability to provide insights into the temporal requirements for specific metabolic functions. Moreover, the use of transposon libraries to infer gene essentiality is complicated by the potential of a population of bacilli containing wild-type alleles to compensate in *trans* for loss of a specific function in the corresponding insertion mutant(s). Systems that allow conditional knockout (or knockdown) of target genes by promoter replacement or regulated protein degradation through the use of tetracycline-responsive genetic elements (Ehrt et al. 2005) have provided a powerful solution to this problem, enabling confirmation of inferred essentiality under a variety of conditions in vitro, as well as precise determinations of the stage of infection at which particular metabolic functions are critical for survival in vivo (Blumenthal et al. 2010; Wei et al. 2011; Kim et al. 2013). For the same reasons, conditional mutants are also very useful in validating putative drug targets (Blumenthal et al. 2010; Kolly et al. 2014), as well as in enabling assessments of the vulnerability of the mycobacterial cell to partial disruption of a specific function (Wei et al. 2011). In addition, the intrinsic resistance of *M. tuberculosis* to most antibiotic compounds has suggested the utility of applying conditional mutants in novel approaches such as target-based whole-cell screening (Lechartier et al. 2014); for example, a conditional knockdown of pantothenate synthase, *panC*, was recently used to identify potential small-molecule inhibitors of the essential vitamin B_5 biosynthetic pathway (Abrahams et al. 2012).

As noted elsewhere (Beste and McFadden 2010; Rhee 2013), an inherent weakness of all genetic manipulations is that the phenotype of the resulting mutant might reflect the loss of a function(s), which cannot be predicted by genetic or bioinformatic analyses. In addition, evidence from other bacterial systems indicates that metabolic networks are robust and tolerate perturbations via compensatory and regulatory mechanisms that are often mediated at multiple levels through complex protein networks (Ishii et al. 2007). The absence of a discernible phenotype at the cellular level might, therefore, obscure the underlying metabolic adjustment necessary to maintain homeostasis. Attempts to circumvent these limitations are increasingly reliant on the so-called "metabolomics" approaches, which do not require genetic manipulation of mycobacterial gene function, but instead depend on the ability to detect, and quantify, specific molecules (metabolites) that can provide detailed information about the metabolic state of the bacillus at a specific instant (i.e., a snapshot of the biochemical makeup of the cell). By definition, the instantaneous cellular composition is a function of the regulatory and other metabolic pathways whose combined activities have yielded the observed state; for this reason, metabolomics is complementary to other approaches such as proteomics, lipidomics, and transcriptomics, and combinations of these techniques can be harnessed to generate true systems biology data (Galagan et al. 2013).

Owing to the considerable technical challenges (Boshoff and Lun 2010), metabolomics has been most profitably applied during growth of *M. tuberculosis* under defined conditions in vitro (de Carvalho et al. 2010a; Beste et al. 2011, 2013; Watanabe et al. 2011), although there is increasing use of metabolite profiling to identify biomarkers of infection in experimental models as well as clinical specimens (Shin et al. 2011; du Preez and Loots 2013; Zhou et al. 2013; Mahapatra et al. 2014). As noted above, these techniques have proved especially useful in enabling key insights into central carbon metabolism in *M. tuberculosis* and, in addition to investigating known pathways, have revealed cryptic biochemical functions. For example, activity-based metabolomic profiling has enabled functional annotation of conserved and hypothetical proteins such as D,L-glycerol 3-phosphate phosphatase, whose presence in the genome implies that *M. tuberculosis* has the metabolic machinery to catabolize glycerophospholipids (Larrouy-Maumus et al. 2013), as well as 2-hydroxy-3-oxoadipate synthase (de Carvalho et al. 2010b). Similarly, pathway profiling established that the primary function of the *igr* operon is to degrade the 2′-propanoate side chain of cholesterol (Thomas et al. 2011).

Metabolomic analyses have also been used to identify potential biomarkers of disease. Experimental models, including mice and guinea pigs (Shin et al. 2011; Somashekar et al. 2012), have established that *M. tuberculosis* infection has a profound impact on host metabolism, and these observations have been reiterated in clinical samples where differential metabolite profiles have been used to distinguish uninfected controls from latently infected patients as well as those with active disease (Weiner et al. 2012b; Zhou et al. 2013). Of special interest is the identification of kynurenine as a defining metabolite of active TB (Weiner et al. 2012b), because this is the product of the indoleamine-2,3-dioxygenase-catalyzed degradation of tryptophan that, as detailed above, recent work has implicated in the host antimycobacterial response (Zhang et al. 2013b). Other approaches include the analysis of sputum for both mycobacterial and host markers of disease (du Preez and Loots 2013), as well as the development of urinary metabolite signatures to track the response to chemotherapy (Mahapatra et al. 2014). In addition, differential metabolite profiles have been investigated as a method to speciate pathogenic and nonpathogenic mycobacteria (Olivier and Loots 2012) and to investigate the impact of drug resistance mutations on bacterial physiology (Bisson et al. 2012; Loots 2014), as discussed further below.

TB DRUG DISCOVERY AND *M. tuberculosis* METABOLISM

Targeting Mycobacterial Metabolism

The metabolic capacity of an obligate pathogen such as *M. tuberculosis* is critical to drug discovery for interrelated reasons: First, it determines which metabolic pathways or functions are essential for pathogenesis, and so might represent preferred antibiotic targets; and, second, it influences predictions around the prospective efficacy of any new drug or drug combination because redundant function, or the potential for alternative metabolic pathways or states, could render a potent in vitro compound useless in disease-relevant conditions. The risk of redundant (or alternative) function is exacerbated by the fact that approximately one-quarter of the *M. tuberculosis* genome lacks functional annotation (Lew et al. 2013; Slayden et al. 2013). Moreover, consistent with the inferred evolution of *M. tuberculosis* as specialist pathogen from an ancestral generalist environmental *Mycobacterium* (Stinear et al. 2008; McGuire et al. 2012), genes annotated on the basis of close homology with orthologs in other organisms can encode proteins that have evolved completely novel and/or additional functions. Compelling examples include the recently identified aspartate (Gouzy et al. 2013) and vitamin B_{12} (Gopinath et al. 2013b) transporters, as well as the multiple subunits of the pyruvate dehydrogenase complex, which were almost entirely misannotated (Rhee et al. 2011) and include the *dlaT*-encoded dihydrolipoamide acyltransferase (Tian et al. 2005b) and *lpd*-encoded lipoamide dehydrogenase (Venugopal et al. 2011). For this reason, functional annotation of the *M. tuberculosis* genome remains a critical research priority (Slayden et al. 2013).

As noted above, investigations of metabolic capacity in *M. tuberculosis* have been framed largely within the context of drug discovery, with a particular focus on the identification of vital (essential) genes or pathways as potential targets. The "essential gene lists" derived in the landmark studies of Christopher Sassetti, Eric Rubin, and colleagues (Sassetti et al. 2003; Sassetti and Rubin 2003), refined in a series of subsequent iterations exploring different infection models (Rengarajan et al. 2005; Brodin et al. 2010; Griffin et al. 2011; Zhang et al. 2013b), have been routinely applied as a starting criterion in target selection and prioritization (Warner and Mizrahi 2012). In turn, this has motivated efforts to develop in vitro growth models that more closely resemble the host environments encountered by *M. tuberculosis* (Franzblau et al. 2012; Dartois and Barry 2013). These studies have catalogued a range of carbon sources (Baek et al. 2011), pH values (Vandal et al. 2008), and oxygen tensions (Cho et al. 2007) in which the bacillus is able to survive and, in most cases, replicate, even in the presence of applied stimuli such as oxidative and nitrosative stresses (de Carvalho et al. 2011; Gold et al. 2012). In addition, alternative screens have been developed against bacilli contained within macrophages (Christophe et al. 2009; Stanley et al. 2014) or grown under conditions that are predicted to obtain during host infection (de Carvalho et al. 2009; Franzblau et al. 2012; Gold et al. 2012).

An instructive example of the direct impact of growth medium composition on drug efficacy was provided by the identification of the pyrimidine-imidazole class of compounds that, despite impressive in vitro potency against *M. tuberculosis*, were inactive in vivo owing to the fact that their inhibitory activity was dependent on metabolic poisoning of bacilli grown in media containing glycerol (Pethe et al. 2010). To counter this effect, most in vitro screening algorithms now use more than carbon source (Franzblau et al. 2012). Nevertheless, determining the in vivo availability of specific lipids, amino acids, cofactors, and trace metals remains critical for antibiotic discovery, as there are a number of cases in which the unexpected ability of different bacteria to scavenge essential nutrients from the host has precluded further development of very promising lead compounds as clinic candidates (Brinster et al. 2009). In addition, there is strong evidence for the impact of metabolic state on drug efficacy; for example, the bactericidal activity of bedaquiline, an ATP synthase inhibitor, is significantly enhanced during growth of *M. tuberculosis* on nonfermentable energy sources such as lipids, which limit the ability of the bacillus to generate ATP via glycolysis (Koul et al. 2014).

Current TB drug screening programs are characterized by significant redundancy in the nature of the compounds screened, as well as the putative targets, with mutations in a handful of "promiscuous" cell wall–associated proteins (e.g., DprE1, MmpL3, and QcrB) accounting for a large proportion of resistance phenotypes (Goldman 2013). There are, however, promising examples of the potential to inhibit other metabolic functions. These include the identification of sulfonamides and rhodanines that, respectively, target lipoamide dehydrogenase (Bryk et al. 2013) and dihydrolipoamide acyltransferase (Bryk et al. 2008), components of both the mycobacterial pyruvate dehydrogenase and peroxynitrite reductase complexes and, therefore, critical for intermediary metabolism as well as oxidative and nitrosative defense (Tian et al. 2005a; Shi and Ehrt 2006; Venugopal et al. 2011). Alternative approaches include the development of ATP-competitive inhibitors of enzymatic activities that are essential for active replication and/or hypoxia-induced nonreplication (Wolfe et al. 2013), as well as small molecules to disrupt biotin biosynthesis (Shi et al. 2011) or posttranslational biotinylation that is essential for protein function (Duckworth et al. 2011).

Mycobacterial Metabolism and Drug Efficacy

Altering key environmental variables can impact the mycobacterial growth rate, triggering a shift to an alternative metabolic state (Beste et al. 2005) that, in turn, can impact susceptibility to specific drugs. For example, growth arrest owing to a variety of stresses thought to prevail during host infection, including hypoxia, iron limitation, and low pH, has been associated with a metabolic shift in *M. tuberculosis* that directs carbon away from the TCA cycle and into the biosynthesis of triacyglycerol, which accumulates in the cytosol (Baek et al. 2011). The resulting metabolic shutdown renders *M. tuberculosis* tolerant to a number of antibiotics and so suggests a direct link between bacterial metabolic state and observed drug efficacy. This effect is reproduced during intracellular infection as well; under hypoxic conditions, *M. tuberculosis*–infected macrophages accumulate lipid droplets, which the bacilli import and assimilate into their own triacylglycerol stores (Daniel et al. 2011). Consistent with in vitro observations (Baek et al. 2011), the ability to use host-derived lipids is dependent on functional triacylglycerol synthase, Tgs1 (Daniel et al. 2011). Moreover, sputum samples from TB patients contain a subpopulation of nonreplicating bacilli loaded with triacylglycerol lipid bodies (Garton et al. 2008), raising the possibility that this state might impact early events in bacillary transmission and host colonization (Woolhiser et al. 2007; Bacon et al. 2014).

Although direct evidence is lacking for the relevance of a nonreplicating state to the extended duration of anti-TB therapy, there is consensus that confining assessments of inhibitory activities to actively replicating bacilli in media comprising rich mixtures of carbon sources under aerobic conditions prejudices the outcome of compound screens (Dartois and Barry 2013; Goldman 2013). As a result, there has been considerable interest in the development of simulated microenvironmental conditions, which elicit a state of "nonreplicating persistence." For example, the combination of reactive nitrogen intermediates, acid, hypoxia, and butyrate as sole carbon source has identified agents active against both replicating and nonreplicating *M. tuberculosis* (de Carvalho et al. 2011; Gold et al. 2012), whereas a carbon starvation model also yielded novel small molecules that are active against metabolically quiescent bacilli (Grant et al. 2013). It is worth noting that, in the latter study, a comparison of the activities of a panel of hit compounds across three different in vitro models of hypoxia and nonreplicating persistence revealed differences in efficacy, suggesting that the phenotypically tolerant state conceals potentially significant variations in the underlying bacterial physiology, a disturbing possibility that requires further investigation.

The Metabolic Response to Drug Treatment

Metabolomics has the potential to provide pharmacokinetic and pharmacodynamic information from the treated mycobacterial cell (de Carvalho et al. 2011; Chakraborty et al. 2013). For this reason, these techniques have been especially useful in determining the systems-level impact of drug treatment on *M. tuberculosis* physiology, providing key insights into the mechanisms of action of new (de Carvalho et al. 2011; Halouska et al. 2012) and even established (Halouska et al. 2013; Prosser and de Carvalho 2013) anti-TB drugs. For example, it was generally assumed that the second-line anti-TB drug, *para*-aminosalicylic acid (PAS), competitively inhibits the essential dihydropteroate synthase in folate metabolism by acting as a mimetic of the natural enzyme substrate, p-aminobenzoate. However, recent analyses have instead established that PAS is a prodrug (Chakraborty et al. 2013) whose active product, a hydroxyl dihydrofolate antimetabolite, inhibits the activity of another essential enzyme in folate metabolism, dihydrofolate reductase (Zheng et al. 2013).

In a complementary approach, systems-level analyses have been increasingly applied to investigate mycobacterial mechanisms of resistance to anti-TB drugs (Kumar et al. 2013), as well as to elucidate the effect of common drug-resistance mutations on bacillary physiology and cell function and, by implication, pathogenesis (Bisson et al. 2012; du Preez and Loots 2012; Loots 2014). For example, proteomic profiling of *M. tuberculosis* isolates resistant to kanamycin and amikacin implicated putative iron homeostatic proteins as well as proteins of unknown function in the metabolic adaptation of mutants resistant to the major second-line aminoglycosides (Kumar et al. 2013). Moreover, comparative proteomics of clinical rifampicin-resistant isolates has revealed differences in the expression profiles of specific *rpoB* mutants of the *Mtb* Haarlem and Beijing lineages compared with corresponding drug-susceptible counterparts (Bisson et al. 2012). Of special interest, distinct alterations were identified in the biosynthesis and regulation of phthiocerol dimycocerosate, a methyl-branched fatty acid that has been implicated in mycobacterial virulence (Jackson et al. 2007). In related analyses of in vitro–selected rifampicin-resistant mutants with distinct *rpoB* mutations, the investigators were able to differentiate the respective *rpoB* mutants from one other as well as the parental strain based on fatty acid composition (du Preez and Loots 2012). Moreover, follow-up work from the same laboratory suggests that a metabolic shift in isoniazid-resistant mutants ameliorates the increased vulnerability to oxidative stress that is consequent on *katG* mutations (Loots 2014). In combination, these results hint at a potential physiological effect of resistance that might be independent of drug selection (Koch et al. 2014); however, further research is required to test this hypothesis.

FUTURE RESEARCH

The increasing availability of whole-genome sequence data has enabled crucial insights into the evolution, epidemiology, population structure, and diversity of *M. tuberculosis* and related pathogenic and nonpathogenic mycobacteria (Ford et al. 2012). In addition to identifying unexpected genome plasticity in *M. tuberculosis* (Domenech et al. 2010; Weiner et al. 2012a; Shitikov et al. 2014), these analyses have established that chromosomal rearrangements and point mutations drive the genetic adaptation of *M. tuberculosis* within its narrow ecological niche. Some nonsynonymous mutations and insertion–deletion events represent known drug-resistance alleles (Farhat et al. 2013; Zhang et al. 2013a; Casali et al. 2014) or are likely to be inactivating (Tsolaki et al. 2004; Keating et al. 2005; Warner et al. 2007); for the majority of genomic mutations and rearrangements, however, predicting the impact of specific polymorphisms on the function of the encoded proteins remains a major challenge (Golby et al. 2013; Rose et al. 2013) and is exacerbated where multiple mutations differentiate the strain of interest from the parental isolate. Moreover, evidence of a functional consequence of a synonymous single-nucleotide polymorphism reinforces the complexity of inferring the relative "importance" (and impact) of observed genomic mutations from sequence data alone (Golby et al. 2013).

One possible approach to functional analysis has been suggested by recent work that used metabolomic footprinting to investigate the adaptation of clonal isolates of *Pseudomonas aeruginosa* collected serially during long-term infections of cystic fibrosis patients (Behrends et al. 2013). This study revealed metabolic adaptations during long-term colonization, including decreased acetate production and evolution of systems for amino acid scavenging. For pathogenic mycobacteria, there have been promising attempts to adapt a commercial platform (Biolog Phenotype Microarray) to generate phenotypic profiles based on the differential abilities of individual lineages and/or strains to use a variety of defined nutrient sources during growth in vitro (Khatri et al. 2013). It seems likely, though, that the development of methods to assign genotype–phenotype correlations, including the impact of mutations on the host–pathogen interaction, for large strain panels will be an active area of future research.

As noted elsewhere (Rhee et al. 2011), the profound disconnection between in vitro growth models and the in vivo life cycle of *M. tuberculosis* as obligate pathogen represents a critical limitation on current attempts to understand the impact of mycobacterial metabolism on the host–pathogen interaction; whereas experimental models of *M. tuberculosis* pathogenesis are largely designed to investigate the ability of the organism to persist under a variety of imposed stresses such as hypoxia, low pH, and nutrient limitation (each of which can induce a state of nonreplication), metabolic and physiological processes are analyzed almost exclusively during active aerobic growth at maximal rates. It will be necessary, therefore, to explore the metabolic state of *M. tuberculosis* in the in vitro systems that recapitulate some of these stresses (Beste and McFadden 2010; Boshoff and Lun 2010; Rhee et al. 2011), including those that allow tighter regulation of the mycobacterial replication rate (Beste et al. 2005). In addition, the development of nonhuman primate models, including macaque (Lin et al. 2013; Mattila et al. 2013) and marmoset (Via et al. 2013), offers the prospect of experimentally tractable in vivo systems for the application of metabolomic analyses in combination with other "omics" techniques to generate true systems biology insight (Galagan et al. 2013). The parallel generation of advanced in silico models that incorporate data from a range of experimental models will be critical to interpret the emerging data and to the generation of translational algorithms that could enable predictions of metabolic states in clinical disease (Bonde et al. 2011), as well as for comparative analyses of the differential metabolic capacities of mycobacterial species and lineages (Lofthouse et al. 2013).

Space constraints dictated that many important aspects of metabolism were ignored in this review. Paramount among these are the signals and signaling mechanisms that regulate metabolic adaptations to different host environments, as well as the transcriptional and posttranslational events that enable the mycobacterial metabolic network to tolerate the perturbations that must inevitably be encountered during host infection. There is increasing evidence that noncoding RNAs are key to the regulation and function of certain metabolic pathways in *M. tuberculosis* (Arnvig et al. 2011; Golby et al. 2013; Li et al. 2013). Moreover, recent observations that specific intergenic regions are essential for mycobacterial survival (Zhang et al. 2012) or are involved in the emergence of drug resistance (Zhang et al. 2013a) hint at a further level of regulation that remains largely unexplored. Metabolic state can also be regulated by other factors; for example, data from *E. coli* suggest that growth-rate dependent alterations in mRNA stability modulate tricarboxylic cycle activity (Esquerre et al. 2013). The possibility, therefore, that the unusually stable transcripts (Rustad et al. 2013) characteristic of a slow-growing pathogen have evolved for specific regulatory functions is likely to be tested in future investigations.

The historical term for TB was "consumption" (Schwenk and Macallan 2000), which eloquently encapsulated the physical effects of the disease on the afflicted patient during its terminal stages. Although I have highlighted some of the consequences of *M. tuberculosis* infection for host function, particularly those relating to the accumulation of fatty acid stores in infected macrophages, the precise mechanisms mediating the observed metabolic dysfunction in TB disease are poorly understood. Therefore, although considerable effort is spent on developing host-directed therapies targeting immune functions, recent evidence (Gouzy et al. 2013; Zhang et al. 2013b) suggests that a deeper understanding of the metabolic factors that influence the outcome of the *M. tuberculosis*–host interaction might offer a profitable source of novel anti-TB interventions.

ACKNOWLEDGMENTS

I thank Krishnamoorthy Gopinath for useful discussions, Raju Mukherjee and Vinayak Singh for some helpful suggestions, and Valerie Mizrahi for critical review of the manuscript. Work in the Molecular Mycobacteriology Research Unit is enabled by core financial support from the South African Medical Research Council, the National Research Foundation (NRF) of South Africa, and the University of Cape Town. Research on vitamin B_{12} metabolism is funded by the NRF South Africa (grant number CPRR13091339569) and a Senior International Research Scholar's grant (to V. Mizrahi).

REFERENCES

*Reference is also in this subject collection.

Abrahams GL, Kumar A, Savvi S, Hung AW, Wen S, Abell C, Barry CE 3rd, Sherman DR, Boshoff HI, Mizrahi V. 2012. Pathway-selective sensitization of *Mycobacterium tuberculosis* for target-based whole-cell screening. *Chem Biol* **19:** 844–854.

Agarwal N, Lamichhane G, Gupta R, Nolan S, Bishai WR. 2009. Cyclic AMP intoxication of macrophages by a *Mycobacterium tuberculosis* adenylate cyclase. *Nature* **460:** 98–102.

* Alderwick LJ, Harrison J, Lloyd GS, Birch HL. 2014. The mycobacterial cell wall—Peptidoglycan and arabinogalactan. *Cold Spring Harb Perspect Med* doi: 10.1101/cshperspect.a021113.

Arnvig KB, Comas I, Thomson NR, Houghton J, Boshoff HI, Croucher NJ, Rose G, Perkins TT, Parkhill J, Dougan G, et al. 2011. Sequence-based analysis uncovers an abundance of non-coding RNA in the total transcriptome of *Mycobacterium tuberculosis*. *PLoS Pathog* **7:** e1002342.

Bacon J, Alderwick LJ, Allnutt JA, Gabasova E, Watson R, Hatch KA, Clark SO, Jeeves RE, Marriott A, Rayner E, et al. 2014. Non-replicating *Mycobacterium tuberculosis* elicits a reduced infectivity profile with corresponding modifications to the cell wall and extracellular matrix. *PLoS ONE* **9:** e87329.

Baek SH, Li AH, Sassetti CM. 2011. Metabolic regulation of mycobacterial growth and antibiotic sensitivity. *PLoS Biol* **9:** e1001065.

Barrios-Payan J, Saqui-Salces M, Jeyanathan M, Alcantara-Vazquez A, Castanon-Arreola M, Rook G, Hernandez-Pando R. 2012. Extrapulmonary locations of *Mycobacterium tuberculosis* DNA during latent infection. *J Infect Dis* **206:** 1194–1205.

Barry CE 3rd, Boshoff HI, Dartois V, Dick T, Ehrt S, Flynn J, Schnappinger D, Wilkinson RJ, Young D. 2009. The spectrum of latent tuberculosis: Rethinking the biology and intervention strategies. *Nat Rev Microbiol* **7:** 845–855.

Baruch M, Belotserkovsky I, Hertzog BB, Ravins M, Dov E, McIver KS, Le Breton YS, Zhou Y, Chen CY, Hanski E. 2014. An extracellular bacterial pathogen modulates host metabolism to regulate its own sensing and proliferation. *Cell* **156:** 97–108.

Baughn AD, Garforth SJ, Vilcheze C, Jacobs WR Jr., 2009. An anaerobic-type α-ketoglutarate ferredoxin oxidoreductase completes the oxidative tricarboxylic acid cycle of *Mycobacterium tuberculosis*. *PLoS Pathog* **5:** e1000662.

Behrends V, Ryall B, Zlosnik JE, Speert DP, Bundy JG, Williams HD. 2013. Metabolic adaptations of *Pseudomonas aeruginosa* during cystic fibrosis chronic lung infections. *Environ Microbiol* **15:** 398–408.

Berg IA, Filatova LV, Ivanovsky RN. 2002. Inhibition of acetate and propionate assimilation by itaconate via propionyl-CoA carboxylase in isocitrate lyase-negative purple bacterium *Rhodospirillum rubrum*. *FEMS microbiology letters* **216:** 49–54.

Beste DJ, McFadden J. 2010. System-level strategies for studying the metabolism of *Mycobacterium tuberculosis*. *Mol Biosyst* **6:** 2363–2372.

Beste DJ, Peters J, Hooper T, Avignone-Rossa C, Bushell ME, McFadden J. 2005. Compiling a molecular inventory for *Mycobacterium bovis* BCG at two growth rates: Evidence for growth rate-mediated regulation of ribosome biosynthesis and lipid metabolism. *J Bacteriol* **187:** 1677–1684.

Beste DJ, Bonde B, Hawkins N, Ward JL, Beale MH, Noack S, Noh K, Kruger NJ, Ratcliffe RG, McFadden J. 2011. ^{13}C metabolic flux analysis identifies an unusual route for pyruvate dissimilation in mycobacteria which requires isocitrate lyase and carbon dioxide fixation. *PLoS Pathog* **7:** e1002091.

Beste DJ, Noh K, Niedenfuhr S, Mendum TA, Hawkins ND, Ward JL, Beale MH, Wiechert W, McFadden J. 2013. ^{13}C-flux spectral analysis of host-pathogen metabolism reveals a mixed diet for intracellular *Mycobacterium tuberculosis*. *Chem Biol* **20:** 1012–1021.

Bisson GP, Mehaffy C, Broeckling C, Prenni J, Rifat D, Lun DS, Burgos M, Weissman D, Karakousis PC, Dobos K. 2012. Upregulation of the phthiocerol dimycocerosate biosynthetic pathway by rifampin-resistant, *rpoB* mutant *Mycobacterium tuberculosis*. *J Bacteriol* **194:** 6441–6452.

Blumenthal A, Trujillo C, Ehrt S, Schnappinger D. 2010. Simultaneous analysis of multiple *Mycobacterium tuberculosis* knockdown mutants in vitro and in vivo. *PLoS ONE* **5:** e15667.

Bonde BK, Beste DJ, Laing E, Kierzek AM, McFadden J. 2011. Differential producibility analysis (DPA) of transcriptomic data with metabolic networks: Deconstructing the metabolic response of *M. tuberculosis*. *PLoS Comput Biol* **7:** e1002060.

Boshoff HI, Barry CE 3rd. 2005. Tuberculosis—Metabolism and respiration in the absence of growth. *Nat Rev Microbiol* **3:** 70–80.

Boshoff HI, Lun DS. 2010. Systems biology approaches to understanding mycobacterial survival mechanisms. *Drug Discov Today Dis Mech* **7:** e75–e82.

Botella H, Peyron P, Levillain F, Poincloux R, Poquet Y, Brandli I, Wang C, Tailleux L, Tilleul S, Charriere GM, et al. 2011. Mycobacterial P_1-type ATPases mediate resistance to zinc poisoning in human macrophages. *Cell Host Microbe* **10:** 248–259.

Brinster S, Lamberet G, Staels B, Trieu-Cuot P, Gruss A, Poyart C. 2009. Type II fatty acid synthesis is not a suitable antibiotic target for Gram-positive pathogens. *Nature* **458:** 83–86.

Brodin P, Poquet Y, Levillain F, Peguillet I, Larrouy-Maumus G, Gilleron M, Ewann F, Christophe T, Fenistein D, Jang J, et al. 2010. High content phenotypic cell-based visual screen identifies *Mycobacterium tuberculosis* acyltrehalose-containing glycolipids involved in phagosome remodeling. *PLoS Pathog* **6:** e1001100.

Bryk R, Gold B, Venugopal A, Singh J, Samy R, Pupek K, Cao H, Popescu C, Gurney M, Hotha S, et al. 2008. Selective killing of nonreplicating mycobacteria. *Cell Host Microbe* **3:** 137–145.

Bryk R, Arango N, Maksymiuk C, Balakrishnan A, Wu YT, Wong CH, Masquelin T, Hipskind P, Lima CD, Nathan C. 2013. Lipoamide channel-binding sulfonamides selectively inhibit mycobacterial lipoamide dehydrogenase. *Biochemistry* **52:** 9375–9384.

Casali N, Nikolayevskyy V, Balabanova Y, Harris SR, Ignatyeva O, Kontsevaya I, Corander J, Bryant J, Parkhill J, Nejentsev S, et al. 2014. Evolution and transmission of drug-resistant tuberculosis in a Russian population. *Nat Genet* **46:** 279–286.

Chakraborty S, Gruber T, Barry CE 3rd, Boshoff HI, Rhee KY. 2013. Para-aminosalicylic acid acts as an alternative substrate of folate metabolism in *Mycobacterium tuberculosis*. *Science* **339:** 88–91.

Chambers MA, Williams A, Gavier-Widen D, Whelan A, Hall G, Marsh PD, Bloom BR, Jacobs WR, Hewinson RG. 2000. Identification of a *Mycobacterium bovis* BCG auxotrophic mutant that protects guinea pigs against *M. bovis* and hematogenous spread of *Mycobacterium tuberculosis* without sensitization to tuberculin. *Infect Immun* **68:** 7094–7099.

Cho SH, Warit S, Wan B, Hwang CH, Pauli GF, Franzblau SG. 2007. Low-oxygen-recovery assay for high-throughput screening of compounds against nonreplicating *Mycobacterium tuberculosis*. *Antimicrob Agents Chemother* **51:** 1380–1385.

Christophe T, Jackson M, Jeon HK, Fenistein D, Contreras-Dominguez M, Kim J, Genovesio A, Carralot JP, Ewann F, Kim EH, et al. 2009. High content screening identifies decaprenyl-phosphoribose 2′ epimerase as a target for intracellular antimycobacterial inhibitors. *PLoS Pathog* **5:** e1000645.

Cole ST, Brosch R, Parkhill J, Garnier T, Churcher C, Harris D, Gordon SV, Eiglmeier K, Gas S, Barry CE 3rd, et al. 1998. Deciphering the biology of *Mycobacterium tuberculosis* from the complete genome sequence. *Nature* **393:** 537–544.

Comas I, Chakravartti J, Small PM, Galagan J, Niemann S, Kremer K, Ernst JD, Gagneux S. 2010. Human T cell epitopes of *Mycobacterium tuberculosis* are evolutionarily hyperconserved. *Nat Genet* **42:** 498–503.

Comas I, Coscolla M, Luo T, Borrell S, Holt KE, Kato-Maeda M, Parkhill J, Malla B, Berg S, Thwaites G, et al. 2013. Out-of-Africa migration and Neolithic coexpansion of *Mycobacterium tuberculosis* with modern humans. *Nat Genet* **45:** 1176–1182.

Daniel J, Maamar H, Deb C, Sirakova TD, Kolattukudy PE. 2011. *Mycobacterium tuberculosis* uses host triacylglycerol to accumulate lipid droplets and acquires a dormancy-like phenotype in lipid-loaded macrophages. *PLoS Pathog* **7:** e1002093.

Dartois V. 2014. The path of anti-tuberculosis drugs: From blood to lesions to mycobacterial cells. *Nat Rev Microbiol* **12:** 159–167.

Dartois V, Barry CE 3rd. 2013. A medicinal chemists' guide to the unique difficulties of lead optimization for tuberculosis. *Bioorg Med Chem Lett* **23:** 4741–4750.

de Carvalho LP, Lin G, Jiang X, Nathan C. 2009. Nitazoxanide kills replicating and nonreplicating *Mycobacterium tuberculosis* and evades resistance. *J Med Chem* **52:** 5789–5792.

de Carvalho LP, Fischer SM, Marrero J, Nathan C, Ehrt S, Rhee KY. 2010a. Metabolomics of *Mycobacterium tuberculosis* reveals compartmentalized co-catabolism of carbon substrates. *Chem Biol* **17:** 1122–1131.

de Carvalho LP, Zhao H, Dickinson CE, Arango NM, Lima CD, Fischer SM, Ouerfelli O, Nathan C, Rhee KY. 2010b. Activity-based metabolomic profiling of enzymatic function: Identification of Rv1248c as a mycobacterial 2-hydroxy-3-oxoadipate synthase. *Chem Biol* **17:** 323–332.

de Carvalho LP, Darby CM, Rhee KY, Nathan C. 2011. Nitazoxanide disrupts membrane potential and intrabacterial pH homeostasis of *Mycobacterium tuberculosis*. *ACS Med Chem Lett* **2:** 849–854.

Domenech P, Kolly GS, Leon-Solis L, Fallow A, Reed MB. 2010. Massive gene duplication event among clinical isolates of the *Mycobacterium tuberculosis* W/Beijing family. *J Bacteriol* **192:** 4562–4570.

du Preez I, Loots D. 2012. Altered fatty acid metabolism due to rifampicin-resistance conferring mutations in the *rpoB* gene of *Mycobacterium tuberculosis*: Mapping the potential of pharmaco-metabolomics for global health and personalized medicine. *Omics* **16:** 596–603.

du Preez I, Loots DT. 2013. New sputum metabolite markers implicating adaptations of the host to *Mycobacterium tuberculosis*, and vice versa. *Tuberculosis (Edinb)* **93:** 330–337.

Duckworth BP, Geders TW, Tiwari D, Boshoff HI, Sibbald PA, Barry CE 3rd, Schnappinger D, Finzel BC, Aldrich CC. 2011. Bisubstrate adenylation inhibitors of biotin protein ligase from *Mycobacterium tuberculosis. Chem Biol* **18:** 1432–1441.

Ehrt S, Guo XV, Hickey CM, Ryou M, Monteleone M, Riley LW, Schnappinger D. 2005. Controlling gene expression in mycobacteria with anhydrotetracycline and Tet repressor. *Nucleic Acids Res* **33:** e21.

Eoh H, Rhee KY. 2013. Multifunctional essentiality of succinate metabolism in adaptation to hypoxia in *Mycobacterium tuberculosis. Proc Natl Acad Sci* **110:** 6554–6559.

Ernst JD. 2012. The immunological life cycle of tuberculosis. *Nat Rev Immunol* **12:** 581–591.

Esquerre T, Laguerre S, Turlan C, Carpousis AJ, Girbal L, Cocaign-Bousquet M. 2013. Dual role of transcription and transcript stability in the regulation of gene expression in *Escherichia coli* cells cultured on glucose at different growth rates. *Nucleic Acids Res* **42:** 2460–2472.

Eum SY, Kong JH, Hong MS, Lee YJ, Kim JH, Hwang SH, Cho SN, Via LE, Barry CE 3rd. 2010. Neutrophils are the predominant infected phagocytic cells in the airways of patients with active pulmonary TB. *Chest* **137:** 122–128.

Farhat MR, Shapiro BJ, Kieser K, Sultana R, Jacobson KR, Victor TC, Warren RM, Streicher EM, Calver A, Sloutsky A, et al. 2013. Genomic analysis identifies targets of convergent positive selection in drug resistant *Mycobacterium tuberculosis. Nat Genet* **45:** 1183–1189.

Ford CB, Lin PL, Chase MR, Shah RR, Iartchouk O, Galagan J, Mohaideen N, Ioerger TR, Sacchettini JC, Lipsitch M, et al. 2011. Use of whole genome sequencing to estimate the mutation rate of *Mycobacterium tuberculosis* during latent infection. *Nat Genet* **43:** 482–486.

Ford C, Yusim K, Ioerger T, Feng S, Chase M, Greene M, Korber B, Fortune S. 2012. *Mycobacterium tuberculosis*—Heterogeneity revealed through whole genome sequencing. *Tuberculosis (Edinb)* **92:** 194–201.

Franzblau SG, DeGroote MA, Cho SH, Andries K, Nuermberger E, Orme IM, Mdluli K, Angulo-Barturen I, Dick T, Dartois V, et al. 2012. Comprehensive analysis of methods used for the evaluation of compounds against *Mycobacterium tuberculosis. Tuberculosis (Edinb)* **92:** 453–488.

Galagan JE, Minch K, Peterson M, Lyubetskaya A, Azizi E, Sweet L, Gomes A, Rustad T, Dolganov G, Glotova I, et al. 2013. The *Mycobacterium tuberculosis* regulatory network and hypoxia. *Nature* **499:** 178–183.

Garton NJ, Waddell SJ, Sherratt AL, Lee SM, Smith RJ, Senner C, Hinds J, Rajakumar K, Adegbola RA, Besra GS, et al. 2008. Cytological and transcript analyses reveal fat and lazy persister-like bacilli in tuberculous sputum. *PLoS Med* **5:** e75.

Gill WP, Harik NS, Whiddon MR, Liao RP, Mittler JE, Sherman DR. 2009. A replication clock for *Mycobacterium tuberculosis. Nat Med* **15:** 211–214.

Golby P, Nunez J, Witney A, Hinds J, Quail MA, Bentley S, Harris S, Smith N, Hewinson RG, Gordon SV. 2013. Genome-level analyses of *Mycobacterium bovis* lineages reveal the role of SNPs and antisense transcription in differential gene expression. *BMC Genomics* **14:** 710.

Gold B, Pingle M, Brickner SJ, Shah N, Roberts J, Rundell M, Bracken WC, Warrier T, Somersan S, Venugopal A, et al. 2012. Nonsteroidal anti-inflammatory drug sensitizes *Mycobacterium tuberculosis* to endogenous and exogenous antimicrobials. *Proc Natl Acad Sci* **109:** 16004–16011.

Goldman RC. 2013. Why are membrane targets discovered by phenotypic screens and genome sequencing in *Mycobacterium tuberculosis*? *Tuberculosis (Edinb)* **93:** 569–588.

Gopinath K, Moosa A, Mizrahi V, Warner DF. 2013a. Vitamin B_{12} metabolism in *Mycobacterium tuberculosis. Future Microbiol* **8:** 1405–1418.

Gopinath K, Venclovas C, Ioerger TR, Sacchettini JC, McKinney JD, Mizrahi V, Warner DF. 2013b. A vitamin B_{12} transporter in *Mycobacterium tuberculosis. Open Biol* **3:** 120175.

Gordhan BG, Smith DA, Alderton H, McAdam RA, Bancroft GJ, Mizrahi V. 2002. Construction and phenotypic characterization of an auxotrophic mutant of *Mycobacterium tuberculosis* defective in L-arginine biosynthesis. *Infect Immun* **70:** 3080–3084.

Gouzy A, Larrouy-Maumus G, Wu TD, Peixoto A, Levillain F, Lugo-Villarino G, Gerquin-Kern JL, de Carvalho LP, Poquet Y, Neyrolles O. 2013. *Mycobacterium tuberculosis* nitrogen assimilation and host colonization require aspartate. *Nat Chem Biol* **9:** 674–676.

Gouzy A, Larrouy-Maumus G, Bottai D, Levillain F, Dumas A, Wallach JB, Caire-Brandli I, de Chastellier C, Wu TD, Poincloux R, et al. 2014. *Mycobacterium tuberculosis* exploits asparagine to assimilate nitrogen and resist acid stress during Infection. *PLoS Pathog* **10:** e1003928.

Grant SS, Kawate T, Nag PP, Silvis MR, Gordon K, Stanley SA, Kazyanskaya E, Nietupski R, Golas A, Fitzgerald M, et al. 2013. Identification of novel inhibitors of nonreplicating *Mycobacterium tuberculosis* using a carbon starvation model. *ACS Chem Biol* **8:** 2224–2234.

Griffin JE, Gawronski JD, Dejesus MA, Ioerger TR, Akerley BJ, Sassetti CM. 2011. High-resolution phenotypic profiling defines genes essential for mycobacterial growth and cholesterol catabolism. *PLoS Pathog* **7:** e1002251.

Griffin JE, Pandey AK, Gilmore SA, Mizrahi V, McKinney JD, Bertozzi CR, Sassetti CM. 2012. Cholesterol catabolism by *Mycobacterium tuberculosis* requires transcriptional and metabolic adaptations. *Chem Biol* **19:** 218–227.

Halouska S, Fenton RJ, Barletta RG, Powers R. 2012. Predicting the in vivo mechanism of action for drug leads using NMR metabolomics. *ACS Chem Biol* **7:** 166–171.

Halouska S, Fenton RJ, Zinniel DK, Marshall DD, Barletta RG, Powers R. 2013. Metabolomics analysis identifies D-alanine-D-alanine ligase as the primary lethal target of D-cycloserine in mycobacteria. *J Proteome Res* **13:** 1065–1076.

Hawn TR, Matheson AI, Maley SN, Vandal O. 2013. Host-directed therapeutics for tuberculosis: Can we harness the host? *Microbiol Mol Biol Rev* **77:** 608–627.

Hernandez-Pando R, Jeyanathan M, Mengistu G, Aguilar D, Orozco H, Harboe M, Rook GA, Bjune G. 2000. Persistence of DNA from *Mycobacterium tuberculosis* in superficially normal lung tissue during latent infection. *Lancet* **356:** 2133–2138.

Hingley-Wilson SM, Sambandamurthy VK, Jacobs WR Jr., 2003. Survival perspectives from the world's most successful pathogen, *Mycobacterium tuberculosis. Nat Immunol* **4:** 949–955.

Hinshelwood S, Stoker NG. 1992. Cloning of mycobacterial histidine synthesis genes by complementation of a *Myco-*

bacterium smegmatis auxotroph. *Mol Microbiol* **6:** 2887–2895.

Hu Y, Movahedzadeh F, Stoker NG, Coates AR. 2006. Deletion of the *Mycobacterium tuberculosis* α-crystallin-like *hspX* gene causes increased bacterial growth in vivo. *Infect Immun* **74:** 861–868.

Ishii N, Nakahigashi K, Baba T, Robert M, Soga T, Kanai A, Hirasawa T, Naba M, Hirai K, Hoque A, et al. 2007. Multiple high-throughput analyses monitor the response of *E. coli* to perturbations. *Science* **316:** 593–597.

* Jackson M. 2014. The mycobacterial cell envelope—Lipids. *Cold Spring Harb Perspect Med* **4:** a021105.

Jackson M, Stadthagen G, Gicquel B. 2007. Long-chain multiple methyl-branched fatty acid-containing lipids of *Mycobacterium tuberculosis*: Biosynthesis, transport, regulation and biological activities. *Tuberculosis (Edinb)* **87:** 78–86.

Jain M, Petzold CJ, Schelle MW, Leavell MD, Mougous JD, Bertozzi CR, Leary JA, Cox JS. 2007. Lipidomics reveals control of *Mycobacterium tuberculosis* virulence lipids via metabolic coupling. *Proc Natl Acad Sci* **104:** 5133–5138.

Jayaswal S, Kamal MA, Dua R, Gupta S, Majumdar T, Das G, Kumar D, Rao KV. 2010. Identification of host-dependent survival factors for intracellular *Mycobacterium tuberculosis* through an siRNA screen. *PLoS Pathog* **6:** e1000839.

Kalscheuer R, Weinrick B, Veeraraghavan U, Besra GS, Jacobs WR Jr., 2010. Trehalose-recycling ABC transporter LpqY-SugA-SugB-SugC is essential for virulence of *Mycobacterium tuberculosis*. *Proc Natl Acad Sci* **107:** 21761–21766.

Kaplan G, Post FA, Moreira AL, Wainwright H, Kreiswirth BN, Tanverdi M, Mathema B, Ramaswamy SV, Walther G, Steyn LM, et al. 2003. *Mycobacterium tuberculosis* growth at the cavity surface: A microenvironment with failed immunity. *Infect Immun* **71:** 7099–7108.

Karakousis PC, Williams EP, Bishai WR. 2008. Altered expression of isoniazid-regulated genes in drug-treated dormant *Mycobacterium tuberculosis*. *J Antimicrob Chemother* **61:** 323–331.

Keating LA, Wheeler PR, Mansoor H, Inwald JK, Dale J, Hewinson RG, Gordon SV. 2005. The pyruvate requirement of some members of the *Mycobacterium tuberculosis* complex is due to an inactive pyruvate kinase: Implications for in vivo growth. *Mol Microbiol* **56:** 163–174.

Khatri B, Fielder M, Jones G, Newell W, Abu-Oun M, Wheeler PR. 2013. High throughput phenotypic analysis of *Mycobacterium tuberculosis* and *Mycobacterium bovis* strains' metabolism using biolog phenotype microarrays. *PLoS ONE* **8:** e52673.

Kim MJ, Wainwright HC, Locketz M, Bekker LG, Walther GB, Dittrich C, Visser A, Wang W, Hsu FF, Wiehart U, et al. 2010. Caseation of human tuberculosis granulomas correlates with elevated host lipid metabolism. *EMBO Mol Med* **2:** 258–274.

Kim JH, O'Brien KM, Sharma R, Boshoff HI, Rehren G, Chakraborty S, Wallach JB, Monteleone M, Wilson DJ, Aldrich CC, et al. 2013. A genetic strategy to identify targets for the development of drugs that prevent bacterial persistence. *Proc Natl Acad Sci* **110:** 19095–19100.

Kjer-Nielsen L, Patel O, Corbett AJ, Le Nours J, Meehan B, Liu L, Bhati M, Chen Z, Kostenko L, Reantragoon R, et al. 2012. MR1 presents microbial vitamin B metabolites to MAIT cells. *Nature* **491:** 717–723.

Koch A, Mizrahi V, Warner DF. 2014. The impact of drug resistance on *Mycobacterium tuberculosis* physiology: What can we learn from rifampicin? *Emerg Microb Infect* **3:** e17.

Kolly GS, Boldrin F, Sala C, Dhar N, Hartkoorn RC, Ventura M, Serafini A, McKinney JD, Manganelli R, Cole ST. 2014. Assessing the essentiality of the decaprenyl-phospho-D-arabinofuranose pathway in *Mycobacterium tuberculosis* using conditional mutants. *Mol Microbiol* **92:** 194–211.

Koul A, Vranckx L, Dhar N, Gohlmann HW, Ozdemir E, Neefs JM, Schulz M, Lu P, Mortz E, McKinney JD, et al. 2014. Delayed bactericidal response of *Mycobacterium tuberculosis* to bedaquiline involves remodelling of bacterial metabolism. *Nat Commun* **5:** 3369.

Kumar D, Rao KV. 2011. Regulation between survival, persistence, and elimination of intracellular mycobacteria: A nested equilibrium of delicate balances. *Microbes Infect* **13:** 121–133.

Kumar D, Nath L, Kamal MA, Varshney A, Jain A, Singh S, Rao KV. 2010. Genome-wide analysis of the host intracellular network that regulates survival of *Mycobacterium tuberculosis*. *Cell* **140:** 731–743.

Kumar B, Sharma D, Sharma P, Katoch VM, Venkatesan K, Bisht D. 2013. Proteomic analysis of *Mycobacterium tuberculosis* isolates resistant to kanamycin and amikacin. *J Proteomics* **94:** 68–77.

Larrouy-Maumus G, Biswas T, Hunt DM, Kelly G, Tsodikov OV, de Carvalho LP. 2013. Discovery of a glycerol 3-phosphate phosphatase reveals glycerophospholipid polar head recycling in *Mycobacterium tuberculosis*. *Proc Natl Acad Sci* **110:** 11320–11325.

Larsen MH, Biermann K, Chen B, Hsu T, Sambandamurthy VK, Lackner AA, Aye PP, Didier P, Huang D, Shao L, et al. 2009. Efficacy and safety of live attenuated persistent and rapidly cleared *Mycobacterium tuberculosis* vaccine candidates in non-human primates. *Vaccine* **27:** 4709–4717.

Lechartier B, Rybniker J, Zumla A, Cole ST. 2014. Tuberculosis drug discovery in the post-post-genomic era. *EMBO Mol Med* **6:** 158–168.

Lee W, VanderVen BC, Fahey RJ, Russell DG. 2013. Intracellular *Mycobacterium tuberculosis* exploits host-derived fatty acids to limit metabolic stress. *J Biol Chem* **288:** 6788–6800.

Lew JM, Mao C, Shukla M, Warren A, Will R, Kuznetsov D, Xenarios I, Robertson BD, Gordon SV, Schnappinger D, et al. 2013. Database resources for the tuberculosis community. *Tuberculosis (Edinb)* **93:** 12–17.

Li SK, Ng PK, Qin H, Lau JK, Lau JP, Tsui SK, Chan TF, Lau TC. 2013. Identification of small RNAs in *Mycobacterium smegmatis* using heterologous Hfq. *RNA* **19:** 74–84.

Lin PL, Rodgers M, Smith L, Bigbee M, Myers A, Bigbee C, Chiosea I, Capuano SV, Fuhrman C, Klein E, et al. 2009. Quantitative comparison of active and latent tuberculosis in the cynomolgus macaque model. *Infect Immun* **77:** 4631–4642.

Lin PL, Ford CB, Coleman MT, Myers AJ, Gawande R, Ioerger T, Sacchettini J, Fortune SM, Flynn JL. 2013. Sterilization of granulomas is common in active and latent tuberculosis despite within-host variability in bacterial killing. *Nat Med* **20:** 75–79

Lofthouse EK, Wheeler PR, Beste DJ, Khatri BL, Wu H, Mendum TA, Kierzek AM, McFadden J. 2013. Systems-based approaches to probing metabolic variation within the *Mycobacterium tuberculosis* complex. *PLoS ONE* **8:** e75913.

Loots DT. 2014. An altered *Mycobacterium tuberculosis* metabolome induced by *katG* mutations resulting in isoniazid resistance. *Antimicrob Agents Chemother* **58:** 2144–2149.

Lowe DM, Redford PS, Wilkinson RJ, O'Garra A, Martineau AR. 2012. Neutrophils in tuberculosis: Friend or foe? *Trends Immunol* **33:** 14–25.

Mahapatra S, Hess AM, Johnson JL, Eisenach KD, DeGroote MA, Gitta P, Joloba ML, Kaplan G, Walzl G, Boom WH, et al. 2014. A metabolic biosignature of early response to anti-tuberculosis treatment. *BMC Infect Dis* **14:** 53.

Marrero J, Rhee KY, Schnappinger D, Pethe K, Ehrt S. 2010. Gluconeogenic carbon flow of tricarboxylic acid cycle intermediates is critical for *Mycobacterium tuberculosis* to establish and maintain infection. *Proc Natl Acad Sci* **107:** 9819–9824.

Marrero J, Trujillo C, Rhee KY, Ehrt S. 2013. Glucose phosphorylation is required for *Mycobacterium tuberculosis* persistence in mice. *PLoS Pathog* **9:** e1003116.

Mattila JT, Ojo OO, Kepka-Lenhart D, Marino S, Kim JH, Eum SY, Via LE, Barry CE 3rd, Klein E, Kirschner DE, et al. 2013. Microenvironments in tuberculous granulomas are delineated by distinct populations of macrophage subsets and expression of nitric oxide synthase and arginase isoforms. *J Immunol* **191:** 773–784.

McAdam RA, Weisbrod TR, Martin J, Scuderi JD, Brown AM, Cirillo JD, Bloom BR, Jacobs WR Jr., 1995. In vivo growth characteristics of leucine and methionine auxotrophic mutants of *Mycobacterium bovis* BCG generated by transposon mutagenesis. *Infect Immun* **63:** 1004–1012.

McGuire AM, Weiner B, Park ST, Wapinski I, Raman S, Dolganov G, Peterson M, Riley R, Zucker J, Abeel T, et al. 2012. Comparative analysis of mycobacterium and related actinomycetes yields insight into the evolution of *Mycobacterium tuberculosis* pathogenesis. *BMC Genomics* **13:** 120.

McKinney JD, Honer zu Bentrup K, Munoz-Elias EJ, Miczak A, Chen B, Chan WT, Swenson D, Sacchettini JC, Jacobs WR Jr., Russell DG. 2000. Persistence of *Mycobacterium tuberculosis* in macrophages and mice requires the glyoxylate shunt enzyme isocitrate lyase. *Nature* **406:** 735–738.

Michelucci A, Cordes T, Ghelfi J, Pailot A, Reiling N, Goldmann O, Binz T, Wegner A, Tallam A, Rausell A, et al. 2013. Immune-responsive gene 1 protein links metabolism to immunity by catalyzing itaconic acid production. *Proc Natl Acad Sci* **110:** 7820–7825.

Molle V, Kremer L. 2010. Division and cell envelope regulation by Ser/Thr phosphorylation: *Mycobacterium* shows the way. *Mol Microbiol* **75:** 1064–1077.

Munoz-Elias EJ, McKinney JD. 2005. *Mycobacterium tuberculosis* isocitrate lyases 1 and 2 are jointly required for *in vivo* growth and virulence. *Nat Med* **11:** 638–644.

Munoz-Elias EJ, McKinney JD. 2006. Carbon metabolism of intracellular bacteria. *Cell Microbiol* **8:** 10–22.

Munoz-Elias EJ, Upton AM, Cherian J, McKinney JD. 2006. Role of the methylcitrate cycle in *Mycobacterium tuberculosis* metabolism, intracellular growth, and virulence. *Mol Microbiol* **60:** 1109–1122.

O'Garra A, Redford PS, McNab FW, Bloom CI, Wilkinson RJ, Berry MP. 2013. The immune response in tuberculosis. *Annu Rev Immunol* **31:** 475–527.

Olivier I, Loots D. 2012. A metabolomics approach to characterise and identify various Mycobacterium species. *J Microbiol Methods* **88:** 419–426.

Owens CP, Chim N, Graves AB, Harmston CA, Iniguez A, Contreras H, Liptak MD, Goulding CW. 2013. The *Mycobacterium tuberculosis* secreted protein Rv0203 transfers heme to membrane proteins MmpL3 and MmpL11. *J Biol Chem* **288:** 21714–21728.

Pandey AK, Sassetti CM. 2008. Mycobacterial persistence requires the utilization of host cholesterol. *Proc Natl Acad Sci* **105:** 4376–4380.

Parish T. 2003. Starvation survival response of *Mycobacterium tuberculosis*. *J Bacteriol* **185:** 6702–6706.

Parish T, Smith DA, Kendall S, Casali N, Bancroft GJ, Stoker NG. 2003. Deletion of two-component regulatory systems increases the virulence of *Mycobacterium tuberculosis*. *Infect Immun* **71:** 1134–1140.

Pavelka MS Jr., Chen B, Kelley CL, Collins FM, Jacobs WR Jr., 2003. Vaccine efficacy of a lysine auxotroph of *Mycobacterium tuberculosis*. *Infect Immun* **71:** 4190–4192.

Pethe K, Sequeira PC, Agarwalla S, Rhee K, Kuhen K, Phong WY, Patel V, Beer D, Walker JR, Duraiswamy J, et al. 2010. A chemical genetic screen in *Mycobacterium tuberculosis* identifies carbon-source-dependent growth inhibitors devoid of in vivo efficacy. *Nat Commun* **1:** 57.

Peyron P, Vaubourgeix J, Poquet Y, Levillain F, Botanch C, Bardou F, Daffe M, Emile JF, Marchou B, Cardona PJ, et al. 2008. Foamy macrophages from tuberculous patients' granulomas constitute a nutrient-rich reservoir for *M. tuberculosis* persistence. *PLoS Pathog* **4:** e1000204.

Prosser GA, de Carvalho LP. 2013. Metabolomics reveal D-alanine: D-alanine ligase as the target of D-cycloserine in *Mycobacterium tuberculosis*. *ACS Med Chem Lett* **4:** 1233–1237.

Qualls JE, Subramanian C, Rafi W, Smith AM, Balouzian L, DeFreitas AA, Shirey KA, Reutterer B, Kernbauer E, Stockinger S, et al. 2012. Sustained generation of nitric oxide and control of mycobacterial infection requires argininosuccinate synthase 1. *Cell Host Microbe* **12:** 313–323.

Rengarajan J, Bloom BR, Rubin EJ. 2005. Genome-wide requirements for *Mycobacterium tuberculosis* adaptation and survival in macrophages. *Proc Natl Acad Sci* **102:** 8327–8332.

Rhee K. 2013. Minding the gaps: Metabolomics mends functional genomics. *EMBO Rep* **14:** 949–950.

Rhee KY, de Carvalho LPS, Bryk R, Ehrt S, Marrero J, Park SW, Schnappinger D, Venugopal A, Nathan C. 2011. Central carbon metabolism in *Mycobacterium tuberculosis*: An unexpected frontier. *Trends Microbiol* **19:** 307–314.

Rohde KH, Veiga DF, Caldwell S, Balazsi G, Russell DG. 2012. Linking the transcriptional profiles and the physiological states of *Mycobacterium tuberculosis* during an extended intracellular infection. *PLoS Pathog* **8:** e1002769.

Rose G, Cortes T, Comas I, Coscolla M, Gagneux S, Young DB. 2013. Mapping of genotype-phenotype diversity among clinical isolates of *Mycobacterium tuberculosis* by sequence-based transcriptional profiling. *Genome Biol Evol* **5:** 1849–1862.

Russell DG. 2011. *Mycobacterium tuberculosis* and the intimate discourse of a chronic infection. *Immunol Rev* **240:** 252–268.

Rustad TR, Minch KJ, Brabant W, Winkler JK, Reiss DJ, Baliga NS, Sherman DR. 2013. Global analysis of mRNA stability in *Mycobacterium tuberculosis*. *Nucleic Acids Res* **41:** 509–517.

Sambandamurthy VK, Derrick SC, Jalapathy KV, Chen B, Russell RG, Morris SL, Jacobs WR Jr, 2005. Long-term protection against tuberculosis following vaccination with a severely attenuated double lysine and pantothenate auxotroph of *Mycobacterium tuberculosis*. *Infect Immun* **73:** 1196–1203.

Sampson SL, Dascher CC, Sambandamurthy VK, Russell RG, Jacobs WR Jr, Bloom BR, Hondalus MK. 2004. Protection elicited by a double leucine and pantothenate auxotroph of *Mycobacterium tuberculosis* in guinea pigs. *Infect Immun* **72:** 3031–3037.

Sampson SL, Mansfield KG, Carville A, Magee DM, Quitugua T, Howerth EW, Bloom BR, Hondalus MK. 2011. Extended safety and efficacy studies of a live attenuated double leucine and pantothenate auxotroph of *Mycobacterium tuberculosis* as a vaccine candidate. *Vaccine* **29:** 4839–4847.

Sassetti CM, Rubin EJ. 2003. Genetic requirements for mycobacterial survival during infection. *Proc Natl Acad Sci* **100:** 12989–12994.

Sassetti CM, Boyd DH, Rubin EJ. 2003. Genes required for mycobacterial growth defined by high density mutagenesis. *Mol Microbiol* **48:** 77–84.

Savvi S, Warner DF, Kana BD, McKinney JD, Mizrahi V, Dawes SS. 2008. Functional characterization of a vitamin B_{12}-dependent methylmalonyl pathway in *Mycobacterium tuberculosis*: Implications for propionate metabolism during growth on fatty acids. *J Bacteriol* **190:** 3886–3895.

Schnappinger D, Ehrt S, Voskuil MI, Liu Y, Mangan JA, Monahan IM, Dolganov G, Efron B, Butcher PD, Nathan C, et al. 2003. Transcriptional adaptation of *Mycobacterium tuberculosis* within macrophages: Insights into the phagosomal environment. *J Exp Med* **198:** 693–704.

Schwegmann A, Brombacher F. 2008. Host-directed drug targeting of factors hijacked by pathogens. *Sci Signal* **1:** re8.

Schwenk A, Macallan DC. 2000. Tuberculosis, malnutrition and wasting. *Curr Opin Clin Nutr Metab Care* **3:** 285–291.

Shi S, Ehrt S. 2006. Dihydrolipoamide acyltransferase is critical for *Mycobacterium tuberculosis* pathogenesis. *Infect Immun* **74:** 56–63.

Shi C, Geders TW, Park SW, Wilson DJ, Boshoff HI, Abayomi O, Barry CE 3rd, Schnappinger D, Finzel BC, Aldrich CC. 2011. Mechanism-based inactivation by aromatization of the transaminase BioA involved in biotin biosynthesis in *Mycobaterium tuberculosis*. *J Am Chem Soc* **133:** 18194–18201.

Shimono N, Morici L, Casali N, Cantrell S, Sidders B, Ehrt S, Riley LW. 2003. Hypervirulent mutant of *Mycobacterium tuberculosis* resulting from disruption of the mce1 operon. *Proc Natl Acad Sci* **100:** 15918–15923.

Shin JH, Yang JY, Jeon BY, Yoon YJ, Cho SN, Kang YH, Ryu do H, Hwang GS. 2011. ^{1}H NMR-based metabolomic profiling in mice infected with *Mycobacterium tuberculosis*. *J Proteome Res* **10:** 2238–2247.

Shitikov EA, Bespyatykh JA, Ischenko DS, Alexeev DG, Karpova IY, Kostryukova ES, Isaeva YD, Nosova EY, Mokrousov IV, Vyazovaya AA, et al. 2014. Unusual large-scale chromosomal rearrangements in *Mycobacterium tuberculosis* Beijing B0/W148 cluster isolates. *PLoS ONE* **9:** e84971.

Singh V, Jamwal S, Jain R, Verma P, Gokhale R, Rao KV. 2012. *Mycobacterium tuberculosis*-driven targeted recalibration of macrophage lipid homeostasis promotes the foamy phenotype. *Cell Host Microbe* **12:** 669–681.

Slayden RA, Jackson M, Zucker J, Ramirez MV, Dawson CC, Crew R, Sampson NS, Thomas ST, Jamshidi N, Sisk P, et al. 2013. Updating and curating metabolic pathways of TB. *Tuberculosis (Edinb)* **93:** 47–59.

Smith DA, Parish T, Stoker NG, Bancroft GJ. 2001. Characterization of auxotrophic mutants of *Mycobacterium tuberculosis* and their potential as vaccine candidates. *Infect Immun* **69:** 1142–1150.

Smith PM, Howitt MR, Panikov N, Michaud M, Gallini CA, Bohlooly YM, Glickman JN, Garrett WS. 2013. The microbial metabolites, short-chain fatty acids, regulate colonic T_{reg} cell homeostasis. *Science* **341:** 569–573.

Somashekar BS, Amin AG, Tripathi P, MacKinnon N, Rithner CD, Shanley CA, Basaraba R, Henao-Tamayo M, Kato-Maeda M, Ramamoorthy A, et al. 2012. Metabolomic signatures in guinea pigs infected with epidemic-associated W-Beijing strains of *Mycobacterium tuberculosis*. *J Proteome Res* **11:** 4873–4884.

Stanley SA, Barczak AK, Silvis MR, Luo SS, Sogi K, Vokes M, Bray MA, Carpenter AE, Moore CB, Siddiqi N, et al. 2014. Identification of host-targeted small molecules that restrict intracellular *Mycobacterium tuberculosis* growth. *PLoS Pathog* **10:** e1003946.

Stinear TP, Seemann T, Harrison PF, Jenkin GA, Davies JK, Johnson PD, Abdellah Z, Arrowsmith C, Chillingworth T, Churcher C, et al. 2008. Insights from the complete genome sequence of *Mycobacterium marinum* on the evolution of *Mycobacterium tuberculosis*. *Genome Res* **18:** 729–741.

Strelko CL, Lu W, Dufort FJ, Seyfried TN, Chiles TC, Rabinowitz JD, Roberts MF. 2011. Itaconic acid is a mammalian metabolite induced during macrophage activation. *J Am Chem Soc* **133:** 16386–16389.

Supply P, Marceau M, Mangenot S, Roche D, Rouanet C, Khanna V, Majlessi L, Criscuolo A, Tap J, Pawlik A, et al. 2013. Genomic analysis of smooth tubercle bacilli provides insights into ancestry and pathoadaptation of *Mycobacterium tuberculosis*. *Nat Genet* **45:** 172–179.

Tannahill GM, Curtis AM, Adamik J, Palsson-McDermott EM, McGettrick AF, Goel G, Frezza C, Bernard NJ, Kelly B, Foley NH, et al. 2013. Succinate is an inflammatory signal that induces IL-1β through HIF-1α. *Nature* **496:** 238–242.

Thomas ST, VanderVen BC, Sherman DR, Russell DG, Sampson NS. 2011. Pathway profiling in *Mycobacterium tuberculosis*: Elucidation of cholesterol-derived catabolite and enzymes that catalyze its metabolism. *J Biol Chem* **286:** 43668–43678.

Tian J, Bryk R, Itoh M, Suematsu M, Nathan C. 2005a. Variant tricarboxylic acid cycle in *Mycobacterium tuberculosis*: Identification of α-ketoglutarate decarboxylase. *Proc Natl Acad Sci* **102:** 10670–10675.

Tian J, Bryk R, Shi S, Erdjument-Bromage H, Tempst P, Nathan C. 2005b. *Mycobacterium tuberculosis* appears to lack α-ketoglutarate dehydrogenase and encodes pyruvate dehydrogenase in widely separated genes. *Mol Microbiol* **57:** 859–868.

Timm J, Post FA, Bekker LG, Walther GB, Wainwright HC, Manganelli R, Chan WT, Tsenova L, Gold B, Smith I, et al. 2003. Differential expression of iron-, carbon-, and oxygen-responsive mycobacterial genes in the lungs of chronically infected mice and tuberculosis patients. *Proc Natl Acad Sci* **100:** 14321–14326.

Tsolaki AG, Hirsh AE, DeRiemer K, Enciso JA, Wong MZ, Hannan M, Goguet de la Salmoniere YO, Aman K, Kato-Maeda M, Small PM. 2004. Functional and evolutionary genomics of *Mycobacterium tuberculosis*: Insights from genomic deletions in 100 strains. *Proc Natl Acad Sci* **101:** 4865–4870.

Tullius MV, Harmston CA, Owens CP, Chim N, Morse RP, McMath LM, Iniguez A, Kimmey JM, Sawaya MR, Whitelegge JP, et al. 2011. Discovery and characterization of a unique mycobacterial heme acquisition system. *Proc Natl Acad Sci* **108:** 5051–5056.

* Uhía I, Williams KJ, Shahrezaei V, Robertson BD. 2014. *Mycobacterial growth. Cold Spring Harb Perspect Med* doi: 10.1101/cshperspect.a021097.

Vandal OH, Pierini LM, Schnappinger D, Nathan CF, Ehrt S. 2008. A membrane protein preserves intrabacterial pH in intraphagosomal *Mycobacterium tuberculosis*. *Nat Med* **14:** 849–854.

Ventura M, Rieck B, Boldrin F, Degiacomi G, Bellinzoni M, Barilone N, Alzaidi F, Alzari PM, Manganelli R, O'Hare HM. 2013. GarA is an essential regulator of metabolism in *Mycobacterium tuberculosis*. *Mol Microbiol* **90:** 356–366.

Venugopal A, Bryk R, Shi S, Rhee K, Rath P, Schnappinger D, Ehrt S, Nathan C. 2011. Virulence of *Mycobacterium tuberculosis* depends on lipoamide dehydrogenase, a member of three multienzyme complexes. *Cell Host Microbe* **9:** 21–31.

Via LE, Lin PL, Ray SM, Carrillo J, Allen SS, Eum SY, Taylor K, Klein E, Manjunatha U, Gonzales J, et al. 2008. Tuberculous granulomas are hypoxic in guinea pigs, rabbits, and nonhuman primates. *Infect Immun* **76:** 2333–2340.

Via LE, Weiner DM, Schimel D, Lin PL, Dayao E, Tankersley SL, Cai Y, Coleman MT, Tomko J, Paripati P, et al. 2013. Differential virulence and disease progression following *Mycobacterium tuberculosis* complex infection of the common marmoset (*Callithrix jacchus*). *Infect Immun* **81:** 2909–2919.

Wagner D, Maser J, Lai B, Cai Z, Barry CE 3rd, Honer Zu Bentrup K, Russell DG, Bermudez LE. 2005. Elemental analysis of *Mycobacterium avium*-, *Mycobacterium tuberculosis*-, and *Mycobacterium smegmatis*-containing phagosomes indicates pathogen-induced microenvironments within the host cell's endosomal system. *J Immunol* **174:** 1491–1500.

Wagner T, Bellinzoni M, Wehenkel A, O'Hare HM, Alzari PM. 2011. Functional plasticity and allosteric regulation of α-ketoglutarate decarboxylase in central mycobacterial metabolism. *Chem Biol* **18:** 1011–1020.

Warner DF, Mizrahi V. 2008. Physiology of *Mycobacterium tuberculosis*. In *Tuberculosis handbook*, Vol. 1 (ed. Rubin EJ, Kaufmann SHE), pp. 53–59. Wiley-VCH, Weinheim, Germany.

Warner DF, Mizrahi V. 2012. Approaches to target identification and validation for tuberculosis drug discovery: A UCT perspective. *S Afr Med J* **102:** 457–460.

Warner DF, Savvi S, Mizrahi V, Dawes SS. 2007. A riboswitch regulates expression of the coenzyme B_{12}-independent methionine synthase in *Mycobacterium tuberculosis*: Implications for differential methionine synthase function in strains H37Rv and CDC1551. *J Bacteriol* **189:** 3655–3659.

Watanabe S, Zimmermann M, Goodwin MB, Sauer U, Barry CE 3rd, Boshoff HI. 2011. Fumarate reductase activity maintains an energized membrane in anaerobic *Mycobacterium tuberculosis*. *PLoS Pathog* **7:** e1002287.

Wei JR, Krishnamoorthy V, Murphy K, Kim JH, Schnappinger D, Alber T, Sassetti CM, Rhee KY, Rubin EJ. 2011. Depletion of antibiotic targets has widely varying effects on growth. *Proc Natl Acad Sci* **108:** 4176–4181.

Weiner B, Gomez J, Victor TC, Warren RM, Sloutsky A, Plikaytis BB, Posey JE, van Helden PD, Gey van Pittius NC, Koehrsen M, et al. 2012a. Independent large scale duplications in multiple *M. tuberculosis* lineages overlapping the same genomic region. *PLoS ONE* **7:** e26038.

Weiner J 3rd, Parida SK, Maertzdorf J, Black GF, Repsilber D, Telaar A, Mohney RP, Arndt-Sullivan C, Ganoza CA, Fae KC, et al. 2012b. Biomarkers of inflammation, immunosuppression and stress with active disease are revealed by metabolomic profiling of tuberculosis patients. *PLoS ONE* **7:** e40221.

Wheeler PR, Ratledge C. 1994. Metabolism of *Mycobacterium tuberculosis*. In *Tuberculosis: Pathogenesis, protection, and control* (ed. Bloom BR), pp. 353–385. American Society for Microbiology, Washington, DC.

Williams M, Mizrahi V, Kana BD. 2014. Molybdenum cofactor: A key component of *Mycobacterium tuberculosis* pathogenesis? *Crit Rev Microbiol* **40:** 18–29.

Wolfe LM, Veeraraghavan U, Idicula-Thomas S, Schurer S, Wennerberg K, Reynolds R, Besra GS, Dobos KM. 2013. A chemical proteomics approach to profiling the ATP-binding proteome of *Mycobacterium tuberculosis*. *Mol Cell Proteomics* **12:** 1644–1660.

Woolhiser L, Tamayo MH, Wang B, Gruppo V, Belisle JT, Lenaerts AJ, Basaraba RJ, Orme IM. 2007. In vivo adaptation of the Wayne model of latent tuberculosis. *Infect Immun* **75:** 2621–2625.

Zhang YJ, Ioerger TR, Huttenhower C, Long JE, Sassetti CM, Sacchettini JC, Rubin EJ. 2012. Global assessment of genomic regions required for growth in *Mycobacterium tuberculosis*. *PLoS Pathog* **8:** e1002946.

Zhang H, Li D, Zhao L, Fleming J, Lin N, Wang T, Liu Z, Li C, Galwey N, Deng J, et al. 2013a. Genome sequencing of 161 *Mycobacterium tuberculosis* isolates from China identifies genes and intergenic regions associated with drug resistance. *Nat Genet* **45:** 1255–1260.

Zhang YJ, Reddy MC, Ioerger TR, Rothchild AC, Dartois V, Schuster BM, Trauner A, Wallis D, Galaviz S, Huttenhower C, et al. 2013b. Tryptophan biosynthesis protects mycobacteria from CD4 T-cell-mediated killing. *Cell* **155:** 1296–1308.

Zheng J, Rubin EJ, Bifani P, Mathys V, Lim V, Au M, Jang J, Nam J, Dick T, Walker JR, et al. 2013. *para*-Aminosalicylic acid is a prodrug targeting dihydrofolate reductase in *Mycobacterium tuberculosis. J Biol Chem* **288:** 23447–23456.

Zhou A, Ni J, Xu Z, Wang Y, Lu S, Sha W, Karakousis PC, Yao YF. 2013. Application of ^{1}H NMR spectroscopy-based metabolomics to sera of tuberculosis patients. *J Proteome Res* **12:** 4642–4649.

Genetic Approaches to Facilitate Antibacterial Drug Development

Dirk Schnappinger

Department of Microbiology and Immunology, Weill Cornell Medical College, New York, New York 10065

Correspondence: dis2003@med.cornell.edu

Very few chemically novel agents have been approved for antibacterial chemotherapies during the last 50 yr. Yet new antibacterial drugs are needed to reduce the impact on global health of an increasing number of drug-resistant infections, including highly drug-resistant forms of tuberculosis. This review discusses how genetic approaches can be used to study the mechanism of action of whole-cell screening hits and facilitate target-driven strategies for antimicrobial drug development.

Many classes of antibiotics in clinical use today stem from the golden age of antibiotic discovery, which had its most productive period from 1940 to 1960 (Davies 2006; Silver 2011). These drugs are one of the reasons why most bacterial infections can be cured with a few pills, generally without side effects, within a couple of weeks. It is thus easy to forget that bacterial infections have remained a major cause of preventable deaths in developing countries and continue to exert a profound impact on human health. The relative paucity of novel antibacterials discovered after 1960 coincided with the appearance and contributed to the spread of drug-resistant bacterial infections. When resistant to not only one, but multiple drugs, such infections threaten to erode a cornerstone of modern health care.

Tuberculosis (TB) is a prime example of how treatment has succeeded in developed countries while meeting frequent failure in the developing nations. Treatment failure contributed to the reemergence of a thought-to-be-conquered disease that now constitutes as a major public health threat. First-line treatment of TB consists of drugs originally identified during the golden age of antibiotic discovery. Together with social changes, these drugs contributed to a drastic reduction of TB cases in Europe and North America while continuing to kill millions in Africa and Asia. Drug-resistant *Mycobacterium tuberculosis* (*Mtb*) appeared shortly after the introduction of TB chemotherapy and evolved into extremely drug-resistant *Mtb*, which threatens the TB control programs worldwide. Therefore, the need for new therapies for treatment of this deadly disease remains unchanged since the preantibiotic era. This review discusses how genetic approaches can facilitate the development of drugs for such new therapies.

GENETICS AND CLASSICAL WHOLE-CELL SCREENING

Whole-cell screening (WCS)-based antibacterial drug discovery begins with identifying small

Cite this article as *Cold Spring Harb Perspect Med* doi: 10.1101/cshperspect.a021139

molecules (hits) that inhibit bacterial growth. This inhibitor-first approach provided the foundation of the golden age of antibacterial drug discovery and remains the only development strategy that has delivered antibacterial drugs to the clinic (Brotz-Oesterhelt and Sass 2010). This includes all first-in-class drug candidates currently under clinical development for the treatment of TB (Lechartier et al. 2014). The superior success rate of inhibitor-first strategies is not unique to antibacterial drug development as phenotypic screening has been more productive than target-driven approaches across a spectrum of diseases (Swinney and Anthony 2011).

Several features contribute to the success of classical WCS. These screens allow for selective investment into the chemical structures that can overcome the major challenge of antibacterial drug development: ability to penetrate the bacterial cell envelope. Furthermore, WCS provides an opportunity to discover compounds that inhibit growth by diverse mechanisms, including those that engage multiple targets. The drawback is that the mechanism of all hits remains to be determined.

Whereas it is not required to understand a drug candidate's mechanism of action (MOA) to obtain regulatory approval for use in humans, knowing how a compound exerts its biological function during development is desirable for several reasons. First, many WCS hits act in a nonspecific manner (e.g., as alkylating agents or detergents) and therefore cannot be developed into drugs (Payne et al. 2007; Roemer and Boone 2013). Second, not all hits that are toxic to the host have to be discarded as toxicity need not necessarily result from a compound's antibacterial activity. Antibacterial activity and toxicity are linked if they both stem from inhibition of the same target, for example, an enzyme that is conserved in both the pathogen and the host. Such compounds are not suited for further development. However, in cases in which the mechanism of toxicity differs from that of bacterial growth inhibition, chemical modifications can sometimes eliminate a compound's toxicity without compromising its antibacterial activity. Third, after identifying the target, the structure activity relationship (SAR) of the compound can be explored in more detail. Fourth, and perhaps most importantly, the antibacterial MOA of a compound is a determinant of its in vivo potency. This is exemplified by recently identified pyrimidine-imidazoles, which were active against *Mtb* in vitro, had appropriate pharmacokinetic properties, but showed no potency in *Mtb*-infected mice (Pethe et al. 2013). The activity of these molecules relied on the presence of glycerol, which is used in many standard liquid media, but it is not a physiological carbon source. Therefore, lack of in vivo potency in these pyrimidine-imidazoles was mechanism-based, leaving no path to develop these compounds further.

The potential for discovering other compounds with MOAs that intrinsically have no in vivo potency (here referred to as *novip* compounds) is significant because screening media can, at best, only mimic some of the environments encountered during an infection. More often, they create a physiological context that is quite different from that within the host as many standard media contain nutrients *Mtb* cannot obtain from the host in the provided form (e.g., iron) (Rodriguez and Smith 2006), cannot obtain from the host at all (e.g., biotin) (Sassetti and Rubin 2003; Woong Park et al. 2011), and lack nutrients that *Mtb* is apparently able to scavenge from the host (e.g., NAD precursors) (Boshoff et al. 2008). These differences can cause some mutations to either result in death of *Mtb* in vitro but not during infections (e.g., mutations in *nadA* [Boshoff et al. 2008]) or prevent growth during infections but not in standard media (e.g., mutations required to scavenge iron from the host [Rodriguez and Smith 2006]). One conceptually straightforward strategy to reduce the risk of identifying *novip* compounds is to screen against intracellular *Mtb* (Christophe et al. 2009). However, such screening procedures can also reveal genes that are required ex vivo but not during an infection (Munoz-Elias et al. 2006). Furthermore, *Mtb* induces a complex and dynamic pathology and can be found in multiple different intracellular and extracellular locations (Barry et al. 2009; Dartois and Barry 2013). Some of these locations permit the pathogen to replicate, whereas others may restrict its growth and yet allow its persistence. Therefore, it seems impossible to design screening conditions that mimic the pathophysiological context of an *Mtb* infection in humans well enough to completely bias against *novips*. The best insurance against MOA-based attrition is therefore a solid understanding of a compound's MOA.

Genetic Strategies for Studying the MOA of Bioactive Small Molecules' RNA Profiling

A cell's genome-wide RNA profile is defined by the abundance of the total RNA produced at a given time. Taking snapshots of these profiles became straightforward after DNA microarrays were invented (Schena et al. 1995; Lashkari et al. 1997), and they can now be reported with even higher resolution by sequencing total RNA extracts (Nagalakshmi et al. 2008; Wilhelm et al. 2008; Arnvig and Young 2012). The foremost study to show the use of genome-wide RNA profiling for characterizing the MOA of bioactive molecules was performed with the anesthetic dyclonine (Hughes et al. 2000). Hughes et al. collected *Saccharomyces cerevisiae* RNA profiles induced by hundreds of different genetic or chemical treatments. This generated a compendium of reference profiles to which the RNA profile induced by dyclonine could be compared. Pattern matching algorithms revealed that dyclonine caused changes similar to those induced by mutations in the ergosterol pathway. This suggested that dyclonine inhibited sterol biosynthesis and follow-up experiments confirmed the sterol isomerase Erg2p as a target of dyclonine. This pattern matching approach, as illustrated in Figure 1, has since been used to uncover targets and the MOA of many other antimicrobial compounds (Brazas and Hancock 2005; Smith et al. 2010; Wecke and Mascher 2011). Indeed, *Mtb* microarrays were first used to study the effect of isoniazid on the RNA profile of *Mtb* (Wilson et al. 1999). Hundreds of compound-induced RNA profiles were reported 5 yr later in a landmark study by Boshoff et al. (2004). These profiles helped to investigate a variety of antimycobacterial small molecules, including capreomycin (Fu and Shinnick 2007), isoniazid (Karakousis et al. 2008), PA-824 (Manjunatha et al. 2009), an inhibitor of menaquinone production (Dhiman et al. 2009), β-lactams (Slayden and Belisle 2009), vancomycin (Provvedi et al. 2009), the benzothioazinone, BTZ043 (Makarov et al. 2009), the natural product chelerythrine (Liang et al. 2011), thioridazine (Thorsing et al. 2013), and

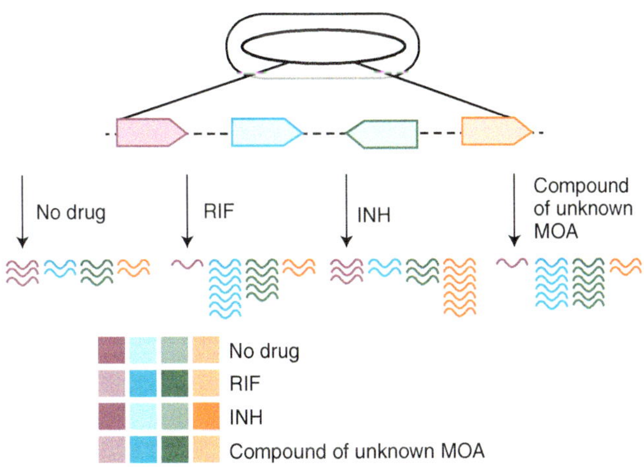

Figure 1. RNA profiling. RNA molecules produced by four genes of the *Mtb* genome with and without drug treatment are represented as colored lines. The color of the squares depicted below the RNA molecules reflects their abundance, with darker colors identifying more abundant RNAs. The fictional data here would suggest that the compound of unknown MOA functions in a manner similar to RIF.

several other WCS hits (Stanley et al. 2013; Wang et al. 2013).

The principal limitations of RNA profiling are twofold. First, these profiles fail to identify the direct target of a compound as they only reveal the biological pathway(s) that respond to the drug. In part, this is because inhibition of different proteins can produce similar RNA profiles, such as in situations in which the proteins form a complex or are required for the same metabolic pathway. Second, the profiles (and other pattern matching approaches) are most informative for compounds, which induce a signature similar to the compounds with a known MOA. Specific predictions are difficult to make for compounds with an entirely novel MOA as appropriate reference profiles are lacking in such cases. This drawback can be overcome by enriching the reference compendium with RNA profiles from genetically defined mutants (Hughes et al. 2000; Mnaimneh et al. 2004; Freiberg et al. 2005). Unfortunately, too few such profiles are available for *Mtb* to apply this principle to facilitate the analysis of antimycobacterial compounds.

Even for relatively small bacterial genomes, genome-wide RNA profiles consist of thousands of individual measurements. This complexity offers the potential to generate unique signatures for many bioactive small molecules while making it difficult to identify the most informative RNAs. The amount of data generated by RNA profiling is not only large, but more importantly, the biological responses to growth perturbation are often complex. This foremost applies to RNA profiles collected at time points or at drug concentrations that impact the abundance of hundreds of RNAs. The nonspecific stress responses contained in such profiles can mask a compound-specific response. Reducing the treatment time and/or drug concentration often simplifies the analysis of bioactive molecules by RNA profiling. Furthermore, the ability of genome-wide RNA analyses to detect minute changes in any single gene coupled with a highly dynamic transcriptional response prevalent in bacteria increases the existing complexity by severalfold. Therefore, obtaining very similar RNA profiles in two apparently identical experiments can be a challenge. Description of all experimental details, strict standardization, and avoidance of procedural changes of gene expression (as can occur, for example, by centrifugation of live *Mtb*) are therefore crucial for producing informative RNA profiles.

Selection and Identification of Resistance Mutations

The first indication that bedaquiline (BDQ, formerly known as TMC207 and originally published as R207910) prevents the growth of *Mtb* by inhibiting the adenosine triphosphate (ATP) synthase was provided by the mutants selected for their ability to grow in the presence of BDQ (Andries et al. 2005). Whole-genome sequencing of these BDQ-resistant strains revealed point mutations in *atpE*, which encodes subunit c of ATP synthase. Genetic and biochemical studies further established that BDQ inhibits ATP synthesis by binding to AtpE, thus confirming ATP synthase as a direct target (Koul et al. 2007). Selecting for resistance followed by whole-genome sequencing (Fig. 2A) has identified mutations that permit growth in the presence of several other small molecules with antimycobacterial activities. Examples include mutations in genes involved in respiration (*qcrB*) (Abrahams et al. 2012b; Pethe et al. 2013), fatty acid synthesis (*inhA*) (Hartkoorn et al. 2012), protein synthesis (*aspS*) (Ioerger et al. 2013), protein secretion (*eccB3*) (Ioerger et al. 2013), polyketide biosynthesis (*pks13*) (Ioerger et al. 2013; Wilson et al. 2013), mycolic acid transport (*mmpL3*) (Grzegorzewicz et al. 2012; La Rosa et al. 2012; Stanley et al. 2012; Tahlan et al. 2012; Ioerger et al. 2013; Remuinan et al. 2013), and arabinogalactan synthesis (*dprE1*) (Christophe et al. 2009; Makarov et al. 2009; Magnet et al. 2010; Stanley et al. 2012; Wang et al. 2013).

Resistance mutations can directly identify high-value drug targets. Selection and identification of such mutations requires no target-specific assay development, can be fast, and is comprehensive as it surveys the entire genome. However, this approach is not without limitations and fails when a resistant strain cannot be

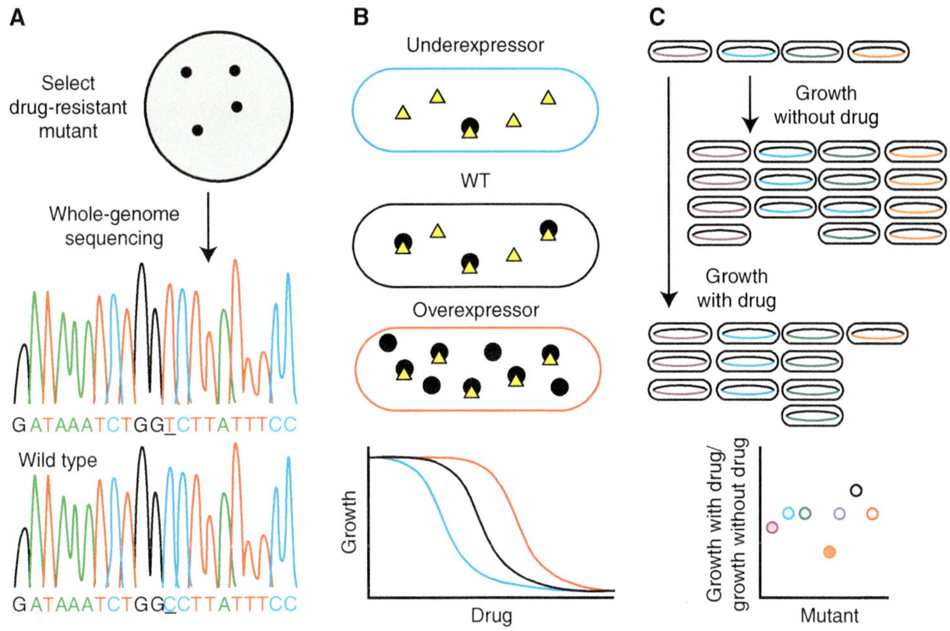

Figure 2. Forward and reverse genetic approaches to investigate small molecule MOAs. (*A*) Selection of resistant mutants. Mutants that are resistant to the compound are selected on agar plates supplemented with the compound of interest. The mutations present in these resistant isolates are identified by whole-genome sequencing. (*B*) Under/over-expression. Reducing or increasing the expression of a candidate target (black circles) can either decrease or increase the MIC of a compound (yellow triangle) inhibiting the target. (*C*) Phenotyping pooled mutants. Mutants are labeled with a genetic barcode and their fitness is analyzed in a competitive growth experiment. This principle can be applied to deletion mutants, underexpressors, overexpressors, or a mix of these strains. The orange-label mutant shows increased sensitivity to the tested drug; the black-labeled mutant (which is only shown in the graph) shows decreased sensitivity.

obtained. Furthermore, alteration of the target responsible for the growth inhibitory effect of a small molecule constitutes only one of the several mechanisms by which mutations can impart resistance. Alternatively, methods such as chemical inactivation, efflux, or failure to transform an inactive prodrug into its active derivative can form the basis of resistance. The knowledge of mutation frequencies that cause resistance by these mechanisms proves highly useful to determine the value of a compound. A high frequency of resistance owing to such mechanisms significantly devalues the compound. However, this knowledge rarely plays a role in defining a compound's MOA. Nevertheless, in scenarios in which a mutation can be mapped to a true target, resistance mutation provides one of the simplest ways to define a compound's MOA.

Linking Small Molecules to Candidate Targets by Increasing or Reducing Gene Activity

To be *directly* involved in the MOA of a bioactive small molecule, a protein has to physically interact with that small molecule. That a candidate protein has the potential for such an interaction within live bacteria can be confirmed indirectly by showing an immediate correlation between the protein's abundance and the minimal inhibitor concentration required to inhibit growth (MIC) (Fig. 2B). This type of experiment has helped to clarify the MOA of INH (isoniazid), which was debated to impair one of two enzymes involved in fatty acid biosynthesis, InhA or KasA. Strains that overexpressed these proteins were analyzed for their susceptibilities to INH and the KasA inhibitor thiolactomycin (TLM). Overexpression of InhA increased the MIC of INH but did not change the MIC of TLM; overexpression of KasA had the opposite effect (Larsen et al. 2002). These results supported the view that InhA and KasA are primary targets of INH and TLM, respectively. Similar overexpression studies have often been performed with *Mycobacterium smegmatis* in which the MOA of different inhibitors was linked to one or more targets, including D-cycloserine to alanine racemase (Alr) and D-ala-D-ala ligase (Ddl) (Feng and Barletta 2003), platensimycin to KasA and KasB (Brown et al. 2009), ethambutol to the arabinosyltransferases EmbB and EmbC (Goude et al. 2009), and certain diphenylurea compounds to inosine monophosphate dehydrogenase (Olaleye et al. 2010; Usha et al. 2011).

In mycobacteria, overexpression has primarily been used to evaluate the role of specific candidate target proteins for compound activity, but it can also provide a means to find candidate targets for a compound with an entirely unknown MOA. To achieve this, libraries of overexpression clones are systematically screened for those that improve growth in the presence of the inhibitor. Such a screen, which used an ordered library of overexpression clones for all essential *Escherichia coli* genes, identified the lipoprotein chaperon, LolA, as a candidate target of the novel antibacterial compound, MAC12343. Biochemical studies confirmed that MAC12343 binds LolA and perturbs lipoprotein trafficking (Pathania et al. 2009). Similar overexpression libraries are under construction for *Mtb* and will hopefully be available soon.

A complication of overexpression screens, especially when using random libraries, is the frequent isolation of efflux pumps. These pumps increase resistance by lowering the intracellular concentration of the compound under investigation, and their isolation does not reveal a compound's MOA. Difficult to interpret MIC shifts can also occur if the candidate target belongs to a protein family of which several members are encoded in the same genome. If the inhibitor binding site is conserved, overexpression of any member of such a protein family will increase the MIC even when only one family member is the physiological target. This has been discussed for inosine-5′-monophosphate (IMP) dehydrogenases (GuaB1/2/3) (Usha et al. 2011), ketoacyl-ACP synthases (KasA/B) (Brown et al. 2009), and methionine aminopeptidases (MapA/B) (Olaleye et al. 2010). In some of these cases, the MIC may have increased because the overproduced protein sequestered the inhibitor from its physiological target.

As target overexpression should increase a compound's MIC, so should target underexpression decrease the MIC (Fig. 2B). This was indeed observed for several conditional *M. smegmatis* knockdown mutants described recently. Underexpression of gyrase subunit A (GyrA, target of quinolones [Sugino et al. 1977], Alr [Caceres et al. 1997], dihydrofolate reductase [DHFR, target of trimethoprim] [Schweitzer et al. 1990], RNA polymerase subunit B [RpoB, target of RIF] [Lancini et al. 1969]), and protein biotin ligase (BirA, target of BioAMS [Duckworth et al. 2011]) sensitized *M. smegmatis* to ciprofloxacin, D-cycloserine, trimethoprim, RIF, and BioAMS, respectively (Duckworth et al. 2011; Kim et al. 2010; Wei et al. 2011). Similar observations were made with *Mtb*, in which partial genetic inactivation of the biotin synthesis enzyme BioA or DHFR increased its susceptibility toward the novel inhibitors of these enzymes (Shi et al. 2011; Kumar et al. 2012). For many of these mutants, it was also shown that they were most strongly sensitized to inhibitors of the partially depleted protein. These and other data (Giaever et al. 1999; DeVito et al. 2002; Lum et al. 2004; Yin et al. 2004; Donald et al. 2009; Abrahams et al. 2012a; Ollinger et al. 2012) confirmed that partial depletion of an in vitro essential protein often causes compound-specific MIC shifts and can thus provide information on the MOA of a bioactive small molecule. However, as is the case for overexpression, underexpression studies by themselves are not sufficient to claim the underproduced protein as the MIC determining target of an inhibitor, as underexpression could also decrease the MIC by sensitizing other enzymes in the same pathway to chemical inhibition.

That underexpression nevertheless provides a powerful tool for identifying candidate targets is apparent from work with *S. cerevisiae*. Construction of underexpressors is relatively straightforward in *S. cerevisiae* and is often achieved with deletion of one gene copy. Such heterozygous deletion strains are available for almost all *S. cerevisiae* genes including those that are essential for normal growth. This mutant collection has been used extensively to study the MOA of bioactive small molecules by drug-induced haploinsufficiency profiling (HIP). HIP measures the effect of sublethal drug concentrations on the relative growth rates of individual mutants (Fig. 2C). Primarily, these studies confirmed that the mutants of known targets of antimicrobial agents are among those most susceptible to growth inhibition by the respective drug (Giaever et al. 1999, 2004; Lum et al. 2004) and were later implemented in identification of novel candidate targets for established drugs. This included the rRNA processing exosome, which was predicted by HIP (Giaever et al. 2004; Lum et al. 2004) and confirmed by various experiments (Fang et al. 2004; Hoskins and Scott Butler 2007; Hoskins and Butler 2008; Kammler et al. 2008) to be involved in the MOA of the anticancer drug 5-fluorouracil. In the opportunistic pathogen *Candida albicans,* HIP helped to identify the guanine monophosphate synthase (Rodriguez-Suarez et al. 2007), a fatty acid desaturase (Xu et al. 2009), and poly(A) polymerase (Jiang et al. 2008) as targets of novel inhibitors. Experiments conceptually similar to HIP have been performed in bacteria where gene expression can be efficiently reduced by antisense RNAs (Donald et al. 2009; Huber et al. 2009; Xu et al. 2010). Unfortunately, antisense RNAs have only rarely been efficient in *Mtb.* Currently, the generation of a large collection of *Mtb* underexpressors depends on approaches that require homologous recombination during mutant construction, such as transcriptional or proteolytic silencing (Ehrt et al. 2005; Wei et al. 2011).

WCS hits are growth inhibitory by definition and thus should primarily target the essential gene products. Nevertheless, mutations in nonessential genes often modulate a compound's activity. Evidence for this came from several studies including those that used the *E. coli* Keio collection. This library contains almost 4000 mutants each of which has a single gene deleted. Of these 4000 mutants, 283 showed greater sensitivity than wild type to at least one of the 14 different antibiotics tested (Tamae et al. 2008; Liu et al. 2010). Whereas some strains were more susceptible to several classes of antibiotics, others were only sensitized to compounds with the same MOA (Girgis et al. 2009; Liu et al. 2010). The drug sensitivity profiles of the latter mutants can be used to classify a compound's MOA with strategies similar to those implemented in RNA profiling. The discriminative power of these profiles can be enriched with mutations that decrease antibiotic susceptibility, which in *E. coli* are as frequent as those that increase susceptibility (Girgis et al. 2009).

The homozygous deletion mutants in *S. cerevisiae* are equivalent to the *E. coli* Keio mutants. Chemical profiling of such mutants (homozygous deletion profiling, HOP) has been particularly useful for compounds whose primary target is not a protein. For example, HOP of ~4700 *S. cerevisiae* mutants revealed that fitness defects caused by deletion of genes involved in DNA repair or in survival during DNA damage can be diagnostic for DNA-damaging agents. In fact, the profiles of these mutants were distinct for chemicals that damage DNA by different mechanisms as they could distinguish compounds that generate interstrand cross-links from those that do not (Lee et al. 2005). The interpretation of HOP experiments can be facilitated by data from genetic interaction studies. Two genes are defined as interacting if the phenotype of their double mutant deviates from the expected phenotypes of the two single gene mutants (Dixon et al. 2009). In *S. cerevisiae*, many such digenic interactions have been defined. These interactions are valuable for analyses of bioactive small molecules as the genetic interaction profile of a gene can be similar to the HOP profile of a small molecule and thus link the small molecule to the respective gene (Parsons et al. 2004, 2006; Costanzo et al. 2010).

FACILITATING TARGET-BASED DRUG DISCOVERY

Target-based approaches typically begin with a screen for inhibitors of a purified enzyme. Unfortunately, most inhibitors identified in several high-throughput screenings (HTSs) against bacterial enzymes had no activity against live bacteria (Payne et al. 2007). Nevertheless, target-based approaches have their own advantages. Primarily, MOA studies are more straightforward for a target-based approach than for WCS hits. For example, a bisubstrate inhibitor (Bio-AMS) designed to inactivate the protein biotin ligase (BirA) was recently found to inhibit the growth of *Mtb*. The study conducted by Duckworth et al. (2011) examined the impact of Bio-AMS on growth and biotinylation of proteins in *M. smegmatis* and *Mtb*. As expected, the activity of BioAMS (but not of INH or ethambutol) against *Mtb* and *M. smegmatis* directly correlated with expression of BirA, and growth inhibition coincided with the depletion of biotinylated proteins. Together, these straightforward observations confirmed BirA as the primary target of BioAMS (Duckworth et al. 2011). The second main advantage of target-based approaches is that they can survey a much larger chemical space than what can be covered in phenotypic screens, especially if fragment-based approaches are included (Scott et al. 2012). This is significant because the physicochemical properties of most molecules in a typical WCS library are different from those of known antibacterials (Brotz-Oesterhelt and Sass 2010).

The Power and Limits of Genetic Target Validation

Choosing a poor target will doom a target-based drug discovery program from the start, yet this might become obvious only after years of work and millions of dollars have been invested. Identifying appropriate targets is thus crucial. Ideally, the selected protein should be (1) conserved among all isolates of the targeted pathogen(s), (2) susceptible to inhibition by a small molecule, (3) different enough from any human homolog to allow development of low toxicity inhibitors, (4) amenable to biochemical HTS, and (5) required for bacterial growth (or survival) in a manner that its partial inactivation suffices to improve a patient's health. Showing that a target fulfills all these criteria requires a small-molecule inhibitor that is safe for use in humans (i.e., a drug). Trying to develop drugs against new targets, therefore, always bears the additional risk that comes from working against a target that is yet to be fully validated. This additional risk applies to inhibitors identified from either WCS or biochemical screens and is one of the factors causing the high rate of attrition of compounds with entirely novel MOAs (Kola and Landis 2004).

Druggability assessments evaluate potential binding pockets by computational or chemical methods (Perot et al. 2010; Barelier and Krimm 2011; Fauman et al. 2011); sequence conservation—within bacteria and between bacterial and human homologs—can be assessed with genome sequence data. An important contribution of genetics to the evaluation of potential targets is its ability to determine the importance of a potential target for growth and survival. The most complete source for this information stems from transposon mutagenesis. Many of the genes that *Mtb* requires to grow normally in vitro (Sassetti et al. 2001, 2003), in macrophages (Rengarajan et al. 2005), or in mouse spleens (Sassetti and Rubin, 2003) were defined by *tra*nsposon *s*ite *h*ybridization (TraSH). TraSH uses DNA microarrays to simultaneously map and analyze the phenotypic consequences of thousands of transposon insertions. Recently, Tn-seq, which uses next-generation DNA sequencing instead of microarrays, has improved these analyses by providing single-nucleotide resolution and a larger dynamic range (Griffin et al. 2012; Zhang et al. 2012, 2013). TraSH and Tn-seq have contributed more to the phenotypic characterization of gene functions in *Mtb* than any other genetic approach. However, they are not ideal to validate gene products as targets for drug development for two reasons. First, TraSH and Tn-seq can identify in vitro essential genes, but neither approach generates mutants for such genes that could be analyzed under a variety of conditions. In the same manner as WCS can identify *novip* compounds, genetic screens can identify *novip* targets (i.e., targets whose inactivation kills *Mtb* under a specific in vitro condition but does not prevent persistence or even growth in animals or humans). It is therefore important to evaluate the role of a gene product for survival under a variety of conditions including those that induce nonreplicating persistence. For genes that *Mtb* requires to grow under standard laboratory conditions, which are among the most attractive targets for drug development, these analyses require conditional knockdown mutants.

The construction of conditional knockdown mutants in *Mtb* became possible with the development of chemically controlled genetic switches for mycobacteria (Schnappinger and Ehrt 2014). Many of the switches developed for mycobacteria depend on placing the gene of interest downstream from a modified promoter so that its transcription can be regulated by a tetracycline repressor and a tetracycline derivative (Blokpoel et al. 2005; Carroll et al. 2005; Ehrt et al. 2005; Klotzsche et al. 2009; Boldrin et al. 2010). These regulatory systems facilitated the analyses of several genes in *Mtb* (Schnappinger and Ehrt 2014), but they depend on secondary events, most notably cell division, to deplete the protein of interest. They are therefore less suited to study the importance of gene functions for survival of nonreplicating *Mtb*. Analyses of nonreplicating bacteria can be performed more efficiently with regulatory systems that directly increase protein turnover. In *Mtb*, this can be achieved by modifying a gene's 3′ end so that it encodes the sequence of the DAS+4 degradation tag (Kim et al. 2010). Conditionality is achieved by controlling the expression of a protein (SspB) that activates the degradation tag. Recently, transcriptional and proteolytic modes of regulation have been combined in a dual-control (DUC) switch, which can achieve efficient and robust gene inactivation in growing and nonreplicating *Mtb* (Kim et al. 2013). Application of the DUC switch to analyses of the NAD synthetase (NadE) identified this enzyme to be essential for survival of both replicating and nonreplicating bacteria. Its inactivation was further sufficient to rapidly eliminate culturable bacteria from mouse lungs and spleens during acute and chronic infections (Kim et al. 2013). Essentiality of NadE for viability of *Mtb* under all conditions tested so far strongly suggests that this enzyme is also required for growth and survival under most (if not all) conditions that *Mtb* encounters in humans. Whether it allows the development of small-molecule inhibitors that would be safe for use in humans remains to be shown.

The second limitation of TraSH and Tn-seq is that they do not allow measurement of the extent to which a gene product needs to be inactivated to impair growth. Although the impact of a transposon insertion on gene function can vary with its insertion site, the phenotypes reported by TraSH/Tn-seq are often attributable to insertions that create a null allele. Complete inactivation of a protein in live bacteria is rarely, if ever, achieved by small molecules. The phenotypes that are caused by complete deletion are thus less relevant to evaluating a new target for drug development than those that result from its partial depletion. All other factors being equal, a protein that needs to be inactivated by >90% (or less) is a more attractive target than one that needs to be inhibited by 90% before growth is inhibited. That vulnerability of mycobacteria to partial depletion indeed varies among different essential proteins was first shown in *M. smegmatis*. For example, HIV-protease-induced degradation depleted *M. smegmatis* of >97% of DHFR and Alr, but this depletion only slowed growth down. In contrast, even modest depletion of RpoB was sufficient to stop growth entirely (Wei et al. 2011). Unfortunately, the extent of functional inactivation that is necessary to impair the growth of *Mtb* is known only for a few proteins, including BioA and PptT, which are required for the synthesis of biotin and polyketides, respectively. *Mtb* is not particularly vulnerable to partial inactivation of either enzyme, as both require to be depleted by >90% to affect growth (Woong Park et al. 2011; Leblanc et al. 2012). Applying conditional gene inactivation systems to the characterization of more genes will hopefully identify proteins that need to be depleted >90% to stop *Mtb* from growing.

Target-Directed WCS

Classical WCS often requires complex studies to define the MOA of hits; biochemical screens rarely identify inhibitors that can penetrate the bacterial cell envelope. Both difficulties can be overcome with target-directed WCS. The principle of this approach was first established in *Staphylococcus aureus*. Overexpression of a *fabF* antisense RNA caused the 5′ end of the *fabF* mRNA to be degraded. This decreased the expression of FabF, an enzyme required for fatty acid biosynthesis, and increased the sensitivity of *S. aureus* to FabF inhibitors (Young et al. 2006). Agar diffusion assays were then used to screen small-molecule libraries against wild-type *S. aureus* and the FabF underexpressor. Molecules that were more active against the underexpressor included platencin and platensimycin, two novel inhibitors of fatty acid biosynthesis with broad-spectrum activity against Gram-positive bacteria (Wang et al. 2006, 2007; Jayasuriya et al. 2007; Fischbach and Walsh 2009). In *Mtb,* transcriptional repression instead of antisense RNA has been used to generate mutants expressing lower than wild-type levels of pantothenate synthase (PanC), diaminopimelate decarboxylase (LysA), isocitrate lyase (Icl1), or the type I signal peptidase (LepB). In addition, these recently constructed mutants show target-specific changes in their susceptibility to different small-molecule inhibitors (Abrahams et al. 2012a; Ollinger et al. 2012). WCS with these strains promises to identify new inhibitors that are able to reach the cytoplasm of *Mtb* and inhibit a desired target.

CONCLUDING REMARKS

None of the approaches discussed in this review existed during the golden age of antibiotic discovery, and antibacterial drug discovery can be pursued without them. However, modern genetics can help improve a process that has delivered few novel molecular entities during the last 50 yr. One important contribution would be to help reduce late-stage attrition (i.e., failure in clinical trials). The cost of introducing a new drug to the market varies between US$500 and 2000 million (Adams and Brantner 2006; Paul et al. 2010). Late-stage attrition can therefore drain the resources of commercially unattractive areas, like antibacterial drug development, and cause them to fail entirely over a long period of time. The two main causes of late-stage attrition are lack of safety and efficacy in people (Kola and Landis 2004; Bennani 2012). Predicting clinical efficacy will remain imprecise. However, if we understand the MOA of the drug candidates that are being tested in the clinic, it should be possible to avoid trials with chemically different compounds that fail for the same mechanistic reasons. The genetic approaches discussed here have helped to characterize the MOA of several antibacterial compounds. However, the MOA of many antibacterials is complex and new insights are still gained into the MOA of drugs that have been in clinical use for decades (Chakraborty et al. 2013). No single approach will therefore be sufficient to define the MOA of most antibacterials. Studies that combine several approaches—for example, underexpression, overexpression, resistance selection, and biochemical studies (Huber et al. 2009)—promise to be the most successful. Drug candidates with novel MOAs are attractive because they could improve TB chemotherapy fundamentally (e.g., by reducing its duration). But they bear a higher risk of late-stage failure if they inactivate targets that have not yet been clinically validated. Measuring the effects that can be achieved by inactivating such novel targets (e.g., by genetic means) in a variety of assays, including animal models, seems prudent.

Second, genetics can also contribute to drug development by providing single-gene underexpressors that help increase the sensitivity of WCS and bias hits toward a desired target. Underexpressors can furthermore be used in a secondary assay to evaluate biochemical HTS hits. This distinguishes compounds that penetrate the bacterial cell envelope poorly (and are not active against wild type but active against an underexpressor) from those that do not penetrate at all (and are active neither against wild type nor the underexpressor). Such compounds could be starting points for medicinal chemistry efforts to improve compound efficacy against wild-type

 Cite this article as *Cold Spring Harb Perspect Med* doi: 10.1101/cshperspect.a021139

bacteria, which could expand the chemical space into the area that is effective against bacteria and underrepresented in most screening libraries.

ACKNOWLEDGMENTS

I thank Kathryn O'Brien, Shipra Grover, and Sabine Ehrt for critically reading the manuscript. I am grateful for past and present support from the National Institutes of Health, the Bill & Melinda Gates Foundation, The Wellcome Trust, and the Ellison Medical Foundation.

REFERENCES

Abrahams GL, Kumar A, Savvi S, Hung AW, Wen S, Abell C, Barry CE III, Sherman DR, Boshoff HI, Mizrahi V. 2012a. Pathway-selective sensitization of *Mycobacterium tuberculosis* for target-based whole-cell screening. *Chem Biol* **19:** 844–854.

Abrahams KA, Cox JA, Spivey VL, Loman NJ, Pallen MJ, Constantinidou C, Fernandez R, Alemparte C, Remuinan MJ, Barros D, et al. 2012b. Identification of novel imidazo[1,2-a]pyridine inhibitors targeting *M. tuberculosis* QcrB. *PloS ONE* **7:** e52951.

Adams CP, Brantner VV. 2006. Estimating the cost of new drug development: Is it really 802 million dollars? *Health Aff (Millwood)* **25:** 420–428.

Andries K, Verhasselt P, Guillemont J, Gohlmann HW, Neefs JM, Winkler H, Van Gestel J, Timmerman P, Zhu M, Lee E, et al. 2005. A diarylquinoline drug active on the ATP synthase of *Mycobacterium tuberculosis. Science* **307:** 223–227.

Arnvig K, Young D. 2012. Non-coding RNA and its potential role in *Mycobacterium tuberculosis* pathogenesis. *RNA Biol* **9:** 427–436.

Barelier S, Krimm I. 2011. Ligand specificity, privileged substructures and protein druggability from fragment-based screening. *Curr Opin Chem Biol* **15:** 469–474.

Barry CE III, Boshoff HI, Dartois V, Dick T, Ehrt S, Flynn J, Schnappinger D, Wilkinson RJ, Young D. 2009. The spectrum of latent tuberculosis: Rethinking the biology and intervention strategies. *Nat Rev Microbiol* **7:** 845–855.

Bennani YL. 2012. Drug discovery in the next decade: Innovation needed ASAP. *Drug Discov Today* **17:** S31–S44.

Blokpoel MC, Murphy HN, O'Toole R, Wiles S, Runn ES, Stewart GR, Young DB, Robertson BD. 2005. Tetracycline-inducible gene regulation in mycobacteria. *Nucleic Acids Res* **33:** e22.

Boldrin F, Casonato S, Dainese E, Sala C, Dhar N, Palu G, Riccardi G, Cole ST, Manganelli R. 2010. Development of a repressible mycobacterial promoter system based on two transcriptional repressors. *Nucleic Acids Res* **38:** e134.

Boshoff HI, Myers TG, Copp BR, McNeil MR, Wilson MA, Barry CE III. 2004. The transcriptional responses of *Mycobacterium tuberculosis* to inhibitors of metabolism: Novel insights into drug mechanisms of action. *J Biol Chem* **279:** 40174–40184.

Boshoff HI, Xu X, Tahlan K, Dowd CS, Pethe K, Camacho LR, Park TH, Yun CS, Schnappinger D, Ehrt S, et al. 2008. Biosynthesis and recycling of nicotinamide cofactors in *Mycobacterium tuberculosis.* An essential role for NAD in nonreplicating bacilli. *J Biol Chem* **283:** 19329–19341.

Brazas MD, Hancock RE. 2005. Using microarray gene signatures to elucidate mechanisms of antibiotic action and resistance. *Drug Discov Today* **10:** 1245–1252.

Brotz-Oesterhelt H, Sass P. 2010. Postgenomic strategies in antibacterial drug discovery. *Future Microbiol* **5:** 1553–1579.

Brown AK, Taylor RC, Bhatt A, Futterer K, Besra GS. 2009. Platensimycin activity against mycobacterial β-ketoacyl-ACP synthases. *PloS ONE* **4:** e6306.

Caceres NE, Harris NB, Wellehan JF, Feng Z, Kapur V, Barletta RG. 1997. Overexpression of the D-alanine racemase gene confers resistance to D-cycloserine in *Mycobacterium smegmatis. J Bacteriol* **179:** 5046–5055.

Carroll P, Muttucumaru DG, Parish T. 2005. Use of a tetracycline-inducible system for conditional expression in *Mycobacterium tuberculosis* and *Mycobacterium smegmatis. Appl Environ Microbiol* **71:** 3077–3084.

Chakraborty S, Gruber T, Barry CE III, Boshoff HI, Rhee KY. 2013. Para-aminosalicylic acid acts as an alternative substrate of folate metabolism in *Mycobacterium tuberculosis. Science* **339:** 88–91.

Christophe T, Jackson M, Jeon HK, Fenistein D, Contreras-Dominguez M, Kim J, Genovesio A, Carralot JP, Ewann F, Kim EH, et al. 2009. High content screening identifies decaprenyl-phosphoribose 2′ epimerase as a target for intracellular antimycobacterial inhibitors. *PLoS Pathog* **5:** e1000645.

Costanzo M, Baryshnikova A, Bellay J, Kim Y, Spear ED, Sevier CS, Ding H, Koh JL, Toufighi K, Mostafavi S, et al. 2010. The genetic landscape of a cell. *Science* **327:** 425–431.

Dartois V, Barry CE III. 2013. A medicinal chemists' guide to the unique difficulties of lead optimization for tuberculosis. *Bioorg Med Chem Lett* **23:** 4741–4750.

Davies J. 2006. Where have all the antibiotics gone? *Can J Infect Dis Med Microbiol* **17:** 287–290.

DeVito JA, Mills JA, Liu VG, Agarwal A, Sizemore CF, Yao Z, Stoughton DM, Cappiello MG, Barbosa MD, Foster LA, et al. 2002. An array of target-specific screening strains for antibacterial discovery. *Nat Biotechnol* **20:** 478–483.

Dhiman RK, Mahapatra S, Slayden RA, Boyne ME, Lenaerts A, Hinshaw JC, Angala SK, Chatterjee D, Biswas K, Narayanasamy P, et al. 2009. Menaquinone synthesis is critical for maintaining mycobacterial viability during exponential growth and recovery from non-replicating persistence. *Mol Microbiol* **72:** 85–97.

Dixon SJ, Costanzo M, Baryshnikova A, Andrews B, Boone C. 2009. Systematic mapping of genetic interaction networks. *Annu Rev Genet* **43:** 601–625.

Donald RG, Skwish S, Forsyth RA, Anderson JW, Zhong T, Burns C, Lee S, Meng X, LoCastro L, Jarantow LW, et al. 2009. A *Staphylococcus aureus* fitness test platform for mechanism-based profiling of antibacterial compounds. *Chem Biol* **16:** 826–836.

Duckworth BP, Geders TW, Tiwari D, Boshoff HI, Sibbald PA, Barry CE III, Schnappinger D, Finzel BC, Aldrich CC. 2011. Bisubstrate adenylation inhibitors of biotin protein ligase from *Mycobacterium tuberculosis*. *Chem Biol* **18:** 1432–1441.

Ehrt S, Guo XV, Hickey CM, Ryou M, Monteleone M, Riley LW, Schnappinger D. 2005. Controlling gene expression in mycobacteria with anhydrotetracycline and Tet repressor. *Nucleic Acids Res* **33:** e21.

Fang F, Hoskins J, Butler JS. 2004. 5-fluorouracil enhances exosome-dependent accumulation of polyadenylated rRNAs. *Mol Cell Biol* **24:** 10766–10776.

Fauman EB, Rai BK, Huang ES. 2011. Structure-based druggability assessment—Identifying suitable targets for small molecule therapeutics. *Curr Opin Chem Biol* **15:** 463–468.

Feng Z, Barletta RG. 2003. Roles of *Mycobacterium smegmatis* D-alanine:D-alanine ligase and D-alanine racemase in the mechanisms of action of and resistance to the peptidoglycan inhibitor D-cycloserine. *Antimicrob Agents Chemother* **47:** 283–291.

Fischbach MA, Walsh CT. 2009. Antibiotics for emerging pathogens. *Science* **325:** 1089–1093.

Freiberg C, Fischer HP, Brunner NA. 2005. Discovering the mechanism of action of novel antibacterial agents through transcriptional profiling of conditional mutants. *Antimicrob Agents Chemother* **49:** 749–759.

Fu LM, Shinnick TM. 2007. Genome-wide exploration of the drug action of capreomycin on *Mycobacterium tuberculosis* using Affymetrix oligonucleotide GeneChips. *J Infect* **54:** 277–284.

Giaever G, Shoemaker DD, Jones TW, Liang H, Winzeler EA, Astromoff A, Davis RW. 1999. Genomic profiling of drug sensitivities via induced haploinsufficiency. *Nat Genet* **21:** 278–283.

Giaever G, Flaherty P, Kumm J, Proctor M, Nislow C, Jaramillo DF, Chu AM, Jordan MI, Arkin AP, Davis RW. 2004. Chemogenomic profiling: Identifying the functional interactions of small molecules in yeast. *Proc Natl Acad Sci* **101:** 793–798.

Girgis HS, Hottes AK, Tavazoie S. 2009. Genetic architecture of intrinsic antibiotic susceptibility. *PloS ONE* **4:** e5629.

Goude R, Amin AG, Chatterjee D, Parish T. 2009. The arabinosyltransferase EmbC is inhibited by ethambutol in *Mycobacterium tuberculosis*. *Antimicrob Agents Chemother* **53:** 4138–4146.

Griffin JE, Pandey AK, Gilmore SA, Mizrahi V, McKinney JD, Bertozzi CR, Sassetti CM. 2012. Cholesterol catabolism by *Mycobacterium tuberculosis* requires transcriptional and metabolic adaptations. *Chem Biol* **19:** 218–227.

Grzegorzewicz AE, Pham H, Gundi VA, Scherman MS, North EJ, Hess T, Jones V, Gruppo V, Born SE, Kordulakova J, et al. 2012. Inhibition of mycolic acid transport across the *Mycobacterium tuberculosis* plasma membrane. *Nat Chem Biol* **8:** 334–341.

Hartkoorn RC, Sala C, Neres J, Pojer F, Magnet S, Mukherjee R, Uplekar S, Boy-Rottger S, Altmann KH, Cole ST. 2012. Towards a new tuberculosis drug: Pyridomycin—Nature's isoniazid. *EMBO Mol Med* **4:** 1032–1042.

Hoskins J, Butler JS. 2008. RNA-based 5-fluorouracil toxicity requires the pseudouridylation activity of Cbf5p. *Genetics* **179:** 323–330.

Hoskins J, Scott Butler J. 2007. Evidence for distinct DNA- and RNA-based mechanisms of 5-fluorouracil cytotoxicity in *Saccharomyces cerevisiae*. *Yeast* **24:** 861–870.

Huber J, Donald RG, Lee SH, Jarantow LW, Salvatore MJ, Meng X, Painter R, Onishi RH, Occi J, Dorso K, et al. 2009. Chemical genetic identification of peptidoglycan inhibitors potentiating carbapenem activity against methicillin-resistant *Staphylococcus aureus*. *Chem Biol* **16:** 837–848.

Hughes TR, Marton MJ, Jones AR, Roberts CJ, Stoughton R, Armour CD, Bennett HA, Coffey E, Dai H, He YD, et al. 2000. Functional discovery via a compendium of expression profiles. *Cell* **102:** 109–126.

Ioerger TR, O'Malley T, Liao R, Guinn KM, Hickey MJ, Mohaideen N, Murphy KC, Boshoff HI, Mizrahi V, Rubin EJ, et al. 2013. Identification of new drug targets and resistance mechanisms in *Mycobacterium tuberculosis*. *PloS ONE* **8:** e75245.

Jayasuriya H, Herath KB, Zhang C, Zink DL, Basilio A, Genilloud O, Diez MT, Vicente F, Gonzalez I, Salazar O, et al. 2007. Isolation and structure of platencin: A FabH and FabF dual inhibitor with potent broad-spectrum antibiotic activity. *Angew Chem Int Ed Engl* **46:** 4684–4688.

Jiang B, Xu D, Allocco J, Parish C, Davison J, Veillette K, Sillaots S, Hu W, Rodriguez-Suarez R, Trosok S, et al. 2008. PAP inhibitor with in vivo efficacy identified by *Candida albicans* genetic profiling of natural products. *Chem Biol* **15:** 363–374.

Kammler S, Lykke-Andersen S, Jensen TH. 2008. The RNA exosome component hRrp6 is a target for 5-fluorouracil in human cells. *Mol Cancer Res* **6:** 990–995.

Karakousis PC, Williams EP, Bishai WR. 2008. Altered expression of isoniazid-regulated genes in drug-treated dormant *Mycobacterium tuberculosis*. *J Antimicrob Chemother* **61:** 323–331.

Kim JH, Wei JR, Wallach JB, Robbins RS, Rubin EJ, Schnappinger D. 2010. Protein inactivation in mycobacteria by controlled proteolysis and its application to deplete the beta subunit of RNA polymerase. *Nucleic Acids Res* **39:** 2210–2220.

Kim JH, O'Brien KM, Sharma R, Boshoff HI, Rehren G, Chakraborty S, Wallach JB, Monteleone M, Wilson DJ, Aldrich CC, et al. 2013. A genetic strategy to identify targets for the development of drugs that prevent bacterial persistence. *Proc Natl Acad Sci* **110:** 19095–19100.

Klotzsche M, Ehrt S, Schnappinger D. 2009. Improved tetracycline repressors for gene silencing in mycobacteria. *Nucleic Acids Res* **37:** 1778–1788.

Kola I, Landis J. 2004. Can the pharmaceutical industry reduce attrition rates? *Nat Rev Drug Discov* **3:** 711–715.

Koul A, Dendouga N, Vergauwen K, Molenberghs B, Vranckx L, Willebrords R, Ristic Z, Lill H, Dorange I, Guillemont J, et al. 2007. Diarylquinolines target subunit c of mycobacterial ATP synthase. *Nat Chem Biol* **3:** 323–324.

Kumar A, Zhang M, Zhu L, Liao RP, Mutai C, Hafsat S, Sherman DR, Wang MW. 2012. High-throughput screening and sensitized bacteria identify an *M. tuberculosis* dihydrofolate reductase inhibitor with whole cell activity. *PloS ONE* **7:** e39961.

La Rosa V, Poce G, Canseco JO, Buroni S, Pasca MR, Biava M, Raju RM, Porretta GC, Alfonso S, Battilocchio C, et al. 2012. MmpL3 is the cellular target of the antitubercular pyrrole derivative BM212. *Antimicrob Agents Chemother* **56:** 324–331.

Lancini G, Pallanza R, Silvestri LG. 1969. Relationships between bactericidal effect and inhibition of ribonucleic acid nucleotidyltransferase by rifampicin in *Escherichia coli* K-12. *J Bacteriol* **97:** 761–768.

Larsen MH, Vilcheze C, Kremer L, Besra GS, Parsons L, Salfinger M, Heifets L, Hazbon MH, Alland D, Sacchettini JC, et al. 2002. Overexpression of inhA, but not kasA, confers resistance to isoniazid and ethionamide in *Mycobacterium smegmatis, M. bovis* BCG and *M. tuberculosis. Mol Microbiol* **46:** 453–466.

Lashkari DA, DeRisi JL, McCusker JH, Namath AF, Gentile C, Hwang SY, Brown PO, Davis RW. 1997. Yeast microarrays for genome wide parallel genetic and gene expression analysis. *Proc Natl Acad Sci* **94:** 13057–13062.

Leblanc C, Prudhomme T, Tabouret G, Ray A, Burbaud S, Cabantous S, Mourey L, Guilhot C, Chalut C. 2012. 4′-Phosphopantetheinyl transferase PptT, a new drug target required for *Mycobacterium tuberculosis* growth and persistence in vivo. *PLoS Pathog* **8:** e1003097.

Lechartier B, Rybniker J, Zumla A, Cole ST. 2014. Tuberculosis drug discovery in the post-post-genomic era. *EMBO Mol Med* **6:** 158–168.

Lee W, St Onge RP, Proctor M, Flaherty P, Jordan MI, Arkin AP, Davis RW, Nislow C, Giaever G. 2005. Genome-wide requirements for resistance to functionally distinct DNA-damaging agents. *PLoS Genet* **1:** e24.

Liang J, Zeng F, Guo A, Liu L, Guo N, Li L, Jin J, Wu X, Liu M, Zhao D, et al. 2011. Microarray analysis of the chelerythrine-induced transcriptome of *Mycobacterium tuberculosis. Curr Microbiol* **62:** 1200–1208.

Liu A, Tran L, Becket E, Lee K, Chinn L, Park E, Tran K, Miller JH. 2010. Antibiotic sensitivity profiles determined with an *Escherichia coli* gene knockout collection: Generating an antibiotic bar code. *Antimicrob Agents Chemother* **54:** 1393–1403.

Lum PY, Armour CD, Stepaniants SB, Cavet G, Wolf MK, Butler JS, Hinshaw JC, Garnier P, Prestwich GD, Leonardson A, et al. 2004. Discovering modes of action for therapeutic compounds using a genome-wide screen of yeast heterozygotes. *Cell* **116:** 121–137.

Magnet S, Hartkoorn RC, Szekely R, Pato J, Triccas JA, Schneider P, Szantai-Kis C, Orfi L, Chambon M, Banfi D, et al. 2010. Leads for antitubercular compounds from kinase inhibitor library screens. *Tuberculosis* **90:** 354–360.

Makarov V, Manina G, Mikusova K, Mollmann U, Ryabova O, Saint-Joanis B, Dhar N, Pasca MR, Buroni S, Lucarelli AP, et al. 2009. Benzothiazinones kill *Mycobacterium tuberculosis* by blocking arabinan synthesis. *Science* **324:** 801–804.

Manjunatha U, Boshoff HI, Barry CE. 2009. The mechanism of action of PA-824: Novel insights from transcriptional profiling. *Commun Integr Biol* **2:** 215–218.

Mnaimneh S, Davierwala AP, Haynes J, Moffat J, Peng WT, Zhang W, Yang X, Pootoolal J, Chua G, Lopez A, et al. 2004. Exploration of essential gene functions via titratable promoter alleles. *Cell* **118:** 31–44.

Munoz-Elias EJ, Upton AM, Cherian J, McKinney JD. 2006. Role of the methylcitrate cycle in *Mycobacterium tuberculosis* metabolism, intracellular growth, and virulence. *Mol Microbiol* **60:** 1109–1122.

Nagalakshmi U, Wang Z, Waern K, Shou C, Raha D, Gerstein M, Snyder M. 2008. The transcriptional landscape of the yeast genome defined by RNA sequencing. *Science* **320:** 1344–1349.

Olaleye O, Raghunand TR, Bhat S, He J, Tyagi S, Lamichhane G, Gu P, Zhou J, Zhang Y, Grosset J, et al. 2010. Methionine aminopeptidases from *Mycobacterium tuberculosis* as novel antimycobacterial targets. *Chem Biol* **17:** 86–97.

Ollinger J, O'Malley T, Ahn J, Odingo J, Parish T. 2012. Inhibition of the sole type I signal peptidase of *Mycobacterium tuberculosis* is bactericidal under replicating and nonreplicating conditions. *J Bacteriol* **194:** 2614–2619.

Parsons AB, Brost RL, Ding H, Li Z, Zhang C, Sheikh B, Brown GW, Kane PM, Hughes TR, Boone C. 2004. Integration of chemical-genetic and genetic interaction data links bioactive compounds to cellular target pathways. *Nat Biotechnol* **22:** 62–69.

Parsons AB, Lopez A, Givoni IE, Williams DE, Gray CA, Porter J, Chua G, Sopko R, Brost RL, Ho CH, et al. 2006. Exploring the mode-of-action of bioactive compounds by chemical-genetic profiling in yeast. *Cell* **126:** 611–625.

Pathania R, Zlitni S, Barker C, Das R, Gerritsma DA, Lebert J, Awuah E, Melacini G, Capretta FA, Brown ED. 2009. Chemical genomics in *Escherichia coli* identifies an inhibitor of bacterial lipoprotein targeting. *Nat Chem Biol* **5:** 849–856.

Paul SM, Mytelka DS, Dunwiddie CT, Persinger CC, Munos BH, Lindborg SR, Schacht AL. 2010. How to improve R&D productivity: The pharmaceutical industry's grand challenge. *Nat Rev Drug Discov* **9:** 203–214.

Payne DJ, Gwynn MN, Holmes DJ, Pompliano DL. 2007. Drugs for bad bugs: Confronting the challenges of antibacterial discovery. *Nat Rev Drug Discov* **6:** 29–40.

Perot S, Sperandio O, Miteva MA, Camproux AC, Villoutreix BO. 2010. Druggable pockets and binding site centric chemical space: A paradigm shift in drug discovery. *Drug Discov Today* **15:** 656–667.

Pethe K, Bifani P, Jang J, Kang S, Park S, Ahn S, Jiricek J, Jung J, Jeon HK, Cechetto J, et al. 2013. Discovery of Q203, a potent clinical candidate for the treatment of tuberculosis. *Nat Med* **19:** 1157–1160.

Provvedi R, Boldrin F, Falciani F, Palu G, Manganelli R. 2009. Global transcriptional response to vancomycin in *Mycobacterium tuberculosis. Microbiology* **155:** 1093–1102.

Remuinan MJ, Perez-Herran E, Rullas J, Alemparte C, Martinez-Hoyos M, Dow DJ, Afari J, Mehta N, Esquivias J, Jimenez E, et al. 2013. Tetrahydropyrazolo[1,5-*a*]pyrimidine-3-carboxamide and *N*-benzyl-6′,7′-dihydrospiro [piperidine-4,4'-thieno[3,2-*c*]pyran] analogues with bactericidal efficacy against *Mycobacterium tuberculosis* targeting MmpL3. *PloS One* **8:** e60933.

Rengarajan J, Bloom BR, Rubin EJ. 2005. Genome-wide requirements for *Mycobacterium tuberculosis* adaptation and survival in macrophages. *Proc Natl Acad Sci* **102:** 8327–8332.

Rodriguez GM, Smith I. 2006. Identification of an ABC transporter required for iron acquisition and virulence in *Mycobacterium tuberculosis*. *J Bacteriol* **188:** 424–430.

Rodriguez-Suarez R, Xu D, Veillette K, Davison J, Sillaots S, Kauffman S, Hu W, Bowman J, Martel N, Trosok S, et al. 2007. Mechanism-of-action determination of GMP synthase inhibitors and target validation in *Candida albicans* and *Aspergillus fumigatus*. *Chem Biol* **14:** 1163–1175.

Roemer T, Boone C. 2013. Systems-level antimicrobial drug and drug synergy discovery. *Nat Chem Biol* **9:** 222–231.

Sassetti CM, Rubin EJ. 2003. Genetic requirements for mycobacterial survival during infection. *Proc Natl Acad Sci* **100:** 12989–12994.

Sassetti CM, Boyd DH, Rubin EJ. 2001. Comprehensive identification of conditionally essential genes in mycobacteria. *Proc Natl Acad Sci* **98:** 12712–12717.

Sassetti CM, Boyd DH, Rubin EJ. 2003. Genes required for mycobacterial growth defined by high density mutagenesis. *Mol Microbiol* **48:** 77–84.

Schena M, Shalon D, Davis RW, Brown PO. 1995. Quantitative monitoring of gene expression patterns with a complementary DNA microarray. *Science* **270:** 467–470.

Schnappinger D, Ehrt S. 2014. Regulated expression systems for mycobacteria and their applications. *Microbiol Spectr* **2:** doi: 10.1128/microbiolspec.MGM1122-0018-2013.

Schweitzer BI, Dicker AP, Bertino JR. 1990. Dihydrofolate reductase as a therapeutic target. *FASEB J* **4:** 2441–2452.

Scott DE, Coyne AG, Hudson SA, Abell C. 2012. Fragment-based approaches in drug discovery and chemical biology. *Biochemistry* **51:** 4990–5003.

Shi C, Geders TW, Park SW, Wilson DJ, Boshoff HI, Abayomi O, Barry CE III, Schnappinger D, Finzel BC, Aldrich CC. 2011. Mechanism-based inactivation by aromatization of the transaminase BioA involved in biotin biosynthesis in *Mycobacterium tuberculosis*. *J Am Chem Soc* **133:** 18194–18201.

Silver LL. 2011. Challenges of antibacterial discovery. *Clin Microbiol Rev* **24:** 71–109.

Slayden RA, Belisle JT. 2009. Morphological features and signature gene response elicited by inactivation of FtsI in *Mycobacterium tuberculosis*. *J Antimicrob Chemother* **63:** 451–457.

Smith AM, Ammar R, Nislow C, Giaever G. 2010. A survey of yeast genomic assays for drug and target discovery. *Pharmacol Ther* **127:** 156–164.

Stanley SA, Grant SS, Kawate T, Iwase N, Shimizu M, Wivagg C, Silvis M, Kazyanskaya E, Aquadro J, Golas A, et al. 2012. Identification of novel inhibitors of *M. tuberculosis* growth using whole cell based high-throughput screening. *ACS Chem Biol* **7:** 1377–1384.

Stanley SA, Kawate T, Iwase N, Shimizu M, Clatworthy AE, Kazyanskaya E, Sacchettini JC, Ioerger TR, Siddiqi NA, Minami S, et al. 2013. Diarylcoumarins inhibit mycolic acid biosynthesis and kill *Mycobacterium tuberculosis* by targeting FadD32. *Proc Natl Acad Sci* **110:** 11565–11570.

Sugino A, Peebles CL, Kreuzer KN, Cozzarelli NR. 1977. Mechanism of action of nalidixic acid: Purification of *Escherichia coli* nalA gene product and its relationship to DNA gyrase and a novel nicking-closing enzyme. *Proc Natl Acad Sci* **74:** 4767–4771.

Swinney DC, Anthony J. 2011. How were new medicines discovered? *Nat Rev Drug Discov* **10:** 507–519.

Tahlan K, Wilson R, Kastrinsky DB, Arora K, Nair V, Fischer E, Barnes SW, Walker JR, Alland D, Barry CE III, et al. 2012. SQ109 targets MmpL3, a membrane transporter of trehalose monomycolate involved in mycolic acid donation to the cell wall core of *Mycobacterium tuberculosis*. *Antimicrob Agents Chemother* **56:** 1797–1809.

Tamae C, Liu A, Kim K, Sitz D, Hong J, Becket E, Bui A, Solaimani P, Tran KP, Yang H, et al. 2008. Determination of antibiotic hypersensitivity among 4,000 single-gene-knockout mutants of *Escherichia coli*. *J Bacteriol* **190:** 5981–5988.

Thorsing M, Klitgaard JK, Atilano ML, Skov MN, Kolmos HJ, Filipe SR, Kallipolitis BH. 2013. Thioridazine induces major changes in global gene expression and cell wall composition in methicillin-resistant *Staphylococcus aureus* USA300. *PloS ONE* **8:** e64518.

Usha V, Gurcha SS, Lovering AL, Lloyd AJ, Papaemmanouil A, Reynolds RC, Besra GS. 2011. Identification of novel diphenyl urea inhibitors of Mt-GuaB2 active against *Mycobacterium tuberculosis*. *Microbiology* **157:** 290–299.

Wang J, Soisson SM, Young K, Shoop W, Kodali S, Galgoci A, Painter R, Parthasarathy G, Tang YS, Cummings R, et al. 2006. Platensimycin is a selective FabF inhibitor with potent antibiotic properties. *Nature* **441:** 358–361.

Wang J, Kodali S, Lee SH, Galgoci A, Painter R, Dorso K, Racine F, Motyl M, Hernandez L, Tinney E, et al. 2007. Discovery of platencin, a dual FabF and FabH inhibitor with in vivo antibiotic properties. *Proc Natl Acad Sci* **104:** 7612–7616.

Wang F, Sambandan D, Halder R, Wang J, Batt SM, Weinrick B, Ahmad I, Yang P, Zhang Y, Kim J, et al. 2013. Identification of a small molecule with activity against drug-resistant and persistent tuberculosis. *Proc Natl Acad Sci* **110:** E2510–E2517.

Wecke T, Mascher T. 2011. Antibiotic research in the age of omics: From expression profiles to interspecies communication. *J Antimicrob Chemother* **66:** 2689–2704.

Wei JR, Krishnamoorthy V, Murphy K, Kim JH, Schnappinger D, Alber T, Sassetti CM, Rhee KY, Rubin EJ. 2011. Depletion of antibiotic targets has widely varying effects on growth. *Proc Natl Acad Sci* **108:** 4176–4181.

Wilhelm BT, Marguerat S, Watt S, Schubert F, Wood V, Goodhead I, Penkett CJ, Rogers J, Bahler J. 2008. Dynamic repertoire of a eukaryotic transcriptome surveyed at single-nucleotide resolution. *Nature* **453:** 1239–1243.

Wilson M, DeRisi J, Kristensen HH, Imboden P, Rane S, Brown PO, Schoolnik GK. 1999. Exploring drug-induced alterations in gene expression in *Mycobacterium tuberculosis* by microarray hybridization. *Proc Natl Acad Sci* **96:** 12833–12838.

Wilson R, Kumar P, Parashar V, Vilcheze C, Veyron-Churlet R, Freundlich JS, Barnes SW, Walker JR, Szymonifka MJ, Marchiano E, et al. 2013. Antituberculosis thiophenes define a requirement for Pks13 in mycolic acid biosynthesis. *Nat Chem Biol* **9:** 499–506.

Woong Park S, Klotzsche M, Wilson DJ, Boshoff HI, Eoh H, Manjunatha U, Blumenthal A, Rhee K, Barry CE III, Aldrich CC, et al. 2011. Evaluating the sensitivity of *My-*

cobacterium tuberculosis to biotin deprivation using regulated gene expression. *PLoS Pathog* **7:** e1002264.

Xu D, Sillaots S, Davison J, Hu W, Jiang B, Kauffman S, Martel N, Ocampo P, Oh C, Trosok S, et al. 2009. Chemical genetic profiling and characterization of small-molecule compounds that affect the biosynthesis of unsaturated fatty acids in *Candida albicans*. *J Biol Chem* **284:** 19754–19764.

Xu HH, Trawick JD, Haselbeck RJ, Forsyth RA, Yamamoto RT, Archer R, Patterson J, Allen M, Froelich JM, Taylor I, et al. 2010. *Staphylococcus aureus* TargetArray: Comprehensive differential essential gene expression as a mechanistic tool to profile antibacterials. *Antimicrob Agents Chemother* **54:** 3659–3670.

Yin D, Fox B, Lonetto ML, Etherton MR, Payne DJ, Holmes DJ, Rosenberg M, Ji Y. 2004. Identification of antimicrobial targets using a comprehensive genomic approach. *Pharmacogenomics* **5:** 101–113.

Young K, Jayasuriya H, Ondeyka JG, Herath K, Zhang CW, Kodali S, Galgoci A, Painter R, Brown-Driver V, Yamamoto R, et al. 2006. Discovery of FabH/FabF inhibitors from natural products. *Antimicrob Agents Chemother* **50:** 519–526.

Zhang YJ, Ioerger TR, Huttenhower C, Long JE, Sassetti CM, Sacchettini JC, Rubin EJ. 2012. Global assessment of genomic regions required for growth in *Mycobacterium tuberculosis*. *PLoS Pathog* **8:** e1002946.

Zhang YJ, Reddy MC, Ioerger TR, Rothchild AC, Dartois V, Schuster BM, Trauner A, Wallis D, Galaviz S, Huttenhower C, et al. 2013. Tryptophan biosynthesis protects mycobacteria from CD4 T-cell-mediated killing. *Cell* **155:** 1296–1308.

Tuberculosis Drug Development: History and Evolution of the Mechanism-Based Paradigm

Sumit Chakraborty[1,2] and Kyu Y. Rhee[1,2]

[1]Division of Infectious Diseases, Department of Medicine, Weill Cornell Medical College, New York, New York 10021

[2]Department of Microbiology and Immunology, Weill Cornell Medical College, New York, New York 10021

Correspondence: kyr9001@med.cornell.edu

Modern tuberculosis (TB) chemotherapy is widely viewed as a crowning triumph of anti-infectives research. However, only one new TB drug has entered clinical practice in the past 40 years while drug resistance threatens to further destabilize the pandemic. Here, we review a brief history of TB drug development, focusing on the evolution of mechanism(s)-of-action studies and key conceptual barriers to rational, mechanism-based drugs.

History recounts streptomycin and para-aminosalicylic acid (PAS) among the first clinical antibiotics developed. Both showed activity against *Mycobacterium tuberculosis* (*Mtb*) and were followed in rapid succession by isoniazid, pyrazinamide, cycloserine, ethionamide, ethambutol, and rifampicin, among others (Barry 2011; Zumla et al. 2013). Together, these advances transformed tuberculosis (TB) from a predictably fatal disease to a curable disease. However, current TB chemotherapies remain far from optimal. TB remains the leading bacterial cause of deaths worldwide, and drug resistance has emerged as a problem of singular importance (Nathan 2009; Russell et al. 2010; Raviglione et al. 2012).

Somewhat unexpectedly, efforts to restock this once celebrated medicine chest have faltered. The causes for this are multifactorial (IDSA 2004; Payne et al. 2007; Zumla et al. 2014). However, mounting evidence has implicated a growing inadequacy of existing tools and approaches (Nathan 2004; Nathan et al. 2008). Although technologically advanced, anti-infectives research remains rooted in the same empirical paradigm that first gave rise to penicillin. While this paradigm was initially reinforced by its delivery of all major classes of clinical antibiotics, its productivity has since waned. We believe that this early success fostered an unintended dissociation between our ability to develop antibiotics and understanding of their mechanisms. Rational, or mechanism-based, paradigms have thus lagged behind.

Here, we review existing knowledge of the mechanisms of current TB drugs and emerging experimental agents. We focus specifically on (1) the frontline agents isoniazid, pyrazinamide, ethambutol, and rifampicin, because of their clinical importance and legacy in the history of

Cite this article as *Cold Spring Harb Perspect Med* doi: 10.1101/cshperspect.a021147

anti-infectives development and (2) bedaquiline because of its role as the first new clinically approved TB drug developed in the past 40 years. However, rather than providing an exhaustive recitation of the literature, which has been extensively cataloged elsewhere (Zhang 2005; Barry 2011; Zumla et al. 2013), we review key findings that informed our current understanding of drug mechanisms and the historical contexts in which they were discovered. By doing so, we highlight recurrent themes that have guided past and current TB drug development efforts and yet unaddressed barriers in the path toward more rational mechanism-based approaches.

HISTORICAL PERSPECTIVES ON TB DRUG DEVELOPMENT

Isoniazid (INH)

Isoniazid (INH) (isonicotinic acid hydrazide) (Fig. 1(1)) is arguably among the most clinically successful and extensively studied TB drugs ever developed (Vilcheze and Jacobs 2007). However, although once synonymous with TB chemotherapy and prophylaxis, INH has paradoxically become a defining feature of the current multidrug-resistant (MDR) and extensively drug-resistant (XDR) epidemic. Historical details of its discovery and studies around its antimycobacterial activities, however, are probably far less well appreciated.

INH was first synthesized in 1912. However, its antitubercular activity was only later discovered en route to the synthesis of amithiozone or thioacetazone (*p*-acetaminobenzaldehyde thiosemicarbazone), a pyridine-based thiosemicarbazone that was being developed in an effort to improve on the tuberculostatic activity of sulfathiazole, first reported by Domagk (Fox 1952; Long 1958). Whereas amithiozone was found to be tuberculostatic in vitro and therapeutically abandoned due to untoward gastrointestinal, allergic, and hematologic toxicities in patients, INH was found to be vastly superior to all other antitubercular compounds tested in vitro and in animals at the time, including closely related nicotinic acid and hydrazine derivatives (Fig. 1). In addition to its potency, INH was found to exhibit remarkable selectivity for mycobacteria, with activity against strains resistant to streptomycin, PAS, and amithiozone (Long 1958).

Numerous in vitro studies soon showed that INH exhibited activity against *Mtb* only when

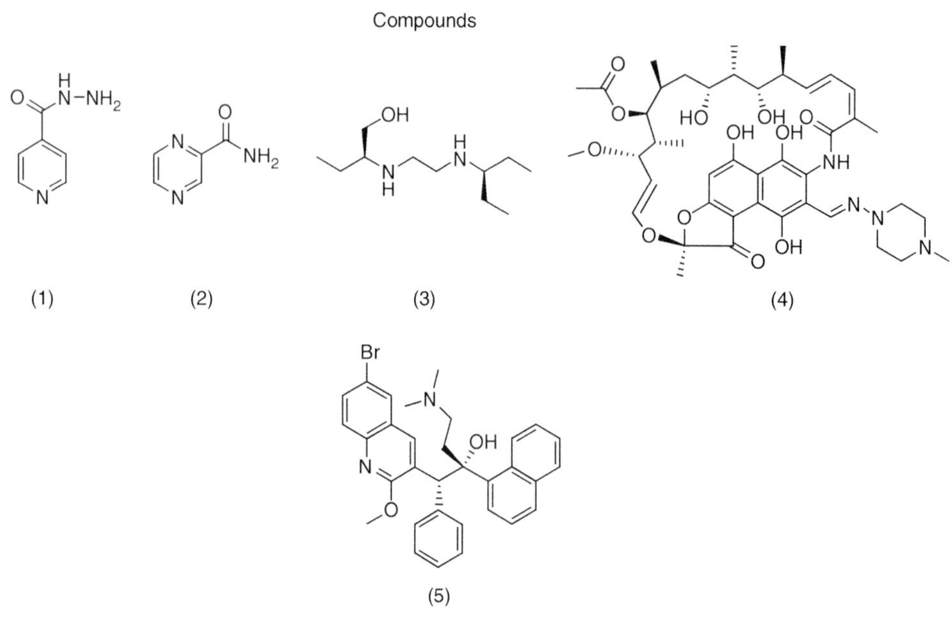

Figure 1. Antitubercular compounds.

replicating and that this activity was preceded by a highly reproducible, although still unexplained, delay of approximately a generation and a half (1–4 d duration). During this period (the initial 16–24 h of exposure), it was noted that INH-susceptible bacilli accumulated ^{14}C-labeled INH that could not be washed away while resistant or dead bacilli did not, and this fixation was accompanied by a loss of its acid fastness and morphologic changes such as surface wrinkling and bulging (*vide supra*).

Concurrent studies by Chorine (1945) serendipitously reported that the structurally related pyridine, nicotinamide, exhibited activity against *Mtb* in vitro and in infected guinea pigs, prompting a litany of studies examining the potential antimetabolic activity of INH (Chorine 1945; Fox 1952; Long 1958; Vilcheze and Jacobs 2007). These studies revealed reductions in NAD levels in INH-treated bacilli but failed to deliver evidence of its direct misincorporation into NAD, whereas the more closely related species nicotinic acid was found to exhibit only weak in vitro activity and no activity in guinea pigs. Notwithstanding, INH was found to induce numerous changes in the biochemical composition and activity of *Mtb*. These included selective effects on its extractable lipids, accumulations of soluble disaccharide trehalose and hexose phosphates, and reductions in respiratory activity. Pope further showed that the activity of INH could be antagonized by the addition of pyridoxine (a precursor of the pyridoxal phosphate cofactor required for many decarboxylation and transamination reactions) and the α-ketoacids, α-ketoglutarate and pyruvate. Although still unexplained, this antagonism was particularly remarkable as pyridoxine also appeared to paradoxically resensitize resistant strains to INH (Boone and Woodward 1953; Pope 1953, 1956; Long 1958).

Serendipity aside, progress toward a functional understanding of the mechanism of action of INH was catalyzed by INH-resistant isolates that were recovered in vitro and in vivo, either following treatment of experimentally infected animals or from the sputum of TB patients, almost immediately after the discovery of INH itself. Work by Middlebrook specifically showed that most INH resistance was accompanied by defects in catalase activity (Middlebrook 1954). Saroja and Gopinathan subsequently showed that INH sensitivity could be restored on transfer of a genetic locus from an INH-sensitive strain of *Mycobacterium smegmatis* encoding a catalase-like activity (manifest, at the time, as resistance to hydrogen peroxide) (Saroja and Gopinathan 1973). Together, these findings introduced the concept that INH might function as a prodrug. Work by Zhang and colleagues later extended these findings to *Mtb*, with the discovery of the *katG*-encoded catalase-peroxidase, which was found to harbor point mutations and deletions in INH-resistant clinical isolates and shown to be sufficient to restore INH susceptibility in resistant strains. Follow-up biochemical studies showed that KatG activates INH by conversion to a range of chemically reactive intermediates, including an isonicotinoyl radical (Johnsson and Schultz 1994; Wilming and Johnsson 1999; Lei et al. 2000), first hypothesized by Winder (1960). Of interest, INH was biochemically also shown to be a potent inhibitor of KatG (Marcinkeviciene et al. 1995).

Adopting a similar approach, Jacobs and colleagues isolated and genetically characterized mutants of *M. smegmatis* resistant to INH and ethionamide (a closely related analog) but exhibiting wild-type levels of catalase activity and susceptibility to other antitubercular compounds (Banerjee et al. 1994). These studies identified a gene named *inhA*, that showed >40% identity to proteins involved in fatty acid biosynthesis in *Escherichia coli* and *Salmonella typhimurium*. These mutants were found to harbor a missense mutation (S94A) that conferred an order of magnitude increase in resistance but could be corrected on allelic exchange with a wild-type copy of the *inhA* gene. High-level resistance could conversely be achieved by overexpressing the wild-type *inhA* gene on a multicopy plasmid. Biochemical studies showed that InhA was a NADH-dependent enoyl-ACP (acyl carrier protein) reductase of the fatty acid synthase type II (FASII) system (Dessen et al. 1995; Quemard et al. 1995; Marrakchi et al. 2000), involved in mycolic acid biosynthesis.

Moreover, these studies showed that INH could inhibit InhA activity in cell-free lysates but that this inhibition was reduced in *inhA* mutant strains.

Using methods of specialized genetic transduction, Jacobs et al. finally showed that the S94A mutation was sufficient to confer coresistance to both the phenotypic and mycolic acid inhibitory activities of INH and ETH at clinically relevant levels of INH (Vilcheze et al. 2006). Together, these findings helped elucidate the significance of (1) decades-long observations reporting INH's effects on acid-fastness (Barclay et al. 1954; Koch-Weser et al. 1955), which was later found to be caused by the unique dye-binding properties of the mycolic acids covalently linked to the 5′-hydroxyl groups of the arabinogalactan polymer of the mycobacterial cell wall (McNeil et al. 1991); (2) the demonstration that isoniazid inhibited the synthesis of mycolic acids in *Mtb* (Winder and Collins 1970; Winder et al. 1970) and its correlation with viability (Takayama et al. 1972); and (3) the specific inhibitory effect of isoniazid on the synthesis of saturated fatty acids greater than 26 carbons (Wang and Takayama 1972; Takayama et al. 1975; Davidson and Takayama 1979).

Building on this work, structural studies of the orthologous enoyl reductase of *E. coli* revealed the presence of a covalent NAD inhibitor species tightly bound to the same proposed region associated with INH resistance in InhA (Baldock et al. 1996). These studies paved the way for the unifying discovery by Rozwarski et al. (1998) that INH did not bind directly to InhA but, instead, as a covalent adduct with NAD. This INH-NAD species was shown to act as a potent, long residence time inhibitor of InhA (Lei et al. 2000; Nguyen et al. 2002; Rawat et al. 2003; Vilcheze et al. 2006). The current working model of the INH mechanism thus proposes that INH is a prodrug activated by the catalase-peroxidase KatG which gives rise to a diverse array of INH-derived radicals and adducts, some of which are capable of killing *Mtb* by potently inhibiting its ability to synthesize mycolic acids. The identities, quantities, and extent to which additional INH-derived species produced by KatG may also synergize with and/or contribute to the remarkable whole-cell potency of INH itself, however, remains to be elucidated.

Pyrazinamide (PZA)

As previously described, pyrazinamide (PZA) (Fig. 1(2)) emerged as an outgrowth of research conducted by Vital Chorine who discovered the ability of subcutaneous nicotinamide to prolong survival of *Mtb*-infected guinea pigs (Chorine 1945). Motivated by this finding, PZA emerged from Lederle Laboratories of American Cynamid as the most active pyrazine analog of nicotinamide tested in mice (Malone et al. 1952). Somewhat unexpectedly, however, PZA was found to lack activity under typical in vitro culture conditions, instead requiring incubation at an acidic pH (e.g., 5.5) similar to that associated with active inflammation (McDermott and Tompsett 1954). However, even under such conditions, PZA showed only bacteriostatic activity with minimum growth inhibitory concentrations (MIC) ranging from 6 to 50 μg mL^{-1} and minimal bactericidal concentrations (MBC) of >1000 μg mL^{-1} (Zhang and Mitchison 2003). This dissociation was further emphasized by the subsequent discovery of PZA's unique treatment shortening (or sterilizing) activity in animals and patients at achieved serum concentrations generally at or below its in vitro MICs (Ellard 1969). Studies of PZA's mechanism(s) of action have thus been hindered by fundamental limitations in the ability to faithfully model its therapeutic activities in vitro.

Limitations notwithstanding, studies of PZA's mechanism(s) of action, like INH, were driven by the in vitro characterization of PZA-resistant strains. McDermott and colleagues showed that, like INH, PZA is a prodrug but activated by an amidase, later found to be encoded by the gene *pncA,* whose ortholog in the closely related and naturally PZA-resistant vaccine strain *Mycobacterium bovis* BCG (Bacillus Calmette–Guérin) was found to harbor an inactivating missense mutation (Konno et al. 1967; Scorpio and Zhang 1996). Moreover, transformation of BCG or *pncA*-defective *Mtb* strains was shown to restore or confer in vitro susceptibility to PZA (Scorpio et al. 1997; Zhang et al. 1999; Boshoff and Mizrahi 2000). Curiously, mutations associated with PZA resistance apart from those mapping to *pncA* have been only rarely described, and attempts to isolate mutants resistant to POA have been unsuccessful. Meticulous biochemical studies by Zhang and colleagues nonetheless showed that in vitro susceptibility to PZA was associated with an intracellular accumulation of its activated form, pyrazinoic acid (POA), as revealed by high rates of POA efflux and the natural resistance of the amidase-proficient mycobacterial species, *M. smegmatis* (Zhang et al. 1999). This accumulation was associated with a dissipation of mycobacterial membrane potential, although the causal significance of this effect remains unresolved (Zhang et al. 2003). More recent affinity-based studies of POA identified several additional high-affinity binding targets. Prominent among these was a subunit of the 30S ribosome, named RpsA, which plays a critical role in a specialized process termed trans-translation which involves the rescue of stalled ribosomes and has been shown to be critical for stress survival and virulence of other pathogens (Shi et al. 2011b). Reflecting the uncertain fidelity of current in vitro models, however, it remains unclear which, if any, of the foregoing findings pertain to the unique sterilizing activity of PZA.

Ethambutol (EMB)

Like PZA, ethambutol (2,2′ ethylenediimino-di-1-butanol) (Fig. 1(3)) was first discovered at Lederle Laboratories of American Cynamid and tested immediately in animals following the discovery of its remarkable stereospecific activity (Thomas et al. 1961; Shepherd et al. 1966). Comparison of all stereoisomers specifically showed that the *dextro* (*S,S*) form was 12 times more active than the *meso* form, whereas the *levo* form was entirely inactive, raising the possibility of a discrete macromolecular target (Thomas et al. 1961). However, its small size and simple structure provided few clues.

Early biochemical studies nonetheless showed that ethambutol (EMB) was rapidly taken up by both replicating and nonreplicating mycobacteria but active only against replicating bacilli, where it was found to impair glycerol metabolism as well as RNA synthesis (Forbes et al. 1962, 1965; Kuck et al. 1963). Subsequent biochemical studies (isotopic-labeling studies and analysis of cellular sugar content) showed that EMB induced an almost immediate accumulation of the major intermediate of arabinogalactan biosynthesis, β-D-arabinofuranosyl-1-monophosphodecaprenol, followed by the sequential accumulation of trehalose mono- and dimycolates and inhibition of mycolic acid incorporation into the cell wall (Takayama et al. 1979; Kilburn et al. 1981; Takayama and Kilburn 1989; Mikusova et al. 1995; Blanchard 1996; Goude et al. 2009). These findings suggested that the primary inhibitory effect of EMB lay at the polymerization of the mycobacterial cell wall arabinan.

As for the case with INH and PZA, this prediction was genetically confirmed with the in vitro generation of EMB-resistant strains and characterization of EMB-resistant clinical isolates, both of which were found to map to a cluster of genes (*embCAB*) associated with arabinogalactan biosynthesis (Belanger et al. 1996; Telenti et al. 1997). Curiously, however, evidence of a specific molecular target remains lacking as even the most common mutations associated with EMB resistance (such as EmbB306) have been also found in clinically susceptible isolates, whereas both EmbB and EmbC encoded arabinosyltransferases are predicted integral membrane proteins that have proven refractory to biochemical study (Safi et al. 2008; Srivastava et al. 2009; Shi et al. 2011a; Guerrero et al. 2013). Studies of EMB resistance have proven similarly challenging to interpret in that high-level resistance, which had been traditionally used as a marker of potential primary targets, was only observed in the setting of multiple mutations (Safi et al. 2013).

Primary target aside, early work by Peets and colleagues showed that the growth inhibitory activity of, and recovery from, EMB treatment could be specifically ameliorated (and often accompanied by MIC shifts of as much as 16-fold) by addition of either the polyamine spermidine or magnesium (but not amino acids, nucleotides, Zn, or Mn) (Forbes et al. 1965). More precise understanding of both its primary and downstream effects thus awaits further investigation.

Rifampicin

Rifampicin (Fig. 1(4)) is a semisynthetic derivative of a natural product ansamycin, which was originally discovered as an antimicrobial activity in the conditioned media of the soil bacterium *Nocardia mediterranei* termed rifamycins (named after a popular French movie about jewel heists). Remarkably, the only component of this extract (termed rifamycin B) that could be isolated in pure crystalline form was a minor (5% − 10%) species with comparatively weak activity that was serendipitously noted to gain activity on incubation in oxygenated aqueous solution. Detailed chemical studies soon showed that this activation was due to a reversible oxidation of a "quinonoid-like" core followed by hydrolytic loss of a glycolic acid moiety, giving rise to the far more active rifamycins S and SV (the latter of which was found to show potent activity against *Mtb*). The discovery of this structure-activity relationship (SAR) provided the first evidence for a potentially specific biologic mode of action that, in conjunction with the poor bioavailability of rifamycin SV, motivated a heroic chemical campaign to develop a more potent and orally bioavailable compound. These efforts culminated in the introduction of rifampicin in the 1960s with detailed knowledge of key molecular determinants of its activity (e.g., ansa chain C21 and C23 hydroxyl groups and C1 and C8 phenols among others) (Sensi 1983; Marriner et al. 2011).

Armed with this knowledge, concurrent studies of protein and nucleic acid biosynthesis revealed that rifampicin specifically inhibited RNA synthesis and, with the identification of RNA polymerase, its molecular mode of inhibition (Wehrli and Staehelin 1971). The study of rifampicin-resistant mutants later confirmed that this inhibition, in fact, accounted for its antitubercular activity as >96% of all resistance mutations could be mapped to an 81-nucleotide region in the coding sequence of the β subunit of RNA polymerase responsible for rifampicin binding (Levin and Hatfull 1993; Telenti et al. 1993).

Bedaquiline (BDQ)

Apart from being the only clinical drug to be approved for the treatment of TB in >40 yr, bedaquiline (BDQ) (previously known as TMC207 and R207910) (Fig. 1(5)) is also the first FDA-approved drug to have been developed in the modern era of molecular sciences (Cohen 2013). BDQ was discovered in a high-throughput phenotypic screen for compounds active against the saprophytic mycobacteria, *M. smegmatis*, and subsequently shown to demonstrate activity against *M. bovis* BCG and *Mtb* (Andries et al. 2005). Early SAR studies of closely related congeners revealed its activity was stereoselective, such that the (*R*,*S*) stereoisomer was the most potent with MICs against *Mtb* ranging from 4 to 70 ng/mL, whereas the (*S*,*R*) isomer exhibited MICs of 0.35–8.8 μg/mL (Andries et al. 2005; Koul et al. 2007). This stereoselectivity suggested the existence of a specific binding target. Remarkably, BDQ was also discovered to also show activity against hypoxic, nonreplicating *Mtb* (Rao et al. 2008). Apart from its potency, BDQ was also found to show an unusually slow time-dependent killing such that only bacteriostatic activity was observed during the first 3–4 d but was then followed by a bactericidal phase with a 4 $\log_{10}$ reduction in measurable colony-forming units by day 14 (Koul et al. 2014).

Insight into the functional target of BDQ first emerged with the generation of resistant mutants followed by whole-genome resequencing. These studies identified mutations in the *atpE* gene encoding the membrane bound c subunit of F_0ATP synthase, which were independently confirmed through comparative sequence analyses of naturally BDQ-susceptible and -resistant mycobacteria, and BDQ-selected resistant *Mtb* strains (Andries et al. 2005; Huitric et al. 2007, 2010). Interestingly, sequence comparisons to the orthologous mitochondrial ATP synthase revealed an alanine-to-methionine substitution at position 63 that was hypothesized to explain the apparent 20,000-fold selectivity of binding to the *Mtb* over mammalian enzyme (Haagsma et al. 2009). Biochemical studies nonetheless showed accompanying reductions in bacterial ATP levels, lending orthogonal evidence for the role of ATP synthase in its mechanism (Andries et al. 2005; Koul et al. 2007, 2014; Rao et al. 2008). Affinity purification-based efforts to identify binding partners (using an amine analog of BDQ immobilized to a sepharose resin) resulted in the identification of α and β subunits of ATP synthase from the total membrane fraction of *M. smegmatis*, although the c subunit was not recovered, perhaps because of its high hydrophobicity (Koul et al. 2007). Interestingly, however, a recent study of resistant mutants from clinical isolates showed that ~38% of mutations were unrelated to the ATP synthase operon (Huitric et al. 2010). Thus, although the available data suggests that BDQ targets ATP synthase, it is possible that additional targets remain to be identified.

RETROSPECTIVE VIEWS ON MECHANISM-BASED STUDIES AND CONCLUSIONS

Looking back, it is interesting to note that as the tools used to develop and study antibiotics have steadily increased in scale and precision, our understanding of their mechanisms has somewhat paradoxically shrunken in scope. Indeed, early studies of antibiotic mechanisms largely consisted in broad phenotypic and biochemical characterizations of antimicrobial activity. The advent of genetic tools and approaches, however, fostered a systematic shift toward organism-wide, but gene-specific, views of drug activity. This shift was largely driven by the successful use of drug resistance as a functional "loss-of-function" window into the targets and mechanisms of INH (InhA), rifampicin (RNA polymerase β subunit), and BDQ (ATP synthase). This same experimental shift, however, was also accompanied by a limited appreciation of the only partial intersection between drug activity and resistance, and operational shift toward more empirical definitions of drug targets and mechanisms based on the genes and/or functions whose dysregulation affected activity. Although functionally powerful for its genome-wide scope, this shift had the unintended consequence of conceptually constraining drug activity to a single best target and mechanism of action because of its experimental proclivity to select for and focus on isolated genes and/or proteins.

Defined by their ability to suppress or kill bacteria, most antibiotics act through the inhibition of biochemical networks, and elicit maladaptive phenotypes that, although experimentally simple to assay, are no less complex than their adaptive physiologic counterparts. Their mechanisms of action are thus likely, if not certain, to be mediated through an equally complex array of factors, whose identities, quantitative contributions, and interactions have only been partially elucidated.

Looking ahead, it is encouraging to see growing recognition of the complexity of antibiotic action and the advent of new level technologies and disciplines to help respond to this challenge. One current area of potential promise is the rapidly emerging field of metabolomics. Metabolomics is the youngest of systems-level disciplines, defined as the global study of metabolites in a biological system under a given set of conditions (Saghatelian and Cravatt 2005; van der Werf et al. 2005, 2007; Patti et al. 2012). Because metabolites are the biochemical fuel of all physiologic processes, metabolomic approaches offer a global biochemical window into the physiologic composition and state of a given cell. From a pharmacologic point of view, metabolomic readouts offer direct biochemical insights into the intrabacterial "pharmacokinetic" fates and "pharmacodynamic" actions of a given compound within *Mtb* (de Carvalho et al. 2010, 2011; Pethe et al. 2010; Chakraborty et al. 2013). Although technologically advanced, current antibiotic development efforts rest heavily, if not exclusively, on the use of indirect bacteriologic or genetic readouts or in vitro measurements of enzyme activity as the primary measures of compound activity. Although valuable, these same tools and readouts have left critical ambiguities. For example, in elucidating the structure-activity relationship of a given compound, it is difficult, if not impossible, to determine the extent to which the activity of a given compound is mediated by its ability to accumulate within a bacterial cell, its biochemical affinity for a specific target, and/or its biotransformation into one or more bioactive species. Direct biochemical readouts of a compound's intrabacterial "pharmacokinetic" fates and "pharmacodynamic" actions thus represent a major unmet scientific need of direct pharmacologic relevance. In a recent study, Chakraborty and colleagues reported one such application of metabolomic technologies using PAS, a close structural analog and competitive in vitro inhibitor of the folate biosynthetic enzyme dihydropteroate synthase (DHPS) (Chakraborty et al. 2013). Using this platform, the investigators showed that, contrary to longstanding inferences, PAS inhibited *Mtb* by functioning as a replacement substrate, rather than inhibitor, that, in turn, gave rise to dysfunctional folate analogs. In contrast, far more potent sulfonamide-based competitive inhibitors of *Mtb*'s DHPS (sulfamethoxazole, sulfaniliamide, and diaminodiphenylsulfone) were shown to lack growth-inhibitory activity because of their rapid intrabacterial inactivation, rather than failure to penetrate its notoriously thick and hydrophobic envelope. These studies thus not only showed the highly unpredictable intrabacterial fates of two well-studied antibiotics, but more importantly revised our fundamental understanding of their accompanying activities (or lack thereof). Metabolomics not withstanding, it remains important to recognize that no one approach is likely to prove sufficient to predictably determine the target and/or mechanism of any antibiotic. It is thus likely that rational mechanism-based drug development will emerge only with a continued expansion and integration of systems-level approaches.

ACKNOWLEDGMENTS

We apologize that many papers could not be discussed owing to the lack of space. The authors gratefully acknowledge the support of the Bill and Melinda Gates Foundation TB Drug Accelerator Program and National Institutes of Health for funding.

REFERENCES

Andries K, Verhasselt P, Guillemont J, Gohlmann HW, Neefs JM, Winkler H, Van Gestel J, Timmerman P, Zhu M, Lee E, et al. 2005. A diarylquinoline drug active on the ATP synthase of *Mycobacterium tuberculosis*. *Science* **307:** 223–227.

Baldock C, Rafferty JB, Sedelnikova SE, Baker PJ, Stuitje AR, Slabas AR, Hawkes TR, Rice DW. 1996. A mechanism of drug action revealed by structural studies of enoyl reductase. *Science* **274:** 2107–2110.

Banerjee A, Dubnau E, Quemard A, Balasubramanian V, Um KS, Wilson T, Collins D, de Lisle G, Jacobs WR Jr. 1994. *inhA*, a gene encoding a target for isoniazid and ethionamide in *Mycobacterium tuberculosis*. *Science* **263:** 227–230.

Barclay WR, Koch-Weser D, Ebert RH. 1954. Mode of action of isoniazid. II. *Am Rev Tuberc* **70:** 784–792.

Barry CE. 2011. Lessons from seven decades of antituberculosis drug discovery. *Curr Top Med Chem* **11:** 1216–1225.

Belanger AE, Besra GS, Ford ME, Mikusova K, Belisle JT, Brennan PJ, Inamine JM. 1996. The *embAB* genes of *Mycobacterium avium* encode an arabinosyl transferase involved in cell wall arabinan biosynthesis that is the target for the antimycobacterial drug ethambutol. *Proc Natl Acad Sci* **93:** 11919–11924.

Blanchard JS. 1996. Molecular mechanisms of drug resistance in *Mycobacterium tuberculosis*. *Annu Rev Biochem* **65:** 215–239.

Boone IU, Woodward KT. 1953. Relationship of pyridoxine and its derivatives to the mechanism of action of isoniazid. *Proc Soc Exp Biol Med* **84:** 292–296.

Boshoff HI, Mizrahi V. 2000. Expression of *Mycobacterium smegmatis* pyrazinamidase in *Mycobacterium tuberculosis* confers hypersensitivity to pyrazinamide and related amides. *J Bacteriol* **182:** 5479–5485.

Chakraborty S, Gruber T, Barry CE III, Boshoff HI, Rhee KY. 2013. Para-aminosalicylic acid acts as an alternative substrate of folate metabolism in *Mycobacterium tuberculosis*. *Science* **339:** 88–91.

Chorine V. 1945. Action de l'amide nicotinique sur les bacilles du genre mycobcaterium. *C R Hebd Seances Acad Sci* **220:** 150–151.

Cohen J. 2013. Infectious disease. Approval of novel TB drug celebrated—With restraint. *Science* **339:** 130.

Davidson LA, Takayama K. 1979. Isoniazid inhibition of the synthesis of monounsaturated long-chain fatty acids in *Mycobacterium tuberculosis* H37Ra. *Antimicrob Agents Chemother* **16:** 104–105.

de Carvalho LP, Fischer SM, Marrero J, Nathan C, Ehrt S, Rhee KY. 2010. Metabolomics of *Mycobacterium tuberculosis* reveals compartmentalized co-catabolism of carbon substrates. *Chem Biol* **17:** 1122–1131.

de Carvalho LP, Darby CM, Rhee KY, Nathan C. 2011. Nitazoxanide disrupts membrane potential and intrabacterial pH homeostasis of *Mycobacterium tuberculosis*. *ACS Med Chem Lett* **2:** 849–854.

Dessen A, Quemard A, Blanchard JS, Jacobs WR Jr, Sacchettini JC. 1995. Crystal structure and function of the isoniazid target of *Mycobacterium tuberculosis*. *Science* **267:** 1638–1641.

Ellard GA. 1969. Absorption, metabolism and excretion of pyrazinamide in man. *Tubercle* **50:** 144–158.

Forbes M, Kuck NA, Peets EA. 1962. Mode of action of ethambutol. *J Bacteriol* **84:** 1099–1103.

Forbes M, Kuck NA, Peets EA. 1965. Effect of ethambutol on nucleic acid metabolism in *Mycobacterium smegmatis* and its reversal by polyamines and divalent cations. *J Bacteriol* **89:** 1299–1305.

Fox HH. 1952. The chemical approach to the control of tuberculosis. *Science* **116:** 129–134.

Goude R, Amin AG, Chatterjee D, Parish T. 2009. The arabinosyltransferase EmbC is inhibited by ethambutol in *Mycobacterium tuberculosis. Antimicrob Agents Chemother* **53:** 4138–4146.

Guerrero E, Lemus D, Yzquierdo S, Vilchez G, Munoz M, Montoro E, Takiff H. 2013. Association between embB mutations and ethambutol resistance in *Mycobacterium tuberculosis* isolates from Cuba and the Dominican Republic: Reproducible patterns and problems. *Rev Argent Microbiol* **45:** 21–26.

Haagsma AC, Abdillahi-Ibrahim R, Wagner MJ, Krab K, Vergauwen K, Guillemont J, Andries K, Lill H, Koul A, Bald D. 2009. Selectivity of TMC207 towards mycobacterial ATP synthase compared with that towards the eukaryotic homologue. *Antimicrob Agents Chemother* **53:** 1290–1292.

Huitric E, Verhasselt P, Andries K, Hoffner SE. 2007. In vitro antimycobacterial spectrum of a diarylquinoline ATP synthase inhibitor. *Antimicrob Agents Chemother* **51:** 4202–4204.

Huitric E, Verhasselt P, Koul A, Andries K, Hoffner S, Andersson DI. 2010. Rates and mechanisms of resistance development in *Mycobacterium tuberculosis* to a novel diarylquinoline ATP synthase inhibitor. *Antimicrob Agents Chemother* **54:** 1022–1028.

Infectious Diseases Society of America (IDSA). 2004. Bad bugs, no drugs: As antibiotic R&D stagnates, a public health crisis brews.

Johnsson K, Schultz PG. 1994. Mechanistic studies of the oxidation of isoniazid by the catalase-peroxidase from *Mycobacterium tuberculosis. J Am Chem Soc* **116:** 7425–7426.

Kilburn JO, Takayama K, Armstrong EL, Greenberg J. 1981. Effects of ethambutol on phospholipid metabolism in *Mycobacterium smegmatis. Antimicrob Agents Chemother* **19:** 346–348.

Koch-Weser D, Barclay WR, Ebert RH. 1955. The influence of isoniazid and streptomycin on acid-fastness, tetrazolium reduction, growth, and survival of tubercle bacilli. *Am Rev Tuberc* **71:** 556–565.

Konno K, Feldmann FM, McDermott W. 1967. Pyrazinamide susceptibility and amidase activity of tubercle bacilli. *Am Rev Respir Dis* **95:** 461–469.

Koul A, Dendouga N, Vergauwen K, Molenberghs B, Vranckx L, Willebrords R, Ristic Z, Lill H, Dorange I, Guillemont J, et al. 2007. Diarylquinolines target subunit c of mycobacterial ATP synthase. *Nat Chem Biol* **3:** 323–324.

Koul A, Vranckx L, Dhar N, Gohlmann HW, Ozdemir E, Neefs JM, Schulz M, Lu P, Mortz E, McKinney JD, et al. 2014. Delayed bactericidal response of *Mycobacterium tuberculosis* to bedaquiline involves remodelling of bacterial metabolism. *Nat Commun* **5:** 3369.

Kuck NA, Peets EA, Forbes M. 1963. Mode of action of ethambutol on *Mycobacterium tuberculosis*, strain H37R V. *Am Rev Respir Dis* **87:** 905–906.

Lei B, Wei CJ, Tu SC. 2000. Action mechanism of antitubercular isoniazid. Activation by *Mycobacterium tuberculosis* KatG, isolation, and characterization of inha inhibitor. *J Biol Chem* **275:** 2520–2526.

Levin ME, Hatfull GF. 1993. *Mycobacterium smegmatis* RNA polymerase: DNA supercoiling, action of rifampicin and mechanism of rifampicin resistance. *Mol Microbiol* **8:** 277–285.

Long ER, ed. 1958. *The chemistry and chemotherapy of tuberculosis*, 3rd ed. Williams & Wilkins, Baltimore.

Malone L, Schurr A, Lindh H, Mc KD, Kiser JS, Williams JH. 1952. The effect of pyrazinamide (aldinamide) on experimental tuberculosis in mice. *Am Rev Tuberc* **65:** 511–518.

Marcinkeviciene JA, Magliozzo RS, Blanchard JS. 1995. Purification and characterization of the *Mycobacterium smegmatis* catalase-peroxidase involved in isoniazid activation. *J Biol Chem* **270:** 22290–22295.

Marrakchi H, Laneelle G, Quemard A. 2000. InhA, a target of the antituberculous drug isoniazid, is involved in a mycobacterial fatty acid elongation system, FAS-II. *Microbiology* **146:** 289–296.

Marriner GA, Nayyar A, Uh E, Wong SY, Mukherjee T, Via LE, Carroll M, Edwards RL, Gruber TD, Choi I, et al. 2011. The medicinal chemistry of tuberculosis chemotherapy. *Top Med Chem* **7:** 47–124.

McDermott W, Tompsett R. 1954. Activation of pyrazinamide and nicotinamide in acidic environments in vitro. *Am Rev Tuberc* **70:** 748–754.

McNeil M, Daffe M, Brennan PJ. 1991. Location of the mycolyl ester substituents in the cell walls of mycobacteria. *J Biol Chem* **266:** 13217–13223.

Middlebrook G. 1954. Isoniazid-resistance and catalase activity of tubercle bacilli; a preliminary report. *Am Rev Tuberc* **69:** 471–472.

Mikusova K, Slayden RA, Besra GS, Brennan PJ. 1995. Biogenesis of the mycobacterial cell wall and the site of action of ethambutol. *Antimicrob Agents Chemother* **39:** 2484–2489.

Nathan C. 2004. Antibiotics at the crossroads. *Nature* **431:** 899–902.

Nathan C. 2009. Taming tuberculosis: A challenge for science and society. *Cell Host Microbe* **5:** 220–224.

Nathan C, Gold B, Lin G, Stegman M, de Carvalho LP, Vandal O, Venugopal A, Bryk R. 2008. A philosophy of anti-infectives as a guide in the search for new drugs for tuberculosis. *Tuberculosis (Edinb)* **88:** S25–S33.

Nguyen M, Quemard A, Broussy S, Bernadou J, Meunier B. 2002. Mn(III) pyrophosphate as an efficient tool for studying the mode of action of isoniazid on the InhA protein of *Mycobacterium tuberculosis. Antimicrob Agents Chemother* **46:** 2137–2144.

Patti GJ, Yanes O, Siuzdak G. 2012. Innovation: Metabolomics: The apogee of the omics trilogy. *Nat Rev Mol Cell Biol* **13:** 263–269.

Payne DJ, Gwynn MN, Holmes DJ, Pompliano DL. 2007. Drugs for bad bugs: Confronting the challenges of antibacterial discovery. *Nat Rev Drug Discov* **6:** 29–40.

Pethe K, Sequeira PC, Agarwalla S, Rhee K, Kuhen K, Phong WY, Patel V, Beer D, Walker JR, Duraiswamy J, et al. 2010. A chemical genetic screen in *Mycobacterium tuberculosis* identifies carbon-source-dependent growth inhibitors devoid of in vivo efficacy. *Nat Commun* **1:** 57.

Pope H. 1953. Antagonism of isoniazid by certain metabolites. *Am Rev Tuberc* **68:** 938–939.

Pope H. 1956. The neutralization of isoniazid activity in *Mycobacterium tuberculosis* by certain metabolites. *Am Rev Tuberc* **73:** 735–747.

Quemard A, Sacchettini JC, Dessen A, Vilcheze C, Bittman R, Jacobs WR Jr, Blanchard JS. 1995. Enzymatic characterization of the target for isoniazid in *Mycobacterium tuberculosis. Biochemistry* **34:** 8235–8241.

Rao SP, Alonso S, Rand L, Dick T, Pethe K. 2008. The protonmotive force is required for maintaining ATP homeostasis and viability of hypoxic, nonreplicating *Mycobacterium tuberculosis. Proc Natl Acad Sci* **105:** 11945–11950.

Raviglione M, Marais B, Floyd K, Lonnroth K, Getahun H, Migliori GB, Harries AD, Nunn P, Lienhardt C, Graham S, et al. 2012. Scaling up interventions to achieve global tuberculosis control: Progress and new developments. *Lancet* **379:** 1902–1913.

Rawat R, Whitty A, Tonge PJ. 2003. The isoniazid-NAD adduct is a slow, tight-binding inhibitor of InhA, the *Mycobacterium tuberculosis* enoyl reductase: Adduct affinity and drug resistance. *Proc Natl Acad Sci* **100:** 13881–13886.

Rozwarski DA, Grant GA, Barton DH, Jacobs WR Jr, Sacchettini JC. 1998. Modification of the NADH of the isoniazid target (InhA) from *Mycobacterium tuberculosis. Science* **279:** 98–102.

Russell DG, Barry CE III, Flynn JL. 2010. Tuberculosis: What we don't know can, and does, hurt us. *Science* **328:** 852–856.

Safi H, Sayers B, Hazbon MH, Alland D. 2008. Transfer of embB codon 306 mutations into clinical *Mycobacterium tuberculosis* strains alters susceptibility to ethambutol, isoniazid, and rifampin. *Antimicrob Agents Chemother* **52:** 2027–2034.

Safi H, Lingaraju S, Amin A, Kim S, Jones M, Holmes M, McNeil M, Peterson SN, Chatterjee D, Fleischmann R, et al. 2013. Evolution of high-level ethambutol-resistant tuberculosis through interacting mutations in decaprenylphosphoryl-β-D-arabinose biosynthetic and utilization pathway genes. *Nat Genet* **45:** 1190–1197.

Saghatelian A, Cravatt BF. 2005. Global strategies to integrate the proteome and metabolome. *Curr Opin Chem Biol* **9:** 62–68.

Saroja D, Gopinathan KP. 1973. Transduction of isoniazid susceptibility-resistance and streptomycin resistance in mycobacteria. *Antimicrob Agents Chemother* **4:** 643–645.

Scorpio A, Zhang Y. 1996. Mutations in pncA, a gene encoding pyrazinamidase/nicotinamidase, cause resistance to the antituberculous drug pyrazinamide in tubercle bacillus. *Nat Med* **2:** 662–667.

Scorpio A, Lindholm-Levy P, Heifets L, Gilman R, Siddiqi S, Cynamon M, Zhang Y. 1997. Characterization of pncA mutations in pyrazinamide-resistant *Mycobacterium tuberculosis. Antimicrob Agents Chemother* **41:** 540–543.

Sensi P. 1983. History of the development of rifampin. *Rev Infect Dis* **5:** S402–S406.

Shepherd RG, Baughn C, Cantrall ML, Goodstein B, Thomas JP, Wilkinson RG. 1966. Structure-activity studies leading to ethambutol, a new type of antituberculous compound. *Ann N Y Acad Sci* **135:** 686–710.

Shi D, Li L, Zhao Y, Jia Q, Li H, Coulter C, Jin Q, Zhu G. 2011a. Characteristics of embB mutations in multidrug-resistant *Mycobacterium tuberculosis* isolates in Henan, China. *J Antimicrob Chemother* **66:** 2240–2247.

Shi W, Zhang X, Jiang X, Yuan H, Lee JS, Barry CE III, Wang H, Zhang W, Zhang Y. 2011b. Pyrazinamide inhibits trans-translation in *Mycobacterium tuberculosis. Science* **333:** 1630–1632.

Srivastava S, Ayyagari A, Dhole TN, Nyati KK, Dwivedi SK. 2009. emb Nucleotide polymorphisms and the role of embB306 mutations in *Mycobacterium tuberculosis* resistance to ethambutol. *Int J Med Microbiol* **299:** 269–280.

Takayama K, Kilburn JO. 1989. Inhibition of synthesis of arabinogalactan by ethambutol in *Mycobacterium smegmatis. Antimicrob Agents Chemother* **33:** 1493–1499.

Takayama K, Wang L, David HL. 1972. Effect of isoniazid on the in vivo mycolic acid synthesis, cell growth, and viability of *Mycobacterium tuberculosis. Antimicrob Agents Chemother* **2:** 29–35.

Takayama K, Schnoes HK, Armstrong EL, Boyle RW. 1975. Site of inhibitory action of isoniazid in the synthesis of mycolic acids in *Mycobacterium tuberculosis. J Lipid Res* **16:** 308–317.

Takayama K, Armstrong EL, Kunugi KA, Kilburn JO. 1979. Inhibition by ethambutol of mycolic acid transfer into the cell wall of Mycobacterium smegmatis. *Antimicrob Agents Chemother* **16:** 240–242.

Telenti A, Imboden P, Marchesi F, Lowrie D, Cole S, Colston MJ, Matter L, Schopfer K, Bodmer T. 1993. Detection of rifampicin-resistance mutations in *Mycobacterium tuberculosis. Lancet* **341:** 647–650.

Telenti A, Philipp WJ, Sreevatsan S, Bernasconi C, Stockbauer KE, Wieles B, Musser JM, Jacobs WR Jr. 1997. The emb operon, a gene cluster of *Mycobacterium tuberculosis* involved in resistance to ethambutol. *Nat Med* **3:** 567–570.

Thomas JP, Baughn CO, Wilkinson RG, Shepherd RG. 1961. A new synthetic compound with antituberculous activity in mice: Ethambutol (dextro-2,2′-(ethylenediimino)-di-l-butanol). *Am Rev Respir Dis* **83:** 891–893.

van der Werf MJ, Jellema RH, Hankemeier T. 2005. Microbial metabolomics: Replacing trial-and-error by the unbiased selection and ranking of targets. *J Ind Microbiol Biotechnol* **32:** 234–252.

van der Werf MJ, Overkamp KM, Muilwijk B, Coulier L, Hankemeier T. 2007. Microbial metabolomics: Toward a platform with full metabolome coverage. *Anal Biochem* **370:** 17–25.

Vilcheze C, Jacobs WR Jr. 2007. The mechanism of isoniazid killing: Clarity through the scope of genetics. *Annu Rev Microbiol* **61:** 35–50.

Vilcheze C, Wang F, Arai M, Hazbon MH, Colangeli R, Kremer L, Weisbrod TR, Alland D, Sacchettini JC, Jacobs WR Jr. 2006. Transfer of a point mutation in *Mycobacterium tuberculosis* inhA resolves the target of isoniazid. *Nat Med* **12:** 1027–1029.

Wang L, Takayama K. 1972. Relationship between the uptake of isoniazid and its action on in vivo mycolic acid synthesis in *Mycobacterium tuberculosis*. *Antimicrob Agents Chemother* **2:** 438–441.

Wehrli W, Staehelin M. 1971. Actions of the rifamycins. *Bacteriol Rev* **35:** 290–309.

Wilming M, Johnsson K. 1999. Spontaneous formation of the bioactive form of the tuberculosis drug isoniazid. *Angew Chem Int Ed Engl* **38:** 2588–2590.

Winder F. 1960. Catalase and peroxidase in mycobacteria. Possible relationship to the mode of action of isoniazid. *Am Rev Respir Dis* **81:** 68–78.

Winder FG, Collins PB. 1970. Inhibition by isoniazid of synthesis of mycolic acids in *Mycobacterium tuberculosis*. *J Gen Microbiol* **63:** 41–48.

Winder FG, Collins P, Rooney SA. 1970. Effects of isoniazid on mycolic acid synthesis in *Mycobacterium tuberculosis* and on its cell envelope. *Biochem J* **117:** 27P.

Zhang Y. 2005. The magic bullets and tuberculosis drug targets. *Annu Rev Pharmacol Toxicol* **45:** 529–564.

Zhang Y, Mitchison D. 2003. The curious characteristics of pyrazinamide: A review. *Int J Tuberc Lung Dis* **7:** 6–21.

Zhang Y, Scorpio A, Nikaido H, Sun Z. 1999. Role of acid pH and deficient efflux of pyrazinoic acid in unique susceptibility of *Mycobacterium tuberculosis* to pyrazinamide. *J Bacteriol* **181:** 2044–2049.

Zhang Y, Wade MM, Scorpio A, Zhang H, Sun Z. 2003. Mode of action of pyrazinamide: Disruption of *Mycobacterium tuberculosis* membrane transport and energetics by pyrazinoic acid. *J Antimicrob Chemother* **52:** 790–795.

Zumla A, Nahid P, Cole ST. 2013. Advances in the development of new tuberculosis drugs and treatment regimens. *Nat Rev Drug Discov* **12:** 388–404.

Zumla AI, Gillespie SH, Hoelscher M, Philips PP, Cole ST, Abubakar I, McHugh TD, Schito M, Maeurer M, Nunn AJ. 2014. New antituberculosis drugs, regimens, and adjunct therapies: Needs, advances, and future prospects. *Lancet Infect Dis* **14:** 327–340.

The Tuberculosis Drug Discovery and Development Pipeline and Emerging Drug Targets

Khisimuzi Mdluli, Takushi Kaneko, and Anna Upton

Global Alliance for TB Drug Development, New York, New York 10005

Correspondence: khisi.mdluli@tballiance.org

The recent accelerated approval for use in extensively drug-resistant and multidrug-resistant-tuberculosis (MDR-TB) of two first-in-class TB drugs, bedaquiline and delamanid, has reinvigorated the TB drug discovery and development field. However, although several promising clinical development programs are ongoing to evaluate new TB drugs and regimens, the number of novel series represented is few. The global early-development pipeline is also woefully thin. To have a chance of achieving the goal of better, shorter, safer TB drug regimens with utility against drug-sensitive and drug-resistant disease, a robust and diverse global TB drug discovery pipeline is key, including innovative approaches that make use of recently acquired knowledge on the biology of TB. Fortunately, drug discovery for TB has resurged in recent years, generating compounds with varying potential for progression into developable leads. In parallel, advances have been made in understanding TB pathogenesis. It is now possible to apply the lessons learned from recent TB hit generation efforts and newly validated TB drug targets to generate the next wave of TB drug leads. Use of currently underexploited sources of chemical matter and lead-optimization strategies may also improve the efficiency of future TB drug discovery. Novel TB drug regimens with shorter treatment durations must target all subpopulations of *Mycobacterium tuberculosis* existing in an infection, including those responsible for the protracted TB treatment duration. This review summarizes the current TB drug development pipeline and proposes strategies for generating improved hits and leads in the discovery phase that could help achieve this goal.

INTRODUCTION AND CURRENT DRUG DEVELOPMENT PIPELINE

The goal of tuberculosis (TB) drug discovery and development is to achieve TB drugs and drug regimens that are well understood and superior to those available today in their efficacy, speed of action, safety and tolerability, ease of use for all patient populations, and accessibility. An ideal new regimen should be rapidly bactericidal and possess potent sterilizing activity to achieve stable cure in a shorter time period than the typical 6 mo required for the current standard of care for drug-sensitive TB. To achieve a significantly shorter duration of therapy, it is expected that a regimen would need to kill all subpopulations of *Mycobacterium tuberculosis* (*Mtb*) that exist in clinical TB and are thought

Cite this article as *Cold Spring Harb Perspect Med* doi: 10.1101/cshperspect.a021154

to vary in replication rate. In addition, new regimens should include drugs that show novel mechanisms of action (MOA) to ensure effectiveness against strains that are resistant to existing TB drugs. The regimens should also be well tolerated and possess absorption, distribution, metabolism, and excretion (ADME) properties suitable for coadministration with anti-HIV (human immunodeficiency virus) agents and appropriate for once-a-day oral dosing, optimally within a fixed-dose combination. It is also imperative that new drugs be available at relatively low cost to remain accessible to all high-burden countries.

The TB drug development pipeline can be viewed on the frequently updated website of the Stop TB Partnership's Working Group for New TB Drugs (www.newtbdrugs.org). Strategies recently used in TB drug development include reevaluation of existing TB drugs to optimize their utility; repurposing of drugs registered for non-TB indications as components of TB drug combinations; development of improved analogs of compounds or drugs with some known but limited value for TB; and development of novel chemical entities with new modes of action against TB. TB drugs are delivered as combinations with at least three compounds to prevent resistance development and reap the efficacy benefits of different compound classes or modes of action. Evaluation of new TB drugs is therefore as part of regimens from clinical Phase II onward.

The current global TB drug development pipeline includes four compounds under evaluation for active pulmonary TB in Phase III clinical trials. Two of these four compounds, the fluoroquinolones, moxifloxacin and gatifloxacin, are being investigated as part of 4-mo regimens, combined with first-line TB drugs, for drug-sensitive TB. The other two, bedaquiline (a diarylquinoline) and delamanid (a nitroimidazole), are being evaluated as additions to background therapy for MDR-TB. Another nitroimidazole, PA-824, is poised to enter Phase III clinical trials as part of a novel drug combination with moxifloxacin and pyrazinamide, in which it will be evaluated as a 4-mo regimen against drug-sensitive TB and as a 4- or 6-month regimen against MDR-TB. Earlier in development, a variety of approaches to novel regimen development are ongoing. PA-824 and bedaquiline, both novel chemical entities, are under evaluation in Phase II as part of novel drug combinations that include the first-line TB drug pyrazinamide as well as the repurposed drugs moxifloxacin and clofazimine. A number of ongoing studies will evaluate members of the well-known anti-TB class, the rifamycins (rifampicin and rifapentine in this case), in regimens for drug-sensitive TB. Besides the nitroimidazoles and diarylquinolines, two other novel chemical classes are being developed for TB—the ethylenediamines (represented by SQ109) and the oxazolidinones (linezolid, sutezolid, and AZD5847). Notably, a gap currently exists in Phase I with no known ongoing studies of new candidate TB drugs at that stage of development. The paucity of new chemical classes represented (and hence distinct modes of action and utility against drug-resistant and drug-sensitive disease) underscores the need for diverse, well-resourced discovery efforts to increase the flow to development to account for attrition and to plug the Phase I gap.

TB Drug Discovery

Recent advances in understanding the molecular biology of *Mtb* have been significant, driven largely by the whole-genome sequencing of the bacterium in 1998 (Cole et al. 1998). Knowledge of the complete *Mtb* genome sequence enabled scientists to establish the number of essential genes both in vitro and in vivo (Sassetti and Rubin 2003; Sassetti et al. 2003), to study genome-wide DNA microarrays for patterns of gene expression under various growth conditions (Sherman et al. 2001; Schnappinger et al. 2003; Rustad et al. 2008; Zhang et al. 2012), and to more rapidly identify targets of new compounds via identification of the mutated genes of compound-resistant mutants (Abrahams et al. 2012a; La Rosa et al. 2012; Ioerger et al. 2013; Remiuinan et al. 2013). The use of elegant gene knockdown techniques has allowed in vitro and in vivo validation of potential drug targets by showing the effect of the depletion of a specific target (Wei et al. 2011; Woong et al. 2011).

There is limited commercial potential for new TB drugs, and therefore, this indication has not been an area of intense activity. In addition, the recent exodus of much of the pharmaceutical industry from antibacterial drug discovery has proven to be a loss for TB drug research and development, as the TB field no longer benefits from drug candidates being developed against other bacteria. Fortunately, some government and nongovernment organizations have taken the initiative to fill this gap, with a turning point occurring with the creation of a number of not-for-profit product-development partnerships (PDPs), such as the Global Alliance for TB Drug Development (TB Alliance) that formed in 2000. Since then, several additional consortia have formed, including the TB Drug Accelerator, the Lilly Early TB Drug Discovery Initiative, and More Medicines for TB (MM4TB) and Orchid, both funded by the European Commission. Academic and government laboratories are also involved in translational medicine of basic research to TB drug discovery, mostly funded by the National Institutes of Health (NIH) and the Bill and Melinda Gates Foundation. The TB field has recently experienced some positive developments with the approval of bedaquiline (TMC-207, Sirturo from Janssen), by the U.S. Food and Drug Administration (FDA) at the end of 2012 (http://www.fda.gov/NewsEvents/Newsroom/PressAnnouncements/ucm33695.htm) (and by EMA in March of 2014), and delamanid (OPC-67683, Deltyba from Otsuka) by the European Medicines Agency (EMA) in December of 2013 (http://online.wsj.com/article/PR-CO-20131125-900844.html), both indicated for MDR-TB. However, the current drug discovery pipeline (http://www.newtbdrugs.org/pipeline-discovery.php) provides little substrate for the development of drastic treatment-shortening drug regimens that will truly change the TB treatment paradigm.

In this review, we focus on the lessons learned from screening efforts of the recent past and how these can be applied for greater future success. We then highlight the lead-generation efforts and TB drug targets that we believe to be the most promising and worthy of more attention. Specifically, we discuss advances in screening technologies that are expected to produce the next generation of progressable hits against *Mtb*, highlighting the potential for natural products as a source for novel hits, and mechanism- or structure-based drug discovery approaches for the generation of anti-TB leads. We then focus on a selection of novel drug targets that have been recently validated such that their inhibition should eliminate *persisters* (a subpopulation of organisms in an infection that is phenotypically resistant to killing by most drugs and thought to be responsible for protracted treatment durations and relapse) and contribute to treatment shortening in novel regimens.

THE CURRENT STATUS AND RECENT HISTORY IN HIT/LEAD GENERATION FOR TB

Screening Efforts

As in the antibacterial field in general, despite significant effort being expended on *Mtb* target-based biochemical screens (Payne et al. 2007), no TB drug or drug candidate has emerged from these efforts to date. Problems with target-based screens include their propensity to identify hits with potency against the target but that do not inhibit bacterial growth because target inhibition does not translate into bacterial killing for a variety of reasons, including poor penetration and efflux. Conversely, whole-cell screening has yielded notable successes for TB drug discovery. As a consequence, it has become the mainstay of TB hit generation. *Mtb* whole-cell screening is an approach in which compound libraries are screened for their ability to inhibit bacterial growth. These screens have been performed against both replicating and nonreplicating *Mtb* under a variety of culture conditions in an effort to identify compounds that can kill the multiple subpopulations of *Mtb* that exist in an infection. Whole-cell screening has the advantage that it is not target-specific, thus, it enables screening against the organism's entire set of potential targets at once. Results of such a screen, which effectively allows the organism's physiology to inform discovery efforts, yield accessible targets and sensitive pathways that would otherwise be unpredicted. This approach also overcomes cell-penetration and cell-efflux issues (i.e., getting and keeping compounds in cells) of target-based screens. However, whole-cell screening is not without its challenges. For example, target identification can be problematic, and if not successful, it can limit the ability to quickly improve the potency of hit compounds. A good example of whole-cell screening success is the compound TMC-207 (Andries et al. 2005); other examples include a diarylcoumarin series that targets the acyl–acyl carrier protein synthetase activity of FadD32 (Kawate et al. 2013; Stanley et al. 2013) and the indolcarboxamides NITD-304 and NITD-349, presumed to inhibit MmpL3 from the sequencing of resistant mutants (Rao et al. 2013). All of these compounds were subsequently shown to be efficacious in vivo against murine TB.

Perhaps the earliest publically accessible whole-cell screening results were from the NIH's effort to acquire and test compounds against *Mtb* (Tuberculosis Antimicrobial Acquisition and Coordinating Facility, TAACF) (Ananthan et al. 2009; Maddry et al. 2009). More recently, several pharmaceutical companies have performed phenotypic screens; for example, GSK recently reported a set of 177 *Mtb*-active compounds (Ballell et al. 2013). Some hits were further investigated in the hit-to-lead phase and have been made public (Abrahams et al. 2012b). The Novartis Institute of Tropical Diseases (NITD) has published results of a hit-to-lead program based on their selected series (Kondreddi et al. 2013; Yokokawa et al. 2013). AstraZeneca has also performed phenotypic screening and published some results (Ramanchandran et al. 2013). Similar screens against *Mtb* are under way by members of the TB Drug Accelerator (TBDA) consortium and MM4TB, among others.

The whole-cell screens published thus far largely used standardized aerobic culture conditions that favor replicating *Mtb*. More recently, specialized whole-cell screens have been performed, including those that use culture conditions considered relevant to in vivo infection *Mtb* inside host cells. The expectations are that these screens will identify inhibitors that will be active in vivo and against persisters. Screens against *Mtb* in macrophages have been successful (Christophe et al. 2010); the late preclinical compound Q203 is one example. It is an imidazo[1,2-a]pyridine-3-carboxamide derivative that targets QcrB, a component of the CytBC1 complex of the respiratory chain (Pethe et al. 2013). Interestingly, this series was also discovered through screens under standard culture conditions and for inhibitors of ATP homeostasis under nonreplicating conditions (Mak et al. 2012). Other cell-based specialized screens recently reported include those for inhibitors of ATP or pH homeostasis (Darby et al. 2013) and against engineered *Mtb* strains with modulated expression of pantothenate synthetase (Kumar et al. 2013). These screens are an improvement over the simple phenotypic screens because inhibitors against particular targets, pathways, or processes already proven essential for TB are likely to be discovered via a whole-cell approach, thus combining the advantages of validated targets with whole-cell screening. Because most of the whole-cell screens against *Mtb* were undertaken in the last 5–10 yr, it may be of some use to analyze the hits that emerged as well as the screens that identified them. Some interesting phenomena are emerging.

First, structurally identical or closely related compounds have been identified as hits many times over by various organizations; these compounds are listed in Table 1. Some examples include imidazo[1,2-a]pyridine-3-carboxamides (e.g., Q203) that were shown to kill *Mtb* by at least four different phenotypic screens performed by various organizations (Abrahams et al. 2012b; Mak et al. 2012; Moraski et al. 2011, 2012); tetrahydropyrazolo[1,5-a]pyrimidine-3-carboxamides were selected as hits in at least three different screens (Maddry et al. 2009); and urea analogs containing an adamantyl group or a norbonanylmethylene group were identified as hits in two different screens (Ananthan et al. 2009; Brown et al. 2011; Scherman et al. 2012). The redundant identification of these hits may reflect the similarity of both the

Table 1. Structurally identical or closely related compounds have been identified as hits many times over by various organizations as listed below

Series	Structures	Investigating organization(s)
Imidazo[1,2-a]pyridine-3-carboxamides	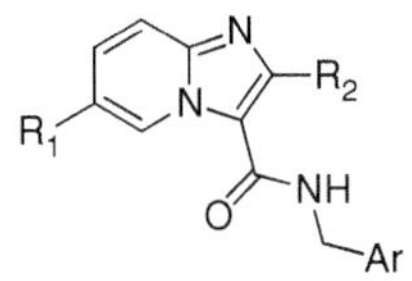	University of Notre Dame Institut Pasteur Korea, Quro National Institutes of Health, Novartis Institute of Tropical Diseases GlaxoSmithKline
Tetrahydropyrazolo[1,5-a]pyrimidine-3-carboxamides	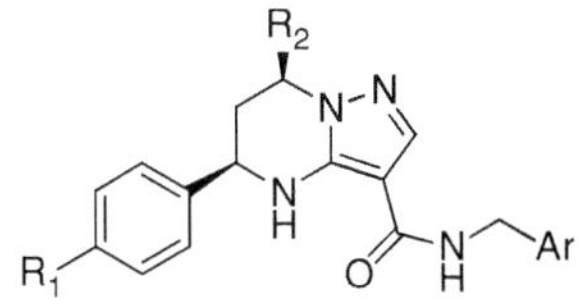	Tuberculosis Antimicrobial Acquisition and Coordination Facility GlaxoSmithKline Novartis Institute of Tropical Diseases
Adamantyl ureas	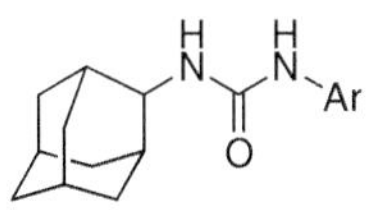	Colorado State University Tuberculosis Antimicrobial Acquisition and Coordination Facility
Indole-2-carboxamides	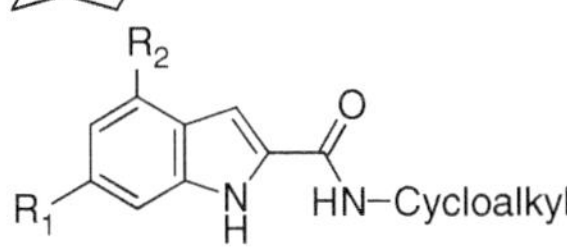	Novartis Institute of Tropical Diseases University of Illinois at Chicago GlaxoSmithKline

libraries of the various organizations and the screening methods.

Second, the same recurring mechanistic targets have been identified for different hits. Representative promiscuous targets are summarized in Table 2. For example, at least five structurally divergent chemical series were shown to have the same target, DprE1, an enzyme involved in isomerization of decaprenylphosphoryl-β-d-ribose to decaprenylphosphoryl-β-d-arabinose, an important cell wall component (Batt et al. 2012). Similarly, structurally divergent compounds were shown to share MmpL3 as the predominant resistant determinant; MmpL3 is a cell membrane transporter of trehalose monomycolate (Grzegorzewicsz et al. 2012a). The exclusivity of MmpL3 as a target of many of the observed hits has been challenged recently and it remains to be debated at present (Li et al. 2014).

The reasons for the same mechanistic targets are not clear, but it may be that these are the most accessible and vulnerable targets under the screening conditions used, and they are mainly cell surface or membrane-bound proteins; the phenomenon of lipophilic compounds and membrane-localized targets has been pointed out in two recent review articles (Stanley et al. 2012; Goldman 2013). The main argument Stanley and Goldman present is that lipophilic compounds may partition and concentrate in the membranes higher than in the intracellular environment. These observations are a reminder that the methodology and conditions of a screen determine the results and the hits identified. Researchers thus may have to rethink their screens and the compound libraries they use because the lipophilic and high-molecular-weight properties of certain hits may preclude successful subsequent downstream development. It is also the case that highly lipophilic and high-molecular-weight compounds that target membrane-localized targets seem to correlate with the potential for hepatotoxicity (Chen et al. 2013), mitochondrial dysfunction (Naven et al. 2013), and nonspecific interactions (Tarcsay and Keseru 2013). They also affect pharmaceutical development owing to the lack of solubility and difficulty in formulation. The fact that bedaquiline (TMC-207), with a cLogP value of 7.3, was successfully developed amply shows that such a compound can be developed, even though the hurdles are high. Various measures can be used to correct this

Table 2. Representative promiscuous targets

Target	Compound	Structure
DprE1	BTZ043	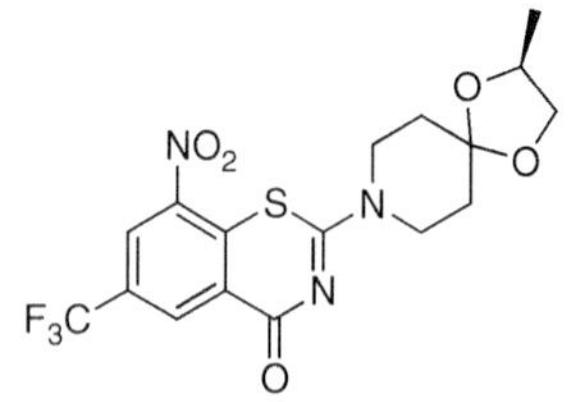
	DNB1	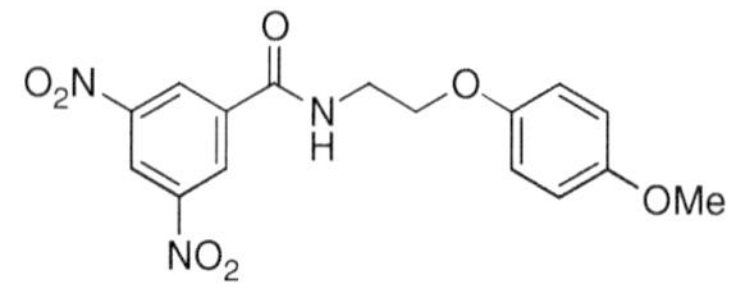
	TAACF377790	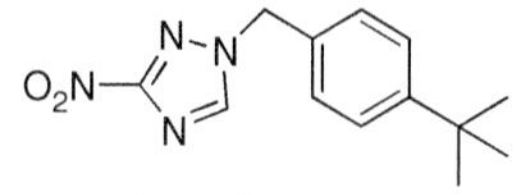
	TCA1	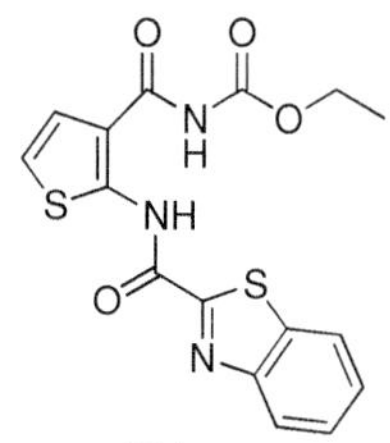
	Azaindoles	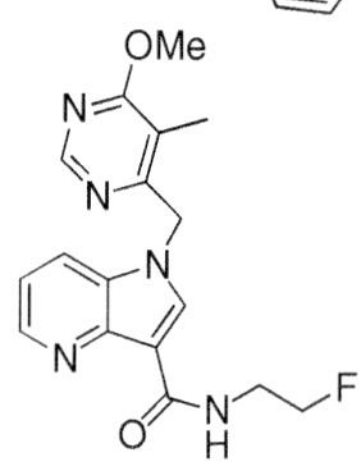
MmpL3	BM212	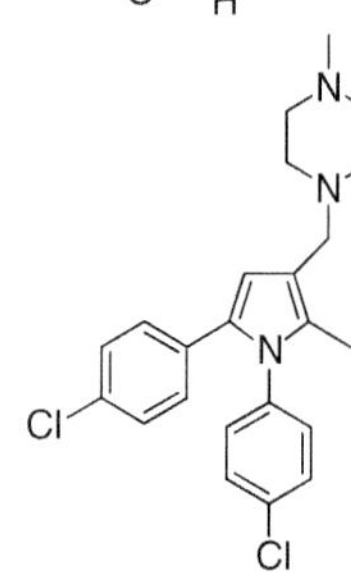
	AU1235	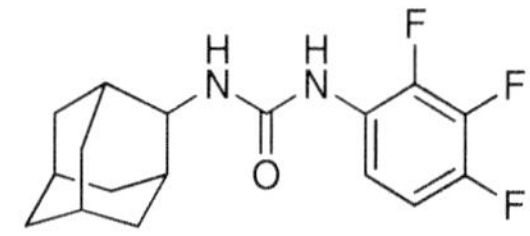
	C215	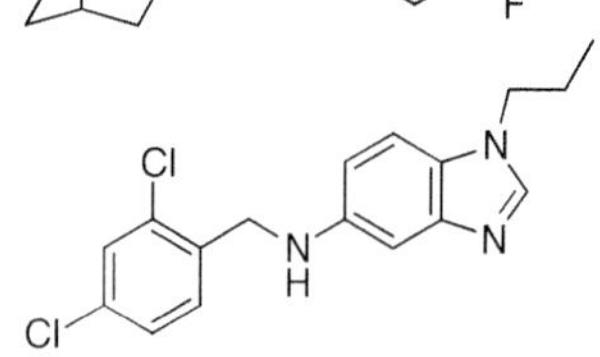

Continued

Table 2. *Continued*

Target	Compound	Structure
	THPP	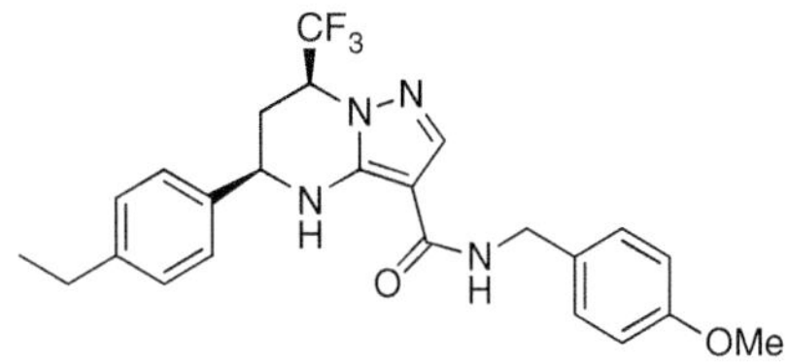
	Spiro	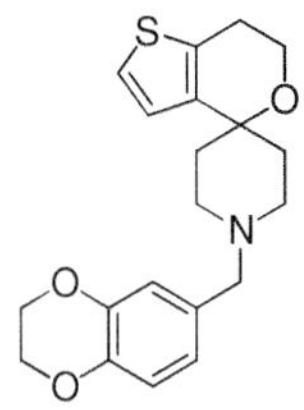
	SQ109	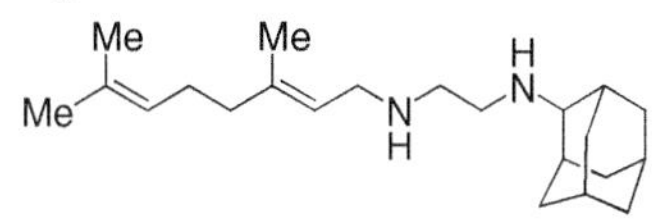
	NITD-304	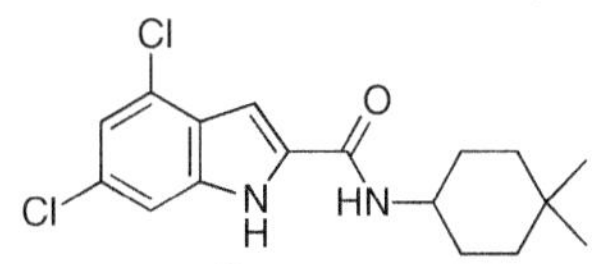
QcrB	Imidazo[1,2-a]pyridine	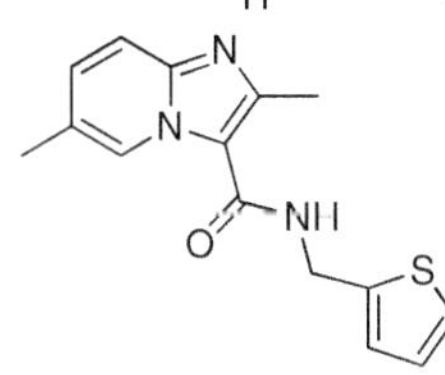
	Q203	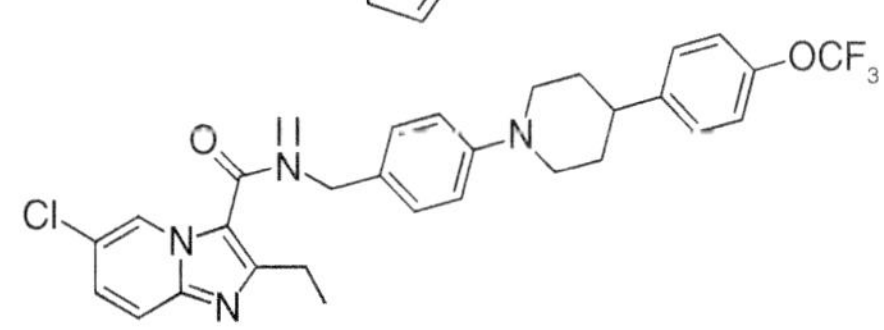

problem. For example, hits with preferred physicochemical properties should be prioritized over higher-potency hits with poor properties, and methods should be established to accurately determine the drug concentrations in various cellular compartments. To that point, a recently reported method for measuring the intracellular compound levels in *Mycobacterium smegmatis* may be useful in linking intracellular compound levels to bacterial killing (Bhat et al. 2013).

Third, instead of the completely nontarget-specific whole-cell screens, target-specific, whole-cell screens using specialized strains that focus on a specific in vivo validated target, pathway, or process should be performed. Such screens should be designed to use the current knowledge of the most sensitive targets—including for persisters—the transport functions (Sarathy et al. 2012), and the porin systems of *Mtb* (Siroy et al. 2008) that can be exploited to transport drugs and avoid efflux.

Fourth, smaller libraries with preferred physicochemical properties should be used. For example, NITD scientists recently screened a library of small and polar compounds, with promising results (U. Manjunatha, P. Smith, et al., pers. comm.).

Fifth, CPZN-45 (Ishizaki et al. 2013), spectinamides, and macrolides are successful chemical series in lead optimization derived from natural products. This suggests that use of natural products as a potential source for novel leads against *Mtb* should be revisited. New potential natural product leads are discussed below.

Underexploited Methods of Lead Generation

Natural Products

It is of interest to note among the four first-line TB drugs (rifampicin, isoniazid, pyrazinamide, and ethambutol) and six series of the second-line TB drugs (aminoglycosides, capreomycin-class polypeptides, fluoroquinolones, cycloserine, and para-aminosalicylic acid), at least four of them are derived from natural products (rifampicin, aminoglycosides, polypeptides, and cycloserine). The utility of natural products and natural product–derived compounds in antibacterial research is well-documented (Newman and Cragg 2012; Brown et al. 2014). Natural products are said to cover a wider chemical space compared with combinatorial library compounds (Feher and Schmidt 2003). This is important especially in view of the identification of frequent hits of synthetic compounds mentioned in the preceding section. Nevertheless, the drug discovery effort in the natural product area still seems to lag behind reflecting the general trend in the pharmaceutical industry, which has mostly retreated from the natural product discovery area 10–20 years ago. There are excellent recent reviews on antitubercular compounds derived from natural products (Singh et al. 2011; Garcia et al. 2012; Guzman et al. 2012; Salomon and Schmidt 2012; Kirst 2013). Here, we highlight some recent notable examples that may prove to be useful leads for TB drug discovery (Fig. 1).

Thuggacin A, isolated from the fermentation broth of the myxobacterium *Sorangium cellulosum*, is active against *Mtb* with an minimum inhibitory concentration (MIC) of 8.0 µg/mL and an MOA believed to be inhibition of the *Mtb* respiratory chain—a target of great interest at present (Steinmetz et al. 2007; Irschik et al. 2007). Ergosterol peroxide, isolated from the leaves of *Radermachera boniana*, has an MIC of 1.5 µg/mL; although it has an unusual peroxide moiety, it appears to have a reasonable selectivity, because its cytotoxicity against Vero cells is greater than 86 µg/mL (Truong et al. 2011). Trichodermin A, isolated from a fungus from marine sponges, has an *Mtb* MIC of 0.12 µg/mL under both aerobic and hypoxic conditions (Pruksakorn et al. 2010); it has been shown to be active against nonreplicating mycobacteria and its MOA to be inhibition of ATP synthesis (Pruksakorn et al. 2011). Another peptide natural product, lariatin A, shows a potent inhibitory activity against *Mtb*, with an MIC of 0.39 µg/mL (Iwatsuki et al. 2007). Isolated from the soil bacterium *Rhodococcus jostii*, lariatin A forms an unusual "lasso" structure in which its tail passes through a ring structure; its MOA is speculated to be inhibition of cell wall biosynthesis (Iwatsuki et al. 2006). A thiostrepton-class compound isolated from *Nocardia pseudobrasiliensis*, nocardithiocin is highly potent against *Mtb*, with an MIC ranging from 0.025 to 1.56 µg/mL. A known natural product, pyridomycin was recently shown to have the same MOA as isoniazid (i.e., inhibition of *Mtb* InhA, the enoyl-ACP reductase involved in mycolic acid biosynthesis) (Hartkoorn et al. 2012); structural studies indicate that this compound blocks both the cofactor- and substrate-binding pockets (Hartkoorn et al. 2013). As discussed below, all of the inhibitors of *Mtb* ClpP proteases to date are natural products or natural product–derived analogs.

These examples indicate natural products; although mostly neglected by current efforts caused by cost and other factors, they remain a relevant source of leads for TB drug development. As mentioned above, natural products occupy a chemical space that is very different from that covered by the various small molecules currently being screened within most pharmaceutical company libraries. Although medicinal chemistry to improve ADME and toxicity properties of an initial natural product hit may be challenging, such compounds can provide novel templates and indicate vulnerable targets for simplified, smaller, more developable

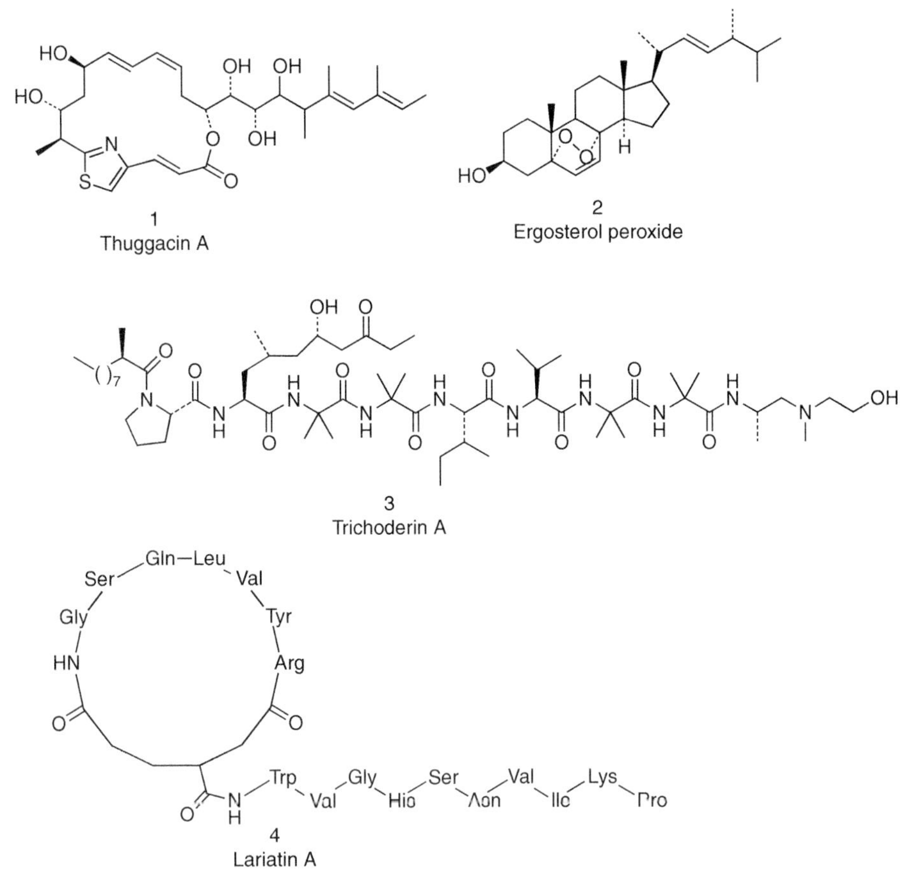

Figure 1. Recent notable examples of natural and natural-derived products that provide leads for TB drug discovery.

analogs. Natural products discovered for non-*Mtb* bacteria may also be a source of future anti TB leads. Because of the recent accumulation of knowledge in biosynthetic genes of secondary metabolites, information on culture conditions to generate secondary metabolites, and isolation of underexplored organisms, the science of natural products is poised to make a great contribution to TB drug discovery when it is combined with advances in analytical chemistry and chemoinformatics (Li and Vederas 2009; Wright 2014).

Mechanism- and Structure-Based Drug Design

There are numerous examples of mechanism- or structure-based drug designs (Finn 2012) in TB research, only some of which will be mentioned here. An interesting case of structure-guided design is the recently reported malate synthase (GlcB) inhibitors that are analogs of phenyl-dikitoacids, designed based on the enzyme X-ray crystal structure. One analog showed efficacy against murine TB, as discussed in the section on targets below (Krieger et al. 2012). FASII enoyl-ACP reductase (InhA) is the well-validated target of the TB drug isoniazid and has been a target of rational drug design (Pan and Tonge 2012). Based on the methylthiazole compounds discovered at GSK (Ballell Pages et al. 2010; Castro Pichel et al. 2012), scientists at AstraZeneca have published their investigation of the binding mode of these agents to InhA (Shirude et al. 2013). This is part of an effort to discover direct InhA inhibitors that, unlike isoniazid, do not require activation by KatG (Encinas et al. 2014). Defective KatG activation is the dominant resistance determinant in isoniazid-resistant *Mtb* clinical isolates.

Another approach to modern drug design, fragment-based drug discovery, has recently succeeded in generating inhibitors of *Mtb* pantothenate synthetase (Pts) (Silvestre et al. 2013). In this study, 1250 fragments were initially screened by a thermal-shift method and nuclear magnetic resonance (NMR) experiments. The initial 39 hits were further characterized by isothermal titration calorimetry and X-ray crystallography to further categorize them into fragments binding at the adenine pocket, those binding at the pantoate pocket, and a fragment binding deep in the pantoate pocket. One fragment has been elaborated to provide potent inhibitors of Pts (Hung et al. 2009).

EMERGING TARGETS

Targeting *Mtb* Iron Acquisition and Storage

Iron is an essential nutrient for all living organisms, including pathogenic bacteria in an infection, but the mammalian immune system uses various methods to restrict a pathogen's access to iron (Doherty 2007). Various mammalian proteins are involved in iron homeostasis, and their effect on the immune system is discussed in an excellent review (Johnson and Wessling-Resnick 2012); they include hepcidin, lactoferrin, siderocalin, haptoglobin, hemopexin, Nramp1, ferroportin, and the transferrin receptor, which underscores the importance of this nutrient in the host–pathogen relationship. Iron is sequestered in the human body by intracellular ferritin and extracellular transferrin (Weinberg 1999). During infection, *Mtb* localizes inside host macrophages (Kauffmann 2004), where it has access to transferrin-bound iron. *Mtb* secretes two classes of siderophores, mycobactins (Rodriguez 2006) and carboxymycobactins (Ratledge and Dover 2000), to bind iron, obstructing it from the mammalian iron-binding proteins, and then internalizes the iron-laden siderophores through its receptors.

Iron Acquisition

It was recently shown that *mbtE* deletion mutants are unable to synthesize mycobactins and are attenuated for growth in vitro, macrophages, and guinea pigs, highlighting the importance of mycobactin biosynthesis for the growth and virulence of *Mtb* and establishing this pathway as a potential target for the TB drug development (Reddy et al. 2013). Mycobactin analogs that inhibited MbtA, another mycobactin biosynthesis enzyme, have shown in vitro *Mtb* activity superior to first-line TB drugs (Neres et al. 2008).

Deletion mutants of *Mtb* lacking *irtA* and *irtB* are attenuated in human macrophages and mouse lungs (Rodriguez and Smith 2006). *IrtAB* genes encode the ABC transporter IrtAB involved in the efficient transport and usage of iron from Fe-carboxymycobactin in *Mtb*. The *irtAB* genes are located in a chromosomal region previously shown to contain genes regulated by iron and the major iron regulator IdeR.

Mutants of Esx-3, a secretion system that works in concert with the ItrAB ABC transport system to take up iron-laden siderophores, have been shown to be severely impaired for growth in macrophages, indicating Esx-3 as another potential drug target in iron acquisition (Seigrist et al. 2009). A novel siderophore-export system consisting of MmpS4/MmpL4 and MmpS5/MmpL5 was recently identified in *Mtb* by Wells et al. (2013), and an *mmpS4/S5* deletion mutant was shown to be attenuated in mouse infection models, indicating siderophore efflux as a potential drug target (Wells and Jones 2013). These investigators further showed that *Mtb* recycles its siderophores to enable efficient iron use and that disrupting this process causes the intracellular accumulation of deferrated siderophores, which poisons *Mtb* (Jones et al. 2014). This suggests that novel drugs targeting inactivation of siderophore export and recycling would deliver a one-two punch to *Mtb* by reducing its capacity to take up iron and by siderophore-mediated self-poisoning, making siderophore secretion a better target than siderophore biosynthesis because inhibition of siderophore biosynthesis is easily over-

 Cite this article as *Cold Spring Harb Perspect Med* doi: 10.1101/cshperspect.a021154

come by *Mtb* using heme (Jones and Niederweis 2011).

An *Mtb* heme-uptake system has been defined (Tullius et al. 2011) that consists of the secreted protein Rv0203 and the transmembrane proteins MmpL3 and MmpL11. Recent experiments showed that Rv0203 transfers heme to both MmpL3 and MmpL11 during *Mtb* heme uptake (Owens et al. 2013), making these proteins potential targets for TB drugs.

Iron Storage

Although iron acquisition is required for the growth and virulence of *Mtb*, it seems that proper iron storage within the pathogen is just as crucial. Excess free iron becomes toxic, catalyzing the production of reactive oxygen radicals that could lead to oxidative damage. *Mtb* has two iron storage proteins, bacterioferritin (BfrA) (Gupta et al. 2008) and a ferritin-like protein (BfrB) (McMath et al. 2010), which have been shown to be essential for *Mtb* protection against oxidative stress, growth in macrophages, and virulence in guinea pigs (Reddy et al. 2012). *Mtb* lacking ferritin suffers from iron-mediated toxicity, is unable to persist in mice, and is highly susceptible to killing by antibiotics (Pandey and Rodriguez 2012), showing that endogenous oxidative stress can enhance antibiotic killing.

Various investigators have targeted siderophores for the development of novel TB drugs. One approach has been to develop agents that directly inhibit enzymes involved in siderophore synthesis (Engelhart and Aldrich 2013). Another approach targets the iron-dependent regulator protein (IdeR) that represses siderophore synthesis genes and virulence factors when sustainable iron levels have been achieved (Mai et al. 2011); dysregulation of IdeR would lead to excess iron and oxidative damage or reduce virulence and enhance bacterial killing. The structural basis for iron activation and IdeR binding to DNA has been recently reported, and these insights have enabled the structure-based design of agents that target IdeR function. Small peptides that either enhance IdeR repression or inhibit IdeR dimerization show that IdeR activity can be rationally modulated (Monfeli and Beeson 2007).

The totality of the data reported here indicates that the biosynthesis, transport, and utilization of siderophores are potential targets for *Mtb* drug discovery, as *Mtb* survival and virulence seem to be directly related to iron availability. Indeed, the host already uses iron metabolism against pathogens: siderocalins are host proteins that sequester iron-laden siderophores (Holmes et al. 2005) as a defense mechanism.

Targeting MmpL

The *Mtb* genome contains 13 genes that encode 12 RND (resistance, nodulation, and cell division) proteins designated *mycobacterial membrane protein large* (MmpL). RND proteins transport a variety of cationic, anionic, or neutral compounds, including various drugs, heavy metals, aliphatic and aromatic solvents, bile salts, fatty acids, detergents, and dyes, across the cytoplasmic membrane (Paulsen et al. 1996; Putman et al. 2000). In a heroic attempt to decipher the role of MmpL proteins in *Mtb*, mutant strains inactivated in 11 *mmpL* genes were generated (Domenech et al. 2005). Susceptibilities to a variety of drugs were unaffected in all the MmpL-deficient strains. One gene, *MmpL3*, was shown to be essential for growth, and mutants in four genes, *MmpL4*, *MmpL7*, *MmpL8*, or *MmpL11*, were attenuated in mice. The role of MmpL7 in virulence is likely explained by the findings that this polypeptide is required for the transport of phthiocerol dimycocerosate (PDIM), a known virulence factor, to the cell surface (Cox et al. 1999; Jain and Cox 2005). MmpL8 was found to be involved in sulfatide biogenesis and virulence (Domenech et al. 2004), and an *Mtb* mutant with disruptions in *mmpL4*, *mmpL5*, *mmpL7*, *mmpL8*, *mmpL10*, and *mmpL11* showed significant attenuation in mice (Lamichhane et al. 2005). As discussed above, Wells et al. (2013) recently showed the direct involvement of MmpL4 and MmpL5 in siderophore export; the involvement of MmpL3 and MmpL11 in heme uptake has also been shown, thus establishing the importance of these proteins in iron homeostasis and as potential targets for TB drug development. MmpL3, the only MmpL protein that has been shown to be essential, has also been shown to be the resistance determinant for a variety of unrelated drug candidates currently being evaluated (Grzegorzewicz et al. 2012a; Tahlan et al. 2012), as well as to be involved in the transport of mycolic acids across the cell membrane onto the cell surface (Grzegorzewicz et al. 2012a). Efflux of azole antibiotics in *Mtb* has been associated with mutations in *Rv0678*, which transcriptionally regulates the efflux system encoded by the *mmpS5–mmpL5* efflux system (Milano et al. 2009).

The above studies clearly indicate the importance of this protein family for growth, transport of vital cell wall components with some involvement in virulence, and perhaps the efflux of small molecules that are toxic to the bacterial cell. It is therefore interesting to imagine a single molecule that might inhibit a variety of MmpL proteins and potentially affect growth, virulence, and sensitivity to other drugs. This would be reminiscent of β-lactam antibiotics that target penicillin-binding proteins and affect peptidoglycan biosynthesis and sensitivity to other drugs. A concerted search for such an inhibitor might uncover a natural product capable of such if MmpLs are as important in soil-dwelling mycobacteria. MmpLs are membrane proteins and may thus be more accessible for targeting than cytosolic enzymes, a potential explanation for the various compounds with reported associations with MmpL3. More studies are required to determine if different MmpLs are important under different in vivo conditions and their potential involvement in pathogenesis and drug efflux in the various environments of the diseased lung.

Targeting Cholesterol Metabolism

Mounting evidence suggests that *Mtb* uses the host's cholesterol as a source of carbon and energy during infection. Strains defective in cholesterol transport or degradation are attenuated in activated macrophages, and *Mtb* requires several genes involved in cholesterol catabolism for full virulence in animal models (Pandey and Sassetti 2008; Chang et al. 2009; Yam et al. 2009; Nesbitt et al. 2010). It is unclear what carbon source for *Mtb* is most important during an infection, but host cholesterol use by *Mtb* has been shown (Van der Geize et al. 2007; Miner et al. 2009) and appears to be particularly important during the chronic phase of infection (Chang et al. 2009). Host cholesterol has been shown to be involved in a human *Mtb* infection (Kim et al. 2010), and high levels of cholesterol in the diet have been shown to significantly enhance the bacterial burden in the lung (Schafer et al. 2009). Specifically, cholesterol is required for phagocytosis of mycobacteria by macrophages (Gatfield and Pieters 2000; Peyron et al. 2000).

The intracellular growth operon, the *igr* locus, encodes enzymes of cholesterol catabolism in the *Mtb* genome (Chang et al. 2007) the primary function of which is the degradation of the 2′-propanoate side chain. Inactivation of the *igr* operon results in reduced *Mtb* growth on cholesterol alone or in combination with glycerol, indicating that cholesterol or its metabolites are toxic to the *igr* mutants. The *igr* locus encodes a cytochrome P450 (*cyp125*), two acyl-CoA dehydrogenases (*fadE28* and *fadE29*), two conserved hypothetical proteins (*Rv3541-2c*), and a putative lipid-carrier protein; the locus is essential for growth in macrophages and critical in the chronic phase of infection (Thomas et al. 2011). An enzyme encoded by *fadA5* has been described that catalyzes the thiolysis of acetoacetyl-CoA and is required for growth on cholesterol and virulence in the late stages of an infection (Nesbitt et al. 2010).

The other phase of cholesterol catabolism in *Mtb* is the degradation of the A–D rings. The 3-ketosteroid 9α-hydroxylase (KshAB) has been identified as a virulence factor involved in cholesterol ring degradation (Capyk et al. 2011). In a seminal study using bioinformatics, it was shown that 51 rhodococcal genes specifically expressed during growth on cholesterol were conserved within an 82-gene cluster in *Mtb* and that mycobacteria grown on cholesterol up-regulate *hsaC* and *kshA* (Van der Geize et al. 2007). Transposon mutagenesis studies suggested that the genes encoding HsaA and HsaD are essential for intracellular survival of *Mtb* in human macrophages (Rengarajan et al. 2005). HsaC, an iron-dependent extradiol dioxygenase, has been shown to be a virulence determinant in guinea pigs that influences dissemination, persistence, and the extent of disease pathology (Yam et al. 2009). Interestingly, cholesterol metabolism was shown to be lethal to an *hsaC Mtb* mutant, consistent with catechol toxicity. HsaD, the cholesterol meta-cleavage product (MCP) hydrolase (Lack et al. 2010), has been associated with the survival of *Mtb* in macrophages (Rengarajan et al. 2005). HsaAB, an enzyme that transforms 3-HSA to 3,4-DHSA in cholesterol catabolism, has also been identified (Dresen et al. 2010). Also, FadD3 has been shown to be a 3aα-H-4α (3′-propanoate)-7aβ-methylhexahydro-1,5-indanedione (HIP)–CoA synthetase that initiates catabolism of steroid rings C and D after side-chain degradation is complete (Casabon et al. 2013).

The rhodococcal Mce4 system is required for steroid uptake and is up-regulated on growth on cholesterol (Mohn et al. 2008). On this basis, it was predicted that all Mce4 systems are steroid transporters and that in *Mtb*, they transport cholesterol during an infection. Indeed, the involvement of the *Mtb mce4*-encoded transport system in cholesterol import has been shown, and *mce4*-deleted mutants have been shown to be severely attenuated in both macrophages and mouse infection models, establishing cholesterol import and metabolism as potential therapeutic targets (Senaratne et al. 2008).

From the above experimental data, it seems that although cholesterol catabolism by *Mtb* is important during infection, if ineffectively metabolized, cholesterol may be toxic to the pathogen. Importantly, both phenomena can be exploited for TB drug discovery, for drugs that inhibit cholesterol metabolism or those that inhibit enzymes which remove the toxic intermediates of cholesterol metabolism. In contrast to these observations, it was recently reported that cholesterol is not required as a nutritional source during infection (Yang et al. 2011).

Targeting the *Mtb* ClpP Protease

The ClpP proteases (cutinase-like proteins, chaperon-linked proteases, or caseinolytic proteases) have been of interest as drug targets because the antibacterial activity of an ADEP, an acyl depsipeptide that binds the Clp protease of *Bacillus subtilis*, was shown (Brotz-Oesterhelt et al. 2005). Clp proteases are conserved proteases involved in the degradation of damaged, poorly formed, and unfolded proteins.

Mtb encodes two ClpP homologs, ClpP1 and ClpP2, which form a self-compartmentalized protease consisting of two heptameric rings stacked on top of each other, enclosing a catalytic chamber. Within the chamber, which can be reached through two axial pores, each of the 14 identical monomers possesses a serine protease active site (Ingvarsson et al. 2007). To gain activity, the ClpP protease multimer associates with hexameric rings of Clp ATPases forming the proteolytic complex. The ATPase subunits (ClpC1 and ClpC2) are responsible for recognition, unfolding, and translocation of peptides into the ClpP degradation chamber. The resulting structure is the chamber in which the active sites are sequestered from the cytoplasm to exclude native proteins and control access to the proteolytic chamber.

It was recently shown that ClpC1 is the protein target of the natural product antibiotic cyclomarin in *Mtb* and that interference with the function of the ClpC1 ATPase with this noncompetitive small molecule is bactericidal in actively growing and in hypoxic nongrowing mycobacteria (Schmitt et al. 2011). The frequency of spontaneous mutations rendering *Mtb* resistant to cyclomarin was extremely low, and the *clpC1* gene could be shown to be essential for *Mtb* growth, a strong indication that interference with ClpC1 is a promising approach for the development of new antitubercular therapies.

A recent *Mtb* global transcriptional analysis identified approximately 100 genes involved in resumption of replication on reaeration following hypoxia, which included a transcription factor, the Clp protease gene regulator ortholog ClgR (Sherrid et al. 2010). *Mtb* ClgR was shown to activate the transcription of at least 10 genes, including four that encode protease systems (ClpP1/C, ClpP2/C, PtrB, and HtrA-like protease Rv1043c) and three that encode chaperones (Acr2, ClpB, and the chaperonin Rv3269). *clgR* deletion mutants were attenuated for growth in macrophages and for controlling the phagosomal pH, compared with wild-type organisms (Estorninho et al. 2010).

Recent studies have shown that ClpP1 and ClpP2 are essential for growth and form a mixed complex that degrades missense and prematurely terminated peptides, as depletion of the protease specifically led to growth reduction in the presence of antibiotics that increase errors in translation. A recent study confirmed that ClpP1 is essential for *Mtb* growth in vitro and that the previously described ClpP activators (acyldepsipeptides [ADEPs], discussed below) are active against *Mtb* (Ollinger et al. 2012). *Mtb* ClpP has thus been validated as a drug target that could be exploited because of its novel mechanism—in the presence of ADEPs—of bacterial killing. It has been shown that ADEP binding leads to a change of ClpP structure, allowing access of unfolded proteins to the proteolytic chamber in the absence of the regulatory Clp ATPases (Kirstein et al. 2009), thus effectively dysregulating this protease system and leading to unregulated proteolysis and bacterial death. It was recently shown that ADEP4-activated ClpP becomes nonspecific in its proteolytic activity and kills *Staphylococcus aureus* persisters by degrading more than 400 proteins, causing cells to self-digest (Conlon et al. 2013). A similarly efficacious dysregulator of *Mtb* ClpP would represent a truly novel mechanism of sterilizing chronically infected lungs, contribute to shortening of treatment durations in novel TB drug regimens, and be effective against resistant disease.

A recent report has described lassomycin, an antibiotic that was specifically bactericidal against both replicating and nonreplicating *Mtb* (Gavrish et al. 2014). Lassomycin was found to bind to the ClpC1 ATPase complex and stimulate its ATPase activity, and it was its uncoupling of ATPase from proteolytic activity that accounted for the bactericidal activity.

Alternatively, a structurally diverse series of β-lactone inhibitors has been shown to form a covalent adduct at the ClpP2 catalytic serine and inhibit *Mtb* growth (Compton et al. 2013). This finding provides yet another pharmacological validation of the ClpP protease as a potential drug target, but in this case, the mechanism is by inhibition of ClpP instead of by dysregulating ClpP activity as occurs with acyldepsipeptides.

Targeting Central Carbon Metabolism

Mtb adapts its metabolism to the environmental conditions to which it is exposed (Rhee et al. 2011). Several metabolic enzymes have been validated as drug targets; the multifunctionality of some of these enzymes makes them of particular interest.

The enzymes of the glyoxylate shunt, isocitrate lyase (ICL) (Honer et al. 1999) and malate synthase (GlcB) (Smith et al. 2003), have long been and remain of interest to TB drug discovery. The glyoxylate shunt serves to bypass the two CO_2^- generating steps of the tricarboxylic acid (TCA) cycle when carbon is limiting, including during growth on fatty acids. ICL-deficient *Mtb* cannot establish an infection in mice (McKinney et al. 2000; Munoz-Elias and McKinney 2005), and *icl* is up-regulated during infection (Timm et al. 2003). Although this suggests reliance on this pathway and subsistence on fatty acids in vivo, the importance of ICL may result from its several roles—ICL in the glyoxylate shunt, methyl-ICL in the methylcitrate cycle of propionyl-coA metabolism (Gould et al. 2006; Munoz-Elias et al. 2006), ICL in ATP homeostasis during adaptation to slow growth (Gengenbacher et al. 2010), and ICL in succinate generation for proton motive force (PMF) maintenance under hypoxia (Eoh and Rhee 2013). Perhaps owing to the small polar active site of ICL (Sharma et al. 2000), only weakly efficacious ICL inhibitors have been reported to date (Kraty and Vinsova 2012). Efforts continue to target ICL, including via target-based whole-cell screening (Abrahams et al. 2012a). Conversely, novel, efficacious phenyl-diketo acid inhibitors of *Mtb* GlcB were recently discovered (Krieger et al. 2012). As for ICL, GlcB appears to play unexpected metabolic roles in carbohydrate and cholesterol metabolism—another example of the metabolic flexibility of *Mtb* (de Carvalho et al. 2010; Beste et al. 2011; Griffin et al. 2011).

Like ICL, phosphoenolpyruvate carboxykinase (PEPCK) is required by *Mtb* for growth on fatty acids and survival in rodents (Liu et al. 2003; Marrero et al. 2010), and it is induced during infection (Timm et al. 2003). PEPCK catalyzes the first committed step of gluconeogenesis, by which sugars are synthesized from TCA intermediates during growth on fatty acids (Mukhopadhyay et al. 2001). As with ICL, the importance of PEPCK in vivo suggests subsistence on fatty acids. However, the glycolytic enzyme glucokinase is also required for survival of *Mtb* in mice (Marrero et al. 2013), suggesting a requirement for metabolism of carbohydrates during late infection. No drug discovery efforts have been reported yet against these interesting targets.

Two better explored targets are lipoamide dehydrogenase (Lpd) and dihydrolipoamide acyltransferase (DlaT). DlaT and Lpd function as components of pyruvate dehydrogenase, which supplies glycolysis-derived acetyl-CoA to the TCA cycle (Tian et al. 2005). Both are also components of the *Mtb* peroxynitrite reductase/peroxidase, which functions to resist host-reactive nitrogen intermediates (Bryk et al. 2000,2002). Lpd also functions within branched-chain amino acid metabolism, perhaps explaining the more profound attenuation for growth in mice on disruption of *lpdC* compared with *dlaT* (Shi and Ehrt 2006; Venogopal et al. 2011). Efforts to target both Lpd (Bryk et al. 2010) and DlaT are ongoing, the latter motivated by the demonstration that DlaT-deficient *Mtb* fails to establish an infection in guinea pigs (Bryk et al. 2008). Discovery efforts focused on DlaT have identified inhibitors that are selectively active against nonreplicating *Mtb*.

Finally, the maltosyltransferase GlgE was recently identified as a target of interest (Kalscheuer and Jacobs 2010). This enzyme participates in a pathway from trehalose to α-glucan, and GlgE-deficient *Mtb* dies in vitro and in mice caused by accumulation of its toxic substrate, maltose-1-phosphate. This pathway also shows a synthetic lethal interaction with the glucosyltransferase Rv3032, suggesting that synergistic TB drugs may be discovered by targeting components of these pathways.

Targeting Energy Generation: Inhibitors of the Respiratory Chain and ATP Synthesis

ATP synthesis and PMF generation are among the best-validated *Mtb* drug targets owing to the clinical successes of the ATP synthase inhibitor TMC207 (bedaquiline, Sirturo) (Andries et al. 2005; Diacon et al. 2009) and the cornerstone TB drug pyrazinamide, which disrupts the PMF (Zhang et al. 2003). PMF and ATP homeostasis are required by replicating and nonreplicating *Mtb*, under a variety of conditions (Koul et al. 2008; Rao et al. 2008), and efforts to target these processes include pathway screens using membrane particles, cell-based screens for ATP homeostasis disruptors, target-based screens, and repurposing of existing drugs known to inhibit this pathway.

Mtb operates a branched respiratory chain, the components of which operate variably, depending on the environment (Kana et al. 2001; Matsoso et al. 2005; Weinstein et al. 2005; Small et al. 2013). A menaquinone pool is reduced by NADH dehydrogenase (Ndh, provided by a 14-subunit NdhI complex and single subunit NdhII) and succinate:menaquinone oxidoreductase (Sdh). Electrons flow from the menaquinone pool to a quinol oxidase (cytochrome *bd* oxidase) or to a cytochrome *bc1*–*aa3* oxidoreductase supercomplex wherein a *bc1* *c*-type cytochrome reductase transfers electrons to the terminal *aa3*-type oxidase. Both oxidases use molecular oxygen as the terminal electron acceptor. In the absence of respiration, *Mtb* maintains the PMF and ATP synthesis using secreted succinate generated by fumarate reductase (Watanabe et al. 2011) and/or produced by ICL.

TB drug discovery efforts have focused on NdhII, encoded in *Mtb* by *ndh* and *ndhA*. The phenothiazines (a class of central nervous system drugs) have anti-*Mtb* activity in vitro and in vivo (Amarai et al. 1996; Bettencourt et al.

2000), and their *Mtb* target is NdhII (Warman et al. 2013), pharmacologically validating this enzyme. In addition, the leprosy drug clofazimine, which is efficacious against murine TB, targets NdhII as part of its mode of action (Yano et al. 2011). The existence of transposon mutants of *ndhA* but not *ndh* (McAdam et al. 2002) suggests the relative importance of the *ndh*-encoded component of NdhII. However, a novel compound identified through a screen for ATP synthesis inhibitors appears to target NdhA (Ioerger et al. 2013). The importance of NdhI and Sdh for *Mtb* energy metabolism is not fully understood, although recent evidence suggests a crucial role for Sdh under hypoxia (Eoh and Rhee 2013).

The biosynthesis of menaquinone is expected to be critical under aerobic and hypoxic conditions (Dhiman et al. 2009; Kurosu and Crick 2009). Menaquinone is synthesized from chorismate by a series of at least eight enzymes. Of these, MenC, MenD, and MenE appear to be essential in vitro (Sassetti and Rubin 2003). A recent report of anti-*Mtb* MenB inhibitors cites a personal communication from C.M. Sassetti that MenB is essential (Li et al. 2011). A report on MenA inhibitors active against replicating and nonreplicating *Mtb* mentioned an unpublished demonstration (by D. Schnappinger) that MenA is essential for growth of *Mtb* in mice, providing genetic validation for MenA and menaquinone biosynthesis in general as a drug target (Debnath et al. 2012). Target-based efforts are ongoing against *Mtb* MenA (Kurosu et al. 2007; Kurosu and Crick 2009), MenB, and MenE (Lu et al. 2012).

The cytochrome *b* subunit (QcrB) of the cytochrome *bc1-aa3* complex has recently emerged as a target of interest. Previous studies (Sassetti and Rubin 2003) indicated that QcrB is essential and that the *aa3*-type cytochrome *c* oxidase is important for aerobic growth, although the less bioenergetically favorable cytochrome *bd* oxidase is more important for microaerobic growth (Kana et al. 2001). However, disruption of *Mtb* cytochrome *c* maturation results in only impaired growth in vitro and in mice, which is partially compensated for by induction of cytochrome *bd* oxidase (Small et al. 2013). This suggests a role for cytochrome *bd* oxidase during aerobic growth and in infection and suggests limited target vulnerability of the cytochrome *bc1* complex. Despite this, the QcrB inhibitor, Q203, shows potent efficacy against murine TB. Q203 and other compounds confirmed or presumed to inhibit QcrB are described in more detail above (Mak et al. 2012a,b). Although *Mtb* QcrB is pharmacologically validated, further efficacy profiling of QcrB inhibitors is ongoing.

Following generation of the PMF, ATP synthesis occurs via F_0F_1 ATP synthase. Its *c* subunit is the target of the diarylquinoline TMC207. Efforts to target ATP synthase are limited by its complex nature. However, cell-based (Mak et al. 2012a) or membrane particle–based screens for ATP synthesis inhibitors may identify new series targeting ATP synthase.

ROS and NOS Generation

Although somewhat controversial (Keren et al. 2013), one hypothesis states that all bactericidal antibiotics kill bacteria by generating reactive oxygen or nitrogen species (ROS/RNS) (Dwyer et al. 2009). Recently, it was shown that a relatively small change (20%) in dissolved oxygen can affect killing of bacterial persiters (Grant et al. 2012), a subpopulation of bacteria in an infection that is phenotypically resistant to killing by most antibiotics but still sensitive, however, to high quantities of radicals. This observation can be critical for killing *Mtb* in granulomas, which have hypoxic cores (Via et al. 2008). Drugs such as clofazimine, PA-824, and delamanid have been shown to generate ROS and/or RNS (Singh et al. 2008; Yano et al. 2011), which is presumably the mechanism for their activity against *Mtb*. Recently, the function of the *Mtb* deazaflavin-dependent nitroreductase (Ddn), an enzyme that activates PA-824, has been hypothesized to be what provides *Mtb* protection from oxidative stress and bactericidal agents (Gurumurthy et al. 2013); the authors of the report noted that Ddn mutants defective in the formation of deazaflavin were hypersensitive to isoniazid, moxifloxacin, and clofazimine. This suggests that any agent that can inhibit Ddn or deazaflavin biosynthesis could synergize with existing anti-TB drugs. Thus, novel mechanisms to generate ROS/NOS at sufficiently high concentrations should be investigated as potential novel therapy for TB, as long as they do not cause oxidative damage to the host cells (Domann 2013).

CONCLUDING REMARKS

A robust global TB drug discovery portfolio is crucial to achieving the goal of new, simpler, shorter, better TB drug regimens useful for all patient populations. The current status of anti-TB lead generation is much improved compared with the situation 10–15 years ago. However, it is still slow and drastically lacking in success; significant changes are needed to produce novel regimens with efficacy against drug-resistant TB and shorter treatment durations. A review of the processes that have led to the current global pipeline suggests a few solutions that could be used to improve the situation and produce better, more easily developable leads. Smaller, targeted compound libraries with favorable physicochemical properties should be used for hit generation; hits with preferred physicochemical properties should be prioritized over higher-potency hits with poor properties; hits with improved cell penetration and with activity against multiple subpopulations of *Mtb* should be prioritized. When possible, leads that can penetrate caseum and have efficacy within hypoxic lesions should be prioritized, and natural products should be revisited to allow the identification of currently unexplored chemical matter.

In addition, structure- and fragment-based approaches should be used wherever practicable. Instead of either target-based biochemical screening or whole-cell-based screening, whole-cell-based, target-specific screens using specialized strains that focus on in-vivo-validated targets, pathways, or processes should be performed. Such screens should be designed using what is currently known about the various bacterial populations in the infected lung; the nature and metabolic properties of the organisms in an infection, including persisters; their transport systems and porins that could be exploited for drug uptake; and the most sensitive targets at the different stages of the disease. Such vulnerable pathways and processes might include the in-vivo-validated iron acquisition and storage pathways; central carbon, cholesterol, and energy metabolism pathways; the MmpL transport systems; and the Clp protease system. Nevertheless, because both knowledge of the biology of *Mtb* remains incomplete (Orme 2014) and the nature of clinical TB is so complex, any current screening approach necessarily remains limited. Multiple subpopulations of bacteria, differing in their replication rate and metabolic state, exist in an infection in the multiple and changing environments of the tuberculous lung (Lin et al. 2014). Any one set of screening conditions is thus unlikely to include key features of all of these environments, and few individual targets and pathways are likely crucial to all physiological states of the organism and disease (Dartois and Barry 2013). It is unlikely that any in-vitro- or even mouse-based screen will select and identify compound series with sufficient exposure for efficacy in necrotic, hypoxic, and cavitary lesions (Kjellsson et al. 2012), or eliminate viable but nonculturable (VBNC) (Pai et al. 2000; Manina and McKinney 2013) organisms.

Yet, we believe that combining the lessons learned from recent and ongoing TB drug discovery efforts with emerging technologies and an evolving understanding of *Mtb* biology should provide a path toward safer, novel regimens with greater treatment shortening potential.

ACKNOWLEDGMENTS

We acknowledge the various collaborators and funders of the TB Alliance.

REFERENCES

Abrahams GL, Kumar A, Savvi S, Hung AW, Wen S, Abell C, Barry CE III, Sherman DR, Boshoff HI, Mizrahi V. 2012a. Pathway-selective sensitization of *Mycobacterium tuberculosis* for target-based whole-cell screening. *Chem Biol* **19:** 844–854.

Abrahams KA, Cox JA, Spivey VL, Loman NJ, Pallen MJ, Constantinidou C, Fernández R, Alemparte C, Remuiñán MJ, Barros D, et al. 2012b. Identification of novel imidazo[1,2-a]pyridine inhibitors targeting *M. tuberculosis* QcrB. *PLoS ONE* **7:** e52951.

Amaral L, Kristiansen JE, Abebe LS, Millett W. 1996. Inhibition of the respiration of multi-drug resistant clinical isolates of *Mycobacterium tuberculosis* by thioridazine: Potential use for initial therapy of freshly diagnosed tuberculosis. *J Antimicrob Chemother* **38:** 1049–1053.

Ananthan S, Faaleolea ER, Goldman RC, Hobrath JV, Kwong CD, Laughon BE, Maddry JA, Mehta A, Rasmussen L, Reynolds RC, et al. 2009. High-throughput screening for inhibitors of *Mycobacterium tuberculosis* H37Rv. *Tuberculosis (Edinb)* **89:** 334–353.

Andries K, Verhasselt P, Guillemont J, Göhlmann HW, Neefs JM, Winkler H, Van Gestel J, Timmerman P, Zhu M, Lee E, et al. 2005. A diarylquinoline drug active on the ATP synthase of *Mycobacterium tuberculosis*. *Science* **307:** 223–227.

Ballell L, Bates RH, Young RJ, Alvarez-Gomez D, Alvarez-Ruiz E, Barroso V, Blanco D, Crespo B, Escribano J, González R, et al. 2013. Fueling open-source drug discovery: 177 Small-molecule leads against tuberculosis. *ChemMedChem* **8:** 313–321.

Ballell Pages L, Castro Pichel J, Fernandez Menendez R, Fernandez Velando EP, Gonzalez Del Valle S, Mendoza Losana A, Wolfendale MJ. 2010. (Pyrazol-3-yl)-1,3,4-thiadiazole-2-amine and(Pyrazol-3-yl)-1,3,4-thiazole-2-amine compounds. PCT publication No. WO 2010/118852 A1.

Batt SM, Jabeen T, Bhowruth V, Quill L, Lund PA, Eggeling L, Alderwick LJ, Fütterer K, Besra GS. 2012. Structural basis of inhibition of *Mycobacterium tuberculosis* DprE1 by benzothiazinone inhibitors. *Proc Natl Acad Sci* **109:** 11354–11359.

Beste DJ, Bonde B, Hawkins N, Ward JL, Beale MH, Noack S, Nöh K, Kruger NJ, Ratcliffe RG, McFadden J. 2011. ^{13}C Metabolic flux analysis identifies an unusual route for pyruvate dissimilation in mycobacteria which requires isocitrate lyase and carbon dioxide fixation. *PLoS Pathog* **7:** e1002091.

Bettencourt MV, Bosne-David S, Amaral L. 2000. Comparative in vitro activity of phenothiazines against multidrug-resistant *Mycobacterium tuberculosis*. *Int J Antimicrob Agents* **16:** 69–71.

Bhat J, Narayan A, Venkatraman J, Chatterji M. 2013. LC-MS based assay to measure intracellular compound levels in *Mycobacterium smegmatis*: Linking compound levels to cellular potency. *J Microbiol Methods* **94:** 152–158.

Brötz-Oesterhelt H, Beyer D, Kroll HP, Endermann R, Ladel C, Schroeder W, Hinzen B, Raddatz S, Paulsen H, Henninger K, et al. 2005. Dysregulation of bacterial proteolytic machinery by a new class of antibiotics. *Nat Med* **11:** 1082–1087.

Brown JR, North EJ, Hurdle JG, Morisseau C, Scarborough JS, Sun D, Korduláková J, Scherman MS, Jones V, Grzegorzewicz A, et al. 2011. The structure-activity relationship of urea derivatives as anti-tuberculosis agents. *Bioorg Med Chem* **19:** 5585–5595.

Brown DG, Lister T, May-Dracka TL. 2014. New natural products as new leads forantibacterial drug discovery. *Bioorg Med Chem Lett* **24:** 413–418.

Bryk R, Griffin P, Nathan C. 2000. Peroxynitrite reductase activity of bacterial peroxiredoxins. *Nature* **407:** 211–215.

Bryk R, Lima CD, Erdjument-Bromage H, Tempst P, Nathan C. 2002. Metabolic enzymes of mycobacteria linked to antioxidant defense by a thioredoxin-like protein. *Science* **295:** 1073–1077.

Bryk R, Gold B, Venugopal A, Singh J, Samy R, Pupek K, Cao H, Popescu C, Gurney M, Hotha S, et al. 2008. Selective killing of nonreplicating mycobacteria. *Cell Host Microbe* **3:** 137–145.

Bryk R, Arango N, Venugopal A, Warren JD, Park YH, Patel MS, Lima CD, Nathan C. 2010. Triazaspirodimethoxybenzoyls as selective inhibitors of mycobacterial lipoamide dehydrogenase. *Biochemistry* **49:** 1616–1627.

Capyk JK, Casabon I, Gruninger R, Strynadka NC, Eltis LD. 2011. Activity of 3-ketosteroid 9α-hydroxylase (KshAB) indicates cholesterol side chain and ring degradation occur simultaneously in *Mycobacterium tuberculosis*. *J Biol Chem* **286:** 40717–40724.

Casabon I, Crowe AM, Liu J, Eltis LD. 2013. FadD3 is an acyl-CoA synthetase that initiates catabolism of cholesterol rings C and D in actinobacteria. *Mol Microbiol* **87:** 269–283.

Castro Pichel J, Fernandez Menendez R, Fernandez Velando EP, Gonzalez Del Valle S, Mallo-Rubio A. 2012. 3-Aminopyrazole derivatives useful against tuberculosis. PCT publication No. WO2012/049161.

Chang JC, Harik NS, Liao RP, Sherman DR. 2007. Identification of mycobacterial genes that alter growth and pathology in macrophages and in mice. *J Infect Dis* **196:** 788–795.

Chang JC, Miner MD, Pandey AK, Gill WP, Harik NS, Sassetti CM, Sherman DR. 2009. igr Genes and *Mycobacterium tuberculosis* cholesterol metabolism. *J Bacteriol* **191:** 5232–5239.

Chen M, Borlak J, Tong W. 2013. High lipophilicity and high daily dose of oral medications are associated with significant risk for drug-induced liver injury. *Hepatology* **58:** 388–396.

Christophe T, Ewann F, Jeon HK, Cechetto J, Brodin P. 2010. High-content imaging of *Mycobacterium tuberculosis*-infected macrophages: An in vitro model for tuberculosis drug discovery. *Future Med Chem* **2:** 1283–1293.

Cole ST, Brosch R, Parkhill J, Garnier T, Churcher C, Harris D, Gordon SV, Eiglmeier K, Gas S, Barry CE III, et al. 1998. Deciphering the biology of *Mycobacterium tuberculosis* from the complete genome sequence. *Nature* **393:** 537–544.

Compton CL, Schmitz KR, Sauer RT, Sello JK. 2013. Antibacterial activity of and resistance to small molecule inhibitors of the ClpP peptidase. *ACS Chem Biol* **8:** 2669–2677.

Conlon BP, Nakayasu ES, Fleck LE, LaFleur MD, Isabella VM, Coleman K, Leonard SN, Smith RD, Adkins JN, Lewis K. 2013. Activated ClpP kills persisters and eradicates a chronic biofilm infection. *Nature* **503:** 365–370.

Cox JS, Chen B, McNeil M, Jacobs WR Jr. 1999. Complex lipid determines tissue-specific replication of *Mycobacterium tuberculosis* in mice. *Nature* **402:** 79–83.

Darby CM, Ingólfsson HI, Jiang X, Shen C, Sun M, Zhao N, Burns K, Liu G, Ehrt S, Warren JD, et al. 2013. Whole cell screen for inhibitors of pH homeostasis in *Mycobacterium tuberculosis*. *PLoS ONE* **8:** e68942.

Dartois V, Barry CE III. 2013. A medicinal chemists' guide to the unique difficulties of lead optimization for tuberculosis. *Bioorg Med Chem Lett* **23:** 4741–4750.

Debnath J, Siricilla S, Wan B, Crick DC, Lenaerts AJ, Franzblau SG, Kurosu M. 2012. Discovery of selective menaquinone biosynthesis inhibitors against *Mycobacterium tuberculosis*. *J Med Chem* **55:** 3739–3755.

de Carvalho LP, Fischer SM, Marrero J, Nathan C, Ehrt S, Rhee KY. 2010. Metabolomics of *Mycobacterium tuberculosis* reveals compartmentalized co-catabolism of carbon substrates. *Chem Biol* **17:** 1122–1131.

Dhiman RK, Mahapatra S, Slayden RA, Boyne ME, Lenaerts A, Hinshaw JC, Angala SK, Chatterjee D, Biswas K, Narayanasamy P, et al. 2009. Menaquinone synthesis is critical for maintaining mycobacterial viability during exponential growth and recovery from non-replicating persistence. *Mol Microbiol* **72:** 85–97.

Diacon AH, Pym A, Grobusch M, Patientia R, Rustomjee R, Page-Shipp L, Pistorius C, Krause R, Bogoshi M, Churchyard G, et al. 2009. The diarylquinoline TMC207 for multidrug-resistant tuberculosis. *N Engl J Med* **360:** 2397–2405.

Doherty CP. 2007. Host-pathogen interactions: The role of iron. *J Nutr* **137:** 1341–1344.

Domann FE. 2013. Aberrant free radical biology is a unifying theme in the etiology and pathogenesis of major human diseases. *Int J Mol Sci* **14:** 8491–8495.

Domenech P, Reed MB, Dowd CS, Manca C, Kaplan G, Barry CE III. 2004. The role of MmpL8 in sulfatide biogenesis and virulence of *Mycobacterium tuberculosis*. *J Biol Chem* **279:** 21257–21265.

Domenech P, Reed MB, Barry CE III. 2005. Contribution of the *Mycobacterium tuberculosis* MmpL protein family to virulence and drug resistance. *Infect Immun* **73:** 3492–3501.

Dresen C, Lin LY, D'Angelo I, Tocheva EI, Strynadka N, Eltis LD. 2010. A flavin-dependent monooxygenase from *Mycobacterium tuberculosis* involved in cholesterol catabolism. *J Biol Chem* **285:** 22264–22275.

Dwyer DJ, Kohanski MA, Collins JJ. 2009. Role of reactive oxygen species in antibiotic action and resistance. *Curr Opin Microbiol* **12:** 482–489.

Encinas L, O'Keefe H, Neu M, Remuiñán MJ, Patel AM, Guardia A, Davie CP, Pérez-Macías N, Yang H, Convery MA, et al. 2014. Encoded library technology as a source of hits for the discovery and lead optimization of a potent and selective class of bactericidal direct inhibitors of *Mycobacterium tuberculosis* InhA. *J Med Chem* **57:** 1276–1288.

Engelhart CA, Aldrich CC. 2013. Synthesis of chromone, quinolone, and benzoxazinone sulfonamide nucleosides as conformationally constrained inhibitors of adenylating enzymes required for siderophore biosynthesis. *J Org Chem* **78:** 7470–7481.

Eoh H, Rhee KY. 2013. Multifunctional essentiality of succinate metabolism in adaptation to hypoxia in *Mycobacterium tuberculosis*. *Proc Natl Acad Sci* **110:** 6554–6559.

Estorninho M, Smith H, Thole J, Harders-Westerveen J, Kierzek A, Butler RE, Neyrolles O, Stewart GR. 2010. ClgR regulation of chaperone and protease systems is essential for *Mycobacterium tuberculosis* parasitism of the macrophage. *Microbiology* **156:** 3445–3455.

Feher M, Schmidt JM. 2003. Property distributions: Differences between drugs, natural products, and molecules from combinatorial chemistry. *J Chem Inf Comput Sci* **43:** 218–227.

Finn J. 2012. Application of SBDD to the discovery of new antibacterial drugs. *Methods Mol Biol* **841:** 291–319.

García A, Bocanegra-García V, Palma-Nicolás JP, Rivera G. 2012. Recent advances in antitubercular natural products. *Eur J Med Chem* **49:** 1–23.

Gatfield J, Pieters J. 2000. Essential role for cholesterol in entry of mycobacteria into macrophages. *Science* **288:** 1647–1650.

Gavrish E, Sit CS, Cao S, Kandror O, Spoering A, Peoples A, Ling L, Fetterman A, Hughes D, Bissell A, et al. 2014. Lassomycin, a ribosomally synthesized cyclic peptide, kills *Mycobacterium tuberculosis* by targeting the ATP-dependent protease ClpC1P1P2. *Chem Biol* **21:** 509–518.

Gengenbacher M, Rao SP, Pethe K, Dick T. 2010. Nutrient-starved, non-replicating *Mycobacterium tuberculosis* requires respiration, ATP synthase and isocitrate lyase for maintenance of ATP homeostasis and viability. *Microbiology* **156:** 81–87.

Goldman RC. 2013. Why are membrane targets discovered by phenotypic screens and genome sequencing in *Mycobacterium tuberculosis*? *Tuberculosis (Edinb)* **93:** 569–588.

Gould TA, van de Langemheen H, Muñoz-Elías EJ, McKinney JD, Sacchettini JC. 2006. Dual role of isocitrate lyase 1 in the glyoxylate and methylcitrate cycles in *Mycobacterium tuberculosis*. *Mol Microbiol* **61:** 940–947.

Grant SS, Kaufmann BB, Chand NS, Haseley N, Hung DT. 2012. Eradication of bacterial persisters with antibiotic-generated hydroxyl radicals. *Proc Natl Acad Sci* **109:** 12147–12152.

Griffin JE, Gawronski JD, Dejesus MA, Ioerger TR, Akerley BJ, Sassetti CM. 2011. High-resolution phenotypic profiling defines genes essential for mycobacterial growth and cholesterol catabolism. *PLoS Pathog* **7:** e1002251.

Grzegorzewicz AE, Pham H, Gundi VA, Scherman MS, North EJ, Hess T, Jones V, Gruppo V, Born SE, Korduláková J, et al. 2012a. Inhibition of mycolic acid transport across the *Mycobacterium tuberculosis* plasma membrane. *Nat Chem Biol* **8:** 334–341.

Grzegorzewicz AE, Korduláková J, Jones V, Born SE, Belardinelli JM, Vaquié A, Gundi VA, Madacki J, Slama N, Laval F, et al. 2012b. A common mechanism of inhibition of the *Mycobacterium tuberculosis* mycolic acid biosynthetic pathway by isoxyl and thiacetazone. *J Biol Chem* **287:** 38434–38441.

Gupta V, Gupta RK, Khare G, Salunke DM, Tyagi AK. 2008. Cloning, expression, purification, crystallization and preliminary X-ray crystallographic analysis of bacterioferritin A from *Mycobacterium tuberculosis*. *Acta Crystallogr Sect F Struct Biol Cryst Commun* **64:** 398–401.

Gurumurthy M, Rao M, Mukherjee T, Rao SP, Boshoff HI, Dick T, Barry CE III, Manjunatha UH. 2013. A novel F(420)-dependent anti-oxidant mechanism protects *Mycobacterium tuberculosis* against oxidative stress and bactericidal agents. *Mol Microbiol* **87:** 744–755.

Guzman JD, Gupta A, Bucar F, Gibbons S, Bhakta S. 2012. Antimycobacterials from natural sources: Ancient times, antibiotic era and novel scaffolds. *Front Biosci (Landmark Ed)* **17:** 1861–1881.

Hartkoorn RC, Sala C, Neres J, Pojer F, Magnet S, Mukherjee R, Uplekar S, Boy-Röttger S, Altmann KH, Cole ST. 2012. Towards a new tuberculosis drug: Pyridomycin—Nature's isoniazid. *EMBO Mol Med* **4:** 1032–1042.

Hartkoorn RC, Pojer F, Read JA, Gingell H, Neres J, Horlacher OP, Altmann KH, Cole ST. 2013. Pyridomycin bridges the NADH- and substrate-binding pockets of the enoyl reductase InhA. *Nat Chem Biol* **10:** 96–98.

Holmes MA, Paulsene W, Jide X, Ratledge C, Strong RK. 2005. Siderocalin (Lcn 2) also binds carboxymycobactins, potentially defending against mycobacterial infections through iron sequestration. *Structure* **13:** 29–41.

Höner Zu Bentrup K, Miczak A, Swenson DL, Russell DG. 1999. Characterization of activity and expression of isocitrate lyase in *Mycobacterium avium* and *Mycobacterium tuberculosis*. *J Bacteriol* **181:** 7161–7167.

Hung AW, Silvestre HL, Wen S, Ciulli A, Blundell TL, Abell C. 2009. Application of fragment growing and fragment linking to the discovery of inhibitors of *Mycobacterium tuberculosis* pantothenate synthetase. *Angew Chem Int Ed Engl* **48:** 8452–8456.

Ingvarsson H, Maté MJ, Högbom M, Portnoï D, Benaroudj N, Alzari PM, Ortiz-Lombardía M, Unge T. 2007. Insights into the inter-ring plasticity of caseinolytic proteases from the X-ray structure of *Mycobacterium tuberculosis* ClpP1. *Acta Crystallogr D Biol Crystallogr* **63:** 249–259.

Ioerger TR, O'Malley T, Liao R, Guinn KM, Hickey MJ, Mohaideen N, Murphy KC, Boshoff HI, Mizrahi V, Rubin EJ, et al. 2013. Identification of new drug targets and resistance mechanisms in *Mycobacterium tuberculosis*. *PLoS ONE* **8:** e75245.

Irschik H, Reichenbach H, Höfle G, Jansen R. 2007. The thuggacins, novel antibacterial macrolides from *Sorangium cellulosum* acting against selected Gram-positive bacteria. *J Antibiot (Tokyo)* **60:** 733–738.

Ishizaki Y, Hayashi C, Inoue K, Igarashi M, Takahashi Y, Pujari V, Crick DC, Brennan PJ, Nomoto A. 2013. Inhibition of the first step in synthesis of the mycobacterial cell wall core, catalyzed by the GlcNAc-1-phosphate transferase WecA, by the novel caprazamycin derivative CPZEN-45. *J Biol Chem* **288:** 30309–30319.

Iwatsuki M, Tomoda H, Uchida R, Gouda H, Hirono S, Omura S. 2006. Lariatins, antimycobacterial peptides produced by *Rhodococcus sp.* K01-B0171, have a lasso structure. *J Am Chem Soc* **128:** 7486–7491.

Iwatsuki M, Uchida R, Takakusagi Y, Matsumoto A, Jiang CL, Takahashi Y, Arai M, Kobayashi S, Matsumoto M, Inokoshi J, et al. 2007. Lariatins, novel anti-mycobacterial peptides with a lasso structure, produced by *Rhodococcus jostii* K01-B0171. *J Antibiot (Tokyo)* **60:** 357–363.

Jain M, Cox JS. 2005. Interaction between polyketide synthase and transporter suggests coupled synthesis and export of virulence lipid in *M. tuberculosis*. *PLoS Pathog* **1:** e2.

Johnson EE, Wessling-Resnick M. 2012. Iron metabolism and the innate immune response to infection. *Microbes Infect* **14:** 207–216.

Jones CM, Niederweis M. 2011. *Mycobacterium tuberculosis* can utilize heme as an iron source. *J Bacteriol* **193:** 1767–1770.

Jones CM, Wells RM, Madduri AV, Renfrow MB, Ratledge C, Moody DB, Niederweis M. 2014. Self-poisoning of *Mycobacterium tuberculosis* by interrupting siderophore recycling. *Proc Natl Acad Sci* **111:** 1945–1950.

Kalscheuer R, Jacobs WR Jr. 2010. The significance of GlgE as a new target for tuberculosis. *Drug News Perspect* **23:** 619–624.

Kana BD, Weinstein EA, Avarbock D, Dawes SS, Rubin H, Mizrahi V. 2001. Characterization of the cydAB-encoded cytochrome bd oxidase from *Mycobacterium smegmatis*. *J Bacteriol* **183:** 7076–7086.

Kauffmann SHE. 2004. New issues in tuberculosis. *Ann Rheum Dis* **63:** 1150–1156.

Kawate T, Iwase N, Shimizu M, Stanley SA, Wellington S, Kazyanskaya E, Hung DT. 2013. Synthesis and structure-activity relationships of phenyl-substituted coumarins with anti-tubercular activity that target FadD32. *Bioorg Med Chem Lett* **23:** 6052–6059.

Keren I, Wu Y, Inocencio J, Mulcahy LR, Lewis K. 2013. Killing by bactericidal antibiotics does not depend on reactive oxygen species. *Science* **339:** 1213–1216.

Kim MJ, Wainwright HC, Locketz M, Bekker LG, Walther GB, Dittrich C, Visser A, Wang W, Hsu FF, Wiehart U, et al. 2010. Caseation of human tuberculosis granulomas correlates with elevated host lipid metabolism. *EMBO Mol Med* **2:** 258–274.

Kirst HA. 2013. Developing new antibacterials through natural product research. *Expert Opin Drug Discov* **8:** 479–493.

Kirstein J, Hoffmann A, Lilie H, Schmidt R, Rübsamen-Waigmann H, Brötz-Oesterhelt H, Mogk A, Turgay K. 2009. The antibiotic ADEP reprogrammes ClpP, switching it from a regulated to an uncontrolled protease. *EMBO Mol Med* **1:** 37–49.

Kjellsson MC, Via LE, Goh A, Weiner D, Low KM, Kern S, Pillai G, Barry CE III, Dartois V. 2012. Pharmacokinetic evaluation of the penetration of antituberculosis agents in rabbit pulmonary lesions. *Antimicrob Agents Chemother* **56:** 446–457.

Kondreddi RR, Jiricek J, Rao SPS, Lakshminarayana SB, Camacho LR, Rao R, Herve M, Bifani P, Ma NL, Kuhen K, et al. 2013. Design, synthesis, and biological evaluation of indole-2-carboxamides: A promising class of antituberculosis agents. *J Med Chem* **56:** 8849–8859.

Koul A, Vranckx L, Dendouga N, Balemans W, Van den Wyngaert I, Vergauwen K, Göhlmann HW, Willebrords R, Poncelet A, Guillemont J, et al. 2008. Diarylquinolines are bactericidal for dormant mycobacteria as a result of disturbed ATP homeostasis. *J Biol Chem* **283:** 25273–25280.

Krátký M, Vinšová J. 2012. Advances in mycobacterial isocitrate lyase targeting and inhibitors. *Curr Med Chem* **19:** 6126–6137.

Krieger IV, Freundlich JS, Gawandi VB, Roberts JP, Gawandi VB, Sun Q, Owen JL, Fraile MT, Huss SI, Lavandera JL, et al. 2012. Structure-guided discovery of phenyl-diketo acids as potent inhibitors of *M. tuberculosis* malate synthase. *Chem Biol* **19:** 1556–1567.

Kumar A, Casey A, Odingo J, Kesicki EA, Abrahams G, Vieth M, Masquelin T, Mizrahi V, Hipskind PA, Sherman DR, et al. 2013. A high-throughput screen against pantothenate synthetase (PanC) identifies 3-biphenyl-4-cyano-pyrrole-2-carboxylic acids as a new class of inhibitor with activity against *Mycobacterium tuberculosis*. *PLoS ONE* **8:** e72786.

Kurosu M, Crick DC. 2009. MenA is a promising drug target for developing novel lead molecules to combat *Mycobacterium tuberculosis*. *Med Chem* **5:** 197–207.

Kurosu M, Narayanasamy P, Biswas K, Dhiman R, Crick DC. 2007. Discovery of 1,4-dihydroxy-2-naphthoate prenyltransferase inhibitors: New drug leads for multidrug-resistant Gram-positive pathogens. *J Med Chem* **50:** 3973–3974.

Lack NA, Yam KC, Lowe ED, Horsman GP, Owen RL, Sim E, Eltis LD. 2010. Characterization of a carbon-carbon hydrolase from *Mycobacterium tuberculosis* involved in cholesterol metabolism. *J Biol Chem* **285:** 434–443.

Lamichhane G, Tyagi S, Bishai WR. 2005. Designer arrays for defined mutant analysis to detect genes essential for survival of *Mycobacterium tuberculosis* in mouse lungs. *Infect Immun* **73:** 2533–2540.

La Rosa V, Poce G, Canseco JO, Buroni S, Pasca MR, Biava M, Raju RM, Porretta GC, Alfonso S, Battilocchio C, et al. 2012. MmpL3 is the cellular target of the antitubercular pyrrole derivative BM212. *Antimicrob Agents Chemother* **56:** 324–331.

Li JW, Vederas JC. 2009. Drug discovery and natural products: End of an era or an endless frontier? *Science* **325:** 161–165.

Li X, Liu N, Zhang H, Knudson SE, Li HJ, Lai CT, Simmerling C, Slayden RA, Tonge PJ. 2011. CoA Adducts of 4-Oxo-4-Phenylbut-2-enoates: Inhibitors of MenB from the *M. tuberculosis* menaquinone biosynthesis pathway. *ACS Med Chem Lett* **2:** 818–823.

Li K, Schurig-Briccio LA, Feng X, Upadhyay A, Pujari V, Lechartier B, Fontes FL, Yang H, Rao G, Zhu W, et al. 2014. Multitarget drug discovery for tuberculosis and other infectious diseases. *J Med Chem* **57:** 3126–3139.

Lin PL, Ford CB, Coleman MT, Myers AJ, Gawande R, Ioerger T, Sacchettini J, Fortune SM, Flynn JL. 2014. Sterilization of granulomas is common in active and latent tuberculosis despite within-host variability in bacterial killing. *Nat Med* **20:** 75–79.

Liu K, Yu J, Russell DG. 2003. pckA-Deficient *Mycobacterium bovis* BCG shows attenuated virulence in mice and in macrophages. *Microbiology* **149:** 1829–1835.

Lu XI, Zhou R, Sharma I, Li X, Kumar G, Swaminathan S, Tonge PJ, Tan DS. 2012. Stable analogues of OSB-AMP: Potent inhibitors of MenE, the *o*-succinatebenzoate-CoA synthetase from bacterial menaquinone biosynthesis. *Chembiochem* **13:** 129–136.

Maddry JA, Ananthan S, Goldman RC, Hobrath JV, Kwong CD, Maddox C, Rasmussen L, Reynolds RC, Secrist JA III, Sosa MI, et al. 2009. Antituberculosis activity of the molecular libraries screening center network library. *Tuberculosis (Edinb)* **89:** 354–363.

Mai D, Jones J, Rodgers JW, Hartman JL IV, Kutsch O, Steyn AJ. 2011. A screen to identify small molecule inhibitors of protein-protein interactions in mycobacteria. *Assay Drug Dev Technol* **9:** 299–310.

Mak PA, Rao SP, Ping Tan M, Lin X, Chyba J, Tay J, Ng SH, Tan BH, Cherian J, Duraiswamy J, et al. 2012a. A high-throughput screen to identify inhibitors of ATP homeostasis in non-replicating *Mycobacterium tuberculosis*. *ACS Chem Biol* **7:** 1190–1197.

Manina G, McKinney JD. 2013. A single-cell perspective on non-growing but metabolically active (NGMA) bacteria. *Curr Top Microbiol Immunol* **374:** 135–161.

Marrero J, Rhee KY, Schnappinger D, Pethe K, Ehrt S. 2010. Gluconeogenic carbon flow of tricarboxylic acid cycle intermediates is critical for *Mycobacterium tuberculosis* to establish and maintain infection. *Proc Natl Acad Sci* **107:** 9819–9824.

Marrero J, Trujillo C, Rhee KY, Ehrt S. 2013. Glucose phosphorylation is required for *Mycobacterium tuberculosis* persistence in mice. *PLoS Pathog* **9:** e1003116.

Matsoso LG, Kana BD, Crellin PK, Lea-Smith DJ, Pelosi A, Powell D, Dawes SS, Rubin H, Coppel RL, Mizrahi V. 2005. Function of the cytochrome *bc1-aa3* branch of the respiratory network in mycobacteria and network adaptation occurring in response to its disruption. *J Bacteriol* **187:** 6300–6308.

McAdam RA, Quan S, Smith DA, Bardarov S, Betts JC, Cook FC, Hooker EU, Lewis AP, Woollard P, Everett MJ, et al. 2002. Characterization of a *Mycobacterium tuberculosis* H37Rv transposon library reveals insertions in 351 ORFs and mutants with altered virulence. *Microbiology* **148:** 2975–2986.

McKinney JD, Höner zu Bentrup K, Muñoz-Elías EJ, Miczak A, Chen B, Chan WT, Swenson D, Sacchettini JC, Jacobs WR Jr, Russell DG. 2000. Persistence of *Mycobacterium tuberculosis* in macrophages and mice requires the glyoxylate shunt enzyme isocitrate lyase. *Nature* **406:** 735–738.

McMath LM, Habel JE, Sankaran B, Yu M, Hung LW, Goulding CW. 2010. Crystallization and preliminary X-ray crystallographic analysis of a *Mycobacterium tuberculosis* ferritin homolog, BfrB. *Acta Crystallogr Sect F Struct Biol Cryst Commun* **66:** 1657–1661.

Milano A, Pasca MR, Provvedi R, Lucarelli AP, Manina G, Ribeiro AL, Manganelli R, Riccardi G. 2009. Azole resistance in *Mycobacterium tuberculosis* is mediated by the MmpS5-MmpL5 efflux system. *Tuberculosis (Edinb)* **89:** 84–90.

Miner MD, Chang JC, Pandey AK, Sassetti CM, Sherman DR. 2009. Role of cholesterol in *Mycobacterium tuberculosis* infection. *Indian J Exp Biol* **47:** 407–411.

Mohn WW, van der Geize R, Stewart GR, Okamoto S, Liu J, Dijkhuizen L, Eltis LD. 2008. The actinobacterial mce4 locus encodes a steroid transporter. *J Biol Chem* **283:** 35368–35374.

Monfeli RR, Beeson C. 2007. Targeting iron acquisition by *Mycobacterium tuberculosis*. *Infect Disord Drug Targets* **7:** 213–220.

Moraski GC, Markley LD, Hipskind PA, Boshoff H, Cho S, Franzblau SG, Miller MJ. 2011. Advent of Imidazo[1,2-a]pyridine-3-carboxamides with potent multi- and extended drug resistant antituberculosis activity. *ACS Med Chem Lett* **2:** 466–470.

Moraski GC, Markley LD, Chang M, Cho S, Franzblau SG, Hwang CH, Boshoff H, Miller MJ. 2012. Generation and exploration of new classes of antitubercular agents: The optimization of oxazolines, oxazoles, thiazolines, thiazoles to imidazo[1,2-a]pyridines and isomeric 5,6-fused scaffolds. *Bioorg Med Chem* **20:** 2214–2220.

Muñoz-Elías EJ, McKinney JD. 2005. *Mycobacterium tuberculosis* isocitrate lyases 1 and 2 are jointly required for in vivo growth and virulence. *Nat Med* **11:** 638–644.

Muñoz-Elías EJ, Upton AM, Cherian J, McKinney JD. 2006. Role of the methylcitrate cycle in *Mycobacterium tuberculosis* metabolism, intracellular growth, and virulence. *Mol Microbiol* **60:** 1109–1122.

Mukhopadhyay B, Concar EM, Wolfe RS. 2001. A GTP-dependent vertebrate-type phosphoenolpyruvate carboxykinase from *Mycobacterium smegmatis*. *J Biol Chem* **276:** 16137–16145.

Naven RT, Swiss R, Klug-McLeod J, Will Y, Greene N. 2013. The development of structure-activity relationships for mitochondrial dysfunction: Uncoupling of oxidative phosphorylation. *Toxicol Sci* **131:** 271–278.

Neres J, Labello NP, Somu RV, Boshoff HI, Wilson DJ, Vannada J, Chen L, Barry CE III, Bennett EM, Aldrich CC. 2008. Inhibition of siderophore biosynthesis in *Mycobacterium tuberculosis* with nucleoside bisubstrate analogues: Structure-activity relationships of the nucleobase domain of 5′-*O*-[*N*-(salicyl)sulfamoyl]adenosine. *J Med Chem* **51:** 5349–5370.

Nesbitt NM, Yang X, Fontán P, Kolesnikova I, Smith I, Sampson NS, Dubnau E. 2010. A thiolase of *Mycobacterium tuberculosis* is required for virulence and production of androstenedione and androstadienedione from cholesterol. *Infect Immun* **78:** 275–282.

Newman DJ, Cragg GM. 2012. Natural products as sources of new drugs over the 30 years from 1981 to 2010. *J Nat Prod* **75:** 311–335.

Ollinger J, O'Malley T, Kesicki EA, Odingo J, Parish T. 2012. Validation of the essential ClpP protease in *Mycobacterium tuberculosis* as a novel drug target. *J Bacteriol* **194:** 663–668.

Orme IM. 2014. A new unifying theory of the pathogenesis of tuberculosis. *Tuberculosis (Edinb)* **94:** 8–14.

Owens CP, Chim N, Graves AB, Harmston CA, Iniguez A, Contreras H, Liptak MD, Goulding CW. 2013. The *Mycobacterium tuberculosis* secreted protein Rv0203 transfers heme to membrane proteins MmpL3 and MmpL11. *J Biol Chem* **288:** 21714–21728.

Pai SR, Actor JK, Sepulveda E, Hunter RL Jr, Jagannath C. 2000. Identification of viable and non-viable *Mycobacterium tuberculosis* in mouse organs by directed RT-PCR for antigen 85B mRNA. *Microb Pathog* **28:** 335–342.

Pan P, Tonge PJ. 2012. Targeting InhA, the FASII enoyl-ACP reductase: SAR studies on novel inhibitor scaffolds. *Curr Top Med Chem* **12:** 672–693.

Pandey AK, Sassetti CM. 2008. Mycobacterial persistence requires the utilization of host cholesterol. *Proc Natl Acad Sci* **105:** 4376–4380.

Pandey R, Rodriguez GM. 2012. A ferritin mutant of *Mycobacterium tuberculosis* is highly susceptible to killing by antibiotics and is unable to establish a chronic infection in mice. *Infect Immun* **80:** 3650–3659.

Paulsen IT, Brown MH, Skurray RA. 1996. Proton-dependent multidrug efflux systems. *Microbiol Rev* **60:** 575–608.

Payne DJ, Gwynn MN, Holmes DJ, Pompliano DL. 2007. Drugs for bad bugs: Confronting the challenges of antibacterial discovery. *Nat Rev Drug Discov* **6:** 29–40.

Pethe K, Bifani P, Jang J, Kang S, Park S, Ahn S, Jiricek J, Jung J, Jeon HK, Cechetto J, et al. 2013. Discovery of Q203, a potent clinical candidate for the treatment of tuberculosis. *Nat Med* **19:** 1157–1160.

Peyron P, Bordier C, N'Diaye EN, Maridonneau-Parini I. 2000. Nonopsonic phagocytosis of *Mycobacterium kansasii* by human neutrophils depends on cholesterol and is mediated by CR3 associated with glycosylphosphatidylinositol-anchored proteins. *J Immunol* **165:** 5186–5191.

Pruksakorn P, Arai M, Kotoku N, Vilchèze C, Baughn AD, Moodley P, Jacobs WR Jr, Kobayashi M. 2010. Trichoderins, novel aminolipopeptides from a marine sponge-derived *Trichoderma sp.*, are active against dormant mycobacteria. *Bioorg Med Chem Lett* **20:** 3658–3663.

Pruksakorn P, Arai M, Liu L, Moodley P, Jacobs WR Jr, Kobayashi M. 2011. Action-mechanism of trichoderin A, an anti-dormant mycobacterial aminolipopeptide from marine sponge-derived *Trichoderma sp. Biol Pharm Bull* **34:** 1287–1290.

Putman M, van Veen HW, Konings WN. 2000. Molecular properties of bacterial multidrug transporters. *Microbiol Mol Biol Rev* **64:** 672–693.

Ramachandran S, Panda M, Mukherjee K, Choudhury NR, Tantry SJ, Kedari CK, Ramachandran V, Sharma S, Ramya VK, Guptha S, et al. 2013. Synthesis and structure activity relationship of imidazo[1,2-a]pyridine-8-carboxamides as a novel antimycobacterial lead series. *Bioorg Med Chem Lett* **23:** 4996–5001.

Rao SP, Alonso S, Rand L, Dick T, Pethe K. 2008. The proton motive force is required for maintaining ATP homeostasis and viability of hypoxic, nonreplicating *Mycobacterium tuberculosis*. *Proc Natl Acad Sci* **105:** 11945–11950.

Rao SP, Lakshminarayana SB, Kondreddi RR, Herve M, Camacho LR, Bifani P, Kalapala SK, Jiricek J, Ma NL, Tan BH, et al. 2013. Indolcarboxamide is a preclinical candidate for treating multidrug-resistant tuberculosis. *Sci Transl Med* **5:** 214ra168.

Ratledge C, Dover LG. 2000. Iron metabolism in pathogenic bacteria. *Annu Rev Microbiol* **54:** 881–941.

Reddy PV, Puri RV, Khera A, Tyagi AK. 2012. Iron storage proteins are essential for the survival and pathogenesis of *Mycobacterium tuberculosis* in THP-1 macrophages and the guinea pig model of infection. *J Bacteriol* **194:** 567–575.

Reddy PV, Puri RV, Chauhan P, Kar R, Rohilla A, Khera A, Tyagi AK. 2013. Disruption of mycobactin biosynthesis leads to attenuation of *Mycobacterium tuberculosis* for growth and virulence. *J Infect Dis* **208:** 1255–1265.

Remuiñán MJ, Pérez-Herrán E, Rullás J, Alemparte C, Martínez-Hoyos M, Dow DJ, Afari J, Mehta N, Esquivias J, Jiménez E, et al. 2013. Tetrahydropyrazolo[1,5-a]pyrimidine-3-carboxamide and *N*-benzyl-6′,7′-dihydrospiro-[piperidine-4,4′-thieno[3,2-c]pyran] analogues with bactericidal efficacy against *Mycobacterium tuberculosis* targeting MmpL3. *PLoS ONE* **8:** e60933.

Rengarajan J, Bloom BR, Rubin EJ. 2005. Genome-wide requirements for *Mycobacterium tuberculosis* adaptation and survival in macrophages. *Proc Natl Acad Sci* **102:** 8327–8332.

Rhee KY, de Carvalho LP, Bryk R, Ehrt S, Marrero J, Park SW, Schnappinger D, Venugopal A, Nathan C. 2011. Central carbon metabolism in *Mycobacterium tuberculosis*: An unexpected frontier. *Trends Microbiol* **19:** 307–314.

Rodriguez GM. 2006. Control of iron metabolism in *Mycobacterium tuberculosis*. *Trends Microbiol* **14:** 320–327.

Rodriguez GM, Smith I. 2006. Identification of an ABC transporter required for iron acquisition and virulence in *Mycobacterium tuberculosis*. *J Bacteriol* **188:** 424–430.

Rustad TR, Harrell MI, Liao R, Sherman DR. 2008. The enduring hypoxic response of *Mycobacterium tuberculosis*. *PLoS ONE* **30:** e1502.

Salomon CE, Schmidt LE. 2012. Natural products as leads for tuberculosis drug development. *Curr Top Med Chem* **12:** 735–765.

Sarathy JP, Dartois V, Lee EJ. 2012. The role of transport mechanisms in *Mycobacterium tuberculosis* drug resistance and tolerance. *Pharmaceuticals (Basel)* **5:** 1210–1235.

Sassetti CM, Rubin EJ. 2003. Genetic requirements for mycobacterial survival during infection. *Proc Natl Acad Sci* **100:** 12989–12994.

Sassetti CM, Boyd DH, Rubin EJ. 2003. Genes required for mycobacterial growth defined by high density mutagenesis. *Mol Microbiol* **48:** 77–84.

Schafer G, Guler R, Murray G, Brombacher F, Brown GD. 2009. The role of scavenger receptor B1 in infection with *Mycobacterium tuberculosis* in a murine model. *PLoS ONE* **4:** e8448.

Scherman MS, North EJ, Jones V, Hess TN, Grzegorzewicz AE, Kasagami T, Kim IH, Merzlikin O, Lenaerts AJ, Lee RE, et al. 2012. Screening a library of 1600 adamantyl ureas for anti-*Mycobacterium tuberculosis* activity in vitro and for better physical chemical properties for bioavailability. *Bioorg Med Chem* **20:** 3255–3262.

Schmitt EK, Riwanto M, Sambandamurthy V, Roggo S, Miault C, Zwingelstein C, Krastel P, Noble C, Beer D, Rao SP, et al. 2011. The natural product cyclomarin kills *Mycobacterium tuberculosis* by targeting the ClpC1 subunit of the caseinolytic protease. *Angew Chem Int Ed Engl* **50:** 5889–5891.

Schnappinger D, Ehrt S, Voskuil MI, Liu Y, Mangan JA, Monahan IM, Dolganov G, Efron B, Butcher PD, Nathan C, et al. 2003. Transcriptional adaptation of *Mycobacterium tuberculosis* within macrophages: Insights into the phagosomal environment. *J Exp Med* **198:** 693–704.

Senaratne RH, Sidders B, Sequeira P, Saunders G, Dunphy K, Marjanovic O, Reader JR, Lima P, Chan S, Kendall S, et al. 2008. *Mycobacterium tuberculosis* strains disrupted in mce3 and mce4 operons are attenuated in mice. *J Med Microbiol* **57:** 164–170.

Sharma V, Sharma S, Hoener zu Bentrup K, McKinney JD, Russell DG, Jacobs WR Jr, Sacchettini JC. 2000. Structure of isocitrate lyase, a persistence factor of *Mycobacterium tuberculosis*. *Nat Struct Biol* **7:** 663–668.

Sherman DR, Voskuil M, Schnappinger D, Liao R, Harrell MI, Schoolnik GK. 2001. Regulation of the *Mycobacterium tuberculosis* hypoxic response gene encoding α-crystallin. *Proc Natl Acad Sci* **98:** 7534–7539.

Sherrid AM, Rustad TR, Cangelosi GA, Sherman DR. 2010. Characterization of a Clp protease gene regulator and the reaeration response in *Mycobacterium tuberculosis*. *PLoS ONE* **5:** e11622.

Shi S, Ehrt S. 2006. Dihydrolipoamide acyltransferase is critical for *Mycobacterium tuberculosis* pathogenesis. *Infect Immun* **74:** 56–63.

Shirude PS, Madhavapeddi P, Naik M, Murugan K, Shinde V, Nandishaiah R, Bhat J, Kumar A, Hameed S, Holdgate G, et al. 2013. Methyl-thiazoles: A novel mode of inhibition with the potential to develop novel inhibitors targeting InhA in *Mycobacterium tuberculosis*. *J Med Chem* **56:** 8533–8542.

Siegrist MS, Unnikrishnan M, McConnell MJ, Borowsky M, Cheng TY, Siddiqi N, Fortune SM, Moody DB, Rubin EJ. 2009. Mycobacterial Esx-3 is required for mycobactin-mediated iron acquisition. *Proc Natl Acad Sci* **106:** 18792–18797.

Silvestre HL, Blundell TL, Abell C, Ciulli A. 2013. Integrated biophysical approach to fragment screening and validation for fragment-based lead discovery. *Proc Natl Acad Sci* **110:** 12984–12989.

Singh SB, Young K, Miesel L. 2011. Screening strategies for discovery of antibacterial natural products. *Expert Rev Anti Infect Ther* **9:** 589–613.

Singh R, Munjunatha U, Boshoff HI, Ha YH, Niyomrattanakit P, Ledwidge R, Dowd CS, Lee IY, Kim P, Zhang L, et al. 2008. PA-824 kills nonreplicating *Mycobacterium tuberculosis* by intracellular NO release. *Science* **322:** 1392–1395.

Siroy A, Mailaender C, Harder D, Koerber S, Wolschendorf F, Danilchanka O, Wang Y, Heinz C, Niederweis M. 2008. Rv1698 of *Mycobacterium tuberculosis* represents a new class of channel-forming outer membrane proteins. *J Biol Chem* **283:** 17827–17837.

Small JL, Park SW, Kana BD, Ioerger TR, Sacchettini JC, Ehrt S. 2013. Perturbation of cytochrome c maturation reveals adaptability of the respiratory chain in *Mycobacterium tuberculosis*. *MBio* **4:** e0047513.

Smith CV, Huang CC, Miczak A, Russell DG, Sacchettini JC, Höner zu Bentrup K. 2003. Biochemical and structural studies of malate synthase from *Mycobacterium tuberculosis*. *J Biol Chem* **278:** 1735–1743.

Stanley SA, Grant SS, Kawate T, Iwase N, Shimizu M, Wivagg C, Silvis M, Kazyanskaya E, Aquadro J, Golas A, et al. 2012. Identification of novel inhibitors of *M. tuberculosis* growth using whole cell based high-throughput screening. *ACS Chem Biol* **7:** 1377–1384

Stanley SA, Kawate T, Iwase N, Shimizu M, Clatworthy AE, Kazyanskaya E, Sacchettini JC, Ioerger TR, Siddiqi NA, Minami S, et al. 2013. Diarylcoumarins inhibit mycolic acid biosynthesis and kill *Mycobacterium tuberculosis* by targeting FadD32. *Proc Natl Acad Sci* **110:** 11565–11570.

Steinmetz H, Irschik H, Kunze B, Reichenbach H, Höfle G, Jansen R. 2007. Thuggacins, macrolide antibiotics active against *Mycobacterium tuberculosis*: Isolation from myxobacteria, structure elucidation, conformation analysis and biosynthesis. *Chemistry* **13:** 5822–5832.

Tahlan K, Wilson R, Kastrinsky DB, Arora K, Nair V, Fischer E, Barnes SW, Walker JR, Alland D, Barry CE III, et al. 2012. SQ109 targets MmpL3, a membrane transporter of trehalose monomycolate involved in mycolic acid donation to the cell wall core of *Mycobacterium tuberculosis*. *Antimicrob Agents Chemother* **56:** 1797–1809.

Tarcsay Á, Keserű GM. 2013. Contributions of molecular properties to drug promiscuity. *J Med Chem* **56:** 1789–1795.

Thomas ST, VanderVen BC, Sherman DR, Russell DG, Sampson NS. 2011. Pathway profiling in *Mycobacterium tuberculosis*: Elucidation of cholesterol-derived catabolite and enzymes that catalyze its metabolism. *J Biol Chem* **286:** 43668–43678.

Tian J, Bryk R, Shi S, Erdjument-Bromage H, Tempst P, Nathan C. 2005. *Mycobacterium tuberculosis* appears to lack alpha-ketoglutarate dehydrogenase and encodes pyruvate dehydrogenase in widely separated genes. *Mol Microbiol* **57:** 859–868.

Timm J, Post FA, Bekker LG, Walther GB, Wainwright HC, Manganelli R, Chan WT, Tsenova L, Gold B, Smith I, et al. 2003. Differential expression of iron-, carbon-, and oxygen-responsive mycobacterial genes in the lungs of chronically infected mice and tuberculosis patients. *Proc Natl Acad Sci* **100:** 14321–14326.

Truong NB, Pham CV, Doan HT, Nguyen HV, Nguyen CM, Nguyen HT, Zhang HJ, Fong HH, Franzblau SG, Soejarto DD, et al. 2011. Antituberculosis cycloartane triterpenoids from *Radermachera boniana*. *J Nat Prod* **74:** 1318–1322.

Tullius MV, Harmston CA, Owens CP, Chim N, Morse RP, McMath LM, Iniguez A, Kimmey JM, Sawaya MR, Whitelegge JP, et al. 2011. Discovery and characterization of a unique mycobacterial heme acquisition system. *Proc Natl Acad Sci* **108:** 5051–5056.

Van der Geize R, Yam K, Heuser T, Wilbrink MH, Hara H, Anderton MC, Sim E, Dijkhuizen L, Davies JE, Mohn WW, et al. 2007. A gene cluster encoding cholesterol catabolism in a soil actinomycete provides insight into *Mycobacterium tuberculosis* survival in macrophages. *Proc Natl Acad Sci* **104:** 1947–1952.

Venugopal A, Bryk R, Shi S, Rhee K, Rath P, Schnappinger D, Ehrt S, Nathan C. 2011. Virulence of *Mycobacterium tuberculosis* depends on lipoamide dehydrogenase, a member of three multienzyme complexes. *Cell Host Microbe* **9:** 21–31.

Via LE, Lin PL, Ray SM, Carrillo J, Allen SS, Eum SY, Taylor K, Klein E, Manjunatha U, Gonzales J, et al. 2008. Tuberculous granulomas are hypoxic in guinea pigs, rabbits, and nonhuman primates. *Infect Immun* **76:** 2333–2340.

Warman AJ, Rito TS, Fisher NE, Moss DM, Berry NG, O'Neill PM, Ward SA, Biagini GA. 2013. Antitubercular pharmacodynamics of phenothiazines. *J Antimicrob Chemother* **68:** 869–880.

Watanabe S, Zimmermann M, Goodwin MB, Sauer U, Barry CE III, Boshoff HI. 2011. Fumarate reductase activity maintains an energized membrane in anaerobic *Mycobacterium tuberculosis*. *PLoS Pathog* **7:** e1002287.

Wei JR, Krishnamoorthy V, Murphy K, Kim JH, Schnappinger D, Alber T, Sassetti CM, Rhee KY, Rubin EJ. 2011. Depletion of antibiotic targets has widely varying effects on growth. *Proc Natl Acad Sci* **108:** 4176–4181.

Weinberg ED. 1999. Iron loading and disease surveillance. *Emerg Infect Dis* **5:** 346–352.

Weinstein EA, Yano T, Li LS, Avarbock D, Avarbock A, Helm D, McColm AA, Duncan K, Lonsdale JT, Rubin H. 2005. Inhibitors of type II NADH:menaquinone oxidoreductase represent a class of antitubercular drugs. *Proc Natl Acad Sci* **102:** 4548–4553.

Wells RM, Jones CM, Xi Z, Speer A, Danilchanka O, Doornbos KS, Sun P, Wu F, Tian C, Niederweis M. 2013. Discovery of a siderophore export system essential for virulence of *Mycobacterium tuberculosis*. *PLoS Pathog* **9:** e1003120.

Woong Park S, Klotzsche M, Wilson DJ, Boshoff HI, Eoh H, Manjunatha U, Blumenthal A, Rhee K, Barry CE III, Aldrich CC, et al. 2011. Evaluating the sensitivity of *Mycobacterium tuberculosis* to biotin deprivation using regulated gene expression. *PLoS Pathog* **7:** e1002264.

Wright GD. 2014. Something old, something new: Revisiting natural products in antibiotic drug discovery. *Can J Microbiol* **60:** 147–154.

Xuequan L, Zhou R, Sharma I, Li X, Kumar G, Swaminathan S, Tonge PF, Tan DS. 2012. Stable analogues of OSB-AMP: Potent inhibitors of MenE, the *o*-succinylbenzoate-CoA synthetase from bacterial menaquinone. Biosynthesis. *Chembiochem* **13:** 129–136.

Yam KC, D'Angelo I, Kalscheuer R, Zhu H, Wang JX, Snieckus V, Ly LH, Converse PJ, Jacobs WR Jr, Strynadka N, et al. 2009. Studies of a ring-cleaving dioxygenase illuminate the role of cholesterol metabolism in the pathogenesis of *Mycobacterium tuberculosis*. *PLoS Pathog* **5:** e1000344.

Yang X, Gao J, Smith I, Dubnau E, Sampson NS. 2011. Cholesterol is not an essential source of nutrition for *Mycobacterium tuberculosis* during infection. *J Bacteriol* **193:** 1473–1476.

Yano T, Kassovska-Bratinova S, Teh JS, Winkler J, Sullivan K, Isaacs A, Schechter NM, Rubin H. 2011. Reduction of clofazimine by mycobacterial type 2 NADH:quinone oxidoreductase: A pathway for the generation of bactericidal levels of reactive oxygen species. *J Biol Chem* **286:** 10276–10287.

Yokokawa F, Wang G, Chan WL, Ang SH, Wong J, Ma I, Rao SPS, Manjunatha U, Lakshminarayana SB, Herve M, et al. 2013. Discovery of tetrahydropyrazolopyrimidine carboxamide derivatives as potent and orally active novel anti-tubercular agents. *ACS Chem Lett* **4:** 451–455.

Zhang Y, Wade MM, Scorpio A, Zhang H, Sun Z. 2003. Mode of action of pyrazinamide: Disruption of *Mycobacterium tuberculosis* membrane transport and energetics by pyrazinoic acid. *J Antimicrob Chemother* **52:** 790–795.

Zhang YJ, Ioerger TR, Huttenhower C, Long JE, Sassetti CM, Sacchettini JC, Rubin EJ. 2012. Global assessment of genomic regions required for growth in *Mycobacterium tuberculosis*. *PLoS Pathog* **8:** e1002946.

Pharmacologic Considerations in Use and Development of Antituberculosis Drugs

Geraint Davies

Institutes of Infection and Global Health and of Translational Medicine, University of Liverpool, Liverpool L69 7BE, United Kingdom

Correspondence: gdavies@liv.ac.uk

Rational development and deployment of antituberculosis drugs depend on a comprehensive understanding of the pharmacokinetics and pharmacodynamics that underlie their clinical behavior. Successful implementation of a pharmacokinetic–pharmacodynamic approach faces difficulties that, although not unique to tuberculosis as a therapeutic area, in combination pose a significant scientific challenge. In recent years, a multidisciplinary response combining new technological and analytical approaches has begun to directly address many of these issues, shedding light on some previously poorly understood aspects of drug distribution and response. These advances have important implications for optimization of existing and development of novel drug regimens, putting quantitative pharmacology at the heart of preclinical and early drug development.

Pharmacology is the key scientific discipline that underpins rational development and deployment of drugs, from the preclinical to postmarketing phases of the drug life cycle and across the dimensions of efficacy and toxicity. The pharmacological approach and attitude is generic, providing a framework within which the subject matter–specific elements of a therapeutic problem can be assembled, analyzed, and more completely understood. Implementing such an integrated approach in practice has always been challenging, however, and nowadays draws heavily on advanced quantitative approaches, such as mathematical and statistical modeling and systems biology. At the macro scale, these tools have been successfully applied to understanding real-life population variability in drug response, incorporating the insights of pharmacogenetics, and facilitating better predictions of dosing regimens and outcomes in clinical trials (Zhang et al. 2006). At the micro scale, the growing and fruitful interface between systems biology and pharmacology offers a new mode of incorporating the explosion of mechanistic information generated by postgenomic technologies into such models, capturing complicated or unexpected drug behavior that may otherwise appear perplexing (Mager et al. 2002; Vicini and van der Graaf 2013).

From a pharmacologic perspective, the therapy of tuberculosis (TB) presents numerous practical and intellectual challenges. From a pharmacokinetic (PK) standpoint the need for combination therapy with multiple agents, many of them prodrugs acting at clinically inaccessible sites on an organism with limited

Cite this article as *Cold Spring Harb Perspect Med* doi: 10.1101/cshperspect.a021170

membrane permeability and potential for efflux, generates uncertainty about therapeutic drug concentrations at the site of action, which are usually the key drivers of drug action. From a pharmacodynamic (PD) perspective, added to the difficulty of selective toxicity when dealing with both host and pathogen is the repertoire of survival responses that *Mycobacterium tuberculosis* shows under drug pressure, which may be broadly characterized as resistance or persistence. These physiological changes have been noted in vitro and in animal models to result in complex, subpopulation- and drug-specific pharmacodynamic patterns, which are not easily captured by simple models (Davies 2010). However, despite these obvious problems, the value of a rigorous pharmacologically oriented approach to TB therapy has been convincingly shown in recent years, and developments in the field give grounds for increasing confidence that a more quantitative and integrated approach incorporating pharmacological concepts will become routine in the future (Davies and Nuermberger 2008). This article reviews these ideas and their application to date in tuberculosis with the hope that they will become better embedded across the range of disciplines that will be collectively required to make real improvements in tuberculosis treatment.

GENERAL CONCEPTS

Although of intrinsic interest in addressing the basic consideration of whether a compound is sufficiently drug-like to be useful in humans, the significance of PK parameters can only really be understood in terms of the relationship of drug concentrations to pharmacodynamics. A classic statement of unified and general PK–PD principles was provided by Jusko et al. (1995) (Fig. 1). This schema captures the key elements of drug action and also allows for a more mechanistic perspective to develop from an initially more empirical approach in a way that can be applied to the preclinical and clinical contexts. Pharmacokinetics acts as the driver or "forcing function" of the PK–PD system, with the linkage to pharmacodynamics mediated by the binding affinity of the drug to the target, the properties of the target (biosignal), and the downstream consequences of target binding (transduction). The emphasis on distribution of drug to the "biophase" at the site of action and allowance for possible differences in the nature of and binding to the target are important features of this general model highly relevant to tuberculosis, although in some important cases these aspects may be as yet poorly characterized (Zhang and Mitchison 2003). In addition, the nature of the observed phenotypic

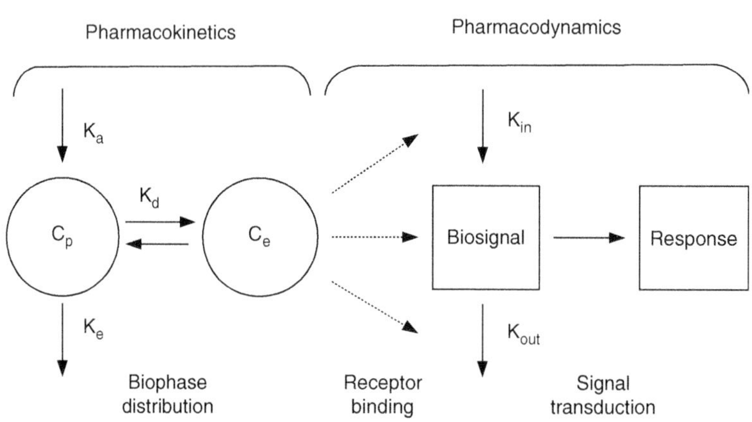

Figure 1. Components of pharmacokinetic–pharmacodynamic models. Determinants of drug action include pharmacokinetics (systemic absorption [K_a] and elimination [K_e] of drug distribution of a biophase [K_d]) and pharmacodynamics (direct binding to or inhibition or stimulation of production [K_{in}] or removal [K_{out}] of a mediator biosignal, and transduction of the response). (Modified from Jusko et al. 1995.)

 Cite this article as *Cold Spring Harb Perspect Med* doi: 10.1101/cshperspect.a021170

response, typically inhibition of cell growth or cell death, and the precise molecular pathways that lead to it following binding of the drug to its target remain highly active research areas (Kohanski et al. 2010; Kim et al. 2013).

PHARMACOKINETICS

Pharmacokinetics deals with the mechanisms and variability of absorption, distribution, metabolism, and excretion of drugs. The PK properties of first- and second-line antituberculosis drugs are very diverse, reflecting almost the whole spectrum of physicochemical and metabolic possibilities (Global Alliance for TB Drug Development 2008; Koul et al. 2011). In fact, the current TB pharmacopoeia still includes drugs that proved to be of key historical importance in our understanding of the major routes of drug metabolism and interaction. Early studies of the wide clinical variability of elimination of isoniazid led to the recognition of the *N*-acetylation pathway (Johnson 1954), whereas the serious drug interactions provoked by rifampicin helped to clarify the metabolic control of hepatic mixed function microsomal oxidases and interactions with drug transport mechanisms (Chen and Raymond 2006). This diversity of PK properties is important to consider in the construction of the combination regimens that are necessary for successful treatment of TB and in combining these with modern antiretroviral therapy in HIV-coinfected patients (Dooley et al. 2012). Some existing and new antituberculosis drugs such as rifapentine, clofazimine, bedaquiline, and delaminid have relatively undesirable PK properties such as bioavailability problems, very high protein binding and prolonged half-lives which may result in complex formulation, dosing, and coadministration issues. In extreme cases, the result may be a combination regimen composed of drugs that have poorly matched PK parameters. This situation may sometimes be of clinical importance. Rifapentine-based regimens, which rely on isoniazid as the sole companion drug in the continuation phase of treatment, are vulnerable to failure of treatment with the emergence of rifamycin monoresistance in HIV-infected individuals (Vernon et al. 1999). In addition, the risk of failure may be related to acetylator status and consequently pharmacokinetic exposure to isoniazid (Weiner et al. 2003). This phenomenon appears to support the interpretation that it is mismatching of the elimination half-lives of the two drugs resulting in periods of functional monotherapy during treatment that promotes the acquisition of resistance. However, this phenomenon has also been observed with other rifamycins with less extreme mismatching (Nettles et al. 2004; Li et al. 2005; Weiner et al. 2005), and some recent in vitro experiments appear to challenge this concept as a general mechanism (Srivastava et al. 2011), suggesting that pharmacokinetics, as measured in plasma at least, may not be the only explanation. Variability of the PK parameters of particular drugs among individuals and its clinical consequences has long been debated among TB pharmacologists. Reports of very variable plasma concentrations from PK studies or therapeutic drug monitoring programs are common in the literature, although there is currently no global overview of the extent of this variability or its determinants (Peloquin et al. 1997; McIlleron et al. 2006; Njiland et al. 2006; Requena-Méndez et al. 2012). Such individual reports should be interpreted with some caution, because numerous factors including the details of the study protocol and bioanalytical methods may affect the estimates considerably, whereas in most cases the likely clinical impact is difficult to assess directly in terms of the PK–PD relationship. Most traditional pharmacokinetic studies were not explicitly designed to assess impact on efficacy, and only a few claim to have been able to show an impact on clinical outcomes (Chideya et al. 2009; Burhan et al. 2013). One recent such study, however, used classification and regression tree methods to identify critical thresholds for treatment success for each drug contained in the first-line regimen. It appeared that the greater the number of drugs in the regimen for which plasma concentrations fell below these thresholds, the higher was the risk of treatment failure or relapse (Pasipanodya et al. 2013). The investigators suggested that this could be interpreted as supporting the concept of interindividual variability in pharmacokinetics as the primary driver of ineffective therapy and of the development of resistance. However, the study was based on a relatively small number of patients with an unusually high rate of poor outcomes. Further studies of this kind using sparser sampling strategies on larger numbers of patients would be necessary to reliably validate these interesting results. Using a different approach, the only meta-analysis of published PK data attempted to date focused on studies that reported isonaizid acetylator status, concluding that in general rapid acetylator phenotype was associated with poorer outcomes (Pasipanodya et al. 2012).

Although plasma concentrations of drugs may in principle bear some useful relationship to drug efficacy, such a link is likely to be indirect. The usual site of disease in tuberculosis is the lung parenchyma, and the pathology of the disease results in a variety of physicochemical environments ranging from normal tissue to heavy inflammatory infiltrates to areas of dense, poorly vascularized caseous necrosis into which drug penetration is believed to be poor. Given the variety of properties of TB drugs, a number of which are weakly basic and/or prodrugs, intrapulmonary distribution is thus likely to be complex. Until recently little information was available on drug concentrations in the biophase at the site of action. Small bronchoscopy studies have evaluated the ratio of concentrations of first-line drugs at around the time of peak plasma concentrations in epithelial lining fluid and alveolar cells, concluding that in general drug penetration is adequate at these sites (Conte et al. 2001, 2002, 2004). Because the vast majority of *Mycobacterium tuberculosis* (MTB) organisms are, however, located in areas of diseased lung, these findings may not be very pertinent to the critical biophase concentration. Recently, use of ^{11}C labeled drugs and PET-CT (positron emission tomography-computed tomography) imaging in a primate model of disease has enabled a clearer picture to be obtained, suggesting that pulmonary uptake of first-line drugs results in tissue concentrations generally similar to or higher than that found in plasma and three- to 10-fold higher than the typical minimum inhibitory concentrations (Liu et al. 2010). An alternative approach has made use of a rabbit model of disease and postmortem tissue PK measurements to specifically study the distribution of first-line drugs and moxifloxacin into a variety of lesions as well as macroscopically normal lung tissue (Kjellsson et al. 2012). Using a modeling approach to analyze this relatively sparse data, the investigators were able to study the expected PK exposure in tissue relative to that in plasma. Interestingly, exposure achieved in lesions was lower than in plasma for most of the drugs studied, with the exception of moxifloxacin for which it was approximately twofold higher. Label-free MALDI (matrix-assisted laser desorption/ionization) mass spectrometric imaging has also been used to study the temporospatial distribution of moxifloxacin into pulmonary lesions in the same rabbit model (Prideaux et al. 2011). These data appear to confirm that moxifloxacin may accumulate homogenously within lesions with appreciable time delay in elimination, again generating at least twofold higher exposures overall, whereas the other drugs studied either did not penetrate the lesions or were equilibrated/eliminated much more rapidly. The methods described here remain to be fully developed but offer some hope that meaningful measurements of antituberculosis drugs in the biophase can be obtained, at least in animal models, and could in principle result in more precise estimates of the true PK–PD relationship.

Developments in pharmacogenomic technologies have also been applied to the study of interindividual pharmacokinetic variability in TB. The paradigm case is isoniazid, for which extensive studies of polymorphism at the NAT-2 locus have been performed in various geographical populations. The frequency of mutant alleles is clearly a strong determinant of the distribution of isoniazid exposure in any given population, and this parameter has been directly linked to the early bactericidal activity (EBA) attributable to the drug (Donald et al. 2004). Variability in the pattern and diversity of PD response in the early days of therapy may therefore be strongly influenced by this locus. Rifampicin shows almost as much PK variability as isoniazid, but the explanation may be more complex and has been more difficult to link to pharmacodynamics. Rifampicin is a substrate and an inducer of numerous drug metabolizing enzymes and drug transporters (Williamson et al. 2013). Recently, the hepatic enzymes that may be responsible for its metabolism have been more clearly characterized with both a human hepatic carboxyesterase (CES1) (Zhu et al. 2008) and arylacetamide deacetylase (AADAC) possibly playing a significant role (Shimizu et al. 2012; Nakajima et al. 2011). Single-nucleotide polymorphisms (SNPs) are known to exist in both loci but have not yet been extensively studied in relation to rifampicin and other rifamycins. SNPs in the hepatic organic anion uptake transporter gene SLCO1B1 have also been linked to rifampicin exposure in two clinical studies (Weiner et al. 2010; Chigutsa et al. 2011). This transporter controls hepatic uptake of rifampicin and the relevant null alleles are widely distributed in African populations, perhaps providing a basis for the low exposures observed in some African PK studies. The interplay between the various possible determinants described here in the control of PK variability in rifamycins remains to be fully elucidated. Furthermore the complex and possibly bidirectional drug–drug interactions that can result mean that pharmacological considerations loom large in codevelopment of combined TB–HIV treatment strategies that include rifamycins (Dooley et al. 2012).

These problems of potentially unreliable or highly variable drug delivery have begun to be addressed by nanoformulation strategies with a focus on the inhalational route of administration. The possibility of simultaneously reducing systemic exposure and achieving higher and more sustained drug concentrations in the lungs and perhaps alveolar macrophages seems to promise reduced toxicity and greater efficacy, especially for those drugs with particularly poor physicochemical/PK properties and/or problematic toxicities such as the injectables currently required for treatment of multidrug-resistant (MDR) TB. Recent studies suggest that a dry powder porous nanoparticle-aggregate particle (PNAP) format may be well suited for this purpose and the technology has been successfully applied to capreomycin, rifampicin, and PA-824 in animal models (Garcia-Contreras et al. 2007; Sung et al. 2009a,b). A number of other promising nanoformulation approaches are also available for this purpose (Pandey et al. 2003; Zahoor et al. 2005), whereas other groups have instead used subcutaneous or intravenous liposomal or niosomal formulations to target the pulmonary compartment (Adams et al. 1999; El-Ridy et al. 2007). Alternatively, using nanodispersion or nanoparticle techniques it may be possible to obtain oral formulations of drugs previously only delivered by injection (Pandey and Khuller 2007). Although much work remains to be performed in this area, these technologies have considerable potential to overcome some of the current limitations of drug delivery in tuberculosis.

PHARMACODYNAMICS

Traditionally the study of pharmacodynamics in tuberculosis in vitro and in vivo has leaned heavily on the measurement of inhibition of growth of MTB organisms. From a practical perspective this is simpler and less time-consuming than attempting to measure definitive killing, but it raises the important issue of whether assays and clinical methods in current use faithfully represent the kind of PD activity required for long-term cure of the disease. The range of end points used in clinical trials suggests that a useful distinction should be drawn between drugs that effectively reduce bacillary load during the early phases of treatment, preventing death and the emergence of resistance, and those that appear to have their critical activity later on and that prevent treatment failure and relapse (Lienhardt and Davies 2010). This broad clinical distinction between "bactericidal activity" and "sterilizing activity" has been increasingly interpreted in terms of drug action against qualitatively different subpopulations of organisms, a hypothesis first put forward by Canetti (1962) and Mitchison (1979). Although the precise defining characteristics of these subpopulations of organisms remain an open question, most researchers now recognize that assays directed at log-phase in vitro organisms alone are likely to be an unreliable tool for drug screening and development and that assays that incorporate at least some of the conditions pertaining in the host such as hypoxia, low PH, and alternative carbon sources are essential (Franzblau et al. 2012). Another important development has been the development and adaptation to tuberculosis of in vitro systems that can simulate dynamic PK-like patterns of drug exposure rather than the static concentrations typically used. Such systems are able to assist in defining the nature of the PK–PD relationship in relation to efficacy and resistance (Gumbo et al. 2004, 2007) and have been implemented using altered growth conditions, which may relate to in vivo physiological states (Gumbo et al. 2009). Recent work has resulted in altered recommendations for susceptibility testing and dosing (Gumbo 2010; Srivastava et al. 2011). Whether and which of these assays correlate with "sterilizing activity" remain unknown, however. In the clinical context, methods to directly differentiate between the qualitatively different states of MTB observed in vitro are in their infancy, although there have been some advances in recent years. Several different methods of measuring bacillary load in clinical specimens are now in use, which may informally represent these different states enabling more precise evaluation of drug activity against them in clinical trials. In addition to colony counting on solid media, liquid culture systems are now being increasingly deployed in clinical trial laboratories (Diacon et al. 2010b), whereas molecular methods such as Xpert (Kayigire et al. 2013) and other real-time polymerase chain reaction (PCR) methods directed at various mRNA or rRNA targets (Honeyborne et al. 2011) can in principle give an estimate of bacillary load that is less dependent on the growth characteristics of those organisms. Most recently, the discovery of several resuscitation promotion factors in MTB has enabled development of a method of enhancing liquid culture, apparently also revealing organisms not quantified by routine methods (Mukamolova et al. 2009). These new technologies raise the possibility of a more sophisticated PD model than is currently in use, which could be more reliable in terms of interpretation (Fig. 2) (Davies 2010). This interplay between our increasing understanding of mycobacterial physiology and drug action in vitro and the laboratory and analytical methods used in early phase clinical trials is absolutely essential to improve our ability to differentiate those drugs that are truly sterilizing from those that simply reduce bacillary load.

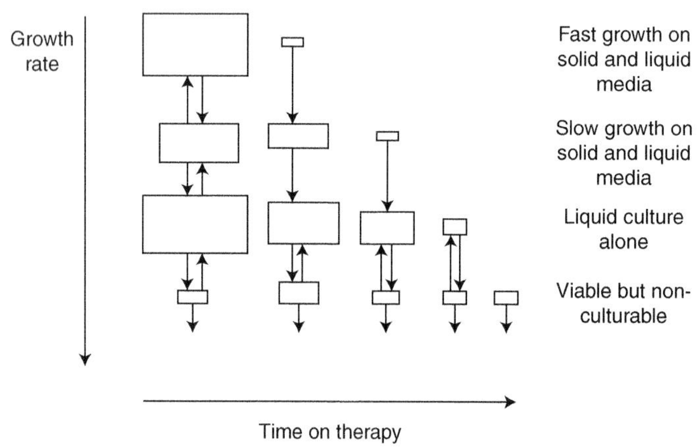

Figure 2. Simplified scheme of a transition pharmacodynamic model for tuberculosis treatment. Boxes represent the size of subpopulations with arrows representing possible transitions between them. Each subpopulation has a defined death rate, which has been omitted for clarity, with the exception of the viable but nonculturable population at the bottom of the figure. As therapy proceeds, subpopulations are sequentially eliminated according to their characteristics.

Currently all clinical drug development programs include a small, usually dose-ranging study of EBA. Although the possible problems of interpretation of such studies have been outlined above, historical EBA studies have been important because they established the possibility of PK–PD analysis in tuberculosis, where previously the development process had been much more informal and heavily dependent on animal experiments (Donald et al. 2003). The paradigm case of isoniazid was the first time that the dose–response and concentration–response relationships incorporating pharmacogenetic variability had been fully defined in humans for any tuberculosis drug (Donald et al. 1997, 2004). The idea was successfully applied to other classes of drugs including rifamycins and fluoroquinolones (Sirgel et al. 2005; Johnson et al. 2006; Diacon et al. 2007). These efforts have been of particular interest because they have shown that changes in physicochemical properties and intrinsic activity among members of each class may markedly affect the EBA. In particular, recognition that the dose–response curves for rifampicin and rifapentine remained incomplete as measured by EBA and that AUC/MIC (area under the curve/minimum inhibitory concentration) ratios achieved in humans compared unfavorably with those achieved in animals, led to new efforts to repurpose and optimize these drugs using modern PK–PD methods. The advent of completely new classes of drugs has also been instructive. The two drugs recently licensed for MDR TB, bedaquiline and delaminid, both show EBA that appears poor by comparison with isoniazid (Rustomjee et al. 2008a; Diacon et al. 2011), whereas clearly adding important activity in the context of MDR TB regimens (Diacon et al. 2009; Gler et al. 2012). More important in the case of bedaquiline, the pattern of pharmacodynamic response reflects the mechanism of action of the drug (depletion of ATP) and is time dependent, creating a mirror image of the response expected based on repeated studies of control regimens based on isoniazid (Diacon et al. 2013). Finally, dose-ranging EBA studies for PA-824 were repeated when EBA was initially observed to be low and not increasing with dose (Diacon et al. 2010a, 2012a). In fact, PA-824 monotherapy outperformed a standard multidrug control regimen, and the lack of dose–response was attributable to selection of dose ranges that animal studies suggested exceeded the maximum response. These new findings argue that although useful information can be derived from EBA studies, they must be carefully interpreted in the context of existing knowledge of the pharmacology of the drug and relevant preclinical findings.

Although the definitive measure of "sterilizing activity" remains relapse of disease after treatment is stopped, often combined with treatment failure at the end of treatment, several groups have attempted to extend the quantitative EBA approach using longer periods of sampling during the first three months when bacteriological measures are still available to provide information on response. Although culture conversion at fixed time points such as two months is currently regarded as the best available candidate surrogate end point for treatment failure/relapse, this is largely because it is supported by historical experience (Food and Drug Administration 2013). The reasonable predictive performance of two-month culture as assessed over these trials (Phillips et al. 2013; Wallis et al. 2013) is undermined by its inflexibility and relative lack of power. To fully capitalize on information from early bacteriological biomarkers, it has been necessary to adopt a more sophisticated statistical modeling approach, of a type more familiar to PK–PD scientists than clinical trialists. Using the full profile of repeated bacteriological measurements during treatment it is possible to get a fuller appreciation of the progress of treatment and perhaps more importantly the pattern of PD response. Initial empirical approaches based on colony counting data from current first-line regimens described a characteristically biphasic PD pattern with the elimination rate of sputum organisms (Davies et al. 2006; Rustomjee et al. 2008b). However, novel regimens have presented diverse patterns of response, necessitating more flexible approaches capable of capturing and yet comparing these qualitatively different profiles (Diacon et al. 2012b). More recently, simple models of elimination fitted to liquid culture data have been developed (Martineau et al. 2011; Chigutsa et al. 2013). Changes in time to positivity in MGIT (Mycobacteria Growth Indicator Tube) appear to be similar in magnitude and variability to those observed with colony counting (Diacon et al. 2010b). An appropriate model for these data appears, however, to be monophasic, perhaps related to decontamination of specimens during laboratory processing. Changes in elimination rate in such models appear capable of predicting long-term outcome in individual patients (Sloan et al. 2013). Finally, a similar approach has been used to model 16S rRNA measurements (Honeyborne et al. 2011). These modeling approaches to early phase clinical trials are gradually gaining wider acceptance and promise to revolutionize the way that early phase development of combination regimens is performed in tuberculosis (Diacon et al. 2012b). However, larger cohorts with appropriate long-term follow-up and relating to a broader range of drug regimens will be needed to establish their reliability in relation to the two-month culture conversion end point.

SYSTEMS PHARMACOLOGY

The emerging discipline of systems pharmacology aims to harness the wealth of new information made available from postgenomic technologies to understand mechanisms of drug response and toxicity in greater detail. A number of groups have developed systems models incorporating the recent explosion of molecular data from MTB, but they have so far largely been used to deepen our understanding of global cellular processes under different growth conditions (Beste and McFadden 2010; Fang et al. 2010; Galagan et al. 2013). However, such models are ideal tools to study the perturbations induced by drug pressure and the robustness of the whole organism or particular physiological pathways to their ramifications, such as postantibiotic effect and cell death (Raman et al. 2009; Fang et al. 2011). In addition, the possibility of representing critical parts of these system models as a subsystem of a multiscale PK–PD model (Goutelle et al. 2011) may be important for drug regimens with specific or unusual mechanisms of action, the results of which could be measured in vivo (e.g., bedaquiline). Incorporation of such information may be of overriding importance in correctly understanding what it is that generates empirically different patterns of PD response in vitro or in vivo and what the implications are for clinical outcome.

CONCLUDING REMARKS

Improving how antituberculosis drugs are used and developed depends on a complete understanding of their pharmacology, construed in the broadest possible sense. Although tuberculosis poses some specific challenges, advances in recent years have resulted in a fruitful multidisciplinary response that has significantly changed our understanding of the therapeutics of the disease and how best to develop new combinations of drugs. It is only by intelligently integrating and using information relating to all aspects of the PK–PD relationship that important biological and clinical phenomena can be usefully incorporated and their implications for drug development and deployment clearly understood. The pharmacological concepts and tools described here are an effective means of promoting that understanding across the diverse disciplines that will contribute to better future treatments for tuberculosis.

REFERENCES

Adams LB, Sinha I, Franzblau SG, Krahenbuhl JL, Mehta RT. 1999. Effective treatment of acute and chronic murine tuberculosis with liposome-encapsulated clofazimine. *Antimicrob Agents Chemother* **43:** 1638–1643.

Beste DJV, McFadden J. 2010. System-level strategies for studying the metabolism of *Mycobacterium tuberculosis*. *Mol Biosyst* **6:** 2363–2372.

Burhan E, Ruesen C, Ruslami R, Ginanjar A, Mangunnegoro H, Ascobat P, Donders R, van Crevel R, Aarnoutse R. 2013. Isoniazid, rifampin, and pyrazinamide plasma concentrations in relation to treatment response in Indonesian pulmonary tuberculosis patients. *Antimicrob Agents Chemother* **57:** 3614–3619.

Canetti G. 1962. The eradication of tuberculosis: Theoretical problems and practical solutions. *Tubercle* **43:** 301–321.

Chen J, Raymond K. 2006. Roles of rifampicin in drug-drug interactions: Underlying molecular mechanisms involving the nuclear pregnane X receptor. *Ann Clin Microbiol Antimicrob* **5:** 3.

Chideya S, Winston CA, Peloquin CA, Bradford WZ, Hopewell PC, Wells CD, Reingold AL, Kenyon TA, Moeti TL, Tappero JW. 2009. Isoniazid, rifampin, ethambutol, and pyrazinamide pharmacokinetics and treatment outcomes among a predominantly HIV-infected cohort of adults with tuberculosis from Botswana. *Clin Infect Dis* **48:** 1685–1694.

Chigutsa E, Visser ME, Swart EC, Denti P, Pushpakom S, Egan D, Holford NHG, Smith PJ, Maartens G, Owen A, et al. 2011. The *SLCO1B1* rs4149032 polymorphism is highly prevalent in South Africans and is associated with reduced rifampin concentrations: Dosing implications. *Antimicrob Agents Chemother* **55:** 4122–4127.

Chigutsa E, Patel K, Denti P, Visser M, Maartens G, Kirkpatrick CMJ, McIlleron H, Karlsson MO. 2013. A time-to-event pharmacodynamic model describing treatment response in patients with pulmonary tuberculosis using days to positivity in automated liquid mycobacterial culture. *Antimicrob Agents Chemother* **57:** 789–795.

Conte JE Jr, Golden JA, Kipps J, Lin ET, Zurlinden E. 2001. Effects of AIDS and gender on steady-state plasma and intrapulmonary ethambutol concentrations. *Antimicrob Agents Chemother* **45:** 2891–2896.

Conte JE, Golden JA, McQuitty M, Kipps J, Duncan S, McKenna E, Zurlinden E. 2002. Effects of gender, AIDS, acetylator status on intrapulmonary concentrations of isoniazid. *Antimicrob Agents Chemother* **46:** 2358–2364.

Conte JE, Golden JA, Kipps JE, Lin ET, Zurlinden E. 2004. Effect of sex and AIDS status on the plasma and intrapulmonary pharmacokinetics of rifampicin. *Clin Pharmacokinet* **43:** 395–404.

Davies GR. 2010. Early clinical development of anti-tuberculosis drugs: Science, statistics and sterilizing activity. *Tuberc Edinb Scotl* **90:** 171–176.

Davies GR, Nuermberger EL. 2008. Pharmacokinetics and pharmacodynamics in the development of anti-tuberculosis drugs. *Tuberculosis (Edinb)* **88:** S65–S74.

Davies GR, Brindle R, Khoo SH, Aarons LJ. 2006. Use of nonlinear mixed-effects analysis for improved precision of early pharmacodynamic measures in tuberculosis treatment. *Antimicrob Agents Chemother* **50:** 3154–3156.

Diacon AH, Patientia RF, Venter A, van Helden PD, Smith PJ, McIlleron H, Maritz JS, Donald PR. 2007. Early bactericidal activity of high-dose rifampin in patients with pulmonary tuberculosis evidenced by positive sputum smears. *Antimicrob Agents Chemother* **51:** 2994–2996.

Diacon AH, Pym A, Grobusch M, Patientia R, Rustomjee R, Page-Shipp L, Pistorius C, Krause R, Bogoshi M, Churchyard G, et al. 2009. The diarylquinoline TMC207 for multidrug-resistant tuberculosis. *N Engl J Med* **360:** 2397–2405.

Diacon AH, Dawson R, Hanekom M, Narunsky K, Maritz SJ, Venter A, Donald PR, van Niekerk C, Whitney K, Rouse DJ, et al. 2010a. Early bactericidal activity and pharmacokinetics of PA-824 in smear-positive tuberculosis patients. *Antimicrob Agents Chemother* **54:** 3402–3407.

Diacon AH, Maritz JS, Venter A, van Helden PD, Andries K, McNeeley DF, Donald PR. 2010b. Time to detection of the growth of *Mycobacterium tuberculosis* in MGIT 960 for determining the early bactericidal activity of antituberculosis agents. *Eur J Clin Microbiol Infect Dis* **29:** 1561–1565.

Diacon AH, Dawson R, Hanekom M, Narunsky K, Venter A, Hittel N, Geiter LJ, Wells CD, Paccaly AJ, Donald PR. 2011. Early bactericidal activity of delamanid (OPC-67683) in smear-positive pulmonary tuberculosis patients. *Int J Tuberc Lung Dis* **15:** 949–954.

Diacon AH, Dawson R, du Bois J, Narunsky K, Venter A, Donald PR, van Niekerk C, Erondu N, Ginsberg AM, Becker P, et al. 2012a. Phase II dose-ranging trial of the early bactericidal activity of PA-824. *Antimicrob Agents Chemother* **56:** 3027–3031.

Diacon AH, Dawson R, von Groote-Bidlingmaier F, Symons G, Venter A, Donald PR, van Niekerk C, Everitt D, Winter H, Becker P, et al. 2012b. 14-day bactericidal activity of PA-824, bedaquiline, pyrazinamide, and moxifloxacin combinations: A randomised trial. *Lancet* **380:** 986–993.

Diacon AH, Dawson R, Von Groote-Bidlingmaier F, Symons G, Venter A, Donald PR, Conradie A, Erondu N, Ginsberg AM, Egizi E, et al. 2013. Randomized dose-ranging study of the 14-day early bactericidal activity of bedaquiline (TMC207) in patients with sputum microscopy smear-positive pulmonary tuberculosis. *Antimicrob Agents Chemother* **57:** 2199–2203.

Donald P, Sirgel F, Botha F, Seifart H, Parkin D, Vandenplas M. 1997. The early bactericidal activity of isoniazid related to its dose size in pulmonary tuberculosis. *Am J Respir Crit Care Med* **156:** 895–900.

Donald P, Sirgel F, Venter A, Parkin D, Seifart H, van de Wal B, Maritz J, Fourie P. 2003. Early bactericidal activity of antituberculosis agents. *Expert Rev Anti Infect Ther* **1:** 141–155.

Donald P, Sirgel F, Venter A, Parkin D, Seifart H, van de Wal B, Werely C, van Helden P, Maritz J. 2004. The influence of human *N*-acetyltransferase genotype on the early bactericidal activity of isoniazid. *Clin Infect Dis* **39:** 1425–1430.

Dooley KE, Kim PS, Williams SD, Hafner R. 2012. TB and HIV therapeutics: Pharmacology research priorities. *AIDS Res Treat* **2012:** 1–9.

El-Ridy MS, Mostafa DM, Shehab A, Nasr EA, Abd El-Alim S. 2007. Biological evaluation of pyrazinamide liposomes for treatment of *Mycobacterium tuberculosis*. *Int J Pharm* **330:** 82–88.

Fang X, Wallqvist A, Reifman J. 2010. Development and analysis of an in vivo-compatible metabolic network of *Mycobacterium tuberculosis*. *BMC Syst Biol* **4:** 160.

Fang X, Wallqvist A, Reifman J. 2011. Modeling synergistic drug inhibition of *Mycobacterium tuberculosis* growth in murine macrophages. *Mol Biosyst* **7:** 2622–2636.

Food and Drug Administration. 2013. *Guidance for industry. Pulmonary tuberculosis: Developing drugs for treatment, Draft Guidance*. FDA, Silver Spring, MD.

Franzblau SG, DeGroote MA, Cho SH, Andries K, Nuermberger E, Orme IM, Mdluli K, Angulo-Barturen I, Dick T, Dartois V, et al. 2012. Comprehensive analysis of methods used for the evaluation of compounds against *Mycobacterium tuberculosis*. *Tuberculosis (Edinb)* **92:** 453–488.

Galagan JE, Minch K, Peterson M, Lyubetskaya A, Azizi E, Sweet L, Gomes A, Rustad T, Dolganov G, Glotova I, et al. 2013. The *Mycobacterium tuberculosis* regulatory network and hypoxia. *Nature* **499:** 178–183.

Garcia-Contreras L, Fiegel J, Telko MJ, Elbert K, Hawi A, Thomas M, VerBerkmoes J, Germishuizen WA, Fourie PB, Hickey AJ, et al. 2007. Inhaled large porous particles of capreomycin for treatment of tuberculosis in a guinea pig model. *Antimicrob Agents Chemother* **51:** 2830–2836.

Gler MT, Skripconoka V, Sanchez-Garavito E, Xiao H, Cabrera-Rivero JL, Vargas-Vasquez DE, Gao M, Awad M, Park S-K, Shim TS, et al. 2012. Delamanid for multidrug-resistant pulmonary tuberculosis. *N Engl J Med* **366:** 2151–2160.

Global Alliance for TB Drug Development. 2008. Handbook of anti-tuberculosis agents. *Tuberculosis (Edinb)* 88: 1–169.

Goutelle S, Bourguignon L, Jelliffe RW, Conte JE Jr, Maire P. 2011. Mathematical modeling of pulmonary tuberculosis therapy: Insights from a prototype model with rifampin. *J Theor Biol* **282:** 80–92.

Gumbo T. 2010. New susceptibility breakpoints for first-line antituberculosis drugs based on antimicrobial pharmacokinetic/pharmacodynamic science and population pharmacokinetic variability. *Antimicrob Agents Chemother* **54:** 1484–1491.

Gumbo T, Louie A, Deziel M, Parsons L, Salfinger M, Drusano G. 2004. Selection of a moxifloxacin dose that suppresses drug resistance in *Mycobacterium tuberculosis* by use of an in vitro pharmacodynamic infection model and mathematical modelling. *J Infect Dis* **190:** 1642–1651.

Gumbo T, Louie A, Liu W, Ambrose P, Bhavnani S, Brown D, Drusano G. 2007. Isoniazid's bactericidal activity ceases because of the emergence of resistance, not depletion of *Mycobacterium tuberculosis* in the log phase of growth. *J Infect Dis* **195:** 194–201.

Gumbo T, Dona CSWS, Meek C, Leff R. 2009. Pharmacokinetics-pharmacodynamics of pyrazinamide in a novel in vitro model of tuberculosis for sterilizing effect: A paradigm for faster assessment of new antituberculosis drugs. *Antimicrob Agents Chemother* **53:** 3197–3204.

Honeyborne I, McHugh TD, Phillips PPJ, Bannoo S, Bateson A, Carroll N, Perrin FM, Ronacher K, Wright L, van Helden PD, et al. 2011. Molecular bacterial load assay, a culture-free biomarker for rapid and accurate quantification of sputum *Mycobacterium tuberculosis* bacillary load during treatment. *J Clin Microbiol* **49:** 3905–3911.

Johnson W. 1954. Biological acetylation of isoniazid. *Nature* **174:** 744–745.

Johnson JL, Hadad DJ, Boom WH, Daley CL, Peloquin CA, Eisenach KD, Jankus DD, Debanne SM, Charlebois ED, Maciel E, et al. 2006. Early and extended early bactericidal activity of levofloxacin, gatifloxacin and moxifloxacin in pulmonary tuberculosis. *Int J Tuberc Lung Dis* **10:** 605–612.

Jusko WJ, Ko HC, Ebling WF. 1995. Convergence of direct and indirect pharmacodynamic response models. *J Pharmacokinet Biopharm* **23:** 5–8; discussion 9–10.

Kayigire XA, Friedrich SO, Venter A, Dawson R, Gillespie SH, Boeree MJ, Heinrich N, Hoelscher M, Diacon AH, Pan African Consortium for the Evaluation of Anti-tuberculosis Antibiotics. 2013. Direct comparison of Xpert MTB/RIF assay with liquid and solid mycobacterial culture for quantification of early bactericidal activity. *J Clin Microbiol* **51:** 1894–1898.

Kim J-H, O'Brien KM, Sharma R, Boshoff HIM, Rehren G, Chakraborty S, Wallach JB, Monteleone M, Wilson DJ, Aldrich CC, et al. 2013. A genetic strategy to identify targets for the development of drugs that prevent bacterial persistence. *Proc Natl Acad Sci* **110:** 19095–19100.

Kjellsson MC, Via LE, Goh A, Weiner D, Low KM, Kern S, Pillai G, Barry CE 3rd, Dartois V. 2012. Pharmacokinetic evaluation of the penetration of antituberculosis agents in rabbit pulmonary lesions. *Antimicrob Agents Chemother* **56:** 446–457.

Kohanski MA, DePristo MA, Collins JJ. 2010. Sublethal antibiotic treatment leads to multidrug resistance via radical-induced mutagenesis. *Mol Cell* **37:** 311–320.

Koul A, Arnoult E, Lounis N, Guillemont J, Andries K. 2011. The challenge of new drug discovery for tuberculosis. *Nature* **469:** 483–490.

Lienhardt C, Davies G. 2010. Methodological issues in the design of clinical trials for the treatment of multidrug-resistant tuberculosis: Challenges and opportunities. *Int J Tuberc Lung Dis* **14:** 528–537.

Li J, Munsiff S, Driver C, Sackoff J. 2005. Relapse and acquired rifampin resistance in HIV-infected patients with tuberculosis treated with rifampin- or rifbutin-based regimens in New York City, 1997–2000. *Clin Infect Dis* **41:** 83–91.

Liu L, Xu Y, Shea C, Fowler JS, Hooker JM, Tonge PJ. 2010. Radiosynthesis and bioimaging of the tuberculosis chemotherapeutics isoniazid, rifampicin and pyrazinamide in baboons. *J Med Chem* **53:** 2882–2891.

Mager D, Wyska E, Jusko W. 2002. Diversity of mechanism-based pharmacodynamic models. *Drug Metab Dispos* **31:** 510–518.

Martineau AR, Timms PM, Bothamley GH, Hanifa Y, Islam K, Claxton AP, Packe GE, Moore-Gillon JC, Darmalingam M, Davidson RN, et al. 2011. High-dose vitamin D_3 during intensive-phase antimicrobial treatment of pulmonary tuberculosis: A double-blind randomised controlled trial. *Lancet* **377:** 242–250.

McIlleron H, Wash P, Burger A, Norman J, Folb P, Smith P. 2006. Determinants of rifampicin, isoniazid, pyrazinamide and ethambutol pharmacokinetics in a cohort of tuberculosis patients. *Antimicrob Agents Chemother* **50:** 1170–1177.

Mitchison D. 1979. Basic mechanisms of chemotherapy. *Chest* **76:** 771–781.

Mukamolova GV, Turapov O, Malkin J, Woltmann G, Barer MR. 2009. Resuscitation promoting factors reveal an occult population of tubercle bacilli in sputum. *Am J Respir Crit Care Med* http://www.ncbi.nlm.nih.gov/pubmed/19875686 (Accessed November 27, 2009).

Nakajima A, Fukami T, Kobayashi Y, Watanabe A, Nakajima M, Yokoi T. 2011. Human arylacetamide deacetylase is responsible for deacetylation of rifamycins: Rifampicin, rifabutin, and rifapentine. *Biochem Pharmacol* **82:** 1747–1756.

Nettles R, Mazo D, Alwood K, Gachuchi R, Maltas G, Wendel K, Cronin W, Hooper N, Bishai W, Sterling T. 2004. Risk factors for relapse and acquired rifamycin resistance after directly observed tuberculosis treatment: A comparison by HIV serostatus and rifamycin use. *Clin Infect Dis* **38:** 731–736.

Njiland H, Ruslami R, Stalenhoef J, Nelwan E, Alisjahbana B, Nelwan R, van der Ven A, Danusantoso H, Aarnoutse R, van Crevel R. 2006. Exposure to rifampicin is strongly reduced in patients with tuberculosis and type 2 diabetes. *Clin Infect Dis* **43:** 848–854.

Pandey R, Khuller GK. 2007. Nanoparticle-based oral drug delivery system for an injectable antibiotic—Streptomycin. Evaluation in a murine tuberculosis model. *Chemotherapy* **53:** 437–441.

Pandey R, Sharma A, Zahoor A, Sharma S, Khuller GK, Prasad B. 2003. Poly (DL-lactide-co-glycolide) nanoparticle-based inhalable sustained drug delivery system for experimental tuberculosis. *J Antimicrob Chemother* **52:** 981–986.

Pasipanodya JG, Srivastava S, Gumbo T. 2012. Meta-analysis of clinical studies supports the pharmacokinetic variability hypothesis for acquired drug resistance and failure of antituberculosis therapy. *Clin Infect Dis* **55:** 169–177.

Pasipanodya JG, McIlleron H, Burger A, Wash PA, Smith P, Gumbo T. 2013. Serum drug concentrations predictive of pulmonary tuberculosis outcomes. *J Infect Dis* **208:** 1464–1473.

Peloquin CA, Jaresko GS, Yong CL, Keung AC, Bulpitt AE, Jelliffe RW. 1997. Population pharmacokinetic modeling of isoniazid, rifampin, and pyrazinamide. *Antimicrob Agents Chemother* **41:** 2670–2679.

Phillips PPJ, Fielding K, Nunn AJ. 2013. An evaluation of culture results during treatment for tuberculosis as surrogate endpoints for treatment failure and relapse. *PloS ONE* **8:** e63840.

Prideaux B, Dartois V, Staab D, Weiner DM, Goh A, Via LE, Barry CE 3rd, Stoeckli M. 2011. High-sensitivity MALDI-MRM-MS imaging of moxifloxacin distribution in tuberculosis-infected rabbit lungs and granulomatous lesions. *Anal Chem* **83:** 2112–2118.

Raman K, Vashisht R, Chandra N. 2009. Strategies for efficient disruption of metabolism in *Mycobacterium tuberculosis* from network analysis. *Mol Biosyst* **5:** 1740–1751.

Requena-Méndez A, Davies G, Ardrey A, Jave O, López-Romero SL, Ward SA, Moore DAJ. 2012. Pharmacokinetics of rifampin in Peruvian tuberculosis patients with and without comorbid diabetes or HIV. *Antimicrob Agents Chemother* **56:** 2357–2363.

Rustomjee R, Diacon AH, Allen J, Venter A, Reddy C, Patientia RF, Mthiyane TCP, De Marez T, van Heeswijk R, Kerstens R, et al. 2008a. Early bactericidal activity and pharmacokinetics of the diarylquinoline TMC207 in treatment of pulmonary tuberculosis. *Antimicrob Agents Chemother* **52:** 2831–2835.

Rustomjee R, Lienhardt C, Kanyok T, Davies GR, Levin J, Mthiyane T, Reddy C, Sturm AW, Sirgel FA, Allen J, et al. 2008b. A Phase II study of the sterilising activities of ofloxacin, gatifloxacin and moxifloxacin in pulmonary tuberculosis. *Int J Tuberc Lung Dis* **12:** 128–138.

Shimizu M, Fukami T, Kobayashi Y, Takamiya M, Aoki Y, Nakajima M, Yokoi T. 2012. A novel polymorphic allele of human arylacetamide deacetylase leads to decreased enzyme activity. *Drug Metab Dispos* **40:** 1183–1190.

Sirgel FA, Fourie PB, Donald PR, Padayatchi N, Rustomjee R, Levin J, Roscigno G, Norman J, McIlleron H, Mitchison DA. 2005. The early bactericidal activities of rifampin and rifapentine in pulmonary tuberculosis. *Am J Respir Crit Care Med* **172:** 128–135.

Sloan D, Mwandumba H, Guwende C, Chipungu G, Butterworth A, Dutton J, Heyderman R, Corbett E, Khoo S, Davies G. 2013. Intensive phase bacillary elimination predicts clinical outcome in HIV^+ and HIV^- Malawian adults with smear positive pulmonary TB. In *Conference on Retroviruses and Opportunistic Infections 2013*, Atlanta, GA. Abstract 858.

Srivastava S, Sherman C, Meek C, Leff R, Gumbo T. 2011. Pharmacokinetic mismatch does not lead to emergence of isoniazid- or rifampin-resistant *Mycobacterium tuberculosis* but to better antimicrobial effect: A new paradigm for antituberculosis drug scheduling. *Antimicrob Agents Chemother* **55:** 5085–5089.

Sung JC, Garcia-Contreras L, Verberkmoes JL, Peloquin CA, Elbert KJ, Hickey AJ, Edwards DA. 2009a. Dry powder nitroimidazopyran antibiotic PA-824 aerosol for inhalation. *Antimicrob Agents Chemother* **53:** 1338–1343.

Sung JC, Padilla DJ, Garcia-Contreras L, Verberkmoes JL, Durbin D, Peloquin CA, Elbert KJ, Hickey AJ, Edwards DA. 2009b. Formulation and pharmacokinetics of self-assembled rifampicin nanoparticle systems for pulmonary delivery. *Pharm Res* **26:** 1847–1855.

Vernon A, Burman W, Benator D, Khan A, Bozeman L. 1999. Acquired rifamycin monoresistance in patients with HIV-related tuberculosis treated with once-weekly rifapentine and isoniazid. Tuberculosis trials consortium. *Lancet* **353:** 1843–1847.

Vicini P, van der Graaf PH. 2013. Systems pharmacology for drug discovery and development: Paradigm shift or flash in the pan? *Clin Pharmacol Ther* **93:** 379–381.

Wallis RS, Wang C, Meyer D, Thomas N. 2013. Month 2 culture status and treatment duration as predictors of tuberculosis relapse risk in a meta-regression model. *PloS ONE* **8:** e71116.

Weiner M, Burman W, Vernon A, Benator D, Peloquin CA, Khan A, Weis S, King B, Shah N, Hodge T. 2003. Low isoniazid concentrations and outcome of tuberculosis treatment with once-weekly isoniazid and rifapentine. *Am J Respir Crit Care Med* **167:** 1341–1347.

Weiner M, Benator D, Burman W, Peloquin CA, Khan A, Vernon A, Jones B, Silva-Trigo C, Zhao Z, Hodge T. 2005. Association between acquired rifamycin resistance and the pharmacokinetics of rifabutin and isoniazid among patients with HIV and tuberculosis. *Clin Infect Dis* **40:** 1481–1491.

Weiner M, Peloquin C, Burman W, Luo C-C, Engle M, Prihoda TJ, Mac Kenzie WR, Bliven-Sizemore E, Johnson JL, Vernon A. 2010. Effects of tuberculosis, race, and human gene SLCO1B1 polymorphisms on rifampin concentrations. *Antimicrob Agents Chemother* **54:** 4192–4200.

Williamson B, Dooley KE, Zhang Y, Back DJ, Owen A. 2013. Induction of influx and efflux transporters and cytochrome P450 3A4 in primary human hepatocytes by rifampin, rifabutin, and rifapentine. *Antimicrob Agents Chemother* **57:** 6366–6369.

Zahoor A, Sharma S, Khuller G. 2005. Inhalable alginate nanoparticles as antitubercular drug carriers against experimental tuberculosis. *Int J Antimicrob Agents* **26:** 298–303.

Zhang Y, Mitchison D. 2003. The curious characteristics of pyrazinamide: A review. *Int J Tuberc Lung Dis* **7:** 6–21.

Zhang L, Sinha V, Forgue ST, Callies S, Ni L, Peck R, Allerheiligen SRB. 2006. Model-based drug development: The road to quantitative pharmacology. *J Pharmacokinet Pharmacodyn* **33:** 369–393.

Zhu H-J, Patrick KS, Yuan H-J, Wang J-S, Donovan JL, DeVane CL, Malcolm R, Johnson JA, Youngblood GL, Sweet DH, et al. 2008. Two *CES1* gene mutations lead to dysfunctional carboxylesterase 1 activity in man: Clinical significance and molecular basis. *Am J Hum Genet* **82:** 1241–1248.

Diversity and Evolution of *Mycobacterium tuberculosis:* Moving to Whole-Genome-Based Approaches

Stefan Niemann[1,2] and Philip Supply[3,4,5,6]

[1]Molecular Mycobacteriology, Forschungszentrum Borstel, Leibniz-Zentrum für Medizin und Biowissenschaften, 23845 Borstel, Germany

[2]German Center for Infection Research (DZIF), partner site Borstel, 23845 Borstel, Germany

[3]Institut National de la Santé et de la Recherche Medicalé (INSERM) U1019, 59019 Lille, France

[4]Centre National de la Recherche Scientifique (CNRS) UMR 8204, 59019 Lille, France

[5]Institut Pasteur de Lille, Center for Infection and Immunity of Lille, 59019 Lille, France

[6]Université Lille Nord de France, 59019 Lille, France

Correspondence: sniemann@fz-borstel.de; philip.supply@pasteur-lille.fr

Genotyping of clinical *Mycobacterium tuberculosis* complex (MTBC) strains has become a standard tool for epidemiological tracing and for the investigation of the local and global strain population structure. Of special importance is the analysis of the expansion of multidrug (MDR) and extensively drug-resistant (XDR) strains. Classical genotyping and, more recently, whole-genome sequencing have revealed that the strains of the MTBC are more diverse than previously anticipated. Globally, several phylogenetic lineages can be distinguished whose geographical distribution is markedly variable. Strains of particular (sub)-lineages, such as Beijing, seem to be more virulent and associated with enhanced resistance levels and fitness, likely fueling their spread in certain world regions. The upcoming generalization of whole-genome sequencing approaches will expectedly provide more comprehensive insights into the molecular and epidemiological mechanisms involved and lead to better diagnostic and therapeutic tools.

With an estimated 100 million new infections, 8.5 million new notified cases, and 1.5 million deaths yearly, tuberculosis (TB) is still a vivid, major public health problem globally (Dye and Williams 2010; Diel et al. 2013).

Among well-known socioepidemiological factors favoring the spread of the disease are bad living conditions (e.g., poverty, malnutrition), war, and displacement, as well as the widespread breakdown of social and TB control systems. Especially in countries of sub-Saharan Africa, the situation is aggravated by high coinfection rates with HIV (Corbett et al. 2003; Dye and Williams 2010). On the pathogen's side, drug-resistant and multidrug-resistant (MDR; resistance at least to isoniazid [INH] and rifampicin [RMP]) *Mycobacterium tuberculosis* strains have emerged worldwide and pose a serious threat for TB control (Dye and Williams 2010; Gandhi et al. 2010). High rates of resistant

Cite this article as *Cold Spring Harb Perspect Med* doi: 10.1101/cshperspect.a021188

and MDR TB have especially been reported in former Eastern USSR republics such as Azerbaijan and Uzbekistan (Dye and Williams 2010; Gandhi et al. 2010). Even more worrisome is the emergence of a barely treatable form of TB—namely, extensively drug-resistant TB (XDR TB), which is defined as MDR plus additional resistance to any fluoroquinolone and at least one of three injectable drugs (i.e., amikacin, kanamycin, or capreomycin). The detection and prevention of the spread of these most dangerous forms of TB is particularly important.

A successful control of the disease is based on several components that range from rapid and accurate diagnostics and effective therapy to the detection of recent transmission chains and outbreaks. Precise knowledge of the actual epidemiological situation is crucial for the optimization of local and global TB control measures and the early detection of changes in dynamics (e.g., the enhanced spread of MDR strains in particular regions [Niemann et al. 2010]). For example, recent studies show that, in addition to ineffective therapy, recent transmission is a key factor fostering the MDR epidemic (Pardini et al. 2009; Niemann et al. 2010).

For disclosing such transmission events, as well as longitudinal outbreaks and transmission hot spots, effective genotyping of clinical MTBC isolates at the strain level is the key. In so-called molecular epidemiological studies, genotyping is used in addition to classical epidemiological approaches, such as contact-tracing investigations, to decipher recent transmission chains and identify epidemiological links (Barnes and Cave 2003). Classical genotyping can be performed using a variety of techniques that interrogate different classes of genetic markers and generate either strain-specific banding patterns (IS*6110* DNA fingerprint), bar code–like signals (spoligotyping), or numerical patterns (24 locus-MIRU-VNTR typing) (Schurch and van Soolingen 2012). However, thanks to rapid improvements in next-generation sequencing (NGS) technologies, comparison of nearly complete genome sequences of *M. tuberculosis* strains is progressively becoming the ultimate approach of choice, providing the maximal resolution power especially needed for resolving complex outbreak situations (Roetzer et al. 2013; Walker et al. 2013a). Epidemiological inferences are made based on the logical assumption that isolates from patients from the same clonal transmission chain have identical genotyping results/identical or nearly identical genome sequences, whereas isolates from unrelated patients are nonclonal and have different genotyping results/significantly different genome sequences. At population level, strains with identical/nearly identical molecular results are grouped in clusters that are indicative for possible cases of recent transmission (reviewed in Barnes and Cave 2003; Schurch and van Soolingen 2012).

In addition, *M. tuberculosis* genotyping and, more recently, whole-genome sequencing have provided fascinating new insights into the population structure and long-term evolution of the pathogen and the relationship between the strain genetic background, the human host populations, and disease characteristics (Hirsh et al. 2004; Gagneux et al. 2006a; Wirth et al. 2008; Comas et al. 2013). A number of studies showed that although the bulk of the pathogen's population is highly clonal (Sreevatsan et al. 1997; Supply et al. 2003; Hirsh et al. 2004), several main phylogenetic lineages coexist with a marked differential geographic distribution, suggesting close coevolution with the human host (Hershberg et al. 2008; Wirth et al. 2008; Comas et al. 2013; Supply et al. 2013). Moreover, increasing evidence suggests that the underlying genetic diversity has a significant impact on the pathogenicity and immunogenicity of individual strains (reviewed in Gagneux and Small 2007). This is thus changing the classical paradigm of TB, in which host (e.g., immune status) and environmental factors (e.g., duration and intensity of exposure to infection) were contemplated as major/sole factors driving the outcome of the infection, whereas the pathogen's diversity was considered unimportant (Gagneux and Small 2007).

In the following sections, molecular epidemiology using classical genotyping and whole-genome sequencing will be considered first, as this discipline intrinsically focuses on limited genetic variation and short-term evolutionary scales, with usual time spans ranging from months to years. The second part will consider the diversity and evolution of the pathogen at larger evolutionary and global population scales.

MOLECULAR EPIDEMIOLOGY BY CLASSICAL GENOTYPING

In molecular epidemiology, research or public health questions range from the analysis of exogenous reinfection (e.g., in hospitals) to the analysis of particular outbreaks and population-based longitudinal epidemiological studies (Small et al. 1993a,b, 1994; Aznar et al. 1995; Barnes et al. 1996; Golub et al. 2001; Diel et al. 2002; Allix-Beguec et al. 2008c). Because the timescale considered is relatively short and before the advent of NGS, molecular epidemiology has focused on the analysis of changes driven by specific, highly polymorphic genetic markers.

IS*6110* DNA fingerprinting has been the standard genotyping technique for more than a decade (van Embden et al. 1993). The technique is based on the detection of the insertion element IS*6110*, which is present in variable copy numbers and positions in the genomes of clinical isolates (McAdam et al. 1990; Cave et al. 1991; Mazurek et al. 1991). Thus, IS*6110* DNA fingerprinting generates highly variable banding patterns that provide high-resolution power for distinguishing different strains (Fig. 1). The use of a common, dedicated analysis software (e.g., Bionumerics), the creation of large genotyping databases (Heersma et al. 1998), and the international agreement on standardization (van Embden et al. 1993) led to worldwide application of this approach for molecular epidemiological analysis.

However, because IS*6110* DNA fingerprinting—relying on Southern blot analysis—is labor intensive and requires large amounts of DNA

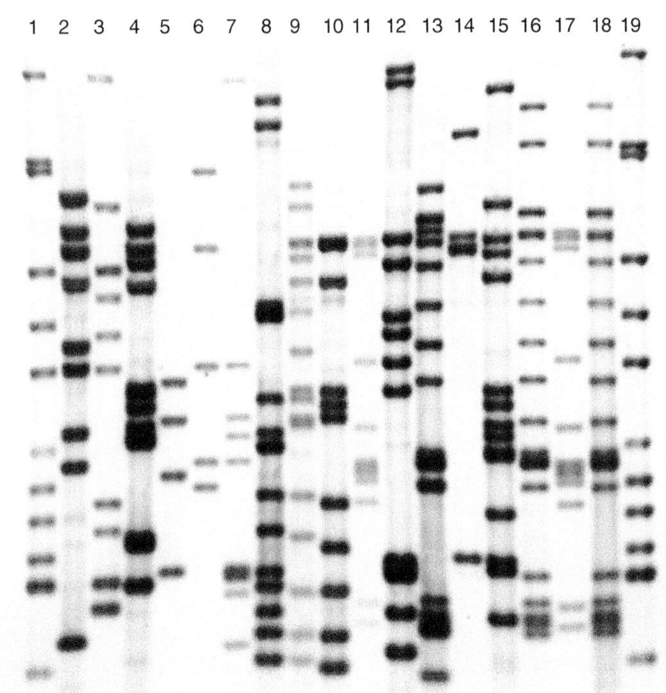

Figure 1. IS*6110* DNA fingerprints of 19 *Mycobacterium tuberculosis* complex strains. *Pvu*II-digested chromosomal DNA was separated on a 1% agarose gel, transferred via vacuum blot on a nylon membrane, and hybridized with a 245-bp internal PCR fragment of IS*6110*. Lanes *1* and *19*, reference strain Mt.14323; lanes *2–18*, diverse clinical *M. tuberculosis* complex isolates.

purified from well-grown cultures, different alternative techniques based on polymerase chain reaction (PCR) have been evaluated.

The first PCR-based method that has reached global application is spoligotyping. This technique is based on the reverse blot detection of 43 variable spacer sequences in the direct repeat (DR) region that is present in virtually all MTBC isolates (Kamerbeek et al. 1997). As the presence or absence of these spacer sequences is variable among strains, spoligotyping is generating variable bar code–like patterns that can be used for discrimination of clinical isolates (Fig. 2) (Kamerbeek et al. 1997). However, compared with IS*6110* DNA fingerprinting and 24-locus MIRU-VNTR typing (see below), spoligotyping has a clearly much lower-resolution power for discriminating MTBC isolates. Thus, in molecular epidemiological studies, it should be used in combination with another, high-resolution method (Barnes and Cave 2003; Prodinger 2007).

The second PCR-based method that has reached worldwide application is MIRU-VNTR typing, which is significantly more effective. This method is based on the analysis of variable numbers of tandem repeats (VNTR) of genetic elements including mycobacterial interspersed repetitive units (MIRUs), which are mostly intergenic. After identification and use of different markers (Supply et al. 1997; Frothingham and Meeker-O'Connell 1998; Smittipat and Palittapongarnpim 2000; Supply et al. 2000; Mazars et al. 2001; Le Fleche et al. 2002; Roring et al. 2002; Skuce et al. 2002; Warren et al. 2004), a 24-locus-based format has been internationally standardized for typing of *M. tuberculosis* (Supply et al. 2006). The sizes of the amplicons obtained from the 24 markers are determined after electrophoretic analysis on agarose gels or on multicapillary DNA sequencers, after individual or multiplexed amplification of the target loci, respectively. The use of a DNA sequencer allows for faster, semiautomated analysis (amplicon sizing and allele calling) of the generated data (Supply et al. 2006). Importantly, regardless of the version used, the final typing result is the same and consists of a portable 24-number genotype, corresponding to the number of repeat units found in each locus. This portability allowed the development of large databases and versatile web-based tools for online analysis of MIRU-VNTR and spoligotyping data, including a universal nomenclature system, such as the MIRU-VNTRPlus (Allix-Beguec et al. 2008b; Weniger et al. 2010) and the SIT-VIT databases (Demay et al. 2012).

The rate of genetic drift of MIRU-VNTR markers in *M. tuberculosis* strains in actual transmission chains and within infected patients has been carefully calibrated by analyzing hundreds of isolates from genetically diverse clusters with proven epidemiological links and sets of clonal serial isolates (Savine et al. 2002; Supply et al. 2006), as well as clonal isolates from an extended longitudinal outbreak spanning 15 years (Allix-Beguec et al. 2014). As only scarce single-locus variations were observed among

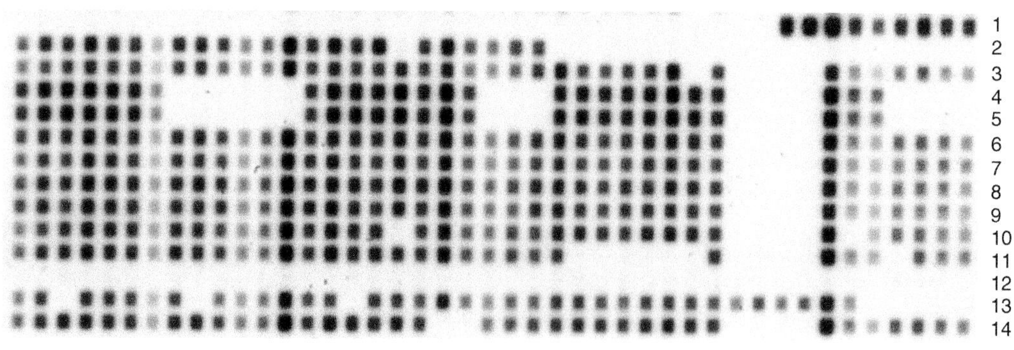

Figure 2. Spoligotyping patterns of 13 *Mycobacterium tuberculosis* complex strains. Lanes *1–11*, clinical *M. tuberculosis* complex isolates; *12*, no DNA; *13*, *Mycobacterium bovis* BCG; *14*, *M. tuberculosis* H37Rv.

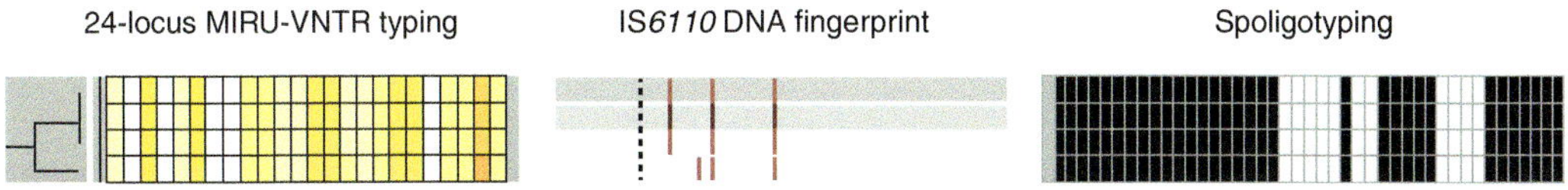

Figure 3. Analysis of four *Mycobacterium tuberculosis* complex strains with IS*6110* DNA fingerprinting, 24-locus MIRU-VNTR typing, and spoligotyping. Strains are ordered in a tree based on the similarity of their 24-locus MIRU-VNTR typing results. MIRU-VNTR alleles are color-coded. Note the concordant one-locus change by MIRU-VNTR typing and the one-band change by IS*6110* fingerprinting, and the conserved spoligotypes among the four isolates, illustrating the higher-resolution power of the two former versus the latter methods.

such clonal isolates, a cluster suggestive of clonal transmission is defined based on strict conservation of the 24 alleles among clinical isolates. Such cluster analysis based on 24 loci, optionally combined with spoligotyping, was shown to provide a close to similar predictive value as IS*6110* fingerprinting for tracing TB transmission in several Western Europe countries or settings (e.g., Oelemann et al. 2007; Allix-Beguec et al. 2008a; Bidovec-Stojkovic et al. 2011; Roetzer et al. 2011; de Beer et al. 2013) (Fig. 3).

However, 24-locus MIRU-VNTR typing lacks resolution power for accurately discriminating closely related clones, which often compose populations of Beijing strains predominating in some world regions. A consensus set of four additional, hypervariable MIRU-VNTR loci has been recently defined that, when used in complement to standard 24-locus-based MIRU-VNTR typing, substantially improves the resolution power on Beijing strain populations and still retains sufficient clonal stability to follow epidemic spread of a particular strain over time (Allix-Beguec et al. 2014).

MOLECULAR EPIDEMIOLOGY BY WHOLE-GENOME SEQUENCING

Although classical genotyping methods target highly variable genetic elements, they only interrogate a small fraction of the genome. Therefore, they can intrinsically not capture microevolution potentially occurring in other genomic regions. In contrast, NGS-based approaches give access to nearly complete genome sequences. The extended use of such approaches for research and epidemiological control has become possible through the rapid improvements and quickly increasing affordability of NGS technologies. So-called benchtop NGS systems (e.g., Illumina MiSeq) can be integrated in a routine workflow, with a throughput adapted to a normal microbiological laboratory (Koser et al. 2012a; Walker et al. 2013b). In addition, commercially available easy-to-use kits for DNA library preparation and sample multiplexing now require only low amounts of genomic DNA, which limits the time needed for culturing the slow growing mycobacteria.

Several studies showed that, in accordance with the wider spectrum of analysis to detect genetic variation, whole-genome-based approaches provide more resolution power than classical genotyping (e.g., 24-locus MIRU-VNTR typing and IS*6110* fingerprinting) (Niemann et al. 2009; Schurch et al. 2010; Roetzer et al. 2013; Walker et al. 2013a). In particular, whole-genome sequence analysis allows for a more precise distinction of isolates belonging to a specific recent transmission chain from other, closely but not directly related isolates, which is especially useful to resolve complex outbreak situations (Gardy et al. 2011; Roetzer et al. 2013; Walker et al. 2013a). In such situations, the phylogenetic trees based on the obtained genome-wide single-nucleotide polymorphism (SNP) data of the isolates correlate much better with the available epidemiological data and the spatiotemporal distribution patterns of the corresponding TB cases, compared with trees based on classical typing data (Roetzer et al. 2013; Walker et al. 2013a) (Fig. 4). In addition to a better time-dependent signal, the higher resolution offered by whole-genome-based analysis also provides other valuable information. For example, the presence of a par-

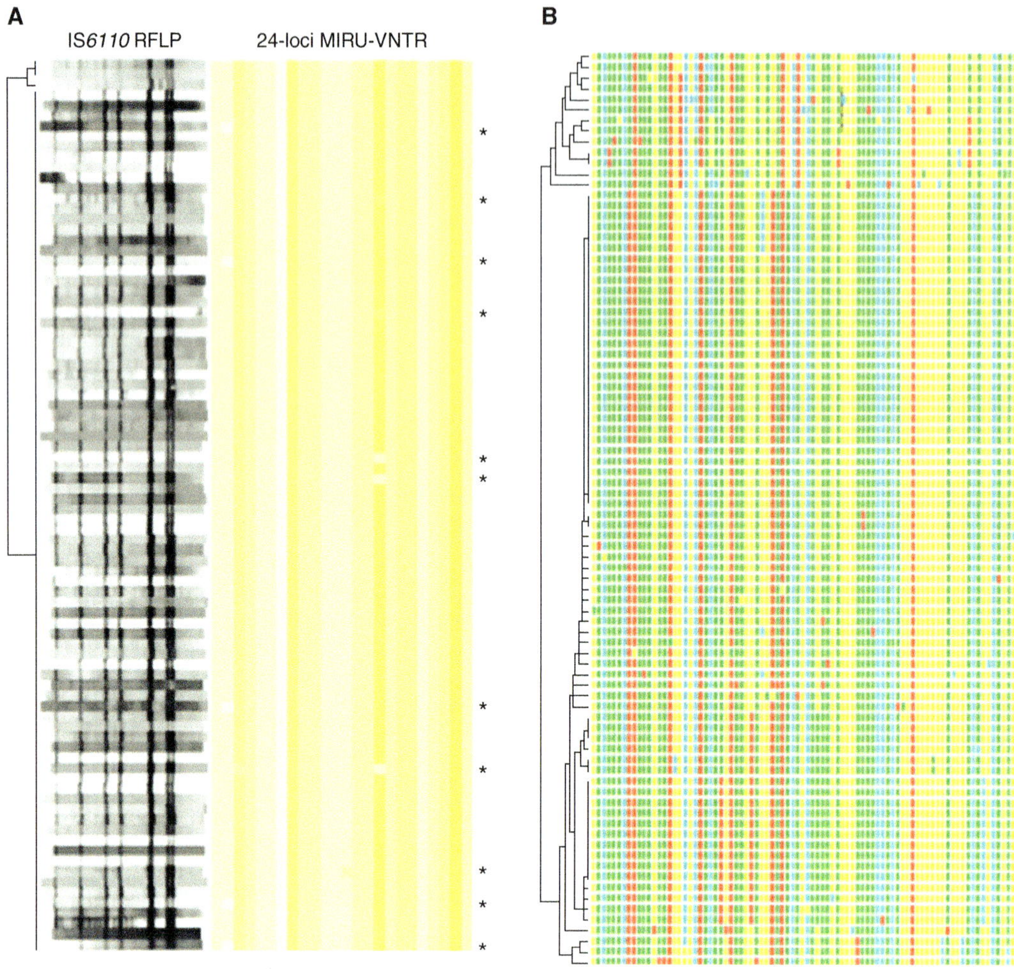

Figure 4. Discrimination of 86 outbreak strains based on IS*6110* DNA fingerprint patterns, 24-locus MIRU-VNTR typing, and 85 single-nucleotide polymorphisms (SNPs) detected by next-generation sequencing (NGS) (Roetzer et al. 2013). IS*6110* band positions were normalized to enable mutual comparison of all isolate fingerprints. The strains are ordered in UPGMA (unweighted pair group method with arithmetic mean)—a tree based on the similarity of the IS*6110* DNA fingerprint patterns (*A*) or concatenated SNP sequences (*B*). MIRU-VNTR alleles are color-coded with yellow shading, with cutoffs ranging from 0 (white) to 35 (red) repeat units. Single-locus differences in 24-locus MIRU-VNTR genotypes are indicated by asterisks. Concatenated SNP sequences are likewise color-coded. Note the largely clustered isolates by IS*6110* fingerprinting and MIRU-VNTR typing, contrasting with the resolution into smaller clusters or singletons by NGS-based SNP analysis.

ticularly contagious case (i.e., a superspreader), leading to multiple secondary cases, can be detected by the observation of star-like topologies in the phylogenetic tree, where clonal variants only differing by a few SNPs and corresponding to secondary cases branch directly from a central node, representing the same single source case. Furthermore, the identification of vacant nodes in the tree topology is predictive of undiagnosed cases in the population. The unidirectional accumulation of SNPs allows a more clear-cut association of new cases to particular previous cases in a longitudinal outbreak, thus allowing for more targeted contact tracing investigations (Roetzer et al. 2013; Walker et al. 2013a). This is of special utility for the precise determination of the source cases for patient isolates of particular importance such as MDR isolates.

To identify and delineate recent transmission chains based on whole-genome sequences, a key parameter to calibrate is the level of genome-wide variation that occurs in *M. tuberculosis* strains within and between infected individuals over time. In different studies, the observed levels of divergence between such longitudinal isolates collected from chronically infected patients or from epidemiologically linked cases virtually never exceeded three to five SNPs, which thus defines a cutoff range for predicting recent transmission (Schurch et al. 2010; Roetzer et al. 2013; Walker et al. 2013a). The calculated mean rate of change in DNA sequence was approximately 0.5 SNPs per genome per year, providing thus a quantitative estimate of the short-term evolution rate of *M. tuberculosis* in the human host population (Roetzer et al. 2013; Walker et al. 2013a). Interestingly, this rate nicely matches the mutation rate estimated for *M. tuberculosis* in a macaque infection model (Ford et al. 2011).

Compared with classical genotyping, another major advantage of whole-genome sequencing is that it simultaneously provides direct and valuable information for predicting drug resistance, as well as highly precise phylogenetic identification (Koser et al. 2013). This combination of such diagnostic and epidemiological information in a single assay is a great benefit, especially for *M. tuberculosis*, for which early detection of drug resistance is important. Analysis based on whole-genome sequencing goes far beyond conventional molecular tests, focusing on known selected mutations in hot spot regions of genes involved in resistance to first and second line antituberculous drugs. In principle, whole-genome sequencing captures most, if not all, the gene sequences determining the so-called *M. tuberculosis* resistome, which thus allows interrogation of the entire spectrum of known mutations associated with drug resistance (Koser et al. 2012b; Roetzer et al. 2013). Moreover, whole-genome sequencing at high depth enables us to detect the emergence and coexistence of different drug-resistance-conferring mutations before selection and fixation of a final mutant, in possible combination with compensatory mutations (Sun et al. 2012; Merker et al. 2013). Such detection is of clinical relevance as the coexistence of wild-type and mutant subpopulations resulting in heteroresistance might confound the current phenotypic and molecular drug-resistance tests (Sun et al. 2012; Merker et al. 2013), as well as conclusions on transmission or secondary acquisition of drug resistance.

Although NGS-based molecular tracing of *M. tuberculosis* has a clearly vast potential, its generalized use is still hampered by some remaining challenges. Despite rapid cost decreases, NGS analyses still remains too costly for many microbial/mycobacteriological laboratories. In addition, the bioinformatics analysis and interpretation of the data require adapted computer and data storage infrastructure. In contrast to classical genotyping, technical and analytical modalities (e.g., the precise delimitation of the genome sequence that is taken into account in the analysis; the minimal sequence coverage) have not yet been standardized with the consequence that data sets generated by different laboratories are not yet directly comparable. Universal databases are not yet available (e.g., for multicentric longitudinal epidemiological studies and surveillance). For optimal prediction of drug resistance, although some databasing tools are already available such as TBDReaMDB (Sandgren et al. 2009), more comprehensive and well-curated databases are needed to better and more quantitatively correlate genetic data with drug susceptibility phenotypes. These challenges are being addressed by large international consortia (e.g., http://patho-ngen-trace.eu/), to accelerate the implementation of NGS-based epidemiology and diagnostics.

GLOBAL DIVERSITY AND EVOLUTION OF *M. tuberculosis*

A substantial part of what we know today about the diversity of the MTBC initially stems from molecular epidemiological surveys, which explored the pathogen's population structure in various countries for contextual molecular epidemiological interpretations. The use of IS*6110* fingerprinting, MIRU-VNTR typing, and spoligotyping lead to the recognition of distinct families or groups of closely related strains and genotypes predominating in different world regions. One of the first and most emblematic examples is the report of strains with particular, closely related IS*6110* fingerprints prevalent in East Asian countries, and particularly in the region of Beijing, China, leading to their designation as Beijing strains (van Soolingen et al. 1995). Other groups of strains were also recognized in other geographic regions, also by other genetic markers, and were therefore assumed to represent different clonal lineages (e.g., Kremer et al. 1999; Sola et al. 2001; Supply et al. 2001). As a result, databases that compile spoligotyping (Brudey et al. 2006; Demay et al. 2012) and 24-locus MIRU-VNTR typing data collected worldwide (i.e., MIRU-VNTRPlus [Allix-Beguec et al. 2008b; Weniger et al. 2010]) currently offer maybe the best qualitative view on the global diversity of the MTBC population. As of early 2014, SITVIT counts more than 7000 different spoligotypes (http://www.pasteur-guadeloupe.fr:8081/SITVIT_ONLINE/description.jsp#), and MIRUVNTR*plus* more than 14,000 different MIRU-VNTR types (based on the 15 most discriminatory loci; http://www.miru-vntrplus.org/MIRU/types15.faces). SpolDB/SITVIT data provide a vision of the geographic distribution of the main spoligotype signatures (defined by the presence/absence of some of the 43 spacers interrogated by spoligotyping) (Filliol et al. 2003; Brudey et al. 2006; Demay et al. 2012), known to reflect to a certain degree the main clonal lineages defined by more orthodox phylogenetic markers (see below). However, although analysis of MIRU-VNTR typing data complemented by detection of spoligotype signatures is of high predictive value for classifying isolates into lineages (Cardoso Oelemann et al. 2011), spoligotyping and, to a lesser extent, MIRU-VNTR typing data both show homoplasy, which makes them not optimal for phylogenetic reconstruction (Comas et al. 2009).

Therefore, the phylogenetic structure of the MTBC described below has essentially been established by exploitation of classical phylogenetic markers (i.e., sequence-based [Sreevatsan et al. 1997; Baker et al. 2004; Gutierrez et al. 2005; Hershberg et al. 2008] and comparative genomics-based [Cole et al. 1998; Brosch et al. 2002; Fleischmann et al. 2002; Gutacker et al. 2002; Garnier et al. 2003; Hirsh et al. 2004; Filliol et al. 2006; Gagneux et al. 2006a; Gutacker et al. 2006; Comas et al. 2010, 2013a; Homolka et al. 2012; Supply et al. 2013]), including analysis of SNPs, regions of genomic differences (RDs)/large sequence polymorphisms (LSPs), and whole-genome sequences.

Compared with other bacteria, the MTBC population is genetically highly compact and essentially clonal with no significant evidence of interstrain horizontal gene transfer and/or recombination (Supply et al. 2003; Hirsh et al. 2004; Comas et al. 2013) (except for *Mycobacterium canettii*, see below). A recent whole-genome phylogeny based on 259 strains that represent the global diversity of the MTBC identified around 34.000 polymorphic sites with pairwise distances of no more than approximately 2000 SNPs separating any MTBC strain (Comas et al. 2013). This compactness, as well as the vertical inheritance of most RDs, LSPs, and SNPs (with very low levels of homoplastic variants), indicates that this whole population results from recent clonal expansion, probably from a few or a single common ancestor(s) (Sreevatsan et al. 1997; Brosch et al. 2002; Hirsh et al. 2004). Despite the relative limitation in genetic diversity of classical MTBC strains, seven main lineages of human strains (including *M. tuberculosis* sensu stricto, in lineages 1–4 and 7, as well as *M. africanum* in lineages 5 and 6), as well as one branch of animal strains, can be clearly distinguished (Fig. 5) (Hirsh et al. 2004; Gagneux et al. 2006a; Comas et al. 2013).

Consistent with the differential geographic distribution of the different genotype groups or families defined by classical genotyping markers (see above), the different human-adapted lineages are remarkably associated with the particular, sympatric human population groups that carry them. This association is apparent both at a global level, when analyzing isolates from pa-

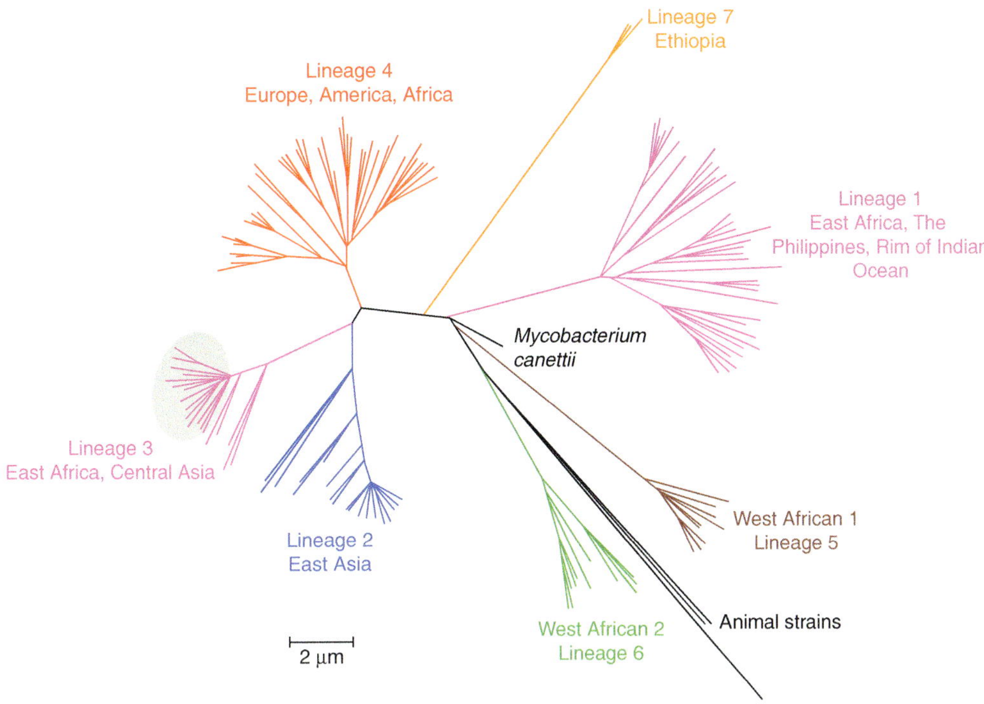

Figure 5. Whole-genome-based phylogeny of 219 isolates of all major MTBC lineages according to Comas et al. (2013). Major lineages are depicted by specific colors. (Image courtesy of Inaki Comas.)

tients living on different continents, and often at a local level as well, when analyzing isolates from residents of a particular cosmopolitan setting originating from different countries (Hirsh et al. 2004; Gagneux et al. 2006a). In the latter case, this association remains visible even when TB transmission takes place in the country of residence, outside the geographic region of origin. This could reflect the non–mutually exclusive contribution of social factors limiting contacts between different host population groups in the studied settings and biological factors including adaptation of *M. tuberculosis* lineages to different host populations (Hirsh et al. 2004; Gagneux et al. 2006a). The role of social factors is suggested (e.g., a contrario by the observation of a weaker association between lineages and host populations in situations or places favoring everyday contacts between human population groups [Varghese et al. 2013]). The hypothesis of biological adaptation is likewise supported by the observation that the association between a pathogen's lineages and host population groups appears disrupted in immunodeficient patients (Gagneux et al. 2006a; Fenner et al. 2013).

The notion of host-adapted genotypes is also suggested by the structuration of the animal strain branch that correlates with host ranges of the different corresponding strains. Although classical *Mycobacterium bovis* strains can be found in a range of mammalian species (cow, badger, wild boar, deer, lion, etc.), the strains of other variant MTBC members show a clearly restricted and specific host range, such as *Mycobacterium microti* (vole), *Mycobacterium caprae* (goat), *Mycobacterium pinnipedii* (seal), and *Mycobacterium orygis* (oryx). Therefore, and because of the conservation of >99% at the nucleotide level among the genomes of the animal and human strains (higher than the genetic threshold usually considered for defining different bacterial species), the different MTBC members (and lineages) may be regarded as a series of so-called ecotypes, occupying distinct niches, instead of different species (Smith et al. 2006, 2009).

The association and possible adaptation of pathogen lineages to particular host populations suggest parallel evolution between the pathogen and its host. For the human strain lineages, such coevolution is supported by several lines of evidence. For example, the observation that the most deeply rooted lineages (lineages 5 and 6) are found exclusively in Africa suggests an African origin for the MTBC (Comas et al. 2013). Similarities that exist between the phylogeny and the geographic distribution of the MTBC strains and that of the main human mitochondrial haplogroups suggest parallel divergence between the pathogen and its host (Comas et al. 2013). Of note, such similarities were not so clear when an MTBC phylogeny was compared with that of human Y chromosome data; however, the latter comparison did not take into account the frequencies of geographic distribution of the MTBC strains to define strain phylogeographical lineages (Pepperell et al. 2013). Also in favor of parallel evolution is the strikingly matching demographic changes, detected by analysis of both MTBC genotyping and whole-genome sequence data, suggesting expansion of the pathogen population coinciding with the human population densification/expansion at the Neolithic period or at the industrialization period two or three centuries ago (Wirth et al. 2008; Comas et al. 2013; Pepperell et al. 2013). Furthermore, recent tests of alternative models using MTBC whole-genome sequence data with initial points calibrated against several key dates in human evolution suggested a striking correlation between dating of splits of specific MTBC lineages and estimated dates of major migratory movements (i.e., lineage 1 alias Indo-Oceanic and the early dispersal around the Indian Ocean; lineage 2-4 including Eurasian lineages vs. the later dispersal throughout Eurasia). Interestingly, the long-term genome genome-wide evolution rate estimated posteriorly on this basis was much lower than the short-term mutation rate of 0.5 SNP per year and per genome based on longitudinal isolates from outbreak or chronically infected patients (Comas et al. 2013) (see above). Although it was proposed that *M. tuberculosis* was mostly under relaxed purifying selection (Hershberg et al. 2008), this difference between short-term and long-term rates might reflect the increased effect over time of fixation or removal of SNPs by natural selection (Namouchi et al. 2012; Comas et al. 2013). In accordance with this idea, the proportion of nonsynonymous versus synonymous mutations was found to be much lower in *M. canettii* than among classical MTBC members, which is compatible with an even longer time during which the evolutionary early-branching *M. canettii* was exposed to purifying selection (Supply et al. 2013).

An African origin for the MTBC is also supported by genotyping (van Soolingen et al. 1997; Fabre et al. 2004; Gutierrez et al. 2005) and whole-genome sequence data (Supply et al. 2013) indicating that *M. canettii* represents the earliest evolutionary branch of the tubercle bacilli. *M. canettii*, also named smooth tubercle bacilli (STB) and/or *Mycobacterium prototuberculosis*, regroups special TB clinical isolates, which have a distinctive smooth colony phenotype on culture media. In contrast to classical MTBC members, *M. canettii* strains are highly recombinogenic (i.e., nonclonal) and show much higher numbers of SNPs in their genomes (up to approximately 60,000 SNPs). Strikingly, most of the *M. canettii* isolates have been obtained from patients living or having lived in East Africa. Together with the earlier branching of *M. canettii*, this geographic restriction thus also points to an African origin of the MTBC. The fact that the strains from these early branching TB bacilli have all been isolated from human cases argues against the hypothesis of a zoonotic origin of the MTBC, consistently with the evolutionary scenarios based on analysis of LSPs or MIRU-VNTR markers (Brosch et al. 2002; Wirth et al. 2008). These data also suggest a coexistence between the pathogen and its human host that predated the clonal emergence of the classical members of the MTBC (Gutierrez et al. 2005; Brisse et al. 2006; Supply et al. 2013).

The hypothesis of a stable longitudinal host–pathogen coevolution that resulted in MTBC lineage-specific pathobiological characteristics (Homolka et al. 2010; Brites and Gagneux 2012) is further supported by the identification of human immunity-related gene variants that appear to protect from infection with a particular MTBC genotype (e.g., Intemann et al. 2009; Thye et al. 2011).

PATHOBIOLOGICAL IMPACT OF THE GENOMIC DIVERSITY

Although the genetic diversity of the MTBC is relatively low, one key finding is that roughly two-thirds of the SNPs found in clinical isolates are nonsynonymous and thus potentially have functional consequences (Sreevatsan et al. 1997; Hershberg et al. 2008). There is increasing evidence that this genomic diversity may influence important pathobiological properties, such as the transmissibility and virulence of the MTBC strains, as well as the immune responses and clinical pictures that they evoke (reviewed in Gagneux and Small 2007). Such an influence has been indicated by field studies looking at epidemiological or clinical correlates of transmissibility and virulence of strains from different lineages (e.g., de Jong et al. 2006, 2008; Kong et al. 2007; Caws et al. 2008; Rakotosamimanana et al. 2010) or by detecting lineage-specific differences in virulence-related features, mycobacterial transcriptomic responses, or cytokine induction patterns in animal or cellular infection models (Lopez et al. 2003; Homolka et al. 2010; Portevin et al. 2011; Reiling et al. 2013).

One of the most marked differences in pathogenicity among MTBC strains was observed for *M. canettii* isolates, which consistently are the most divergent and early branching tubercle bacilli compared with the rest of the population. In mouse infection models, *M. canettii* isolates showed lower virulence/persistence compared with *M. tuberculosis*. These findings led to the conclusion that the MTBC emerged from an ancestral *M. canettii*–like pool of mycobacteria by gain of as yet unknown persistence and virulence mechanisms, which favored its subsequent clonal radiation worldwide (Supply et al. 2013).

Specific pathobiological properties of the Beijing/East Asian lineage (alias lineage 2) are also intensively studied. Indeed, a number of reports suggest their selective spread in certain regions of the world, frequently (but not always) in association with drug resistance (e.g., Cowley et al. 2008; Niemann et al. 2010; reviewed in Glynn et al. 2002; Parwati et al. 2010). This spread has been proposed to result from several potential selective advantages. Among different possible causes, conflicting evidence based on mouse infection models and molecular epidemiological studies exists for a potential role of Bacillus Calmette–Guérin (BCG) vaccination, which has been hypothesized to be less protective against Beijing strains and thus induce an escape favoring the selective spread of these strains (Lopez et al. 2003; Tsenova et al. 2005; Jeon et al. 2008; Ordway et al. 2011). Higher virulence and, for example, an elicited immune response skewed toward a less protective Th1 response have also been indicated for some Beijing strains investigated using animal infection models (Lopez et al. 2003; Dormans et al. 2004; Manca et al. 2004; Reed et al. 2004). However, recent data suggested differences in pathogenicity and other properties such as transmissibility at Beijing sublineage level (Kato-Maeda et al. 2010; Kato-Maeda et al. 2012), thus suggesting more complex associations between strain genetic background and phenotypes than previously thought.

Still relatively little is known about the genetic polymorphisms that could explain these (sub)lineage-specific phenotypic differences. For example, the production of a phenolic glycolipid by an intact *pks15-1* gene in some Beijing strains has been shown to modulate the early host cytokine response in vitro, which may explain the induction of a suboptimal Th1 response mentioned above, but this production does not in itself confer increased virulence (Sinsimer et al. 2008). Beijing strains classified as "modern" also constitutively up-regulate the DosR regulon, involved in adaption for survival during periods of nonreplicating persistence in vitro. Such up-regulation was proposed to provide selective advantages in conditions encountered during chronic or latent phases of infection (Reed et al. 2007). A frameshift mutation has been identified in these Beijing strains, in the gene encoding the DosT sensor kinase putatively interacting with DosR in a corresponding two-component regulatory system. However, this mutation is not directly responsible for the constitutive up-regulation of the DosR regulon (Fallow et al. 2010). Along the same lines, a massive gene duplication event spanning 350 kb and including the *dosR* region was detected among some but not all sublineages of modern Beijing strains, which can thus not in itself explain the constitutive up-regulation of the DosR regulon by the modern Beijing strains (Domenech et al. 2010).

Increasing knowledge is being gained regarding the molecular mechanisms underlying the association between drug resistance and strain genetic background. There is some evidence, however strongly debated (Werngren and Hoffner 2003; Werngren 2013), for a higher mutation rate of strains of the East Asian/Beijing (sub)lineage compared with the strains, leading to increased rate of drug resistance acquisition in vitro, as well as a predicted higher probability of multidrug resistance in TB patients infected with these strains (de Steenwinkel et al. 2012; Ford et al. 2013). Although specific SNPs have been identified in Beijing strains in genes involved in DNA replication, recombination, and repair, none of these polymorphisms has yet been shown to confer increased mutability in *M. tuberculosis* (Mestre et al. 2011). Another factor that likely plays a major role is the interplay between the fitness cost associated to drug resistance mutations, acquisition of compensatory mutations, and, more generally, influence of epistasis, defined as the phenotypic interaction between mutations affecting different regions of a same protein or different gene products involved in a same or linked metabolic pathway(s) (Muller et al. 2013). For example, high-fitness-cost mutations in *katG*, the 16S rRNA, or *rpoB*, causing resistance to isoniazid, aminoglycosides, or rifampicin, respectively, have been found to be associated with compensatory mutations in the regulatory region of *ahpC* (Gagneux et al. 2006b; Hazbon et al. 2006), other regions of the 16S rRNA (Shcherbakov et al. 2010), or *rpoA* or *rpoC* (Casali et al. 2012; Comas et al. 2012). More than 30% of the MDR clinical isolates from Abkhazia/Georgia, Uzbekistan, and Kazakhstan, which are the countries with the highest incidence of MDR TB worldwide, were found to harbor mutations in *rpoA* or *rpoC* putatively compensating for *rpoB* mutations (Comas et al. 2012). Such configurations of mutations were especially found in Beijing strains that predominate in these regions, and are correlated with high molecular clustering of the corresponding isolates, thus suggesting increased transmissibility as a result of drug resistance associated to an increased fitness. Such epistatic interaction may plausibly be influenced by the genetic background of specific (sub)lineages or strains, which could offer more or less favorable arrays of preexisting mutations for compensating the cost of an emerging drug resistance mutation (Muller et al. 2013). As mentioned above, coemergence of drug resistance and compensatory mutations have also been observed by deep genome sequencing of *M. tuberculosis* populations isolated from TB patients during development of drug resistance (Sun et al. 2012; Merker et al. 2013).

CONCLUDING REMARKS

Recently accumulated data have contributed to change previous dogmas on the diversity of the pathogen and on the origin of the disease and have provided as well fascinating, new insights into the parallel evolution of *M. tuberculosis* and its human host. At the same time, these data also indicate that complex interactions probably underpin the links between the strain genetic background, drug resistance, and other features of biomedical interest. Integrative approaches coupling whole-genome sequencing to transcriptomic analysis, epidemiological analysis, and biological characterization are expected to provide the power needed to identify the determinants involved.

REFERENCES

Allix-Beguec C, Fauville-Dufaux M, Supply P. 2008a. Three-year population-based evaluation of standardized mycobacterial interspersed repetitive-unit-variable-number tandem-repeat typing of *Mycobacterium tuberculosis*. *J Clin Microbiol* **46:** 1398–1406.

Allix-Beguec C, Harmsen D, Weniger T, Supply P, Niemann S. 2008b. Evaluation and strategy for use of MIRU-VNTR*plus*, a multifunctional database for online analysis of genotyping data and phylogenetic identification of *Mycobacterium tuberculosis* complex isolates. *J Clin Microbiol* **46:** 2692–2699.

Allix-Beguec C, Supply P, Wanlin M, Bifani P, Fauville-Dufaux M. 2008c. Standardised PCR-based molecular epidemiology of tuberculosis. *Eur Respir J* **31:** 1077–1084.

Allix-Beguec C, Wahl C, Hanekom M, Nikolayevskyy V, Drobniewski F, Maeda S, Campos-Herrero I, Mokrousov I, Niemann S, Kontsevaya I, et al. 2014. Proposal of a consensus set of hypervariable mycobacterial interspersed repetitive-unit-variable-number tandem-repeat loci for subtyping of *Mycobacterium tuberculosis* Beijing isolates. *J Clin Microbiol* **52:** 164–172.

Aznar J, Safi H, Romero J, Alejo A, Gracia A, Palomares JC. 1995. Nosocomial transmission of tuberculosis infection in pediatrics wards. *Pediatr Infect Dis J* **14:** 44–48.

Baker L, Brown T, Maiden MC, Drobniewski F. 2004. Silent nucleotide polymorphisms and a phylogeny for *Mycobacterium tuberculosis*. *Emerg Infect Dis* **10:** 1568–1577.

Barnes PF, Cave MD. 2003. Molecular epidemiology of tuberculosis. *N Engl J Med* **349:** 1149–1156.

Barnes PF, el-Hajj H, Preston-Martin S, Cave MD, Jones BE, Otaya M, Pogoda J, Eisenach KD. 1996. Transmission of tuberculosis among the urban homeless. *JAMA* **275:** 305–307.

Bidovec-Stojkovic U, Zolnir-Dovc M, Supply P. 2011. One year nationwide evaluation of 24-locus MIRU-VNTR genotyping on Slovenian *Mycobacterium tuberculosis* isolates. *Respir Med* **105:** S67–S73.

Brisse S, Supply P, Brosch R, Vincent V, Gutierrez MC. 2006. 'A re-evaluation of *M. prototuberculosis*': Continuing the debate. *PLoS Pathog* **2:** e95.

Brites D, Gagneux S. 2012. Old and new selective pressures on *Mycobacterium tuberculosis*. *Infect Genet Evol* **12:** 678–685.

Brosch R, Gordon SV, Marmiesse M, Brodin P, Buchrieser C, Eiglmeier K, Garnier T, Gutierrez C, Hewinson G, Kremer K, et al. 2002. A new evolutionary scenario for the *Mycobacterium tuberculosis* complex. *Proc Natl Acad Sci* **99:** 3684–3689.

Brudey K, Driscoll JR, Rigouts L, Prodinger WM, Gori A, Al-Hajoj SA, Allix C, Aristimuno L, Arora J, Baumanis V, et al. 2006. *Mycobacterium tuberculosis* complex genetic diversity: Mining the fourth international spoligotyping database (SpolDB4) for classification, population genetics and epidemiology. *BMC Microbiol* **6:** 23.

Cardoso Oelemann M, Gomes HM, Willery E, Possuelo L, Batista Lima KV, Allix-Beguec C, Locht C, Goguet de la Salmoniere YO, Gutierrez MC, Suffys P, et al. 2011. The forest behind the tree: Phylogenetic exploration of a dominant *Mycobacterium tuberculosis* strain lineage from a high tuberculosis burden country. *PLoS ONE* **6:** e18256.

Casali N, Nikolayevskyy V, Balabanova Y, Ignatyeva O, Kontsevaya I, Harris SR, Bentley SD, Parkhill J, Nejentsev S, Hoffner SE, et al. 2012. Microevolution of extensively drug-resistant tuberculosis in Russia. *Genome Res* **22:** 735–745.

Cave MD, Eisenach KD, McDermott PF, Bates JH, Crawford JT. 1991. IS6110: Conservation of sequence in the *Mycobacterium tuberculosis* complex and its utilization in DNA fingerprinting. *Mol Cell Probes* **5:** 73–80.

Caws M, Thwaites G, Dunstan S, Hawn TR, Lan NT, Thuong NT, Stepniewska K, Huyen MN, Bang ND, Loc TH, et al. 2008. The influence of host and bacterial genotype on the development of disseminated disease with *Mycobacterium tuberculosis*. *PLoS Pathog* **4:** e1000034.

Cole ST, Brosch R, Parkhill J, Garnier T, Churcher C, Harris D, Gordon SV, Eiglmeier K, Gas S, Barry CE, 3rd, et al. 1998. Deciphering the biology of *Mycobacterium tuberculosis* from the complete genome sequence. *Nature* **393:** 537–544.

Comas I, Homolka S, Niemann S, Gagneux S. 2009. Genotyping of genetically monomorphic bacteria: DNA sequencing in *Mycobacterium tuberculosis* highlights the limitations of current methodologies. *PLoS ONE* **4:** e7815.

Comas I, Chakravartti J, Small PM, Galagan J, Niemann S, Kremer K, Ernst JD, Gagneux S. 2010. Human T cell epitopes of *Mycobacterium tuberculosis* are evolutionarily hyperconserved. *Nat Genet* **42:** 498–503.

Comas I, Borrell S, Roetzer A, Rose G, Malla B, Kato-Maeda M, Galagan J, Niemann S, Gagneux S. 2012. Whole-genome sequencing of rifampicin-resistant *Mycobacterium tuberculosis* strains identifies compensatory mutations in RNA polymerase genes. *Nat Genet* **44:** 106–110.

Comas I, Coscolla M, Luo T, Borrell S, Holt KE, Kato-Maeda M, Parkhill J, Malla B, Berg S, Thwaites G, et al. 2013. Out-of-Africa migration and Neolithic coexpansion of *Mycobacterium tuberculosis* with modern humans. *Nat Genet* **45:** 1176–1182.

Corbett EL, Watt CJ, Walker N, Maher D, Williams BG, Raviglione MC, Dye C. 2003. The growing burden of tuberculosis: Global trends and interactions with the HIV epidemic. *Arch Intern Med* **163:** 1009–1021.

Cowley D, Govender D, February B, Wolfe M, Steyn L, Evans J, Wilkinson RJ, Nicol MP. 2008. Recent and rapid emergence of W-Beijing strains of *Mycobacterium tuberculosis* in Cape Town, South Africa. *Clin Infect Dis* **47:** 1252–1259.

de Beer JL, van Ingen J, de Vries G, Erkens C, Sebek M, Mulder A, Sloot R, van den Brandt AM, Enaimi M, Kremer K, et al. 2013. Comparative study of IS*6110* restriction fragment length polymorphism and variable-number tandem-repeat typing of *Mycobacterium tuberculosis* isolates in the Netherlands, based on a 5-year nationwide survey. *J Clin Microbiol* **51:** 1193–1198.

de Jong BC, Hill PC, Brookes RH, Gagneux S, Jeffries DJ, Otu JK, Donkor SA, Fox A, McAdam KP, Small PM, et al. 2006. *Mycobacterium africanum* elicits an attenuated T cell response to early secreted antigenic target, 6 kDa, in patients with tuberculosis and their household contacts. *J Infect Dis* **193:** 1279–1286.

de Jong BC, Hill PC, Aiken A, Awine T, Antonio M, Adetifa IM, Jackson-Sillah DJ, Fox A, Deriemer K, Gagneux S, et al. 2008. Progression to active tuberculosis, but not transmission, varies by *Mycobacterium tuberculosis* lineage in The Gambia. *J Infect Dis* **198:** 1037–1043.

de Steenwinkel JE, ten Kate MT, de Knegt GJ, Kremer K, Aarnoutse RE, Boeree MJ, Verbrugh HA, van Soolingen

D, Bakker-Woudenberg IA. 2012. Drug susceptibility of *Mycobacterium tuberculosis* Beijing genotype and association with MDR TB. *Emerg Infect Dis* **18:** 660–663.

Demay C, Liens B, Burguiere T, Hill V, Couvin D, Millet J, Mokrousov I, Sola C, Zozio T, Rastogi N. 2012. SITVITWEB—A publicly available international multimarker database for studying *Mycobacterium tuberculosis* genetic diversity and molecular epidemiology. *Infect Genet Evol* **12:** 755–766.

Diel R, Schneider S, Meywald-Walter K, Ruf CM, Rusch-Gerdes S, Niemann S. 2002. Epidemiology of tuberculosis in Hamburg, Germany: Long-term population-based analysis applying classical and molecular epidemiological techniques. *J Clin Microbiol* **40:** 532–539.

Diel R, Loddenkemper R, Zellweger JP, Sotgiu G, D'Ambrosio L, Centis R, van der Werf MJ, Dara M, Detjen A, Gondrie P, et al. 2013. Old ideas to innovate tuberculosis control: Preventive treatment to achieve elimination. *Eur Respir J* **42:** 785–801.

Domenech P, Kolly GS, Leon-Solis L, Fallow A, Reed MB. 2010. Massive gene duplication event among clinical isolates of the *Mycobacterium tuberculosis* W/Beijing family. *J Bacteriol* **192:** 4562–4570.

Dormans J, Burger M, Aguilar D, Hernandez-Pando R, Kremer K, Roholl P, Arend SM, van Soolingen D. 2004. Correlation of virulence, lung pathology, bacterial load and delayed type hypersensitivity responses after infection with different *Mycobacterium tuberculosis* genotypes in a BALB/c mouse model. *Clin Exp Immunol* **137:** 460–468.

Dye C, Williams BG. 2010. The population dynamics and control of tuberculosis. *Science* **328:** 856–861.

Fabre M, Koeck JL, Le Fleche P, Simon F, Herve V, Vergnaud G, Pourcel C. 2004. High genetic diversity revealed by variable-number tandem repeat genotyping and analysis of *hsp65* gene polymorphism in a large collection of "*Mycobacterium canettii*" strains indicates that the *M. tuberculosis* complex is a recently emerged clone of "*M. canettii*". *J Clin Microbiol* **42:** 3248–3255.

Fallow A, Domenech P, Reed MB. 2010. Strains of the East Asian (W/Beijing) lineage of *Mycobacterium tuberculosis* are DosS/DosT-DosR two-component regulatory system natural mutants. *J Bacteriol* **192:** 2228–2238.

Fenner L, Egger M, Bodmer T, Furrer H, Ballif M, Battegay M, Helbling P, Fehr J, Gsponer T, Rieder HL, et al. 2013. HIV infection disrupts the sympatric host–pathogen relationship in human tuberculosis. *PLoS Genet* **9:** e1003318.

Filliol I, Driscoll JR, van Soolingen D, Kreiswirth BN, Kremer K, Valetudie G, Dang DA, Barlow R, Banerjee D, Bifani PJ, et al. 2003. Snapshot of moving and expanding clones of *Mycobacterium tuberculosis* and their global distribution assessed by spoligotyping in an international study. *J Clin Microbiol* **41:** 1963–1970.

Filliol I, Motiwala AS, Cavatore M, Qi W, Hazbon MH, Bobadilla del Valle M, Fyfe J, Garcia-Garcia L, Rastogi N, Sola C, et al. 2006. Global phylogeny of *Mycobacterium tuberculosis* based on single nucleotide polymorphism (SNP) analysis: Insights into tuberculosis evolution, phylogenetic accuracy of other DNA fingerprinting systems, and recommendations for a minimal standard SNP set. *J Bacteriol* **188:** 759–772.

Fleischmann RD, Alland D, Eisen JA, Carpenter L, White O, Peterson J, DeBoy R, Dodson R, Gwinn M, Haft D, et al. 2002. Whole-genome comparison of *Mycobacterium tuberculosis* clinical and laboratory strains. *J Bacteriol* **184:** 5479–5490.

Ford CB, Lin PL, Chase MR, Shah RR, Iartchouk O, Galagan J, Mohaideen N, Ioerger TR, Sacchettini JC, Lipsitch M, et al. 2011. Use of whole genome sequencing to estimate the mutation rate of *Mycobacterium tuberculosis* during latent infection. *Nat Genet* **43:** 482–486.

Ford CB, Shah RR, Maeda MK, Gagneux S, Murray MB, Cohen T, Johnston JC, Gardy J, Lipsitch M, Fortune SM. 2013. *Mycobacterium tuberculosis* mutation rate estimates from different lineages predict substantial differences in the emergence of drug-resistant tuberculosis. *Nat Genet* **45:** 784–790.

Frothingham R, Meeker-O'Connell WA. 1998. Genetic diversity in the *Mycobacterium tuberculosis* complex based on variable numbers of tandem DNA repeats. *Microbiology* **144:** 1189–1196.

Gagneux S, Small PM. 2007. Global phylogeography of *Mycobacterium tuberculosis* and implications for tuberculosis product development. *Lancet Infect Dis* **7:** 328–337.

Gagneux S, DeRiemer K, Van T, Kato-Maeda M, de Jong BC, Narayanan S, Nicol M, Niemann S, Kremer K, Gutierrez MC, et al. 2006a. Variable host–pathogen compatibility in *Mycobacterium tuberculosis*. *Proc Natl Acad Sci* **103:** 2869–2873.

Gagneux S, Long CD, Small PM, Van T, Schoolnik GK, Bohannan BJ. 2006b. The competitive cost of antibiotic resistance in *Mycobacterium tuberculosis*. *Science* **312:** 1944–1946.

Gandhi NR, Nunn P, Dheda K, Schaaf HS, Zignol M, van Soolingen D, Jensen P, Bayona J. 2010. Multidrug-resistant and extensively drug-resistant tuberculosis: A threat to global control of tuberculosis. *Lancet* **375:** 1830–1843.

Gardy JL, Johnston JC, Ho Sui SJ, Cook VJ, Shah L, Brodkin E, Rempel S, Moore R, Zhao Y, Holt R, et al. 2011. Whole-genome sequencing and social-network analysis of a tuberculosis outbreak. *N Engl J Med* **364:** 730–739.

Garnier T, Eiglmeier K, Camus JC, Medina N, Mansoor H, Pryor M, Duthoy S, Grondin S, Lacroix C, Monsempe C, et al. 2003. The complete genome sequence of *Mycobacterium bovis*. *Proc Natl Acad Sci* **100:** 7877–7882.

Glynn JR, Whiteley J, Bifani PJ, Kremer K, van Soolingen D. 2002. Worldwide occurrence of Beijing/W strains of *Mycobacterium tuberculosis*: A systematic review. *Emerg Infect Dis* **8:** 843–849.

Golub JE, Cronin WA, Obasanjo OO, Coggin W, Moore K, Pope DS, Thompson D, Sterling TR, Harrington S, Bishai WR, et al. 2001. Transmission of *Mycobacterium tuberculosis* through casual contact with an infectious case. *Arch Intern Med* **161:** 2254–2258.

Gutacker MM, Smoot JC, Migliaccio CA, Ricklefs SM, Hua S, Cousins DV, Graviss EA, Shashkina E, Kreiswirth BN, Musser JM. 2002. Genome-wide analysis of synonymous single nucleotide polymorphisms in *Mycobacterium tuberculosis* complex organisms: Resolution of genetic relationships among closely related microbial strains. *Genetics* **162:** 1533–1543.

Gutacker MM, Mathema B, Soini H, Shashkina E, Kreiswirth BN, Graviss EA, Musser JM. 2006. Single-nucleotide polymorphism–based population genetic analysis of *Mycobacterium tuberculosis* strains from 4 geographic sites. *J Infect Dis* **193:** 121–128.

Gutierrez MC, Brisse S, Brosch R, Fabre M, Omais B, Marmiesse M, Supply P, Vincent V. 2005. Ancient origin and gene mosaicism of the progenitor of *Mycobacterium tuberculosis*. *PLoS Pathog* **1:** e5.

Hazbon MH, Brimacombe M, Bobadilla del Valle M, Cavatore M, Guerrero MI, Varma-Basil M, Billman-Jacobe H, Lavender C, Fyfe J, Garcia-Garcia L, et al. 2006. Population genetics study of isoniazid resistance mutations and evolution of multidrug-resistant *Mycobacterium tuberculosis*. *Antimicrob Agents Chemother* **50:** 2640–2649.

Heersma HF, Kremer K, van Embden JD. 1998. Computer analysis of IS*6110* RFLP patterns of *Mycobacterium tuberculosis*. *Methods Mol Biol* **101:** 395–422.

Hershberg R, Lipatov M, Small PM, Sheffer H, Niemann S, Homolka S, Roach JC, Kremer K, Petrov DA, Feldman MW, et al. 2008. High functional diversity in *Mycobacterium tuberculosis* driven by genetic drift and human demography. *PLoS Biol* **6:** e311.

Hirsh AE, Tsolaki AG, DeRiemer K, Feldman MW, Small PM. 2004. Stable association between strains of *Mycobacterium tuberculosis* and their human host populations. *Proc Natl Acad Sci* **101:** 4871–4876.

Homolka S, Niemann S, Russell DG, Rohde KH. 2010. Functional genetic diversity among *Mycobacterium tuberculosis* complex clinical isolates: Delineation of conserved core and lineage-specific transcriptomes during intracellular survival. *PLoS Pathog* **6:** e1000988.

Homolka S, Projahn M, Feuerriegel S, Ubben T, Diel R, Nubel U, Niemann S. 2012. High resolution discrimination of clinical *Mycobacterium tuberculosis* complex strains based on single nucleotide polymorphisms. *PLoS ONE* **7:** e39855.

Intemann CD, Thye T, Niemann S, Browne EN, Amanua Chinbuah M, Enimil A, Gyapong J, Osei I, Owusu-Dabo E, Helm S, et al. 2009. Autophagy gene variant IRGM -261T contributes to protection from tuberculosis caused by *Mycobacterium tuberculosis* but not by *M. africanum* strains. *PLoS Pathog* **5:** e1000577.

Jeon BY, Derrick SC, Lim J, Kolibab K, Dheenadhayalan V, Yang AL, Kreiswirth B, Morris SL. 2008. *Mycobacterium bovis* BCG immunization induces protective immunity against nine different *Mycobacterium tuberculosis* strains in mice. *Infect Immun* **76:** 5173–5180.

Kamerbeek J, Schouls L, Kolk A, van Agterveld M, van Soolingen D, Kuijper S, Bunschoten A, Molhuizen H, Shaw R, Goyal M, et al. 1997. Simultaneous detection and strain differentiation of *Mycobacterium tuberculosis* for diagnosis and epidemiology. *J Clin Microbiol* **35:** 907–914.

Kato-Maeda M, Kim EY, Flores L, Jarlsberg LG, Osmond D, Hopewell PC. 2010. Differences among sublineages of the East-Asian lineage of *Mycobacterium tuberculosis* in genotypic clustering. *Int J Tuberc Lung Dis* **14:** 538–544.

Kato-Maeda M, Shanley CA, Ackart D, Jarlsberg LG, Shang S, Obregon-Henao A, Harton M, Basaraba RJ, Henao-Tamayo M, Barrozo JC, et al. 2012. Beijing sublineages of *Mycobacterium tuberculosis* differ in pathogenicity in the guinea pig. *Clin Vaccine Immunol* **19:** 1227–1237.

Kong Y, Cave MD, Zhang L, Foxman B, Marrs CF, Bates JH, Yang ZH. 2007. Association between *Mycobacterium tuberculosis* Beijing/W lineage strain infection and extrathoracic tuberculosis: Insights from epidemiologic and clinical characterization of the three principal genetic groups of *M. tuberculosis* clinical isolates. *J Clin Microbiol* **45:** 409–414.

Koser CU, Ellington MJ, Cartwright EJ, Gillespie SH, Brown NM, Farrington M, Holden MT, Dougan G, Bentley SD, Parkhill J, et al. 2012a. Routine use of microbial whole genome sequencing in diagnostic and public health microbiology. *PLoS Pathog* **8:** e1002824.

Koser CU, Feuerriegel S, Summers DK, Archer JA, Niemann S. 2012b. Importance of the genetic diversity within the *Mycobacterium tuberculosis* complex for the development of novel antibiotics and diagnostic tests of drug resistance. *Antimicrob Agents Chemother* **56:** 6080–6087.

Koser CU, Bryant JM, Becq J, Torok ME, Ellington MJ, Marti-Renom MA, Carmichael AJ, Parkhill J, Smith GP, Peacock SJ. 2013. Whole-genome sequencing for rapid susceptibility testing of *M. tuberculosis*. *N Engl J Med* **369:** 290–292.

Kremer K, van Soolingen D, Frothingham R, Haas WH, Hermans PW, Martin C, Palittapongarnpim P, Plikaytis BB, Riley LW, Yakrus MA, et al. 1999. Comparison of methods based on different molecular epidemiological markers for typing of *Mycobacterium tuberculosis* complex strains: Interlaboratory study of discriminatory power and reproducibility. *J Clin Microbiol* **37:** 2607–2618.

Le Fleche P, Fabre M, Denoeud F, Koeck JL, Vergnaud G. 2002. High resolution, on-line identification of strains from the *Mycobacterium tuberculosis* complex based on tandem repeat typing. *BMC Microbiol* **2:** 37.

Lopez B, Aguilar D, Orozco H, Burger M, Espitia C, Ritacco V, Barrera L, Kremer K, Hernandez-Pando R, Huygen K, et al. 2003. A marked difference in pathogenesis and immune response induced by different *Mycobacterium tuberculosis* genotypes. *Clin Exp Immunol* **133:** 30–37.

Manca C, Reed MB, Freeman S, Mathema B, Kreiswirth B, Barry CE 3rd, Kaplan G. 2004. Differential monocyte activation underlies strain-specific *Mycobacterium tuberculosis* pathogenesis. *Infect Immun* **72:** 5511–5514.

Mazars E, Lesjean S, Banuls AL, Gilbert M, Vincent V, Gicquel B, Tibayrenc M, Locht C, Supply P. 2001. High-resolution minisatellite-based typing as a portable approach to global analysis of *Mycobacterium tuberculosis* molecular epidemiology. *Proc Natl Acad Sci* **98:** 1901–1906.

Mazurek GH, Cave MD, Eisenach KD, Wallace RJ Jr, Bates JH, Crawford JT. 1991. Chromosomal DNA fingerprint patterns produced with IS*6110* as strain-specific markers for epidemiologic study of tuberculosis. *J Clin Microbiol* **29:** 2030–2033.

McAdam RA, Hermans PW, van Soolingen D, Zainuddin ZF, Catty D, van Embden JD, Dale JW. 1990. Characterization of a *Mycobacterium tuberculosis* insertion sequence belonging to the IS3 family. *Mol Microbiol* **4:** 1607–1613.

Merker M, Kohl TA, Roetzer A, Truebe L, Richter E, Rusch-Gerdes S, Fattorini L, Oggioni MR, Cox H, Varaine F, et al. 2013. Whole genome sequencing reveals complex evolution patterns of multidrug-resistant *Mycobacterium tuberculosis* Beijing strains in patients. *PLoS ONE* **8:** e82551.

Mestre O, Luo T, Dos Vultos T, Kremer K, Murray A, Namouchi A, Jackson C, Rauzier J, Bifani P, Warren R, et al. 2011. Phylogeny of *Mycobacterium tuberculosis* Beijing strains constructed from polymorphisms in genes involved in DNA replication, recombination and repair. *PLoS ONE* **6:** e16020.

Muller B, Borrell S, Rose G, Gagneux S. 2013. The heterogeneous evolution of multidrug-resistant *Mycobacterium tuberculosis*. *Trends Genet* **29:** 160–169.

Namouchi A, Didelot X, Schock U, Gicquel B, Rocha EP. 2012. After the bottleneck: Genome-wide diversification of the *Mycobacterium tuberculosis* complex by mutation, recombination, and natural selection. *Genome Res* **22:** 721–734.

Niemann S, Koser CU, Gagneux S, Plinke C, Homolka S, Bignell H, Carter RJ, Cheetham RK, Cox A, Gormley NA, et al. 2009. Genomic diversity among drug sensitive and multidrug resistant isolates of *Mycobacterium tuberculosis* with identical DNA fingerprints. *PLoS ONE* **4:** e7407.

Niemann S, Diel R, Khechinashvili G, Gegia M, Mdivani N, Tang YW. 2010. *Mycobacterium tuberculosis* Beijing lineage favors the spread of multidrug-resistant tuberculosis in the Republic of Georgia. *J Clin Microbiol* **48:** 3544–3550.

Oelemann MC, Diel R, Vatin V, Haas W, Rusch-Gerdes S, Locht C, Niemann S, Supply P. 2007. Assessment of an optimized mycobacterial interspersed repetitive-unit-variable-number tandem-repeat typing system combined with spoligotyping for population-based molecular epidemiology studies of tuberculosis. *J Clin Microbiol* **45:** 691–697.

Ordway DJ, Shang S, Henao-Tamayo M, Obregon-Henao A, Nold L, Caraway M, Shanley CA, Basaraba RJ, Duncan CG, Orme IM. 2011. *Mycobacterium bovis* BCG-mediated protection against W-Beijing strains of *Mycobacterium tuberculosis* is diminished concomitant with the emergence of regulatory T cells. *Clin Vaccine Immunol* **18:** 1527–1535.

Pardini M, Niemann S, Varaine F, Iona E, Meacci F, Orru G, Yesilkaya H, Jarosz T, Andrew P, Barer M, et al. 2009. Characteristics of drug-resistant tuberculosis in Abkhazia (Georgia), a high-prevalence area in Eastern Europe. *Tuberculosis (Edinb)* **89:** 317–324.

Parwati I, van Crevel R, van Soolingen D. 2010. Possible underlying mechanisms for successful emergence of the *Mycobacterium tuberculosis* Beijing genotype strains. *Lancet Infect Dis* **10:** 103–111.

Pepperell CS, Casto AM, Kitchen A, Granka JM, Cornejo OE, Holmes EC, Birren B, Galagan J, Feldman MW. 2013. The role of selection in shaping diversity of natural *M. tuberculosis* populations. *PLoS Pathog* **9:** e1003543.

Portevin D, Gagneux S, Comas I, Young D. 2011. Human macrophage responses to clinical isolates from the *Mycobacterium tuberculosis* complex discriminate between ancient and modern lineages. *PLoS Pathog* **7:** e1001307.

Prodinger WM. 2007. Molecular epidemiology of tuberculosis: Toy or tool? A review of the literature and examples from Central Europe. *Wien Klin Wochenschr* **119:** 80–89.

Rakotosamimanana N, Raharimanga V, Andriamandimby SF, Soares JL, Doherty TM, Ratsitorahina M, Ramarokoto H, Zumla A, Huggett J, Rook G, et al. 2010. Variation in gamma interferon responses to different infecting strains of *Mycobacterium tuberculosis* in acid-fast bacillus smear-positive patients and household contacts in Antananarivo, Madagascar. *Clin Vaccine Immunol* **17:** 1094–1103.

Reed MB, Domenech P, Manca C, Su H, Barczak AK, Kreiswirth BN, Kaplan G, Barry CE, 3rd. 2004. A glycolipid of hypervirulent tuberculosis strains that inhibits the innate immune response. *Nature* **431:** 84–87.

Reed MB, Gagneux S, Deriemer K, Small PM, Barry CE, 3rd. 2007. The W-Beijing lineage of *Mycobacterium tuberculosis* overproduces triglycerides and has the DosR dormancy regulon constitutively upregulated. *J Bacteriol* **189:** 2583–2589.

Reiling N, Homolka S, Walter K, Brandenburg J, Niwinski L, Ernst M, Herzmann C, Lange C, Diel R, Ehlers S, et al. 2013. Clade-specific virulence patterns of *Mycobacterium tuberculosis* complex strains in human primary macrophages and aerogenically infected mice. *mBio* **30:** e00250-13.

Roetzer A, Schuback S, Diel R, Gasau F, Ubben T, di Nauta A, Richter E, Rusch-Gerdes S, Niemann S. 2011. Evaluation of *Mycobacterium tuberculosis* typing methods in a 4-year study in Schleswig-Holstein, Northern Germany. *J Clin Microbiol* **49:** 4173–4178.

Roetzer A, Diel R, Kohl TA, Ruckert C, Nubel U, Blom J, Wirth T, Jaenicke S, Schuback S, Rusch-Gerdes S, et al. 2013. Whole genome sequencing versus traditional genotyping for investigation of a *Mycobacterium tuberculosis* outbreak: A longitudinal molecular epidemiological study. *PLoS Med* **10:** e1001387.

Roring S, Scott A, Brittain D, Walker I, Hewinson G, Neill S, Skuce R. 2002. Development of variable-number tandem repeat typing of *Mycobacterium bovis*: Comparison of results with those obtained by using existing exact tandem repeats and spoligotyping. *J Clin Microbiol* **40:** 2126–2133.

Sandgren A, Strong M, Muthukrishnan P, Weiner BK, Church GM, Murray MB. 2009. Tuberculosis drug resistance mutation database. *PLoS Med* **6:** e2.

Savine E, Warren RM, van der Spuy GD, Beyers N, van Helden PD, Locht C, Supply P. 2002. Stability of variable-number tandem repeats of mycobacterial interspersed repetitive units from 12 loci in serial isolates of *Mycobacterium tuberculosis*. *J Clin Microbiol* **40:** 4561–4566.

Schurch AC, van Soolingen D. 2012. DNA fingerprinting of *Mycobacterium tuberculosis*: From phage typing to whole-genome sequencing. *Infect Genet Evol* **12:** 602–609.

Schurch AC, Kremer K, Kiers A, Daviena O, Boeree MJ, Siezen RJ, Smith NH, van Soolingen D. 2010. The tempo and mode of molecular evolution of *Mycobacterium tuberculosis* at patient-to-patient scale. *Infect Genet Evol* **10:** 108–114.

Shcherbakov D, Akbergenov R, Matt T, Sander P, Andersson DI, Bottger EC. 2010. Directed mutagenesis of *Mycobacterium smegmatis* 16S rRNA to reconstruct the in-vivo evolution of aminoglycoside resistance in *Mycobacterium tuberculosis*. *Mol Microbiol* **77:** 830–840.

Sinsimer D, Huet G, Manca C, Tsenova L, Koo MS, Kurepina N, Kana B, Mathema B, Marras SA, Kreiswirth BN, et al. 2008. The phenolic glycolipid of *Mycobacterium tubercu-*

losis differentially modulates the early host cytokine response but does not in itself confer hypervirulence. *Infect Immun* **76:** 3027–3036.

Skuce RA, McCorry TP, McCarroll JF, Roring SM, Scott AN, Brittain D, Hughes SL, Hewinson RG, Neill SD. 2002. Discrimination of *Mycobacterium tuberculosis* complex bacteria using novel VNTR-PCR targets. *Microbiology* **148:** 519–528.

Small PM, McClenny NB, Singh SP, Schoolnik GK, Tompkins LS, Mickelsen PA. 1993a. Molecular strain typing of *Mycobacterium tuberculosis* to confirm cross-contamination in the mycobacteriology laboratory and modification of procedures to minimize occurrence of false-positive cultures. *J Clin Microbiol* **31:** 1677–1682.

Small PM, Shafer RW, Hopewell PC, Singh SP, Murphy MJ, Desmond E, Sierra MF, Schoolnik GK. 1993b. Exogenous reinfection with multidrug-resistant *Mycobacterium tuberculosis* in patients with advanced HIV infection. *N Engl J Med* **328:** 1137–1144.

Small PM, Hopewell PC, Singh SP, Paz A, Parsonnet J, Ruston DC, Schecter GF, Daley CL, Schoolnik GK. 1994. The epidemiology of tuberculosis in San Francisco. A population-based study using conventional and molecular methods. *N Engl J Med* **330:** 1703–1709.

Smith NH, Gordon SV, de la Rua-Domenech R, Clifton-Hadley RS, Hewinson RG. 2006. Bottlenecks and broomsticks: The molecular evolution of *Mycobacterium bovis*. *Nat Rev Microbiol* **4:** 670–681.

Smith NH, Hewinson RG, Kremer K, Brosch R, Gordon SV. 2009. Myths and misconceptions: The origin and evolution of *Mycobacterium tuberculosis*. *Nat Rev Microbiol* **7:** 537–544.

Smittipat N, Palittapongarnpim P. 2000. Identification of possible loci of variable number of tandem repeats in *Mycobacterium tuberculosis*. *Tuber Lung Dis* **80:** 69–74.

Sola C, Filliol I, Legrand E, Mokrousov I, Rastogi N. 2001. *Mycobacterium tuberculosis* phylogeny reconstruction based on combined numerical analysis with IS*1081*, IS*6110*, VNTR, and DR-based spoligotyping suggests the existence of two new phylogeographical clades. *J Mol Evol* **53:** 680–689.

Sreevatsan S, Pan X, Stockbauer KE, Connell ND, Kreiswirth BN, Whittam TS, Musser JM. 1997. Restricted structural gene polymorphism in the *Mycobacterium tuberculosis* complex indicates evolutionarily recent global dissemination. *Proc Natl Acad Sci* **94:** 9869–9874.

Sun G, Luo T, Yang C, Dong X, Li J, Zhu Y, Zheng H, Tian W, Wang S, Barry CE III, et al. 2012. Dynamic population changes in *Mycobacterium tuberculosis* during acquisition and fixation of drug resistance in patients. *J Infect Dis* **206:** 1724–1733.

Supply P, Magdalena J, Himpens S, Locht C. 1997. Identification of novel intergenic repetitive units in a mycobacterial two-component system operon. *Mol Microbiol* **26:** 991–1003.

Supply P, Mazars E, Lesjean S, Vincent V, Gicquel B, Locht C. 2000. Variable human minisatellite-like regions in the *Mycobacterium tuberculosis* genome. *Mol Microbiol* **36:** 762–771.

Supply P, Lesjean S, Savine E, Kremer K, van Soolingen D, Locht C. 2001. Automated high-throughput genotyping for study of global epidemiology of *Mycobacterium tuberculosis* based on mycobacterial interspersed repetitive units. *J Clin Microbiol* **39:** 3563–3571.

Supply P, Warren RM, Banuls AL, Lesjean S, Van Der Spuy GD, Lewis LA, Tibayrenc M, Van Helden PD, Locht C. 2003. Linkage disequilibrium between minisatellite loci supports clonal evolution of *Mycobacterium tuberculosis* in a high tuberculosis incidence area. *Mol Microbiol* **47:** 529–538.

Supply P, Allix C, Lesjean S, Cardoso-Oelemann M, Rusch-Gerdes S, Willery E, Savine E, de Haas P, van Deutekom H, Roring S, et al. 2006. Proposal for standardization of optimized mycobacterial interspersed repetitive unit-variable-number tandem repeat typing of *Mycobacterium tuberculosis*. *J Clin Microbiol* **44:** 4498–4510.

Supply P, Marceau M, Mangenot S, Roche D, Rouanet C, Khanna V, Majlessi L, Criscuolo A, Tap J, Pawlik A, et al. 2013. Genomic analysis of smooth tubercle bacilli provides insights into ancestry and pathoadaptation of *Mycobacterium tuberculosis*. *Nat Genet* **45:** 172–179.

Thye T, Niemann S, Walter K, Homolka S, Intemann CD, Chinbuah MA, Enimil A, Gyapong J, Osei I, Owusu-Dabo E, et al. 2011. Variant G57E of mannose binding lectin associated with protection against tuberculosis caused by *Mycobacterium africanum* but not by *M. tuberculosis*. *PLoS ONE* **6:** e20908.

Tsenova L, Ellison E, Harbacheuski R, Moreira AL, Kurepina N, Reed MB, Mathema B, Barry CE, 3rd, Kaplan G. 2005. Virulence of selected *Mycobacterium tuberculosis* clinical isolates in the rabbit model of meningitis is dependent on phenolic glycolipid produced by the bacilli. *J Infect Dis* **192:** 98–106.

van Embden JD, Cave MD, Crawford JT, Dale JW, Eisenach KD, Gicquel B, Hermans P, Martin C, McAdam R, Shinnick TM, et al. 1993. Strain identification of *Mycobacterium tuberculosis* by DNA fingerprinting: Recommendations for a standardized methodology. *J Clin Microbiol* **31:** 406–409.

van Soolingen D, Qian L, de Haas PE, Douglas JT, Traore H, Portaels F, Qing HZ, Enkhsaikan D, Nymadawa P, van Embden JD. 1995. Predominance of a single genotype of *Mycobacterium tuberculosis* in countries of east Asia. *J Clin Microbiol* **33:** 3234–3238.

van Soolingen D, Hoogenboezem T, de Haas PE, Hermans PW, Koedam MA, Teppema KS, Brennan PJ, Besra GS, Portaels F, Top J, et al. 1997. A novel pathogenic taxon of the *Mycobacterium tuberculosis* complex, Canetti: Characterization of an exceptional isolate from Africa. *Int J Syst Bacteriol* **47:** 1236–1245.

Varghese B, Supply P, Allix-Beguec C, Shoukri M, Al-Omari R, Herbawi M, Al-Hajoj S. 2013. Admixed phylogenetic distribution of drug resistant *Mycobacterium tuberculosis* in Saudi Arabia. *PLoS ONE* **8:** e55598.

Walker TM, Ip CL, Harrell RH, Evans JT, Kapatai G, Dedicoat MJ, Eyre DW, Wilson DJ, Hawkey PM, Crook DW, et al. 2013a. Whole-genome sequencing to delineate *Mycobacterium tuberculosis* outbreaks: A retrospective observational study. *Lancet Infect Dis* **13:** 137–146.

Walker TM, Monk P, Grace Smith E, Peto TE. 2013b. Contact investigations for outbreaks of *Mycobacterium tuberculosis*: Advances through whole genome sequencing. *Clin Microbiol Infect* **19:** 796–802.

Warren RM, Victor TC, Streicher EM, Richardson M, van der Spuy GD, Johnson R, Chihota VN, Locht C, Supply P, van

Helden PD. 2004. Clonal expansion of a globally disseminated lineage of *Mycobacterium tuberculosis* with low IS6110 copy numbers. *J Clin Microbiol* **42:** 5774–5782.

Weniger T, Krawczyk J, Supply P, Niemann S, Harmsen D. 2010. MIRU-VNTRplus: A web tool for polyphasic genotyping of *Mycobacterium tuberculosis* complex bacteria. *Nucleic Acids Res* **38:** W326–W331.

Werngren J. 2013. *Mycobacterium tuberculosis* Beijing type mutation frequency. *Emerg Infect Dis* **19:** 522.

Werngren J, Hoffner SE. 2003. Drug-susceptible *Mycobacterium tuberculosis* Beijing genotype does not develop mutation-conferred resistance to rifampin at an elevated rate. *J Clin Microbiol* **41:** 1520–1524.

Wirth T, Hildebrand F, Allix-Beguec C, Wolbeling F, Kubica T, Kremer K, van Soolingen D, Rusch-Gerdes S, Locht C, Brisse S, et al. 2008. Origin, spread and demography of the *Mycobacterium tuberculosis* complex. *PLoS Pathog* **4:** e1000160.

Host-Directed Therapies for Tuberculosis

David M. Tobin

Department of Molecular Genetics and Microbiology, Center for Microbial Pathogenesis, Center for AIDS Research, Duke University School of Medicine, Durham, North Carolina 27710

Correspondence: david.tobin@duke.edu

Host-directed therapies are a relatively new and promising approach to treatment of tuberculosis. Modulation of specific host immune pathways, including those that impact inflammation and immunopathology, can limit mycobacterial infection and pathology, both in cell culture and in animal models. This review explores a range of host pathways and drugs, some already approved for clinical use that have the potential to provide new adjunctive therapies for tuberculosis. Drugs targeting host processes may largely avoid the development of bacterial antibiotic resistance, a major public health concern for tuberculosis. However, these drugs may also have generally increased risk for side effects on the host. Understanding the specific mechanisms by which these drugs act and the relationship of these mechanisms to *Mycobacterium tuberculosis* pathogenesis will be critical in selecting appropriate host-directed therapy. Overall, these host-directed compounds provide a novel strategy for anti-tuberculosis therapy.

Frustrated by the limitations of traditional antimycobacterial therapies, researchers in the tuberculosis (TB) community have focused on the possibility of modulating the host immune response as adjunctive therapy. Particularly in the case of multidrug-resistant (MDR) or extensively drug-resistant TB (XDR-TB), host-directed therapies provide a largely untapped approach as adjunctive anti-TB therapies, either to directly increase the ability of the host immune system to effectively eliminate mycobacteria or to limit collateral tissue damage associated with infection that can result in morbidity and mortality. New attention has focused on exploring host-directed therapies, and there has been a spike in reviews articulating fundamental principles; each aspect of the host response can conceivably be modulated in a way that maximizes bacterial killing while minimizing inflammatory tissue damage (Hawn et al. 2013; Zumla et al. 2013, 2014; Kaufmann et al. 2014; Wilkinson 2014). These approaches are still somewhat speculative, and there are only a few actively used host-directed drugs in the field. However, there is growing sentiment that alternative approaches are needed and that manipulation of host immunity coupled to a greater understanding of biological mechanisms hold new promise in the anti-TB armamentarium. Many compounds under active investigation have already been approved by the United States Food and Drug Administration (FDA) and thus might lead to accelerated clinical trials and implementation.

Cite this article as *Cold Spring Harb Perspect Med* doi: 10.1101/cshperspect.a021196

ADVANTAGES TO HOST-DIRECTED APPROACHES

Antibiotic resistance is a major public health concern for TB, even for effectively administered therapeutics, and MDR-TB and XDR-TB are serious problems worldwide (Shah et al. 2007; Gandhi et al. 2010; WHO 2010). In part, this is because of long therapies that sometimes are not completed (Castelnuovo 2010). In addition and despite the long generation time of *Mycobacterium tuberculosis (Mtb)*, there is consistent accumulation of alleles that confer resistance to a variety of drugs during the course of a human infection (Sacchettini et al. 2008). Antibiotic-resistant alleles classically involve mutation of a direct antibiotic target and arise relatively frequently, in spite of the long generation time of *Mtb*, and may also arise from increased expression of membrane transporters (Ioerger et al. 2013). Studies based on whole-genome sequencing in cynomolgus macaques revealed an in vivo mutation rate on the order of 10^{-10} mutations per bacterial generation (Ford et al. 2011). Notably, mutation rates were comparable in latent disease, and DNA lesions identified suggested that oxidative damage might be a driving force increasing mutational load in vivo. Furthermore, East Asian lineage strains had close to a 10-fold increase in mutation rate relative to standard strains from the Euro-American lineage (Ford et al. 2013). Via whole-genome sequencing of an outbreak strain in humans, the mutation rate in active TB was similar, but latent TB was reduced (Colangeli et al. 2014). In any event, the number of antibiotic-resistant strains is burgeoning and can lead to rapid depletion of options for physicians and health care workers and the development of circulating drug-resistant strains (Gandhi et al. 2006). In theory, host-directed therapies bypass many of the problems associated with pathogen-directed therapies (Schwegmann and Brombacher 2008). They offer to potentiate existing immune defenses against *Mtb* or evoke new ones. Because host therapies target host proteins, it is much less likely that bacteria will generate a mutation that directly abrogates compound binding.

HOST-DIRECTED THERAPIES IN CLINICAL HUMAN TRIALS OR PRECLINICAL ANIMAL STUDIES

Anti-Inflammatory Therapies

So far, most host-directed therapies are still theoretical. One major exception is the use of broadly acting corticosteroids. TB infections in humans induce classic inflammatory responses (Kaufmann and Dorhoi 2013), and, as in other infectious diseases, it is the balance between immunopathology and insufficient inflammation that may determine disease severity and outcome (Casadevall and Pirofski 2003). Broadly acting glucocorticoids, such as dexamethasone and prednisone, have been used in a number of trials and are the standard-of-care for some severe forms of TB. They represent a relatively accessible and inexpensive approach to limiting inflammation, which can be a prime cause of morbidity and mortality. They have proved particularly effective in cases of TB meningitis (Schoeman et al. 1997; Thwaites et al. 2004; Prasad and Singh 2008) and have been adopted as standard-of-care for TB pericarditis and meningitis (Hakim et al. 2000; Mayosi et al. 2002; Thwaites et al. 2009). A recent meta-analysis of clinical trials using corticosteroids showed a 17% reduction in mortality across 41 clinical trials (Critchley et al. 2013).

The detrimental effects of inflammation in the human host are crystallized in TB-IRIS (immune reconstitution inflammatory syndrome), a paradoxical worsening of TB and inflammatory symptoms with reconstitution of the immune system associated with highly active antiretroviral therapy (HAART) (Dhasmana et al. 2008; Meintjes et al. 2008). A randomized controlled trial for adjunctive prednisone showed amelioration of symptoms for TB-IRIS (Meintjes et al. 2010). More generally, the morbidity associated with the inflammatory symptoms of IRIS reflects a generally detrimental inflammatory state that can be induced by TB infection (Marais et al. 2009). It remains to be investigated, as described below, whether corticosteroids could be generally beneficial in pulmonary TB, or perhaps among a subset of cases with particularly high levels of inflammation.

As host-directed therapies, however, these more general suppressors of inflammation may lead to secondary complications including immunosuppression. Knowing the basic biology of mycobacterial pathogenesis, as heterogeneous as that might be, may guide the search for more effective and specific host-directed therapies.

Modulation of Inflammation by Phosphodiesterase Inhibitors

cAMP plays a key role in both inflammation and tumor necrosis factor (TNF) production, as cAMP produced in host cells can lead to modulation of TNF levels. Therefore, cAMP levels are tightly regulated by host phosphodiesterases (PDEs). However, bacterial adenylyl cyclases can promote cAMP production in host cells (Agarwal et al. 2009). Based on the effectiveness of thalidomide in treating severe leprosy reactions (erythema nodosum leprosum), it was proposed that the modulation of extreme inflammation/TNF levels via thalidomide might be host-beneficial (Corral and Kaplan 1999). Thalidomide has been used in clinical pediatric trials of adjunctive therapy for TB meningitis, and the limitation of TNF production is thought to be key (Schoeman et al. 2000, 2004). However, the extreme teratogenic properties of thalidomide make it particularly dangerous (Kim and Scialli 2011), and other modulators of TNF-mediated pathologies in TB would be preferable.

One promising host-directed approach is the set of PDE inhibitors that appear to act directly on host cAMP levels. The PDE4 inhibitor CC-3052, a thalidomide analog, increased the effectiveness of isoniazid in a mouse model through reduced TNF production (Koo et al. 2011; Subbian et al. 2011a,b). Similarly, in two different mouse models, the FDA-approved PDE3 inhibitor cilostazol, which inhibits a separate class of PDEs reduced time to sterilization during antibiotic short course therapy by 1 mo (from 6 mo) (Maiga et al. 2012). Inhibition of PDE4 in a mouse model by different drugs resulted in worse outcomes in mice, but this may also be consistent with increased growth in the PDE-inhibited environment (the PDE4 inhibitor CC-3052 in rabbits was shown to result in slightly increased burden as monotherapy) and may suggest that adjunctive use could still benefit the host (Maiga et al. 2013). Fundamentally, these therapies aim to restrict immunopathology arising from TNF excess while allowing many of the antimycobacterial properties of host cells to remain intact.

Eicosanoid Modulation

Intriguingly, cAMP levels also impinge directly on production of host eicosanoids, lipid mediators of inflammation that are increasingly recognized as important modulators of the host immune response in mycobacterial infection. Eicosanoids may be central to the control of inflammatory responses during infection with pathogenic mycobacteria. The balance of these pro- and anti-inflammatory lipid mediators may lead to either uncontrolled inflammation or insufficient production of protective inflammatory mediators.

Virulent mycobacteria induce production of anti-inflammatory lipoxins, including Lipoxin A_4 (LXA_4) during high-dose mouse infections and in cell culture macrophage infections (Bafica et al. 2005; Chen et al. 2008; Divangahi et al. 2009). LXA_4 favors necrotic cell death in cell culture models in part by limiting production of PGE_2, which is required for plasma membrane repair and membrane integrity (Chen et al. 2008; Divangahi et al. 2009). By promoting necrotic cell death, LXA_4 and the limitation of PGE_2 production drive bacterial expansion to the detriment of the host.

In a mouse high-dose infection model, protection was noted for *Mtb*-infected mice deficient in *Alox5*, the gene encoding the enzyme responsible for both production of the LTA_4 intermediate upstream of the proinflammatory eicosanoid LTB_4 and important in the production of the anti-inflammatory lipoxin LXA_4 (Bafica et al. 2005). The ability of zileuton, a clinically used asthma drug, to block lipoxin production was suggested initially as a host-directed therapy that might improve TB outcomes (Bafica et al. 2005).

In the zebrafish-*Mycobacterium marinum* model, a forward genetic screen for susceptibility loci identified the enzyme Lta4h as critical in controlling mycobacterial disease. Namely, when the *lta4h* gene was mutated, the LTA_4 intermediate was shunted to anti-inflammatory lipoxins, and this lipoxin excess was found to modulate TNF levels, thereby limiting the ability of the host to restrict mycobacterial infection (Tobin et al. 2010, 2012).

How relevant are these findings in mammalian and zebrafish models to human disease? In two human cohorts, one in Vietnam and one in Nepal, there was an association of heterozygosity at the *LTA4H* locus with disease severity, in both TB meningitis and leprosy (Tobin et al. 2010). Two copies of a functional, high-activity promoter variant led to excess inflammation, presumably caused by excess production of proinflammatory, TNF-promoting eicosanoids, such as LTB4. In contrast, two copies of the low-activity promoter variant altered the balance into what is thought to be an excessively anti-inflammatory state (Tobin et al. 2012). Remarkably, in a retrospective analysis of a randomly controlled trial for adjunctive dexamethasone therapy in TB meningitis, the entirety of the beneficial effect was associated with the group of high-activity homozygotes, whereas the low-activity homozygotes derived no benefit from adjunctive therapy (Thwaites et al. 2004; Tobin et al. 2012). These findings led to a model in which balanced inflammation was optimal, and which predicted that different genotypes drove more severe disease for fundamentally different reasons (Fig. 1).

Eicosanoids, with their well-known roles in inflammation and their emerging roles in TB pathogenesis, thus provide an important host-specific target. The findings at the level of innate immunity extend also to downstream effects on the adaptive immune response, with impaired antigen cross-presentation, suggesting that the eicosanoids control mycobacterial infection at a number of levels (Divangahi et al. 2010).

In the high inflammatory state, LTA4H excess leads to increased TNF levels and engages a pathway of programmed necrosis in zebrafish macrophages (Tobin et al. 2012). Although higher TNF levels lead to early improved control of infection in individual macrophages, RIP1/RIP3-mediated necroptosis ultimately leads to necroptotic cell death that liberates the infecting mycobacteria to grow extracellularly, relatively unrestrained (Roca and Ramakrishnan 2013). In a thorough genetic analysis, the generation of mitochondrial reactive oxygen species was shown to lead initially to increased intracellular killing of mycobacteria, but then to macrophage necroptotic cell death via two parallel pathways—ceramide production mediated through acid sphingomyelinase and regulation of mitochondrial cyclophilin D (Roca and Ramakrishnan 2013). By understanding these processes in molecular detail, two host-directed, clinically approved drugs targeting each of these pathways were shown to rescue the hypersusceptibility induced by high TNF levels. Desipramine targets acid sphingomyelinase (Elojeimy et al. 2006). Alisporivir, currently in phase III clinical trials, targets cyclophilin D interactions with the mitochondrial permeability transition pore complex, a crucial step in mitochondrial destruction (Vandenabeele et al. 2010; Quarato et al. 2012). Because TNF initially promotes increased intracellular control, combination of higher TNF levels with inhibition of programmed necrosis resulted in a transformation of a more severe disease phenotype to greater resistance (Roca and Ramakrishnan 2013).

Finally, modulation of PGE_2 itself in the context of interleukin-1 (IL-1)-deficient mice and type I interferon (IFN) induction provides a promising host-directed therapy. In a mouse infection model using mice deficient in IL-1 signaling or with excess type I IFN production, conditions that may be particularly relevant to patients with more severe disease (Mayer-Barber et al. 2011), zileuton and PGE_2 administration had host-beneficial effects (Mayer-Barber et al. 2014). Inhibition of the enzyme 5-lipooxygenase (5-LO) via the asthma drug zileuton, is proposed to shunt eicosanoid production toward increased PGE_2 production, which in the context of high-inflammatory states driven by type I IFNs, can suppress detrimental type I IFN production, partially rescues mortality, and reduces bacterial burden (Mayer-Barber et al. 2014). Thus, multiple clinically approved drugs that act on eicosanoid balance and displayed in

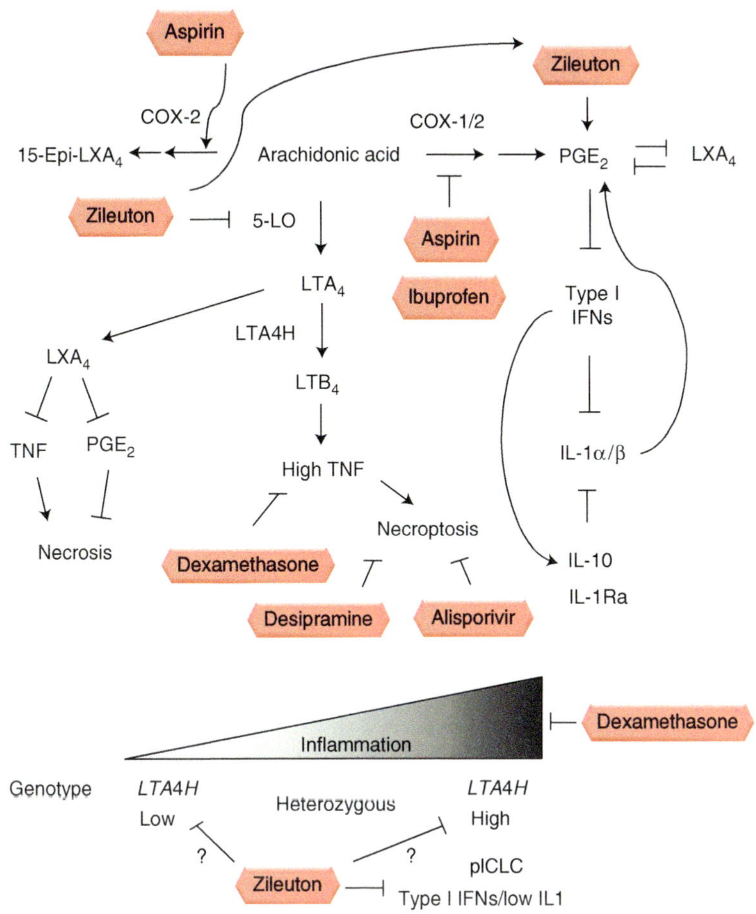

Figure 1. Schematic of opportunities for host-directed therapies modulating eicosanoid balance. Clinically approved drugs that modulate eicosanoid production and that have been tested in animal models of mycobacterial infection are shown in boxes. Some drugs, such as aspirin, may act at multiple points in the eicosanoid pathway, whereas others, such as zileuton, may result in shunting effects. *Bottom* panel depicts human genotypes associated in a Vietnamese cohort with increased or decreased production of LTA4H and differential responsiveness to dexamethasone adjunctive therapy as well as a mouse model of disease in IL-1 pathway-deficient mice or animals with elevated type I interferons.

Figure 1 appear to have potential as host-directed therapies. Moreover, many of the host-directed therapies described above have genotype-specific effects that depend on eicosanoid balance in zebrafish, mice, and humans.

Nonsteroidal Anti-Inflammatory Drugs

Aspirin is a well-tested and effective administered drug with low risk in adults. In addition to its effect as a COX-1/COX-2 inhibitor that limits production of prostaglandins, it has been shown to modify COX-2 to produce the aspirin-triggered lipoxins (Claria and Serhan 1995), potent proresolving lipids that have in vivo effects on neutrophil recruitment and inflammatory cytokines (Morris et al. 2009). In addition to modulating inflammation through classical COX-dependent inhibition of prostaglandins, it may actively promote the proresolving signals mediated by lipoxins, and it has been used as a therapy in the zebrafish model of hyperinflammatory states during mycobacterial infection (Tobin et al. 2012). In the case of TB driven by hyperinflammatory genotypes or status, the production of these lipoxins may exert proresolving effects and limit disease pathology. However, in the case of insufficient inflammation, the effects may be different in skewing the balance of PGE_2 and LXA_4. In a mouse model with a predominant type I INF response, for example, PGE_2 amplification is thought to promote host survival in the context of a type I INF predominant innate immune response, and so aspirin might have unwanted effects under conditions that recapitulate this model (Mayer-Barber et al. 2014). Two clinical trials assessing the effect of aspirin on TB meningitis outcomes were inconclusive, with one trial suggesting a significant benefit ($p = 0.03$) of adjunctive therapy on survival. However, it would be interesting to examine the effects of adjunctive aspirin administration on different genotypes and inflammatory states, given what literature on eicosanoid balance has suggested (Misra et al. 2010; Schoeman et al. 2011).

Additionally, using the C3HeB/FeJ mouse model of TB (Pan et al. 2005), in which caseation necrosis occurs, ibuprofen treatment given as a monotherapy starting 4 wk postinfection reduced burden and increased survival (Vilaplana et al. 2013). The precise basis of these effects, other than a hypothesized suppression of detrimental inflammation, remains to be seen. Future studies could address if reducing hyperinflammatory damage is sufficient or if research should focus on specific pathways engaged, including the eicosanoids and aspirin-triggered lipoxins.

Imatinib

As noted with therapies to modulate eicosanoids, the straightest line to host-directed therapy may be to identify drugs that are already FDA-approved. One promising example from this work comes from use of the ABL tyrosine kinase inhibitor imatinib mesylate, known commercially as Gleevec. Previously, it had been shown that imatinib was able to inhibit poxvirus pathogenesis via limitation of actin motility of the cell-associated enveloped virions (Reeves et al. 2005). In mycobacterial infections with both *Mtb* and the closely related *M. marinum*, there appear to be both cell autonomous and cell nonautonomous beneficial effects of inhibition, with inhibition of ABL resulting in increased killing and promoting acidification of the mycobacterial phagosome (Napier et al. 2011; Bruns et al. 2012). Mice treated with imatinib had fewer granuloma lesions and less bacterial load in infected organs, for both *Mtb* and *M. marinum* infections (Napier et al. 2011). When coadministered with first-line drugs, imatinib had a synergistic therapeutic effect (Napier et al. 2011). In addition, monocytes from imatinib-treated patients showed more acidic vacuoles by LysoSensor staining (Bruns et al. 2012). As Gleevec is soon to be off patent, this may be an effective and viable therapy for cases of both drug-resistant and drug-susceptible *Mtb*.

Alteration of Lipid Metabolism

Statins provide an interesting additional avenue for a host-directed therapy, as widely used drugs that have proven safe and effective (Ray et al. 2010). Parihar et al. (2014) have shown increased promotion of phagosome maturation and autophagy via reduction of cholesterol levels, both processes that are thought to be host-beneficial in the context of mycobacterial infection. Because mycobacteria hijack host cholesterol as a carbon source on IFN-γ activation (Pandey and Sassetti 2008; Griffin et al. 2012), limitation of cholesterol levels may also influence bacterial persistence, although it is unclear to what extent altering these levels would have a meaningful effect on disease progression in humans. Epidemiological studies of TB susceptibility or progression among individuals taking statins have not yet been achieved, in part owing to largely nonoverlapping populations.

Pathogenic mycobacteria are thus able to reprogram lipid balance within host cells for their own benefit. Notably, in addition to animal models, this has been observed in human lung tissue in profiling of laser-capture microdissections of human caseating granulomas from resected lung (Kim et al. 2010) and in decreased phagosomal lipolysis (Podinovskaia et al. 2013). Virulent but not avirulent *Mtb* (as well as Bacillus Calmette–Guérin [BCG]) reprograms lipid balance within infected macrophages in cell culture, leading to a foamy cell phenotype with extensive lipid droplets that is thought to benefit the infecting bacterium (D'Avila et al. 2006; Singh et al. 2012; Podinovskaia et al. 2013). During infection, glycolysis is shifted toward ketone body synthesis, and the product D-3-hydroxybutyrate (DHB) then activates the G-protein-coupled receptor GPR109A; this then leads to a feedback mechanism that promotes cAMP signaling and limits lipolysis (Singh et al. 2012). By targeting this pathway with mepenzolate bromide, a GPR109A inhibitor, bacterial burden was reduced in cell culture and in mouse in vivo models (Singh et al. 2012).

Other pathways controlling lipid composition are also targets for intervention. PPAR-γ is a canonical ligand-activated nuclear receptor that modulates fatty acid metabolism and storage as well as playing previously underappreciated roles in macrophage immune response (Kiss et al. 2013). Notably, in the generation of foamy macrophages, which have high levels of PPAR-γ expression, *Mtb* and manLAM activate PPAR-γ through a mannose receptor-dependent pathway, and knockdown in human macrophages or inhibition leads to decreased mycobacterial growth (Almeida et al. 2009; Rajaram et al. 2010). Knockdown of either PPAR-γ or testicular receptor 4 (TR4) resulted in reduced bacterial burden in macrophages, with modulation of CD36, IL-10 production, and phagolysosome fusion as possible mechanisms (Mahajan et al. 2012). There are at least three FDA-approved compounds pioglitazone, rosiglitazone, and treprostinil with activity directed at PPAR-γ (Kiss et al. 2013; Rask-Andersen et al. 2014). Finally, other nuclear receptors such as TR4, which may be activated by keto-mycolic acid, may also play important roles in mediating foamy macrophage formation (Mahajan et al. 2012; Dkhar et al. 2014). Thus, these candidate compounds and others modulating these pathways also provide prospective adjunctive therapies.

Vitamin D

Vitamin D has long been proposed to have important host-beneficial effects in TB, including immunomodulatory effects. In human macrophages, TLR2-mediated or INF-γ-mediated activation of cyp27b1 leads to conversion of 25-hydroxyvitamin D3 (25(OH)D3) to bioactive 1,25-dihydroxyvitamin D3 (Liu et al. 2006; Krutzik et al. 2008; Fabri et al. 2011). In contrast to rodent models, the primary antimycobacterial effector function on TLR stimulation of this conversion event lies in the generation of antimicrobial peptides (Liu et al. 2006). IFN-γ antimicrobial activity can be mediated through activation of CYP27B1. More recently, 1,25-dihydroxyvitamin D (1,25D) was shown to enhance IL-1β transcription in macrophages and induce antimicrobial peptide production in cocultured lung epithelial cells (Verway et al. 2013). Finally, vitamin D has been shown to induce autophagy in cell culture via production of LL-37 (Yuk et al. 2009) (see autophagy section below), thus linking to an additional host-protective process that might also contribute to bacterial control in vivo. In addition to its antimicrobial effects on the host macrophage, subgroup analysis of a clinical trial showed that vitamin D as an adjunctive therapy may reduce hyperinflammatory responses and thus may contribute in multiple ways to improved outcomes (Coussens et al. 2012).

Because this is an inexpensive intervention, it is a particularly appealing host-directed therapy, and a number of clinical studies, including randomized controlled trials, have been performed. Genetic associations and serum concentration measurements have suggested associations of vitamin D production with susceptibility to TB (Wilkinson et al. 2000; Ustianowski et al. 2005; Wejse et al. 2007). Initially, clinical trials of vitamin D supplementation gave mixed results (Morcos et al. 1998; Nursyam et al. 2006; Wejse et al. 2009). However, in the most extensive clinical trial performed to date, there was no overall statistically significant effect on time to sputum clearance (Martineau et al. 2011). On stratification of the patient population by vitamin D receptor genotype, it was suggested that one class of homozygotes derived benefit from the therapy (Martineau et al. 2011). The functional consequence of this human variant is not known, but it would be interesting to follow up in further and perhaps larger trials, including the use of vitamin D supplementation for investigation of drug-resistant strains of *Mtb*.

IDENTIFICATION OF NEW HOST-DIRECTED THERAPIES

Cell-Culture-Based Screens

Cell-culture-based screens showed in principle that limitation of host gene products can dramatically restrict mycobacterial growth, particularly in cell-autonomous assays. Genome-wide screens, first in *Drosophila* S2 cells using *Mycobacterium fortuitum* with a *Drosophila* RNA interference (RNAi) library (Philips et al. 2005), revealed a number of gene products promoting phagocytosis and restricting bacterial growth. Using *Mtb* infection and a small interfering RNA (siRNA) screen in murine macrophages, first for kinases and phosphatases and then in a genome-wide screen in human macrophages, an important host-based set of genes with resistance phenotypes on inhibition identified wide targets, including autophagic networks (Jayaswal et al. 2010; Kumar et al. 2010). Thus, in principle, host genes that allow mycobacteria to replicate intracellularly could be targeted, although few chemical inhibitors of these hits were well known.

Originally identified in an RNAi cell-culture-based screen for *Salmonella typhimurium* growth restriction, AKT1 inhibition and a host-directed chemical inhibitor of AKT1 were sufficient to limit *Mtb* intracellular growth (Kuijl et al. 2007). Both AKT1 and AKT2 also appeared in one of the host siRNA screens, confirming a role for AKT1 as host-permissive within macrophages and suggesting that its inhibition might be effective as a host-directed therapy (Kumar et al. 2010).

More recently, these screens have evolved to relatively high-throughput chemical screens, often coupled to cellular phenotypes. Using a library of FDA-approved small molecules, combined with an siRNA screen and high-throughput imaging of BCG infection, two compounds were identified that reduced burden and modulated autophagy. Nortriptyline and prochlorperazine edisylate thus represent host-directed drugs that are already approved (Sundaramurthy et al. 2013).

Similarly, Stanley et al. (2014) identified host-targeting small molecules that had no effect on in vitro–grown *Mtb* but restricted bacterial intracellular growth. Known drugs identified included fluoxetine, which induced autophagy in cell culture, and gefitinib, an inhibitor of epidermal growth factor receptor (EGFR), which was also shown to reduce bacterial replication in an in vivo mouse model of acute infection (Stanley et al. 2014).

Here, one of the translational questions is the degree to which cell-culture assays serve as a proxy for the complexity of the human immune response. However, chemical screens in cell culture with FDA-approved compounds may prove to be a powerful shortcut to de novo drug development.

Autophagy

One striking result from many of the cell-culture screens is a significant number of hits involving autophagic pathways (Kumar et al. 2010; Sundaramurthy et al. 2013). Autophagy is thought to play an important role in restriction of a number of intracellular pathogens and is the subject of active research that seeks to target this process for host-directed therapies (Rubinsztein et al. 2012; Shoji-Kawata et al. 2013). In *Mtb* infections, autophagy restricts mycobacterial replication and may be triggered by a number of cues, including IFN-γ and extracellular DNA sensing via STING (stimulator of interferon genes) (Gutierrez et al. 2004; Watson et al. 2012). Induction of IRGM, which is required for control in a mouse model, may drive autophagy in some cases (MacMicking et al. 2003; Singh et al. 2006). Mice deficient in central autophagy pathway components such as ATG5 have both higher bacterial burden and increased inflammation, which appears in a cell-autonomous manner (i.e., is not merely an effect of higher burden)

(Castillo et al. 2012). This suggests that autophagic processes are induced and can limit mycobacterial infections but that they are normally inhibited at least partially by pathogenic mycobacteria and that full induction of autophagy can have dramatic host-beneficial effects.

It remains elusive how these cell-autonomous processes will translate into animal models, when multiple cell types are exposed to a drug. Generally, animals defective in autophagic processes have defects in mycobacterial control, but few whole-animal rescue experiments have been performed.

Protein Kinase as a Potential Host Target

Double-stranded RNA (dsRNA)-dependent protein kinase (PKR) was shown to be an enzyme in which its absence in mice results in improved control of bacterial burden and thus meets a clear notion of a host-directed therapy, and chemical inhibitors are being developed (Bryk et al. 2011; Wu et al. 2012). Again, by targeting these host proteins, overall burden is reduced. New compounds have not yet been examined for off-target effects in whole animals, although proof of principle using a mouse knockout in live animals is a promising beginning.

MODELS OF IMMUNOPATHOLOGY

Cell-culture models, although amenable to higher-throughput experimentation, can be limited to assessing largely cell-autonomous effects on burden. The reality of TB as an in vivo disease implies that models of host are similarly important. However, even well-established versatile models like the mouse can differ in their outcomes depending on strain differences. This has led to the adoption of less genetically and immunologically tractable models that may recapitulate better the full spectrum of physiology and pathology, including primates, guinea pigs, mini-pigs, and rabbits (Flynn 2006). The combination of host-directed therapies with these models will give insights into what may ultimately prove most effective in humans and allows the observation of different cell types in a whole organism.

Neutrophils

Although the tuberculous granuloma is largely defined by the presence of epithelioid macrophages, neutrophils are clearly present at both early and later stages of infection where they play multiple roles (Canetti 1955; Eum et al. 2010). Transcriptional profiling of whole blood revealed a neutrophil-associated signature in active cases (Martineau et al. 2007; Berry et al. 2010). These roles include both host-protective functions—in the zebrafish mycobacterial infection model, they are important in mycobacterial killing within the granuloma through NADPH-oxidase-dependent mechanisms, notably after the initial formation of the granuloma (Yang et al. 2012). However, neutrophil-mediated inflammation appears to play an important host-detrimental role in later infection (Desvignes and Ernst 2009; Nandi and Behar 2011). Epithelial-produced CXCL5 mediates recruitment of CXCR2-positive neutrophils. Knockout mice of either the ligand or receptor are relatively protected in a high-dose mouse infection model (Nouailles et al. 2014). Thus, the balance of sufficient neutrophil function and limitation of immunopathology may be critical. Similarly, in a mouse infection model, deletion of miR-223 leads to dysregulated inflammation and recruitment of neutrophils (Dorhoi et al. 2013). These data suggest that host modulation of microRNAs (miRNAs) might form another basis for host-directed therapies. *Mtb* lipomannan has been shown in macrophages to regulate the balance of proinflammatory and anti-inflammatory miRNAs (mir-155 and mir-125b), respectively, to modulate TNF production (Rajaram et al. 2011). Because of considerable clinical interest in modulation of miRNAs, this might form a future approach, but delivery technologies in humans or in the context of TB require further investigation (Iannaccone et al. 2014).

Matrix Metalloproteases

Matrix metalloproteases, key remodeling enzymes in the human lung, may also play a role in immunopathology of TB. Induced in human

TB and in whole-animal models, MMP-1 is a canonical matrix metalloprotease that is found in the human TB granuloma (Elkington et al. 2011b). Although not present in mice, human MMP-1 expressed transgenically in the mouse drives alveolar destruction in lung granulomas and greater collagen breakdown (Elkington et al. 2011a). Potential routes for modulating the collagenase MMP-1 include a specific collagenase inhibitor, Ro32-3555, currently in trials for rheumatoid arthritis (Hemmings et al. 2001; Elkington et al. 2011b).

Other MMPs may play important roles in tissue-specific choreographed responses in which tissue remodeling occurs and new structures are formed. The mycobacterial granuloma itself is thought to be exploited by infecting bacteria to promote growth initially (Ramakrishnan 2012). Deletion of the matrix metalloprotease MMP-9 has been shown in mouse models to reduce burden and granuloma formation and in zebrafish to be induced in an ESX-1/RD-1-dependent manner to drive granuloma formation via interaction with host epithelial cells (Taylor et al. 2006; Volkman et al. 2010). Inhibition of the MMPs has given equivocal results in cancer trials, suggesting that there may be multiple roles at the level of the whole organism (Overall and Lopez-Otin 2002; Parks et al. 2004), but the specific effects of single MMP knockouts or modulation suggest that these could be important targets for host-directed therapy.

OTHER APPROACHES

Immunotherapy

More expensive, host-directed therapies delivering specific cytokines have been an option and some are undergoing clinical trials. Because the IL-12/IFN-γ axis is so critical in Mendelian susceptibilities to mycobacterial disease as well as promoting restriction of mycobacterial growth in animal and cell culture models, the thought emerged that supplementation of IFN-γ held promise as a host immunotherapy (Abel et al. 2014). Indeed, clinical trials with IFN-γ, particularly for MDR-TB, have >15 yr of experience (Condos et al. 1997; Koh et al. 2004; Dawson et al. 2009).

IL-2 immunotherapy has also been proposed but has met with mixed results (Johnson et al. 1997, 2003).

More recently, there has been interest in potential roles for γδ T cells in enhancing immunity. In a nonhuman primate model, researchers have focused on the γδ immune lineage only present in primates; stimulation with IL-2 and a closely related phosphoantigen to that of *Mtb* (the phosphoantigen Picostim carries a one-carbon difference from mycobacterial (*E*)-4-hydroxy-3-methyl-but-2-enyl pyrophosphate [HMBPP]) results in expansion of protective Vγ2 Vδ2 T cells (Chen et al. 2013). Notably, these effects are seen in animals with preexisting disease. The immunotherapy studies in humans and other primates have all been relatively limited with small, but generally measurable and beneficial effects. Immunotherapy may thus represent a potential treatment for particularly hard-to-treat and severe forms of TB.

Dual Host-Targeting and Antimicrobial Functions

Finally, existing antibiotics may also have additional host-directed effects. Clofazimine has in vitro antimycobacterial effects and has been used in combination therapy for *Mycobacterium leprae* treatment (Arbiser and Moschella 1995). It is in clinical trials for MDR-TB cases, but it may also act through a dual role in modulating the host immune response (Grosset et al. 2013), as it has been suggested to function in part by inducing macrophage apoptosis in the host (Fukutomi et al. 2011). Similarly, existing antimycobacterials such as isoniazid and pyrazinamide may act in part through the induction of host autophagy (Kim et al. 2012). Thus, the strict delineation between host-directed and bacterially directed therapies may not be absolute. More generally, combination effects of drugs on multiple pathways may be important for the full effect of a given drug, particularly when the initial effect is determined empirically and identified in phenotypic screens. Although target identification is critical to understanding the mechanism and to developing new effective compounds, it may be a combination of targets that mediates a full phenotypic effect.

CONCLUDING REMARKS

Only recently embraced by the TB community and funding agencies, the development of host-directed therapies is a promising new and relatively unexplored avenue for attacking a frustratingly intractable disease. However, it is important to note some concerns. In contrast to targeting bacteria directly, whole-animal, wholesale inhibition of host proteins may lead to other consequences. Host proteins may also be used in other contexts, including other organs and other cell types not directly related to mycobacterial infection. Thus, host targeting may have an increased risk for side effects on patients. However, the magic bullet model for TB therapeutics—a drug that targets the bacteria in all of its metabolic states and physiological compartments and is effective in the context of existing public health infrastructure—has clearly not yet been attained. Host-directed therapies open a new trove of possibilities. Repurposing of FDA-approved drugs, some of which show substantial promise in cell-culture models and in in vivo models, may quickly open orthogonal approaches. Choosing among these therapeutic possibilities and fine-tuning them based on a knowledge of mechanism and even host genotypes may result in important new adjunctive therapies that are precisely targeted and highly effective.

ACKNOWLEDGMENTS

The author is grateful to Kim Dohlich for critical reading of this chapter and Ana María Xet-Mull for assistance with figures. The Tobin laboratory is funded through a Mallinckrodt Scholar Award, a Searle Scholar Award, a National Institutes of Health Director's New Innovator Award (1DP2OD008614-01), a Vallee Foundation Young Investigator Award, a Whitehead Scholar Award, and the Duke University Center for AIDS Research (5P30 AI064518).

REFERENCES

Abel L, El-Baghdadi J, Bousfiha AA, Casanova JL, Schurr E. 2014. Human genetics of tuberculosis: A long and winding road. *Philos Trans R Soc Lond B Biol Sci* **369:** 20130428.

Agarwal N, Lamichhane G, Gupta R, Nolan S, Bishai WR. 2009. Cyclic AMP intoxication of macrophages by a *Mycobacterium tuberculosis* adenylate cyclase. *Nature* **460:** 98–102.

Almeida PE, Silva AR, Maya-Monteiro CM, Torocsik D, D'Avila H, Dezso B, Magalhaes KG, Castro-Faria-Neto HC, Nagy L, Bozza PT. 2009. *Mycobacterium bovis* bacillus Calmette-Guerin infection induces TLR2-dependent peroxisome proliferator-activated receptor γ expression and activation: Functions in inflammation, lipid metabolism, and pathogenesis. *J Immunol* **183:** 1337–1345.

Arbiser JL, Moschella SL. 1995. Clofazimine: A review of its medical uses and mechanisms of action. *J Am Acad Dermat* **32:** 241–247.

Bafica A, Scanga CA, Serhan C, Machado F, White S, Sher A, Aliberti J. 2005. Host control of *Mycobacterium tuberculosis* is regulated by 5-lipoxygenase-dependent lipoxin production. *J Clin Invest* **115:** 1601–1606.

Berry MP, Graham CM, McNab FW, Xu Z, Bloch SA, Oni T, Wilkinson KA, Banchereau R, Skinner J, Wilkinson RJ, et al. 2010. An interferon-inducible neutrophil-driven blood transcriptional signature in human tuberculosis. *Nature* **466:** 973–977.

Bruns H, Stegelmann F, Fabri M, Dohner K, van Zandbergen G, Wagner M, Skinner M, Modlin RL, Stenger S. 2012. Abelson tyrosine kinase controls phagosomal acidification required for killing of *Mycobacterium tuberculosis* in human macrophages. *J Immunol* **189:** 4069–4078.

Bryk R, Wu K, Raimundo BC, Boardman PE, Chao P, Conn GL, Anderson E, Cole JL, Duffy NP, Nathan C, et al. 2011. Identification of new inhibitors of protein kinase R guided by statistical modeling. *Bioorg Med Chem Lett* **21:** 4108–4114.

Canetti G. 1955. *The tubercle bacillus in the pulmonary lesion of man: Histobacteriology and its bearing on the therapy of pulmonary tuberculosis*, Springer, New York.

Casadevall A, Pirofski LA. 2003. The damage-response framework of microbial pathogenesis. *Nat Rev Microbiol* **1:** 17–24.

Castelnuovo B. 2010. A review of compliance to anti tuberculosis treatment and risk factors for defaulting treatment in Sub Saharan Africa. *Afr Health Sci* **10:** 320–324.

Castillo EF, Dekonenko A, Arko-Mensah J, Mandell MA, Dupont N, Jiang S, Delgado-Vargas M, Timmins GS, Bhattacharya D, Yang H, et al. 2012. Autophagy protects against active tuberculosis by suppressing bacterial burden and inflammation. *Proc Natl Acad Sci* **109:** E3168–E3176.

Chen M, Divangahi M, Gan H, Shin DS, Hong S, Lee DM, Serhan CN, Behar SM, Remold HG. 2008. Lipid mediators in innate immunity against tuberculosis: Opposing roles of PGE2 and LXA4 in the induction of macrophage death. *J Exp Med* **205:** 2791–2801.

Chen CY, Yao S, Huang D, Wei H, Sicard H, Zeng G, Jomaa H, Larsen MH, Jacobs WR Jr, Wang R, et al. 2013. Phosphoantigen/IL2 expansion and differentiation of

Vγ2Vδ2 T cells increase resistance to tuberculosis in nonhuman primates. *PLoS Pathog* **9:** e1003501.

Claria J, Serhan CN. 1995. Aspirin triggers previously undescribed bioactive eicosanoids by human endothelial cell-leukocyte interactions. *Proc Natl Acad Sci* **92:** 9475–9479.

Colangeli R, Arcus VL, Cursons RT, Ruthe A, Karalus N, Coley K, Manning SD, Kim S, Marchiano E, Alland D. 2014. Whole genome sequencing of *Mycobacterium tuberculosis* reveals slow growth and low mutation rates during latent infections in humans. *PLoS ONE* **9:** e91024.

Condos R, Rom WN, Schluger NW. 1997. Treatment of multidrug-resistant pulmonary tuberculosis with interferon-γ via aerosol. *Lancet* **349:** 1513–1515.

Corral LG, Kaplan G. 1999. Immunomodulation by thalidomide and thalidomide analogues. *Ann Rheum Dis* **58:** I107–I113.

Coussens AK, Wilkinson RJ, Hanifa Y, Nikolayevskyy V, Elkington PT, Islam K, Timms PM, Venton TR, Bothamley GH, Packe GE, et al. 2012. Vitamin D accelerates resolution of inflammatory responses during tuberculosis treatment. *Proc Natl Acad Sci* **109:** 15449–15454.

Critchley JA, Young F, Orton L, Garner P. 2013. Corticosteroids for prevention of mortality in people with tuberculosis: A systematic review and meta-analysis. *Lancet Infect Dis* **13:** 223–237.

D'Avila H, Melo RC, Parreira GG, Werneck-Barroso E, Castro-Faria-Neto HC, Bozza PT. 2006. *Mycobacterium bovis* bacillus Calmette-Guerin induces TLR2-mediated formation of lipid bodies: Intracellular domains for eicosanoid synthesis in vivo. *J Immunol* **176:** 3087–3097.

Dawson R, Condos R, Tse D, Huie ML, Ress S, Tseng CH, Brauns C, Weiden M, Hoshino Y, Bateman E, et al. 2009. Immunomodulation with recombinant interferon-γ1b in pulmonary tuberculosis. *PLoS ONE* **4:** e6984.

Desvignes L, Ernst JD. 2009. Interferon-γ-responsive nonhematopoietic cells regulate the immune response to *Mycobacterium tuberculosis*. *Immunity* **31:** 974–985.

Dhasmana DJ, Dheda K, Ravn P, Wilkinson RJ, Meintjes G. 2008. Immune reconstitution inflammatory syndrome in HIV-infected patients receiving antiretroviral therapy: Pathogenesis, clinical manifestations and management. *Drugs* **68:** 191–208.

Divangahi M, Chen M, Gan H, Desjardins D, Hickman TT, Lee DM, Fortune S, Behar SM, Remold HG. 2009. *Mycobacterium tuberculosis* evades macrophage defenses by inhibiting plasma membrane repair. *Nat Immunol* **10:** 899–906.

Divangahi M, Desjardins D, Nunes-Alves C, Remold HG, Behar SM. 2010. Eicosanoid pathways regulate adaptive immunity to *Mycobacterium tuberculosis*. *Nat Immunol* **11:** 751–758.

Dkhar HK, Nanduri R, Mahajan S, Dave S, Saini A, Somavarapu AK, Arora A, Parkesh R, Thakur KG, Mayilraj S, et al. 2014. *Mycobacterium tuberculosis* keto-mycolic acid and macrophage nuclear receptor TR4 modulate foamy biogenesis in granulomas: A case of a heterologous and noncanonical ligand-receptor pair. *J Immunol* **193:** 295–305.

Dorhoi A, Iannaccone M, Farinacci M, Fae KC, Schreiber J, Moura-Alves P, Nouailles G, Mollenkopf HJ, Oberbeck-Muller D, Jorg S, et al. 2013. MicroRNA-223 controls susceptibility to tuberculosis by regulating lung neutrophil recruitment. *J Clin Invest* **123:** 4836–4848.

Elkington P, Shiomi T, Breen R, Nuttall RK, Ugarte-Gil CA, Walker NF, Saraiva L, Pedersen B, Mauri F, Lipman M, et al. 2011a. MMP-1 drives immunopathology in human tuberculosis and transgenic mice. *J Clin Invest* **121:** 1827–1833.

Elkington PT, D'Armiento JM, Friedland JS. 2011b. Tuberculosis immunopathology: The neglected role of extracellular matrix destruction. *Sci Transl Med* **3:** 71ps76.

Elojeimy S, Holman DH, Liu X, El-Zawahry A, Villani M, Cheng JC, Mahdy A, Zeidan Y, Bielwaska A, Hannun YA, et al. 2006. New insights on the use of desipramine as an inhibitor for acid ceramidase. *FEBS Lett* **580:** 4751–4756.

Eum SY, Kong JH, Hong MS, Lee YJ, Kim JH, Hwang SH, Cho SN, Via LE, Barry CE., 3rd. 2010. Neutrophils are the predominant infected phagocytic cells in the airways of patients with active pulmonary TB. *Chest* **137:** 122–128.

Fabri M, Stenger S, Shin DM, Yuk JM, Liu PT, Realegeno S, Lee HM, Krutzik SR, Schenk M, Sieling PA, et al. 2011. Vitamin D is required for IFN-γ-mediated antimicrobial activity of human macrophages. *Sci Transl Med* **3:** 104ra102.

Flynn JL. 2006. Lessons from experimental *Mycobacterium tuberculosis* infections. *Microbes Infect* **8:** 1179–1188.

Ford CB, Lin PL, Chase MR, Shah RR, Iartchouk O, Galagan J, Mohaideen N, Ioerger TR, Sacchettini JC, Lipsitch M, et al. 2011. Use of whole genome sequencing to estimate the mutation rate of *Mycobacterium tuberculosis* during latent infection. *Nat Genet* **43:** 482–486.

Ford CB, Shah RR, Maeda MK, Gagneux S, Murray MB, Cohen T, Johnston JC, Gardy J, Lipsitch M, Fortune SM. 2013. *Mycobacterium tuberculosis* mutation rate estimates from different lineages predict substantial differences in the emergence of drug-resistant tuberculosis. *Nat Genet* **45:** 784–790.

Fukutomi Y, Maeda Y, Makino M. 2011. Apoptosis-inducing activity of clofazimine in macrophages. *Antimicrob Agents Chemother* **55:** 4000–4005.

Gandhi NR, Moll A, Sturm AW, Pawinski R, Govender T, Lalloo U, Zeller K, Andrews J, Friedland G. 2006. Extensively drug-resistant tuberculosis as a cause of death in patients co-infected with tuberculosis and HIV in a rural area of South Africa. *Lancet* **368:** 1575–1580.

Gandhi NR, Nunn P, Dheda K, Schaaf HS, Zignol M, van Soolingen D, Jensen P, Bayona J. 2010. Multidrug-resistant and extensively drug-resistant tuberculosis: A threat to global control of tuberculosis. *Lancet* **375:** 1830–1843.

Griffin JE, Pandey AK, Gilmore SA, Mizrahi V, McKinney JD, Bertozzi CR, Sassetti CM. 2012. Cholesterol catabolism by *Mycobacterium tuberculosis* requires transcriptional and metabolic adaptations. *Chem Biol* **19:** 218–227.

Grosset JH, Tyagi S, Almeida DV, Converse PJ, Li SY, Ammerman NC, Bishai WR, Enarson D, Trebucq A. 2013. Assessment of clofazimine activity in a second-line regimen for tuberculosis in mice. *Am J Respir Crit Care Med* **188:** 608–612.

Gutierrez MG, Master SS, Singh SB, Taylor GA, Colombo MI, Deretic V. 2004. Autophagy is a defense mechanism inhibiting BCG and *Mycobacterium tuberculosis* survival in infected macrophages. *Cell* **119:** 753–766.

Hakim JG, Ternouth I, Mushangi E, Siziya S, Robertson V, Malin A. 2000. Double blind randomised placebo controlled trial of adjunctive prednisolone in the treatment of effusive tuberculous pericarditis in HIV seropositive patients. *Heart* **84:** 183–188.

Hawn TR, Matheson AI, Maley SN, Vandal O. 2013. Host-directed therapeutics for tuberculosis: Can we harness the host? *Microbiol Mol Biol Rev* **77:** 608–627.

Hemmings FJ, Farhan M, Rowland J, Banken L, Jain R. 2001. Tolerability and pharmacokinetics of the collagenase-selective inhibitor Trocade in patients with rheumatoid arthritis. *Rheumatology* **40:** 537–543.

Iannaccone M, Dorhoi A, Kaufmann SH. 2014. Host-directed therapy of tuberculosis: What is in it for microRNA? *Expert Opin Ther Targets* **18:** 491–494.

Ioerger TR, O'Malley T, Liao R, Guinn KM, Hickey MJ, Mohaideen N, Murphy KC, Boshoff HI, Mizrahi V, Rubin EJ, et al. 2013. Identification of new drug targets and resistance mechanisms in *Mycobacterium tuberculosis*. *PLoS ONE* **8:** e75245.

Jayaswal S, Kamal MA, Dua R, Gupta S, Majumdar T, Das G, Kumar D, Rao KV. 2010. Identification of host-dependent survival factors for intracellular *Mycobacterium tuberculosis* through an siRNA screen. *PLoS Pathog* **6:** e1000839.

Johnson BJ, Bekker LG, Rickman R, Brown S, Lesser M, Ress S, Willcox P, Steyn L, Kaplan G. 1997. rhuIL-2 adjunctive therapy in multidrug resistant tuberculosis: A comparison of two treatment regimens and placebo. *Tuber Lung Dis* **78:** 195–203.

Johnson JL, Ssekasanvu E, Okwera A, Mayanja H, Hirsch CS, Nakibali JG, Jankus DD, Eisenach KD, Boom WH, Ellner JJ, et al. 2003. Randomized trial of adjunctive interleukin-2 in adults with pulmonary tuberculosis. *Am J Respir Crit Care Med* **168:** 185–191.

Kaufmann SH, Dorhoi A. 2013. Inflammation in tuberculosis: Interactions, imbalances and interventions. *Curr Opin Immunol* **25:** 441–449.

Kaufmann SH, Lange C, Rao M, Balaji KN, Lotze M, Schito M, Zumla AI, Maeurer M. 2014. Progress in tuberculosis vaccine development and host-directed therapies—A state of the art review. *Lancet Respir Med* **2:** 301–320.

Kim JH, Scialli AR. 2011. Thalidomide: The tragedy of birth defects and the effective treatment of disease. *Toxicol Sci* **122:** 1–6.

Kim MJ, Wainwright HC, Locketz M, Bekker LG, Walther GB, Dittrich C, Visser A, Wang W, Hsu FF, Wiehart U, et al. 2010. Caseation of human tuberculosis granulomas correlates with elevated host lipid metabolism. *EMBO Mol Med* **2:** 258–274.

Kim JJ, Lee HM, Shin DM, Kim W, Yuk JM, Jin HS, Lee SH, Cha GH, Kim JM, Lee ZW, et al. 2012. Host cell autophagy activated by antibiotics is required for their effective antimycobacterial drug action. *Cell Host Microbe* **11:** 457–468.

Kiss M, Czimmerer Z, Nagy L. 2013. The role of lipid-activated nuclear receptors in shaping macrophage and dendritic cell function: From physiology to pathology. *J Allergy Clin Immunol* **132:** 264–286.

Koh WJ, Kwon OJ, Suh GY, Chung MP, Kim H, Lee NY, Kim TS, Lee KS. 2004. Six-month therapy with aerosolized interferon-γ for refractory multidrug-resistant pulmonary tuberculosis. *J Korean Med Sci* **19:** 167–171.

Koo MS, Manca C, Yang G, O'Brien P, Sung N, Tsenova L, Subbian S, Fallows D, Muller G, Ehrt S, et al. 2011. Phosphodiesterase 4 inhibition reduces innate immunity and improves isoniazid clearance of *Mycobacterium tuberculosis* in the lungs of infected mice. *PLoS ONE* **6:** e17091.

Krutzik SR, Hewison M, Liu PT, Robles JA, Stenger S, Adams JS, Modlin RL. 2008. IL-15 links TLR2/1-induced macrophage differentiation to the vitamin D-dependent antimicrobial pathway. *J Immunol* **181:** 7115–7120.

Kuijl C, Savage ND, Marsman M, Tuin AW, Janssen L, Egan DA, Ketema M, van den Nieuwendijk R, van den Eeden SJ, Geluk A, et al. 2007. Intracellular bacterial growth is controlled by a kinase network around PKB/AKT1. *Nature* **450:** 725–730.

Kumar D, Nath L, Kamal MA, Varshney A, Jain A, Singh S, Rao KV. 2010. Genome-wide analysis of the host intracellular network that regulates survival of *Mycobacterium tuberculosis*. *Cell* **140:** 731–743.

Liu PT, Stenger S, Li H, Wenzel L, Tan BH, Krutzik SR, Ochoa MT, Schauber J, Wu K, Meinken C, et al. 2006. Toll-like receptor triggering of a vitamin D-mediated human antimicrobial response. *Science* **311:** 1770–1773.

MacMicking JD, Taylor GA, McKinney JD. 2003. Immune control of tuberculosis by IFN-γ-inducible LRG-47. *Science* **302:** 654–659.

Mahajan S, Dkhar HK, Chandra V, Dave S, Nanduri R, Janmeja AK, Agrewala JN, Gupta P. 2012. *Mycobacterium tuberculosis* modulates macrophage lipid-sensing nuclear receptors PPARγ and TR4 for survival. *J Immunol* **188:** 5593–5603.

Maiga M, Agarwal N, Ammerman NC, Gupta R, Guo H, Maiga MC, Lun S, Bishai WR. 2012. Successful shortening of tuberculosis treatment using adjuvant host-directed therapy with FDA-approved phosphodiesterase inhibitors in the mouse model. *PLoS ONE* **7:** e30749.

Maiga M, Ammerman NC, Maiga MC, Tounkara A, Siddiqui S, Polis M, Murphy R, Bishai WR. 2013. Adjuvant host-directed therapy with types 3 and 5 but not type 4 phosphodiesterase inhibitors shortens the duration of tuberculosis treatment. *J Infect Dis* **208:** 512–519.

Marais S, Wilkinson RJ, Pepper DJ, Meintjes G. 2009. Management of patients with the immune reconstitution inflammatory syndrome. *Curr HIV/AIDS Rep* **6:** 162–171.

Martineau AR, Newton SM, Wilkinson KA, Kampmann B, Hall BM, Nawroly N, Packe GE, Davidson RN, Griffiths CJ, Wilkinson RJ. 2007. Neutrophil-mediated innate immune resistance to mycobacteria. *J Clin Invest* **117:** 1988–1994.

Martineau AR, Timms PM, Bothamley GH, Hanifa Y, Islam K, Claxton AP, Packe GE, Moore-Gillon JC, Darmalingam M, Davidson RN, et al. 2011. High-dose vitamin D(3) during intensive-phase antimicrobial treatment of pulmonary tuberculosis: A double-blind randomised controlled trial. *Lancet* **377:** 242–250.

Mayer-Barber KD, Andrade BB, Barber DL, Hieny S, Feng CG, Caspar P, Oland S, Gordon S, Sher A. 2011. Innate and adaptive interferons suppress IL-1α and IL-1β production by distinct pulmonary myeloid subsets during

Mycobacterium tuberculosis infection. *Immunity* **35:** 1023–1034.

Mayer-Barber KD, Andrade BB, Oland SD, Amaral EP, Barber DL, Gonzalez J, Derrick SC, Shi R, Kumar NP, Wei W, et al. 2014. Host-directed therapy of tuberculosis based on interleukin-1 and type I interferon crosstalk. *Nature* **511:** 99–103.

Mayosi BM, Ntsekhe M, Volmink JA, Commerford PJ. 2002. Interventions for treating tuberculous pericarditis. *Cochrane Database Syst Rev* **2002:** CD000526.

Meintjes G, Lawn SD, Scano F, Maartens G, French MA, Worodria W, Elliott JH, Murdoch D, Wilkinson RJ, Seyler C, et al. 2008. Tuberculosis-associated immune reconstitution inflammatory syndrome: Case definitions for use in resource-limited settings. *Lancet Infect Dis* **8:** 516–523.

Meintjes G, Wilkinson RJ, Morroni C, Pepper DJ, Rebe K, Rangaka MX, Oni T, Maartens G. 2010. Randomized placebo-controlled trial of prednisone for paradoxical tuberculosis-associated immune reconstitution inflammatory syndrome. *AIDS* **24:** 2381–2390.

Misra UK, Kalita J, Nair PP. 2010. Role of aspirin in tuberculous meningitis: A randomized open label placebo controlled trial. *J Neurol Sci* **293:** 12–17.

Morcos MM, Gabr AA, Samuel S, Kamel M, el Baz M, el Beshry M, Michail RR. 1998. Vitamin D administration to tuberculous children and its value. *Boll Chim Farm* **137:** 157–164.

Morris T, Stables M, Hobbs A, de Souza P, Colville-Nash P, Warner T, Newson J, Bellingan G, Gilroy DW. 2009. Effects of low-dose aspirin on acute inflammatory responses in humans. *J Immunol* **183:** 2089–2096.

Nandi B, Behar SM. 2011. Regulation of neutrophils by interferon-γ limits lung inflammation during tuberculosis infection. *J Exp Med* **208:** 2251–2262.

Napier RJ, Rafi W, Cheruvu M, Powell KR, Zaunbrecher MA, Bornmann W, Salgame P, Shinnick TM, Kalman D. 2011. Imatinib-sensitive tyrosine kinases regulate mycobacterial pathogenesis and represent therapeutic targets against tuberculosis. *Cell Host Microbe* **10:** 475–485.

Nouailles G, Dorhoi A, Koch M, Zerrahn J, Weiner J, 3rd, Fae KC, Arrey F, Kuhlmann S, Bandermann S, Loewe D, et al. 2014. CXCL5-secreting pulmonary epithelial cells drive destructive neutrophilic inflammation in tuberculosis. *J Clin Invest* **124:** 1268–1282.

Nursyam EW, Amin Z, Rumende CM. 2006. The effect of vitamin D as supplementary treatment in patients with moderately advanced pulmonary tuberculous lesion. *Acta Med Indones* **38:** 3–5.

Overall CM, Lopez-Otin C. 2002. Strategies for MMP inhibition in cancer: Innovations for the post-trial era. *Nat Rev Cancer* **2:** 657–672.

Pan H, Yan BS, Rojas M, Shebzukhov YV, Zhou H, Kobzik L, Higgins DE, Daly MJ, Bloom BR, Kramnik I. 2005. Ipr1 gene mediates innate immunity to tuberculosis. *Nature* **434:** 767–772.

Pandey AK, Sassetti CM. 2008. Mycobacterial persistence requires the utilization of host cholesterol. *Proc Natl Acad Sci* **105:** 4376–4380.

Parihar SP, Guler R, Khutlang R, Lang DM, Hurdayal R, Mhlanga MM, Suzuki H, Marais AD, Brombacher F. 2014. Statin therapy reduces the *Mycobacterium tuberculosis* burden in human macrophages and in mice by enhancing autophagy and phagosome maturation. *J Infect Dis* **209:** 754–763.

Parks WC, Wilson CL, Lopez-Boado YS. 2004. Matrix metalloproteinases as modulators of inflammation and innate immunity. *Nat Rev Immunol* **4:** 617–629.

Philips JA, Rubin EJ, Perrimon N. 2005. *Drosophila* RNAi screen reveals CD36 family member required for mycobacterial infection. *Science* **309:** 1251–1253.

Podinovskaia M, Lee W, Caldwell S, Russell DG. 2013. Infection of macrophages with *Mycobacterium tuberculosis* induces global modifications to phagosomal function. *Cell Microbiol* **15:** 843–859.

Prasad K, Singh MB. 2008. Corticosteroids for managing tuberculous meningitis. *Cochrane Database Syst Rev* **2008:** CD002244.

Quarato G, D'Aprile A, Gavillet B, Vuagniaux G, Moradpour D, Capitanio N, Piccoli C. 2012. The cyclophilin inhibitor alisporivir prevents hepatitis C virus-mediated mitochondrial dysfunction. *Hepatology* **55:** 1333–1343.

Rajaram MV, Brooks MN, Morris JD, Torrelles JB, Azad AK, Schlesinger LS. 2010. *Mycobacterium tuberculosis* activates human macrophage peroxisome proliferator-activated receptor γ linking mannose receptor recognition to regulation of immune responses. *J Immunol* **185:** 929–942.

Rajaram MV, Ni B, Morris JD, Brooks MN, Carlson TK, Bakthavachalu B, Schoenberg DR, Torrelles JB, Schlesinger LS. 2011. *Mycobacterium tuberculosis* lipomannan blocks TNF biosynthesis by regulating macrophage MAPK-activated protein kinase 2 (MK2) and microRNA miR-125b. *Proc Natl Acad Sci* **108:** 17408–17413.

Ramakrishnan L. 2012. Revisiting the role of the granuloma in tuberculosis. *Nat Rev Immunol* **12:** 352–366.

Rask-Andersen M, Masuram S, Schioth HB. 2014. The druggable genome: Evaluation of drug targets in clinical trials suggests major shifts in molecular class and indication. *Annu Rev Pharmacol Toxicol* **54:** 9–26.

Ray KK, Seshasai SR, Erqou S, Sever P, Jukema JW, Ford I, Sattar N. 2010. Statins and all-cause mortality in high-risk primary prevention: A meta-analysis of 11 randomized controlled trials involving 65,229 participants. *Arch Intern Med* **170:** 1024–1031.

Reeves PM, Bommarius B, Lebeis S, McNulty S, Christensen J, Swimm A, Chahroudi A, Chavan R, Feinberg MB, Veach D, et al. 2005. Disabling poxvirus pathogenesis by inhibition of Abl-family tyrosine kinases. *Nat Med* **11:** 731–739.

Roca FJ, Ramakrishnan L. 2013. TNF dually mediates resistance and susceptibility to mycobacteria via mitochondrial reactive oxygen species. *Cell* **153:** 521–534.

Rubinsztein DC, Codogno P, Levine B. 2012. Autophagy modulation as a potential therapeutic target for diverse diseases. *Nat Rev Drug Discov* **11:** 709–730.

Sacchettini JC, Rubin EJ, Freundlich JS. 2008. Drugs versus bugs: In pursuit of the persistent predator *Mycobacterium tuberculosis*. *Nat Rev Microbiol* **6:** 41–52.

Schoeman JF, Van Zyl LE, Laubscher JA, Donald PR. 1997. Effect of corticosteroids on intracranial pressure, computed tomographic findings, and clinical outcome in young children with tuberculous meningitis. *Pediatrics* **99:** 226–231.

Schoeman JF, Springer P, Ravenscroft A, Donald PR, Bekker LG, van Rensburg AJ, Hanekom WA, Haslett PA, Kaplan G. 2000. Adjunctive thalidomide therapy of childhood tuberculous meningitis: Possible anti-inflammatory role. *J Child Neurol* **15:** 497–503.

Schoeman JF, Springer P, van Rensburg AJ, Swanevelder S, Hanekom WA, Haslett PA, Kaplan G. 2004. Adjunctive thalidomide therapy for childhood tuberculous meningitis: Results of a randomized study. *J Child Neurol* **19:** 250–257.

Schoeman JF, Janse van Rensburg A, Laubscher JA, Springer P. 2011. The role of aspirin in childhood tuberculous meningitis. *J Child Neurol* **26:** 956–962.

Schwegmann A, Brombacher F. 2008. Host-directed drug targeting of factors hijacked by pathogens. *Sci Signal* **1:** re8.

Shah NS, Wright A, Bai GH, Barrera L, Boulahbal F, Martin-Casabona N, Drobniewski F, Gilpin C, Havelkova M, Lepe R, et al. 2007. Worldwide emergence of extensively drug-resistant tuberculosis. *Emerg Infect Dis* **13:** 380–387.

Shoji-Kawata S, Sumpter R, Leveno M, Campbell GR, Zou Z, Kinch L, Wilkins AD, Sun Q, Pallauf K, MacDuff D, et al. 2013. Identification of a candidate therapeutic autophagy-inducing peptide. *Nature* **494:** 201–206.

Singh SB, Davis AS, Taylor GA, Deretic V. 2006. Human IRGM induces autophagy to eliminate intracellular mycobacteria. *Science* **313:** 1438–1441.

Singh V, Jamwal S, Jain R, Verma P, Gokhale R, Rao KV. 2012. *Mycobacterium tuberculosis*-driven targeted recalibration of macrophage lipid homeostasis promotes the foamy phenotype. *Cell Host Microbe* **12:** 669–681.

Stanley SA, Barczak AK, Silvis MR, Luo SS, Sogi K, Vokes M, Bray MA, Carpenter AE, Moore CB, Siddiqi N, et al. 2014. Identification of host-targeted small molecules that restrict intracellular *Mycobacterium tuberculosis* growth. *PLoS Pathog* **10:** e1003946.

Subbian S, Tsenova L, O'Brien P, Yang G, Koo MS, Peixoto B, Fallows D, Dartois V, Muller G, Kaplan G. 2011a. Phosphodiesterase-4 inhibition alters gene expression and improves isoniazid-mediated clearance of *Mycobacterium tuberculosis* in rabbit lungs. *PLoS Pathog* **7:** e1002262.

Subbian S, Tsenova L, O'Brien P, Yang G, Koo MS, Peixoto B, Fallows D, Zeldis JB, Muller G, Kaplan G. 2011b. Phosphodiesterase-4 inhibition combined with isoniazid treatment of rabbits with pulmonary tuberculosis reduces macrophage activation and lung pathology. *Am J Pathol* **179:** 289–301.

Sundaramurthy V, Barsacchi R, Samusik N, Marsico G, Gilleron J, Kalaidzidis I, Meyenhofer F, Bickle M, Kalaidzidis Y, Zerial M. 2013. Integration of chemical and RNAi multiparametric profiles identifies triggers of intracellular mycobacterial killing. *Cell Host Microbe* **13:** 129–142.

Taylor JL, Hattle JM, Dreitz SA, Troudt JM, Izzo LS, Basaraba RJ, Orme IM, Matrisian LM, Izzo AA. 2006. Role for matrix metalloproteinase 9 in granuloma formation during pulmonary *Mycobacterium tuberculosis* infection. *Infect Immun* **74:** 6135–6144.

Thwaites GE, Nguyen DB, Nguyen HD, Hoang TQ, Do TT, Nguyen TC, Nguyen QH, Nguyen TT, Nguyen NH, Nguyen TN, et al. 2004. Dexamethasone for the treatment of tuberculous meningitis in adolescents and adults. *N Engl J Med* **351:** 1741–1751.

Thwaites G, Fisher M, Hemingway C, Scott G, Solomon T, Innes J, British Infection S. 2009. British Infection Society guidelines for the diagnosis and treatment of tuberculosis of the central nervous system in adults and children. *J Infect* **59:** 167–187.

Tobin DM, Vary JC Jr, Ray JP, Walsh GS, Dunstan SJ, Bang ND, Hagge DA, Khadge S, King MC, Hawn TR, et al. 2010. The lta4 h locus modulates susceptibility to mycobacterial infection in zebrafish and humans. *Cell* **140:** 717–730.

Tobin DM, Roca FJ, Oh SF, McFarland R, Vickery TW, Ray JP, Ko DC, Zou Y, Bang ND, Chau TT, et al. 2012. Host genotype-specific therapies can optimize the inflammatory response to mycobacterial infections. *Cell* **148:** 434–446.

Ustianowski A, Shaffer R, Collin S, Wilkinson RJ, Davidson RN. 2005. Prevalence and associations of vitamin D deficiency in foreign-born persons with tuberculosis in London. *J Infect* **50:** 432–437.

Vandenabeele P, Galluzzi L, Vanden Berghe T, Kroemer G. 2010. Molecular mechanisms of necroptosis: An ordered cellular explosion. *Nat Rev Mol Cell Biol* **11:** 700–714.

Verway M, Bouttier M, Wang TT, Carrier M, Calderon M, An BS, Devemy E, McIntosh F, Divangahi M, Behr MA, et al. 2013. Vitamin D induces interleukin-1β expression: Paracrine macrophage epithelial signaling controls *M. tuberculosis* infection. *PLoS Pathog* **9:** e1003407.

Vilaplana C, Marzo E, Tapia G, Diaz J, Garcia V, Cardona PJ. 2013. Ibuprofen therapy resulted in significantly decreased tissue bacillary loads and increased survival in a new murine experimental model of active tuberculosis. *J Infect Dis* **208:** 199–202.

Volkman HE, Pozos TC, Zheng J, Davis JM, Rawls JF, Ramakrishnan L. 2010. Tuberculous granuloma induction via interaction of a bacterial secreted protein with host epithelium. *Science* **327:** 466–469.

Watson RO, Manzanillo PS, Cox JS. 2012. Extracellular *M. tuberculosis* DNA targets bacteria for autophagy by activating the host DNA-sensing pathway. *Cell* **150:** 803–815.

Wejse C, Olesen R, Rabna P, Kaestel P, Gustafson P, Aaby P, Andersen PL, Glerup H, Sodemann M. 2007. Serum 25-hydroxyvitamin D in a West African population of tuberculosis patients and unmatched healthy controls. *Am J Clin Nutr* **86:** 1376–1383.

Wejse C, Gomes VF, Rabna P, Gustafson P, Aaby P, Lisse IM, Andersen PL, Glerup H, Sodemann M. 2009. Vitamin D as supplementary treatment for tuberculosis: A double-blind, randomized, placebo-controlled trial. *Am J Respir Crit Care Med* **179:** 843–850.

WHO. 2010. *Multidrug and extensively drug-resistant TB (M/XDR-TB): 2010 global report on surveillance and response.* World Health Organization, Geneva.

Wilkinson RJ. 2014. Host-directed therapies against tuberculosis. *Lancet Respir Med* **2:** 85–87.

Wilkinson RJ, Llewelyn M, Toossi Z, Patel P, Pasvol G, Lalvani A, Wright D, Latif M, Davidson RN. 2000. Influence of vitamin D deficiency and vitamin D receptor polymorphisms on tuberculosis among Gujarati Asians in west London: A case-control study. *Lancet* **355:** 618–621.

Wu K, Koo J, Jiang X, Chen R, Cohen SN, Nathan C. 2012. Improved control of tuberculosis and activation of macrophages in mice lacking protein kinase R. *PLoS ONE* **7:** e30512.

Yang CT, Cambier CJ, Davis JM, Hall CJ, Crosier PS, Ramakrishnan L. 2012. Neutrophils exert protection in the early tuberculous granuloma by oxidative killing of mycobacteria phagocytosed from infected macrophages. *Cell Host Microbe* **12:** 301–312.

Yuk JM, Shin DM, Lee HM, Yang CS, Jin HS, Kim KK, Lee ZW, Lee SH, Kim JM, Jo EK. 2009. Vitamin D3 induces autophagy in human monocytes/macrophages via cathelicidin. *Cell Host Microbe* **6:** 231–243.

Zumla A, Nahid P, Cole ST. 2013. Advances in the development of new tuberculosis drugs and treatment regimens. *Nat Rev Drug Discov* **12:** 388–404.

Zumla AI, Gillespie SH, Hoelscher M, Philips PP, Cole ST, Abubakar I, McHugh TD, Schito M, Maeurer M, Nunn AJ. 2014. New antituberculosis drugs, regimens, and adjunct therapies: Needs, advances, and future prospects. *Lancet Infect Dis* **14:** 327–340.

Comparative Genomics of Mycobacteria: Some Answers, Yet More New Questions

Marcel A. Behr[1,2]

[1]McGill International Tuberculosis Centre, McGill University, Montreal, Quebec H3G 1A4, Canada
[2]Research Institute of the McGill University Health Centre, Montreal, Quebec H3G 1A4, Canada
Correspondence: marcel.behr@mcgill.ca

Comparative genomic studies permit a genus-level perspective on the distinction between environmental mycobacteria and *Mycobacterium tuberculosis*, as well as a species-level assessment of genetic variability within *M. tuberculosis*. Both of these strata of evolutionary analysis serve to generate hypotheses regarding the genomic basis of *M. tuberculosis* virulence. In contrasting lessons from macroevolutionary study and microevolutionary study, one can form predictions about which segments of the genome are likely to be essential for or dispensable for the pathogenesis of tuberculosis. Although some of these predictions have been experimentally verified, notable exceptions challenge the direct link between these virulence factors and the capacity of *M. tuberculosis* to successfully cause disease and propagate between human hosts. These unexpected findings serve as the stimulus for further studies, using genomic comparisons and other approaches, to better define the remarkable success of this recalcitrant pathogen.

Since the first genome sequence of *Mycobacterium tuberculosis* was published in 1998 (Cole et al. 1998), a number of investigators have analyzed and used these data to ask what makes this bacteria particularly effective at causing infection and disease in humans. One attractive approach involves comparing the genome of the reference strain *M. tuberculosis* H37Rv with other related bacteria; in theory, genes that are deleted among bacteria that successfully cause disease are dispensable for full virulence (Tsolaki et al. 2004), whereas genes that have been deleted in strains of low virulence present as candidates for virulence genes (Behr et al. 1999). Although the technologies applied have evolved considerably from late 1990s, the goal of this review is not to focus on the techniques (subtractive hybridization [Mahairas et al. 1996], DNA microarrays [Behr et al. 1999], GeneChips [Salamon et al. 2000], tiling arrays [Leung et al., 2008], whole-genome sequencing [Garnier et al. 2003; Brosch et al. 2007]) but instead to highlight certain key findings that have been confirmed in controlled, experimental studies. Additionally, an attempt will be made to introduce somewhat unexpected observations from comparative genomics that suggest that our understanding of the genomic basis of *M. tuberculosis* pathogenicity might benefit from further investigation.

Cite this article as *Cold Spring Harb Perspect Med* doi: 10.1101/cshperspect.a021204

In terms of strata of investigation, comparative genomics can address microevolution or macroevolution. Because *M. tuberculosis* is strictly a subspecies of the *M. tuberculosis* complex, one can consider genomic differences at the level of (1) variability within *M. tuberculosis* sensu stricto, such as strain–strain differences; (2) variability within the *M. tuberculosis* complex, such as *M. tuberculosis* versus *Mycobacterium bovis*; and (3) variability between *M. tuberculosis* and nontuberculous mycobacteria (NTM), such as *Mycobacterium kansasii* and *Mycobacterium marinum*. In this review, I will comment on each of these levels of variability, citing selectively rather than systemically from the published literature that has accrued in the past two decades of comparative genomic studies.

M. tuberculosis SENSU STRICTO VARIABILITY

The existence of *M. tuberculosis* variability was recognized for more than two decades for molecular epidemiologic studies that exploited DNA differences between isolates to track transmission patterns in space and time (discussed in more detail in Niemann and Supply 2014). Using a number of different genotyping modalities, it has now been robustly shown that there are genetically defined lineages of *M. tuberculosis* (Fig. 1) that differ in their geographic distribution, broadly following the history of human migrations out of Africa toward different regions of the planet. A key pending question is whether these genomically distinct strains of *M. tuberculosis* differ in terms of their ability to infect, cause disease, and transmit across human populations.

A number of papers have experimentally documented *M. tuberculosis* strain differences, in vitro more so than in vivo (Manca et al. 1999, 2001, 2004; Reed et al. 2004, 2007; Barczak et al. 2005; Tsenova et al. 2005; Fallow et al. 2010; Homolka et al. 2010; Krishnan et al. 2011; Reiling et al. 2013). However, a key epidemiologic filter that should not be overlooked is that the bacteria chosen for such studies have all most recently caused clinical disease. Therefore, although we might potentially be exposed to mutants that are unable to cause infection, or we might be infected with mutants that are unable to cause disease, these bacteria will not available for genomic interrogation. When we do comparative genomics of *M. tuberculosis* isolates, we cannot ask about the absolute capacity to cause disease, but rather about relative differences in pathogenicity, *among successful strains*. A further consideration is that when experimentally testing whether certain strains are more or less virulent, many investigators use a murine model that best approximates progressive primary tuberculosis (TB) disease, without latency, reactivation, or chronic cavitary disease. In such a model, one might interpret an earlier time to death as evidence of a more "virulent" strain, which it clearly is, from the vantage of the in-

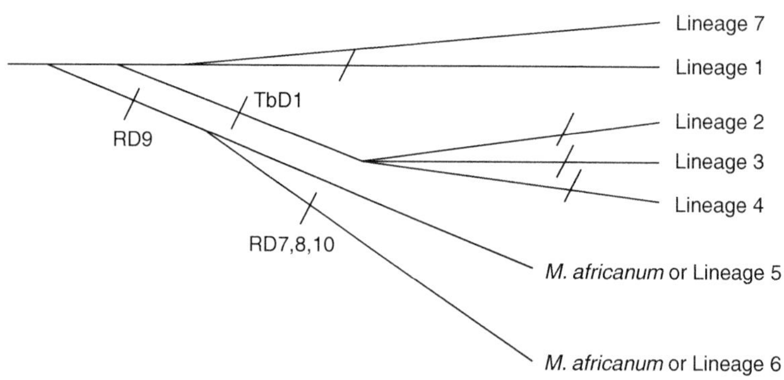

Figure 1. Phylogenetic relationship of *Mycobacterium tuberculosis* lineages. Lineages 5 and 6 were previously named *Mycobacterium africanum*, types 1 and 2, although some authors consider these to be two lineages of human-adapted *M. tuberculosis*. The short lines at right angles to lineages refer to specific genomic deletions.

fected mouse (Reed et al. 2004). However, this laboratory phenotype may be a proxy for lower transmissibility, because invasive, fatal TB is detrimental to the fitness of both the host and the pathogen. Conversely, a strain that is unable to kill the mouse after a prolonged infection might be deemed to have attenuated virulence (Manca et al. 1999), when an alternative interpretation is that this strain is better suited for generating a chronic pulmonary focus in a relatively well host. Thus, before asking whether we can document different between strains in controlled, experimental infections, we need to ask whether the laboratory models we use address the epidemiologic observations of "success" in the field. Whether different strains have a different propensity toward drug resistance and whether this could impart fitness advantages in the face of antibiotic pressures are completely separate matters that are addressed in Niemann and Supply (2014).

Given the preceding considerations, it can be hypothesized that genomic regions that are deleted in isolates from active TB cases might be "dispensable" regions that are not absolutely required for the capacity of the organism to cause transmissible disease. This latter proposition, however, challenges the importance of certain experimentally proven virulence factors. For example, Lineage 4 (or Euro-American) bacteria are incapable of producing phenolic glycolipids (PGLs), a property that has been variably associated with virulence in murine models of disease (Reed et al. 2004; Sinsimer et al. 2008). Yet, Lineage 4 bacilli successfully swept across the Americas, as documented in molecular epidemiologic papers tracking their spread in historical (Pepperell et al. 2011) and modern epidemics (Nguyen et al. 2003). Does this suggest something about the human hosts encountered by these bacteria, or does this imply that *M. tuberculosis* can successfully cause disease without PGLs by altering the expression and/or production of alternative virulence factors? Another example is the *DosR* regulon, so named because of the regulator that controls expression of a defined set of genes upon bacterial exposure to hypoxic conditions (Park et al. 2003). In laboratory investigations, it has been shown that this regulatory response is critical for the capacity of *M. tuberculosis* to endure low oxygen tension (Gautam et al. 2014). Furthermore, the demonstration that some of the proteins coded by *DosR* genes elicit adaptive immune responses in mice and humans suggests that at least some of these proteins are involved in infection, persistence, or the generation of transmissible disease (Leyten et al. 2006; Roupie et al. 2007). Yet, sequence analysis of a Colombian virulent isolate found a 3.6-kB deletion that eliminates two *DosR* genes, *Rv1996* and *Rv1997* (Isaza et al. 2012). Furthermore, transcriptome studies indicate that some of the so-called Beijing strains have lost the fine-tuning ability of the *DosR* regulon and constitutively express these genes instead (Fallow et al. 2010). Again, does this suggest that certain components of the *DosR* regulon are not important in certain people or rather does the genome provide redundant mechanisms to cope with changes in oxygen tension during the infection cycle? If PGLs and *DosR* are not essential for *M. tuberculosis* to cause disease *in natura*, are there unknown virulence mechanisms that remain to be discovered?

The converse approach is to ask which genes are retained in clinical isolates, as there are two possible explanations: Either these genes are situated in regions of the genome that do not accommodate genomic disruption or deletions at these sites are structurally permissible but have been selected against during the thousands of years of *M. tuberculosis*–human coevolution. The list of conserved genes is not readily accessible, in part because most publications detail missing genes and in part because whole-genome sequencing of isolates from around the world is ongoing. Therefore, with one publication, a "conserved" gene today can become a "dispensable" gene tomorrow. However, among a smaller list of genes that appear to be consistently found in isolates to date, it is possible to ask about variability within genes, as has been performed in a study of genes coding for experimentally proven antigenic proteins. This provocative paper found that genes for antigens are less variable than genes defined as "essential genes" in transposon screens (Sassetti and Rubin 2003; Sassetti et al. 2003), and that the motif coding for the epitopes was most conserved (Comas et al. 2010). This finding suggests that *M. tuberculosis* may depend on adaptive immune responses for its capacity to cause disease and/or transmit, such that mutations in these epitopes adversely affect the bacterial life cycle. The notion that *M. tuberculosis* requires the elaboration of a cell-mediate immune response to successfully transmit among humans has received independent support from epidemiologic studies, in which HIV-negative TB patients are more likely to transmit to their contacts than TB patients suffering from coinfection from HIV/AIDS (Corbett et al. 2006).

Beyond providing lists of genes that are variable or conserved, comparative genomics allows one to derive robust phylogenies of lineages that are found around the world, revealing geographic associations of strains over time suggestive of a stable host–pathogen relationship. Settings with more than one strain offer epidemiologists an opportunity to ask whether different major lineages of *M. tuberculosis* behave comparably *in natura*. Although there have been a number of reports in which one or another genomically defined lineage has been particularly successful, it is not always clear whether that particular strain was "good" or "lucky." For instance, an outbreak of TB in an AIDS hospice does not prove a more successful strain when a more likely explanation here would be a cluster of profoundly susceptible hosts (Daley et al. 1992). Furthermore, in many molecular epidemiology studies, the foreign/imported strains were less likely to transmit than the local strain, for a variety of social and behavioral reasons (Alland et al. 1994; Small et al. 1994). Thus, if a molecular epidemiology study investigates bacterial lineage, it can be predicted that the "local" strain may appear to be a risk factor for ongoing transmission, when in fact the apparent association may be confounded by the kinds of people who are infected with this strain. An alternative to looking at bacterial performance in a setting with high transmission is to observe the clinical and public health consequences of different strains that are introduced into a low-transmission setting. In Montreal, Canada, *M. tuberculosis* is imported via immigration from more than 80 countries in the world, whereupon these bacteria encounter a city with very little ongoing transmission (Kulaga et al. 2002). Additionally, all TB patients are managed in a comparable manner through a publicly funded health-care system, with patient care evidently provided blinded to strain identity. By typing isolates according to the major global lineages (Reed et al. 2009), we have found remarkably few differences in clinical outcomes or rates of tuberculin conversions of household contacts (Albanna et al. 2011). Importantly, TB due to the East-Asian/Lineage 2/Beijing strain has not behaved in a discernibly different manner than other strains from around the world, an observation also described in Switzerland (Fenner et al. 2012). Moreover, although we have obtained no evidence whatsoever of a "more virulent" strain in Montreal, in-depth analysis of Lineage 3 (sometimes called East-African-Indian lineage) revealed that these organisms were *less likely* to cause severe disease and that close contacts of patients producing these organisms were *less likely* to have a tuberculin conversion (Albanna et al. 2011). How a strain can propagate despite lower virulence begs a largely theoretical question. One possibility is that strains that evolved in densely populated regions of the world might depend on a high-transmission environment for their propagation. If true, when such a strain is introduced into a low-transmission environment, the relatively reduced virulence is more easily observed. The notion of whether (and how) strains with lesser virulence are able to persist in their host population is reconsidered below in the section on *M. tuberculosis* complex variability.

M. tuberculosis COMPLEX VARIABILITY

The existence of phenotypic differences between the human and the bovine tubercle bacillus was documented in the 19th century. These organisms, subsequently named *M. tuberculosis* and *M. bovis*, were assayed in a comparative virulence assay; both organisms were able to cause disease in guinea pigs but only *M. bovis* was virulent in rabbits (Smith 1898). Subsequent laboratory isolations revealed a collection of related bacteria, of which at least eight are recognized members of the *M. tuberculosis* complex (MTC), complete with a Latin name: *M. tuberculosis*, *Mycobacterium africanum*, *Mycobacterium microtii*, *Mycobacterium mungi*, *Mycobacterium orygis*, *Mycobacterium pinnipedii*, *Mycobacterium caprae*, and *M. bovis*. The dassie bacillus has not been formally named but has a distinct genomic profile that will be detailed below (Mostowy et al. 2004). A single recent isolate from a wild chimpanzee has been subject to genomic study, potentially suggesting either a new lineage, but more such isolates will be required before its situation in the MTC can be affirmed (Coscolla et al. 2013). A group of bacteria called the smooth tubercle bacilli (STB), including *Mycobacterium canetti*, are considered by some to be an out-group and by others to be members of the MTC (Gutierrez et al. 2005; Brisse et al. 2006; Supply et al. 2013). With further sampling of mammalian hosts, in the wild and in zoos, it is possible that new variants of the MTC might be uncovered in coming years.

In terms of genetic differences, a number of platforms have been used to confirm distinct genomic identities of MTC members (Fig. 2) (Brosch et al. 2002; Mostowy et al. 2002). What is harder to establish is the phenotypic basis for these variable host–pathogen relationships. For some of these organisms, the bacteria are not easily obtained for laboratory investigation (Alexander et al. 2010). Even if these were to be obtained and grown to a standard inoculum, with minimal in vitro passage, the kinds of comparative virulence studies conducted by Theobald Smith in the 1890s may not explain how each MTC member causes disease in its own particular host. Therefore, to date, genomic comparisons among the MTC have helped formulate a MTC phylogeny, but linking genomic deletions to a phenotypic effect suffers from many of the same issues raised for *M. tuberculosis* sensu stricto, with the additional complicating factor of the many different hosts involved. Because it is not currently feasible to experimentally complete the in vivo 8 × 8 host–pathogen matrix (i.e., by putting *M. pinnipedii* into dassies, etc.), the explanation for the long-standing associations might be an intimate host–pathogen interaction determined by a specific molecular fit or more trivially by the possibility that dassies have never been exposed to *M. pinnipedii*.

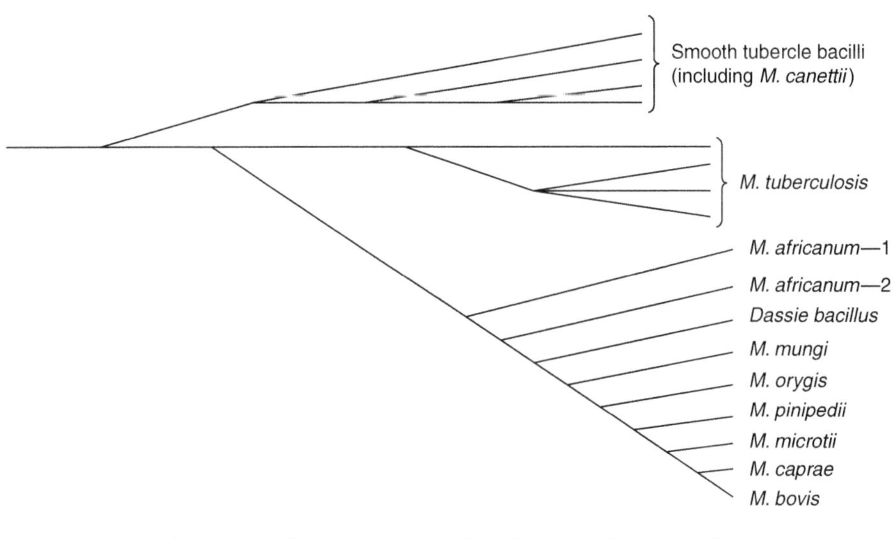

Figure 2. Phylogenetic relationship of *Mycobacterium tuberculosis* complex (MTC) lineages. Here, *Mycobacterium africanum* is clustered with "exotic" members of the MTC based on shared genomic deletions. Only virulent *Mycobacterium bovis* is shown, with *M. bovis* BCG representing a laboratory-adapted strain of *M. bovis*.

As noted before, if a MTC variant lacks a genomic region and is able to successfully transmit within its host species, it can be argued that genes in this deleted region are dispensable for full virulence. Yet, the RD1 locus, now known to code for proteins of the ESX-1 secretion system, has been independently deleted three times in naturally occurring members of the MTC. RD1 was first described as deleted from BCG (Bacillus Calmette–Guérin) vaccines (Mahairas et al. 1996), and this deletion is now accepted to contribute to the safety profile of these live, attenuated strains (Pym et al. 2002; Lewis et al. 2003). Yet, genomic studies have documented that *M. microtii* (Pym et al. 2002) and the dassie bacillus (Mostowy et al. 2004) have distinct deletions in the RD1 locus, such that both bacteria lack the genes *Rv3874-Rv3876*, including *esxB* (coding for CFP-10) and *esxA* (coding for ESAT-6). More recently, a genomic study of the tubercle bacillus associated with disease in mongooses reported a new RD1 deletion, in the organism now named *M. mungi* (Alexander et al. 2010). How can three different MTC members successfully cause disease and transmit among members of their respective mammalian hosts in the absence of the ESX-1 secretion system? Is ESX-1 overrated, or is this virulence system not needed for disease in these hosts? If the latter, what is the common feature of voles, dassies, and mongooses that could explain the convergent deletion of RD1 in their respective tubercle bacilli? In the absence of experimental data, the answer to this question is perforce speculative. One hypothesis notes that voles, dassies, and mongooses are burrowing animals that inhabit spaces with limited ventilation, unlike oryxes, seals, goats, and cattle. Because the life cycle of *M. tuberculosis* involves (1) achieving productive infection in a number of contacts and (2) having a subset of these progress to active, transmissible disease, a bacterium with a reduced attack rate could achieve a transmission index of unity or above as long as it is being spread in a high-transmission environment. If true, this may explain why *M. microtii*, *M. mungi*, and the dassie bacillus are not isolated from human TB cases, unlike *M. pinnipedii* (Thompson et al. 1993), *M. caprae* (Kubica et al. 2003), and *M. bovis* (Evans et al. 2007). Given that TB in humans may be considered a "crowd" disease, the increasing density of human communities over time may also permit a gradual attenuation of virulence of the human-adapted form, potentially explaining why we see reduced transmission of at least one *M. tuberculosis* lineage among immigrants to Montreal.

Because there are limited phenotypic data for the "exotic" members of the MTC, the most phenotypic data on MTC variability derive from the classical comparison of *M. tuberculosis* versus *M. bovis*. In many animal models, *M. bovis* is more "virulent" (Smith 1898; Medina et al. 2006; Nedeltchev et al. 2009), although as mentioned above, the laboratory definition of virulence again may not serve as the most appropriate proxy for bacterial transmissibility. In natural cross-host studies, *M. bovis* does not successfully transmit among human populations; conversely, *M. tuberculosis* has been used as a naturally attenuated vaccine in cattle. Therefore, the notion of greater or lesser virulence has to be framed in a host-specific context. Nonetheless, the observation that *M. bovis* has managed to generate sustained infections in a broader range of hosts (cattle, deer, bison, brush-tailed possums, badgers, East-Asian water buffaloes) suggests some sort of adaptive gain of the veterinary pathogen, as compared with the restricted host distribution of the human variant. As *M. bovis* has a smaller genome, with no unique DNA, it has been inferred that any gain-of-function phenotypes in *M. bovis* must be caused by altered regulation of extant genes (Garnier et al. 2003).

In an attempt to explain the basis for the different behaviors of *M. tuberculosis* and *M. bovis*, our laboratory and others have performed comparative transcriptomics of these organisms, to catalog differences in gene expression (Said-Salim et al. 2006; Rehren et al. 2007). Perhaps the most obvious difference involves a small set of genes under control of the extracytosolic regulator, Sigma factor K (SigK). Previously it had been shown that virulent *M. bovis* and some (but not all) *M. bovis* BCG strains produce high quantities of the antigenic proteins MPT70 and MPT83, with MPT70 production accounting for >10% of the mass of culture filtrate proteins (Harboe and Nagai 1984). In contrast, *M. tuberculosis* does not produce these proteins in vitro, but expression of the genes is seen rapidly after infection (Schnappinger et al. 2003). This offers three "states": *M. tuberculosis* (LOW-INDUCIBLE), *M. bovis* including BCG Russia (ON), and selected BCG including BCG Pasteur (OFF). By transcriptome analysis, we showed that the differential expression of MPT70 and MPT83 across BCG strains was caused by a start mutation in *sigK* that occurred between 1927 and 1931 at the Institut Pasteur (Charlet et al. 2005). Given that the SigK mutation explains BCG differences, we next turned to the *M. tuberculosis–M. bovis* difference, showing that the cognate anti-Sigma K, called the Regulator of SigK (RskA), is mutated in *M. bovis* (Said-Salim et al. 2006). Curiously, *rskA* is also mutated in *M. orygis*, with a distinct, independent mutation also resulting in overexpression of the SigK regulon. The explanation for how two different MTC members have independently achieved constitutive expression of these antigenic proteins remains elusive. In unpublished work (MA Behr and FJ Veyrier, unpubl.), it has been shown that the mutant forms of *rskA* are not simply defective for inhibiting SigK activity; but rather that introduction of $rskA_{bovis}$ or $rskA_{orygis}$ into *M. tuberculosis* activates the SigK regulon, resulting in constitutive production of MPT70 and MPT83, even in the presence of a wild-type RskA. Ongoing work seeks to define the phenotypic consequence of altering the expression of the SigK-controlled genes, with a view to understanding how such an expression change could have been twice selected among MTC species circulating in different mammalian hosts.

Mycobacterium-LEVEL VARIABILITY

The preceding sections focused first on variability between *M. tuberculosis* strains and then variability between MTC species. By "zooming up" one more level, one can ask about the similarities and differences between *M. tuberculosis* and nontuberculosis mycobacteria (NTM). Through sequence analysis of a number of NTM species, it is currently appreciated that the NTM that are genetically most similar to *M. tuberculosis* are *M. marinum* and *M. kansasii* (Fig. 3) (Stinear et al. 2008; Veyrier et al. 2009; Wang and Behr 2014). *M. marinum* has already been used with great success as a model for TB pathogenesis, given the conservation of ESX-1 secretion across organisms (Gao et al. 2004) and the optical advantages of live videomicroscopy for in vivo infection studies (Cosma et al. 2003; Ramakrishnan 2012). The *M. marinum* genome has served as the first out-group to ask what genes are present in *M. tuberculosis* but lacking in NTM species, suggesting the acquisition of new *M. tuberculosis*–specific genes by the ancestor of the MTC, after their common ancestor (Stinear et al. 2008). These findings were supported by an independent compositional analysis of the *M. tuberculosis* genome that also sug-

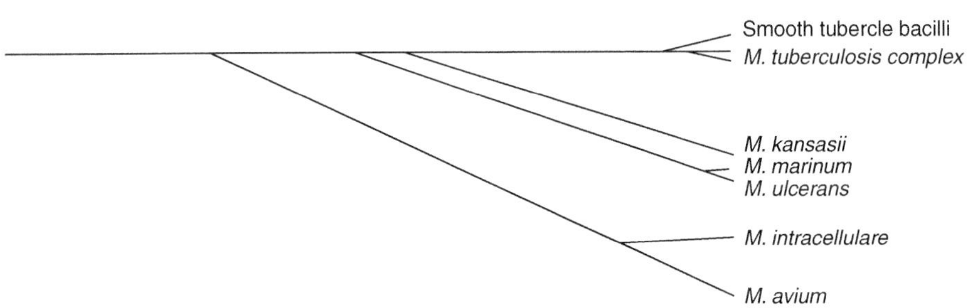

Figure 3. Phylogenetic relationship of slow-growing mycobacterial species, based on multilocus sequence analysis of 20 conserved housekeeping genes (as described in Veyrier et al. 2009). Outside of the *Mycobacterium tuberculosis* complex, the closely nontuberculous mycobacteria are *Mycobacterium kansasii* and the *Mycobacterium marinum-ulcerans* complex, which are organisms that share a number of virulence determinants with *Mycobacterium tuberculosis.*

gested the existence of horizontal gene transfer (HGT) as the certain *M. tuberculosis* genes (Becq et al. 2007).

M. kansasii offers a further perspective on the emergence of *M. tuberculosis* for a number of reasons. Epidemiologically, *M. kansasii* is recognized to be an environmental mycobacterium that can be readily isolated from water sources, but does not spread from person to person. Thus the genome of *M. kansasii* affords a perspective of common mycobacterial survival strategies that are not necessarily selected for the capacity to infect or cause disease. Yet, clinically, *M. kansasii* lung disease can present as right upper lobe cavitary disease that is indistinguishable from TB. This suggests that certain features of the pathogenesis of TB, including inhalation of bacteria into the alveoli and intrapulmonary spread to the lung apices, are not directed by *M. tuberculosis* in a specific manner. Genetically, analysis of 20 housekeeping genes conserved across mycobacterial genomes suggests that *M. kansasii* may be a closer relative of *M. tuberculosis* than *M. marinum* (Veyrier et al. 2009). Based on these considerations, and the shotgun sequence reads for the *M. kansasii* genome, we asked whether the *M. tuberculosis* genome contains genes that lack orthologs in *M. kansasii*, *M. marinum*, and other NTM. Our analysis suggested the stepwise accumulation of genes coincident with the divergent of slow-growing mycobacteria from rapid-growing mycobacteria, and then after the divergence with *M. avium*, the divergence with *M. marinum*, and the divergence with *M. kansasii* (Veyrier et al. 2011). *M. tuberculosis* contains at least 55 coding genes that lack orthologs in all other mycobacteria, with bioinformatic evidence that they were acquired via HGT including the presence of vectors of HGT and differences in the GC content of these putative HGT islands (Veyrier et al. 2009). As there are considerable differences between conserved sequences of *M. tuberculosis* and *M. kansasii*, it cannot be inferred that these are closely related organisms that recently diverged because of HGTelements, as is the case with other pathogens, like *Yersinia pestis*. Rather, the emergence of *M. tuberculosis* has apparently occurred over a protracted period of time, with a number of stepwise additions of HGT islands, which together enabled an environmental mycobacteria to alter its lifestyle to become a committed professional pathogen (Veyrier et al. 2011). At present there are no obvious intermediate hosts that can be assessed to test this model, with the exception of STB. However, the number of STB isolates is small, arguing against an ongoing human epidemic, and their definitive reservoir is presently unknown. Should STB, including *M. canetii*, be isolated from environmental sources, such as water, then common features of the *M. canetii* and *M. kansasii* genomes might point to environmental survival strategies, whereas differences between these organisms and *M. tuberculosis* would point to key pathogen-specific elements. Alternatively, if STB are host-adapted organisms, without an environmental reservoir, then the study of the STB genomes might provide a glimpse into genomic remodeling of an apparently moribund lineage of the tubercle bacillus. More information about the epidemiologic profile and potential sources of exposure of humans with TB due to STB isolates might shed some light on these possibilities.

Beyond looking at differences between *M. tuberculosis* and NTM, the availability of NTM genomes also provides an opportunity to catalog conserved genes. Just as the genes conserved across *M. tuberculosis* isolates suggested selection for these genes to cause disease, the conservation of genes across a broad range of mycobacterial species suggests a selection for these genes to survive and replicate in the various environments these bacteria encounter. From the vantage of TB research, it can be argued that *M. tuberculosis* must survive the first contact with human cells, persist within granulomatous lesions, induce immunopathology, and spread via the airways in aerosols to the next host. Thus, it follows that *M. tuberculosis* must regulate gene expression, protein production, and protein degradation to appropriately adjust to the various conditions encountered during the infectious cycle. From the vantage of NTM research, it can be argued that *M. avium* in a pond must endure much more severe fluctuations in temperature and pH, while withstanding the antimicrobial pressures of a polymicrobial community of pond-dwelling organisms. Thus, it is perhaps not surprising that NTM have larger genomes and more Sigma factors than *M. tuberculosis*. By extension, a number of *M. tuberculosis* "virulence factors" are not specific to the pathogen; to a varying extent, NTM genomes code for the ESX-1 secretion system, PhoP and LprG, among other examples. Although these observations by no means detract from the importance of these systems for the full virulence of *M. tuberculosis*, from the vantage of comparative genomics, the existence of these elements in NTM genomes suggests that these virulence factors cannot on their own explain the remarkable success of *M. tuberculosis* as a human pathogen. Recent findings that a gene island specific to *M. tuberculosis* (Rv3377-78), two genes previously implicated in the modulation of phagosomal acidification (Pethe et al. 2004), produces a novel lipid, called 1-tuberculosinyladenosine (Layre et al. 2014). This finding provides an example of the kinds of investigations that may shed further light on the genesis of *M. tuberculosis*. Further studies of *M. tuberculosis*–specific genes, many of which have currently have unknown or hypothetical functions, might ultimately provide fundamental insights on *M. tuberculosis* as a pathogen and also uncover novel, TB-specific biomarkers for clinical applications.

CONCLUDING REMARKS

After nearly two decades of study, it can be affirmed that comparative genomics helped uncover the ESX-1 secretion system but then challenged whether it is essential for virulence in all members of the MTC. On a microevolutionary scale, comparative genomics has shown that strains of *M. tuberculosis* lacking in PGLs and *DosR* regulon genes are able to cause disease while on a macroevolutionary scale, comparative genomics has shown that a number of virulence factors critical for TB disease are conserved in low-virulence environmental mycobacteria. Thus, there is no single virulence factor yet that is both specific to *M. tuberculosis* and invariant across TB-causing bacteria.

Together these observations beg the question of whether comparative genomics can detect the elusive nature of what makes *M. tuberculosis* such a recalcitrant foe. Just as the human genome has not laid bare what makes people different than chimpanzees, perhaps the *M. tuberculosis* genome is the cornerstone for a different kind of investigation, asking not simply what is present and absent, but how the ensemble is orchestrated, at the levels of transcription, translation, and molecular recycling pathways. Comparative genomics has clearly provided guidance of cataloguing the right bacteria for investigation; misnomers can confound investigation and lead to false hypotheses that can never be confirmed despite the efforts of our trainees. Thus, we now know that *M. avium* is a complex of both pathogenic and nonpathogenic bacteria (Turenne et al. 2007), that *M. marinum* and *Mycobacterium ulcerans* diverged quite recently (Veyrier et al. 2009), and that *M. kansasii* is closely related to *M. tuberculosis* but epidemiologically quite different. We now know that within the MTC there are many variants of the tubercle bacillus that are apparently persisting in symbiotic relationships with their respective hosts. And we now know that within the *M. tuberculosis* sensu stricto, there is also evidence of symbiosis, defined as cohabitation of divergent organisms (Gagneux et al. 2006). Perhaps what is needed next is a global perturbogen, to disrupt the apparently comfortable residence that *M. tuberculosis* has established in one-third of humanity. Whether this can be achieved with existing tools, applied in a scaled-up manner, or achieved with novel approaches, to be derived from other research described in this book, is itself an ongoing question.

REFERENCES

**Reference is also in this collection.*

Albanna AS, Reed MB, Kotar KV, Fallow A, McIntosh FA, Behr MA, Menzies D. 2011. Reduced transmissibility of East African Indian strains of *Mycobacterium tuberculosis*. *PLoS ONE* **6:** e25075.

Alexander KA, Laver PN, Michel AL, Williams M, van Helden PD, Warren RM, Gey van Pittius NC. 2010. Novel *Mycobacterium tuberculosis* complex pathogen, *M. mungi*. *Emerg Infect Dis* **16:** 1296–1299.

Alland D, Kalkut GE, Moss AR, McAdam RA, Hahn JA, Bosworth W, Drucker E, Bloom BR. 1994. Transmission of tuberculosis in New York City. An analysis by DNA fingerprinting and conventional epidemiologic methods. *N Engl J Med* **330:** 1710–1716.

Barczak AK, Domenech P, Boshoff HI, Reed MB, Manca C, Kaplan G, Barry CE III. 2005. In vivo phenotypic dominance in mouse mixed infections with *Mycobacterium tuberculosis* clinical isolates. *J Infect Dis* **192:** 600–606.

Becq J, Gutierrez MC, Rosas-Magallanes V, Rauzier J, Gicquel B, Neyrolles O, Deschavanne P. 2007. Contribution of horizontally acquired genomic islands to the evolution of the tubercle bacilli. *Mol Biol Evol* **24:** 1861–1871.

Behr MA, Wilson MA, Gill WP, Salamon H, Schoolnik GK, Rane S, Small PM. 1999. Comparative genomics of BCG vaccines by whole-genome DNA microarray. *Science* **284:** 1520–1523.

Brisse S, Supply P, Brosch R, Vincent V, Gutierrez MC. 2006. "A re-evaluation of M. prototuberculosis": Continuing the debate. *PLoS Pathog* **2:** e95.

Brosch R, Gordon SV, Marmiesse M, Brodin P, Buchrieser C, Eiglmeier K, Garnier T, Gutierrez C, Hewinson G, Kremer K, et al. 2002. A new evolutionary scenario for the *Mycobacterium tuberculosis* complex. *Proc Natl Acad Sci* **99:** 3684–3689.

Brosch R, Gordon SV, Garnier T, Eiglmeier K, Frigui W, Valenti P, Dos SS, Duthoy S, Lacroix C, Garcia-Pelayo C, et al. 2007. Genome plasticity of BCG and impact on vaccine efficacy. *Proc Natl Acad Sci* **104:** 5596–5601.

Charlet D, Mostowy S, Alexander D, Sit L, Wiker HG, Behr MA. 2005. Reduced expression of antigenic proteins MPB70 and MPB83 in *Mycobacterium bovis* BCG strains due to a start codon mutation in sigK. *Mol Microbiol* **56:** 1302–1313.

Cole ST, Brosch R, Parkhill J, Garnier T, Churcher C, Harris D, Gordon SV, Eiglmeier K, Gas S, Barry CE III, et al. 1998. Deciphering the biology of *Mycobacterium tuberculosis* from the complete genome sequence. *Nature* **393:** 537–544.

Comas I, Chakravartti J, Small PM, Galagan J, Niemann S, Kremer K, Ernst JD, Gagneux S. 2010. Human T cell epitopes of *Mycobacterium tuberculosis* are evolutionarily hyperconserved. *Nat Genet* **42:** 498–503.

Corbett EL, Marston B, Churchyard GJ, De Cock KM. 2006. Tuberculosis in sub-Saharan Africa: Opportunities, challenges, and change in the era of antiretroviral treatment. *Lancet* **367:** 926–937.

Coscolla M, Lewin A, Metzger S, Maetz-Rennsing K, Calvignac-Spencer S, Nitsche A, Dabrowski PW, Radonic A, Niemann S, Parkhill J, et al. 2013. Novel *Mycobacterium tuberculosis* complex isolate from a wild chimpanzee. *Emerg Infect Dis* **19:** 969–976.

Cosma CL, Sherman DR, Ramakrishnan L. 2003. The secret lives of the pathogenic mycobacteria. *Annu Rev Microbiol* **57:** 641–676.

Daley CL, Small PM, Schecter GF, Schoolnik GK, McAdam RA, Jacobs WR Jr, Hopewell PC. 1992. An outbreak of tuberculosis with accelerated progression among persons infected with the human immunodeficiency virus. An analysis using restriction-fragment-length polymorphisms. *N Engl J Med* **326:** 231–235.

Evans JT, Smith EG, Banerjee A, Smith RM, Dale J, Innes JA, Hunt D, Tweddell A, Wood A, Anderson C, et al. 2007. Cluster of human tuberculosis caused by *Mycobacterium bovis*: Evidence for person-to-person transmission in the UK. *Lancet* **369:** 1270–1276.

Fallow A, Domenech P, Reed MB. 2010. Strains of the East Asian (W/Beijing) lineage of *Mycobacterium tuberculosis* are DosS/DosT-DosR two-component regulatory system natural mutants. *J Bacteriol* **192:** 2228–2238.

Fenner L, Gagneux S, Helbling P, Battegay M, Rieder HL, Pfyffer GE, Zwahlen M, Furrer H, Siegrist HH, Fehr J, et al. 2012. *Mycobacterium tuberculosis* transmission in a country with low tuberculosis incidence: Role of immigration and HIV infection. *J Clin Microbiol* **50:** 388–395.

Gagneux S, DeRiemer K, Van T, Kato-Maeda M, de Jong BC, Narayanan S, Nicol M, Niemann S, Kremer K, Gutierrez MC, et al. 2006. Variable host-pathogen compatibility in *Mycobacterium tuberculosis*. *Proc Natl Acad Sci* **103:** 2869–2873.

Gao LY, Guo S, McLaughlin B, Morisaki H, Engel JN, Brown EJ. 2004. A mycobacterial virulence gene cluster extending RD1 is required for cytolysis, bacterial spreading and ESAT-6 secretion. *Mol Microbiol* **53:** 1677–1693.

Garnier T, Eiglmeier K, Camus JC, Medina N, Mansoor H, Pryor M, Duthoy S, Grondin S, Lacroix C, Monsempe C, et al. 2003. The complete genome sequence of *Mycobacterium bovis*. *Proc Natl Acad Sci* **100:** 7877–7882.

Gautam US, Sikri K, Vashist A, Singh V, Tyagi JS. 2014. Essentiality of DevR/DosR interaction with SigA for the dormancy survival program in *Mycobacterium tuberculosis*. *J Bacteriol* **196:** 790–799.

Gutierrez MC, Brisse S, Brosch R, Fabre M, Omais B, Marmiesse M, Supply P, Vincent V. 2005. Ancient origin and gene mosaicism of the progenitor of *Mycobacterium tuberculosis*. *PLoS Pathog* **1:** e5.

Harboe M, Nagai S. 1984. MPB70, a unique antigen of *Mycobacterium bovis* BCG. *Am Rev Respir Dis* **129:** 444–452.

Homolka S, Niemann S, Russell DG, Rohde KH. 2010. Functional genetic diversity among *Mycobacterium tuberculosis* complex clinical isolates: Delineation of conserved core and lineage-specific transcriptomes during intracellular survival. *PLoS Pathog* **6:** e1000988.

Isaza JP, Duque C, Gomez V, Robledo J, Barrera LF, Alzate JF. 2012. Whole genome shotgun sequencing of one Colombian clinical isolate of *Mycobacterium tuberculosis* reveals DosR regulon gene deletions. *FEMS Microbiol Lett* **330:** 113–120.

Krishnan N, Malaga W, Constant P, Caws M, Tran TH, Salmons J, Nguyen TN, Nguyen DB, Daffe M, Young DB, et al. 2011. *Mycobacterium tuberculosis* lineage influences innate immune response and virulence and is associated with distinct cell envelope lipid profiles. *PLoS ONE* **6:** e23870.

Kubica T, Rusch-Gerdes S, Niemann S. 2003. *Mycobacterium bovis* subsp. *caprae* caused one-third of human *M. bovis*-associated tuberculosis cases reported in Germany between 1999 and 2001. *J Clin Microbiol* **41:** 3070–3077.

Kulaga S, Behr M, Musana K, Brinkman J, Menzies D, Brassard P, Kunimoto D, Tannenbaum TN, Thibert L, Joseph L, et al. 2002. Molecular epidemiology of tuberculosis in Montreal. *CMAJ* **167:** 353–354.

Layre E, Lee HJ, Young DC, Jezek MA, Buter J, Minnaard AJ, Annand JW, Fortune SM, Snider BB, Matsunaga I, et al. 2014. Molecular profiling of *Mycobacterium tuberculosis* identifies tuberculosinyl nucleoside products of the virulence-associated enzyme Rv3378c. *Proc Natl Acad Sci* **111:** 2978–2983.

Leung AS, Tran V, Wu Z, Yu X, Alexander DC, Gao GF, Zhu B, Liu J. 2008. Novel genome polymorphisms in BCG vaccine strains and impact on efficacy. *BMC Genomics* **9:** 413.

Lewis KN, Liao RL, Guinn KM, Hickey MJ, Smith S, Behr MA, Sherman DR. 2003. Deletion of RD1 from *Mycobacterium tuberculosis* mimics bacille Calmette–Guerin attenuation. *J Infect Dis* **187:** 117–123.

Leyten EM, Lin MY, Franken KL, Friggen AH, Prins C, van Meijgaarden KE, Voskuil MI, Weldingh K, Andersen P, Schoolnik GK, et al. 2006. Human T-cell responses to 25 novel antigens encoded by genes of the dormancy regulon of *Mycobacterium tuberculosis*. *Microbes Infect* **8:** 2052–2060.

Mahairas GG, Sabo PJ, Hickey MJ, Singh DC, Stover CK. 1996. Molecular analysis of genetic differences between *Mycobacterium bovis* BCG and virulent *M. bovis*. *J Bacteriol* **178:** 1274–1282.

Manca C, Tsenova L, Barry CE III, Bergtold A, Freeman S, Haslett PA, Musser JM, Freedman VH, Kaplan G. 1999. *Mycobacterium tuberculosis* CDC1551 induces a more vigorous host response in vivo and in vitro, but is not more virulent than other clinical isolates. *J Immunol* **162:** 6740–6746.

Manca C, Tsenova L, Bergtold A, Freeman S, Tovey M, Musser JM, Barry CE III, Freedman VH, Kaplan G. 2001. Virulence of a *Mycobacterium tuberculosis* clinical isolate in mice is determined by failure to induce Th1 type immunity and is associated with induction of IFN-α/β. *Proc Natl Acad Sci* **98:** 5752–5757.

Manca C, Reed MB, Freeman S, Mathema B, Kreiswirth B, Barry CE III, Kaplan G. 2004. Differential monocyte activation underlies strain-specific *Mycobacterium tuberculosis* pathogenesis. *Infect Immun* **72:** 5511–5514.

Medina E, Ryan L, LaCourse R, North RJ. 2006. Superior virulence of Mycobacterium bovis over *Mycobacterium tuberculosis* (*Mtb*) for *Mtb*-resistant and *Mtb*-susceptible mice is manifest as an ability to cause extrapulmonary disease. *Tuberculosis (Edinb)* **86:** 20–27.

Mostowy S, Cousins D, Brinkman J, Aranaz A, Behr MA. 2002. Genomic deletions suggest a phylogeny for the *Mycobacterium tuberculosis* complex. *J Infect Dis* **186:** 74–80.

Mostowy S, Cousins D, Behr MA. 2004. Genomic interrogation of the dassie bacillus reveals it as a unique RD1 mutant within the *Mycobacterium tuberculosis* complex. *J Bacteriol* **186:** 104–109.

Nedeltchev GG, Raghunand TR, Jassal MS, Lun S, Cheng QJ, Bishai WR. 2009. Extrapulmonary dissemination of *Mycobacterium bovis* but not *Mycobacterium tuberculosis* in a bronchoscopic rabbit model of cavitary tuberculosis. *Infect Immun* **77:** 598–603.

Nguyen D, Proulx JF, Westley J, Thibert L, Dery S, Behr MA. 2003. Tuberculosis in the Inuit community of Quebec, Canada. *Am J Respir Crit Care Med* **168:** 1353–1357.

* Niemann S, Supply P. 2014. Diversity and evolution of *Mycobacterium tuberculosis*: Moving to whole-genome-based approaches. *Cold Spring Harb Perspect Med* doi: 10.1101/cshperspect.a021188.

Park HD, Guinn KM, Harrell MI, Liao R, Voskuil MI, Tompa M, Schoolnik GK, Sherman DR. 2003. Rv3133c/*dosR* is a transcription factor that mediates the hypoxic response of *Mycobacterium tuberculosis*. *Mol Microbiol* **48:** 833–843.

Pepperell CS, Granka JM, Alexander DC, Behr MA, Chui L, Gordon J, Guthrie JL, Jamieson FB, Langlois-Klassen D, Long R, et al. 2011. Dispersal of *Mycobacterium tuberculosis* via the Canadian fur trade. *Proc Natl Acad Sci* **108:** 6526–6531.

Pethe K, Swenson DL, Alonso S, Anderson J, Wang C, Russell DG. 2004. Isolation of *Mycobacterium tuberculosis* mutants defective in the arrest of phagosome maturation. *Proc Natl Acad Sci* **101:** 13642–13647.

Pym AS, Brodin P, Brosch R, Huerre M, Cole ST. 2002. Loss of RD1 contributed to the attenuation of the live tuberculosis vaccines *Mycobacterium bovis* BCG and *Mycobacterium microti*. *Mol Microbiol* **46:** 709–717.

Ramakrishnan L. 2012. Revisiting the role of the granuloma in tuberculosis. *Nat Rev Immunol* **12:** 352–366.

Reed MB, Domenech P, Manca C, Su H, Barczak AK, Kreiswirth BN, Kaplan G, Barry CE III. 2004. A glycolipid of hypervirulent tuberculosis strains that inhibits the innate immune response. *Nature* **431:** 84–87.

Reed MB, Gagneux S, DeRiemer K, Small PM, Barry CE III. 2007. The W-Beijing lineage of *Mycobacterium tuberculosis* overproduces triglycerides and has the DosR dormancy regulon constitutively upregulated. *J Bacteriol* **189:** 2583–2589.

Reed MB, Pichler VK, McIntosh F, Mattia A, Fallow A, Masala S, Domenech P, Zwerling A, Thibert L, Menzies D, et al. 2009. Major *Mycobacterium tuberculosis* lineages associate with patient country of origin. *J Clin Microbiol* **47:** 1119–1128.

Rehren G, Walters S, Fontan P, Smith I, Zarraga AM. 2007. Differential gene expression between *Mycobacterium bovis* and *Mycobacterium tuberculosis*. *Tuberculosis (Edinb)* **87:** 347–359.

Reiling N, Homolka S, Walter K, Brandenburg J, Niwinski L, Ernst M, Herzmann C, Lange C, Diel R, Ehlers S, et al. 2013. Clade-specific virulence patterns of *Mycobacterium tuberculosis* complex strains in human primary macrophages and aerogenically infected mice. *MBio* **4:** e00250-13.

Roupie V, Romano M, Zhang L, Korf H, Lin MY, Franken KL, Ottenhoff TH, Klein MR, Huygen K. 2007. Immunogenicity of eight dormancy regulon-encoded proteins of *Mycobacterium tuberculosis* in DNA-vaccinated and tuberculosis-infected mice. *Infect Immun* **75:** 941–949.

Said-Salim B, Mostowy S, Kristof AS, Behr MA. 2006. Mutations in *Mycobacterium tuberculosis* Rv0444c, the gene encoding anti-SigK, explain high level expression of MPB70 and MPB83 in *Mycobacterium bovis*. *Mol Microbiol* **62:** 1251–1263.

Salamon H, Kato-Maeda M, Small PM, Drenkow J, Gingeras TR. 2000. Detection of deleted genomic DNA using a semiautomated computational analysis of GeneChip data. *Genome Res* **10:** 2044–2054.

Sassetti CM, Rubin EJ. 2003. Genetic requirements for mycobacterial survival during infection. *Proc Natl Acad Sci* **100:** 12989–12994.

Sassetti CM, Boyd DH, Rubin EJ. 2003. Genes required for mycobacterial growth defined by high density mutagenesis. *Mol Microbiol* **48:** 77–84.

Schnappinger D, Ehrt S, Voskuil MI, Liu Y, Mangan JA, Monahan IM, Dolganov G, Efron B, Butcher PD, Nathan C, et al. 2003. Transcriptional adaptation of *Mycobacterium tuberculosis* within macrophages: Insights into the phagosomal environment. *J Exp Med* **198:** 693–704.

Sinsimer D, Huet G, Manca C, Tsenova L, Koo MS, Kurepina N, Kana B, Mathema B, Marras SA, Kreiswirth BN, et al. 2008. The phenolic glycolipid of *Mycobacterium tuberculosis* differentially modulates the early host cytokine response but does not in itself confer hypervirulence. *Infect Immun* **76:** 3027–3036.

Small PM, Hopewell PC, Singh SP, Paz A, Parsonnet J, Ruston DC, Schecter GF, Daley CL, Schoolnik GK. 1994. The epidemiology of tuberculosis in San Francisco. A population-based study using conventional and molecular methods. *N Engl J Med* **330:** 1703–1709.

Smith T, 1898. A comparative study of bovine tubercle bacilli and of human bacilli from sputum. *J Exp Med* **3:** 451–511.

Stinear TP, Seemann T, Harrison PF, Jenkin GA, Davies JK, Johnson PD, Abdellah Z, Arrowsmith C, Chillingworth T, Churcher C, et al. 2008. Insights from the complete genome sequence of *Mycobacterium marinum* on the evolution of *Mycobacterium tuberculosis*. *Genome Res* **18:** 729–741.

Supply P, Marceau M, Mangenot S, Roche D, Rouanet C, Khanna V, Majlessi L, Criscuolo A, Tap J, Pawlik A, et al. 2013. Genomic analysis of smooth tubercle bacilli provides insights into ancestry and pathoadaptation of *Mycobacterium tuberculosis*. *Nat Genet* **45:** 172–179.

Thompson PJ, Cousins DV, Gow BL, Collins DM, Williamson BH, Dagnia HT. 1993. Seals, seal trainers, and mycobacterial infection. *Am Rev Respir Dis* **147:** 164–167.

Tsenova L, Ellison E, Harbacheuski R, Moreira AL, Kurepina N, Reed MB, Mathema B, Barry CE III, Kaplan G. 2005. Virulence of selected *Mycobacterium tuberculosis* clinical isolates in the rabbit model of meningitis is dependent on phenolic glycolipid produced by the bacilli. *J Infect Dis* **192:** 98–106.

Tsolaki AG, Hirsh AE, DeRiemer K, Enciso JA, Wong MZ, Hannan M, Goguet de la Salmoniere YO, Aman K, Kato-Maeda M, Small PM. 2004. Functional and evolutionary genomics of *Mycobacterium tuberculosis*: Insights from genomic deletions in 100 strains. *Proc Natl Acad Sci* **101:** 4865–4870.

Turenne CY, Wallace R Jr, Behr MA. 2007. *Mycobacterium avium* in the postgenomic era. *Clin Microbiol Rev* **20:** 205–229.

Veyrier F, Pletzer D, Turenne C, Behr MA. 2009. Phylogenetic detection of horizontal gene transfer during the step-wise genesis of *Mycobacterium tuberculosis*. *BMC Evol Biol* **9:** 196.

Veyrier FJ, Dufort A, Behr MA. 2011. The rise and fall of the *Mycobacterium tuberculosis* genome. *Trends Microbio* **19:** 156–161.

Wang J, Behr MA. 2014. Building a better bacillus: The emergence of *Mycobacterium tuberculosis*. *Front Microbiol* **5:** 139.

Global Epidemiology of Tuberculosis

Philippe Glaziou, Charalambos Sismanidis, Katherine Floyd, and Mario Raviglione

HIV/AIDS, Tuberculosis & Malaria, World Health Organization, 1211 Geneva 27, Switzerland

Correspondence: glazioup@who.int

Despite the availability of effective chemotherapy, tuberculosis (TB) killed 1.3 million people in 2012. Alongside HIV, it remains a top cause of death from an infectious disease. Global targets for reductions in the epidemiological burden of TB have been set for 2015 and 2050 within the context of the Millennium Development Goals (MDGs) and by the Stop TB Partnership. Achieving these targets is the focus of national and international efforts in TB control, and showing whether or not they are achieved is of major importance to guide future and sustainable investments. This article provides a short overview of sources of data to estimate TB disease burden; presents estimates of TB incidence, prevalence, and mortality in 2012 and an assessment of progress toward the 2015 targets for reductions in these indicators based on trends since 1990 and projections up to 2015; analyzes trends in TB notifications and in the implementation of the Stop TB Strategy; and considers prospects for elimination of TB after 2015.

Tuberculosis (TB) is likely to have affected humans for most of their history (Holloway et al. 2011; Comas et al. 2013) and remains a major cause of death worldwide despite the discovery of effective and affordable chemotherapy more than 50 years ago. With 1.3 million TB deaths (including TB deaths in HIV positive individuals) in 2012 (WHO 2013a), TB and the human immunodeficiency virus (HIV) are the top causes of death from a single infectious agent worldwide (Lozano et al. 2012; Ortblad et al. 2013). TB is a leading killer among adults in the most economically productive age groups and people living with HIV (Lopez et al. 2006), and even those cured from TB can be left with lifetime sequelae that substantially reduce their quality of life (Miller et al. 2009). Recognition of these facts has kept TB control high on the international public health agenda since the early 1990s (Zumla et al. 2009; Lienhardt et al. 2012a), following years of neglect during the 1980s (Raviglione and Pio 2002).

Evidence that chemotherapy is among the most cost-effective of all health-care interventions (Murray et al. 1991; Dye and Floyd 2006), the catastrophic impact of the HIV epidemic on TB in Africa, and the global concern about the growth of multidrug-resistant TB (MDR-TB) have emphasized the need to improve TB prevention and control. Global targets for reductions in the epidemiological burden of TB have been set for 2015 and 2050 within the context of the Millennium Development Goals (MDGs) and separately by the Stop TB Partnership, a global coalition of stakeholders established to coordinate international efforts

Cite this article as *Cold Spring Harb Perspect Med* doi: 10.1101/cshperspect.a017798

BOX 1. GOALS, TARGET, AND INDICATORS FOR TB CONTROL

Health in the Millennium Development Goals

Goal 6: Combat HIV/AIDS, Malaria, and Other Diseases

Target 6c: Halt and begin to reverse the incidence of malaria and other major diseases
Indicator 6.9: Incidence, prevalence, and death rates associated with TB
Indicator 6.10: Proportion of TB cases detected and cured under DOTS

Stop TB Partnership Targets

By 2005: At least 70% of people with sputum smear-positive TB will be diagnosed (i.e., under the DOTS strategy), and at least 85% will be successfully treated. The targets of a case detection rate of at least 70% and a treatment success rate of at least 85% were first set by the World Health Assembly of WHO in 1991.
By 2015: The global burden of TB (per capita prevalence and death rates) will be reduced by 50% relative to 1990 levels.
By 2050: The global incidence of active TB will be less than one case per million population per year.

(Box 1). The WHO's recommended approach for achieving these targets is the Stop TB Strategy (Raviglione and Uplekar 2006), which comprises best practices in the diagnosis and treatment of patients with active TB, approaches to address major epidemiological and system challenges, and the promotion of research for innovations (Box 2). It was launched in 2006 and underpins the Global Plan 2011–2015, a comprehensive and budgeted plan to reach the global targets (Raviglione 2006b; 2007; Korenromp et al. 2012).

Reaching the 2015 targets has been the focus of national and international efforts in TB control for more than a decade, and the World Health Organization (WHO) has established a Global Task Force on TB Impact Measurement (Dye et al. 2008) to ensure the best possible evaluation of whether or not they are achieved. Every year, WHO publishes estimates of TB incidence, prevalence, and mortality at global, regional, and country levels, along with an analysis of progress toward achievement of global targets (WHO 2013a).

This article provides an overview of sources of data to estimate the burden of disease; presents estimates of the global burden of TB in 2012 and trends in incidence, prevalence, and mortality from 1990 to 2012, with projections up to 2015; analyzes trends in TB notifications and in the implementation of the Stop TB Strategy; and considers prospects for elimination of TB after 2015. Special attention is given to drug-resistant TB, the association of TB with HIV, and TB in children.

GLOBAL MONITORING OF THE BURDEN OF TB

TB incidence has never been measured at the national level because this would require long-term studies among large cohorts of people (hundreds of thousands) at high cost and with challenging logistics. The best approach to estimating TB incidence is from routine surveillance systems in which case reports are more or less complete, such that notifications can be considered a close proxy of incidence. This is possible in settings with universal health-care coverage (Moreno-Serra and Smith 2012; O'Neill et al. 2013), and in which operational research has been used to quantify the small fraction of cases that are treated but not notified to surveillance systems (Van Hest et al. 2008). However, surveillance systems in many countries are not yet capable of providing a direct measure of TB incidence because the numbers of cases who are treated but not notified, or undiagnosed at all, are unknown. The major reasons why cases are missed from official notifica-

BOX 2. STOP TB STRATEGY (Raviglione and Uplekar 2006; World Health Organization 2007)

Vision, Goal, Objectives, and Targets

Vision: A world free of TB

Goal: To dramatically reduce the global burden of TB by 2015 in line with the Millennium Development Goals and the Stop TB Partnership targets

Objectives:

- Achieve universal access to high-quality diagnosis and patient-centered treatment
- Reduce the human suffering and socioeconomic burden associated with TB
- Protect poor and vulnerable populations from TB, TB/HIV, and multidrug-resistant TB
- Support development of new tools and enable their timely and effective use

Targets:

- MDG 6, Target 8: . . .halted by 2015 and begun to reverse the incidence. . . .
- Targets linked to the MDGs and endorsed by the Stop TB Partnership:
  by 2005: detect at least 70% of new sputum smear-positive TB cases and cure at least 85% of these cases
  by 2015: reduce prevalence of and death due to TB by 50% relative to 1990
  by 2050: eliminate TB as a public health problem (less than one case per million population)

Components of the Stop TB Strategy

1. Pursue high-quality DOTS expansion and enhancement
   - Secure political commitment, with adequate and sustained financing
   - Ensure early case detection, and diagnosis through quality-assured bacteriology
   - Provide standardized treatment with supervision, and patient support
   - Ensure effective drug supply and management
   - Monitor and evaluate performance and impact
2. Address TB-HIV, MDR-TB, and the needs of poor and vulnerable populations
   - Scale-up collaborative TB/HIV activities
   - Scale-up prevention and management of multidrug-resistant TB (MDR-TB)
   - Address the needs of TB contacts, and of poor and vulnerable populations
3. Contribute to health system strengthening based on primary health care
   - Help improve health policies, human resource development, financing, supplies, service delivery, and information
   - Strengthen infection control in health services, other congregate settings, and households
   - Upgrade laboratory networks, and implement the Practical Approach to Lung Health (PAL)
   - Adapt successful approaches from other fields and sectors, and foster action on the social determinants of health
4. Engage all care providers
   - Involve all public, voluntary, corporate, and private providers through Public-Private Mix (PPM) approaches
   - Promote use of the International Standards for Tuberculosis Care (ISTC)

Continued

BOX 2. *Continued*

5. Empower people with TB, and communities through partnership
   - Pursue advocacy, communication, and social mobilization
   - Foster community participation in TB care
   - Promote use of the Patients' Charter for Tuberculosis Care
6. Enable and promote research
   - Conduct program-based operational research, and introduce new tools into practice

tion data include laboratory errors (Botha et al. 2008), lack of notification of cases by public (Dye et al. 1999) and private providers (Uplekar et al. 2001), failure of health-care staff to recognize TB signs and symptoms among people accessing health services (Meintjes et al. 2008), and lack of access to health services (Veron et al. 2004). Operational research (such as capture-recapture studies) as well as supporting evidence (such as whether prescriptions for TB drugs are available in the private sector, and practices of staff managing people suspected of having TB in primary health-care facilities) can be used to assess the plausible range of the fraction of cases that are unaccounted for in case notification data (Borgdorff et al. 2004; Cailhol et al. 2005; Baussano et al. 2006; Crofts et al. 2008; Van Hest et al. 2008; WHO 2013a). Duplicated or misclassified records (Bierrenbach et al. 2007), inconsistent case notification data at the subnational level, inconsistent time trends, or inconsistencies with existing knowledge about TB epidemiology (Dye et al. 2007) all contribute to uncertainty about TB incidence estimates obtained from case notification data.

In contrast to incidence, TB prevalence can be directly measured in nationwide population-based surveys in countries with a high burden of TB (Glaziou et al. 2008; WHO 2011c). Since 2002, 19 countries have successfully measured the prevalence of TB disease through such surveys (Hong et al. 1998; Tupasi et al. 1999; Dye et al. 2000; Soemantri et al. 2007; WHO 2013a) including seven in Africa, and 14 more (eight in Africa) have planned to implement a survey by 2015. Repeat surveys conducted about every 10 years allow trends in disease burden to be assessed. Countries that have completed repeat surveys in the last 10 years include Cambodia, China, the Philippines, and Thailand, and repeat surveys are planned in Myanmar and Vietnam (WHO 2013a). Prevalence surveys have proved extremely useful for designing and adapting national TB control program strategies. A large proportion of the global burden of TB as expressed in terms of TB prevalence will be directly measured from population-based surveys by 2015, as opposed to indirectly estimated from statistical modeling.

TB mortality among HIV-negative people can be directly measured using data from national vital registration (VR) systems, provided that these systems have high coverage and causes of death are accurately coded according to the latest revision of the *International classification of diseases* (ICD-10) (Korenromp et al. 2009). Sample VR systems covering representative areas of the country (e.g., China) provide an interim solution. Direct measurements of TB mortality from 123 countries were used in 2012 (WHO 2013a). The parts of the world where there are major gaps in the availability of VR data are the African region and parts of the Southeast Asia region; in the latter, Indonesia is currently building a sample VR system.

TB mortality among HIV-positive people is hard to measure even when national VR systems with standard coding of causes of death are in place, because deaths among HIV-positive people are coded as HIV deaths and contributory causes (such as TB) are generally not reliably recorded. This will need to be corrected to permit a comprehensive assessment of TB mortality, especially in countries with a high prevalence of HIV. In the interim, well-monitored cohorts of HIV-positive people who are enrolled in care and/or autopsy studies provide very useful data on contributory causes of AIDS deaths. Starting in 2013, estimates of TB mortality among HIV-positive people are obtained using models implemented in the Spectrum software (see http://www.futuresinstitute.org/spectrum.aspx) (WHO 2013a).

The incidence of and mortality from MDR-TB can be estimated from periodic surveys or from routine drug-susceptibility testing (DST) if the coverage of patient testing is sufficiently comprehensive (WHO 2013a). The global surveillance of resistance to at least the two most important first-line anti-TB drugs—isoniazid and rifampicin—has been coordinated by WHO since 1994 (Pablos-Mendez et al. 1998; Zignol et al. 2012). Extensively drug-resistant TB (XDR-TB) is defined as MDR-TB plus resistance to the two most effective classes of second-line drugs—the fluoroquinolones and second-line injectable drugs (the aminoglycosides amikacin and kanamycin, and the polypeptide capreomycin) (WHO 2006).

TB EPIDEMIOLOGY

TB is contagious and airborne (Riley 1983). The risk of acquiring *Mycobacterium tuberculosis* infection is essentially determined by exogenous factors. TB is most commonly transmitted from a person with infectious pulmonary TB to others by droplet nuclei, which are aerosolized by coughing, sneezing, or speaking. Other routes of transmission are uncommon and of no epidemiologic significance. The probability of contact with a person who has an infectious form of TB, the intimacy and duration of that contact, the degree of infectiousness of the case, and the shared environment in which the contact takes place are important determinants of the likelihood of transmission. About one-third of the world's population is estimated to have been exposed to TB bacteria and potentially infected (WHO 2013a). Of those infected, only a small proportion will become sick with TB (Vynnycky and Fine 2000; Borgdorff et al. 2011) but people living with HIV, people with weakened immune systems caused by the prolonged use of medicines such as steroids or TNF-α inhibitors, and patients with diabetes, renal insufficiency, and silicosis (among other morbidities) have a much greater risk of falling ill from TB. Among HIV-uninfected the risk of death after 10 years has been variously reported between 53% and 86%, with a weighted mean of 70% (Tiemersma et al. 2011), compared with ~3% of HIV-uninfected treated tuberculosis patients expected to die because of TB (Straetemans et al. 2011). TB is a disease of poverty that thrives where social and economic determinants of ill health prevail, and that affects mostly young adults in their most productive years living in the developing world (WHO 2013a).

Incidence

In 2012, there were an estimated 8.6 million incident cases of TB (range, 8.3 million–9.0 million) in the world, equivalent to 122 cases per 100,000 population. The absolute number of incident cases has been decreasing, albeit slowly, since the early 2000s (WHO 2013a). Most of the estimated cases in 2012 occurred in the WHO regions of Southeast Asia, the western Pacific (58%), and the African region (27%); smaller proportions of cases occurred in the eastern Mediterranean region (8%), the European region (4%), and the region of the Americas (3%). The largest number of incident cases in 2012 was in India (uncertainty range 2.0 million–2.4 million) corresponding to 26% of global cases, China (0.9 million–1.1 million), and South Africa (0.4 million–0.6 million). Of the 8.6 million incident cases, an estimated 0.5 million were children and 2.9 million (2.7–3.1 million) occurred among women.

The incidence rate varies widely among countries (Fig. 1). The lowest rates are found predominantly in high-income countries including most countries in Western Europe, Canada, the United States of America, Australia, and New Zealand. In these countries, the incidence rate is less than 10 cases per 100,000 population. Most countries in the region of the Americas have rates below 50 per 100,000 population and this is the region with the lowest burden

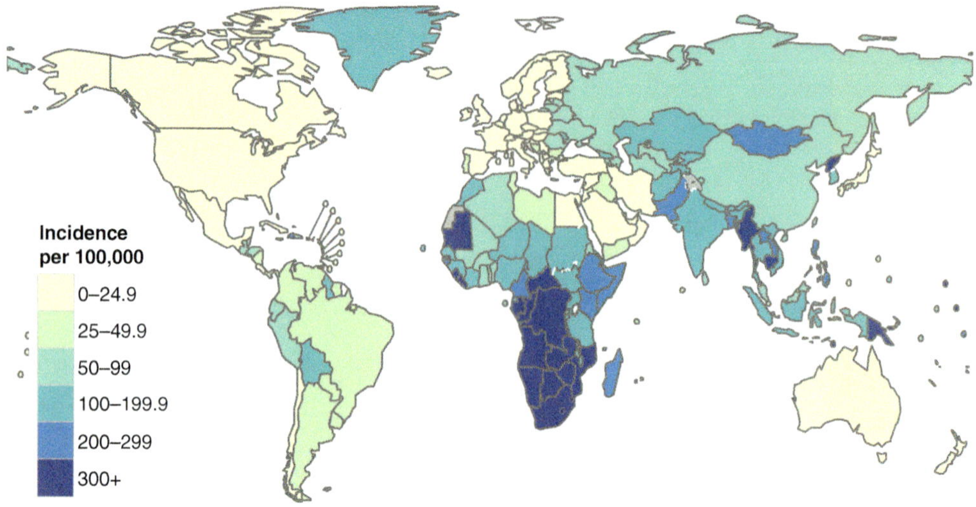

Figure 1. Estimated tuberculosis incidence rates per 100,000 population, 2012.

of TB on average. Countries in the top 10 worldwide in terms of incidence rates are mostly in Africa. In South Africa and Swaziland, the best estimate is that at least one in every 100 people develops TB each year.

Globally, the incidence rate was relatively stable from 1990 up to around 2001, and then started to decrease, achieving the MDG target ahead of the 2015 deadline. Between 2011 and 2012, the rate of decline was 2% (Fig. 2, left panel). This downward trend needs to be sustained to ensure that the MDG target is met in 2015. Incidence rates are also declining in all of six WHO regions, fastest in the European region

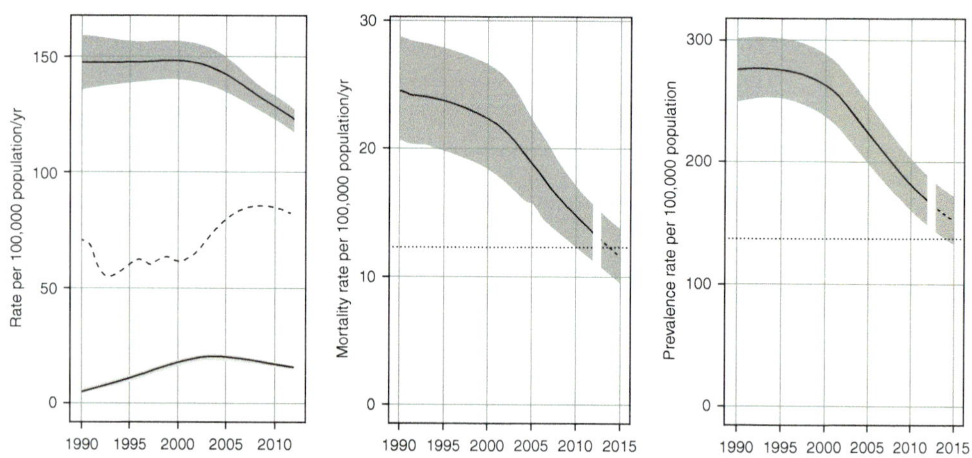

Figure 2. Global trends in estimated TB incidence and estimated TB mortality. (*Left*) Global trends in estimated incidence including HIV-negative and HIV-positive TB (dark gray, *top*) and estimated incidence of HIV-positive TB (light gray, *bottom*). The dashed line shows global trends in case notification rates (all forms of TB). (*Middle*) Global trends in estimated TB mortality excluding TB-associated AIDS deaths. The dotted line represents the Stop TB Partnership targets of halving mortality by 2015 compared with the level of 1990. (*Right*) Global trends in estimated TB prevalence. The dotted line represents the Stop TB Partnership targets of halving prevalence by 2015 compared with the level of 1990. Shaded areas represent uncertainty bands.

 Cite this article as *Cold Spring Harb Perspect Med* doi: 10.1101/cshperspect.a017798

(6.5% per year) and slowest in the eastern Mediterranean and Southeast Asia regions (<1% per year and 2% per year, respectively). Incidence rates have been decreasing since the mid-1990s in the eastern Mediterranean region and since around 2000 in the Southeast Asia region; they peaked around 1997 in the European region and around 2002 in the African region, and have been decreasing since 1990 in the region of the Americas and the western Pacific region.

Mortality

There were an estimated 1.3 million TB deaths in 2012: 940,000 among HIV-negative people and 320,000 among HIV-positive people. These deaths included 410,000 among women and 74,000 among HIV-negative children. Approximately 75% of total TB deaths occurred in the African and South-East Asia Regions in 2012 (both including and excluding TB deaths among HIV-positive people). India and South Africa accounted for about one-third of global TB deaths.

The number of TB deaths per 100,000 population averaged 13 globally in 2012 and 17.6 when TB deaths among HIV-positive people are included. There is considerable variation among countries, ranging from less than one TB death per 100,000 population (examples include most countries in western Europe, Canada, the United States of America, Australia and New Zealand) to more than 40 deaths per 100,000 population in much of the African region as well as three high burden countries (HBCs) in Asia (Bangladesh, Cambodia, and Myanmar).

Globally, mortality rates (excluding deaths among HIV-positive people) have decreased by 45% since 1990 (Fig. 2, central panel); the current forecast suggests that the international target of a 50% reduction in TB mortality by 2015 compared with a baseline of 1990 will be achieved. Mortality rates are declining in all six WHO regions (Fig. 3). The 2015 target has already been surpassed in the region of the Americas (since 2004) and the western Pacific region (since 2002), and may have been reached in the eastern Mediterranean region. Among the other three regions, the Southeast Asia region appears best placed to achieve the target. The resurgence of TB mortality in Eastern European countries during the 1990s can be explained by the major political, economic, and social disruption associated with the breakup of the Soviet Union in 1991 and related failures in TB control and provision of health care (Shilova and Dye 2001).

Prevalence

There were an estimated 12 million prevalent cases (11 million–13 million) of TB in 2012, equivalent to 169 cases per 100,000 population. By 2012, the prevalence rate had decreased 37% globally since 1990 (Fig. 2, right panel). Current forecasts suggest that the Stop TB Partnership target of halving TB prevalence by 2015 compared with a baseline of 1990 will not be met worldwide.

Regionally, prevalence rates are declining in all six WHO regions. The region of the Americas halved the 1990 level of TB prevalence by around 2004, well in advance of the target year of 2015, and the best estimate suggests that the Western Pacific Region achieved the 50% reduction target in 2012. Reaching the 50% reduction target by 2015 appears feasible in the Southeast Asia region and also in the European region with a relatively small acceleration in the current rate of progress. The target appears out of reach in the African and eastern Mediterranean regions. In Africa, prevalence rates increased substantially during the 1990s, and by 2007 were still far above the 1990 level. With limited access to antiretroviral therapy (ART), HIV has probably had a smaller effect on TB prevalence than on incidence because the duration of TB among HIV-infected patients is relatively short: for people with advanced HIV infection, the progression to severe tuberculosis is rapid, with a marked reduction in life expectancy (Corbett et al. 2004).

Case Notifications and Treatment Success

Routine recording and reporting of the numbers of TB cases diagnosed and treated by NTPs and monitoring of treatment outcomes was one

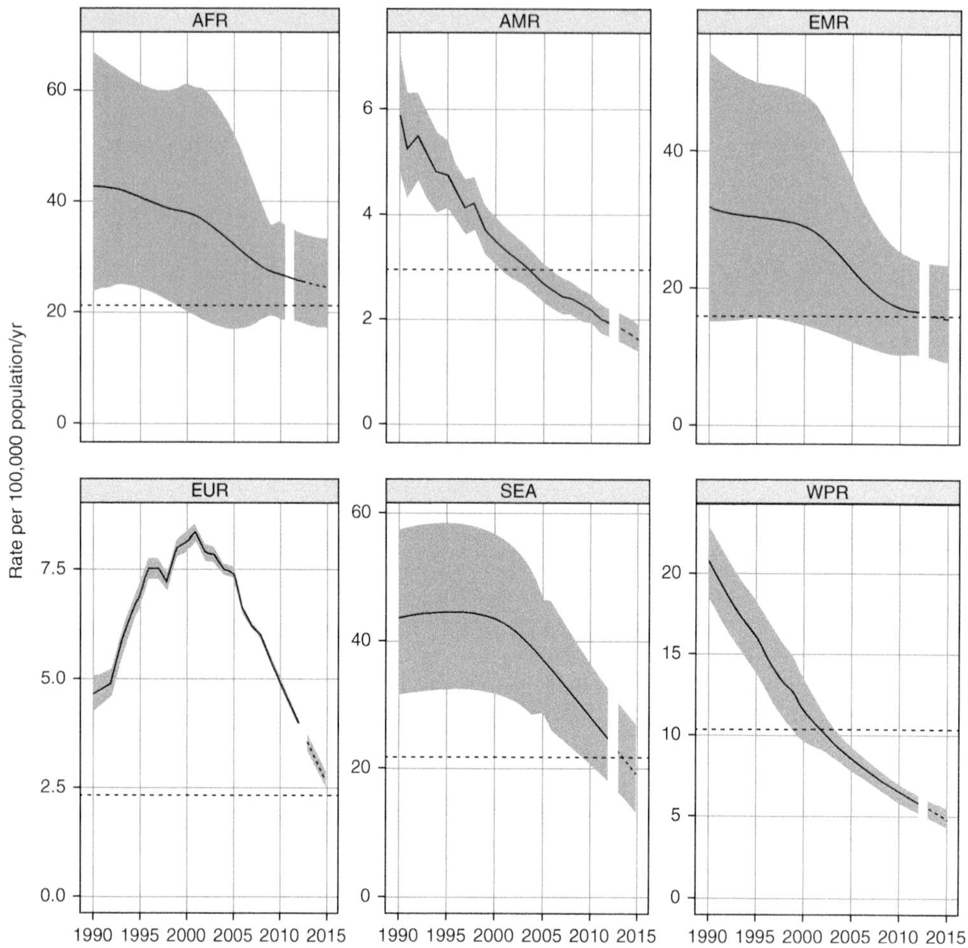

Figure 3. Trends in estimated TB mortality rates excluding HIV during the period 1990–2012 and forecast TB mortality rates 2013–2015 by WHO region. Estimated TB mortality excludes TB deaths among HIV-positive people (which are classified as AIDS deaths). Shaded areas represent uncertainty bands. The horizontal dashed lines represent the Stop TB Partnership target of a 50% reduction in the mortality rate by 2015 compared with 1990. The other dashed lines show projections up to 2015.

of the five components of the global TB strategy (DOTS) launched by WHO in the mid-1990s and it remains a core element of its successor, the *Stop TB Strategy* (Box 2). With the standard definitions of cases and treatment outcomes recommended by WHO and associated recording and reporting framework as a foundation, global monitoring of trends in case notifications and treatment outcomes has been possible since 1995.

In 2012, 6.1 million cases of TB were notified by NTPs and reported to WHO. 5.7 million were individuals newly diagnosed in 2012 and 0.4 million were previously diagnosed TB patients whose treatment regimen was changed. India and China accounted for 39% of notified cases of TB worldwide in 2012, African countries for 23% and the 22 HBCs for 82%. Notifications of TB cases have stabilized in recent years, and in 2012 represented 66% (64%–69%) of estimated incident cases (Fig. 2).

Most cases (88%) were aged 15–64 yr. Children (aged <15 yr) accounted for <10% of notified cases. The sex ratio (M/F) was 1.7, ranging from 1.0 to 2.1 among the six WHO regions. The reasons for higher TB notification rates in men are poorly understood (Ottmani and Uplekar 2008). Possible explanations include biological differences between men and women in certain age groups that affect the risk of being infected as well as the risk of infection progressing to active disease (Thorson et al. 2007), and differences in the societal roles of men and women that influence their risk of exposure to TB and access to care (gender differences) (Connolly and Nunn 1996; Borgdorff et al. 2000; Somma et al. 2008). The observation that TB notification rates tend to be more equal between men and women in countries with a high prevalence of HIV supports the hypothesis of biological differences that can be lessened by immunological suppression caused by HIV, but other nonbiological factors may play a role. Variation in the sex ratio among countries may reflect real differences in epidemiology as well as differential access to health care and use of services linked to the NTP. In some settings (e.g., Afghanistan and the neighboring provinces of Iran and Pakistan), the sex ratio among notified cases is less than one. However, the recent national population-based survey in Pakistan (E Qadeer, R Fatima, S Tahseen, et al., unpubl.) confirmed findings from all other recent prevalence surveys to date that there are more men than women among prevalent TB cases (in Asian surveys conducted since 1990, the sex ratio has been between around 3 and 4), suggesting that women access TB care services linked to the NTP to a greater extent than men in some settings or that disease progression in those settings could be slower on average in women.

Globally, 87% of the new cases in 2011 were successfully treated (Fig. 4). The lowest treatment success rates were in Africa (79%, despite steady improvement since 2006), in the region of the Americas (75%), and in the European region (72%); in the latter case probably because of a high prevalence of multidrug-resistant TB. Treatment success for MDR-TB patients is in general much lower (see below).

The provision of diagnosis and treatment according to the DOTS/Stop TB Strategy has resulted in major achievements in TB care and control. Between 1995 and 2012, 56 million people were successfully treated for TB in countries that had adopted the DOTS/Stop TB Strategy, saving 22 million lives.

HIV-Associated TB

The 8.6 million incident TB cases in 2012 included 1.0 million–1.2 million (12%–14%) among people living with HIV, with a best estimate of 1.1 million (13%). The probability of

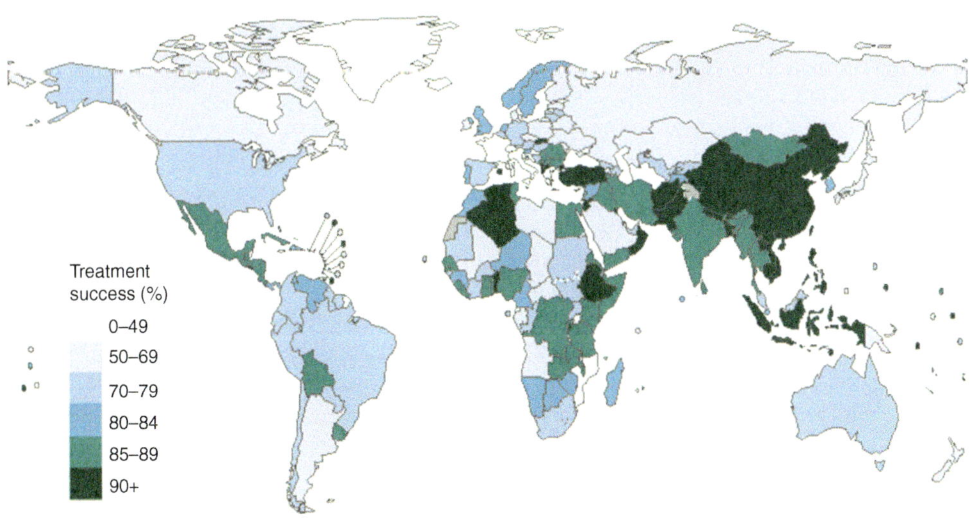

Figure 4. Treatment success rate, 2011 cohort of newly diagnosed TB cases (all forms). Countries shown in white did not report data to WHO for the 2011 cohort.

developing TB among people living with HIV divided by the probability of developing TB among HIV-negative people is the incidence rate ratio (IRR), a measure of the relative risk of TB in HIV-positive individuals compared with HIV-negative individuals. The estimated global IRR in 2012 was 29.6 (27.1–32.1).

The proportion of TB cases coinfected with HIV was highest in countries in the African region. Overall, 37% of TB cases were estimated to be coinfected with HIV in this region, which accounted for 75% of TB cases among people living with HIV worldwide. In parts of southern Africa, >50% of TB cases were coinfected with HIV. The number of people dying from HIV-associated TB has been decreasing since 2003. However, there were still 320,000 deaths from HIV-associated TB in 2012 and further efforts are needed to reduce this burden.

Globally, the percentage of notified TB patients with a documented HIV test result was 46% in 2012. In the African region, 74% of notified TB patients had an HIV test result in 2012. Among the 41 countries with the highest TB/HIV burden, 15 achieved HIV testing levels of ≥85%. There was an encouraging increase in ART coverage among HIV-positive TB patients between 2011 and 2012, from 49% worldwide in 2011 to 57% in 2012. Nonetheless, given the WHO recommendation that all HIV-positive TB patients are eligible for ART, the coverage of ART for HIV-positive TB patients still needs to be greatly improved. Antiretroviral therapy (ART) is expected to play an increasing role in preventing TB deaths as coverage expands (~57% of notified TB cases estimated to be infected with HIV globally were on ART in 2012, compared with 16% in 2010) (Straetemans et al. 2010; Williams et al. 2010; Glaziou et al. 2011; WHO 2013a). ART and INH prophylaxis will also increasingly contribute to prevention of TB in individuals with both HIV infection and latent TB infection.

Multidrug-Resistant TB

Drug resistance, which develops as a result of inadequate treatment creating a selection pressure on spontaneously occurring mutants, complicates the management of TB; MDR- and XDR-TB represent one of the most important challenges in the control of TB worldwide (Raviglione and Uplekar 2006; Migliori et al. 2007a; Velayati et al. 2009; WHO 2011b; Udwadia et al. 2012).

Globally among notified TB cases, an estimated 3.6% of new cases and 20.2% of those previously treated have MDR-TB. Eastern Europe and central Asia have the highest MDR-TB percentage globally (up to 35% among new cases in some oblasts of Russia and Belarus), whereas important data gaps exist in the African region (Fig. 5). There were an estimated 450,000 (300,000–600,000) new cases of MDR-TB in 2012. These emerged either among incident TB cases (primary MDR-TB) or prevalent TB cases currently on treatment (acquired MDR-TB) in 2012. Among new and retreated TB patients known to National TB Programs that could have tested for drug resistance, there were an estimated 300,000 (220,000–380,000) MDR-TB cases in 2012; more than half of these cases were in India, China, and the Russian Federation. Of these 300,000 estimated cases, 94,000 were detected as having MDR-TB and 82% of those started on second-line treatment. However, treatment success globally remains well behind the conventional target of 75% set in the Global Plan to Stop TB (WHO 2011a), at only 48% in the 2010 patient cohort (the latest cohort for which data were available at in 2013, given treatment duration of around 2 years). Finally, deaths from MDR-TB in 2012 were estimated at 170,000 (100,000–240,000). Extensively drug-resistant TB (XDR-TB) has been so far reported from 92 countries world-wide. It is estimated that ~10% of the MDR-TB cases are XDR-TB.

By the end of June 2013, new diagnostics based on molecular techniques had started to be deployed in 88 low- and middle-income countries (WHO 2013a) and 49% of low and middle-income countries had incorporated WHO policy guidance on new diagnostics (Weyer et al. 2013) in their national guidelines. New diagnostics will make it possible for more people with drug-resistant disease to be detected earlier on in the course of their disease, thus improving outcomes.

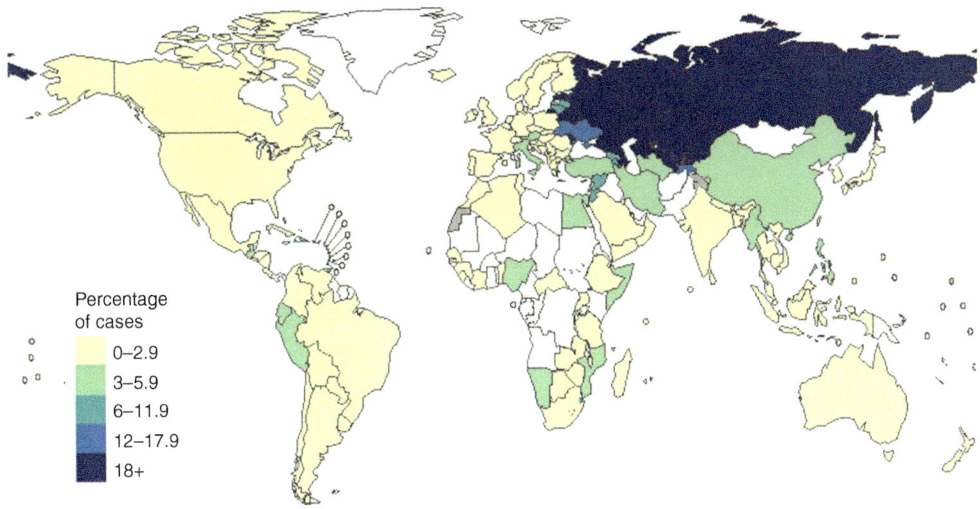

Figure 5. Percentage of new TB cases with MDR-TB, based on the most recent year for which data have been reported, which varies between countries. Countries and territories shown in white have reported no data. In Brazil, Spain, Central African Republic, Russia, Turkmenistan, India, Malaysia, and Indonesia, drug resistance surveillance data was only subnational.

Childhood TB

In 2012, an estimated 530,000 (510,000–550,000) children (aged 15 or less) fell ill with TB representing ~6% of the global burden and there were 74,000 (59,000–90,000) deaths among HIV-negative children (representing ~8% of total TB mortality among HIV-negative people). Out of the ~350,000 TB notifications among children, 70% had pulmonary TB; most of these cases (~80%) were diagnosed without bacteriological confirmation.

The traditionally low prioritization given to mostly noninfectious TB cases among children in overburdened health systems is aggravated by and has contributed to inadequate availability of diagnostic and treatment tools tailored to the needs of children, as well as to limitations in the availability of robust and nationally representative surveillance data. Nonetheless, growing attention to childhood TB in recent years has resulted in the development of clearly articulated actions for all stakeholders to address historical shortcomings. These include (1) strengthening surveillance through better recording and reporting and engagement with the private sector, especially pediatricians; (2) integrating TB screening in existing maternal and child health services, especially in TB endemic settings; and (3) addressing knowledge and research gaps in epidemiology, basic and operational research; and the development of new tools, such as diagnostics, drugs, vaccines (WHO 2013b).

TB PREVENTION AND CONTROL AFTER 2015

Incidence rates comparable with those currently found in low- and middle-income countries with a high burden of TB were recorded in North America and Western Europe as late as the early 20th century. A few of these countries have reliably documented their substantial reductions in case rates for more than 100 years (Styblo et al. 1969). The fastest nationwide declines of ~10% per year occurred in the post-1945 period immediately after the second World War, when continued improvements in living conditions were combined with rapid economic growth, the introduction of effective chemotherapy, and universal (and largely free or not impoverishing) access to health care. Steeper reductions of 16% per year were recorded in two subpopulations with incidence rates 10 times higher than the 2012 global average (Canadian Inuits

[Enarson and Grzybowski 1986] and Alaskan Eskimos [Grzybowski et al. 1976]) in the 1950s and 1960s, thanks to effective treatment programs combined with mass screening and preventive therapy. The current best performers among high-burden countries, such as Cambodia, China, and Rwanda, have recently achieved reductions of ~3%–5% per year and the global decline in incidence is only 2% per year. With current tools, effective TB control should be able to achieve faster reductions in incidence of 5%–10% per year (Dye et al. 2013). The 2050 target of TB elimination is most likely to be achieved if, besides early detection and treatment of active TB cases, latent infection is treated and active disease prevented with either such an easily administered preventive treatment or a new vaccine (Dye and Williams 2008). This will require new and better tools.

To date, only BCG vaccination, provided to >80% of the annual birth cohort, and treatment of active TB using first-line drugs, have been implemented on a large scale (Lonnroth et al. 2010; Raviglione et al. 2012a). With these interventions that result in a global decline of some 2% per year, elimination (less than one case per million population) will not be achieved by 2050 (Lonnroth and Raviglione 2008). A rapid reduction in TB incidence and mortality in excess of what has been achieved historically requires more effective implementation of existing tools and the development and widespread use of a highly effective and safe new vaccine or prophylactic treatment (PT) to prevent reactivation of TB disease among the estimated 2 billion infected people (Dye et al. 1999; WHO 2012b) already. Currently, the only vaccine for TB prevention (BCG) dates from the 1920s and is mainly effective in preventing severe forms of TB in children, whereas its efficacy in the infectious adult forms of TB varies according to settings and populations not resulting in any large-scale protection. The earliest date at which a new vaccine may become available is now estimated as early to mid 2020. Randomized controlled trials of PT have shown that up to 9 mo of daily INH for treatment of latent infection confers 25%–92% protection against developing active TB, with results toward the upper end of this range when patients adhere fully to the treatment regimen (Sterling 2008). Isoniazid, alone or in combination (Sterling et al. 2011), is also a relatively safe drug. Its main side effect, hepatitis, occurs in 1% of patients; however, four to seven treated individuals per 100,000 may develop fatal hepatitis (Millard et al. 1996). The high risk of TB among people coinfected with *M. tuberculosis* and HIV is a reason for promoting much greater use in settings with a high prevalence of HIV (Woldehanna and Volmink 2004; Churchyard et al. 2007). To date, however, PTs with INH or combinations of drugs are not widely used.

First-line treatments that cure ~90% of drug-susceptible cases remain long (6 mo) and are based on drug combinations dating from the 1970s. In mid-2013, there were 12 vaccine candidates for TB prevention in clinical trials and 10 new or repurposed drugs in late phases of clinical development. Two new drugs belonging to two novel classes of antibiotics were approved by strict regulatory authorities in the past 15 mo—the dyarilquinoline, bedaquiline (Diacon et al. 2012) and the nitroimidazole, delamanid (Gler et al. 2012). These two drugs offer hope of better outcomes in severe cases of MDR-TB, but have not yet been tested to shorten treatment of drug-susceptible TB or as preventive treatment. Various new diagnostic tests and methods have been endorsed since 2007, although a point-of-care test remains elusive. Research and development related to new drugs, new diagnostics, and new vaccines has accelerated in recent years (Lonnroth and Raviglione 2008; Ly and McMurray 2008; Pai and O'Brien 2008; Lienhardt et al. 2012a,b; Nicolau et al. 2012; Raviglione et al. 2012a; WHO 2013a).

Besides PT, there is considerable scope to expand interventions to reduce TB-related mortality in HIV-positive people. ART decreases the incidence of TB among people living with HIV (although more research is needed to understand the impact of large scale ART programs on TB epidemics) and reduces mortality. Cotrimoxazole preventive therapy (CPT) for HIV-positive TB patients reduces mortality (Grimwade et al. 2005; Harries et al. 2009). Recent expansion of TB control in areas in which the

Cite this article as *Cold Spring Harb Perspect Med* doi: 10.1101/cshperspect.a017798

prevalence of HIV is high has also exposed a neglect of the basic principles of infection control, in which immunosuppressed patients have been exposed to patients with active TB in clinics and hospitals (Bock et al. 2007; Wells et al. 2007).

Provision of diagnosis and treatment for cases of MDR-TB is mostly confined to the European region, North America, and South Africa (WHO 2013a). Urgent improvements in the provision of services for laboratory culture and DST, new rapid drug susceptibility tests as well as treatment are needed in many countries. The emergence of XDR-TB (Migliori et al. 2007b; Shah et al. 2007) has reinforced the need for updated plans to improve the performance of TB control, including prevention of additional acquisition of resistance, transmission of resistant strains, and the capacity to diagnose and provide adequate treatment for drug-resistant TB (Manissero and Fernandez de la Hoz 2006; Raviglione 2006a; Raviglione and Smith 2007).

In addition to scaling up interventions related to treatment of latent infection, TB/HIV, and MDR-TB, the Stop TB Strategy emphasizes the importance of engaging the full range of health-care providers. These include those in prisons and the armed forces, private clinicians, services provided by nongovernmental organizations, faith-based organizations, and mission services and hospitals, and clinics in the corporate sector (Lonnroth et al. 2004; Ambe et al. 2005; Lonnroth and Uplekar 2005; Floyd et al. 2006; Pantoja et al. 2009). Such engagement can shorten delays to diagnosis and ensure that treatment for all patients (in both the public and the nonstate sector) meets international standards (Hopewell et al. 2006).

As in the immediate post–World War II period, a paradigm shift in the tools available for TB control is now needed, in the context of Universal Health Coverage (WHO 2012a). Incidence would need to decline as fast as 20% per year on average for the elimination target to be achieved by 2050. Wider application of existing interventions combined with development and implementation of new tools is required, as set out in the Stop TB Strategy and the Global Plan to Stop TB (Raviglione 2006b, 2007). In addition, TB control and prevention need to be placed in the wider context of health and development (Dye and Raviglione 2013). The challenge will be to incorporate new tools into TB control practices while also strengthening overall health systems and ensuring wider access to prevention, diagnostic, and treatment. In 2012, WHO initiated work on a new post-2015 global TB strategy that incorporates all of these elements; it is anticipated that the strategy and associated operational guidance will be finalized by 2015.

Recognition that TB depends largely on social and economic determinants of ill health is crucial to achieve full control and elimination. Factors such as smoking, alcohol abuse, diabetes, indoor air pollution, and malnutrition that, like HIV, are impacting on TB epidemiology impeding faster progress toward its control (Lonnroth et al. 2009; Lienhardt et al. 2012a). Preventive strategies may result in remarkable outcomes among certain vulnerable groups, such as people with diabetes and those infected with HIV. Reductions in levels of smoking, alcohol abuse, malnutrition, and indoor air pollution will likely be associated with reduction in TB infection and disease. Ultimately, education, health promotion, universal health coverage (Moreno-Serra and Smith 2012), and poverty-reduction strategies will have an effect on the TB epidemic by removing progressively individuals from the vulnerable pool.

CONCLUSIONS

Major gains were achieved in TB control over the past two decades. Between 1995 and 2012, 22 million lives were saved in countries that had adopted the DOTS/Stop TB Strategy (WHO 2013a) and international TB targets for 2015 will likely be met at the global level (WHO 2013a). Nonetheless, the burden of TB remains high and affects disproportionately poor and disadvantaged populations worldwide (Squire et al. 2006), and whereas the burden of TB is declining, the rate of progress is too slow. The accelerated development of new tools allows for a more optimistic view of the future course of the TB pandemic. A post-2015 global strategy to control TB will necessarily include the successful development and application of new and safe prophylactic treatments and effective vaccines (Raviglione et al. 2012b) administered on a very large scale. While pursuing new tool research and development, global adoption and rapid implementation of the universal health-care agenda and effectively addressing determinants of TB will be the key to accelerating the decline in incidence.

ACKNOWLEDGMENTS

We sincerely thank Matteo Zignol and Dennis Falzon for their contribution to the section on drug-resistant tuberculosis. The World Health Organization (WHO) has graciously granted the authors and publishers permission to publish this material, which remains exclusively vested in WHO.

REFERENCES

Ambe G, Lonnroth K, Dholakia Y, Copreaux J, Zignol M, Borremans N, Uplekar M. 2005. Every provider counts: Effect of a comprehensive public-private mix approach for TB control in a large metropolitan area in India. *Int J Tuberc Lung Dis* **9:** 562–568.

Baussano I, Bugiani M, Gregori D, van Hest R, Borraccino A, Raso R, Merletti F. 2006. Undetected burden of tuberculosis in a low-prevalence area. *Int J Tuberc Lung Dis* **10:** 415–421.

Bierrenbach AL, Stevens AP, Gomes AB, Noronha EF, Glatt R, Carvalho CN, Oliveira Junior JG, Souza Mde F. 2007. [Impact on tuberculosis incidence rates of removal of repeat notification records]. *Revista de saude publica* **41:** 67–76.

Bock NN, Jensen PA, Miller B, Nardell E. 2007. Tuberculosis infection control in resource-limited settings in the era of expanding HIV care and treatment. *J Infect Dis* **196:** S108–S113.

Borgdorff MW, Nagelkerke NJ, Dye C, Nunn P. 2000. Gender and tuberculosis: A comparison of prevalence surveys with notification data to explore sex differences in case detection. *Int J Tuberc Lung Dis* **4:** 123–132.

Borgdorff MW, Glynn JR, Vynnycky E. 2004. Using capture-recapture methods to study recent transmission of tuberculosis. *Int J Epidemiol* **33:** 905–906.

Borgdorff MW, Sebek M, Geskus RB, Kremer K, Kalisvaart N, van Soolingen D. 2011. The incubation period distribution of tuberculosis estimated with a molecular epidemiological approach. *Int J Epidemiol* **40:** 964–970.

Botha E, den Boon S, Lawrence KA, Reuter H, Verver S, Lombard CJ, Dye C, Enarson DA, Beyers N. 2008. From suspect to patient: Tuberculosis diagnosis and treatment initiation in health facilities in South Africa. *Int J Tuberc Lung Dis* **12:** 936–941.

Cailhol J, Che D, Jarlier V, Decludt B, Robert J. 2005. Incidence of tuberculous meningitis in France, 2000: A capture-recapture analysis. *Int J Tuberc Lung Dis* **9:** 803–808.

Churchyard GJ, Scano F, Grant AD, Chaisson RE. 2007. Tuberculosis preventive therapy in the era of HIV infection: Overview and research priorities. *J Infect Dis* **196:** S52–S62.

Comas I, Coscolla M, Luo T, Borrell S, Holt KE, Kato-Maeda M, Parkhill J, Malla B, Berg S, Thwaites G, et al. 2013. Out-of-Africa migration and Neolithic coexpansion of *Mycobacterium tuberculosis* with modern humans. *Nat Genet* **45:** 1176–1182.

Connolly M, Nunn P. 1996. Women and tuberculosis. *World Health Stat Q* **49:** 115–119.

Corbett EL, Charalambous S, Moloi VM, Fielding K, Grant AD, Dye C, De Cock KM, Hayes RJ, Williams BG, Churchyard GJ. 2004. Human immunodeficiency virus and the prevalence of undiagnosed tuberculosis in African gold miners. *Am J Respir Crit Care Med* **170:** 673–679.

Crofts JP, Pebody R, Grant A, Watson JM, Abubakar I. 2008. Estimating tuberculosis case mortality in England and Wales, 2001–2002. *Int J Tuberc Lung Dis* **12:** 308–313.

Diacon AH, Dawson R, von Groote-Bidlingmaier F, Symons G, Venter A, Donald PR, van Niekerk C, Everitt D, Winter H, Becker P, et al. 2012. 14-day bactericidal activity of PA-824, bedaquiline, pyrazinamide, and moxifloxacin combinations: A randomised trial. *Lancet* **380:** 986–993.

Dye C, Floyd K. 2006. Tuberculosis. In *Disease Control Priorities Priorities in Developing Countries* (ed. Jamison DT et al.), pp. 289–309. Oxford University Press, Washington, DC.

Dye C, Raviglione M. 2013. Weigh all TB risks. *Nature* **502:** S13.

Dye C, Williams BG. 2008. Eliminating human tuberculosis in the twenty-first century. *J R Soc Interface* **5:** 653–662.

Dye C, Scheele S, Dolin P, Pathania V, Raviglione MC. 1999. Consensus statement. Global burden of tuberculosis: Estimated incidence, prevalence, and mortality by country. WHO Global Surveillance and Monitoring Project. *JAMA* **282:** 677–686.

Dye C, Fengzeng Z, Scheele S, Williams B. 2000. Evaluating the impact of tuberculosis control: Number of deaths prevented by short-course chemotherapy in China. *Int J Epidemiol* **29:** 558–564.

Dye C, Ottmani S, Laasri L, Bencheikh N. 2007. The decline of tuberculosis epidemics under chemotherapy: A case study in Morocco. *Int J Tuberc Lung Dis* **11:** 1225–1231.

Dye C, Bassili A, Bierrenbach AL, Broekmans JF, Chadha VK, Glaziou P, Gopi PG, Hosseini M, Kim SJ, Manissero D, et al. 2008. Measuring tuberculosis burden, trends, and the impact of control programmes. *Lancet Infect Dis* **8:** 233–243.

Dye C, Glaziou P, Floyd K, Raviglione M. 2013. Prospects for tuberculosis elimination. *Annu Rev Public Health* **34:** 271–286.

Enarson DA, Grzybowski S. 1986. Incidence of active tuberculosis in the native population of Canada. *CMAJ* **134:** 1149–1152.

Floyd K, Arora VK, Murthy KJ, Lonnroth K, Singla N, Akbar Y, Zignol M, Uplekar M. 2006. Cost and cost-effectiveness of PPM-DOTS for tuberculosis control: Evidence from India. *Bull World Health Organ* **84:** 437–445.

Glaziou P, van der Werf MJ, Onozaki I, Dye C, Borgdorff MW, Chiang CY, Cobelens F, Enarson DA, Gopi PG, Holtz TH, et al. 2008. Tuberculosis prevalence surveys: Rationale and cost. *Int J Tuberc Lung Dis* **12:** 1003–1008.

Glaziou P, Floyd K, Korenromp EL, Sismanidis C, Bierrenbach AL, Williams BG, Atun R, Raviglione M. 2011. Lives saved by tuberculosis control and prospects for achieving the 2015 global target for reducing tuberculosis mortality. *Bull World Health Organ* **89:** 573–582.

Gler MT, Skripconoka V, Sanchez-Garavito E, Xiao H, Cabrera-Rivero JL, Vargas-Vasquez DE, Gao M, Awad M, Park SK, Shim TS, et al. 2012. Delamanid for multidrug-resistant pulmonary tuberculosis. *N Engl J Med* **366:** 2151–2160.

Grimwade K, Sturm AW, Nunn AJ, Mbatha D, Zungu D, Gilks CF. 2005. Effectiveness of cotrimoxazole prophylaxis on mortality in adults with tuberculosis in rural South Africa. *AIDS (London, England)* **19:** 163–168.

Grzybowski S, Styblo K, Dorken E. 1976. Tuberculosis in Eskimos. *Tubercle* **57:** S1–S58.

Harries AD, Zachariah R, Lawn SD. 2009. Providing HIV care for co-infected tuberculosis patients: A perspective from sub-Saharan Africa. *Int J Tuberc Lung Dis* **13:** 6–16.

Holloway KL, Henneberg RJ, de Barros Lopes M, Henneberg M. 2011. Evolution of human tuberculosis: A systematic review and meta-analysis of paleopathological evidence. *Homo* **62:** 402–458.

Hong YP, KSJ, Lew WJ, Lee EK, Han YC. 1998. The seventh nationwide tuberculosis prevalence survey in Korea, 1995. *Int J Tuberc Lung Dis* **2:** 27–36.

Hopewell PC, Pai M, Maher D, Uplekar M, Raviglione MC. 2006. International standards for tuberculosis care. *Lancet Infect Dis* **6:** 710–725.

Korenromp EL, Williams BG, Dye C. 2009. The measurement and estimation of tuberculosis mortality. *Int J Tuberc Lung Dis* **13:** 283–303.

Korenromp EL, Glaziou P, Fitzpatrick C, Floyd K, Hosseini M, Raviglione M, Atun R, Williams B. 2012. Implementing the global plan to stop TB, 2011–2015—Optimizing allocations and the Global Fund's contribution: A scenario projections study. *PLoS ONE* **7:** e38816.

Lienhardt C, Glaziou P, Uplekar M, Lonnroth K, Getahun H, Raviglione M. 2012a. Global tuberculosis control: Lessons learnt and future prospects. *Nat Rev Microbiol* **10:** 407–416.

Lienhardt C, Raviglione M, Spigelman M, Hafner R, Jaramillo E, Hoelscher M, Zumla A, Gheuens J. 2012b. New drugs for the treatment of tuberculosis: Needs, challenges, promise, and prospects for the future. *J Infect Dis* **205:** S241–S249.

Lonnroth K, Raviglione M. 2008. Global epidemiology of tuberculosis: Prospects for control. *Semin Respir Crit Care Med* **29:** 481–491.

Lonnroth K, Uplekar M. 2005. Invest in breaking the barriers of public-private collaboration for improved tuberculosis care. *Bull World Health Organ* **83:** 558–559.

Lonnroth K, Uplekar M, Arora VK, Juvekar S, Lan NT, Mwaniki D, Pathania V. 2004. Public-private mix for DOTS implementation: What makes it work? *Bull World Health Organ* **82:** 580–586.

Lonnroth K, Jaramillo E, Williams BG, Dye C, Raviglione M. 2009. Drivers of tuberculosis epidemics: The role of risk factors and social determinants. *Soc Sci Med* **68:** 2240–2246.

Lonnroth K, Castro KG, Chakaya JM, Chauhan LS, Floyd K, Glaziou P, Raviglione MC. 2010. Tuberculosis control and elimination 2010–50: Cure, care, and social development. *Lancet* **375:** 1814–1829.

Lopez AD, Mathers CD, Ezzati M, Jamison DT, Murray CJ. 2006. Global and regional burden of disease and risk factors, 2001: Systematic analysis of population health data. *Lancet* **367:** 1747–1757.

Lozano R, Naghavi M, Foreman K, Lim S, Shibuya K, Aboyans V, Abraham J, Adair T, Aggarwal R, Ahn SY, et al. 2012. Global and regional mortality from 235 causes of death for 20 age groups in 1990 and 2010: A systematic analysis for the Global Burden of Disease Study 2010. *Lancet* **380:** 2095–2128.

Ly LH, McMurray DN. 2008. Tuberculosis: Vaccines in the pipeline. *Expert Rev Vaccines* **7:** 635–650.

Manissero D, Fernandez de la Hoz K. 2006. Surveillance methods and case definition for extensively drug resistant TB (XDR-TB) and relevance to Europe: Summary update. *Euro Surveill* **11:** E061103.1.

Meintjes G, Schoeman H, Morroni C, Wilson D, Maartens G. 2008. Patient and provider delay in tuberculosis suspects from communities with a high HIV prevalence in South Africa: A cross-sectional study. *BMC Infect Dis* **8:** 72.

Migliori GB, De Iaco G, Besozzi G, Centis R, Cirillo DM. 2007a. First tuberculosis cases in Italy resistant to all tested drugs. *Euro Surveill* **12:** E070517.1.

Migliori GB, Loddenkemper R, Blasi F, Raviglione MC. 2007b. 125 years after Robert Koch's discovery of the tubercle bacillus: The new XDR-TB threat. Is "science" enough to tackle the epidemic? *Eur Respir J* **29:** 423–427.

Millard PS, Wilcosky TC, Reade-Christopher SJ, Weber DJ. 1996. Isoniazid-related fatal hepatitis. *West J Med* **164:** 486–491.

Miller TL, McNabb SJ, Hilsenrath P, Pasipanodya J, Weis SE. 2009. Personal and societal health quality lost to tuberculosis. *PLoS ONE* **4:** e5080.

Moreno-Serra R, Smith PC. 2012. Does progress towards universal health coverage improve population health? *Lancet* **380:** 917–923.

Murray CJ, DeJonghe E, Chum HJ, Nyangulu DS, Salomao A, Styblo K. 1991. Cost effectiveness of chemotherapy for pulmonary tuberculosis in three sub-Saharan African countries. *Lancet* **338:** 1305–1308.

Nicolau I, Ling D, Tian L, Lienhardt C, Pai M. 2012. Research questions and priorities for tuberculosis: A survey of published systematic reviews and meta-analyses. *PLoS ONE* **7:** e42479.

O'Neill K, Takane M, Sheffel A, Abou-Zahr C, Boerma T. 2013. Monitoring service delivery for universal health coverage: The Service Availability and Readiness Assessment. *Bull World Health Organ* **91:** 923–931.

Ortblad KF, Lozano R, Murray CJ. 2013. The burden of HIV: Insights from the Global Burden of Disease Study 2010. *AIDS* **27:** 2003–2017.

Ottmani SE, Uplekar MW. 2008. Gender and TB: Pointers from routine records and reports. *Int J Tuberc Lung Dis* **12:** 827–828.

Pablos-Mendez A, Raviglione MC, Laszlo A, Binkin N, Rieder HL, Bustreo F, Cohn DL, Lambregts-van Weezenbeek CS, Kim SJ, Chaulet P, et al. 1998. Global surveillance for antituberculosis-drug resistance, 1994–1997. World Health Organization-International Union against Tuberculosis and Lung Disease Working Group on Anti-Tuberculosis Drug Resistance Surveillance. *N Engl J Med* **338:** 1641–1649.

Pai M, O'Brien R. 2008. New diagnostics for latent and active tuberculosis: State of the art and future prospects. *Semin Respir Crit Care Med* **29:** 560–568.

Pantoja A, Floyd K, Unnikrishnan KP, Jitendra R, Padma MR, Lal SS, Uplekar M, Chauhan LS, Kumar P, Sahu S, et al. 2009. Economic evaluation of public-private mix for tuberculosis care and control, India. Part I. Socio-economic profile and costs among tuberculosis patients. *Int J Tuberc Lung Dis* **13:** 698–704.

Raviglione M. 2006a. XDR-TB: Entering the post-antibiotic era? *Int J Tuberc Lung Dis* **10:** 1185–1187.

Raviglione MC. 2006b. The Global Plan to Stop TB, 2006–2015. *Int J Tuberc Lung Dis* **10:** 238–239.

Raviglione MC. 2007. The new Stop TB Strategy and the Global Plan to Stop TB, 2006–2015. *Bull World Health Organ* **85:** 327.

Raviglione MC, Pio A. 2002. Evolution of WHO policies for tuberculosis control, 1948–2001. *Lancet* **359:** 775–780.

Raviglione MC, Smith IM. 2007. XDR tuberculosis—Implications for global public health. *N Engl J Med* **356:** 656–659.

Raviglione MC, Uplekar MW. 2006. WHO's new Stop TB Strategy. *Lancet* **367:** 952–955.

Raviglione M, Marais B, Floyd K, Lonnroth K, Getahun H, Migliori GB, Harries AD, Nunn P, Lienhardt C, Graham S, et al. 2012a. Scaling up interventions to achieve global tuberculosis control: Progress and new developments. *Lancet* **379:** 1902–1913.

Raviglione M, Zumla A, Marais B, Horton R, Motsoaledi A. 2012b. A sustainable agenda for tuberculosis control and research. *Lancet* **379:** 1077–1078.

Riley RL. 1983. The contagiosity of tuberculosis. *Schweiz Med Wochenschr* **113:** 75–79.

Shah NS, Wright A, Bai GH, Barrera L, Boulahbal F, Martin-Casabona N, Drobniewski F, Gilpin C, Havelkova M, Lepe R, et al. 2007. Worldwide emergence of extensively drug-resistant tuberculosis. *Emerg Infect Dis* **13:** 380–387.

Shilova MV, Dye C. 2001. The resurgence of tuberculosis in Russia. *Philos Trans R Soc Lond B Biol Sci* **356:** 1069–1075.

Soemantri S, Senewe FP, Tjandrarini DH, Day R, Basri C, Manissero D, Mehta F, Dye C. 2007. Three-fold reduction in the prevalence of tuberculosis over 25 years in Indonesia. *Int J Tuberc Lung Dis* **11:** 398–404.

Somma D, Thomas BE, Karim F, Kemp J, Arias N, Auer C, Gosoniu GD, Abouihia A, Weiss MG. 2008. Gender and socio-cultural determinants of TB-related stigma in Bangladesh, India, Malawi and Colombia. *Int J Tuberc Lung Dis* **12:** 856–866.

Squire SB, Obasi A, Nhlema-Simwaka B. 2006. The Global Plan to Stop TB: A unique opportunity to address poverty and the Millennium Development Goals. *Lancet* **367:** 955–957.

Sterling TR. 2008. New approaches to the treatment of latent tuberculosis. *Semin Respir Crit Care Med* **29:** 532–541.

Sterling TR, Villarino ME, Borisov AS, Shang N, Gordin F, Bliven-Sizemore E, Hackman J, Hamilton CD, Menzies D, Kerrigan A, et al. 2011. Three months of rifapentine and isoniazid for latent tuberculosis infection. *N Engl J Med* **365:** 2155–2166.

Straetemans M, Bierrenbach AL, Nagelkerke N, Glaziou P, van der Werf MJ. 2010. The effect of tuberculosis on mortality in HIV positive people: A meta-analysis. *PLoS ONE* **5:** e15241.

Straetemans M, Glaziou P, Bierrenbach AL, Sismanidis C, van der Werf MJ. 2011. Assessing tuberculosis case fatality ratio: A meta-analysis. *PLoS ONE* **6:** e20755.

Styblo K, Meijer J, Sutherland I. 1969. [The transmission of tubercle bacilli: Its trend in a human population]. *Bull World Health Organ* **41:** 137–178.

Thorson A, Long NH, Larsson LO. 2007. Chest X-ray findings in relation to gender and symptoms: A study of patients with smear positive tuberculosis in Vietnam. *Scand J Infect Dis* **39:** 33–37.

Tiemersma EW, van der Werf MJ, Borgdorff MW, Williams BG, Nagelkerke NJ. 2011. Natural history of tuberculosis: Duration and fatality of untreated pulmonary tuberculosis in HIV negative patients: A systematic review. *PLoS ONE* **6:** e17601.

Tupasi TE, Radhakrishna S, Rivera AB, Pascual MLG, Quelapio MI, Co VM, Villa MLA, Beltran G, Legaspi JD, Mangubat NV, et al. 1999. The 1997 nationwide tuberculosis prevalence survey in the Philippines. *Int J Tuberc Lung Dis* **3:** 471–477.

Udwadia ZF, Amale RA, Ajbani KK, Rodrigues C. 2012. Totally drug-resistant tuberculosis in India. *Clin Infect Dis* **54:** 579–581.

Uplekar M, Pathania V, Raviglione M. 2001. Private practitioners and public health: Weak links in tuberculosis control. *Lancet* **358:** 912–916.

Van Hest N, Story A, Grant AD, Antoine D, Crofts JP, Watson JM. 2008. Record-linkage and capture-recapture analysis to estimate the incidence and completeness of reporting of tuberculosis in England 1999–2002. *Epidemiol Infect* **136:** 1606–1616.

Velayati AA, Masjedi MR, Farnia P, Tabarsi P, Ghanavi J, Ziazarifi AH, Hoffner SE. 2009. Emergence of new forms of totally drug-resistant tuberculosis bacilli: Super extensively drug-resistant tuberculosis or totally drug-resistant strains in Iran. *Chest* **136:** 420–425.

Veron LJ, Blanc LJ, Suchi M, Raviglione MC. 2004. DOTS expansion: Will we reach the 2005 targets? *Int J Tuberc Lung Dis* **8:** 139–146.

Vynnycky E, Fine PE. 2000. Lifetime risks, incubation period, and serial interval of tuberculosis. *Am J Epidemiol* **152:** 247–263.

Wells CD, Cegielski JP, Nelson LJ, Laserson KF, Holtz TH, Finlay A, Castro KG, Weyer K. 2007. HIV infection and multidrug-resistant tuberculosis: The perfect storm. *J Infect Dis* **196:** S86–S107.

Weyer K, Mirzayev F, Migliori GB, Van Gemert W, D'Ambrosio L, Zignol M, Floyd K, Centis R, Cirillo DM, Tortoli E, et al. 2013. Rapid molecular TB diagnosis: Evidence, policy making and global implementation of Xpert MTB/RIF. *Eur Respir J* **42:** 252–271.

WHO. 2006. *WHO Global Task Force outlines measures to combat XDR-TB worldwide [Internet]*. WHO, Geneva.

WHO. 2011a. *The Global Plan to Stop TB 2011–2015.*

WHO. 2011b. Towards universal access to diagnosis and treatment of multidrug-resistant and extensively drug-resistant tuberculosis by 2015. *WHO progress report 2011.* (ed. WHO). WHO, Geneva.

WHO ed. 2011c. *Tuberculosis prevalence surveys: A handbook.* World Health Organization, Geneva.

WHO. 2012a. *Health financing for universal coverage.* WHO, Geneva.

WHO. 2012b. *Tuberculosis fact sheet.* WHO, Geneva.

WHO. 2013a. *Global TB report 2013* WHO, Geneva.

WHO. 2013b. *Roadmap for childhood tuberculosis.* (ed. WHO). WHO, Geneva.

Williams BG, Granich R, De Cock KM, Glaziou P, Sharma A, Dye C. 2010. Antiretroviral therapy for tuberculosis control in nine African countries. *Proc Natl Acad Sci* **107:** 19485–19489.

Woldehanna S, Volmink J. 2004. Treatment of latent tuberculosis infection in HIV infected persons. *Cochrane database of systematic reviews (Online)*: CD000171.

World Health Organization. 2007. *Global tuberculosis control: Surveillance, planning, financing.* World Health Organization, Geneva.

Zignol M, van Gemert W, Falzon D, Sismanidis C, Glaziou P, Floyd K, Raviglione M. 2012. Surveillance of anti-tuberculosis drug resistance in the world: An updated analysis, 2007–2010. *Bull World Health Organ* **90:** 111–119D.

Zumla A, Mwaba P, Huggett J, Kapata N, Chanda D, Grange J. 2009. Reflections on the white plague. *Lancet Infect Dis* **9:** 197–202.

Advances in Diagnostic Assays for Tuberculosis

Stephen D. Lawn[1,2]

[1]Department of Clinical Research, Faculty of Infectious and Tropical Diseases, London School of Hygiene and Tropical Medicine, London WC1E 7HT, United Kingdom

[2]The Desmond Tutu HIV Centre, Institute for Infectious Disease and Molecular Medicine, Faculty of Health Sciences, University of Cape Town, Cape Town 7925, South Africa

Correspondence: stephen.lawn@lshtm.ac.uk

Approximately one-third of the global burden of tuberculosis (TB) remains undiagnosed each year and the vast majority of cases of multidrug-resistant TB remain undetected. Many countries still place heavy reliance on outdated technologies that are blunt and ineffective tools for controlling this epidemic. However, during the past 10 years, there has been substantial progress within the TB diagnostics developmental pipeline. Old technologies have been reviewed and improved and new technologies have been developed and evaluated and are now being implemented. This review summarizes these developments and describes the currently available diagnostic tools. Consideration is given to the requirements of future diagnostic tests and how these should be evaluated not only with regard to their diagnostic accuracy and operational feasibility, but ultimately in terms of whether they impact clinical outcomes cost effectively, especially for those most in need.

The global burden of tuberculosis (TB) remains enormous, and the incidence rate is decreasing at just 2% per year (WHO 2013a). Although the reasons underlying this slow progress in TB control are complex, TB diagnostic tools have long been recognized as a critical weakness in the care pathway. It was estimated that of the 8.6 million cases that occurred in 2012, 3.0 million of these were missed by national notification systems. Moreover, just one in five of the 450,000 cases of multidrug-resistant TB (MDR-TB) that occur worldwide each year was detected (WHO 2013a). To accelerate progress toward elimination of TB as a public health problem by 2050, there is a need for major improvements in the diagnostic process and in the microbiological tools that are used (Abu-Raddad et al. 2009).

In low- and middle-income countries, which bear the vast majority of the global burden of disease, heavy reliance is still placed on outdated TB diagnostic tools such as direct sputum smear microscopy, solid culture, and chest radiography. These lack either sufficient sensitivity or specificity, are too slow, or are not available at the periphery of the health system where patients first seek care. Opportunities to intervene early in the disease are lost, and diagnosis based solely on clinical suspicion results in overprescription of TB treatment in some settings.

Whereas rapid and accurate point-of-care assays have greatly simplified the diagnosis of

Cite this article as *Cold Spring Harb Perspect Med* doi: 10.1101/cshperspect.a017806

blood-borne disease such as human immunodeficiency virus type 1 (HIV-1) infection and malaria, no comparable tools exist for TB. TB presents a far greater diagnostic challenge. Diagnostic tools must be able to detect pulmonary and extrapulmonary disease when testing a wide variety of clinical sample types, which may differ substantially in bacillary burden. The ability to reliably distinguish between active TB and latent infection is crucial. To reduce morbidity, mortality, and transmission risk, accurate diagnosis is needed in the early stages of disease when bacillary burden in samples may still be low. Assays should be useful in both adults and children as well as those with immunodeficiency due, for example, to HIV coinfection. The growing threat of drug resistance worldwide (WHO 2013a) means that drug susceptibility testing (DST) must be routinely performed, and the advantages of incorporating this within the initial diagnostic assessment are self-evident.

Appropriate diagnostic assays are required for use at all levels of the health-care system and the community, even in settings with the least developed infrastructure. Obtaining samples and testing them must be safe for the patient, for other patients, for the staff in the health-care environment, and for laboratory staff. Frequent failure of diagnosed TB cases to start TB treatment (MacPherson et al. 2014), often referred to as "initial treatment default," highlights the critical need for same-day diagnosis and treatment initiation. The complexity of these various requirements and the vastly differing settings in which the diagnostic assays need to be used means that it is highly unlikely that a single test will ever be developed, but rather it is likely that a range of different assays will be needed at different levels within the health-care system.

The developmental pipeline for TB diagnostics has received much needed focus in recent years. Old technologies have been reviewed and improved and new ones have been developed, evaluated, and implemented. With a rapidly growing evidence base, the World Health Organization (WHO) has issued 11 separate policy statements between 2007 and 2014 regarding TB diagnosis and diagnostic tools (Table 1). Four of these address sputum smear microscopy. Two statements address culture-based systems for diagnosis and DST, and one addresses the use of line-probe assays (LPAs) for rapid molecular diagnosis of drug resistance. Negative recommendations have also been issued regarding the use of serodiagnostic assays and interferon-γ release assays (IGRAs) for TB diagnosis. Following endorsement in December 2010, WHO issued a policy statement in 2011 on use of the Xpert MTB/RIF automated rapid molecular assay for diagnosis of pulmonary TB and detection of rifampicin resistance. Guidelines on Xpert MTB/RIF were updated in 2013 to incorporate recommendations on use in children and for diagnosis of extrapulmonary TB.

The inverse care law states that the availability of good medical care tends to vary inversely with the need for it in the population served (Hart 1971). This is very true of TB diagnostic capacity. The WHO regions with the greatest burden of TB (Africa and South and Southeast Asia) have the least capacity for TB culture and DST by phenotypic means or by line-probe assay, for example (Table 2). Even though a simple and effective means of improving smear microscopy using light-emitting diode (LED) microscopes was endorsed by WHO in 2011, uptake around the world is still at very low levels (Table 2). Thus, developments in new diagnostic tools and evolution of global policies must be accompanied by effective implementation, especially where the need is greatest.

LABORATORY TECHNOLOGIES

Microscopy and Culture

Microscopy

Light microscopy of sputum smears has been the mainstay of TB diagnosis for more than a century and remains the most common means of case detection with assessment of >80 million patients per year (Perkins 2009). It uses cheap equipment and materials and is relatively rapid. However, it is insensitive and requires significant effort on the part of the laboratory technologist who has to meticulously examine dozens of microscopic fields such that quality

 Cite this article as *Cold Spring Harb Perspect Med* doi: 10.1101/cshperspect.a017806

Table 1. World Health Organization (WHO) policy statements on tuberculosis diagnosis (2007–2013)

Year	Policy	Summary of recommendation	Reference
2007	Definition of a new smear-positive TB case	Can be based on the presence of ≥1 acid-fast bacilli in ≥1 sputum sample in quality-assured laboratories	WHO 2007a
2007	Number of smears for the diagnosis of pulmonary TB	Number of samples tested can be reduced from three to two in quality-assured laboratories	WHO 2007b
2007	Use of liquid culture medium for culture and DST	Use of liquid medium for culture, rapid species identification, and DST recommended in low- and middle-income countries	WHO 2007c
2008	Use of line probe assays	Molecular line probe assays are recommended for rapid screening for MDR-TB	WHO 2008
2011	Same-day diagnosis of TB by microscopy	Recommends a case-finding strategy that examines two consecutive specimens obtained on the same day	WHO 2011a
2011	Noncommercial culture and DST methods to detect MDR-TB	Microscopic observation of drug susceptibility (MODS), nitrate reductase assay (NRA), and colorimetric redox indicator (CRI) are recommended for use in reference laboratories	WHO 2011b
2011	Fluorescent light-emitting diode (LED) microscopy for TB diagnosis	Ziehl-Neelen light microscopy and conventional fluorescence microscopy should be replaced by LED microscopy	WHO 2011c
2011	Commercial serodiagnostic tests for diagnosis of TB	Strong recommendation that existing commercial serological tests for TB are not used for diagnosis of pulmonary or extrapulmonary TB	WHO 2011d
2011	Use of interferon-γ release assays (IGRAs) in low- and middle-income countries	IGRAs should not be used in low- and middle-income countries for the diagnosis of pulmonary or extrapulmonary TB or to replace tuberculin skin testing for diagnosis of latent TB	WHO 2011e
2011	Xpert/RIF for rapid detection of TB and rifampicin resistance	Xpert/RIF should be used as the initial diagnostic test in individuals suspected of MDR-TB or HIV-associated TB; Xpert/RIF may also be used as a follow-on test to microscopy in settings in which HIV and MDR-TB are a lesser concern	WHO 2011f
2013	Xpert MTB/RIF for the diagnosis of pulmonary and extrapulmonary TB in adults and children: policy update	Xpert/RIF should be used as the initial diagnostic test in adults and children suspected of MDR-TB or HIV-associated TB; Xpert should be used as the preferred diagnostic test for CSF samples in those with suspected TB meningitis and may be used as a replacement for testing lymph node and other tissues	WHO 2013b

DST, drug susceptibility testing; CSF, cerebrospinal fluid; MDR-TB, multidrug-resistant TB.

is very operator-dependent. The sensitivity of smear microscopy is limited to detection of samples with greater than 10,000 bacilli per milliliter of sputum. Bacillary concentrations in sputum are typically lower in patients with HIV coinfection, such that the sensitivity of smear microscopy is often ~20% lower in these patients (Gupta et al. 2013). Maintaining functional equipment and proficient microscopists out to the periphery of the health-care system in resource-limited settings has proved challenging. The specificity of microscopy is generally good in high TB burden settings, but it is lower in high-income countries where the proportion of positive sputum smears that is attributable to nontuberculous mycobacterial species is greater.

Two methods have been developed to increase the sensitivity of smear microscopy—sputum processing before preparation of smears

Table 2. Global laboratory tuberculosis diagnostics capacity in 2012 according to World Health Organization (WHO) region

	Burden of TB and MDR-TB			Laboratory capacity, 2012						
WHO Region	Incident TB cases (millions)	Incidence rate/ 100,000 population	MDR-TB (% of new TB cases)	MDR-TB (% of retreatment TB cases)	Smear microscopy laboratories/ 100,000 population	LED microscopy (% labs)	Culture laboratories/ 5 million population	DST laboratories/ 5 million population	LPA laboratories/ 5 million population	Xpert MTB/RIF included in national TB policy (% countries)
African	2.3	255	2.3	11	1.5	6	0.6	0.4	0.3	62%
Americas	0.28	29	2.2	14	2.2	<1	16	0.8	0.2	35%
Eastern Mediterranean	0.67	109	3.5	32	0.8	<1	1.4	0.4	0.1	36%
European	0.36	40	16	45	0.7	2	9.8	4.6	1.8	56%
South and Southeast Asian	3.4	187	2.2	16	1.2	2	0.5	0.2	0.1	64%
Western Pacific	1.6	87	4.7	22	0.5	2	3.4	0.6	0.1	33%
Global	**8.6**	**121**	**3.6**	**20.2**	**1.1**	**2**	**3.8**	**0.9**	**0.3**	**49%**

Data extracted from WHO Global TB Report (WHO 2013a).

MDR-TB, multidrug-resistant TB; LED microscopy, light-emitting diode microscopy; DST, drug susceptibility testing; LPA, line probe assay.

and use of fluorescent staining. Numbers of methods for sputum liquefaction (e.g., using inexpensive household bleach) and concentration (e.g., using centrifugation) have been shown to increase yield (Steingart et al. 2006a). Fluorescence microscopy for *Mycobacterium tuberculosis* was developed 70 years ago and allows slide examination with a medium power (25× – 40×) objective, increasing the speed of reading slides and increasing sensitivity by ~10% with no loss in specificity (Steingart et al. 2006b). A major barrier to use of fluorescence microscopy in resource-limited settings was the high equipment cost and short bulb life. However, this problem has now been overcome by the development of microscopes with ultrabright light-emitting diodes (LEDs), which have low energy requirements (allowing battery operation) and a life span of >10,000 h (Perkins 2009; Minion et al. 2011a). High-performance and inexpensive LED microscopes are now available and are increasingly being used, although the rate of scale-up is slow (Table 2). Development of automated microscopy has resulted in prototype devices, but successful devices have not yet emerged.

The Xpert MTB/RIF has now been implemented nationwide as a replacement for smear microscopy in South Africa, and it is possible that other high-burden countries may also do so in the future. However, paradoxically, smear microscopy is unlikely at present to be replaced as a primary diagnostic screening tool in industrialized countries where detection of nontuberculous mycobacterial species is of greater importance than in resource-limited settings.

Culture-Based Diagnosis Drug Susceptibility Testing

The most sensitive means of detecting *M. tuberculosis* is the culture of processed samples on enriched media. If culture is performed in high-burden countries, this usually uses solid egg-based media (Lowenstein–Jensen or Ogawa) with subsequent visualization of colonies. This requires 6–8 wk to rule out growth because *M. tuberculosis* replicates very slowly. Use of selective liquid media and growth indicator systems increase both the sensitivity and speed of detection. Time to detection is shortest using liquid culture with continuous automated monitoring systems, approximately halving the time to detection compared with culture on solid media (Perkins 2009). The emergence of the global epidemic of drug-resistant TB worldwide during the past decade has emphasized the need for much wider availability of culture for both diagnosis and DST. The most widely used method in resource-limited settings has been indirect DST of positive cultures on solid media, typically taking 2–3 mo. Incorporation of DST into automated liquid culture detection can reduce time to culture and DST results to ~2 wk. In 2007, WHO endorsed the use of liquid culture media and phenotypic DST in low- and middle-income countries (Table 1).

As liquid culture is highly sensitive for growth of a wide range of nontuberculous mycobacteria, including environmental species, rapid and simple species identification is essential. Thus, WHO endorsement of liquid culture also included rapid species identification in solid or liquid culture isolates using a simple, low-cost, lateral-flow test (Capilia TB-Neo, Tauns Laboratories Inc., Japan) that detects the MPT-64 protein specific to *M. tuberculosis* (Hillemann et al. 2005). This has great advantages in terms of speed, simplicity, and cost over previously used phenotypic or genotypic methods of speciation.

Commercially available liquid culture systems have capital and reagent costs that are prohibitive for many resource-limited countries. Moreover, both the specimen processing and culture systems are relatively complex procedures that are challenging to perform outside reference laboratories. Thus, although commercial liquid culture systems and line-probe assays emerged in 2008 as the WHO-recommended gold standard endorsed for rapid detection of MDR-TB (Table 1), their technical complexity, cost, and the requirement for sophisticated laboratory infrastructure have limited their implementation (Table 2). In view of this, several other noncommercial, low-cost methods of culture and DST that require less sophisticated laboratory infrastructure have also been developed.

In 2011, WHO endorsed the use of three of these as an interim solution while capacity for more technically demanding assays was being developed (WHO 2011b). These assays included the microscopic observation of the drug susceptibility (MODS) assay, the nitrate reductase assay (NRA), and the colorimetric redox indicator (CRI) assay. All three rely on detection of growth of *M. tuberculosis* in drug-free and drug-containing media. MODS is a microcolony liquid culture method conducted in 24-well culture plates with microscopic detection of early growth with *M. tuberculosis* through recognition of highly characteristic cord formation using an inverted microscope (Moore et al. 2006). Inclusion of additional TB drug-containing wells allows evaluation of susceptibility to a range of additional drugs. MODS has high accuracy for diagnosis of MDR-TB and provides a result within a mean turnaround time of 10 d (Minion et al. 2010).

The nitrate reductase phenotypic assay is a colorimetric method, which can be used as a direct method on sputum or as an indirect method on cultures (Musa et al. 2005). The assay is based on the ability of *M. tuberculosis* to reduce nitrate, which is detected by a color reaction on solid media. The CRI assay is based on the reduction of a colored indicator added to culture medium in a microtiter plate after exposure of *M. tuberculosis* to anti-TB drugs (Palomino et al. 2007). A simple visual readout is therefore possible.

WHO did not find sufficient evidence in 2011 to endorse the thin-layer agar (TLA) or phage-based assays. The TLA assay works on the same basis as MODS, but it uses drug-free and drug-containing agar with a colorimetric indicator in segmented Petri dishes (Robledo et al. 2008). Phage-based assays rely on mycobacteriophages, which infect *M. tuberculosis* bacilli if they are viable. Thus, detection of replicating bacteriophages in decontaminated specimens in the presence or absence of drug provides a rapid means of assessing drug susceptibility (Kiraz et al. 2007). A commercially available version of this assay (FASTPlaqueTB, Biotec, UK) uses a conventional plaque readout on a lawn of rapidly growing mycobacterial on solid media, giving results within 48 h.

Field experience and operational research are providing an increasing evidence base for these assays as an alternative to commercial liquid culture and DST. Despite comparatively low costs, they remain relatively labor-intensive, requiring preinoculation processing and repeated examinations during incubation. These assays are not as yet being widely implemented.

Nucleic Acid Amplification Tests

Major progress has been made in the rapid molecular detection of *M. tuberculosis* using nucleic acid amplification tests (NAATs). These assays use a range of molecular techniques including polymerase chain reaction (PCR), real-time PCR, isothermal amplification, strain displacement or transcription-mediated amplification, and ligase chain reaction (Drobniewski et al. 2013). These are often combined with highly specific detection systems with hybridization with specific oligonucleotide probes to increased assay specificity. Speed and biosafety are the main advantages as containment is only required for the initial sample processing.

The first generation of assays developed 20 years ago showed excellent performance in terms of speed and specificity. However, although analytic performance was high in laboratory-based evaluations and in studies of smear-positive clinical samples, sensitivity for smear-negative samples was limited, potentially being compromised by the presence of PCR inhibitors or by loss of nucleic acids during sample processing. These initial assays were therefore not widely implemented as they were unable to compete with culture with regard to either sensitivity or DST, and their cost and complexity resulted in their use being largely restricted to high-income countries (Perkins 2009). However, development of newer assays and the growing need for rapid molecular detection of drug-resistant TB have resulted in WHO endorsement of rapid molecular assays in recent years, including line-probe assays and the Xpert MTB/RIF assay (Table 1). Table 3 shows the range of NAATs that were commercially available in 2013 for diagnosis of pulmonary TB directly from sputum samples. These include assays launched 20 years ago to assays only recently marketed.

Table 3. Commercially available nucleic acid amplification tests (NAATs) for diagnosis of pulmonary tuberculosis directly from sputum samples

Manufacturer (country)	Test	Market release	Fully integrated	Dedicated instrument	Throughput	Detection of drug resistance	Intended setting	WHO endorsed	Regulatory approvals
Hologic Genprobe (USA)	AMTD test	1993	No	Yes	50 tests in 5.5 h	No	Reference	No	FDA, CE-IVD
Becton Dickinson (USA)	BD ProbeTec ET Direct TB Assay	1999	No	Yes	150 tests in 8 h	No	Reference	No	CE-IVD
Hain Lifescience (Germany)	GenoType MTBDR*plus*	2008	No	Yes	96 tests per day	Yes (MDR)	Reference	Yes	CE-IVD, CFDA
Hain Lifescience (Germany)	GenoType MTBDR*sl*	2009	No	Yes	96 tests per day	Yes (XDR)	Reference	No	CE-IVD
Roche (USA)	Cobas TaqMan MTB Test	2009	No	Yes	44 tests in 3 h	No	Reference	No	CE-IVD, Health Canada, FDA?
Ustar Biotechnologies (China)	EasyNAT TB	2009	No	No	30 tests per day	No	Peripheral	No	CE-IVD
CapitalBio (China)	Drug Resistance Detection Kit	2009	No	Yes	24–48 tests in 8 h	Yes (XDR)	Reference	No	CE-IVD, CFDA
Cepheid Inc (USA)	Xpert MTB/RIF assay	2009	Yes	Yes	90 min per cartridge module	Yes	Intermediate/ peripheral	Yes	CE-IVD, Health Canada, FDA
CapitalBio (China)	Mycobacteria Real-time PCR	2011	No	No	36 tests in 4 h	No	Reference	No	CE-IVD, CFDA
Seegene (South Korea)	Anyplex II MTB/ MDR/XDR	2012	No	Yes	90 tests in 6 h	Yes (XDR)	Reference	No	CE-IVD, Korean FDA
Eiken (Japan)	Loopamp MTBC Detection Kit	2012	No	Yes	14 tests in 2 h	No	Peripheral	No	CE-IVD, Japan
Epistem (UK)	Genedrive Mycobacterium iD Test-kit	2013	No	Yes	90 min per test device	Yes (MDR)	Peripheral	No	CE-IVD
Molbio (India)	Truelab TB Assay	2013	No	Yes	12 tests in 8 h	No	Peripheral	No	CE-IVD, Indian DCGI
Tosoh Bioscience (Japan)	TRC Rapid M.TB	Unknown	No	Yes	N/A	No	Reference	No	N/A

Data adapted from UNITAID 2013.

CE-IVD, Conformite Europeenne-in vitro diagnostic; FDA, U.S. Food and Drug Administration; CFDA, China Food and Drug Administration; MDR, multidrug resistant; XDR, extensively drug-resistant.

Line Probe Assays

Line probe assays (LPAs) use PCR amplification of DNA sequences that are *M. tuberculosis*-specific and that are sites of mutations that are known to confer drug resistance. Detection uses DNA probes bound to solid membranes and hybridization is detected colorimetrically, producing visible bands that indicate the presence of *M. tuberculosis* and either a sensitive or resistant genotype.

To enhance the capacity for rapid diagnosis of MDR-TB, WHO in 2008 approved the use of LPAs for the rapid molecular detection of drug resistance in smear-positive specimens or culture isolates (WHO 2008). The main commercially available LPAs are the INNO-LiPA Rif.TB assay (Ommunogenetics, Zwijndrecht, Belgium) and, providing detection of both rifampicin and isoniazid resistance mutations, the GenoType MTBDR and MTBDR*plus* assays (Hain LifeScience GmbH, Nehren, Germany) (Morgan et al. 2005; Ling et al. 2008). More recently, the newer MTBDR*plus* version 2.0 assay (Hain Lifescience) has shown improved performance, with sensitivity for sputum smear-negative TB that is similar to that of the Xpert MTB/RIF assay (Barnard et al. 2012; Crudu et al. 2012).

In 2009, the Genotype MTBDR*sl* assay (Hain Lifescience) was released, providing capacity for expanded DST to include second-line drugs (Hillemann et al. 2009). WHO expert review of data concerning this assay in 2012 found moderate test sensitivity for the detection of fluoroquinolone and second-line injectable resistance with high specificity. It was concluded that although the Genotype MTBDR*sl* assay cannot be used as a replacement for conventional phenotypic DST, it does provide a rapid rule-in (but not rule-out) screen for XDR-TB (WHO 2013c). However, because cross-resistance between second-line injectables is incomplete, the assay cannot be used to identify individual drugs to be used for treatment.

Xpert MTB/RIF Assay

GeneXpert (Cepheid Inc, Sunnyvale, CA, USA) is a self-contained, fully integrated and automated cartridge-based diagnostic platform that can be operated with minimal technical expertise (Lawn et al. 2013). The Xpert MTB/RIF cartridges incorporate microfluidics technology and fully automated nucleic acid analysis to purify, concentrate, detect, and identify targeted nucleic acid sequences from unprocessed clinical samples using real-time PCR technology and a molecular beacon detection system (Fig. 1). This permits identification of the *M. tuberculosis complex* within 2 h and simultaneous detection of the presence or absence of mutations that confer rifampicin resistance in the 81-base-pair core region of the *rpoB* gene (Lawn and Nicol 2011). Following initial endorsement in December 2010, WHO issued policy recommendations in 2011 for the use of this assay for diagnosis of pulmonary TB (WHO 2010), and these were updated in 2013 to include diagnosis of TB in children and diagnosis of extrapulmonary TB (WHO 2013b).

Extensive data from around the world are available on the diagnostic accuracy of the Xpert MTB/RIF assay for pulmonary TB (Boehme et al. 2010). Pooled summary estimates of sensitivity for sputum-culture-positive disease show that Xpert MTB/RIF detects approximately nine out of 10 cases with a pooled specificity of 99% (95%CI, 98%–99%) including almost all smear-positive cases and approximately two-thirds of smear-negative cases (Table 4). Despite the high frequency of smear-negative disease, the sensitivity of Xpert MTB/RIF in those with HIV-coinfection was not substantially lower than that in HIV-negative participants (Steingart et al. 2014). Accumulating evidence now supports the role of the Xpert MTB/RIF assay for diagnosis of some forms of extrapulmonary TB (Denkinger et al. 2014). Sensitivity varies according to sample type, whereas specificity is uniformly high across all types. Useful sensitivity is observed when testing biopsies and needle aspirates of lymph nodes, biopsies of other tissues, and cerebrospinal fluid samples (Table 4). However, sensitivity is much more limited when testing pleural fluid samples, leading to WHO recommendations that the assay can be used for diagnosis of TB meningitis and TB in lymph nodes and other tissues (WHO 2013b).

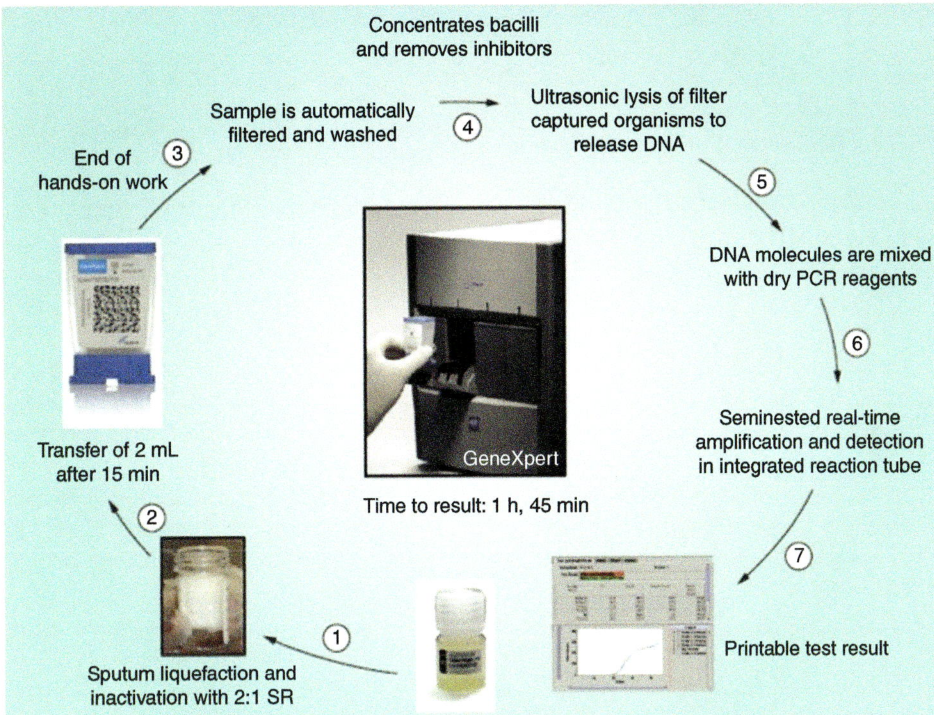

Figure 1. Schematic showing the sequential steps of the Xpert MTB/RIF assay test procedure. SR, sample reagent; PCR, polymerase chain reaction. (Figure reproduced from Lawn and Nicol 2011, with permission from the authors.)

The pooled sensitivity of Xpert MTB/RIF for detection of rifampicin resistance in pulmonary specimens was 95% (Steingart et al. 2014), reflecting the proportion of rifampicin resistance that is mediated by mutations in the target region of the *rpoB* gene. Pooled specificity for rifampicin resistance was suboptimal (98%; 97%–99%), however, which means that in clinical populations with low prevalence of rifampicin-resistant TB, the positive predictive value

Table 4. Pooled summary estimates of the sensitivity of the Xpert MTB/RIF assay for pulmonary and extrapulmonary tuberculosis (TB) compared with a culture reference standard

Sample types	Pooled sensitivity
Respiratory specimens	
Overall	89% (85%–92%)
Smear-positive	98% (97%–99%)
Smear-negative	67% (60%–74%)
Pulmonary TB in HIV-negatives	86% (76%–92%)
Pulmonary TB in HIV-positives	79% (70%–86%)
Nonrespiratory specimens	
Lymph node biopsies or aspirates	83% (71%–91%)
Cerebrospinal fluid	81% (59%–92%)
Pleural fluid	46% (26%–68%)

Data summarized from Steingart et al. 2014 and Denkinger et al. 2014.

of rifampicin-resistant result from Xpert MTB/RIF is limited. Following modification of the assay cartridge and platform software in December 2011, however, data on the performance of the revised G4 version of the cartridge indicate higher specificity for rifampicin resistance (Osman et al. 2014).

The Xpert MTB/RIF assay is now being widely implemented around the world and, in 2011, South Africa took the bold decision to implement this nationwide as a replacement for sputum smear microscopy. Although the Xpert MTB/RIF assay is a substantial advance, it is an imperfect solution. High cost, sophisticated hardware, linkage to a computer, the need for an uninterrupted power supply, annual calibration, module breakdowns, and operator training requirements are all disadvantages in resource-limited settings (Trebucq et al. 2011). Although the assay can be completed within 2 h, same-day diagnosis and treatment initiation are logistically challenging to achieve within overcrowded clinics in resource-limited settings. Economic and logistical issues mean that implementation of this assay will largely be constrained to the laboratory environment and away from the actual clinical interface.

Developmental Automated Rapid Molecular Systems

Fully automated systems that use isothermal amplification at lower operational temperatures have much lower power requirements than the Xpert MTB/RIF assay (Niemz and Boyle 2012; UNITAID 2013). Hand-held battery-powered systems the size of a smart-phone produce PCR product far more rapidly (<30 min) than GeneXpert and therefore may be much more readily used at the point-of-care. A number of new NAATs have been commercially launched, including some that are intended for use in peripheral laboratories (Table 3). It is anticipated that in the coming few years, a number of fully automated multiplexed assays (referred to as "fast-followers") with fully integrated sample processing will emerge to compete with the Xpert MTB/RIF assay, enabling both rapid TB diagnosis and detection of resistance to multiple drugs.

Manual Loop-Mediated Isothermal Amplification Test

Work continues on the development and evaluation of a simplified manual molecular assay for laboratory-based use in resource-limited settings, using loop-mediated isothermal amplification (LAMP) with a simple visual colorimetric readout (George et al. 2011; Mitarai et al. 2011). Rather than requiring repeated heating and cooling cycles used in PCR, such assays can be performed using a simple water bath, making the assay far more amenable to use within resource-limited settings. Expert review by WHO in 2013 of the Loopamp assay (Eiken Chemical Co., Japan) found that this could detect the vast majority of smear-positive samples and approximately half of smear-negative samples (WHO 2013d). However, specificity was insufficient (<95%) for the assay to be recommended as a replacement for smear microscopy and further developmental work is needed, especially to improve specificity.

Antigen Detection

M. tuberculosis antigen detection has long been viewed positively as an option for TB diagnosis as this has the advantage of reflecting mycobacterial burden (active disease rather than latent infection) and not depending on the immune status of the individual. Moreover, analysis of urine rather than sputum samples is a very attractive option as this is simple to collect without generating hazardous bioaerosols, it is safe to handle in the laboratory, it has relatively few bacterial contaminants, and sample quality is unlikely to be highly variable (Peter et al. 2010).

A number of mycobacterial antigens can be detected in the urine of patients with pulmonary TB (Kashino et al. 2008), but the most promising of these to emerge is the cell wall lipopolysaccharide lipoarabinomannan (LAM) (Peter et al. 2010; Lawn 2012). A polyclonal antibody, sandwich enzyme-linked immunosorbent assay (ELISA) for urine LAM has been commercially

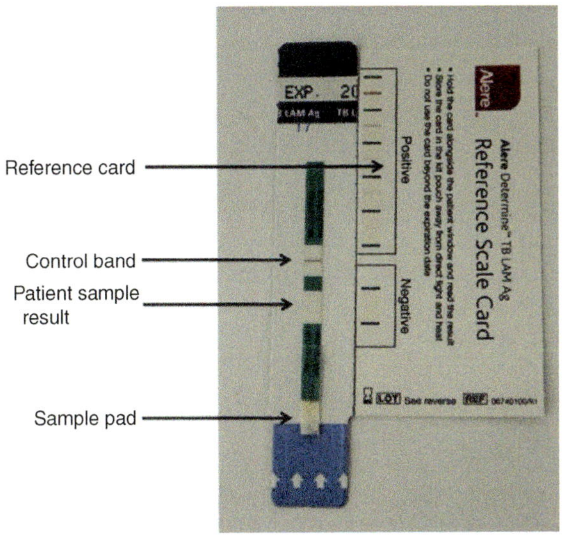

Figure 2. Photograph of a Determine TB-LAM Ag lateral flow test strip. Urine (60 μL) is applied to the sample pad, and after 25–35 min of incubation at room temperature, the control band is checked and the sample test result is read with comparison to the reference card. The presence of a band of sufficient intensity in the sample window indicates the presence of lipoarabinomannan (LAM) in the urine, providing a rapid diagnosis of tuberculosis. (Figure reproduced from Lawn 2012, with permission from the author.)

available for a number of years (Minion et al. 2011b), and more recently, a simple, low-cost, lateral flow version of this assay has been developed and this can be used at the point-of-care (Fig. 2) (Lawn et al. 2012a; Peter et al. 2012).

Multiple studies have shown that the specific niche for this assay is for diagnosis of HIV-associated TB in patients with advanced immunodeficiency (CD4 cell counts <200 cells/μL), such as those being screened in antiretroviral treatment clinics or HIV-infected medical in-patients. Studies from South Africa have reported that among those with the lowest CD4 cell counts, the assay can diagnose between one-half and two-thirds of cases with high specificity within 30 min. Those detected by this assay are likely to have disseminated TB, and growing evidence suggests that the main mechanism underlying the presence of LAM in urine is actual renal involvement with TB following hematogenous seeding (Lawn 2012). This explains why the utility of the assay is restricted to those with advanced immunodeficiency, poor prognostic characteristics, and high mortality risk (Lawn et al. 2012b; Talbot et al. 2012). These are the very patients in whom TB diagnosis and initiation of treatment are most urgent. Studies of the clinical impact of using this assay are awaited. The growing evidence base on this assay is being reviewed by WHO in 2014.

Serological Assays

Serological assays have long been attractive as a prospect for a simple, rapid, low-cost, and non-instrumented assay that uses a finger prick blood sample and can be used in the very lowest tier of the health-care system and community. However, systematic reviews of a large range of commercially available serodiagnostic assays for TB used widely in some parts of the world revealed that they had very limited accuracy and were of no clinical value (Steingart et al. 2007a,b). In 2011, WHO took the unprecedented step of issuing a negative recommendation against the use of currently available assays (WHO 2011d). However, future use of serodiagnostic assays has not been discounted and active research and development are ongoing.

A better understanding of the complex and evolving nature of the humoral immune response during the different stages of infection and disease is needed. The multiplicity of different *M. tuberculosis* exposure, infection, and disease states (Lawn et al. 2011; Young et al. 2009) is likely to be associated with overlapping humoral immune response profiles, such that limited specificity is likely to remain the Achilles heel in high-burden settings. Early tests were based on crude mixtures of antigens that lacked specificity, but now an expanding range of purified immunodominant antigens has been identified (Steingart et al. 2009). Assays using individual antigens are unlikely to have sufficient sensitivity, and so it is likely that combinations of purified antigens will be needed. Sensitivity is usually limited in those with HIV coinfection, although serological responses to certain antigens appear to be preserved in this patient group (Yu et al. 2012). Serological assays have frequently been evaluated in small case-control studies in which highly selected study groups have been recruited, potentially giving a false impression of their accuracy. Much larger prospective studies are needed.

Interferon-γ-Release Assays

Interferon-γ-release assays (IGRAs) detect interferon-γ production by CD4 lymphocytes in the blood of individuals in response to ex vivo stimulation with RD1-encoded *M. tuberculosis*-specific antigens, such as culture filtrate protein-10 (CFP-10) and early secretory antigen-6 (ESAT-6) (Pai et al. 2008). Positive responses indicate immune sensitization by prior exposure to the organism. However, because these assays lack sensitivity among those with active disease and cannot distinguish between active disease and latent infection, these assays should not be used in place of standard diagnostic methods for diagnosing active TB. WHO has specifically recommended that these assays not be used in low- or middle-income countries for diagnosis of active disease or latent infection (WHO 2011d). However, in limited clinical situations such as those in which all microbiological tests are negative and in diagnosis in children, IGRAs can contribute supplementary information as part of a diagnostic work-up (European Centre for Disease Control 2011). However, this role is limited as the assays can neither be used to rule in nor rule out TB.

Other Developmental Assays

When *M. tuberculosis* is actively replicating, volatile organic compounds (VOCs) are released and are detectable in sputum, urine, and breath, thereby potentially forming the basis of a diagnostic assay (UNITAID 2012). As a proof of concept, Giant African Pouch rats can be trained to identify TB in sputum samples by olfaction, but this does not constitute a viable, scalable solution. Thus, a field of diagnostics research is exploring the use of "breathalyzers" and "electronic noses" that detect VOCs using chemical sensors and pattern recognition systems (Bruins et al. 2012; Phillips et al. 2012). The advantages of using such tests to screen for TB would be speed, noninvasiveness, and the lack of need for sample processing. However, to date, early developmental systems have required sophisticated laboratory equipment and highly skilled technicians and have lacked specificity (Phillips et al. 2012). Thus, viable prototypes for routine use have yet to emerge.

DEVELOPING THE IDEAL DIAGNOSTIC TEST

The ideal test for TB would be one that could be performed at the point-of-care, providing immediate results that can be used to reliably inform treatment decisions without the need for further laboratory-based testing. The test should be readily used at all levels of the health-care system, on hospital wards, outpatient clinics, peripheral health posts, mobile medical services, medical outreach teams visiting the remotest locations, and within the patient's home. Standalone diagnostic devices already exist for a range of infectious diseases, including HIV infection, malaria, hepatitis B, syphilis, and Chagas' disease. However, TB diagnosis presents a greater challenge. Unlike many of these diseases, TB is not primarily blood-borne, a wide spectrum of infection and disease states occur, and disease may be caused by very low bacillary numbers and may occur at any anatomic site. Although use of a single test for diagnosis would be ideal, an al-

Table 5. Minimum specifications for a point-of-care diagnostic test for tuberculosis (TB)

Parameter	Minimum specification required
Outcome of testing	Initiation of treatment
Sensitivity in adults (irrespective of HIV status)	Smear-positive, culture-positive PTB: 95% Smear-negative, culture-positive PTB: 60%–80%[a] EPTB: detection preferred but not required
Specificity in adults	Compared with culture: 95%
Sensitivity in children (irrespective of HIV status)	Culture-confirmed PTB and EPTB: 80% Probable PTB and EPTB: 60%
Specificity in children	Compared with culture: 95% In culture-negative probable cases: 90%
Throughput	20 tests per day by a single operator
Waste disposal	Environmentally friendly disposal feasible
Storage and stability	No cold chain required; stable at 30°C for 2 yr
Instrumentation	Maintenance free, robust in tropical climates, acceptable replacement cost, portable (e.g., in backpack), can be battery operated, shock resistant
Operation	Requires minimal instruction
Cost	Less than $10 per test

Data adapted from Lemaire and Casenghi 2010 and McNerney and Daley 2011.

Recommendations of an expert meeting facilitated by Medecins Sans Frontieres (MSF) Access Campaign, Treatment Action Group (TAG), and Partners in Health (PIH) and convened in March 2009.

PTB, pulmonary tuberculosis; EPTB, extrapulmonary tuberculosis.

[a]No consensus reached on lower limit.

ternative approach would be serial testing using a high-sensitivity, low-specificity screening test followed by referral for a definitive test. However, in general, the more complex the screening algorithm, the weaker it is likely to be. If the screening test were simple and low-cost, this might nevertheless provide a suitable approach for screening in very remote communities with poor access to health services.

The specifications of the "ideal" diagnostic test for TB are a subject of debate (McNerney and Daley 2011). Although such a test may never be developed, prespecified desirable characteristics are important for guiding ongoing research and development. Table 5 shows the minimum test specifications that were identified during an expert meeting in 2009, including diagnostic accuracy, issues related to operational feasibility in a range of environments and cost (Lemaire and Casenghi 2010). The Xpert MTB/RIF assay has made progress toward fulfilling some of these goals, including diagnostic accuracy requirements in adults and being made available at a heavily subsidized cost of $9.98 per test in low- and middle-income countries. Drawbacks of the Xpert MTB/RIF assay include the sophisticated diagnostic platform, which is costly, needs to be linked to a computer, is subject to breakdown of the modules, requires annual calibration, has high power requirements, and lacks portability (Lawn et al. 2013). The next-generation rapid molecular devices have much simpler instrumentation, greater speed, and low power requirements (UNITAID 2013) but their diagnostic accuracy remains to be defined. Although these evolving rapid molecular assays offer the prospects of much improved TB diagnosis, they still remain far from the simplicity of a lateral-flow HIV test. Thus, there remains a huge need for ongoing biomarker discovery and research and development of new diagnostic formats (Wallis et al. 2013).

EVALUATIONS OF NEW DIAGNOSTIC TESTS FOR TB

As with any other medical technology, new TB diagnostic assays require thorough evaluation before their implementation into routine practice. The methods and nomenclature for appraising diagnostic accuracy date back to 1947 (Yerushalmy 1947), with 2 × 2 tables being used to derive the familiar indices of sensitivity, specificity, positive and negative predictive values, and likelihood ratios. The laboratory-based analytic performance is often first assessed using specimen banks of clinical samples. Thereafter, diagnostic accuracy studies are conducted in clinical populations, and the Standards for Reporting Diagnostic Accuracy (STARD) statement provides an important framework for the standardized reporting of such studies (Bossuyt et al. 2003). Diagnostic accuracy studies need to be conducted in a wide variety of clinical populations so as to encompass the true spectrum of disease and patients. Systematic reviews and meta-analyses are a critical next step in the synthesis of the findings of these studies, with careful review of the biases inherent in the studies included.

A critical component of diagnostic accuracy studies is a robust reference standard against which to compare the new assay. This is particularly challenging for certain forms of extrapulmonary TB and especially for pediatric TB in which only a limited proportion of disease may be microbiologically proven. There is additional difficulty in which the reference standard and index test are performed on samples from different anatomic compartments. For example, many of the evaluations of the Determine TB-LAM Ag urine LAM assay have used sputum culture as the reference standard despite the fact that a high proportion of true-positive LAM tests occur in patients with either negative sputum tests or no sputum production (Lawn et al. 2014).

Diagnostic accuracy is, however, only one component in the evaluation of diagnostic assays and much else needs to be considered. Factors include patient acceptability, the logistics of the testing procedure, the safety of patients and health-care workers, the precise role of the test within the diagnostic algorithm, the impact of the test on clinical decision-making, impact on health outcomes, cost-effectiveness, and overall cost of implementation. Testing procedures must be patient friendly and take into account the indirect costs that patients often have to bear when making repeated attendances at health clinics. The speed and throughput of the assay, as well as its ease of use within the clinical or laboratory environment, are critical. Biosafety is a vital consideration both during sample collection and running the test.

The final goal of a new diagnostic test is not simply to achieve accurate diagnosis of TB but is rather to achieve a clinical impact (Bossuyt et al. 2012). At the level of the individual patient, the aim is to reduce TB-related morbidity and mortality and, at the community-level, the aim is to reduce TB transmission and the burden of TB. New diagnostic tests have to be evaluated within the context and complexities of the clinical care pathway. In the face of limited sensitivity of TB diagnostic assays, the decision for health-care workers to start or not start TB treatment is not straightforward but rather takes into account a complex array of information in addition to the results of diagnostic tests. Thus, new TB diagnostic tests need to be evaluated in pragmatic randomized trials to assess clinical impact (Dowdy et al. 2012). To take into account the full diagnostic process, these often use a cluster-randomized design, although in certain circumstances, individually randomized trials are the only viable option. Study outcomes may include the diagnostic process (e.g., proportion diagnosed, proportion treated, and time to initiation of treatment) and clinical outcomes (e.g., outcomes of TB treatment and survival). Although assessment of individual outcomes may be achievable, the secondary effects of early TB diagnosis resulting in reduced TB transmission and reduced long-term burden of TB in the community are much more difficult to quantify. Careful context-specific economic analyses are also needed to evaluate cost-effectiveness. In addition, because cost-effectiveness does not denote affordability, budget impact analyses are also needed. Only then can rational choices be made by national Ministries of Health and national TB control program.

CONCLUSIONS

Huge progress has been made in the TB diagnostic developmental pipeline during the past 10 years, resulting in steady evolution of WHO

 Cite this article as *Cold Spring Harb Perspect Med* doi: 10.1101/cshperspect.a017806

policies for TB diagnosis and drug susceptibility testing. Despite this encouraging progress, we remain very far from the much-needed test that allows rapid and accurate diagnosis in unselected patients at the point-of-care, resulting in improved clinical outcomes and reduced TB transmission. Although the current array of technologies that are emerging from the developmental pipeline need to be implemented as effectively as possible, there remains a huge need for ongoing biomarker discovery combined with development of innovative technologies that lead to new and effective tools.

REFERENCES

Abu-Raddad LJ, Sabatelli L, Achterberg JT, Sugimoto JD, Longini IM Jr, Dye C, Halloran ME. 2009. Epidemiological benefits of more-effective tuberculosis vaccines, drugs, and diagnostics. *Proc Natl Acad Sci* **106:** 13980–13985.

Barnard M, Gey van Pittius NC, van Helden PD, Bosman M, Coetzee G, Warren RM. 2012. The diagnostic performance of the genotype MTBDR*plus* version 2 line probe assay is equivalent to that of the Xpert MTB/RIF assay. *J Clin Microbiol* **50:** 3712–3716.

Boehme CC, Nabeta P, Hillemann D, Nicol MP, Shenai S, Krapp F, Allen J, Tahirli R, Blakemore R, Rustomjee R, et al. 2010. Rapid molecular detection of tuberculosis and rifampin resistance. *N Engl J Med* **363:** 1005–1015.

Bossuyt PM, Reitsma JB, Bruns DE, Gatsonis CA, Glasziou PP, Irwig LM, Moher D, Rennie D, de Vet HC, Lijmer JG. 2003. The STARD statement for reporting studies of diagnostic accuracy: Explanation and elaboration. *Ann Intern Med* **138:** W1–W12.

Bossuyt PM, Reitsma JB, Linnet K, Moons KG. 2012. Beyond diagnostic accuracy: The clinical utility of diagnostic tests. *Clin Chem* **58:** 1636–1643.

Bruins M, Rahim Z, Bos A, van de Sande WW, Endtz HP, van Belkum A. 2012. Diagnosis of active tuberculosis by e-nose analysis of exhaled air. *Tuberculosis (Edinb)* **93:** 232–238.

Crudu V, Stratan E, Romancenco E, Allerheiligen V, Hillemann A, Moraru N. 2012. First evaluation of an improved assay for molecular genetic detection of tuberculosis as well as rifampin and isoniazid resistances. *J Clin Microbiol* **50:** 1264–1269.

Denkinger CM, Schumacher SG, Boehme CC, Dendukuri N, Pai M, Steingart KR. 2014. Xpert MTB/RIF assay for the diagnosis of extrapulmonary tuberculosis: A systematic review and meta-analysis. *Eur Respir J* **44:** 435–446.

Dowdy DW, Gounder CR, Corbett EL, Ngwira LG, Chaisson RE, Merritt MW. 2012. The ethics of testing a test: Randomized trials of the health impact of diagnostic tests for infectious diseases. *Clin Infect Dis* **55:** 1522–1526.

Drobniewski F, Nikolayevskyy V, Maxeiner H, Balabanova Y, Casali N, Kontsevaya I, Ignatyeva O. 2013. Rapid diagnostics of tuberculosis and drug resistance in the industrialized world: Clinical and public health benefits and barriers to implementation. *BMC Med* **11:** 190.

European Centre for Disease Control. 2011. Use of interferon-γ release assays in support of TB diagnosis. Stockholm: ECDC, Accessible at: http://ecdc.europa.eu/en/publications/publications/1103_gui_igra.pdf.

George G, Mony P, Kenneth J. 2011. Comparison of the efficacies of loop-mediated isothermal amplification, fluorescence smear microscopy and culture for the diagnosis of tuberculosis. *PLoS ONE* **6:** e21007.

Gupta RK, Lawn SD, Bekker LG, Caldwell J, Kaplan R, Wood R. 2013. Impact of human immunodeficiency virus and CD4 count on tuberculosis diagnosis: Analysis of city-wide data from Cape Town, South Africa. *Int J Tuberc Lung Dis* **17:** 1014–1022.

Hart JT. 1971. The inverse care law. *Lancet* **1:** 405–412.

Hillemann D, Rusch-Gerdes S, Richter E. 2005. Application of the Capilia TB assay for culture confirmation of *Mycobacterium tuberculosis* complex isolates. *Int J Tuberc Lung Dis* **9:** 1409–1411.

Hillemann D, Rusch-Gerdes S, Richter E. 2009. Feasibility of the GenoType MTBDR*sl* assay for fluoroquinolone, amikacin-capreomycin, and ethambutol resistance testing of *Mycobacterium tuberculosis* strains and clinical specimens. *J Clin Microbiol* **47:** 1767–1772.

Kashino SS, Pollock N, Napolitano DR, Rodrigues V Jr, Campos-Neto A. 2008. Identification and characterization of *Mycobacterium tuberculosis* antigens in urine of patients with active pulmonary tuberculosis: An innovative and alternative approach of antigen discovery of useful microbial molecules. *Clin Exp Immunol* **153:** 56–62.

Kiraz N, Et L, Akgun Y, Kasifoglu N, Kiremitci A. 2007. Rapid detection of *Mycobacterium tuberculosis* from sputum specimens using the FASTPlaqueTB test. *Int J Tuberc Lung Dis* **11:** 904–908.

Lawn SD. 2012. Point-of-care detection of lipoarabinomannan (LAM) in urine for diagnosis of HIV-associated tuberculosis: A state of the art review. *BMC Infect Dis* **12:** 103.

Lawn SD, Nicol MP. 2011. Xpert(R) MTB/RIF assay: Development, evaluation and implementation of a new rapid molecular diagnostic for tuberculosis and rifampicin resistance. *Future Microbiol* **6:** 1067–1082.

Lawn SD, Wood R, Wilkinson RJ. 2011. Changing concepts of "latent tuberculosis infection" in patients living with HIV infection. *Clin Dev Immunol* **2011:** 980594.

Lawn SD, Kerkhoff AD, Vogt M, Wood R. 2012a. Diagnostic accuracy of a low-cost, urine antigen, point-of-care screening assay for HIV-associated pulmonary tuberculosis before antiretroviral therapy: Descriptive study. *Lancet Infect Dis* **12:** 201–209.

Lawn SD, Kerkhoff AD, Vogt M, Wood R. 2012b. Clinical significance of lipoarabinomannan detection in urine using a low-cost point-of-care diagnostic assay for HIV-associated tuberculosis. *AIDS* **26:** 1635–1643.

Lawn SD, Mwaba P, Bates M, Piatek A, Alexander H, Marais BJ, Cuevas LE, McHugh TD, Zijenah L, Kapata N, et al. 2013. Advances in tuberculosis diagnostics: The Xpert MTB/RIF assay and future prospects for a point-of-care test. *Lancet Infect Dis* **13:** 349–361.

Lawn SD, Kerkhoff AD, Burton R, Meintjes G. 2014. Underestimation of the incremental diagnostic yield of HIV-associated tuberculosis in studies of the determine TB-LAM Ag urine assay. *AIDS* **28:** 1846–1848.

Lemaire JF, Casenghi M. 2010. New diagnostics for tuberculosis: Fulfilling patient needs first. *J Int AIDS Soc* **13:** 40.

Ling DI, Zwerling AA, Pai M. 2008. GenoType MTBDR assays for the diagnosis of multidrug-resistant tuberculosis: A meta-analysis. *Eur Respir J* **32:** 1165–1174.

MacPherson P, Houben RM, Glynn JR, Corbett EL, Kranzer K. 2014. Pre-treatment loss to follow-up in tuberculosis patients in low- and lower-middle-income countries and high-burden countries: A systematic review and meta-analysis. *Bull World Health Organ* **92:** 126.

McNerney R, Daley P. 2011. Towards a point-of-care test for active tuberculosis: Obstacles and opportunities. *Nat Rev Microbiol* **9:** 204–213.

Minion J, Leung E, Menzies D, Pai M. 2010. Microscopic-observation drug susceptibility and thin layer agar assays for the detection of drug resistant tuberculosis: A systematic review and meta-analysis. *Lancet Infect Dis* **10:** 688–698.

Minion J, Pai M, Ramsay A, Menzies D, Greenaway C. 2011a. Comparison of LED and conventional fluorescence microscopy for detection of acid fast bacilli in a low-incidence setting. *PLoS ONE* **6:** e22495.

Minion J, Leung E, Talbot E, Dheda K, Pai M, Menzies D. 2011b. Diagnosing tuberculosis with urine lipoarabinomannan: Systematic review and meta-analysis. *Eur Respir J* **38:** 1398–1405.

Mitarai S, Okumura M, Toyota E, Yoshiyama T, Aono A, Sejimo A, Azuma Y, Sugahara K, Nagasawa T, Nagayama N, et al. 2011. Evaluation of a simple loop-mediated isothermal amplification test kit for the diagnosis of tuberculosis. *Int J Tuberc Lung Dis* **15:** 1211–1217.

Moore DA, Evans CA, Gilman RH, Caviedes L, Coronel J, Vivar A, Sanchez E, Pinedo Y, Saravia JC, Salazar C, et al. 2006. Microscopic-observation drug-susceptibility assay for the diagnosis of TB. *N Engl J Med* **355:** 1539–1550.

Morgan M, Kalantri S, Flores L, Pai M. 2005. A commercial line probe assay for the rapid detection of rifampicin resistance in *Mycobacterium tuberculosis*: A systematic review and meta-analysis. *BMC Infect Dis* **5:** 62.

Musa HR, Ambroggi M, Souto A, Angeby KA. 2005. Drug susceptibility testing of *Mycobacterium tuberculosis* by a nitrate reductase assay applied directly on microscopy-positive sputum samples. *J Clin Microbiol* **43:** 3159–3161.

Niemz A, Boyle DS. 2012. Nucleic acid testing for tuberculosis at the point-of-care in high-burden countries. *Expert Rev Mol Diagn* **12:** 687–701.

Osman M, Simpson JA, Caldwell J, Bosman M, Nicol MP. 2014. GeneXpert MTB/RIF version G4 for identification of rifampin-resistant tuberculosis in a programmatic setting. *J Clin Microbiol* **52:** 635–637.

Pai M, Zwerling A, Menzies D. 2008. Systematic review: T-cell-based assays for the diagnosis of latent tuberculosis infection: An update. *Ann Intern Med* **149:** 177–184.

Palomino JC, Martin A, Portaels F. 2007. Rapid drug resistance detection in *Mycobacterium tuberculosis*: A review of colourimetric methods. *Clin Microbiol Infect* **13:** 754–762.

Perkins MD. 2009. New diagnostics for tuberculosis. In *Tuberculosis—A comprehensive clinical reference* (ed. Schaaf HS, Zumla A). Elsevier, London.

Peter J, Green C, Hoelscher M, Mwaba P, Zumla A, Dheda K. 2010. Urine for the diagnosis of tuberculosis: Current approaches, clinical applicability, and new developments. *Curr Opin Pulm Med* **16:** 262–270.

Peter JG, Theron G, van Zyl-Smit R, Haripersad A, Mottay L, Kraus S, Binder A, Meldau R, Hardy A, Dheda K. 2012. Diagnostic accuracy of a urine LAM strip-test for TB detection in HIV-infected hospitalised patients. *Eur Respir J* **40:** 1211–1240.

Phillips M, Basa-Dalay V, Blais J, Bothamley G, Chaturvedi A, Modi KD, Pandya M, Natividad MP, Patel U, Ramraje NN, et al. 2012. Point-of-care breath test for biomarkers of active pulmonary tuberculosis. *Tuberculosis (Edinb)* **92:** 314–320.

Robledo J, Mejia GI, Paniagua L, Martin A, Guzman A. 2008. Rapid detection of rifampicin and isoniazid resistance in *Mycobacterium tuberculosis* by the direct thin-layer agar method. *Int J Tuberc Lung Dis* **12:** 1482–1484.

Steingart KR, Ng V, Henry M, Hopewell PC, Ramsay A, Cunningham J, Urbanczik R, Perkins MD, Aziz MA, Pai M. 2006a. Sputum processing methods to improve the sensitivity of smear microscopy for tuberculosis: A systematic review. *Lancet Infect Dis* **6:** 664–674.

Steingart KR, Henry M, Ng V, Hopewell PC, Ramsay A, Cunningham J, Urbanczik R, Perkins M, Aziz MA, Pai M. 2006b. Fluorescence versus conventional sputum smear microscopy for tuberculosis: A systematic review. *Lancet Infect Dis* **6:** 570–581.

Steingart KR, Henry M, Laal S, Hopewell PC, Ramsay A, Menzies D, Cunningham J, Weldingh K, Pai M. 2007a. A systematic review of commercial serological antibody detection tests for the diagnosis of extrapulmonary tuberculosis. *Thorax* **62:** 911–918.

Steingart KR, Henry M, Laal S, Hopewell PC, Ramsay A, Menzies D, Cunningham J, Weldingh K, Pai M. 2007b. Commercial serological antibody detection tests for the diagnosis of pulmonary tuberculosis: A systematic review. *PLoS Med* **4:** e202.

Steingart KR, Dendukuri N, Henry M, Schiller I, Nahid P, Hopewell PC, Ramsay A, Pai M, Laal S. 2009. Performance of purified antigens for serodiagnosis of pulmonary tuberculosis: A meta-analysis. *Clin Vaccine Immunol* **16:** 260–276.

Steingart KR, Schiller I, Horne DJ, Pai M, Boehme CC, Dendukuri N. 2014. Xpert(R) MTB/RIF assay for pulmonary tuberculosis and rifampicin resistance in adults. *Cochrane Database Syst Rev* **1:** CD009593.

Talbot E, Munseri P, Teixeira P, Matee M, Bakari M, Lahey T, von Reyn F. 2012. Test characteristics of urinary lipoarabinomannan and predictors of mortality among hospitalized HIV-infected tuberculosis suspects in Tanzania. *PLoS ONE* **7:** e32876.

Trebucq A, Enarson DA, Chiang CY, Van DA, Harries AD, Boillot F, Detjen A, Fujiwara PI, Graham SM, Monedero I, et al. 2011. Xpert(R) MTB/RIF for national tuberculosis programmes in low-income countries:

When, where and how? *Int J Tuberc Lung Dis* **15:** 1567–1572.

UNITAID. 2012. Tuberculosis diagnostic technology landscape. UNITAID, World Health Organization, Geneva, 2012. Accessible at: http://www.unitaid.eu/images/marketdynamics/publications/UNITAID-Tuberculosis-Landscape_2012.pdf.

UNITAID. 2013. Tuberculosis diagnostics technology and market landscape. 2nd ed. UNITAID, World Health Organization, Geneva. Accessible at: http://www.unitaid.eu/images/marketdynamics/publications/TB-Dx-Landscape_1-Jul-2013.pdf.

Wallis RS, Kim P, Cole S, Hanna D, Andrade BB, Maeurer M, Schito M, Zumla A. 2013. Tuberculosis biomarkers discovery: Developments, needs, and challenges. *Lancet Infect Dis* **13:** 362–372.

World Health Organization. 2007a. TB diagnostics and laboratory strengthening–WHO policy. Definition of a new sputum smear-positive TB cases. World Health Organization, Geneva. Accessible at: http://www.who.int/tb/laboratory/policy_sputum_smearpositive_tb_case/en/index.html.

World Health Organization. 2007b. TB diagnostics and laboratory strengthening–WHO policy. Reduction in the number of smears for the diagnosis of pulmonary TB. WHO, Geneva. Accessible at http://www.who.int/tb/laboratory/policy_diagnosis_pulmonary_tb/en/index.html.

World Health Organization. 2007c. TB diagnostics and laboratory strengthening–WHO policy. The use of liquid medium for culture and DST. WHO, Geneva. Accessible at: http://www.who.int/tb/laboratory/policy_liquid_medium_for_culture_dst/en/index.html.

World Health Organization. 2008. Molecular line probe assays for rapid screening of patients at risk of multidrug-resistant tuberculosis (MDR-TB). Policy statement June 2008. www.who.int/entity/tb/dots/laboratory/lpa_policy.pdf.

World Health Organization 2010. Tuberculosis diagnostics automated DNA test. WHO endorsement and recommendations. World Health Organization, Geneva. Accessible at: http://www.who.int/tb/features archive/xpert_factsheet.pdf.

World Health Organization. 2011a. TB diagnostics and laboratory strengthening–WHO policy. Same-day diagnosis of tuberculosis by microscopy. WHO, Geneva. Accessible at: http://whqlibdoc.who.int/publications/2011/9789241501606_eng.pdf.

World Health Organization. 2011b. TB diagnostics and laboratory strengthening–WHO policy. Noncommerical culture and drug-susceptibility testing methods for screening patients at risk for multidrug-resistant tuberculosis. Accessible at: http://whqlibdoc.who.int/publications/2011/9789241501620_eng.pdf.

World Health Organization. 2011c. TB diagnostics and laboratory strengthening–WHO policy. Fluorescent light-emitting diode (LED) microscopy for diagnosis of tuberculosis. Accessible at: http://whqlibdoc.who.int/publications/2011/9789241501613_eng.pdf.

World Health Organization. 2011d. Commercial serodiagnostic tests of diagnosis of tuberculosis. WHO, Geneva. Accessible at: http://whqlibdoc.who.int/publications/2011/9789241502054_eng.pdf.

World Health Organization. 2011e. Use of tuberculosis interferon-γ release assays (IGRAs) in low- and middle-income countries. WHO, Geneva. Accessible at: http://whqlibdoc.who.int/publications/2011/9789241502672_eng.pdf.

World Health Organization 2011f. Automated real-time nucleic acid amplification technology for rapid and simultaneous detection of tuberculosis and rifampicin resistance: Xpert MTB/RIF System Policy Statement. WHO, Geneva. Accessed on 28th June 2011 at: http://whqlibdoc.who.int/publications/2011/9789241501545_eng.pdf.

World Health Organization. 2013a. Global tuberculosis report. World Health Organization, Geneva. Accessible at the following URL: http://apps.who.int/iris/bitstream/10665/91355/1/9789241564656_eng.pdf.

World Health Organization. 2013b. Xpert MTB/RIF for the diagnosis of pulmonary and extrapulmonary TB in adults and children: Policy update. WHO/HTM/TB/2013.16. WHO, Geneva. Accessible at the following URL: http://apps.who.int/iris/bitstream/10665/112472/1/9789241506335_eng.pdf?ua=1.

World Health Organization. 2013c. The use of molecular line probe assay for the detection of resistance to second-line anti-tuberculosis drugs. Expert group meeting report, Geneva, February 2013. WHO, Geneva. Accessible at: http://apps.who.int/iris/bitstream/10665/78099/1/WHO_HTM_TB_2013.01.eng.pdf.

World Health Organization. 2013d. The use of a commercial loop-mediated isothermal amplification assay (TB-LAMP) for the detection of tuberculosis. Expert group meeting report, Geneva, May 2013. WHO, Geneva. Accessible at: http://apps.who.int/iris/bitstream/10665/83142/1/WHO_HTM_TB_2013.05_eng.pdf.

Yerushalmy J. 1947. Statistical problems in assessing methods of medical diagnosis, with special reference to X-ray techniques. *Public Health Rep* **62:** 1432–1449.

Young DB, Gideon HP, Wilkinson RJ. 2009. Eliminating latent tuberculosis. *Trends Microbiol* **17:** 183–188.

Yu X, Prados-Rosales R, Jenny-Avital ER, Sosa K, Casadevall A, Achkar JM. 2012. Comparative evaluation of profiles of antibodies to mycobacterial capsular polysaccharides in tuberculosis patients and controls stratified by HIV status. *Clin Vaccine Immunol* **19:** 198–208.

Imaging in Tuberculosis

Jamshed B. Bomanji[1], Naraainder Gupta[2], Parveen Gulati[3], and Chandan J. Das[4]

[1]Institute of Nuclear Medicine, T5, University College Hospital, London NW1 2BU, United Kingdom
[2]Department of Radiology, Hospital of University of Pennsylvania, Philadelphia, Pennsylvania 19104
[3]Dr. Gulati Imaging Institute, Hauz Khas, New Delhi, 110016, India
[4]Department of Radiology, All India Institute of Medical Sciences, Ansari Nagar, New Delhi, 110029, India
Correspondence: jamshed.bomanji@uclh.nhs.uk

Despite many advances in both diagnosis and treatment, tuberculosis still remains one of commonest causes of morbidity and mortality from any infectious cause in the world. Although the overall incidence and mortality rate for tuberculosis has decreased over the years, timely and accurate diagnosis of tuberculosis is essential for the health of the patient as well as the public. For the diagnosis of tuberculosis, a high degree of clinical suspicion is required, and this becomes much more important in high-risk populations. Tuberculosis may masquerade as any disease; therefore, tissue and microbiological assessment is sometimes important for establishing the diagnosis. However, in daily practice, the clinician and radiologist should be familiar with the imaging features of pulmonary and extrapulmonary tuberculosis, as well as manifestations of tuberculosis in immunocompromised patients. Imaging provides a very important role in the diagnosis and management of tuberculosis. Although chest X rays remain the basic imaging modality for pulmonary tuberculosis, computed tomography, magnetic resonance imaging, and nuclear medicine techniques, including positron emission tomography/computed tomography, are extremely helpful in the assessment of both pulmonary and extrapulmonary tuberculosis.

The role of imaging in tuberculosis (TB) has shown exponential growth, as in all spheres of medicine. The possibility of a tubercular etiology is often first suggested on an imaging study, particularly in relatively inaccessible sites. In a known case of TB, imaging is often requested to assess the extent of disease, evaluate response to therapy, or detect residual infection after completion of therapy. Imaging also plays a vital role in guiding aspiration and biopsies and provides guidance for therapeutic drainage of pathological fluid collections.

All the imaging modalities, ranging from radiography to combined positron emission tomography/computed tomography (PET-CT), have their role depending on the clinical profile of the patient. Despite the advent of CT, PET-CT, and magnetic resonance imaging (MRI), conventional radiography remains the initial modality for suspected pulmonary TB or for mass screening purposes, and its role in musculoskeletal imaging remains unchallenged. The introduction of digital or computed radiography has enhanced the throughput, with improve-

Cite this article as *Cold Spring Harb Perspect Med* doi: 10.1101/cshperspect.a017814

ment in image quality and reduction of radiation dose to patients. Owing to its high speed and better resolution, CT is the modality of choice for evaluation of thoracic, gastrointestinal, and urogenital TB. Multislice CT has practically replaced conventional barium studies as well as intravenous pyelography. Nephrotoxicity of the contrast media used for CT remains a cause of concern, especially in patients with impaired renal function. Its multiplanar imaging capability and unsurpassed soft tissue contrast resolution make MRI the modality of choice in evaluating central nervous system (CNS) TB. Advancements in MR technology have resulted in expansion of the role of MRI in other parts of body also. PET-CT has the advantage of providing anatomical and metabolic information. It is expected to improve the sensitivity and specificity; however, more studies are required to establish its role in detection, differentiation, and follow-up of TB.

Although any organ of the body can be involved by TB, the lung remains the most commonly involved organ. The imaging appearances of TB may mimic a number of other diseases, and it is imperative to correlate imaging findings with clinical profile and other investigations.

In the following, the imaging appearances of TB are described for five major categories: pulmonary, CNS, abdominal, musculoskeletal, and miscellaneous.

PULMONARY TUBERCULOSIS

Mycobacterium tuberculosis is an airborne organism that reaches the pulmonary alveoli. It has conventionally been divided into primary and postprimary TB (Figs. 1 and 2).

Primary Tuberculosis

Primary TB is due to first-time exposure to mycobacterium bacilli. In TB-endemic regions, primary pulmonary TB often begins early in childhood with the inhalation of the tubercle bacillus (Raviglione and O'Brien 2005); however, it may be seen in adults, especially in developed countries, where the incidence of primary TB in adults has been reported to be 23%–34% (Miller and Miller 1993).

Primary TB may manifest as parenchymal disease, lymphadenopathy, pleural effusion, miliary disease, or any combination thereof. It may also present as lobar or segmental atelectasis. The inspired organism usually settles in the middle and lower lungs or in the anterior segment of the upper lobe, as these are the areas with greatest ventilation (Ghon focus), and extends via lymphatics to mediastinal nodes (Ghon complex). Once a Ghon focus undergoes fibrosis/calcification, it is called a Ranke focus, and, when calcification of lymph nodes occurs, it is called a Ranke complex. On plain radiography of the chest or CT, primary TB manifests as an area of homogeneous parenchymal consolidation, which is usually sublobar and subpleural. Multilobar consolidation is uncommon but can be seen in almost 25% of cases. The consolidation is usually dense; it may show an air bronchogram, especially on CT, and may mimic bacterial consolidation. Lobar or segmental atelectasis is a common radiological manifestation in children, the anterior segment of an upper lobe or the medial segment of the middle lobe commonly being involved. Associated enlarged nodes and poor response to antibiotics may provide clues to the diagnosis. With good immunity, the Ghon lesion usually heals, and a calcified focus seen on the chest radiograph in many adult patients is then the only telltale sign of infection in the remote past.

Enlarged paratracheal or hilar nodes differentiate primary from postprimary TB. Groups of lymph nodes more commonly involved are the hilar, right paratracheal, subcarinal, and aortopulmonary. In the Indian population, the right paratracheal group is the most commonly involved (Garg and Kalra 2010). CT is more sensitive than plain radiography in showing the enlarged nodes. Typically, affected nodes are larger than 2 cm and have low-attenuation centers on contrast CT, representing necrosis (Burrill et al. 2007). Low-density areas on enhanced CT are seen in 60% of the tubercular nodes (Gulati et al. 1994). Gross enlargement of lymph nodes may be seen in TB and may simulate sarcoidosis, lymphoma, or metastatic lymphadenopathy.

Pleural effusion may also be observed, and in some patients, it may be the sole manifesta-

 Cite this article as *Cold Spring Harb Perspect Med* doi: 10.1101/cshperspect.a017814

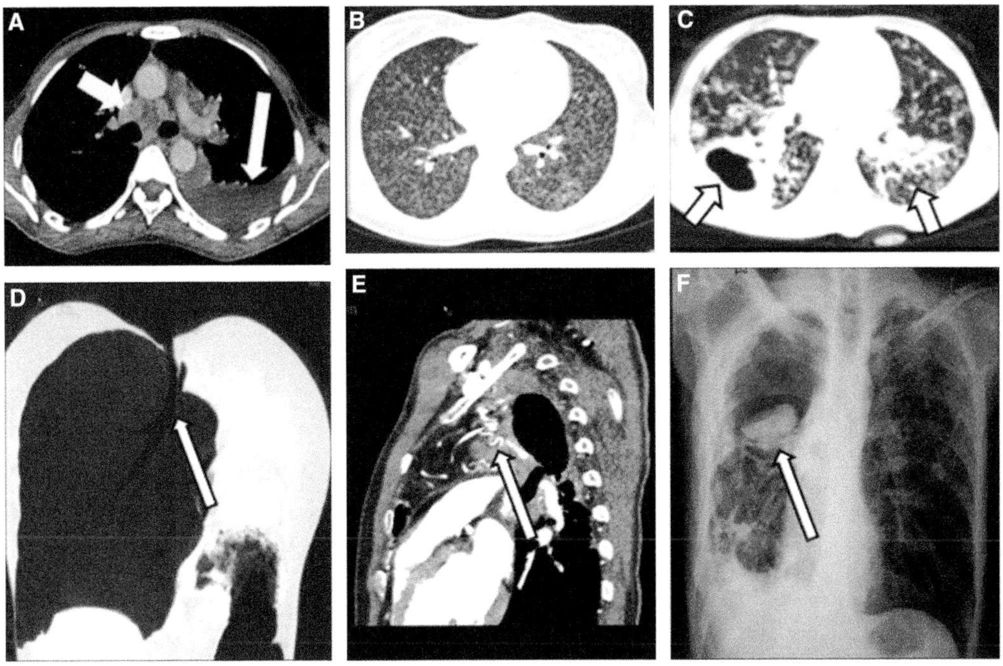

Figure 1. Spectrum of imaging findings in pulmonary tuberculosis (TB). (*A*) Axial computed tomography (CT) section of the mediastinum showing a hypodense subcarinal and precarinal node (short white arrow) and left pleural effusion (long white arrow). (*B*) Axial lung window CT section showing numerous miliary nodules in both lung fields. (*C*) Axial lung window section showing a thick-walled cavity in the right lung (arrow) and numerous centrilobular nodules in the left lung (arrow). (*D*) Coronal minimum intensity projection (MiniP) showing bronchostenosis leading to complete cutoff of the left main bronchus (arrow) and resultant collapse of the left lung. (*E*) Sagittal section of CT angiogram showing numerous tortuous dilated vessels (arrow) in a patient with hemoptysis and a history of TB 20 yr previously. Bronchial artery embolization was performed for this patient. (*F*) Chest radiograph posterioanterior (PA) view showing a dependent aspergilloma in a tubercular cavity in the right upper lobe (arrow).

tion of infection, especially in adult-onset primary TB. It is usually unilateral. Septations may be seen on ultrasound, reflecting the chronic nature of the disease.

With compromised immunity, a progressive primary infection may present as miliary disease. High-resolution CT is more sensitive than plain radiography in detecting such disease. The nodules are 1–3 mm in diameter and are seen in a perivascular and periseptal but random distribution.

Postprimary Tuberculosis

Both reactivation and reinfection with the tubercle bacillus are categorized under postprimary TB. In an adult with a healed remote infection, decreasing immunity may result in reactivation, which has a predilection for apical and posterior segments of the upper lobe and superior segments of the lower lobe. Postprimary TB is seen almost exclusively in adults and is characterized by a predilection for the upper lobe, cavitation, and absence of lymph node enlargement. A poorly defined area of consolidation is the earliest finding. These areas may evolve into more defined reticular or nodular opacities. Cavitation is the sine qua non of postprimary TB. It usually occurs in areas of consolidation with irregular thick walls. Cavitation may progress to endobronchial spread, which results in a typical tree-in-bud distribution of

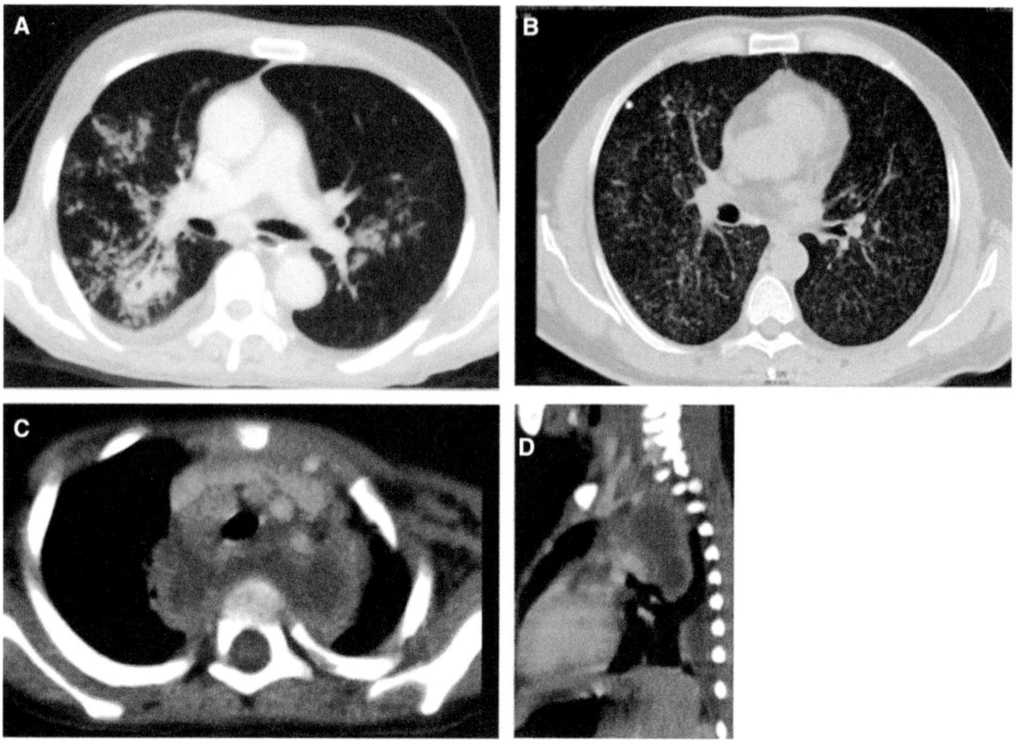

Figure 2. Imaging findings in pulmonary TB. (*A*) Ill-defined parenchymal opacity with cavitation on the right side. Random nodules give a tree-in-bud appearance in both lungs. (*B*) Diffuse miliary mottling in both lungs. Note the calcified granuloma and fibrotic strands on the right side. (*C,D*) Axial and sagittal reconstructions show conglomerate necrotic posterior and superior mediastinal lymphadenopathy displacing the trachea and branches of the arch of aorta anteriorly and extending into the retropharyngeal region, giving an abscess-like appearance.

nodules in addition to cavitation. Pleural effusion, although more common in primary TB, is seen in ~6%–18% of cases of postprimary TB (Woodring et al. 1986). The effusions are usually small and may be loculated. Pleura may be thickened.

The insidious nature of symptoms often causes a delay in diagnosis resulting in extensive disease, which in the long run leads to fibrosis, bronchial stenosis, and bronchiectasis. Bronchiectasis, a common complication of postprimary TB, is a result of a paracicatricial process secondary to pulmonary destruction and fibrosis. A tuberculous cavity with tortuous vessels may result in hemoptysis and secondary formation of aspergillomas or Rasmussen's aneurysm. Persistent communication between the bronchial tree and pleural space caused by TB (bronchopleural fistula) not only is associated with considerable morbidity and mortality but also poses a challenging management problem.

Active or Inactive?

TB makes its presence felt on imaging long after the resolution of disease. Whether or not the infection is active is a question that forever plagues the radiologist. Active disease is in general characterized by the presence of centrilobular nodules, thick-walled cavities, consolidation, miliary nodules, pleural effusions, or necrotic lymphadenopathy. Resolution to thin-walled smooth cavities, fibrosis, and parenchymal, nodal, or pleural calcifications often denotes remote infection. Air fluid level within a cavity may indicate superadded infection. In addition, involvement of the chest wall and osseous structures signifies activity.

Tuberculosis in HIV Patients

HIV patients are more susceptible to TB. Leung et al. (1996) compared the CT scans of HIV-positive and HIV-negative patients with TB and found that the former showed more features resembling primary TB. Radiological manifestations in HIV-associated pulmonary TB have been found to be related to the level of immunosuppression. HIV-seropositive patients with a CD4 T lymphocyte count of $<200/\text{mm}^3$ have a higher incidence of mediastinal or hilar lymph node enlargement, a lower prevalence of cavitation, and more frequent extrapulmonary involvement as compared with HIV patients with a CD4 T lymphocyte count of $>200/\text{mm}^3$ (Goodman 1990; Barnes et al. 1991; Jeong and Lee 2008).

CENTRAL NERVOUS SYSTEM TUBERCULOSIS

Involvement of the CNS produces the most devastating manifestations of the disease (Figs. 3–8). With the global pandemic of HIV infection, the incidence of CNS infections has also increased. CNS involvement may develop during the initial exposure or in the postprimary phase.

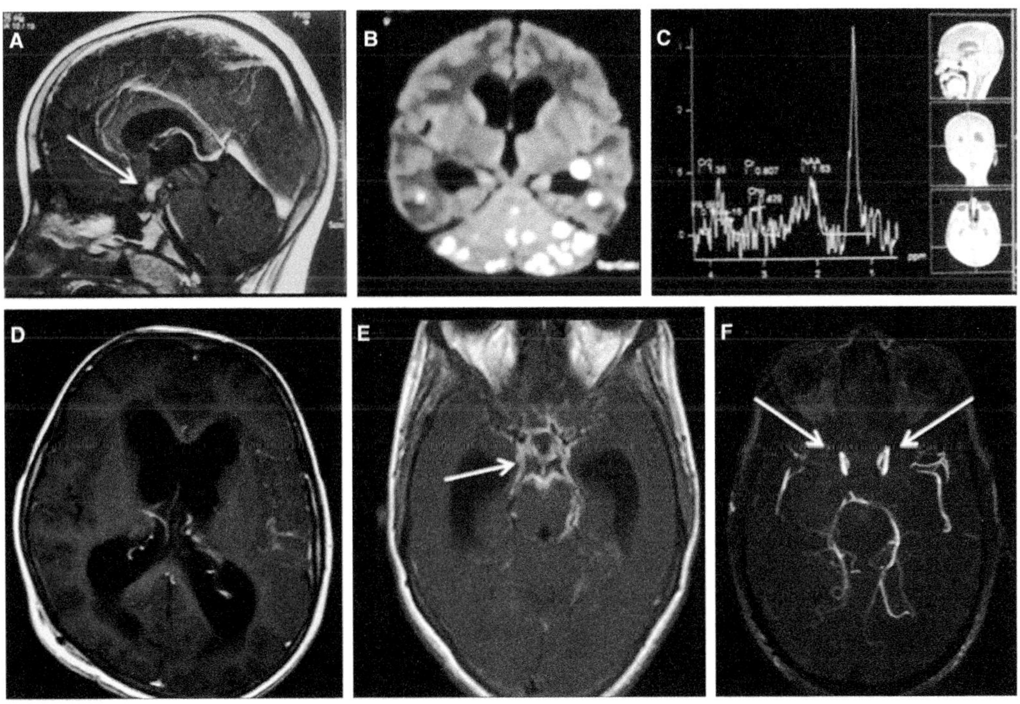

Figure 3. Spectrum of imaging findings in central nervous system tuberculosis. (*A*) Sagittal T1 postgadolinium magnetic resonance (MR) image showing a ring-enhancing tuberculoma (arrow) in the region of the pituitary and hypothalamus in a patient who presented with diabetes insipidus. (*B*) Diffusion-weighted image of the brain showing numerous hyperintense lesions representing tuberculomas, which show central diffusion restriction. (*C*) MR spectroscopy at 135 ppm showing a lipid peak at 1.3 ppm. (*D*) T1 postcontrast axial image showing hydrocephalus as a complication of TB. (*E*) T1 postcontrast image showing basal meningeal enhancement (arrow) in a patient with meningeal TB. (*F*) Postcontrast MR angiogram showing complete absence of takeoff of the anterior cerebral artery and marked attenuation of the middle cerebral arteries (arrows), suggesting tubercular vasculitis. The patient had dense basal exudates.

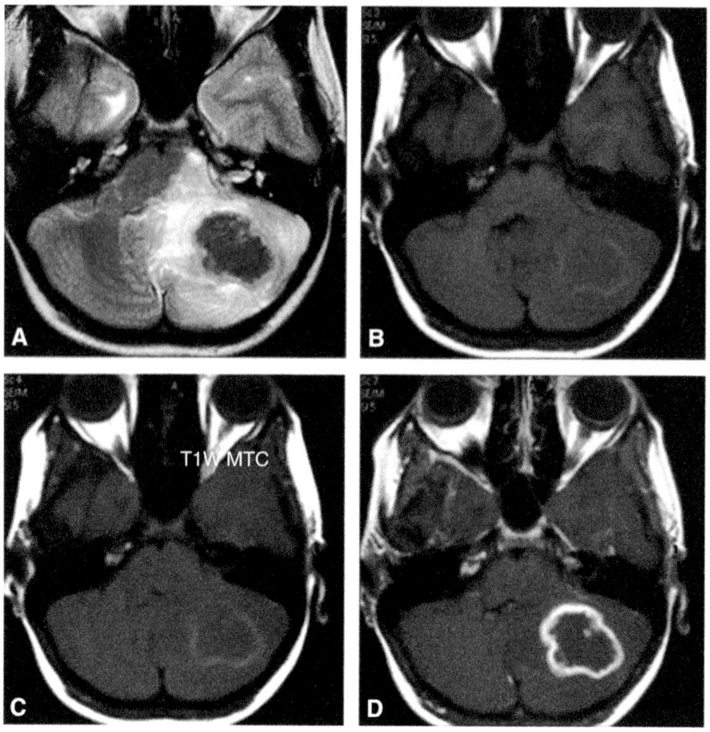

Figure 4. Axial T2 image (*A*) showing a lobulated lesion of low intensity in the left cerebellum with perilesional oedema showing a hyperintense signal. Corresponding T1 (*B*) and magnetization transfer contrast (*C*) images show a peripheral rim of mild hyperintensity with central iso- to hypo-intense signal. Postcontrast scan (*D*) shows rim enhancement with a central nonenhancing area.

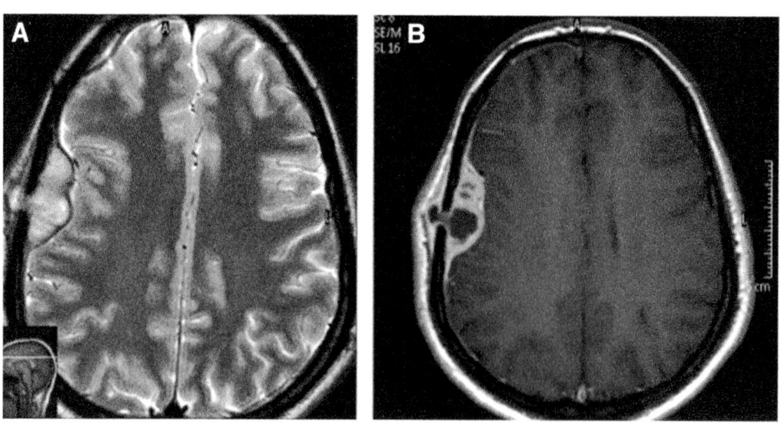

Figure 5. Axial T2 (*A*) and postcontrast axial T1 (*B*) images showing an extradural collection in the right frontoparietal region with extension to the subgaleal region through a focal lytic lesion in the parietal bone—collar stud appearance, tubercular.

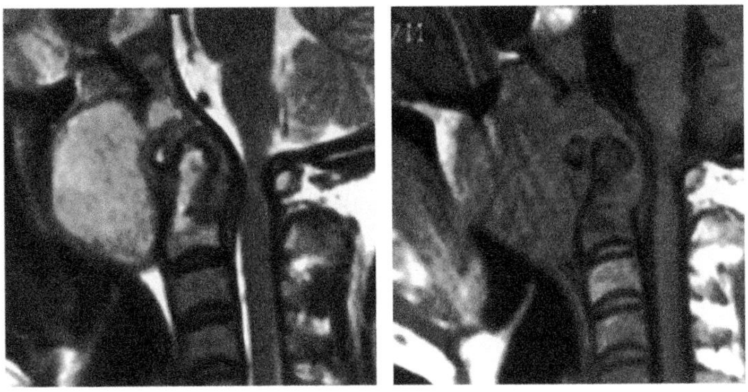

Figure 6. Sagittal T2 and T1 images showing partial destruction with signal alteration of C1–2, especially the dens, with a large prevertebral collection. A thin epidural collection results in compression over the cervicomedullary junction.

Various forms of involvement of the CNS, often coexistent, are observed: parenchymal (Fig. 4), meningeal (meningitis and its sequelae or complications) (Fig. 3), calvarial (Fig. 5), and spinal (Figs. 6–8).

Parenchymal Tuberculosis

The parenchyma may be involved either from direct spread from cerebrospinal fluid (CSF) or through hematogenous dissemination. Indeed, the most commonly involved territories within the brain are the corticomedullary junction and the periventricular region, typical for hematogenous dissemination.

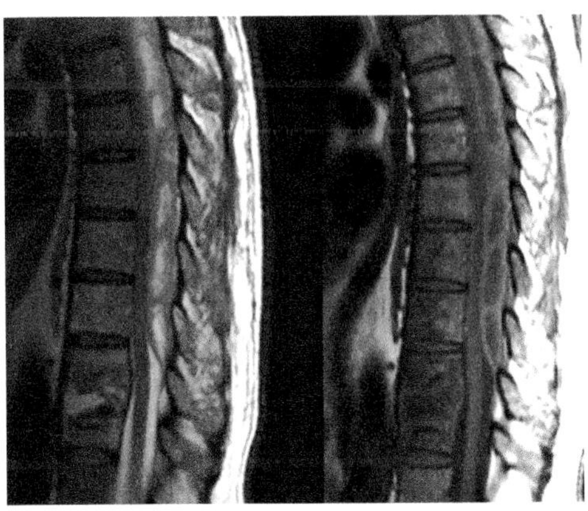

Figure 7. Sagittal T2 and T1 images showing partial destruction with signal alteration of D9–10 and of D7–8 with involvement of the intervening disc. An associated large posterior epidural collection from D9 upward is resulting in moderate to marked compression over the adjacent dorsal cord, which is pushed anteriorly.

Parenchymal involvement is most frequently seen in the form of a tuberculous granuloma (tuberculoma, the classic lesion) (Celso et al. 2009), but it can also be observed in various other forms, including tuberculoma en plaque, tuberculous abscess, cystic tuberculoma, multiple grapelike tuberculoma, microtuberculoma, calcified tuberculoma, and tuberculous encephalopathy. The imaging appearance of tuberculoma on MRI depends on the stage of the tuberculoma. A noncaseating granuloma is hyperintense on T2 and hypointense on T1 and shows solid enhancement. A solid caseating granuloma is hypointense on both T1 and T2, although it may show a T1 hyperintense rim. When liquefaction of the center or caseous necrosis occurs, the center becomes hyperintense on T2. Caseating granulomas show ring enhancement. T1 magnetization transfer images have been described to increase lesion conspicuity. In addition, calculation of the magnetization transfer ratio allows relatively specific diagnosis of tubercular etiology. Central diffusion restriction and lipid peaks on MR spectroscopy are supportive of a diagnosis of tuberculomas. On CT, tuberculomas appear as round or lobulated soft tissue masses with varying attenuation and homogeneous or ring enhancement. A target

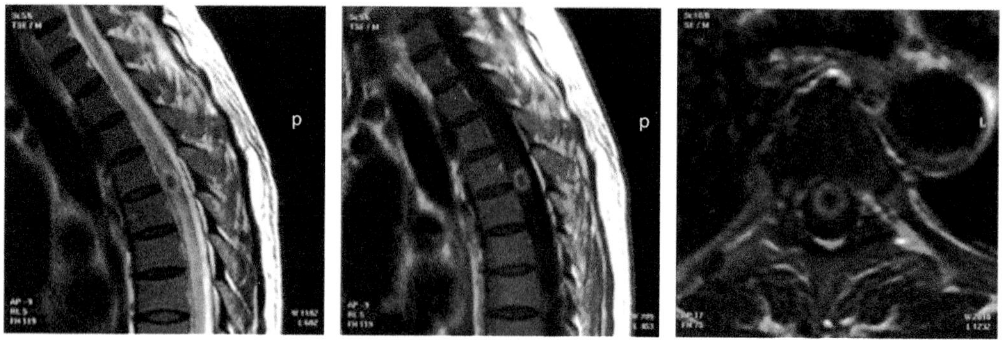

Figure 8. Sagittal T2 and postcontrast sagittal and axial images showing a well-defined intramedullary lesion with a low-intensity signal on T2 and rim enhancement on contrast images. Intramedullary tuberculoma.

sign (i.e., a central calcification or punctate enhancement surrounded by hypoattenuation and ring enhancement on CT [described by Margado and Ruivo 2005]) is suggestive but not diagnostic of tuberculoma. Tuberculomas in the pediatric age group are seen more frequently in cerebellum, whereas in adults they have a predilection for the cerebral hemispheres and basal ganglion. A number of lesions may mimic tuberculoma on routine imaging, including degenerating cysticercus, fungal granuloma, tumors such as lymphomas, and metastases. Newer techniques such as diffusion imaging, spectroscopy, and magnetization transfer imaging may help in differentiating these lesions (Gupta 2002; Patkar et al. 2012).

Tubercular abscess is relatively rare, being seen most often in immunocompromised patients. Abscesses lack epithelioid giant cells and have a wall composed of vascular granulation tissue. Unlike tuberculomas (which have a center of caseous necrosis), abscesses have a core of semiliquid pus with innumerable acid-fast bacilli (AFB)-positive bacilli. On imaging, abscesses are larger than granulomas, are multiloculated and show a T2 hyperintense center with a hypointense periphery. They generally show a thin rim of enhancement, although they sometimes display thick and irregular enhancement. Diffusion-weighted imaging and magnetization transfer imaging may help in differentiating a tubercular from a pyogenic abscess, the former showing low apparent diffusion coefficient and lower magnetization transfer ratio values (Gupta et al. 2001).

Miliary TB is often associated with TB meningitis (Trivedi et al. 2009) and presents as small (<2 mm) foci, which show low-intensity signal on T2 images and homogeneous nodular enhancement after administration of gadolinium.

Encephalopathy is an uncommon complication of cranial TB and is a result of a delayed hypersensitivity reaction to protein in tubercle bacilli. There is resultant extensive damage to white matter, seen on imaging as extensive brain edema (Patkar et al. 2012).

Meningeal Tuberculosis

Meningeal involvement can occur because of either rupture of a subpial granuloma into the CSF space or hematogenous spread from meningeal vessels (Trivedi et al. 2009). Characteristic of TB is the involvement of basal meninges with thick basal exudate. Such exudate is seen in the basal cisterns, sylvian fissure and, rarely, in meninges over the convexity; the cisternal component may result in hydrocephalus and cranial nerve involvement. The basal enhancement, hydrocephalus, tuberculomas, and infarcts are more common in tubercular meningitis than in pyogenic meningitis (Chowdhury et al. 1991; Patkar et al. 2012). Basal exudates show hyperdensity on CT, and lack of suppression of extra-axial CSF spaces may be seen on FLAIR images. Meningeal enhancement, particularly of the basal meninges, may be seen on administration of contrast. Contrast-enhanced MRI is superior to CT for evaluation of meningitis and its sequelae. Magnetization transfer imaging has been found to be useful in assessing the abnormal meninges and in differentiating tubercular from pyogenic meningitis (Patkar et al. 2012).

Diffuse and focal involvement of the dura may also be seen in the form of pachymeningitis, usually caused by a dural-based lesion. Whereas focal pachymeningitis is hypointense on T2, diffuse pachymeningitis shows hyperintensity on T2. Pachymeningitis, however, is a nonspecific finding.

There are a number of sequelae or complications of meningitis, and patients frequently present with complications, the most common of which include hydrocephalus, vasculitis, infarcts, and cranial nerve involvement. Hydrocephalus may be communicating (nonobstructive), noncommunicating (obstructive), or complex. Yadav et al. (2009) reported a high incidence of complex hydrocephalus in tubercular meningitis, resulting in failure of third ventriculostomy in these patients. MRI with recent advancements is superior to CT in evaluating the type of hydrocephalus and flow patterns and in patient follow-up.

Vasculitis occurs as a result of inflammatory changes in the vessels attributable to the basal exudates. Large intracerebral vessels are affected, including the terminal segment of the anterior cerebral artery, the middle cerebral artery, and the proximal anterior cerebral artery. Resulting intimal changes, vasospasm, thrombosis, and formation of mycotic aneurysms lead to large areas of cerebral infarction. The triad of a hydrocephalic pattern, narrowing of the arteries at the base of the brain, and narrowing or occlusion of small or medium-sized arteries with early draining veins on conventional angiography favors tubercular arteritis (Lehrer 1966). Focal segmental or uniform narrowing of large segments, an irregular beaded appearance of vessels, and complete occlusion are the features seen on MR or CT angiograms. MR scores more than CT in showing infarcts and in differentiating acute from chronic infarcts (Shukla et al. 2008). Basal ganglion, thalamus, and internal capsule are the common sites of infarcts in tubercular meningitis/vasculitis (Nair et al. 2009).

Cranial nerve involvement is another important sequela of tubercular meningitis and may be a result of ischemic changes in the nerve, entrapment of the nerve, mass effect on the nerve, or direct involvement of the cranial nerve nuclei by pathology. Chronic changes may lead to fibrosis and permanent functional loss of the affected nerve.

SPINAL TUBERCULOSIS

The spine is the commonest site of osseous involvement by TB. Spondylodiscitis, also known as Pott's disease, is the commonest form; however, it can also manifest as tubercular myelitis, intramedullary tuberculoma, spinal meningitis, arachnoiditis, or epidural abscess.

Spondylodiscitis usually begins in the anterior part of the vertebral body adjacent to end plates, commonly in the lower dorsal and upper lumbar spine (Weaver and Lifeso 1984). Infection then spreads beneath the anterior longitudinal ligament or posterior longitudinal ligament or sometimes through the vertebral endplate. Vertebral body destruction, marrow edema, soft tissue abscesses, hyperintensity, and enhancement of disc and loss of disc height commonly ensue. The infection may spread into the spinal canal, with formation of epidural abscesses that may compress the thecal sac, causing neurological symptoms. Plain radiographs are normal in the early stages. The earliest sign may be demineralization of the endplates with resorption and loss of dense margins. As the disease progresses, radiographs will show progressive vertebral collapse with anterior wedging and gibbus formation. MRI is the most sensitive modality for early diagnosis and follow-up of spinal TB. The earliest sign is marrow edema, seen as hyperintense signal on T2 and STIR (short tau inversion recovery) images. With progression of the disease, MRI shows loss of definition of the endplates and adjoining vertebral bodies with hypointense signal on T1 and hyperintense signal on T2 and STIR images. At this stage, the intervertebral disc shows hyperintense signal on T2 and STIR images with loss of internuclear cleft. With further progression, there is reduction in the intervertebral space, varying degrees of collapse of the vertebrae, and resultant kyphosis. Associated pre- and paravertebral, as well as epidural collection/abscess, is best seen on MRI. The collapsed vertebrae along with the epidural collection/abscess may result in varying degrees of extradural compression, best evaluated on MRI. The cord changes in the form of edema or myelitis are best seen on STIR images. The most common differential diagnosis is pyogenic meningitis, which at times may be difficult to differentiate solely on the basis of imaging. Other conditions that may simulate spinal TB are lymphoma, metastasis, and myeloma. Uncommon presentations include involvement of a solitary vertebra, multifocal skip lesions, isolated neural arch involvement, intramedullary tuberculoma, and isolated tubercular myelitis. Intramedullary tuberculomas show a signal intensity and enhancement pattern similar to those of intracranial tuberculoma (Jena et al. 1991).

Spinal arachnoiditis follows almost the same pathology as cranial meningitis. MRI is the modality of choice for diagnosis of the arachnoiditis, the features consisting of CSF (cerebrospinal fluid) loculations, obliteration of the spinal subarachnoid space, clumping of nerve roots, and adherence to the dura, best seen on T2-weighted sequences. On sagittal sections, an irregular wavy appearance is seen. Axial sections may give the appearance of an empty thecal sac owing to adherence of nerve roots to the dura.

NECK TUBERCULOSIS

Involvement of the neck nodes is a relatively common manifestation in the form of painless cervical lymphadenitis. The enlarged lymph nodes initially may be homogeneous, but they subsequently develop central necrosis seen as central low attenuating areas on CT (Fig. 9) and areas of hyperintense signal on T2 MR images (Tan et al. 2010). Contrast study will show peripheral enhancement. It may, however, be difficult to differentiate involved nodes from necrotic nodes seen in metastatic head and neck squamous cell carcinomas on imaging alone. Extranodal involvement of the other neck structures, such as the larynx, pharynx, and sinonasal cavity, although rare, may be seen; the imaging findings in these cases are, however, nonspecific (Burrill et al. 2007).

ABDOMINAL TUBERCULOSIS

The abdomen is the sixth most common site of extrapulmonary TB (Prakash 2009). There may be involvement of the peritoneum and its reflections, the gastrointestinal tract, the lymphatic system, and solid organs such as the liver (Figs. 10–12).

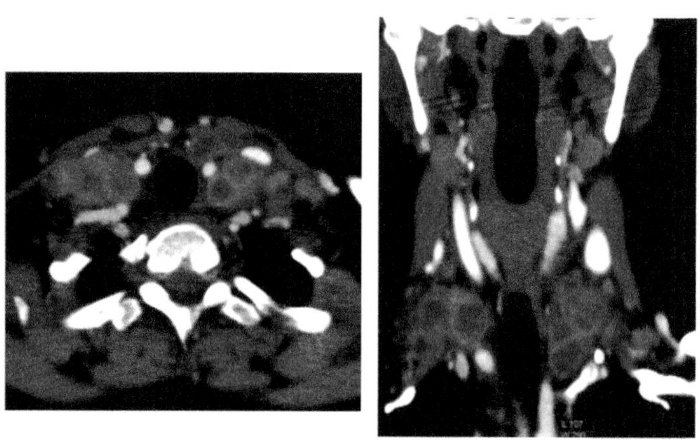

Figure 9. Postcontrast axial and coronal maximum intensity projection (MIP) images showing bilateral large conglomerate necrotic supraclavicular and cervical lymph nodes. Aspiration cytology confirmed tuberculosis.

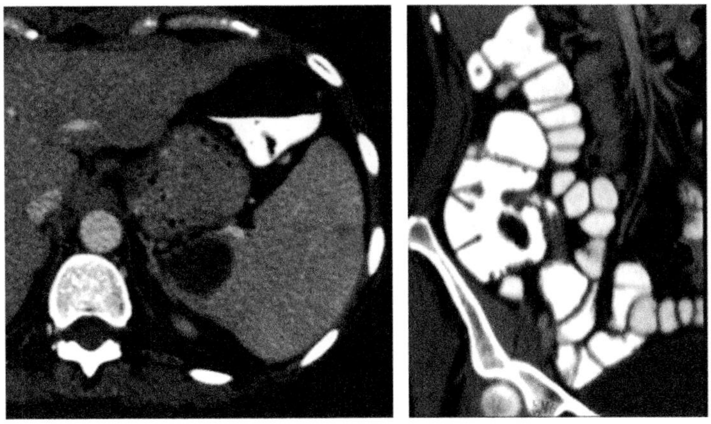

Figure 10. Axial and oblique coronal maximum intensity projection computed tomography images showing a well-defined lesion in the spleen with stricture in the terminal ileum. Note also two more small hypoattenuating lesions in the spleen. Ileal tuberculosis with splenic tubercular abscess.

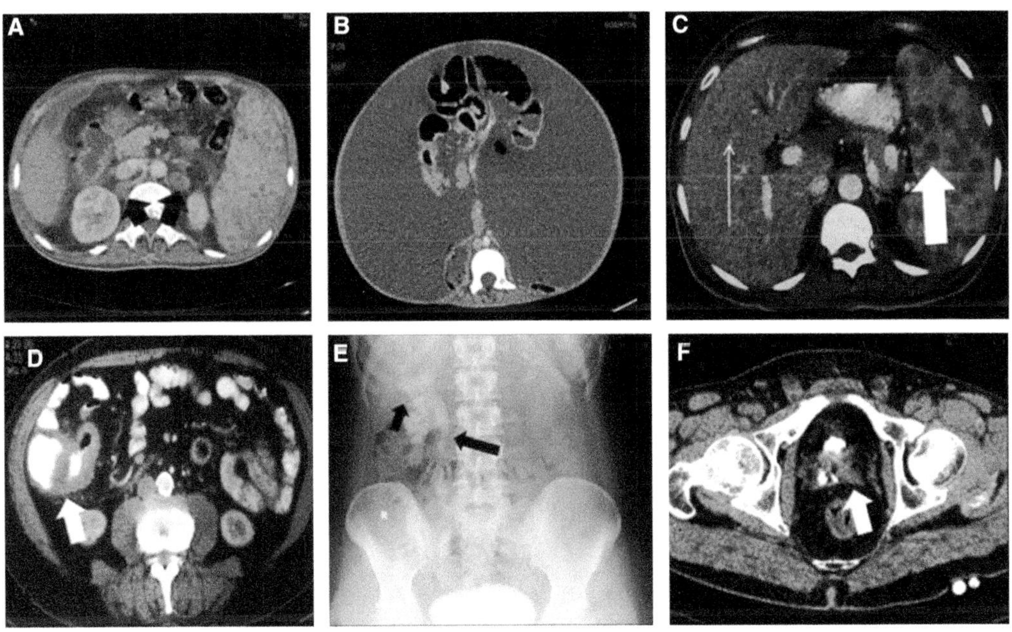

Figure 11. Spectrum of imaging findings in abdominal TB. (*A*) Axial computed tomography (CT) section of abdomen showing retrocaval and retro-aortic hypodense nodes (black arrow). Note splenomegaly and small hypodense lesions in the spleen. (*B*) Axial CT section showing wet tubercular peritonitis with high-density ascites. (*C*) Numerous small hypodense lesions in the liver (thin arrow) and larger hypodense lesions in the spleen (thick arrow) in a patient with disseminated tuberculosis. (*D*) Thickening of the ileo-caecal junction (white arrow). (*E*) KUB (kidney, ureter, bladder) radiograph as part of an intravenous urogram (IVU) study, showing an irregular cavity communicating with an upper pole calyx (short arrow) with stricture and deformation of the upper ureter (long arrow). (*F*) Small-capacity bladder with small amount of contrast within (thimble bladder).

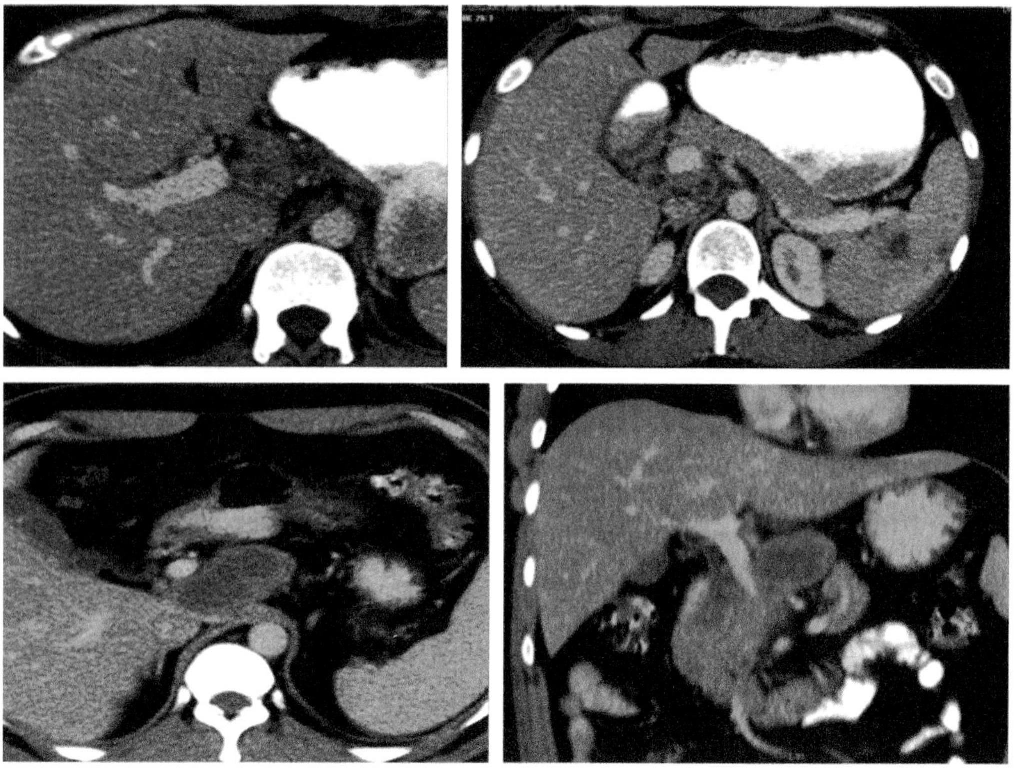

Figure 12. Contrast-enhanced computed tomography scan showing large necrotic lymph node posterior to and compressing the portal vein. Necrotic periportal lymph nodes and a few thick-walled cystic lesions (granulomas) are also seen in the spleen with septa. Tuberculosis was confirmed on histopathology.

Lymphadenopathy

Lymph node enlargement is the most common manifestation of abdominal TB and may or may not be associated with other abdominal organ involvement. Characteristically the nodal involvement reflects the lymphatic drainage of the involved bowel. The appearance of the involvement may range from an increased number of normal-sized nodes to grossly enlarged discrete nodes or a conglomerate with matting. Ultrasound shows a heterogeneous echotexture with a central hypoechoic area, in contrast to the homogeneously hypoechoic nodes seen in lymphoma (Prakash 2009). Abdominal lymph node involvement is best evaluated on CT. Plain scans show low or soft tissue attenuation values. Contrast-enhanced scans may show peripheral enhancement (the central liquefactive portion is nonenhancing) or heterogeneous enhancement and rarely homogeneous enhancement (Suri et al. 1999). MRI also may show different patterns; the appearance is typically hypointense on T1 images, whereas on T2 images, the signal is generally hyperintense or there is a central hyperintense signal with peripheral low-intensity signal. Rarely, hypo- to isointense signal is observed on T1 as well as T2 images (Sinan et al. 2002; Prakash 2009).

Peritoneal Involvement

Peritoneal involvement can occur through hematogenous spread to the peritoneum or via rupture of involved nodes, small bowel lesions, or the fallopian tubes. The imaging appearance has been classified into three types (Tarique et al. 2002).

- Wet—The most common type, characterized by high-density free or loculated ascites. The hyperattenuation on CT may be attributed to the high protein and cellular content.

- Dry—An uncommon type of peritoneal TB characterized by peritoneal caseous nodules and a fibrous reaction.
- Fibrotic—Associated with omental masses, matted bowel loops, and occasionally loculated ascites.

The CT appearance is nonspecific and can also be seen in peritoneal carcinomatosis, mesothelioma, peritonitis, and rarely lymphoma.

Hepatosplenic Involvement

Hepatosplenic involvement is commonly seen in patients with disseminated TB. The lesions may be miliary with innumerable small nodules of 0.5–2 mm (which may or may not be seen on CT but on ultrasound usually present as bright liver or spleen patterns in the form of a diffuse increase in echogenicity). A macronodular form, visualized as large hypoattenuating nodules on CT or hypoechoic lesions on ultrasound, is rare. These lesions may eventually undergo calcification (Burrill et al. 2007). MRI is more sensitive than ultrasound and CT in detecting hepatosplenic TB.

Gastrointestinal Tract Involvement

Any part of the GI tract may get involved, but the most commonly involved segment is the ileocecal region. Esophageal and gastric TB is uncommon but usually seen in association with thoracic TB. Obstruction due to ileocecal TB is most common. Plain radiographs may show enteroliths, with features of obstruction including multiple air fluid levels. Imaging features of small bowel TB will depend on the stage of pathology. Initially, it may be seen as rapid transit of contrast, hypersegmentation, or flocculation of the contrast column, or changes in the contour or mucosal pattern of intestine. Later, there is sclerosis, hypertrophy, and stenosis, resulting in a short stricture or strictures that have smooth but stiff contours and in which mucosal relief has disappeared (Prakash 2009). Multiple strictures with segmental dilatations are a common feature in small bowel TB. Fixity of loops, spiculation, matting, and signs of malabsorption are other features.

The ileocecal region is the area most commonly affected because of physiological stasis, abundant lymphoid tissue, increased rate of absorption in the region, and closer contact of the bacilli with mucosa in this region (Leder and Low 1995). Mural thickening involving both the ileum and the cecum is commonly identified on CT. The thickening is commonly concentric, although when eccentric, it frequently involves the medial cecal wall. Localized lymphadenopathy, surrounding fat stranding and skip lesions in the small bowel are often seen. On barium studies, thickening, spasm, and hypermobility of an incompetent ileocecal valve are considered characteristic. A gaping ileocecal valve with narrowing of the terminal ileum (Fleischner sign) or a narrowed terminal ileum with rapid emptying of the involved segment through a gaping ileocecal valve into a shortened, rigid, obliterated cecum (Stierlin sign) raise the suspicion of ileocecal TB. Shallow mucosal ulceration with elevated margins may also be seen if a double contrast examination is performed (Thoeni and Margulis 1979; Nakano et al. 1992). Retraction of the mesocolon eventually results in a "pulled-up cecum." CT enteroclysis further improves the sensitivity in early diagnosis. At present, MR is not widely performed for evaluation of intestinal TB, but bowel wall changes can be well evaluated with MR enteroclysis. Crohn's disease and lymphoma mimic ileocecal TB and may be difficult to differentiate on imaging alone.

Isolated large bowel involvement is less common and is seen in only about 9% of cases of GI tract TB (Theoni and Margulis 1979) and usually presents as a long or short segment of spiculations, spasm, rigidity, or ulceration.

Adrenal Involvement

Adrenal TB is the commonest cause of the adrenal insufficiency (Addison's disease). Tubercular involvement of adrenal glands on contrast-enhanced CT may be seen as bilateral enlargement of the gland with or without internal necrotic areas or calcification and in later stages, as a small gland with or without calcification (Francis and Korobkin 1997).

GENITOURINARY TUBERCULOSIS

Genitourinary TB is one of the common extrapulmonary manifestations (Fig. 13). The spread is usually hematogenous but may be by direct extension.

Parenchymal TB is usually associated with collecting system involvement and in the initial stage, results in localized tissue edema and vasoconstriction which can be seen on contrast-enhanced CT or MRI as areas of hypoperfusion; however, these findings are nonspecific (Jung et al. 2005). The collecting system is the most commonly involved site. In early stages, papillary necrosis or calyceal deformity occurs, whereas once acute inflammation has resolved, multifocal strictures may be seen (Wang et al. 2003). Erosion of the calyces results in an irregular contour and feathery appearance. Deformation of the collecting system gives rise to characteristic appearances: infundibular stenosis resulting in traction on the renal pelvis (Kerr's kink), deformity of the pelvis causing a "hiked-up" pelvis and complete cut off of the calyx resulting in a phantom calyx. Resultant stasis leads to the production of renal calculi, which today are the most common manifestations of renal TB. Parenchymal scarring and calcification are also seen (Bhalla et al. 2009). Contrast-enhanced CT/CT urography is the most sensitive modality to show early lesions. Depending on the extent of the disease, ultrasound may show alterations in parenchymal echogenicity, well-defined parenchymal lesions, liquefying tubercular cavity, perinephric abscess, or parenchymal calcification. The major role of ultrasound remains the provision of guidance for interventional procedures.

The passage of tubercle bacilli into the collecting system results in involvement of the rest of the genitourinary system as well. The ureters initially respond with atony caused by the baciluria, seen as dilatation. Eventually, irregularities caused by mucosal erosion and scarring are observed, producing a beaded appearance. Severe thickening of the wall in late stages gives rise to a "pipe stem" ureter. If not diagnosed and treated at an early stage, the kidney loses its morphology and may appear as multiple thin-walled cysts or as a multiloculated cyst. Sometimes, inadequately treated TB results in dystrophic calcifications involving the entire kidney, so-called putty kidney (Kim 2000).

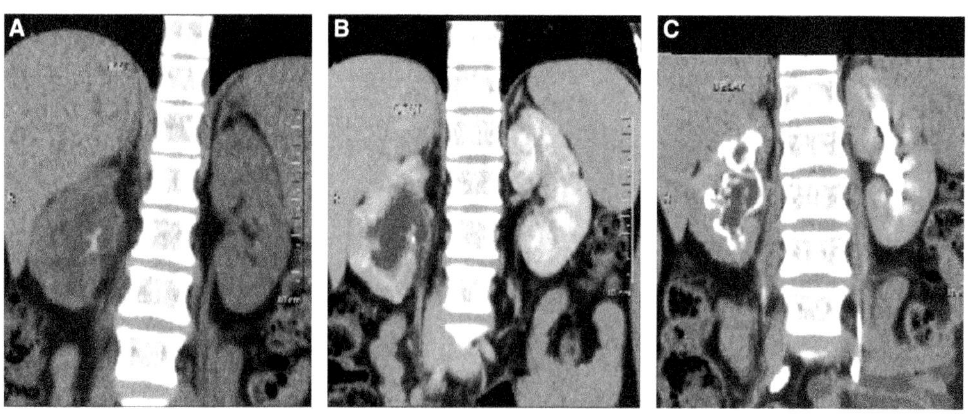

Figure 13. Coronal maximum intensity projection precontrast (*A*) and early (*B*) and delayed (*C*) postcontrast images in a case of renal tuberculosis, showing cortical irregularity of the right kidney with echogenic debris in the collecting system on ultrasound. CT shows calcification within the soft tissue, which is seen as a filling defect on delayed images. Mild hydronephrosis is seen with pelvi-ureteric junction obstruction. Note the thick-walled right ureter.

Large tuberculomas within the bladder wall may present radiologically as filling defects. Scarring results in a thickening of the wall and contracture of the bladder, giving the appearance of a "thimble bladder."

GENITAL TUBERCULOSIS

TB may affect the male as well as the female genital tract via the hematogenous or lymphatic route or via direct extension from the lower urinary tract (Fig. 14).

The epididymis is one of the male genital organs most commonly affected by genital TB. Ultrasound shows a heterogeneous texture with diffuse swelling (Kim 2000; Jung et al. 2005). As at other sites, MRI shows relatively low-intensity signal on T2 images with enlargement. Involvement of the prostate can be in the form of prostatitis or abscess; on ultrasound, the former is seen as low echogenicity and increased vascularity. Prostatic abscess on MRI appears as a peripherally enhancing lesion with radiating, streaky areas of low-intense signal, often called the watermelon skin (Engin et al. 2000; Jung et al. 2005). Prostatic abscesses and periurethral abscesses and fistulas may also result, although relatively uncommon. Urethral strictures are another uncommon manifestation, and when seen, they commonly involve the bulbo-membranous junction (Bhalla et al. 2009). Dystrophic calcification results in long-standing cases. The seminal vesicles and the vas deferens also can be involved by TB, and cross-sectional images show wall thickening, contraction, or intraluminal or wall calcifications (Birnbaum et al. 1990; Kim 2000). In females, the fallopian tubes are the genital organ most often involved. Ascending infection of the female genital tract results in hydrosalpinx and complex tubo-ovarian masses. Ultrasound via the transabdominal and transvaginal routes is very helpful in making the diagnosis, as well as assessing extent. Hydrosalpinx is seen as an aperistaltic, tubular anechoic channel with incomplete septations. Tubo-ovarian masses are seen as a conglomerate mass which is unilocular or multilocular with a thickened wall that may show enhancement on contrast-enhanced MRI. Normal ovarian follicles may sometimes be identified as a part of the mass.

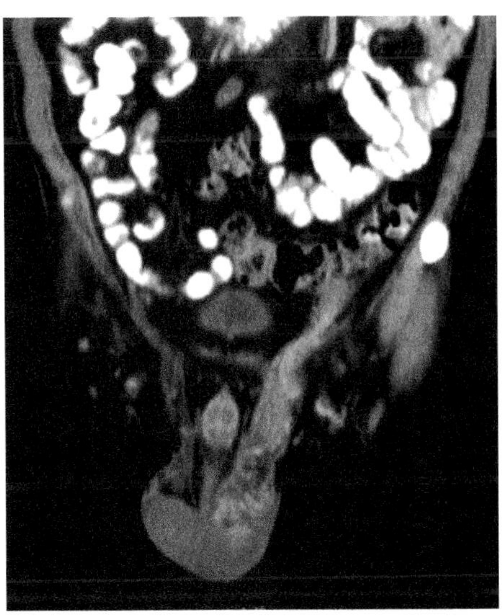

Figure 14. Coronal maximum intensity projection image showing left epididymo-orchitis with left-sided hydrocele. Note the thickened left spermatic cord—funiculitis.

MUSCULOSKELETAL TUBERCULOSIS

Any part of the musculoskeletal system can get involved at any age, but the large weight-bearing joints of the lower limb—hip, knee and ankle—are most commonly involved (Fig. 15). The smaller joints of the foot and hand, shoulder, elbow, and sternoclavicular and sacroiliac joints may also become affected. Isolated tubercular osteomyelitis may affect long as well as short tubular bones. The flat bones such as the skull, ribs, sternum, and iliac bones or bones of the carpus and tarsus, especially the calcaneum, may also be involved (Murray and Jacobson 1997).

Imaging findings in musculoskeletal TB are often nonspecific and only indicative of an infective etiology, rather than of an exact causative organism. Chronicity of the lesion is often the only pointer toward a tubercular etiology. Marked periostitis, sequestra formation, and sclerosis are seen more often in pyogenic infection, whereas transphyseal spread and joint involvement tend to indicate a tubercular etiology.

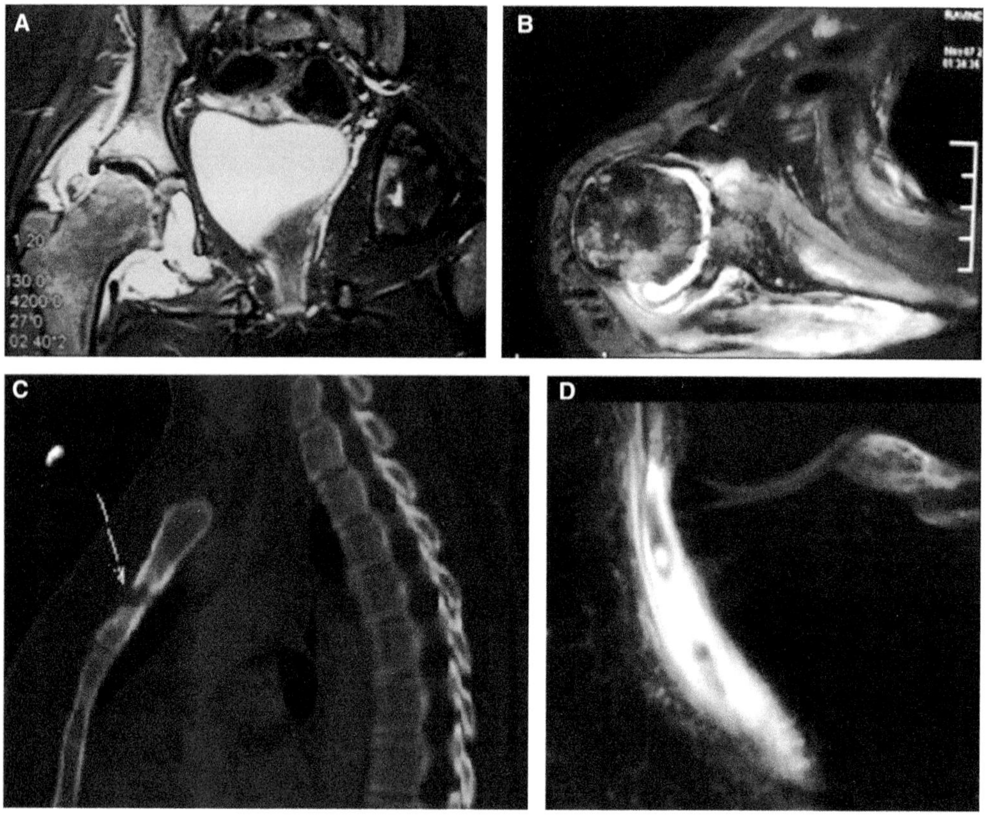

Figure 15. Spectrum of imaging findings in musculoskeletal tuberculosis. (*A*,*B*) Synovial thickening and surrounding bone changes. (*C*) Sagittal MIP CT image showing a lytic lesion in the sternum with surrounding mild sclerosis. (*D*) T1 postgadolinium coronal image showing thickening and enhancement of the medial collateral ligament bursa of the knee as a result of tubercular bursitis.

Plain radiography of the suspected area is the ideal initial modality and, along with the clinical profile, can point toward the diagnosis. In the initial stages, plain radiographs may be normal and further evaluation with MRI, CT, or ultrasound may be required. Because of unsurpassed soft tissue contrast resolution, MRI is the most sensitive modality for early diagnosis and complete delineation of the disease. Conventional T2 and STIR images are most useful. CT has the advantages of showing bony destruction and being capable of guiding interventional procedures. In experienced hands, ultrasound with high-frequency transducers can provide invaluable information about the synovium, tendon sheaths, and bursal spaces and effusions. Isotope scan is sensitive but not specific.

Articular TB is commonly monoarticular and involves large joints. Synovitis, osteopenia, and marginal erosions are seen. Resulting hyperemia may result in the overgrowth of epiphysis in children. In chronic stages, fibrous ankylosis may be seen. Bony ankylosis may also be seen, although this is more common with pyogenic infections. In the initial stages, plain radiographs may show widening of joint space with soft tissue swelling. With progression of the disease process, marginal erosions, smudged and indistinct articular cortex, and still later loss of subchondral bone are seen on radiographs. Phemister's triad of juxta-articular osteoporosis, peripherally located osseous erosions, and gradual narrowing of joint space indicate TB (Harisinghani et al. 2000). MRI scores more than other mo-

 Cite this article as *Cold Spring Harb Perspect Med* doi: 10.1101/cshperspect.a017814

dalities in showing all features of tubercular pathology—synovitis, active and chronic pannus, articular erosions, cartilage destruction, abscesses, tenosynovitis, bursitis, periarticular inflammation, and marrow edema (Sawlani et al. 2003). MRI without gadolinium may not always differentiate fluid from thickened synovium, but after administration of contrast, the synovium shows early enhancement and so can be differentiated from fluid. Ultrasound can differentiate synovial thickening from effusion, the former being hypoechoic and fluid, anechoic.

Tubercular osteomyelitis is usually accompanied by arthritis. Osteopenia with lytic lesions without significant surrounding sclerosis points toward TB. Involvement of the epiphysis across the growth plate is often seen, unlike in pyogenic infection. Short tubular bones may be involved, producing a fusiform soft tissue swelling with associated periostitis. Cystic TB is a distinct form of TB commonly seen in children, leading to cystic lucencies in the bone with minimal surrounding sclerosis.

Tubercular tenosynovitis may be seen, commonly involving tendons of the hand. In the first stage, only a serous exudate is observed. As infection progresses, thickening of the synovium and presence of T2 hyperintense material within synovial fluid are seen, and eventually soft tissue masses form. Tubercular bursitis has also been described and commonly affects sites subjected to frequent trauma. The infected bursa may involve adjacent muscles, joints, tendons, and bones (Jaovisidha et al. 1996).

MISCELLANEOUS

In a country where TB is endemic, like India, the disease may involve locations such as the eyes (Helm and Holland 1993), heart, temporal bone (Moon et al. 1997), and breast, which are otherwise exceedingly rare sites of TB (Fig. 16).

Cardiac TB is rare and generally involves the pericardium. It may present as pericardial effusion or a combination of effusion and constriction (Mayosi et al. 2005). Constrictive pericarditis is seen on imaging as thickened irregular pericardium with or without calcification. Accompanying signs of congestive cardiac failure may be seen. Myocardial TB is extremely rare and presents as a mass-like lesion or a diffuse infiltrative lesion (Jagia et al. 2010; Gulati and Kothari 2011).

TB is also a common cause of otomastoiditis. In a patient with soft tissue in the middle ear and mucosal thickening of the external auditory canal, the relative preservation of walls of the mastoid air cells and scutum without significant sclerosis points toward a tubercular etiology (Rho et al. 2007).

PET-CT Scanning in TB

PET-CT scanning is nonspecific for tumor as well as infectious and inflammatory conditions (Figs. 17 and 18). Therefore, interpretation of any positive fluorine-18 fluorodeoxyglucose (FDG) study should include consideration of benign diseases, including TB, especially in the tubercular endemic regions (Zheng et al. 2011). Soussan et al. (2012) described two distinct patterns of FDG PET activity in pulmonary TB—the pulmonary pattern and the lymphatic pattern. In the pulmonary pattern, FDG uptake was seen within the cavitary or noncavitary consolidation surrounded by micronodules along with mild to moderate tracer uptake within the mediastinal and hilar lymph nodes. In the lymphatic pattern, usually observed in patients with extrapulmonary/systemic symptoms, FDG uptake was seen as extrathoracic involvement. In patients with the lymphatic pattern, hilar and mediastinal lymph nodes were larger and showed higher uptake. Therefore, FDG PET improved specificity, especially in the detection of pulmonary tubercular involvement. Assessment of a single pulmonary nodule in endemic areas returns a high false-positive rate for malignancy (Li et al. 2011). Tubercular pleuritis can be confused with pleural mesothelioma on FDG PET (Yeh et al. 2009). Dual point imaging has been advocated to distinguish between tubercular and malignant lesions but has shown only limited promise (Yen et al. 2008; Razak et al. 2011).

FDG PET-CT has been shown to be useful (Tian et al. 2010b; Yadla et al. 2012) for the assessment of response to treatment in ex-

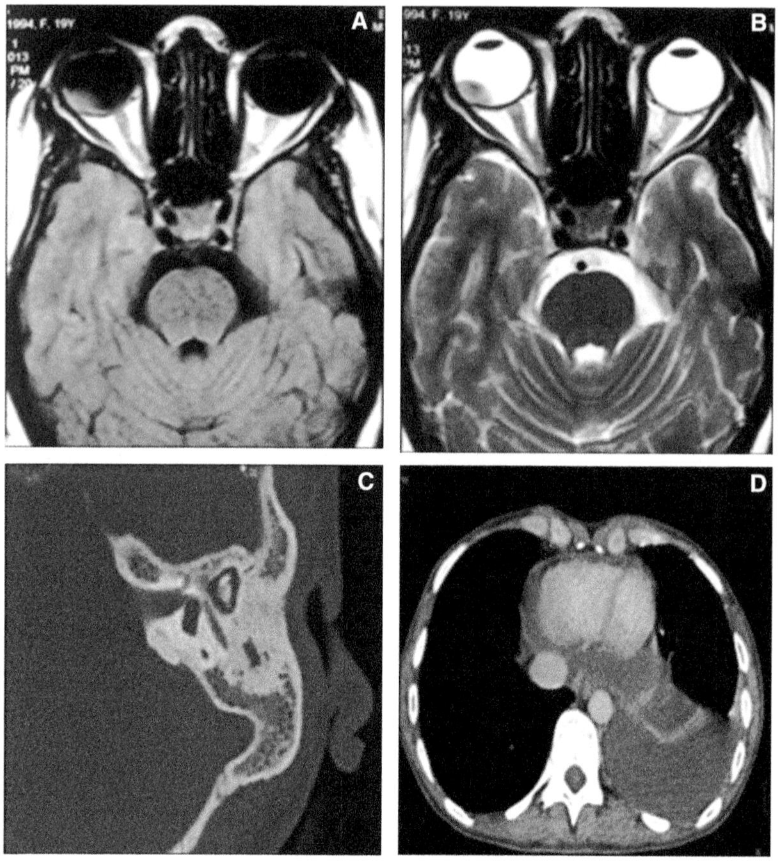

Figure 16. Unusual and miscellaneous sites of involvement. (*A*) T1 axial image and (*B*) T2 axial image of the orbit showing a T1 hyperintense and T2 hypointense mass initially diagnosed on imaging as a choroidal melanoma. The patient had disseminated TB, and the ocular lesion was proven to be a caseating granuloma. (*C*) High-resolution CT of the temporal bone in a patient with tubercular otomastoiditis showing relative preservation of the ossicular chain and mastoid air cells. (*D*) Axial CT image, mediastinal window, showing thickening of the pericardium and pericardial effusion.

trapulmonary TB (Fig. 19), and a decrease of approximately one-third in maximum standardized uptake value (SUV) has been reported at one month (Martinez et al. 2012). In addition, nonresponders can be predicted from the responders on the basis of persistent uptake in the five or more mediastinal lymph node stations and a maximum SUV >10 on delayed dual-point FDG imaging (Sathekge et al. 2011). In patients in whom the majority of lesions are improving on anticarcinogenic treatment but who also display nonresponding FDG-avid lesions, the latter may be of another etiology, including TB (Lee et al. 2011).

Abdominal and peritoneal TB is another presentation of TB in endemic countries. FDG PET-CT shows high false-positive rates in abdominal TB (Shimamoto et al. 2007; Takalkar et al. 2007; Tian et al. 2010a), but the distribution pattern may help in distinguishing peritoneal carcinomatosis from TB (Jeffry et al. 2003). Diffuse hepatosplenic FDG uptake without focal anatomical lesions may be a predictor of TB after lymphoma in these organs (Jeong et al. 2010). FDG PET-CT can detect tubercular involvement of unknown and unexpected sites (including tuberculous arthritis [Fig. 20] and common bile duct, pharyngeal, jejunal, and adrenal TB),

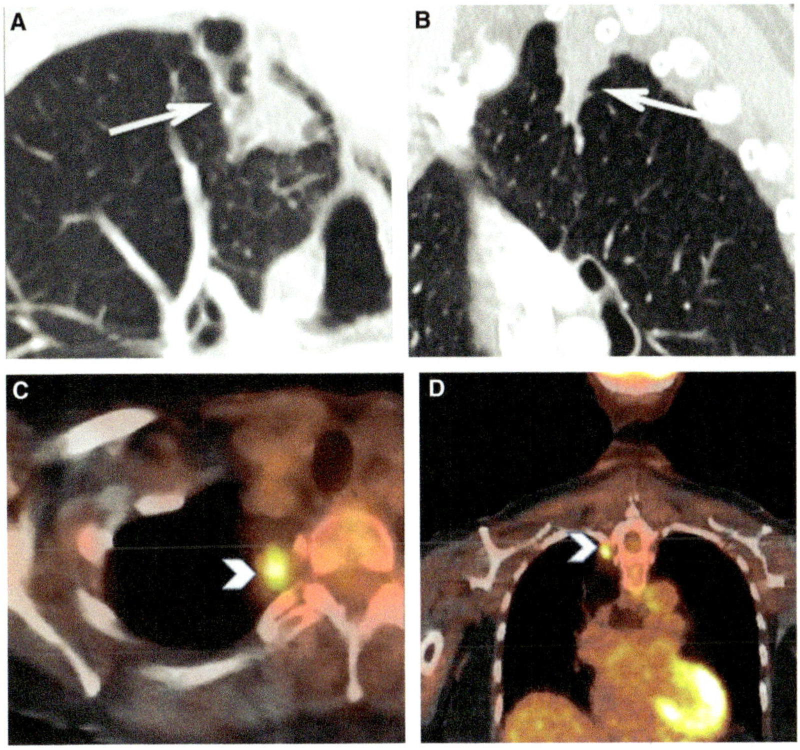

Figure 17. Biopsy-proven FDG-positive tuberculosis. This ex-smoker 72-year-old woman was detected with a mass at the right lung apex on a thyroid ultrasound. (*A*,*B*) Enhanced computed tomography (CT) of the chest showed a 28 × 15-mm ill-defined nodular density abutting the pleura (white arrows). There was no enlarged mediastinal or hilar lymph nodes. (*C*,*D*) Axial and coronal fused PET-CT images show increased tracer uptake with a maximum SUV of 4.0 (white arrowheads). No other FDG-avid lesions were identified. These findings were suspicious for bronchogenic, but a wedge resection pathology of this lesion showed "few acid-fast bacilli seen with necrotizing granulomatous inflammation." No carcinoma was seen. Therefore, this FDG uptake can be seen in active tuberculosis. This patient was subsequently treated with antitubercular treatment.

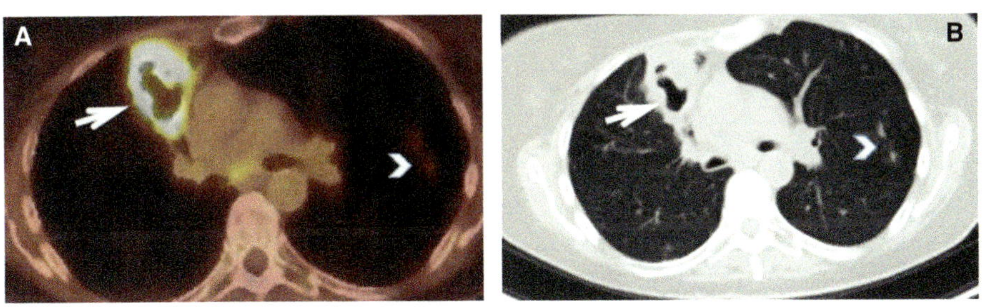

Figure 18. Increased activity in an atypical mycobacterium infection (culture proven). A 70-year-old female with previous computed tomography (CT) changes of atypical mycobacterium underwent PET-CT for follow-up of surgically resected tonsillar squamous cell carcinoma. (*A*,*B*) Peripheral moderate increased FDG uptake (arrow) in a new right lung cavitary lesion with additional two new, tiny lung nodules showing mild increased tracer uptake (arrowhead). The differential diagnosis included metastatic disease, aspiration, and infection including atypical mycobacterium. A bronchoscopically obtained specimen grew atypical mycobacterium.

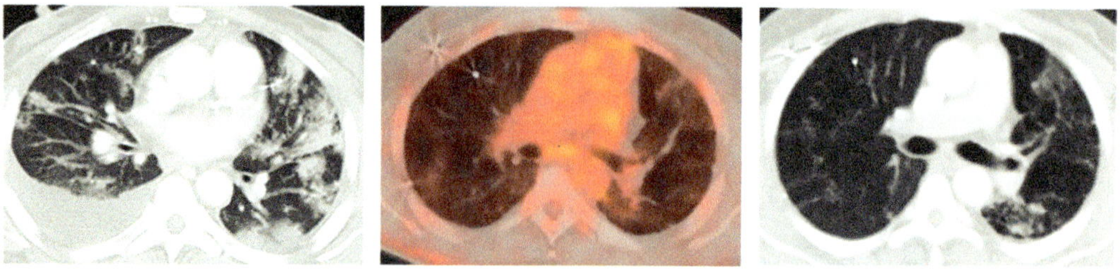

Figure 19. Minimal to no activity in a treated known TB case. A 53-year-old male with known history of lymphoma and culture proven TB was on antitubercular treatment. A computed tomography (CT) section shows patchy consolidations (*left*) that were predominantly in upper lobe distribution. PET-CT after 7 mo (*right*) shows almost total resolution of consolidations, and there is no significant increased tracer uptake in this treated TB (*middle*).

in cases which were initially thought to be malignant (Wang and Lin 2006; Roudaut et al. 2008; Ito et al. 2010; Dong et al. 2013; Wang et al. 2013). HIV-positive patients are at increased risk of malignancy as well as TB, and FDG PET-CT scanning was found not to be useful in distinguishing these three entities (Sathekge et al. 2010).

FDG PET-CT scanning for staging of lung carcinoma is more specific, especially in TB-prevalent areas (Lee et al. 2009). Carbon-11 choline is useful in distinguishing between pulmonary malignancy and TB, but its role in extrapulmonary TB needs further research (Chen et al. 2008).

The authors believe that as more data become available from areas where TB is endemic, owing to the increasing availability and use of FDG PET-CT scanning, there will be emerging specific use of this modality.

SUMMARY

TB is rife in developing countries, but it has also shown increased incidence in developed coun-

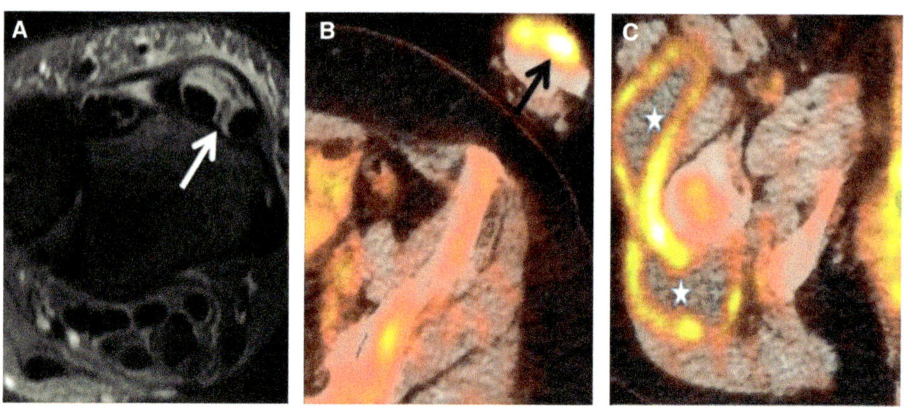

Figure 20. Biopsy-proven left wrist tubercular synovitis and right thigh nontubercular trochanteric bursitis. Nonsmoker 48-year-old female with previous BCG vaccination suffers from rheumatoid arthritis and drug-induced Sjogren's syndrome. She underwent a PET-CT to rule out malignancy. (*A*) Fast relaxation fast spin echo T2-weighted axial section show left wrist extensor compartment tenosynovitis (white arrow). (*B*,*C*) Axial fused PET-CT images show left wrist dorsum uptake (black arrow) and multiloculated collection in the right thigh with peripheral uptake (asterisk). The synovectomy of left wrist showed tuberculosis; however, repeated aspirations and cultures of right thigh collections were negative for fungal and acid-fast bacilli with no growth and therefore attributed to right trochanteric bursitis.

tries because of infection of immunocompromised hosts. TB can involve any organ system in the body, and there is a wide range of imaging features. Whereas diagnosis continues to require a high index of clinical suspicion, imaging has a very important role to play in both the diagnosis and the management of TB. PET-CT is an emerging technology in developing countries, and further data from these countries will assist in formulating exciting indications for this modality along with the already established options of plain radiography, ultrasound, CT, and MRI.

REFERENCES

Barnes PF, Bloch AB, Davidson PT, Snider DE Jr. 1991. Tuberculosis in patients with human immunodeficiency virus infection. *N Engl J Med* **324:** 1644–1650.

Bhalla AS, Gupta AK, Sharma R. 2009. Tubercular infection of the urinary tract. In *Diagnostic radiology genitourinary imaging*, 3rd ed. (ed. Khandelwal N, Chowdhury V, Gupta AK) pp. 120–138. Jaypee Brother Medical, New Delhi, India.

Birnbaum BA, Friedman JP, Lubat E, Megibow AJ, Bosniak MA. 1990. Extrarenal genitourinary tuberculosis: CT appearance of calcified pipe-stem ureter and seminal vesicle abscess. *J Comput Assist Tomogr* **14:** 653–655.

Burrill J, Williams CJ, Bain G, Conder G, Hin AL, Misra RR. 2007. Tuberculosis: A radiological review. *Radiographics* **27:** 1255–1273.

Celso L, da Cruz H Jr, Domingues RC. 2009. Intracranial infections. In *Magnetic resonance imaging of the brain and spine*, 4th ed. (ed. Atlas SW), pp. 929–1026. Lippincott Williams & Wilkins, Philadelphia.

Chen CJ, Yao WJ, Chou CY, Chiu NT, Lee BF, Wu PS. 2008. Peritoneal tuberculosis with elevated serum CA125 mimicking peritoneal carcinomatosis on F-18 FDG-PET/CT. *Ann Nucl Med* **22:** 525–527.

Chowdhury V, Gulati P, Sachdev A, Mittal SK. 1991. Sonography in pyogenic and tubercular meningitis: A comparative study. *Indian J Radiol Imag* **1:** 7–10.

Dong A, Wang Y, Gong J, Zuo C. 2013. FDG PET/CT findings of common bile duct tuberculosis. *Clin Nucl Med* **39:** 67–70.

Engin G, Acunas G, Tunaci M. 2000. Imaging of extrapulmonary tuberculosis. *Radiographics* **20:** 471–488.

Francis IR, Korobkin M. 1997. The incidentally discovered adrenal masses. *Magn Reson Imaging Clin N Am* **5:** 147–164.

Garg MK, Kalra N. 2010. Radiological manifestations of pulmonary tuberculosis. In *Diagnostic radiology*, 3rd ed. (ed. Chowdhury V, Gupta AK, Khandelwal N), pp. 60–68. Jaypee Brother Medical, New Delhi, India.

Goodman PC. 1990. Pulmonary tuberculosis in patients with acquired immunodeficiency syndrome. *J Thorac Imaging* **5:** 38–45.

Gulati GS, Kothari SS. 2011. Diffuse infiltrative cardiac tuberculosis. *Ann Pediatr Cardiol* **4:** 87–89.

Gulati M, Suri S, Kaur G, Jindal SK, Behera D. 1994. CT manifestations of tubercular mediastinal lymphadenopathy. *Indian J Chest Dis Allied Sci* **36:** 3–7.

Gupta RK. 2002. Magnetization transfer MR imaging in central nervous system infections. *Indian J Radiol Imaging* **12:** 51–58.

Gupta RK, Vatsal DK, Hussain N, Chawla S, Prasad KN, Roy R, Kumar R, Jha D, Hussain M. 2001. Differentiation of tuberculous from pyogenic brain abscesses with in vivo proton MR spectroscopy and magnetization transfer MR imaging. *AJNR Am J Neuroradiol* **22:** 1503–1509.

Harisinghani MG, McLoud TC, Shepard JA, Ko JP, Shroff MM, Mueller PR. 2000. Tuberculosis from head to toe. *Radiographics* **20:** 449–470.

Helm CJ, Holland GN. 1993. Ocular tuberculosis. *Surv Ophthalmol* **38:** 229–256.

Ito K, Morooka M, Kubota K. 2010. 18F-FDG PET/CT findings of pharyngeal tuberculosis. *Ann Nucl Med* **24:** 493–496.

Jagia P, Gulati GS, Sharma S. 2010. Imaging in cardiomyopathies. In *Diagnostic radiology*, 3rd ed. (ed. Chowdhury V, Gupta AK, Khandelwal N), pp. 376–383. Jaypee Brother Medical, New Delhi, India.

Jaovisidha S, Chen C, Ryu KN, Siriwongpairat P, Pekanan P, Sartonis DJ, Resnick D. 1996. Tuberculous tenosynovitis and bursitis: Imaging findings in 21 cases. *Radiology* **201:** 507–513.

Jeffry L, Kerrou K, Camatte S, Lelievre L, Metzger U, Robin F, Lecuru F. 2003. Peritoneal tuberculosis revealed by carcinomatosis on CT scan and uptake at FDG-PET. *BJOG* **110:** 1129–1131.

Jena AN, Banerji AK, Tripathi RP, Gulati PK, Jain RK, Khushu S, Sapra ML. 1991. Demonstration of intramedullary tuberculomas by magnetic resonance imaging: A report of two cases. *Br J Radiol* **64:** 555–557.

Jeong YJ, Lee KS. 2008. Pulmonary tuberculosis: Up-to-date imaging and management. *AJR Am J Roentgenol* **191:** 834–844.

Jeong YJ, Sohn MH, Lim ST, Kim DW, Jeong HJ, Chung MJ, Yim CY. 2010. "Hot liver" on 18F-FDG PET/CT imaging in a patient with hepatosplenic tuberculosis. *Eur J Nucl Med Mol Imaging* **37:** 1618–1619.

Jung YY, Kim JK, Cho K. 2005. Genitourinary tuberculosis: Comprehensive sectional imaging. *AJR Am J Roentgenol* **184:** 143–150.

Kim SH. 2000. Genitourinary tuberculosis. In *Clinical urography*, 2nd ed. (ed. Pollack HM, Dyer R, McClennan BL), pp. 1193–1228. Saunders, Philadelphia.

Leder RA, Low VHS. 1995. Tuberculosis of the abdomen. *Radiol Clin North Am* **33:** 691–705.

Lee JW, Kim BS, Lee DS, Chung JK, Lee MC, Kim S, Kang WJ. 2009. 18F-FDG PET/CT in mediastinal lymph node staging of non-small-cell lung cancer in a tuberculosis-endemic country: Consideration of lymph node calcification and distribution pattern to improve specificity. *Eur J Nucl Med Mol Imaging* **36:** 1794–1802.

Lee G, Lee JH, Park SG. 2011. F-18 FDG PET/CT imaging of solitary genital tuberculosis mimicking recurrent lymphoma. *Clin Nucl Med* **36:** 315–316.

Lehrer H. 1966. The angiographic triad in tuberculous meningitis. A radiographic and clinicopathologic correlation. *Radiology* **87:** 829–835.

Leung AN, Brauner MW, Gamsu G, Milika-Cabanne N, Ben Romdhane H, Carette MF, Grenier P. 1996. Pulmonary tuberculosis: Comparison of CT findings in HIV sero positive and HIV sero negative patients. *Radiology* **198:** 687–691.

Li Y, Su M, Li F, Kuang A, Tian R. 2011. The value of (18)F-FDG-PET/CT in the differential diagnosis of solitary pulmonary nodules in areas with a high incidence of tuberculosis. *Ann Nucl Med* **25:** 804–811.

Margado C, Ruivo N. 2005. Imaging meningo-encephalic tuberculosis. *Eur J Radiol* **55:** 188–192.

Martinez V, Castilla-Lievre MA, Guillet-Caruba C, Grenier G, Fior R, Desarnaud S, Boue F. 2012. (18)F-FDG PET/CT in tuberculosis: An early non-invasive marker of therapeutic response. *Int J Tuberc Lung Dis* **16:** 1180–1185.

Mayosi BM, Burgess LJ, Doubell AF. 2005. Heart disease in Africa. *Circulation* **112:** 3608–3616.

Miller WT, Miller WT Jr. 1993. Tuberculosis in the normal host: Radiological findings. *Semin Roentgenol* **28:** 109–118.

Moon WK, Han MH, Chang KH, Im JG, Kim HJ, Sung KJ, Lee HK. 1997. CT and MR imaging of head and neck tuberculosis. *Radiographics* **17:** 391–402.

Murray RO, Jacobson HG. 1997. Skeletal tuberculosis in the radiology of skeletal diseases. In *Exercises in diagnosis*, 2nd ed, pp. 414–426. Churchill Livingstone, Edinburgh.

Nair PP, Kalita J, Kumar S, Misra UK. 2009. MRI pattern of infarcts in basal ganglia region in patients with tuberculous meningitis. *Neuroradiology* **51:** 221–225.

Nakano H, Jaramillo E, Watanabe M, Miyachi I, Takahama K, Itoh M. 1992. Intestinal tuberculosis: Findings on double contrast barium enema. *Gastrointest Radiol* **17:** 108–114.

Patkar D, Narang J, Yanamandala R, Lawande M, Shah G. 2012. Central nervous system tuberculosis: Pathophysiology and imaging findings. *Neuroimag Clin North Am* **22:** 677–705.

Prakash A. 2009. Abdominal tuberculosis. In *Diagnostic radiology gastrointestinal and hepatobiliary imaging*, 3rd ed. (ed. Gupta A, Chowdhury V, Khandelwal N). Jaypee Brother Medical, New Delhi, India.

Raviglione MC, O'Brien RJ. 2005. Tuberculosis. In *Harrison's principles of internal medicine*, 17th ed. (ed. Kasper DL, Barunwald E, Fauci A, et al.), pp. 1006–1021. McGraw-Hill, New York.

Razak HR, Geso M, Abdul Rahim N, Nordin AJ. 2011. Imaging characteristics of extrapulmonary tuberculosis lesions on dual time point imaging (DTPI) of FDG PET/CT. *J Med Imaging Radiat Oncol* **55:** 556–562.

Rho MH, Kim DW, Kim SS, Sung YS, Kwon JS, Lee SW. 2007. Tuberculous otomastoiditis on high-resolution temporal bone CT: Comparison with nontuberculous otomastoiditis with and without cholesteatoma. *AJNR Am J Neuroradiol* **28:** 493–496.

Roudaut N, Malecot JM, Dupont E, Boussion N, Visvikis D, Doucet L, Cheze-Le Rest C. 2008. Adrenal tuberculosis revealed by FDG PET. *Clin Nucl Med* **33:** 821–823.

Sathekge M, Maes A, Kgomo M, Pottel H, Stolz A, Van De Wiele C. 2010. FDG uptake in lymph-nodes of HIV+ and tuberculosis patients: Implications for cancer staging. *Q J Nucl Med Mol Imaging* **54:** 698–703.

Sathekge M, Maes A, Kgomo M, Stoltz A, Van de Wiele C. 2011. Use of 18F-FDG PET to predict response to first-line tuberculostatics in HIV-associated tuberculosis. *J Nucl Med* **52:** 880–885.

Sawlani V, Chandra T, Mishra RN, Aggarwal A, Jain UK, Gujral RB. 2003. MRI features of tuberculosis of peripheral joints. *Clin Radiol* **58:** 755–762.

Shimamoto H, Hamada K, Higuchi I, Tsujihata M, Nonomura N, Tomita Y, Hatazawa J. 2007. Abdominal tuberculosis: Peritoneal involvement shown by F-18 FDG PET. *Clin Nucl Med* **32:** 716–718.

Shukla R, Abbas A, Kumar P, Gupta RK, Jha S, Prasad KN. 2008. Evaluation of cerebral infarction in tuberculous meningitis by diffusion weighted imaging. *J Infect* **57:** 298–306.

Sinan T, Sheikh M, Ramadan S, Sahwney S, Behbehani A. 2002. CT features in abdominal tuberculosis: 20 years experience. *BMC Med Imaging* **2:** 1–7.

Soussan M, Brillet PY, Mekinian A, Khafagy A, Nicolas P, Vessieres A, Brauner M. 2012. Patterns of pulmonary tuberculosis on FDG-PET/CT. *Eur J Radiol* **81:** 2872–2876.

Suri S, Gupta S, Suri R. 1999. Computed tomography in abdominal tuberculosis. *Br J Radiol* **72:** 92–98.

Takalkar AM, Bruno GL, Reddy M, Lilien DL. 2007. Intense FDG activity in peritoneal tuberculosis mimics peritoneal carcinomatosis. *Clin Nucl Med* **32:** 244–246.

Tan CH, Kontoyiannis DP, Viswanathan C, Iyer RB. 2010. Tuberculosis: A benign impostor. *Am J Roentengenol* **194:** 555–561.

Theoni RF, Margullis AR. 1979. Gastrointestinal tuberculosis. *Semin Roentgenol* **14:** 283–294.

Tian G, Xiao Y, Chen B, Guan H, Deng QY. 2010a. Multi-site abdominal tuberculosis mimics malignancy on 18F-FDG PET/CT: Report of three cases. *World J Gastroenterol* **16:** 4237–4242.

Tian G, Xiao Y, Chen B, Xia J, Guan H, Deng Q. 2010b. FDG PET/CT for therapeutic response monitoring in multi-site non-respiratory tuberculosis. *Acta Radiol* **51:** 1002–1006.

Trivedi R, Saksena S, Gupta RK. 2009. Magnetic resonance imaging in central nervous system tuberculosis. *Indian J Radiol Imaging* **19:** 256–265.

Wang HY, Lin WY. 2006. Jejunal tuberculosis: Incidental finding on an FDG-PET scan. *Kaohsiung J Med Sci* **22:** 34–38.

Wang LJ, Wu CF, Wong YC, Chuang CK, Chu SH, Chen CJ. 2003. Imaging findings of urinary tuberculosis on excretory urography and computerized tomography. *J Urol* **169:** 524–528.

Wang JH, Chi CY, Lin KH, Ho MW, Kao CH. 2013. Tuberculous arthritis—Unexpected extrapulmonary tuberculosis detected by FDG PET/CT. *Clin Nucl Med* **38:** e93–e94.

Weaver P, Lifeso R. 1984. The radiological diagnosis of tuberculosis of the adult spine. *Skeletal Radiol* **12:** 178–186.

Woodring JH, Vandiviere HM, Fried AM, Dillon ML, Williams TD, Melvin IG. 1986. Update: The radiographic features of pulmonary tuberculosis. *AJR Am J Roentgenol* **146:** 497–506.

Yadav YR, Mukerji G, Parihar V, Sinha M, Pandey S. 2009. Complex hydrocephalus (combination of communicating and obstructive type): An important cause of failed endoscopic third ventriculostomy. *BMC Res Notes* **2:** 137.

Yadla M, Sivakumar V, Kalawat T. 2012. Assessment of early response to treatment in extrapulmonary tuberculosis: Role of FDG-PET. *Indian J Nucl Med* **27:** 136–137.

Yeh CL, Chen LK, Chen SW, Chen YK. 2009. Abnormal FDG PET imaging in tuberculosis appearing like mesothelioma: Anatomic delineation by CT can aid in differential diagnosis. *Clin Nucl Med* **34:** 815–817.

Yen RF, Chen KC, Lee JM, Chang YC, Wang J, Cheng MF, Lee YC. 2008. 18F-FDG PET for the lymph node staging of non-small cell lung cancer in a tuberculosis-endemic country: Is dual time point imaging worth the effort? *Eur J Nucl Med Mol Imaging* **35:** 1305–1315.

Zheng Z, Pan Y, Guo F, Wei H, Wu S, Pan T, Li J. 2011. Multimodality FDG PET/CT appearance of pulmonary tuberculoma mimicking lung cancer and pathologic correlation in a tuberculosis-endemic country. *South Med J* **104:** 440–445.

Tuberculosis Treatment and Drug Regimens

Giovanni Sotgiu[1], Rosella Centis[2], Lia D'ambrosio[2], and Giovanni Battista Migliori[2]

[1]Clinical Epidemiology and Medical Statistics Unit, Department of Biomedical Sciences, University of Sassari, Research, Medical Education and Professional Development Unit, AOU Sassari 07100, Italy

[2]World Health Organization Collaborating Centre for Tuberculosis and Lung Diseases, Fondazione S. Maugeri, Care and Research Institute, Tradate 21049, Italy

Correspondence: gbmigliori@fsm.it

Tuberculosis is an airborne infectious disease treated with combination therapeutic regimens. Adherence to long-term antituberculosis therapy is crucial for maintaining adequate blood drug level. The emergence and spread of drug-resistant *Mycobacterium tuberculosis* strains are mainly favored by the inadequate medical management of the patients. The therapeutic approach for drug-resistant tuberculosis is cumbersome, because of the poor, expensive, less-effective, and toxic alternatives to the first-line drugs. New antituberculosis drugs (bedaquiline and delamanid) have been recently approved by the health authorities, but they cannot represent the definitive solution to the clinical management of drug-resistant tuberculosis forms, particularly in intermediate economy settings where the prevalence of drug resistance is high (China, India, and former Soviet Union countries). New research and development activities are urgently needed. Public health policies are required to preserve the new and old therapeutic options.

Medical treatment of tuberculosis, together with correct diagnosis, represents a cornerstone in the management and control of tuberculosis. It is relevant from a clinical and public health perspective, as tuberculosis is a serious contagious airborne disease.

Antibiotic treatment, reducing the bacterial load in the lungs, can be helpful to reduce the probability of transmission, along with other public health measures, such as isolation and cough etiquette.

The dramatic change of the epidemiological scenario during the last two decades, as a consequence of the increased incidence of the tuberculosis/HIV (human immunodeficiency virus) coinfection and of drug-resistant forms of tuberculosis, however, significantly complicated the clinical and public health management of the patients and of their contacts.

Currently, clinicians and public health specialists are facing daily problems related to the prescription of less effective and toxic second-line drugs, with frequent pharmacological interactions with antiretroviral drugs or medicines used to treat other comorbidities.

TUBERCULOSIS THERAPY: HISTORY AND RATIONALE

Tuberculosis is an ancient disease; nevertheless, effective drugs were not available for centuries. The preantibiotic therapy was initially repre-

Cite this article as *Cold Spring Harb Perspect Med* doi: 10.1101/cshperspect.a017822

sented by isolation in sanatoria to reduce the probability of *Mycobacterium tuberculosis* transmission to healthy contacts, with rest, adequate nutrition, and sunlight exposure; then, the surgical approach represented the gold standard, after Carlo Forlanini's discovery of the beneficial effects of the artificially induced pneumothorax in 1927 (Rosenblatt 1973; Sakula 1983; Dheda and Migliori 2012).

Only after the discovery of the etiological agent by Robert Koch in 1882 and the identification of the antibacterial activity of penicillin by Alexander Fleming did new experimental activities focused on the evaluation of the efficacy of natural and chemical compounds in animals start (Goldsworthy and McFarlane 2002; Daniel 2006).

The first experimental evidence of the potential efficacy of new antituberculosis drugs was obtained in 1940 when a dapsone-derivative compound, known as promin, was administered to a sample of guinea pigs. However, that sulfonamide was never given to humans (Barry 1964; World Health Organization 2004; Migliori et al. 2011; Sotgiu et al. 2013).

A different destiny awaited streptomycin, a natural substance isolated from *Streptomyces griseus*, which proved its efficacy in animals and then in humans. In 1944, Schatz and Waksman stated that the drug could be prescribed for the treatment of tuberculosis as a consequence of its bactericidal activity. In 1946, the United Kingdom Medical Research Council Tuberculosis Unit showed its short-term 6-mo efficacy in terms of mortality reduction (i.e., from 27% to 7%). However, after 5 yr, no differences were found between those exposed and not exposed to streptomycin as a consequence of the acquired antibiotic resistance (Table 1) (Schatz et al. 1944; Hinshaw and Feldman 1945; Wassersug 1946; Fox et al. 1954, 1999; World Health Organization 2004).

Four years later, the discovery of streptomycin, a new synthetic drug, called para-aminosalicylic acid (PAS), was presented as an alternative drug for the treatment of tuberculosis.

Following the poor results of the monotherapy, in 1952, the first regimen based on the combination of streptomycin, PAS, and isoniazid was proposed. Sir John Crofton with the "Edinburgh method," characterized by the prescription of at least two drugs, showed the efficacy of the combination therapy (Crofton 1960, 1969, 2006; Fox et al. 1999; World Health Organization 2004; Migliori et al. 2011; Sotgiu et al. 2013).

In 1954, pyrazinamide was discovered, but at the prescribed dosages, the rate of hepatic toxicity was significantly high. Ethambutol and rifampicin were introduced in 1961 and 1963, respectively. The duration of therapy varied from 1 to 2 yr. In 1970, trials on regimens including rifampicin showed good results with a therapy of 9 mo, whereas in 1974, the inclusion of rifampicin and pyrazinamide at low dosages demonstrated the efficacy of a 6-mo treat-

Table 1. Antituberculosis drugs

Drug	Mean daily dosage
Isoniazid	5 mg/kg
Rifampicin	10 mg/kg
Ethambutol	15–25 mg/kg
Pyrazinamide	30–40 mg/kg
Streptomycin	15–20 mg/kg
Amikacin	15–20 mg/kg
Kanamycin	15–20 mg/kg
Capreomycin	15–20 mg/kg
Ofloxacin	800 mg
Ciprofloxacin	1000 mg
Gatifloxacin	400 mg
Moxifloxacin	400 mg
Levofloxacin	1000 mg
Ethionamide	15–20 mg/kg
Prothionamide	15–20 mg/kg
Cycloserine	500–1000 mg
Para-aminosalicylic acid	150 mg/kg
Linezolid	600 mg
Clofazimine	200–300 mg
Amoxicillin/ clavulanate	875/125 mg BID or 500/125 mg TID
Clarithromycin	1000 mg
Terizidone	600–900 mg
Thiacetazone	150 mg
Thioridazine	75 mg
Bedaquiline	400 mg (for 2 wk) 200 mg TIW (for 22 wk)
Delamanid	200 mg

BID, twice a day; TID, thrice a day; TIW, thrice a week.

ment (East African/British Medical Research Council 1974; Sensi 1983; Fox et al. 1999; Migliori et al. 2011; Sotgiu et al. 2013).

The Madras study started in India in 1956. It showed the efficacy of the ambulatory treatment and the crucial role of the directly observed treatment for the improvement of the patient's adherence (Table 2) (Dawson et al. 1966; Migliori et al. 2011; Sotgiu et al. 2013).

On the basis of the microbiological characteristics of *M. tuberculosis* (i.e., slow growth and dormancy of some of the bacilli belonging to the bacterial population), numerous scientific contributions showed the efficacy of a long-term and multidrug therapeutic approach to obtain a bacteriological eradication in pulmonary and extrapulmonary sites.

Other factors can contribute to the successful outcome of the antituberculosis therapy, including the chemical features of the infection site. An adequate combination of effective drugs can reduce the probability of failure, relapse, and selection of resistant strains. To achieve those clinical and public health outcomes, it is necessary to prescribe antituberculosis drugs with an adequate dosage, for a specific time of exposure, and whose efficacy has been proved in in vitro tests (i.e., drug-susceptibility testing). In particular, to avoid the emergence of resistant strains, it is necessary to prescribe at least two effective drugs.

Table 2. Historical steps of the antituberculosis treatment

Year	Historical step
1940	Use of promin in guinea pigs
1944–1946	Discovery of streptomycin
1948	Discovery of para-aminosalicylic acid
1952	Streptomycin + para-aminosalicylic acid + isoniazid
1954	Discovery of pyrazinamide
1956	Madras study
1961	Discovery of ethambutol
1963	Discovery of rifampicin
1970	9-mo rifampicin-containing regimens
1974	6-mo rifampicin- and pyrazinamide-containing regimens
2012	Food and Drug Administration approval of bedaquiline
2013	Approval of delamanid by European Regulatory authorities

Duration of drug exposure is different according to the susceptibility of the isolated strains. In general, two different steps in the treatment of tuberculosis can be recognized—initial (or bactericidal) phase and continuation (or sterilizing) phase. During the first step of treatment, mycobacteria with a high replication rate are killed, and, consequently, with the histological pulmonary restoration and the reduction of the inflammation process, symptoms and clinical signs resolve (clinical recovery). From a public health perspective, this phase is crucial because the treated patient becomes noninfectious and the probability of selection of drug-resistant strains decreases (it is directly correlated to the fast-growing bacteria). The continuation phase is oriented to the elimination of semidormant bacteria, whose size is significantly reduced if compared with that at the beginning of the antituberculosis therapy; this quantitative feature, related to the low replication rate, is associated with a low probability of emergence of drug-resistant mycobacteria. In cases of drug-susceptible tuberculosis, two potent medicines are sufficient (e.g., isoniazid and rifampicin) in this phase. On the other hand, the regimen prescribed during the initial phase is more complex: two bactericidal drugs (isoniazid with streptomycin or rifampicin), ethambutol to inhibit monoresistant strains and to reduce the mycobacterial burden, and pyrazinamide, whose action is mainly focused to the semidormant mycobacteria. The intensive phase has a duration of 4 mo, whereas the sterilizing phase has a duration of 2 mo.

On this basis, the choice of the antituberculosis drugs in the different phases is not random but is based on the epidemiology (e.g., resistance rate in a specific setting, probability of having been infected by a contact with drug-resistant tuberculosis) and on the specificity of action of the antituberculosis drugs. The antituberculosis drug armamentarium is characterized by molecules with two main different mechanisms of action—bactericidal effect and sterilizing effect. The first one is crucial in the intensive phase and allows a relevant reduction of the bacterial load; the indirect consequence of this activity is the reduction of the probability of selecting drug-resistant strains. The most important drugs prescribed for that aim are isoniazid, pyrazinamide, rifampicin, and streptomycin. The sterilizing activity is relevant in the initial phase and in the continuation phase, but primarily in the continuation phase because it is oriented to kill mycobacteria in a dormancy state. Antituberculosis drugs deemed helpful in this phase are pyrazinamide and rifampicin.

These general principles are accepted worldwide, and the standardized regimens recommended by the World Health Organization in its guidelines have their roots in this biological rationale (World Health Organization 2004; Migliori et al. 2011; Sotgiu et al. 2013).

The World Health Organization classified antituberculosis drugs into five classes following several criteria, among them their efficacy and their chemical characteristics. The drugs usually prescribed for the drug-susceptible tuberculosis are included in the first class, whereas the drugs with unclear efficacy are included in the fifth class. In particular, the following drugs are integrated in the first class: ethambutol, isoniazid, pyrazinamide, and rifampicin. The second class includes amikacin, capreomycin, kanamycin, and streptomycin; old- and new-generation fluoroquinolones are included in the third class. The antituberculosis drugs in the fourth class are cycloserine, ethionamide, para-aminosalicylic acid, prothionamide, terizidone, and thioacetazone. The fifth class encompasses amoxicillin/clavulanate, clarithromycin, clofazimine, imipenem, and linezolid (World Health Organization 2010).

TREATMENT OF DRUG-SUSCEPTIBLE TUBERCULOSIS (WORLD HEALTH ORGANIZATION 2010)

Individuals diagnosed with a pulmonary form of tuberculosis, not exposed to antituberculosis drugs for >1 mo (i.e., "new cases" of tuberculosis), have to be treated for 6 mo. During the 2-mo intensive phase, patients should be administered a combined regimen including ethambutol, isoniazid, pyrazinamide, and rifampicin. Only isoniazid and rifampicin are prescribed during the 4-mo continuation phase.

Patients should take drugs daily to obtain a clinical and a microbiological cure; however, during the second phase of treatment, thrice per week is allowed, but, in that case, adherence is crucial to avoid reduction of the drugs' blood level and, consequently, the risk of emergence of drugs' resistances.

As mentioned above, a higher efficacy of antituberculosis regimens longer than 6 mo for individuals both with and without HIV infection was not shown; a different scenario has been found in the treatment of the latent tuberculosis infection, in which the duration of the treatment is longer in HIV-infected patients.

Microbiological monitoring of the efficacy of the prescribed regimen is mandatory; sputum smear and culture conversion should be evaluated, particularly at the end of the intensive and continuation phases of treatment.

Previously treated cases (i.e., previous course of antituberculosis drugs for >1 mo) should be managed differently. To prescribe an effective regimen tailored on the phenotypic profile of the mycobacterial isolates, a rapid and conventional drug-susceptibility testing is required before the initiation of therapy. It is crucial to monitor the potential adverse events to avoid the interruption of the prescribed therapy (Table 3).

The World Health Organization recommends the prescription of an empiric regimen for those who are identified as relapsers or defaulters, in case of a low multidrug resistance prevalence—ethambutol, isoniazid, pyrazinamide, rifampicin, and streptomycin in the intensive phase, followed by ethambutol, isoniazid, pyrazinamide, and rifampicin for 30 d; the last 5-mo phase is characterized by ethambutol, isoniazid, and rifampicin, for a total duration of 8 mo (Table 4).

It was clearly shown that the 6-mo regimen is practically 100% effective; after a follow-up period of 2 yr, the relapse rate can range from 0% to 7%. Intermittent regimens proved a similar efficacy, with a slightly higher relapse rate at

Table 3. Main adverse events of the antituberculosis drugs

Drug	Adverse event
Isoniazid Linezolid	Peripheral neuropathy
Bedaquiline Isoniazid Para-aminosalicylic acid Pyrazinamide Rifampicin	Liver dysfunction
Amikacin Amoxicillin/clavulanate Fluoroquinolones Isoniazid kanamycin Rifampicin Streptomycin Thiacetazone	Skin rash
Bedaquiline Pyrazinamide Thiacetazone	Arthromyalgia
Amikacin Capreomycin Kanamycin Streptomycin	Renal dysfunction
Amikacin Capreomycin Kanamycin Streptomycin	Vestibular and auditory dysfunction
Amoxicillin/clavulanate Bedaquiline Clarithromycin Clofazimine Ethionamide Fluoroquinolones Linezolid Prothionamide Para-aminosalicylic acid Terizidone Thiacetazone	Gastrointestinal disorders
Cycloserine Fluoroquinolones Terizidone	Psychosis

2 and 5 yr and a lower proportion of adverse events (World Health Organization 2004).

Extrapulmonary tuberculosis is a paucibacillary disease, and therapeutic regimens are the same as those prescribed for the pulmonary forms. Severe extrapulmonary disease, characterized by the neurological, abdominal, bilateral pleural, pericardial, bone, or joint or systemic involvement, needs four drugs in the intensive phase and sometimes a treatment duration of 9 mo (e.g., in case of neurological involvement). In case of relevant inflammation, the prescription of steroids is recommended. However, the prognosis strictly depends on the precocity of the administration of the antituberculosis drugs (World Health Organization 2004).

TREATMENT OF DRUG-RESISTANT TUBERCULOSIS

The clinical and public health management of drug-resistant tuberculosis is complicated. The therapeutic approach, as well as the prognosis, is significantly associated with the resistance pattern (Falzon et al. 2011; World Health Organization 2011b).

It has been clearly shown that the multidrug resistance (i.e., the resistance in vitro to at least isoniazid and rifampicin) could represent a relevant clinical issue because of the poorest therapeutic armamentarium. The so-called second- and third-line antituberculosis drugs are less efficacious, more toxic, and more expensive than the first-line drugs.

It is straightforward that the adequate treatment of drug-resistant tuberculosis can prevent the emergence of new serious drug-resistant forms, which could have a worst prognosis and less alternative therapeutic options.

Furthermore, another relevant feature of an adequate and early treatment is the low probability of transmission of drug-resistant mycobacterial strains in a specific setting, such as a hospital or a community.

Nevertheless, to obtain a clinical and a microbiological cure, it is mandatory to treat individuals for a long period because of the lesser effectiveness of the second- and third-line drugs. The prolonged exposure to medicines, characterized by a poor safety and tolerability profile, reduces the adherence of the patient. This pathogenetic step could be crucial for the

Table 4. Recommended antituberculosis regimens from World Health Organization

New tuberculosis cases				Previously treated tuberculosis cases			
Intensive phase		Continuation phase		Probability of multidrug-resistant tuberculosis			
					Medium or low (relapse, default)		
Drugs	Duration (mo)	Drugs	Duration (mo)	High (failure)	Drugs (duration, mo)	Drugs (duration, mo)	Drugs (duration, mo)
Ethambutol[a] Isoniazid Pyrazinamide Rifampicin	2	Isoniazid Rifampicin	4	Empirical multidrug-resistant tuberculosis regimen[c]	Ethambutol Isoniazid Pyrazinamide Rifampicin Streptomycin (2)	Ethambutol Isoniazid Pyrazinamide Rifampicin (1)	Ethambutol Isoniazid Rifampicin[c] (5)
Ethambutol[a] Isoniazid Pyrazinamide Rifampicin	2[b]	Ethambutol Isoniazid Rifampicin	4				

[a]Only for noncavitary, smear-negative pulmonary tuberculosis or for extrapulmonary tuberculosis. In tuberculosis meningitis, streptomycin is suggested.
[b]Level of isoniazid resistance among new is elevated and in vitro isoniazid-susceptibility testing is not available.
[c]Changed once drug-susceptibility testing results are available.

emergence of new drug-resistant mycobacterial strains and their spread in the community.

One of the most important points in the management of the drug-resistant strains is the prescription of an efficacious drug regimen, which should be based on the results of the drug-susceptibility testing. The current availability of rapid molecular tests, which can assess the resistances of mycobacterial strains to isoniazid and rifampicin, can allow the administration of an early tailored antituberculosis regimen. In particular, the World Health Organization recently approved an automated nucleic acid amplification test to diagnose tuberculosis disease and to assess mycobacterial resistance to rifampicin (Xpert MTB/RIF System). The rapid identification of a multidrug-resistant case can allow an immediate prescription of an empiric and specific antituberculosis drug regimen. This molecular method might avoid the administration of an inappropriate treatment and, consequently, indirectly favor the clinical recovery of patients and the reduction of their infectiousness (World Health Organization 2011a).

The World Health Organization suggests the prescription of at least four active drugs during the intensive phase. In particular, the backbone of the administered regimen should include pyrazinamide, one of the injectable second-line drugs (amikacin, capreomycin, or kanamycin), a new-generation fluoroquinolone, ethionamide (or prothionamide), and cycloserine (or PAS). Other drugs should be prescribed in case of resistances to one or more of the backbone drugs. The duration of the first phase of the treatment should depend on the culture conversion, but it should last at least 8 mo, whereas the duration of the second phase should be longer than 20 mo.

The World Health Organization guidelines issued in 2011 (WHO 2011b) showed significant differences if compared with those issued in 2008; in particular, the suggested duration of the intensive phase is longer (i.e., 8 vs. 6 mo), as well as the total duration of therapy (i.e., at least 20 mo). If feasible, pyrazinamide should be added up to a backbone regimen of four second-line antituberculosis drugs, in which ethionamide and new-generation fluoroquinolones are the preferred medicines. Furthermore, monthly monitoring of the culture conversion is relevant to assess the efficacy of the prescribed therapy (World Health Organization 2008).

New therapeutic options have been proposed in recent years for the management of the drug-resistant mycobacterial strains, including new molecules and drugs prescribed for other diseases.

Several drugs, approved for infectious diseases other than tuberculosis, showed in vitro and in vivo antimycobacterial activity; among them, imipenem-cilastatin, linezolid, and meropenem-clavulanate have had a relevant role in individuals with drug-resistant tuberculosis in the last few years. The new molecules recently approved or in the last clinical trial phases are bedaquiline (a new diarylquinoline, previously called TMC 207), delamanid (previously called OPC-67683), sutezolid (PNU 100480), and PA-824.

Bedaquiline and delamanid have recently received a marketing approval. Bedaquiline-containing regimens increase by 12 times the probability of culture conversion in multi-drug-resistant tuberculosis cases and prevent the emergence of further resistances to the drugs included in the backbone regimens. It reduces the time to culture conversion in the first 6 mo of exposure (hazard ratio: 2.3). The safety and tolerability profile is good if compared with other antituberculosis drugs (i.e., acne, bilateral hearing impairment, extremity and noncardiac chest pain). However, the frequency of nausea was significantly higher during some clinical trials if compared with that in the control group (Diacon et al. 2009, 2012a,b, 2013; Willyard 2012; Mahajan 2013; World Health Organization 2013b).

Delamanid-containing regimens showed a short- and long-term efficacy in terms of culture conversion. The positive microbiological features are associated with the relevant improvement of a strong epidemiological indicator-like mortality; the proportion of individuals who died after a $\geq$6-mo exposure to delamanid was 1% versus 8% in those not exposed or with a short-term exposure. The percentage of individuals who culture-converted at 2 mo was about 45% versus nearly 30% in the control group. The most important adverse event that occurred in patients exposed to this novel nitroimidazole was QT prolongation, although not associated to relevant cardiac events (Diacon et al. 2011; Gler et al. 2012; Skripconoka et al. 2013).

Other new promising drugs are currently being tested in the phase II and III clinical trials. In particular, sutezolid, belonging to the same chemical family of linezolid, showed its ability in the reduction of the colony forming units (Shaw and Barbachyn 2011; Wallis et al. 2012). The early bactericidal activity showed by PA-824, a new nitroimidazo-oxazine, was superior to that of bedaquiline in the first clinical trials (Diacon et al. 2012a,b; Migliori and Sotgiu 2012).

Antibiotics licensed for bacterial infections other than tuberculosis proved their efficacy in the treatment of the multidrug-resistant and extensively drug-resistant tuberculosis cases.

Linezolid is efficacious but is characterized by several hematological side effects (anemia and/or leucopenia and/or thrombocytopenia), peripheral nervous system problems, and gastrointestinal toxicity. However, it has been proved that the therapeutic monitoring of its blood levels (TDM) can allow a dosage adjustment, followed by the reduction of the probability of occurrence of adverse events. Several pharmacokinetic studies showed that a 600-mg dosage has the best cost/benefit ratio. TDM was helpful in understanding the best dosage to be administered to patients on the basis of the blood drug concentration. It was clear that a daily dosage of 1200 mg is toxic if compared with a 600-mg dosage. On the other hand, a 300-mg daily dosage is less efficacious (Migliori et al. 2009; Sotgiu et al. 2009, 2012; Alffenaar et al. 2010; Koh et al. 2012; Srivastava et al. 2013).

Meropenem-clavulanate and cotrimoxazole showed their efficacy in some observational studies. The former favored sputum smear and culture conversion in >80% of the multidrug-resistant tuberculosis cases (88% and 84%, respectively, in a case-control study) and was associated with an optimal safety profile (De Lorenzo et al. 2013). The latter was evaluated in vitro and in a few cases, and its efficacy needs to be proved in experimental, controlled studies (Forgacs et al. 2009; Huang et al. 2012; Vilchèze and Jacobs 2012). New experimental clinical trials are needed to assess the clinical profile of the new therapeutic options (Grosset et al. 2012; Pontali et al. 2013).

The management of individuals with multidrug-resistant tuberculosis and HIV infection requires the involvement of tuberculosis/HIV specialists. Anti-HIV drugs should be prescribed within 8 mo from the first administration of the antituberculosis drugs. The pill burden is relevant and the adherence of the patients can be significantly affected; furthermore, the toxicity linked to the pharmacological interactions can contribute to reduce the compliance of the patients. In particular, the severity of the hepatic, gastrointestinal, hematological, renal, and central and peripheral nervous system toxicity could interrupt the treatment (Table 5).

A recent systematic review, enrolling 217 patients, whose CD4 cell counts were <200 μL in the majority of cases, showed that individuals exposed to antiretrovirals were more likely to survive (hazard ratio of 0.38) and have a longer median time to death (i.e., 37 mo vs. 11 mo among those not exposed to antiretrovirals). Furthermore, the prescription of antiretroviral drugs was associated with a higher probability of cure (hazard ratio, 3.4). It was proved that the level of immunodeficiency and the mycobacterial resistance pattern do not influence the above-mentioned risks (Arentz et al. 2012).

The concomitant prescription of anti-HIV and antituberculosis drugs does not depend on the severity of the immunodeficiency and then on the CD4 cell counts.

ADHERENCE TO ANTITUBERCULOSIS THERAPY

The efficacy of the combination regimens described above will determine, in addition to bacteriological conversion, a subjective improvement of the patient's clinical conditions. The latter feature may anticipate the microbiological conversion and could be paradoxically dangerous from an individual and a public

Table 5. Main adverse events of the antituberculosis drugs and of the antiretrovirals

Antituberculosis drugs	Antiretroviral drugs	Adverse event
Isoniazid Linezolid	Didanosine Stavudine	Peripheral neuropathy
Bedaquiline Isoniazid Para-aminosalicylic acid Pyrazinamide Rifampicin	Efavirenz Etravirine Maraviroc Nevirapine Ritonavir/protease inhibitors	Liver dysfunction
Amikacin Amoxicillin/clavulanate Fluoroquinolones Isoniazid kanamycin Rifampicin Streptomycin Thiacetazone	Abacavir Efavirenz Etravirine Nevirapine	Skin rash
Bedaquiline Pyrazinamide Thiacetazone	-	Arthromyalgia
Amikacin Capreomycin Kanamycin Streptomycin	Indinavir Tenofovir	Renal dysfuction
Amikacin Capreomycin Kanamycin Streptomycin	-	Vestibular and auditory dysfunction
Amoxicillin/clavulanate Bedaquiline clarithromycin Clofazimine Ethionamide fluoroquinolones linezolid Prothionamide Para-aminosalicylic acid Terizidone Thiacetazone	Didanosine Protease inhibitors Stavudine Zidovudine	Gastrointestinal disorders
Cycloserine fluoroquinolones terizidone	Efavirenz	Psychosis

Data modified from Arentz et al. 2012.

health perspective; patients feeling better might decide to interrupt their treatment.

Several approaches have been proposed to increase patient's adherence. One of the most important is the so-called DOT (i.e., directly observed therapy). The patient takes the prescribed therapy in the presence of a health-care worker (physician or nurse), a social worker, or another person involved in agreement with the local tuberculosis program. The direct observation avoids all the problems associated with self-administration, including compliance with the dosages and time of administration affecting the pharmacokinetic curve of the drugs. In addition, DOT allows rapid management of adverse events related to the drug intake.

Another important tool to enhance adherence is represented by the fixed-dose combination of the antituberculosis drugs. They were introduced in clinical practice at the end of the 1980s, and several advantages were immediately recognized: easy management for the national tuberculosis program and for health staff not fully familiar with antituberculosis drugs and reduced probability of emergence of drug resistances because of the improved patient's adherence. The main disadvantages, intrinsically related to the fixed dose, are the risk of a nonadequate blood level (rare, and limited to patients characterized by a poor intestinal absorption or by a rapid metabolism) and the difficulty in attributing an adverse event to a specific drug.

Another strategic therapeutic approach to improve adherence is represented by the intermittent regimens, whose efficacy was shown in 1964 in Chennai, India. Antituberculosis drugs are administered at intervals of >1 d. The relapse rate is 8% after a follow-up of 2 yr (World Health Organization 2004).

An important role to increase adherence can be played by incentives and enablers (money, food, incentives for transportation, etc.), particularly in resource-limited countries. Poor patients living in rural areas can lose their job and their daily salary because of the medical visits in far urban settings. National tuberculosis programs should identify the geographical areas or the social groups where these nonmedical interventions could be crucial in improving adherence (Tuberculosis Coalition for Technical Assistance 2009).

Last but not least, when health education is adequately provided by health services to the patients and their families, adherence tends to improve.

CONCLUDING REMARKS

The current therapeutic management of drug-susceptible and drug-resistant strains needs to be further improved. The available regimens are characterized by a relevant pill burden, long duration, variable efficacy, safety, and tolerability. The overall treatment success rate is below the recommended World Health Organization proportion of 85%, and, consequently, the drug resistance level increases.

The World Health Organization estimates that a suboptimal proportion of multidrug-resistant cases is presently diagnosed and treated. In 2010, 48% of the detected multidrug-resistant tuberculosis cases were successfully treated. Only 34 countries obtained a treatment success rate ≥75% (World Health Organization 2013a). Even in tuberculosis reference centers, the proportion of treatment success in multidrug-resistant cases does not exceed 50%.

Although the adherence, efficacy, safety, and tolerability profile of the newly available drugs (delamanid and bedaquiline, in particular) appear to be promising, we cannot predict, as of today, their long-term efficacy and the affordability of their use in resource-limited settings. Further research efforts are necessary to identify the potentialities of the new drugs and to understand better how to use them in combination regimens.

These new regimens are ideally able to treat tuberculosis sustained by both drug-susceptible and drug-resistant strains without interfering with antiretroviral drugs, thus allowing a more effective approach against HIV-infected cases.

The new approach adopted to test different drug combinations in parallel can improve the current situation, giving new insights in a shorter period of time.

New research and development activities are requested, along with a preservation of the current therapeutic options. Training and educational activities focused on the rationale use of the antituberculosis drugs are necessary to avoid the dramatic increase of the drug-resistant forms.

National and local public health programs should issue guidance, based on the local epidemiology, to prevent inappropriate management of the new and old antibiotics, as to ensure that all cases of tuberculosis diagnosed and correctly treated, complete their treatment. The risk is to loose the new drugs in much less than the time necessary to develop them.

REFERENCES

Alffenaar JW, van Altena R, Harmelink IM, Filguera P, Molenaar E, Wessels AM, van Soolingen D, Kosterink

JG, Uges DR, van der Werf TS. 2010. Comparison of the pharmacokinetics of two dosage regimens of linezolid in multidrug-resistant and extensively drug-resistant tuberculosis patients. *Clin Pharmacokinet* **49:** 559–565.

Arentz M, Pavlinac P, Kimerling ME, Horne DJ, Falzon D, Schünemann HJ, Royce S, Dheda K, Walson JL, ART study group. 2012. Use of anti-retroviral therapy in tuberculosis patients on second-line anti-TB regimens: A systematic review. *PLoS ONE* **7:** e47370.

Barry VC. 1964. Development of the chemotherapeutic agent for tuberculosis. In *Chemotherapy of tuberculosis* (ed. Barry VC). Butterworths, London.

Crofton J. 1960. Tuberculosis undefeated. *Br Med J* **2:** 679–687.

Crofton J. 1969. Some principles in the chemotherapy of bacterial infections. *Br Med J* **2:** 137–141.

Crofton J. 2006. The MRC randomized trial of streptomycin and its legacy: A view from the clinical front line. *J R Soc Med* **99:** 531–534.

Daniel TM. 2006. The history of tuberculosis. *Respir Med* **100:** 1862–1870.

Dawson JJY, Devadatta S, Fox W, Radhakrishna S, Ramakrishnan CV, Somasundaram PR, Stott H, Tripathy SP, Velu S. 1966. A 5-year study of patients with pulmonary tuberculosis in a concurrent comparison of home and sanatorium treatment for one year with isoniazid plus PAS. *Bull World Health Organ* **34:** 533–551.

De Lorenzo S, Alffenaar JW, Sotgiu G, Centis R, D'Ambrosio L, Tiberi S, Bolhuis MS, van Altena R, Viggiani P, Piana A, et al. 2013. Efficacy and safety of meropenem-clavulanate added to linezolid-containing regimens in the treatment of MDR-/XDR-TB. *Eur Respir J* **41:** 1386–1392.

Dheda K, Migliori GB. 2012. The global rise of extensively drug-resistant tuberculosis: Is the time to bring back sanatoria now overdue? *Lancet* **379:** 773–775.

Diacon AH, Pym A, Grobusch M, Patientia R, Rustomjee R, Page-Shipp L, Pistorius C, Krause R, Bogoshi M, Churchyard G, et al. 2009. The diarylquinoline TMC207 for multidrug-resistant tuberculosis. *N Engl J Med* **360:** 2397–2405.

Diacon AH, Dawson R, Hanekom M, Narunsky K, Venter A, Hittel N, Geiter LJ, Wells CD, Paccaly AJ, Donald PR. 2011. Early bactericidal activity of delamanid (OPC-67683) in smear-positive pulmonary tuberculosis patients. *Int J Tuberc Lung Dis* **15:** 949–954.

Diacon AH, Dawson R, von Groote-Bidlingmaier F, Symons G, Venter A, Donald PR, van Niekerk C, Everitt D, Winter H, Becker P, et al. 2012a. 14-day bactericidal activity of PA-824, bedaquiline, pyrazinamide, and moxifloxacin combinations: A randomised trial. *Lancet* **380:** 986–993.

Diacon AH, Donald PR, Pym A, Grobusch M, Patientia RF, Mahanyele R, Bantubani N, Narasimooloo R, De Marez T, van Heeswijk R, et al. 2012b. Randomized pilot trial of eight weeks of bedaquiline (TMC207) treatment for multidrug-resistant tuberculosis: Long-term outcome, tolerability, and effect on emergence of drug resistance. *Antimicrob Agents Chemother* **56:** 3271–3276.

Diacon AH, Dawson R, du Bois J, Narunsky K, Venter A, Donald PR, van Niekerk C, Erondu N, Ginsberg AM, Becker P, et al. 2012c. Phase II dose-ranging trial of the early bactericidal activity of PA-824. *Antimicrob Agents Chemother* **56:** 3027–3031.

Diacon AH, Dawson R, Von Groote-Bidlingmaier F, Symons G, Venter A, Donald PR, Conradie A, Erondu N, Ginsberg AM, Egizi E, et al. 2013. Randomized dose-ranging study of the 14-day early bactericidal activity of bedaquiline (TMC207) in patients with sputum microscopy smear-positive pulmonary tuberculosis. *Antimicrob Agents Chemother* **57:** 2199–2203.

East African/British Medical Research Council. 1974. Controlled clinical treatment of short course (6 months) regime of chemotherapy for treatment of pulmonary tuberculosis. Third report. *Lancet* **2:** 237–248.

Falzon D, Jaramillo E, Schünemann HJ, Arentz M, Bauer M, Bayona J, Blanc L, Caminero JA, Daley CL, Duncombe C, et al. 2011. WHO guidelines for the programmatic management of drug-resistant tuberculosis: 2011 update. *Eur Respir J* **38:** 516–528.

Forgacs P, Wengenack NL, Hall L, Zimmerman SK, Silverman ML, Roberts GD. 2009. Tuberculosis and trimethoprim-sulfamethoxazole. *Antimicrob Agents Chemother* **53:** 4789–4793.

Fox W, Sutherland I, Daniels M. 1954. A five-year assessment of patients in a controlled trial of streptomycin in pulmonary tuberculosis: Report to the Tuberculosis Chemotherapy Trials Committee of the Medical Research Council. *QJM* **91:** 347–366.

Fox W, Ellard GA, Mitchison DA. 1999. Studies on the treatment of tuberculosis undertaken by the British Medical Research Council tuberculosis units, 1946–1986, with relevant subsequent publications. *Int J Tuberc Lung Dis* **3:** S231–S279.

Gler MT, Skripconoka V, Sanchez-Garavito E, Xiao H, Cabrera-Rivero JL, Vargas-Vasquez DE, Gao M, Awad M, Park SK, Shim TS, et al. 2012. Delamanid for multidrug-resistant pulmonary tuberculosis. *N Engl J Med* **366:** 2151–2160.

Goldsworthy PD, McFarlane AC. 2002. Howard Florey, Alexander Fleming and the fairy tale of penicillin. *Med J Aust* **176:** 176–178.

Grosset JH, Singer TG, Bishai WR. 2012. New drugs for the treatment of tuberculosis: Hope and reality. *Int J Tuberc Lung Dis* **16:** 1005–1014.

Hinshaw HC, Feldman WH. 1945. Streptomycin in the treatment of clinical tuberculosis; a preliminary report. *Proc Staff Meet Mayo Clin* **20:** 313–318.

Huang TS, Kunin CM, Yan BS, Chen YS, Lee SS, Syu W Jr. 2012. Susceptibility of *Mycobacterium tuberculosis* to sulfamethoxazole, trimethoprim and their combination over a 12 year period in Taiwan. *J Antimicrob Chemother* **67:** 633–637.

Koh WJ, Kang YR, Jeon K, Kwon OJ, Lyu J, Kim WS, Shim TS. 2012. Daily 300 mg dose of linezolid for multidrug-resistant and extensively drug-resistant tuberculosis: Updated analysis of 51 patients. *J Antimicrob Chemother* **67:** 1503–1507.

Mahajan R. 2013. Bedaquiline: First FDA-approved tuberculosis drug in 40 years. *Int J Appl Basic Med Res* **3:** 1–2.

Migliori GB, Sotgiu G. 2012. Treatment of tuberculosis: Have we turned the corner? *Lancet* **380:** 955–957.

Migliori GB, Eker B, Richardson MD, Sotgiu G, Zellweger JP, Skrahina A, Ortmann J, Girardi E, Hoffmann H, Besozzi G, et al. 2009. A retrospective TBNET assessment of linezolid safety, tolerability and efficacy in multidrug-resistant tuberculosis. *Eur Respir J* **34:** 387–393.

Migliori GB, Sotgiu G, Centis R, Grzemska M, Falzon D, Getahun H, Raviglione MC. 2011. Antituberculosis therapy and current global guidelines. In *Current & emerging diagnostics, therapeutics & vaccines for tuberculosis* (ed. Kaufmann SHE), pp. 42–63. Future Medicine, London.

Pontali E, Matteelli A, Migliori GB. 2013. Drug-resistant tuberculosis. *Curr Opin Pulm Med* **19:** 266–272.

Rosenblatt MB. 1973. Pulmonary tuberculosis: Evolution of modern therapy. *Bull NY Acad Med* **49:** 163–196.

Sakula A. 1983. Carlo Forlanini, inventor of artificial pneumothorax for treatment of pulmonary tuberculosis. *Thorax* **38:** 326–332.

Schatz A, Bugie E, Waksman SA. 1944. Streptomycin, a substance exhibiting antibiotic activity against Gram-positive and Gram-negative bacteria. *ProcSoc Exp Biol Med* **55:** 66–69.

Shaw KJ, Barbachyn MR. 2011. The oxazolidinones: Past, present, and future. *Ann N Y Acad Sci* **1241:** 48–70.

Sensi P. 1983. History of the development of rifampicin. *Rev Infect Dis* **5:** 402–406.

Skripconoka V, Danilovits M, Pehme L, Tomson T, Skenders G, Kummik T, Cirule A, Leimane V, Kurve A, Levina K, et al. 2013. Delamanid improves outcomes and reduces mortality in multidrug-resistant tuberculosis. *Eur Respir J* **41:** 1393–1400.

Sotgiu G, Lange C, Richardson MD, Matteelli A, Centis R, Eker B, Guenther G, Spanevello A, Migliori GB; TBNET. 2009. Comment on: Daily 300 mg dose of linezolid for the treatment of intractable multidrug-resistant and extensively drug-resistant tuberculosis. *J Antimicrob Chemother* **64:** 879–883.

Sotgiu G, Centis R, D'Ambrosio L, Alffenaar JW, Anger HA, Caminero JA, Castiglia P, De Lorenzo S, Ferrara G, Koh WJ, et al. 2012. Efficacy, safety and tolerability of linezolid containing regimens in treating MDR-TB and XDR-TB: Systematic review and meta-analysis. *Eur Respir J* **40:** 1430–1442.

Sotgiu G, Centis R, D'Ambrosio L, Migliori GB. 2013. Medical treatment of pulmonary tuberculosis. *Eur Respir Society Monograph* **61:** 11–19.

Srivastava S, Peloquin CA, Sotgiu G, Migliori GB. 2013. Therapeutic drug management: Is it the future of multidrug-resistant tuberculosis treatment? *Eur Respir J* **42:** 1449–1453.

Tuberculosis Coalition for Technical Assistance. *International Standards for Tuberculosis Care (ISTC)*, 2nd ed. 2009. Tuberculosis Coalition for Technical Assistance, The Hague.

Vilchèze C, Jacobs WR Jr. 2012. The combination of sulfamethoxazole, trimethoprim, and isoniazid or rifampin is bactericidal and prevents the emergence of drug resistance in *Mycobacterium tuberculosis*. *Antimicrob Agents Chemother* **56:** 5142–5148.

Wallis RS, Jakubiec W, Mitton-Fry M, Ladutko L, Campbell S, Paige D, Silvia A, Miller PF. 2012. Rapid evaluation in whole blood culture of regimens for XDR-TB containing PNU-100480 (sutezolid), TMC207, PA-824, SQ109, and pyrazinamide. *PLoS ONE* **7:** e30479.

Wassersug JD. 1946. Pulmonary tuberculosis. *N Engl J Med* **235:** 220–229.

Willyard C. 2012. Race heats up for first-to-market drugs for resistant tuberculosis. *Nat Med* **18:** 1157.

World Health Organization. 2004. Toman's tuberculosis: Case detection, treatment and monitoring, second edition. WHO, Geneva.

World Health Organization. 2008. Guidelines for the programmatic management of drug-resistant tuberculosis. Emergency update 2008. WHO/HTM/TB/2008.402. WHO, Geneva.

World Health Organization. 2010. The treatment of tuberculosis guidelines. Document WHO/HTM/TB/2009.420. WHO, Geneva.

World Health Organization. 2011a. Automated real-time nucleic acid amplification technology for rapid and simultaneous detection of tuberculosis and rifampicin resistance: Xpert MTB/RIF system. Policy statement. WHO/HTM/TB/2011.4. WHO, Geneva.

World Health Organization. 2011b. Guidelines for the programmatic management of drug-resistant tuberculosis, 2011 update. WHO/HTM/TB/2011.6. WHO, Geneva.

World Health Organization. 2013a. Global tuberculosis report 2013. WHO/HTM/TB/2013.11. WHO, Geneva.

World Health Organization. 2013b. The use of bedaquiline in the treatment of multidrug-resistant tuberculosis: Interim policy guidance. WHO, Geneva.

Diagnosis and Management of Latent Tuberculosis Infection

Laura Muñoz[1,2], Helen R. Stagg[2], and Ibrahim Abubakar[2]

[1]Infectious Diseases Department, Bellvitge University Hospital-IDIBELL, Barcelona 08970, Spain

[2]Research Department of Infection and Population Health, University College London, London WC1E 6JB, United Kingdom

Correspondence: i.abubakar@ucl.ac.uk

The post-2015 World Health Organization global tuberculosis strategy recognizes that elimination requires a focus on reducing the pool of latently infected individuals, an estimated 30% of the global population, from which future tuberculosis cases would be generated. Tackling latent tuberculosis infection requires the identification and treatment of asymptomatic individuals to reduce the risk of progression to active disease. Diagnosis of latent tuberculosis infection is based on the detection of an immune response to *Mycobacterium tuberculosis* antigens using either the tuberculin skin test or interferon-γ release assays. Current treatment requires the use of antibiotics for at least 3 months. In this article, we review the current knowledge of the natural history, immunology, and pathogenesis of latent tuberculosis, describe key population groups for screening and risk assessment, discuss clinical management in terms of diagnosis and preventative treatment, and identify areas for future research.

Latent tuberculosis infection (LTBI) is defined by the detection of a specific immune response to *Mycobacterium tuberculosis* complex (MTC) antigens in a healthy subject (i.e., with no symptoms or signs of active tuberculosis [TB]). As *M. tuberculosis* can only be isolated from humans when it is in an active phase, causing illness, the detection of the presence of LTBI is wholly reliant on indirect measurements of immune reactivity to antigenic challenge.

By evading both innate and adaptive immunity, bacteria of the MTC are able to persist in a dormant phase for several decades, or even for the lifetime of the host. In ~10% of all infected individuals, a LTBI will progress to active replication and cause TB disease. This can be prevented with antibiotic treatment; globally standard regimens are of 6–9-mo duration with a single drug, or at least 3 mo of two antibiotics. Increasing the number of drugs within the regimen increases the potential for consequent adverse events. Given the small proportion of LTBI-positive individuals who develop active TB, the imperfect effectiveness of LTBI treatment and associated its side effects, the critical question is, therefore, who should be targeted for treatment? This question is pertinent because none of the tests currently available are

Cite this article as *Cold Spring Harb Perspect Med* doi: 10.1101/cshperspect.a017830

able to accurately predict future progression. It is widely recognized that the risk of progression is highest in young children, the immunosuppressed, and shortly after infection. Pragmatically, therefore, these individuals should be targeted for LTBI screening and treatment. In most cases, this would lead to an "intention to test is intention to treat" approach, with an exception for close contacts of multidrug-resistant TB cases, in which testing may be used to inform "watchful waiting."

In this article, we review the current knowledge of the natural history and immunology of LTBI, describe key population groups for screening and risk assessment, discuss clinical management in terms of diagnosis and preventative treatment, and finally look to the key fields for future research.

HISTORY (CONCEPT OF DORMANT BACILLI)

Although TB is one of the most ancient diseases, LTBI was only recognized at the end of the 19th century following (1) the accurate description of the morbid anatomy of TB, its clinical evolution, and surrounding circumstances; (2) the first experimental animal models; and (3) the development of essential tools such as the microscope. Soon after the discovery of the causative agent of TB in 1882, Robert Koch created the Koch's fluid ("a glycerine extract of pure cultivations of tubercle bacilli" [Koch 1891]), for use as a live vaccine; it turned out to be an ineffective preventive agent. Koch's fluid, which was given the name of tuberculin, later proved to be a valuable diagnostic tool for active TB in cattle. In the last years of the 19th century, experiments showed that cows with confirmed TB developed a febrile reaction 14–18 h after tuberculin administration. Apparently healthy cows who presented the same systemic reaction were slaughtered; some of the necropsies revealed active tubercles (Mi'fadyean 1891; Martin and Robins 1898). Reactive cattle without tubercles had their positive reaction attributed to dormant TB, as quiescent tuberculous foci were identified in some of the necropsies (Martin and Robins 1898).

Mantoux's description of a new technique to administer tuberculin (the "tuberculin skin test" [TST]) in 1908, together with its improved composition in 1934 (purified protein derivate [PPD]), made its use as a human diagnostic method possible, as systemic reactions were not observed in tested subjects. The first trials that tested tuberculin on TB patients also showed positive results in healthy controls. It was at this time that the notion of latent bacteria or bacillary allergy emerged.

As for preventive purposes, the 20th century saw the introduction of several successful vaccines, and there were great expectations for an effective preparation against TB. In 1902, Behring proposed to use the bacillus isolated from humans for the vaccination of cows. Calmette and Guerin passaged *Mycobacterium bovis*, which has antigenic properties similar to those of the virulent *M. tuberculosis* bacilli and the ability to provoke antibody formation in humans, to obtain the attenuated Bacillus Calmette–Guérin (BCG) strain. BCG was successfully tested in infants exposed to family cases of TB owing to the high mortality usually seen in such infants (72%) (Calmette 1931).

The immunological response to *M. bovis* and *M. tuberculosis* is highly similar, allowing the effective use of BCG as a vaccine and tuberculin as a diagnostic reagent. The proportion of BCG-vaccinated people who have a positive tuberculin skin test (TST) has been reported to vary from 0% to 90% (Wang et al. 2002). These wide differences may depend on dose, the manufacturer of the vaccine, age, and the interval between vaccination and testing. Variation in the cutoff for positivity used during TST testing also explains some of the observed variation. Nevertheless, a positive reaction of >15 mm in someone who was vaccinated >15 yr before is unlikely to be related to BCG vaccination and would likely reflect the presence of TB infection.

Questions were raised about the infectiousness of the tubercle bacilli and how to prevent the spread of the disease. This led to early contact studies surrounding single active cases, with the aim of finding latently infected individuals (positive TST responders but without TB symptoms) and treating them to prevent the development of active TB. Soon after the discovery of streptomycin (1944) and isoniazid (1952) for active TB, the first experiments using isoniazid as a preventive treatment in an animal model were undertaken (1955). Initial clinical trials in humans began in 1957, with results reported in the mid-1960s. During the next few decades, five major randomized trials showed the benefits of isoniazid in preventing active TB.

NATURAL HISTORY AND PATHOGENESIS

Underpinning all attempts at the diagnosis and treatment of LTBI is our understanding of the natural history of TB, particularly the process through which LTBI is established, and the host and bacterial factors influential in determining latency and progression. The most important reservoir of *M. tuberculosis* is humans, whereas cattle are the equivalent host for *M. bovis*. Zoonotic transmission of *M. bovis* was frequent in ancient times; however, pasteurization of milk and the testing of herds decreased the public health impact of *M. bovis* in humans in wealthier countries. Many developing countries continue to observe zoonotic transmission.

Humans with active pulmonary TB currently play the dominant role in the transmission and maintenance of TB. Studies by Flügge in 1899 (Hillier 1903) showed that both dried tuberculous sputum dust and the minute drops coughed out by pulmonary TB patients were capable of surviving for several days while remaining infectious. These tiny particles contain tubercle bacilli inside droplet nuclei, are easily inhaled, and constitute the route of entry and first contact with the healthy subject (Box 1).

Infection

On inhalation, *M. tuberculosis* reaches the main airway and alveoli and faces the first cell-mediated barrier of the innate immune system. Alveolar macrophages phagocytose the pathogen and isolate it through a process of membrane invaginations that finally culminates in phagosome formation. From now on, two contending forces compete for control—the bacterium's struggle for survival and macrophage's attempts to contain the infection.

After phagosome formation, infected macrophages and dendritic cells display *M. tuberculosis* antigens via major histocompatibility complex (MHC) class II molecules. These professional antigen-presenting cells expressing MTC molecules travel to the lymph system and then into local mediastinal lymph nodes, where they will activate $CD4^+$ T-helper cells (Th). These cells regulate the secretion of cytokines via endocrine and paracrine signaling and function in the formation and maintenance of granulomas by means of a proinflammatory response signal cascade (interferon-γ [IFN-γ], interleukin-2 [IL-2], and tumor necrosis factor-α [TNF-α]), which leads to the attraction of mononuclear cells and T lymphocytes. These cell types, together with B lymphocytes and dendritic cells, build up a granuloma, "the hallmark tissue reaction of TB" (Gengenbacher and Kaufmann 2012). Other functions of $CD4^+$ Th cells include activation of $CD8^+$ cytotoxic T cells and B lymphocytes, as well as differentiation into diverse Th cell subtypes.

Depending on the cytokine environment, different types of Th cells will develop. IFN-γ drives Th1 cell production and generates clone

BOX 1. DETERMINANTS OF ACQUISITION OF TB INFECTION

The closeness and duration of contact with a patient with infectious TB (Rieder et al. 2009).

The effective amount of shared air space determined by the level of air circulation and size of the room, which influences effective exposure.

Patients with a higher bacterial load, such as those with cavitatory pulmonary TB and those AFB (acid-fast bacillus) smear positive, transmit TB more efficiently.

The susceptibility of the host.

expansion as well as differentiation into memory cells; on the contrary, IL-10 and IL-4 inhibit their development. Th1 cells regulate cell-mediated immunity and activate natural killer cells through IFN-γ secretion. High levels of IL-4, IL-5, and IL-10 are needed for the differentiation of Th2 cells, their clonal expansion, and generation of memory cells. IFN-γ down-regulates the development of this cell type. Th2 cells are responsible for controlling humoral immunity and activation of B cells into plasma cells.

Adaptive immunity can take as long as 42 d after MTC exposure and infection to be established (Wallgren 1948; Poulsen 1950; Berry et al. 2010). At this point, a large number of activated macrophages are recruited to the site of infection and construct the granuloma, to which lymphocytes, epithelioid, and giant cells are also attracted. By depriving the center of the granuloma of oxygen, the lowering the pH necrosis occurs internally, preventing bacterial replication but enabling dormancy. However, it is likely that some replication still occurs, because without this, isoniazid would not be effective against LTBI, as it is only bactericidal against *replicating M. tuberculosis.*

Macrophages and dendritic cells also transport bacteria to the local lymph nodes during the construction of granulomas, allowing the dispersal of infection, particularly to well-oxygenated areas such as lung apices, suprarenal glands, the brain cortex, and bone and growing joints.

Disease

Only ~10% of infected individuals develop active disease; of these, most will progress in the first 2 years after exposure. There are two possible methods for the development of active disease—an active primary infection, and reactivation of LTBI. Reactivation may occur years after infection in older individuals, usually caused by a failure of the host immune response (Box 2).

IMMUNOLOGY AND PATHOGENESIS

The breadth of information available on the immunology and pathogenesis of LTBI means that the intention of this section is not to comprehensively cover all the available material, but rather to provide a summary of the key concepts to allow readers to better understand the diagnostic and therapeutic management of LTBI.

MTC Factors

M. tuberculosis has a series of tools to enable survival inside the human host. First, a unique cell *wall* structure with high *lipid* content protects the bacterium from the highly acidic pH of the phagosome. Second, it is able to arrest phagosome–lysosome fusion. Third, it interferes in antigen presentation as well as in the normal function of $CD8^+$ T cells, natural killer cells, and the complement attack complex. Fourth, *M. tuberculosis* can resist host-derived antimicrobials (reactive nitrogen and oxygen intermediates).

Host Factors

As described above, the human immune response against the MTC includes both the innate defense system (macrophage and natural killer cells, complement activation, ciliary clearance, and secretions of the main airways) and the adaptive response, comprising both cellular and humoral immunity. T cells are the main component of the cellular response that provides protection against TB and promotes memory response and granuloma formation. Although historically B cells and humoral immunity were not considered to offer any protection, some studies have shown they do contribute to immunological control (Gupta et al. 2012).

The main benefit of the adaptive response is the presence of immunological memory, so that a copy of each antigen found is stored in memory T cells and will lead to a rapid and enhanced response to subsequent encounters with that same antigen. This is the basis for the TST, a delayed-type hypersensitivity reaction caused by cytokines released from previously sensitized T cells when they are exposed to PPD antigens. Although hypersensitivity is linked to protective immunity, protection is not complete. Dif-

 Cite this article as *Cold Spring Harb Perspect Med* doi: 10.1101/cshperspect.a017830

BOX 2. RISK FACTORS

For *M. tuberculosis* Infection

- Children are more prone to primary infection, as their immune system is not yet completely mature.
- Close contacts of persons known or suspected of having active TB.
- Health-care workers, as well as residents and employees of congregate settings whose clients are at increased risk for active TB (correctional facilities, homeless shelters).
- Being born in areas that have a high incidence of active TB.

For Progression of Infection to Active Tuberculosis (TB)

- HIV infection
- Treatment with anti-TNF agents
- Solid organ transplantation
- Immunosuppressive treatment
- End-stage renal disease
- Hematological malignancies
- Head and neck neoplasm
- Gastrectomy
- Silicosis
- Underweight and malnutrition
- Corticosteroid therapy
- Diabetes mellitus
- Untreated fibrotic lesions suggesting previous TB in chest X-ray

Some patients have no obvious predisposing factors and may just be naturally susceptible to progression.

ferent studies have shown that TST-positive reactors are less likely to be reinfected than nonresponders, but there is no way to prevent reactivation without specific treatment.

From 2 to 4 wk after the first encounter between bacteria of the MTC and macrophages, the human host prepares two types of responses. The first one is delayed-type hypersensitivity to tubercle bacilli, which is tissue damaging as it promotes destruction of nonactivated macrophages containing proliferating mycobacterium. The second is a cell-mediated response, which activates macrophages to kill bacteria. There is a dynamic equilibrium between these two responses, which can lead to either TB progression or containment of MTC.

BURDEN IMPORTANCE

In 1993, the World Health Organization (WHO) declared TB to be a global public health emergency, stating that: "Tuberculosis today is humanity's great killer, and it is out of control in many parts of the world. The disease, preventable and treatable, has been grossly neglected and no country is immune to it." The first priority for TB elimination is early diagnosis and treatment of pulmonary TB, to reduce transmission. Subsequent steps include screening for clinically asymptomatic LTBI in high-risk populations. In addition to effective active TB control, the post-2015 WHO global TB strategy recognizes that elimination requires a focus on reducing the pool of latently infected individuals from which future TB cases would be generated.

It is estimated that one-third of the world's population is latently infected with MTC. However, given the 10% progression rate, clinical and public health services must focus their energies primarily on groups at a higher risk of disease. These include recently infected persons, immunocompromised individuals such as HIV (human immunodeficiency virus) patients, anti-TNF and transplant candidates, and household contacts of pulmonary TB cases. Additionally, health-care workers and migrants from high-incidence countries to low-incidence settings may be tested and given preventive treatment.

DIAGNOSTIC TESTS

Introduction

Individuals should not be tested for LTBI unless the responsible clinician has a management plan; "intention to test is intention to treat." The low risk of progression, treatment completion, and effectiveness and the adverse effects of treatment should be taken into account when testing is offered.

As previously stated, there is no way to directly diagnose LTBI, as the MTC cannot be recovered from the host unless active TB is present. An indirect immunological assessment of exposure is made instead by ascertaining the reactivity of host lymphocytes to mycobacterial antigens, either by testing the in vivo response with the TST or in vitro with INF-α release assays (IGRAs).

TST

The TST consists of an intradermal injection of tuberculin. Although a variety of approaches have been used, the Mantoux technique, which is administered on the inner surface of the forearm, is one of the most widely used globally. Tuberculin material can be PPD or RT-23. The standard doses are 5 PPD units (0.1 mL) or 2 RT-23 units, which are equivalent. Both types of tuberculins contain a complex mixture of antigens, including those of *M. bovis*–BCG strains and several antigens of nontuberculous mycobacteria (NTM), as well as *M. tuberculosis* antigens. Tuberculin will stimulate a delayed-type hypersensitivity response via T lymphocytes. A positive TST can be detected by an induration on the site of injection after 48–72 h. The result is the transverse diameter of the induration, which is usually recorded in millimeters. The interpretation of the result should take into account immunosuppression as well as the prevalence of TB in the setting in question—5 mm is considered positive if the patient is immunosuppressed, but it will be considered negative in healthy patients living in high-prevalence areas, for whom a 15-mm cutoff will apply. In some settings, a uniform cutoff of 10 mm is applied. These different and subjective considerations make it difficult to compare TST properties between studies in different countries and populations.

The main limitation of TST is its low specificity because of previous BCG vaccination and NTM infections. There are also other drawbacks in this apparently simple test. In subjects with chronic debilitating conditions or immunosuppression, TST may have a lower sensitivity than in healthy people. It must be administrated and read by trained professionals so as to avoid variability of the results. It also requires two clinical visits, and a positive reaction may interfere with confidentiality issues.

IGRAs

These tests use a blood sample taken from the patient to measure T-cell release of IFN-γ in vitro after stimulation by specific MTC antigens. Two IGRAs have been developed: the QuantiFERON-TB® Gold In-Tube (QFT) (Cellestis Limited, Carnegie, Victoria, Australia) and the T-SPOT.TB® (Oxford Immunotec, Oxford, UK). Both tests use the early secreted antigenic target 6 (ESAT-6) and culture filtrate protein 10 (CFP10), which are encoded by genes located on the region of difference 1 (RD-1) segment of the MTC genome. QFT also includes a third antigen, TB7.7 (RD-11).

QFT is an enzyme-linked immunosorbent-assay (ELISA)-based test performed on whole

 Cite this article as *Cold Spring Harb Perspect Med* doi: 10.1101/cshperspect.a017830

blood. It measures levels of IFN-γ in the supernatant of a cell suspension. The result is easily processed by software and is reported in international units per mL (IU/mL). T-SPOT.TB is an enzyme-linked immunospot assay (ELISPOT) performed on separated T lymphocytes. The result is reported as number of IFN-γ producing T cells.

The main advantage of IGRAs is their specificity, as ESAT-6, CFP10, and TB7.7 are found in the MTC genome, but not in *M. bovis*–BCG, or in the majority of NTMs. Moreover, IGRAs can differentiate a negative result from anergy by means of a positive control, which uses phytohemagglutinin to stimulate production of IFN-γ. In this review, we will talk about IGRAs without distinction, assuming that both QFT and T-SPOT.TB properties are comparable.

Neither TST nor IGRAs are able to detect TB infection in its first stages. Because they measure the adaptive immune response to MTC, an ~8-wk period after infection is required for a reliable result.

There are three notable disadvantages shared by both types of immunologic tests. The first one is their poor positive predictive value (PPV) for progression to active TB. Several studies have tried to correlate the risk of progression to the quantitative response of both in vivo tests (TST measurement) and in vitro tests (i.e., IFN-γ concentration in QFT tubes), but no conclusive results have been found. A recent meta-analysis showed a slightly better PPV with IGRAs compared with TST (2.4% for TST and 6.8% for IGRAs in high-risk groups) for the development of active disease (Diel et al. 2012), i.e., in a group of 100 IGRA-positive subjects tested for LTBI, and left without preemptive treatment, seven individuals would develop TB. However, to date, it is not possible to identify these seven before they progress to active disease. Furthermore, another review concluded that there is little difference between TST and IGRA PPVs (Rangaka et al. 2012), contributing to the WHO deendorsement of the use of IGRAs in developing countries.

The second common disadvantage is the inability of TSTs and IGRAs to distinguish between LTBI and active disease. The WHO has recommended against the use of IGRAs for active TB diagnosis, as a negative result does not rule out disease.

The third issue is that the tests are unable to distinguish recent from remote infection. The response profiles for past and recent infection are not different from each other. Each result must be carefully examined and tailored, as peculiarities of the host may modify sensitivity and specificity of both TST and IGRAs (Abubakar et al. 2013).

Evidence of Diagnostic Accuracy

Sensitivity

Because there is no "gold standard" for LTBI diagnosis, it is not possible to properly measure the sensitivity and specificity of the available diagnostic tests. The only individuals with proven TB infection are active TB patients, from whom bacteria of the MTC can be isolated. Data from a recent meta-analysis of diagnostic tests in TB patients showed a global sensitivity of 0.70 (TST), 0.81 (QFT), and 0.88 (T-SPOT.TB) (Diel et al. 2010). The immune response of latently infected and active TB patients is likely to not be equivalent, as TB itself is a well-known cause of anergy. Thus, sensitivity may be even higher in healthy people. In this population, a negative TST or IGRA rules out TB infection and has an almost 100% negative predictive value (NPV) for progression to active TB. A negative result, however, may not be reliable in other clinical scenarios, such as clinical suspicion of active TB or immunosuppressed patients. Several studies have tested how IGRAs perform in these specific circumstances; IGRAs seem to be less affected by immunosuppression than the TST (Redelman-Sidi and Sepkowitz 2013).

Specificity

Specificity is the main difference between the TST and IGRAs. Tuberculin contains several antigens shared by the MTC, *M. bovis*–BCG, and NTMs; thus, a positive TST does not necessarily equate to TB infection, especially in BCG-vaccinated subjects, among whom a higher proportion of false-positive results can be found. On the contrary, IGRAs have excellent specificity as they use antigens encoded in specific sequences of the MTC genome. Pooled specificity data show a range of 0.86–0.99 for IGRAs versus 0.97 and 0.59 for TST in BCG-vaccinated and non-BCG-vaccinated individuals, respectively (Diel et al. 2010).

Improved specificity prevents the excessive use of treatment to prevent progression, as false-positive results will be excluded. If a group of 1000 healthy recent contacts of pulmonary TB cases were tested by TST, ~50% would test positive and be treated. If an IGRA was used instead, only 30% would be treated, resulting in large savings by preventing unnecessary treatment.

Other Issues: Two Steps versus One Step and Cost-Effectiveness

Data on the cost-effectiveness of the different approaches to LTBI diagnosis are limited because of the paucity of information on predictive values. Individually, it is generally more expensive to test with an IGRA than with a TST. In the community, the better the selection of people at risk of TB for testing, the less unnecessary treatment and fewer adverse events, as well as reduced expenditure on testing and follow-up visits.

Guidance on diagnostic strategies for LTBI in individuals at risk varies considerably between countries. Although there are several discrepancies between guidelines in terms of the TST cutoff for positivity, the repetition of TST (looking for a boosting effect), and the use of one or more types of tests, there is growing evidence on the superiority of IGRAs over the TST in terms of sensitivity and specificity. Given their higher specificity and their at least comparable NPV for reactivation of TB, IGRAs may be preferable to TST for targeting people for preventive treatment. There are very few countries (United States, Spain, and Portugal) where the two-step TST is heeded. This strategy aims to obtain a LTBI diagnosis in older and immunosuppressed patients, in which an initial TST may boost the immune system against an older latent infection that would be evident after the second dose of tuberculin. However, the effectiveness of this second test is usually low, and several studies have reported a nonnegligible proportion of false-positive results, mainly in BCG-vaccinated individuals.

A more widely used two-step approach, usually based on cost-effectiveness analysis, is the application of IGRAs to confirm an initial TST. The rationale for this is that the cheaper and potentially equally sensitive test (TST) is applied first, and the diagnosis is confirmed with an IGRA test. Which strategy (IGRAs in place of TST or as a confirmatory test) is more suitable for testing individuals at risk is unclear, but it will depend on the immune status of the host and the expected prevalence of TB infection in the population tested (Table 1). In immunocompetent individuals, in whom the sensitivity of the two tests can be regarded as roughly comparable, positive IGRA results are expected to also be TST-positive. In this scenario, using IGRAs as a confirmatory test may be appropriate if the expected proportion of infection is low. Conversely, if the expected proportion of infection is high, testing with an IGRA instead of TST may be more cost-saving.

In immunocompromised patients, the use of IGRA plus TST to increase sensitivity may avoid missing some infected subjects at a high risk of progression to active disease. However, the results from several studies in patients about to start biologic therapeutics suggest that screening for LTBI and decisions regarding preventive treatment can be reliably based on IGRAs, irrespective of TST results (Laffitte et al. 2009; Chang et al. 2011; Qumseya et al. 2011; Garcovich et al. 2012; Hsia et al. 2012, 2013; Jung et al. 2012; Mariette et al. 2012; Greveson et al. 2013). Furthermore, the additional cost of undertaking two tests for the limited gain in sensitivity likely means that dual testing may not be cost-effective.

TREATMENT

Drugs—Trial Evidence of Effectiveness

The treatment of LTBI has a long history, starting from the early studies of the 1950s through to modern trials of novel combination regimens

Table 1. Differences between TST and IGRAs according to immune status

	Healthy subjects	Immunosuppressed subjects (including HIV, IMID patients attributable to starting anti-TNF therapy, patients awaiting for transplantation)
First step	**Always rule out active TB** (Clinical history and examination, chest X-ray, and sputum microscopy and culture as well as other tests if extrapulmonary TB is suspected)	
When to test?	Recent infection (contact tracing study) Occupational risk (HCW)	At HIV diagnosis Before the beginning of IS treatment
How do TST perform?	Good sensitivity	Less sensitivity because of weakening condition
	Poor specificity: high proportion of false-positive reactions in BCG-vaccinated subjects Window period (recent infection)	Poor specificity: high proportion of false-positive reactions in BCG-vaccinated subjects No window period needed
How do IGRAs perform?	Good sensitivity	Less sensitivity than in healthy subjects, but better sensitivity than TST
	Good specificity Window period (recent infection)	Good specificity No window period needed
Recommended strategies for LTBI diagnosis and targeting patients for preventive treatment	High TB infection prevalence expected: **IGRA** Low TB infection prevalence expected: two-step strategy **Positive TST followed by an IGRA**	Most guidelines recommend TST AND IGRA to maximize sensitivity; several studies used **ONLY IGRAs** with no issues

TST, tuberculin skin test; IGRA, interferon-γ release assay; HIV, human immunodeficiency virus; IMID, immune-mediated inflammatory disease; TNF, tumor necrosis factor; HCW, health-care workers; IS, immunosuppressive; BCG, Bacillus Calmétte–Guérin.

in high-risk populations. Drugs for treating latent infection should possess sterilizing activity against dormant mycobacteria, as such is the status of bacteria in these patients. As previously described, the very fact that isoniazid is active against LTBI suggests that at least some replication is occurring, as the target of this drug's activity is the inhibition of the synthesis of mycolic acid, required for the mycobacterial cell wall, during replication. Numerous randomized controlled trials and a handful of systematic reviews have shown the safety and efficacy of isoniazid in the general population, HIV-infected individuals, and posttransplant patients for preventing TB reactivation.

Rifampicin, the second proven active drug for LTBI, is a well-known antibiotic with intracellular activity that inhibits the bacterial DNA-dependent RNA polymerase and has been used against other bacterial infections in their latency period.

Globally, it is most common to use 6–9 mo of daily isoniazid monotherapy (dose 300 mg) although recent data suggest that 4 mo of daily rifampicin (dose 600 mg), or 3 mo of combined therapy with isoniazid 300 mg and rifampicin 600 mg may be equally effective (Stagg et al. 2014). A novel regimen consisting of 12 doses of a weekly regimen of rifapentin (900 mg) and high-dose isoniazid (900 mg) has been recently described as effective and is currently used in the United States under directly observed therapy.

The first and major reason for treatment failure, and thus for the development of active TB, is poor medication adherence. Unfortunately, the direct observation of each patient is unaffordable for most countries. LTBI treatments are lengthy, and a close monitoring of subjects is required to ensure high treatment compliance. Several methods for checking treatment compliance have been validated. They include the Eidus-Hamilton test and commercially available reactive strips that can easily detect urine metabolites of isoniazid metabolites. Checking the orange-colored urine of subjects taking rifampicin may also be useful for adherence control.

Adverse Events

The three common treatment regimens are generally well tolerated. Patients must always be told about symptoms that may indicate the development of adverse effects so that they seek care promptly. The most common life-threatening adverse event resulting from isoniazid is liver toxicity. Not only is a clinical assessment needed, but liver function tests are also essential in the third or fourth week of treatment, and then in the second and third month, as well as in the instance of patients reporting hepatitis signs and symptoms. Biochemistry variations on alanine transaminase (ALT) and aspartate transaminase (AST) precede symptoms as indicators of liver damage and that is the reason for testing apparently healthy patients. Another frequent adverse event of isoniazid is peripheral neuropathy, which can easily be prevented with daily pyridoxine.

Patients taking rifamycins can present flu-like symptoms in their first week of treatment. This adverse event is more common in intermittent regimens (i.e., weekly doses).

Hypersensitivity reactions are more frequently related to rifamycins, although they might also be caused by isoniazid. These reactions are mostly seen in the second to fourth week of treatment and consist of a rash and fever, ranging from harmless itching of the skin to severe clinical pictures including Stevens–Johnson syndrome.

Special Issues

Although preventing drug-resistant TB cases is of great concern for clinicians and health authorities, there are no recommended regimens for LTBI treatment of those exposed to multidrug-resistant TB, as there are no sterilizing drugs for dormant bacilli apart from isoniazid and the rifamycins. Guidelines advise only "watchful waiting" of these individuals to assure an early diagnosis in case of the development of active TB. Young children, who are household contacts of multidrug-resistant TB cases, may benefit from prophylactic treatment. This should always be supervised by a physician with knowledge and experience of multidrug-resistant TB prophylactic treatment, based on drug susceptibility results of the index case.

For all LTBI patients diagnosed within a contact study, it is mandatory for the clinician to check the drug susceptibility of the index case and to ensure that the transmitted bacteria are likely to be sensitive to the chosen LTBI treatment regimen.

MANAGEMENT

The most important issue for LTBI management is to properly target candidates for screening and treating, that is, to identify an individual's risk of developing active TB. The main contraindication for LTBI treatment is active TB, and thus the first commitment of the clinician is to rule out the disease through a clinical interview for the specific symptoms of TB and a careful examination of a recent chest X-ray. Medical and nursing staff skilled in treating TB patients and dealing with adverse events of antituberculosis drugs should ideally manage LTBI screening.

Individuals at Risk

Newly Infected Individuals

As mentioned above, the first 2 yr after infection carry the highest risk for developing active disease. For this reason, individuals at risk for MTC infection found to have converted from a negative to a positive result for a LTBI diagnostic test, as well as individuals testing positive after a contact tracing study, will be the most likely to benefit from preventive treatment.

Contact Tracing (Erkens et al. 2010). After diagnosing an individual with pulmonary TB, it is mandatory to get information regarding transmission settings to assign priorities for the investigation. The purpose of conducting a contact examination of a TB case is to evaluate individuals for active TB disease (to find either the source case or secondary cases) so that treatment can be given and further transmission stopped, as well as diagnosing and treating those with LTBI.

Priorities for contact investigation depend on the characteristics of the index case (cavitation on chest X-ray and positive AFB smear sputum are the most infectious), susceptibility and vulnerability of contacts (children under 5 yr and immunocompromised patients are assigned the highest priority), and circumstances of the exposure (household contacts, congregate settings).

All referred contacts should be specifically asked for respiratory symptoms and current general health. Then, a TST or an IGRA (either alone or in a two-step strategy) should be undertaken. Patients with negative results obtained before 8 wk after the end of exposure should have the test repeated so as to avoid false-negative results in the window period.

Subjects reporting any suggestive symptom of TB and all individuals with positive results on the LTBI diagnostic tests should have a chest X-ray to rule out active TB. After TB is excluded, all LTBI patients should be offered treatment with either isoniazid (6 mo), rifampicin (4 mo), or a combined 3-mo regimen with daily isoniazid and rifampicin or weekly isoniazid and rifapentine, with close follow-up. This includes adherence, asking for symptoms attributable to adverse events, and liver function tests, with at least one test before the beginning of treatment and another in 3–4 wk. Further tests may be needed.

Household contacts who are children (or those with a close relationship with the TB patient) should have TB ruled out with a chest X-ray. They should also be started on preventive treatment even though a negative result may be found in the first LTBI test (TST or an IGRA). Children, especially those under 5 yr of age, have an immature immune system that favors both false-negative results and the development of active TB. If active TB has been excluded and a second LTBI diagnostic test remains negative after the window period, treatment can be stopped.

When a child is found to have TB disease, a contact study should be performed around them, because although TB in children is rarely infectious, it is usually a sign of a close contact who is the source case.

Health-Care Workers. An IGRA or TST may be used for persons with occupational exposure to the MTC. If TB infection is systematically tested for and ruled out when the individual commences their new job, and then every 2 yr as long as they remain negative responders, a conversion from negative to positive result may be detected and thus treatment for a recent infection could be offered to prevent TB development.

Immunocompromised Patients

Immunocompromised persons with LTBI are at an increased risk for progression to active TB; treatment of LTBI in this population can reduce this risk.

People Living with HIV. Patients coinfected with HIV and MTC are particularly prone to a reactivation of LTBI and the development of disseminated disease. For this reason, systematic screening for TB infection in individuals newly diagnosed with HIV has been recommended. After ruling out active disease, patients should be tested with either a TST or an IGRA, and those with positive results should receive preventive treatment. Several studies have shown the better performance of IGRAs over TSTs in patients with lower CD4 cells counts (<200 cells/mm^3). These patients should be treated with at least 6 mo of isoniazid 300 mg daily.

Subjects Considered for Anti-TNF Drugs. Individuals diagnosed with immune-mediated inflammatory diseases have an impaired immune system attributable to their disease or its treatment. Those receiving anti-TNF (especially infliximab and adalimumab) are at particular risk for reactivation, as these drugs break up granulomas, which are partially maintained by self-released TNF.

One strategy proposed in candidates to receive anti-TNF is systematically screening for LTBI before treatment begins. How to test this population is still an area of debate in different countries. To ensure the greatest sensitivity, several nations have encouraged the use of both TST and an IGRA and the treatment of any patient with a positive result.

Transplant Candidates. Among solid organ transplant recipients, the risk of developing active TB has been calculated to be 36- to 74-fold higher than in the general population (Singh and Paterson 1998), with lung transplantation being the most risky. Active screening of LTBI is increasingly becoming part of the routine in the check-up of transplant candidates before the surgical procedure.

Patients with end-stage kidney disease and those with advanced liver cirrhosis waiting for kidney and liver transplantation deserve special comment. These two conditions are risk factors for skin test anergy and thus an increased rate of false-negative results in TST. For this reason, an IGRA is preferred to determine which patients should receive LTBI treatment.

Migrants from Endemic Areas Arriving to High-Income Countries

As the majority of TB in migrants arises through the reactivation of infections acquired overseas and developed in the first few years postentry, screening for LTBI in this population on arrival is an essential element of any TB elimination strategy. This group may be a hard-to-reach population, with low rates of returning to have TSTs read; thus, an IGRA test might be preferred. The use of IGRAs can increase test completion rates, so control efforts should focus on those most likely to benefit from further evaluation and treatment.

LOOKING TO THE FUTURE

The control and eventual global elimination of TB would depend on either an effective postexposure vaccine or better tools and drugs to detect and treat LTBI. Current research focused on improving the diagnosis and positive predictive value of LTBI tests ranges from improvements of IGRAs by investigating additional antigens as well as alternative cytokines, to research based on proteomics, transcriptomics, and metabolomics. For example, several ongoing studies in humans are measuring different cytokine profiles (e.g., IFN-γ and IL2) to differentiate active TB and LTBI in vitro, whereas others have focused on transcriptional profiles apparently associated with latently infected individuals who might progress to disease. It is likely that advances in our understanding of latency in TB would be revolutionized in the next decade based on ongoing research in large-population cohorts using these approaches.

New research must also identify treatment regimens that are considerably shorter, more effective, and less toxic. The new rifapentine regimen of only 12 doses has been made possible because of the long half-life of this drug. Future research must consider whether newer drugs with a long half-life, such as bedaquiline, may be used to shorten treatment. Such research must also investigate the adverse effect profile of any new regimen.

REFERENCES

Abubakar I, Stagg HR, Whitworth H, Lalvani A. 2013. How should I interpret an interferon γ release assay result for tuberculosis infection? *Thorax* **68:** 298–301.

Berry MP, Graham CM, McNab FW, Xu Z, Bloch SA, Oni T, Wilkinson KA, Banchereau R, Skinner J, Wilkinson RJ, et al. 2010. An interferon-inducible neutrophil-driven blood transcriptional signature in human tuberculosis. *Nature* **466:** 973–977.

Calmette A. 1931. Preventive vaccination against tuberculosis with BCG. *Proc R Soc Med* **24:** 1481–1490.

Chang B, Park HY, Jeon K, Ahn JK, Cha HS, Koh EM, Kang ES, Koh WJ. 2011. Interferon-γ release assay in the diagnosis of latent tuberculosis infection in arthritis patients treated with tumor necrosis factor antagonists in Korea. *Clin Rheumatol* **30:** 1535–1541.

Diel R, Loddenkemper R, Nienhaus A. 2010. Evidence-based comparison of commercial interferon-γ release assays for detecting active TB. A meta analysis. *Chest* **137:** 952–968.

Diel R, Loddenkemper R, Nienhaus A. 2012. Predictive value of interferon-γ release assays and tuberculin skin testing for progression from latent TB infection to disease state: A meta-analysis. *Chest* **142:** 63–75.

Erkens CGM, Kamphorst M, Abubakar I, Bothamley GH, Chemtob D, Haase W, Migliori GB, Rieder HL, Zellweger JP, Lange C. 2010. Tuberculosis contact investigation in low prevalence countries: A European consensus. *Eur Respir J* **36:** 925–949.

Garcovich S, Ruggeri A, D'Agostino M, Ardito F, De Simone C, Delogu G, Fadda G. 2012. Clinical applicability of Quantiferon-TB-Gold testing in psoriasis patients during long-term anti-TNF-α treatment: A prospective, observational study. *J Eur Acad Dermatol Venereol* **26:** 1572–1576.

Gengenbacher M, Kaufmann SH. 2012. *Mycobacterium tuberculosis:* Success through dormancy. *FEMS Microbiol Rev* **36:** 514–532.

Greveson K, Goodhand J, Capocci S, Woodward S, Murray C, Cropley I, Hamilton M, Lipman M. 2013. Yield and cost effectiveness of mycobacterial infection detection using a simple IGRA-based protocol in UK subjects with inflammatory bowel disease suitable for anti-TNFα therapy. *J Crohn's Colitis* **7:** 412–418.

Gupta A, Kaul A, Tsolaki AG, Kishore U, Bhakta S. 2012. *Mycobacterium tuberculosis:* Immune evasion, latency and reactivation. *Immunobiology* **217:** 363–374.

Hillier A. 1903. The nature of the infectivity of phthisis: A study of the views of Koch, Flügge, and others. *Br Med J* **1:** 593–596.

Hsia EC, Schluger N, Cush JJ, Chaisson RE, Matteson EL, Xu S, Beutler A, Doyle MK, Hsu B, Rahman MU. 2012. Interferon-γ release assay versus tuberculin skin test prior to treatment with golimumab, a human anti-tumor necrosis factor antibody, in patients with rheumatoid arthritis, psoriatic arthritis, or ankylosing spondylitis. *Arthritis Rheum* **64:** 2068–2077.

Hsia EC, Cush JJ, Matteson EL, Beutler A, Doyle MK, Hsu B, Xu S, Rahman MU. 2013. Comprehensive tuberculosis screening program in patients with inflammatory arthritides treated with golimumab, a human anti-tumor necrosis factor antibody, in Phase III clinical trials. *Arthritis Care Res (Hoboken)* **65:** 309–313.

Jung YJ, Lyu J, Yoo B, Lee CK, Kim YG, Yang SK, Byeon JS, Kim KJ, Ye BD, Lee KH, et al. 2012. Combined use of a TST and the T-SPOT®.TB assay for latent tuberculosis infection diagnosis before anti-TNF-α treatment. *Int J Tuberc Lung Dis* **16:** 1300–1306.

Koch R. 1891. A further communication on a remedy for tuberculosis. *Br Med J* **1:** 125–127.

Laffitte E, Janssens JP, Roux-Lombard P, Thielen AM, Barde C, Marazza G, Panizzon RG, Saurat JH. 2009. Tuberculosis screening in patients with psoriasis before antitumour necrosis factor therapy: Comparison of an interferon-γ release assay vs. tuberculin skin test. *Br J Dermatol* **161:** 797–800.

Mariette X, Baron G, Tubach F, Lioté F, Combe B, Miceli-Richard C, Flipo RM, Goupille P, Allez M, Salmon D, et al. 2012. Influence of replacing tuberculin skin test with ex vivo interferon γ release assays on decision to administer prophylactic antituberculosis antibiotics before anti-TNF therapy. *Ann Rheum Dis* **71:** 1783–1790.

Martin CF, Robins GD. 1898. On the diagnostic value of tuberculin. *Br Med J* **1:** 357–359.

Mi'fadyean J. 1891. Experiments with tuberculin on cattle. *Br Med J* **1:** 634–635.

Poulsen A. 1950. Some clinical features of tuberculosis. *Acta Tuberc Scand* **24:** 311–346.

Qumseya BJ, Ananthakrishnan AN, Skaros S, Bonner M, Issa M, Zadvornova Y, Naik A, Perera L, Binion DG. 2011. QuantiFERON-TB Gold testing for tuberculosis screening in an inflammatory bowel disease cohort in the United States. *Inflamm Bowel Dis* **17:** 77–83.

Rangaka MX, Wilkinson KA, Glynn JR, Ling D, Menzies D, Mwansa-Kambafwile J, Fielding K, Wilkinson RJ, Pai M. 2012. Predictive value of interferon-γ release assays for incident active tuberculosis: A systematic review and meta-analysis. *Lancet Infect Dis* **12:** 45–55.

Redelman-Sidi G, Sepkowitz KA. 2013. IFN-γ release assays in the diagnosis of latent tuberculosis infection among immunocompromised adults. *Am J Respir Crit Care Med* **188:** 422–431.

Rieder H, Chen-Yuan C, Gie RP, Enarson D. 2009. General background to clinical tuberculosis. Infection and disease. *Crofton's clinical tuberculosis*, 3rd ed., pp. 1–10. Macmillan, Oxford.

Singh N, Paterson D. 1998. *Mycobacterium tuberculosis* infection in solid-organ transplant recipients: Impact and implications for management. *Clin Infect Dis* **27:** 1266–1277.

Stagg HR, Zenner D, Harris RJ, Muñoz L, Lipman MC, Abubakar I. 2014. Treatment of latent tuberculosis: A network meta-analysis. *Ann Intern Med* (in press).

Wallgren A. 1948. The time-table of tuberculosis. *Tubercle* **29:** 245–251.

Wang L, Turner MO, Elwood RK, Schulzer M, FitzGerald JM. 2002. A meta-analysis of the effect of Bacille Calmette Guérin vaccination on tuberculin skin test measurements. *Thorax* **57:** 804–809.

nificant exposure), making a rapid and accurate diagnosis and initiating effective treatment promptly are central to good patient care and public health TB management. Not only does this alleviate symptoms and reduce mortality for the individual, but it also decreases onward transmission to others and hence impacts on the overall burden of TB.

TB in adults can present in a variety of ways. The lung is the predominant site of TB as infection with *Mycobacterium tuberculosis* (*Mtb*) or other members of the TB complex arises almost exclusively from inhaling droplets containing the bacilli. This may result in symptomatic, primary pulmonary TB disease (usually in children) and in adults, after a variable amount of time in a clinically asymptomatic state of latent TB infection (LTBI), generally as postprimary pulmonary TB. *Mtb* may spread directly from the lungs, via the lymphatics, or the bloodstream, to other body sites causing the various extrapulmonary TB manifestations described in this review.

The location of disease should be documented in all patients. Given that there may be multiple sites involved, it is recommended that at least two, a major and a minor site, when applicable, be recorded. Here, the definitions used are those proposed by a Working Group of the World Health Organization (WHO) and the European Region of the International Union Against Tuberculosis and Lung Disease (IUATLD) for uniform reporting of TB cases (Rieder et al. 1996).

It is important to note that TB can be diagnosed via a number of different clinical pathways and settings. In a low incidence country such as Germany, among more than 25,000 TB cases studied between 1996 and 2000, almost 80% were diagnosed through passive case finding (~62% had symptoms suggesting TB, 16% were diagnosed during investigations for other medical causes, 1% at autopsy) and 19% by active case finding in high-risk groups, particularly in close contacts of infectious patients (Forssbohm 2004). This further reinforces the importance of thinking of TB as a possible cause of a patient's symptoms or signs in clinical practice (Craig et al. 2009).

CLINICAL PRESENTATION AND DIAGNOSIS OF TB

Pulmonary TB

Pulmonary TB is defined as tuberculosis of the lung parenchyma and the tracheobronchial tree only. Primary pulmonary TB should be distinguished from postprimary pulmonary TB, which is the most frequent TB manifestation in adults. The classic clinical features of pulmonary TB include chronic cough, sputum production, appetite loss, weight loss, fever, night sweats, and hemoptysis (Lawn and Zumla 2011). Someone presenting with any of these symptoms should be suspected of having TB. If they are or were known to be in contact with infectious TB, they are even more likely to be suffering from TB (Ait-Khaled et al. 2010.)

Primary Pulmonary TB

In countries with a high TB prevalence, primary pulmonary disease occurs usually in childhood, but where TB is less endemic, it occurs fairly often also in adults. It is characterized by local granulomatous inflammation, usually in the periphery of the lung (Ghon focus), and may be accompanied by ipsilateral lymph node involvement, termed the Ghon complex. The infection is usually asymptomatic but can present as an acute lower respiratory tract infection. The most important clue to the diagnosis is a history of close contact with an infectious TB case. The diagnosis is suspected when a tuberculin skin test or a blood interferon-γ release assay (IGRA) converts to positive, usually 3–8 wk after infection. The chest radiograph may show the Ghon focus/complex (Fig. 1).

Rare primary sites of TB are the alimentary tract caused by swallowing *Mtb*, usually *Mycobacterium bovis*, present in nonpasteurized milk products (de la Rua-Domenech 2006), or after direct cutaneous infection (usually occurring in laboratory personnel) (Menzies et al. 2003). Intravesical Bacillus Calmette–Guérin (BCG) vaccination used to treat localized bladder tumors may occasionally disseminate and present as primary BCG disease (Fig. 2) (Lamm 1992).

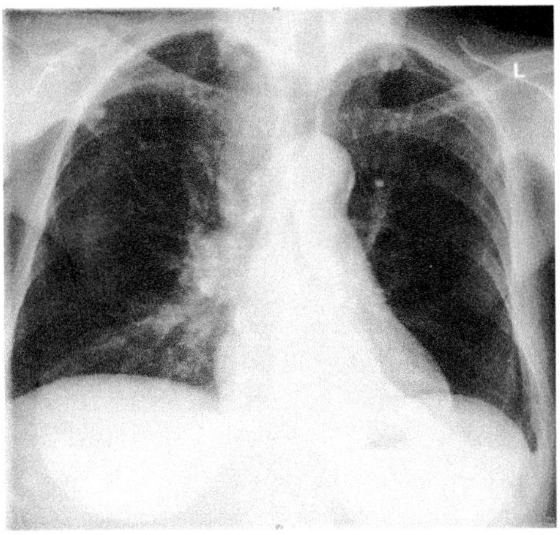

Figure 1. Ghon complex. (Figure reprinted from Fuehner et al. 2007, with permission, from Springer, © 2007.)

Local complications of primary pulmonary TB may result from lymph node enlargement leading to bronchial obstruction. Tuberculous pleurisy can arise early in the course of primary pulmonary TB, either by direct spread from the pulmonary lesion or through hematogenous dissemination.

Rare, serious, early systemic complications caused by blood-borne spread of *Mtb* are miliary TB and meningitis. Many years later, TB of the skeletal or urogenital system and other organs may result (Wallgren 1948).

Postprimary pulmonary TB may follow primary TB. In the generally immunocompetent, there is a lifetime chance of reactivation of the dormant primary complex of 5%–10% (Horsburgh Jr 2004). These estimates were developed before the availability of molecular techniques that can distinguish reactivation from reinfection with another strain of *Mtb*, and it may be that the overall risk is rather less in most people with latent TB infection not exposed again to *Mtb*. The first 2 yr following primary infection are the period of maximal risk of progression. This can be reduced significantly by treating LTBI, which is indicated particularly in high-risk groups (Table 1) (Diel et al. 2013). It is not known why only ~10% of individuals infected with *Mtb* develop active disease. Apart from diverse risk factors such as diabetes, smoking, and chronic renal failure (Hu et al. 2014), several genes have been found to be associated with increased susceptibility to, or resistance against, *Mtb* (Möller et al. 2010).

Erythema nodosum and other skin conditions such as granulomatous panniculitis plus forms of uveitis and polyarthritis (Poncet's disease) are considered to reflect the host immune response to mycobacterial antigen. They can be

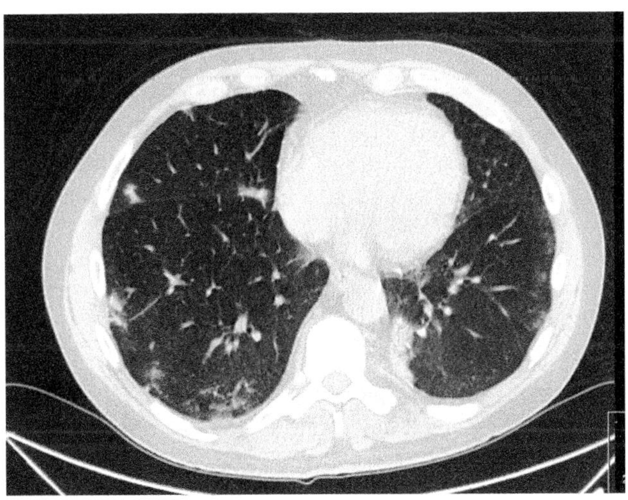

Figure 2. Disseminated BCG disease. Computed tomography (CT) of the chest showing bilateral patchy ground glass shadowing and consolidation in a patient who developed fevers, cough, and positive blood cultures for BCG following treatment with intravesical BCG for bladder carcinoma. (Figure provided by Marc Lipman.)

Table 1. Persons at high risk of progressing from latent to active TB

Recent contact with a TB case
Persons with fibrotic changes on chest radiograph consistent with old TB
HIV-infected persons
Organ transplant recipients
Persons immunosuppressed for other reasons (e.g., taking the equivalent of 15 mg/d of prednisone for >1 mo or taking tumor necrosis factor-α inhibitors)
Recent immigrants (<5 yr) from high prevalence countries
Persons with the following clinical conditions:
Diabetes mellitus
Chronic renal failure
Some hematologic disorders (e.g., leukemia and lymphomas)
Other specific malignancies (e.g., carcinoma of the head or neck and lung)
Gastrectomy and jejunoileal bypass
Silicosis
Injection drug users
Tobacco smokers
Residents and employees of high-risk congregate living facilities (e.g., correctional facilities, nursing homes, homeless shelters, hospitals, and other health-care facilities)
Mycobacteriology laboratory personnel

Data modified from Diel et al. 2013.

seen both during primary infection and at some time distant from presumed infection (Kroot et al. 2007). The features are often nonspecific, and the key clinical issue here is to consider TB as a possible underlying cause of the presentation. This is generally based on determining whether there is a history of exposure or residence in a TB-endemic area. The increasing numbers of individuals who are immunocompromised from infections such as HIV or through medical treatments (and are at much greater risk of developing active TB) make this method of categorization less helpful than previously.

Postprimary Pulmonary TB

Postprimary TB of the lungs is the prevailing TB manifestation in adults (in 60%–80%) (Public Health England 2014). It can occur many years after exposure to an individual with infectious TB and may be provoked by temporary or permanent immunological impairment. Males are more often affected than females (Borgdorff et al. 2000).

The most frequent symptoms of active disease are fever, anorexia or reduced appetite, weight loss, night sweats, anemia, and persistent cough (i.e., lasting >14 d) (TB CARE 2014) usually productive of purulent and/or blood-stained sputum. Occasionally, patients complain of localized thoracic pain attributable to accompanying pleural inflammation. In extensive and long-lasting pulmonary disease, patients may report breathlessness. Hemoptysis is usually the result of cavitating lung disease causing erosion of pulmonary blood vessels (Fig. 3).

Hoarseness can occur if there is laryngeal involvement. Patients with laryngeal and tracheobronchial (Fig. 4) TB may have *Mtb* in sputum despite a normal chest X-ray, although in general, the radiograph will suggest the possible diagnosis (Bhat et al. 2009).

Tuberculoma of the lung should be considered as part of the differential diagnosis in mass lesions presenting in individuals with a history of exposure to *Mtb* (Fig. 5).

The physical signs of TB are not specific. Auscultation often does not show any pathological breath sounds or may reveal crackles, wheezing, or bronchial breathing (which is

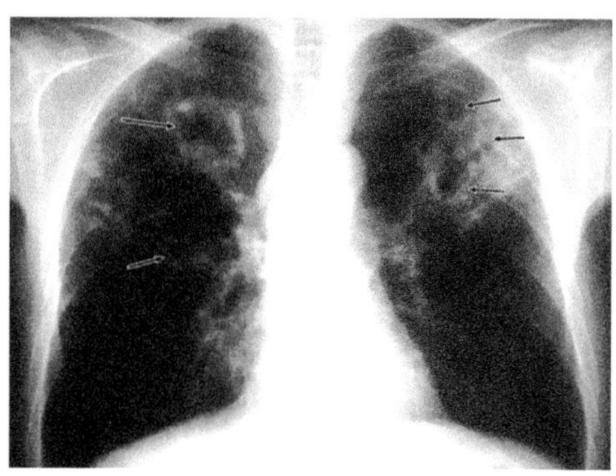

Figure 3. Cavitating tuberculosis presenting with hemoptysis (note arrows indicating cavities). (Figure reprinted from Fuehner et al. 2007, with permission, from Springer, © 2007.)

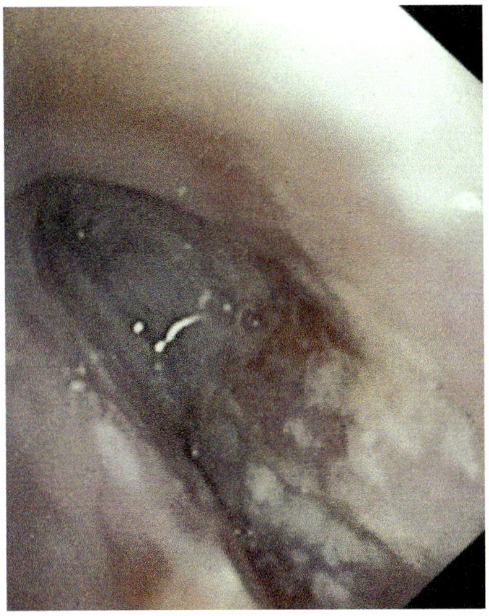

Figure 4. TB in the mucosa of the left main bronchus. Histology and culture from biopsy were positive for *Mtb*. (Figure provided by Robert Loddenkemper.)

termed amphoric when related to the movement of air within a cavity). The radiographic features vary from very discrete infiltrates to extensive and bilateral changes with multiple cavities characteristic of TB. Usually, the changes are more pronounced in the upper lobes. The differential diagnosis of cavitation includes other infections as well as malignant and inflammatory lung diseases (Table 2).

There are no specific blood tests that aid the diagnosis of TB. Patients will have a profile that reflects their general state of health and nutrition. They may or may not be anemic and have moderately elevated inflammatory markers such as C-reactive protein. However, all of these measures are highly variable (Breen et al. 2008a). The following blood tests are recommended generally as baseline assessments rather than for any specific value in TB diagnosis. These include kidney and liver function, blood sugar, hemoglobin, white cell and differential counts, platelet count, and C-reactive protein (or ESR). It is recommended that routine HIV and hepatitis B and C testing be performed and vitamin D blood levels measured, as patients are invariably deficient (Blasi and Matteelli 2013).

The presentation of HIV-associated pulmonary TB can mimic that seen in the HIV uninfected. This is generally found in subjects with relatively well-preserved immunity (manifest as blood CD4 counts >350 cells/μL) (Cain et al. 2010). However, the associated immune dysregulation in most individuals with active TB and HIV coinfection means that although symptoms may be similar, patients can also present with very nonspecific although severe systemic features (e.g., weight loss, night sweats, and fever) and minimal specific respiratory complaints (Breen et al. 2008a).

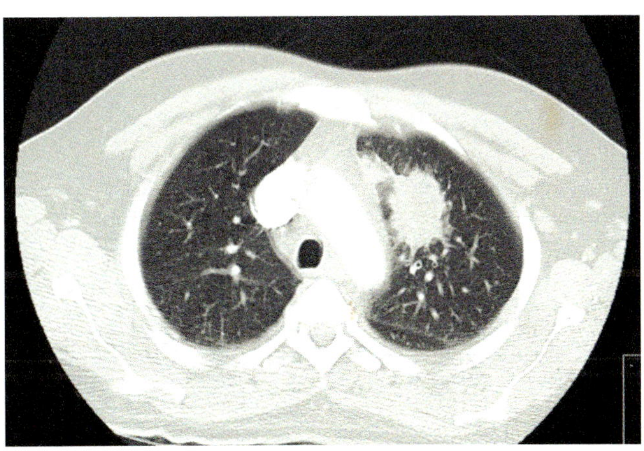

Figure 5. Lung tuberculoma. Initially thought to be a primary lung cancer, bronchoscopic biopsy showed acid-fast bacilli on smear. Culture grew *Mtb*. (Figure provided by Marc Lipman.)

Table 2. Differential diagnosis of pulmonary cavitation

Cause	Examples
Infection	Tuberculosis
	Acute bacterial, e.g., *Staphylococcus aureus*, *Klebsiella pneumoniae*
	Subacute/chronic bacterial (e.g., *Nocardia* sp, melidoidosis, actinomycosis)
	Fungal (e.g., cryptococcosis, coccidiodomycosis)
	Infected pneumatocele
Malignancy	Primary lung cancer (e.g., non–small cell squamous)
	Pulmonary metastases
Inflammatory	Sarcoidosis
	Wegener's granulomatous angiitis
	Rheumatoid arthritis
Vascular	Pulmonary infarct
Congenital	Sequestered lung; bronchogenic cyst

The radiology of HIV TB is discussed in more detail elsewhere. However, an important point to note is that parenchymal cavitation is less likely in individuals with low blood CD4 counts. Extrapulmonary manifestations (including mediastinal nodal disease and pleural effusions) are also more common in HIV coinfection (Lawn and Zumla 2011).

The lack of cavities means that sputum samples in HIV-associated pulmonary TB are often smear-negative. This is despite individuals having in fact a very high mycobacterial burden (Elliott et al. 1993; Crump et al. 2012; Huang et al. 2014). Indeed, sputum cultures are generally positive as frequently in HIV-infected as -uninfected subjects. The importance of obtaining samples from other body fluids and locations cannot be overemphasized. This should include mycobacterial blood and urine cultures. Given that HIV-associated TB is often multisite, general radiological evaluation (including computed tomography [CT] chest, abdomen, and pelvis or equivalent investigations, e.g., abdominal ultrasound) may identify other areas of pathology that are amenable to diagnostic aspiration or biopsy. The high mycobacterial burden associated with HIV means that often urine antigen tests such as the cell wall component lipoarabinnoman (available in commercially produced kits) may be positive in patients with very low blood CD4 counts (<100 cells/μL). These offer, therefore, an alternative approach to TB diagnosis in advanced HIV infection (Lawn et al. 2013).

In many clinical settings, HIV is diagnosed at the same time as TB (Rice et al. 2013). This mainly follows the pattern of presentation with clinical TB, which then results in an HIV test. However, the use of antiretroviral therapy in an individual at risk of TB can lead to an unmasking paradoxical reaction (which is part of the immune reconstitution inflammatory syndrome, IRIS) (Breen et al. 2005). These are typically highly inflammatory presentations, in which individuals develop intense systemic symptoms and new onset signs and radiological changes within a matter of days.

Although the underlying mechanism has not been fully elucidated, it appears to arise as a consequence of a host immune response directed against a (generally foreign) persistent antigen. Mycobacteria fulfill this role well, although so do other chronic intracellular organisms such as fungi. Hence, a presentation of apparent unmasking TB must be investigated comprehensively. Samples should be sent for cytology, histology, and bacterial, fungal, and mycobacterial cultures to avoid diagnostic confusion and inappropriate treatment.

Sputum sampling is a key step in the diagnosis of TB. Attempts should be made to obtain at least two sputum samples from individuals with suspected TB (including extrapulmonary TB, which is often associated with positive sputum cultures despite few reported symptoms) (Parimon et al. 2008). Good-quality sputum samples should be obtained. It is standard to ask for three samples, although evidence suggests that two may strike a better balance in terms of value (Mase et al. 2007). These are generally requested to be provided first thing in the morning (i.e., at a time when individuals are most productive). However, in an ambulatory setting, this can result in delay, and often there is utility in obtaining samples in one day (e.g., in the morning and afternoon).

Should an individual be unable to produce sputum spontaneously, many centers will perform induced sputum using hypertonic saline (generally between 3% and 7% concentration). This technique is quick (in total taking <1 h), relatively inexpensive, and not as invasive as a bronchoscopy. It also has a good yield (Brown et al. 2007). However, this is operator-dependent, and the procedure requires experienced technicians to ensure that optimal samples are obtained.

Sputum induction creates a considerable aerosol of potentially infectious material (Dooley et al. 1990). It should therefore be performed in a setting where infection control is of a high standard, or there is minimal risk of transmission to others, e.g., induction performed in an open air setting, away from others.

Should sputum induction be unavailable or unsuccessful, flexible bronchoscopy with bronchoalveolar lavage is indicated. This procedure has the advantage of being able to sample specific sites (and hence in theory improve the recovery from, e.g., localized disease or a cavity) (Schoch et al. 2007). A good-quality sample, which is promptly set up for mycobacterial culture, has a high diagnostic yield (Breen et al. 2008b). This is important because the procedure is associated with significant up-front capital cost, and potential risk to both patients and health-care workers.

Bronchoscopic procedures also enable aspiration and biopsies to be performed. This includes both lung tissue (bronchial biopsies) and needle aspiration under either direct vision or using ultrasound (EBUS) (Navani et al. 2011).

Pulmonary samples can be assessed using acid-fast bacilli (AFB) smear, nucleic acid amplification techniques such as GeneXpert, mycobacterial culture, or cytological analysis. AFB sputum smear is the most long standing, although it is fairly insensitive (requiring at least 5×10^3 bacilli per mL for detection). Molecular diagnostics are equally rapid, more sensitive, and also currently more expensive. They can also detect genetic resistance to antituberculosis drugs (Boehme et al. 2011), and with modification they might distinguish between live and dead bacilli (Honeyborne et al. 2011).

Culture techniques are still regarded as the gold standard. Liquid fluorometric systems are faster than solid media and more sensitive (Dhillon et al. 2014). However, they are also expensive and require skilled personnel to use them. At present, they are not routinely available worldwide for all patient samples that are obtained for suspected TB.

Extrapulmonary Tuberculosis

Extrapulmonary tuberculosis (EPTB) occurs in 10%–42% of adult TB patients depending on race or ethnic background, age, presence or absence of underlying disease, genotype of the *Mtb* strain, and immune status (Caws et al. 2008) (Table 3). EPTB is defined as TB affecting any site other than the lung. Sometimes it is accompanied by pulmonary disease (Public Health England 2014). It can affect any organ in the body and has numerous clinical manifestations, and thus requires a high index of clinical suspicion (Zumla et al. 2013). EPTB can occur many years after exposure. In addition to systemic fea-

Table 3. Frequency of bacteriological culture confirmation of *Mtb* complex among reported tuberculosis cases by site of disease, Germany, 1996–2000

	Culture confirmation		
	Present	Absent	Total
Total	18,501 (70%)	7801	26,302
Pulmonary	15,134 (73%)	5493	20,627
Extrapulmonary	3367 (59%)	2308	5675
Lymphatic, peripheral	859 (51%)	826	1685
Lymphatic, intrathoracic	223 (39%)	352	575
Pleural	579 (55%)	470	1049
Genitourinary	746 (78%)	212	958
Osteoarticular	326 (71%)	131	457
Miliary	126 (69%)	58	184
Meningeal	91 (68%)	42	133
Peritoneal	65 (56%)	51	116
Cutaneous	70 (61%)	45	115
Other	282 (70%)	121	403

[1]Data modified from Forssbohm et al. 2008.
[2]Data are presented as *n* or *n* (%).

tures, patients with EPTB may complain of symptoms related to the involved site/organ. In contrast to pulmonary TB, females are more often affected (one exception to this being pleurisy) (Forssbohm et al. 2008) (Fig. 6). The differences in the proportion of EPTB by area of origin are remarkable. Patients from Africa and Asia are generally far more likely to present with EPTB than those from Germany (Forssbohm et al. 2008); genetic factors may explain some of these differences (Fernando et al. 2007). HIV and other conditions that markedly impair host immunity have led to an increase in extrapulmonary disease. This reflects an inability to contain *Mtb*, and hence dissemination, with positive cultures from a number of body sites, often occurs. The diagnosis can require biopsy and/or surgical removal.

Lymph Node TB

Intrathoracic Lymph Node TB

Intrathoracic lymph node TB is relatively more frequent in children than in adults, usually in association with primary pulmonary TB. It may be noted on the chest radiograph as mediastinal enlargement, sometimes associated with calcification (Fig. 7). The use of CT scanning has shown the relative insensitivity of chest radiographs.

Often, enlarged lymph nodes are present only on one side of the mediastinum, although they may be bilateral. The lymph nodes may become so large that they cause bronchial obstruction and collapse of an adjacent region of the lung. If they perforate into the bronchial tract, this may result in sublobar or lobar pneumonia (Fig. 8). The differential diagnosis includes other infectious etiologies such as nontuberculosis mycobacteria (NTM) and fungal infection, malignancy (lymphoma, lung cancer), sarcoidosis, and silicosis.

The diagnosis can be established by bronchoscopy (Chung and Lee 2000) (Fig. 9), which may be used also as an adjunctive therapeutic measure by removing obstructing intrabronchial lesions or by placement of an intrabronchial stent (Lee et al. 2010). If hilar or mediastinal intrathoracic lymph node involvement is the sole TB manifestation, transbronchial needle aspiration ("blind" TBNA or under ultrasound guidance as EBUS) or mediastinoscopy may establish the etiology. Rapid molecular diagnostic methods have been successfully applied to EBUS-derived lymph node samples (Dhasmana et al. 2014). This provides the op-

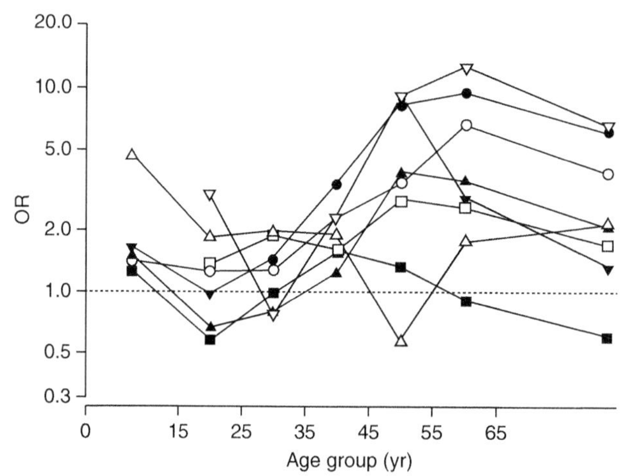

Figure 6. Age-specific female-to-male odds ratio (OR) of having extrapulmonary TB compared with pulmonary TB by site of extrapulmonary TB, Germany 1996–2000. Solid circle, lymphatic, peripheral; open circle, lymphatic intrathoracic; solid square, pleural; open square, genitourinary; solid triangle, osteoarticular; inverted solid triangle, meningeal; inverted open triangle, peritoneal. (Figure reprinted from Forssbohm et al. 2008, with permission, from the European Respiratory Society, © 2008.)

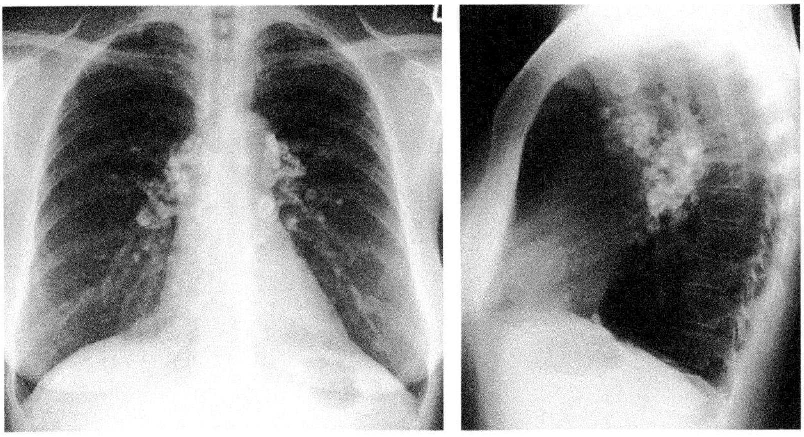

Figure 7. Silicotuberculosis. (Figure reprinted from Fuehner et al. 2007, with permission, from Springer, © 2007.)

portunity to confirm clinically suspected disease promptly and also to obtain samples for drug sensitivity testing.

Extrathoracic Lymph Node TB

Extrathoracic lymph node TB is one of the most frequent EPTB manifestations in adults. In Germany, for example, it accounts for 30% of EPTB (Forssbohm et al. 2008). In most cases, the cervical/supraclavicular (Fig. 10), and more rarely the axillary or inguinal, lymph nodes are in volved.

At first, the lymph nodes are firm, painless, and not warm (Fig. 10), but they may later become fluctuant, matted together, and inflamed. If not treated, they may perforate through the skin and create nonhealing fistulas.

The differential diagnosis includes other infectious etiologies such as NTM and fungal infection, malignancy (lymphoma, [lung] cancer), and sarcoidosis. The diagnosis is established by needle aspiration, occasionally by surgical biopsy.

Tuberculous Pleurisy

Tuberculous pleurisy is one of the most frequent EPTB manifestations. In Germany, it accounts for 19% of EPTB cases (Forssbohm et al. 2008).

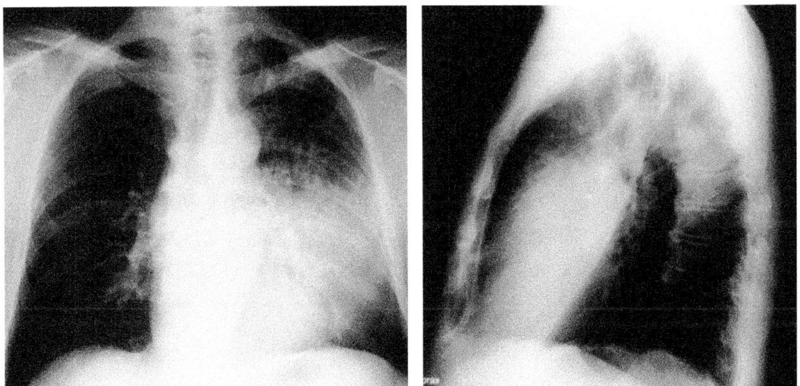

Figure 8. Pneumonia of left upper lobe (lingula) caused by lymph node perforation. (Figure provided by Robert Loddenkemper.)

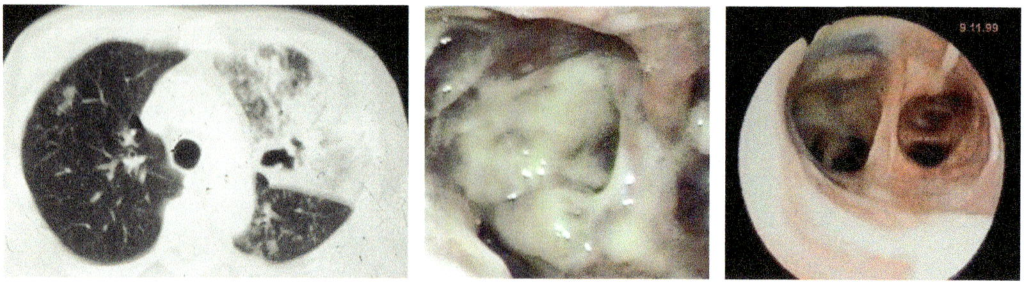

Figure 9. CT of the chest and bronchoscopy showing lymph node perforation, before and after treatment for TB. (Figure provided by Robert Loddenkemper.)

It is more frequent (15%–90%) in HIV coinfection, being seen in patients with higher blood CD4 counts (Gopi et al. 2007). As with pulmonary TB, and contrary to other forms of EPTB, males are more often affected than females. Usually, it occurs in the young; however, in countries with a low TB incidence, pleural disease may develop at older ages as well.

It can present acutely with high fever or as a subacute/chronic illness. Clinical features may start with pleuritic chest pain (dry pleurisy), but the predominant symptom, caused by pleural effusion, is breathlessness. Physical signs of effusion are dullness on percussion and reduced breath sounds at the affected site. The size of the effusion can vary between very small to almost complete involvement of the hemithorax; it is rarely bilateral (Fig. 11). Pulmonary TB changes are present in the minority, but studies have shown that in up to 20%, *Mtb* can be found in sputum (Parimon et al. 2008).

The differential diagnosis includes all causes of pleural effusion. The diagnosis is established by investigation of the pleural fluid and/or by pleural biopsies (closed-needle biopsies or thoracoscopic biopsies [Light 2010]). The diagnosis of pleural TB is hampered by its paucibacillary nature (Chegou et al. 2008). Less than 10% of pleural fluids are smear-positive, and culture is positive in only ~30% (20%–50%) of cases. However, in HIV-positive patients, the fluid is much more likely to be smear- and culture-positive for *Mtb* if the CD4 count is <100 cells/μL (Heydermann et al. 1998). The

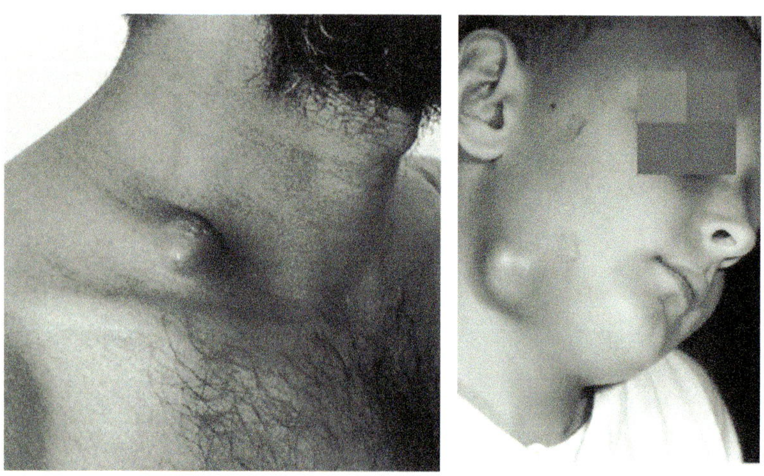

Figure 10. Extrathoracic lymph node disease. (*Left* figure, provided by the authors; *right* figure, reprinted from Siemon 2007, with permission, from Springer, © 2007.)

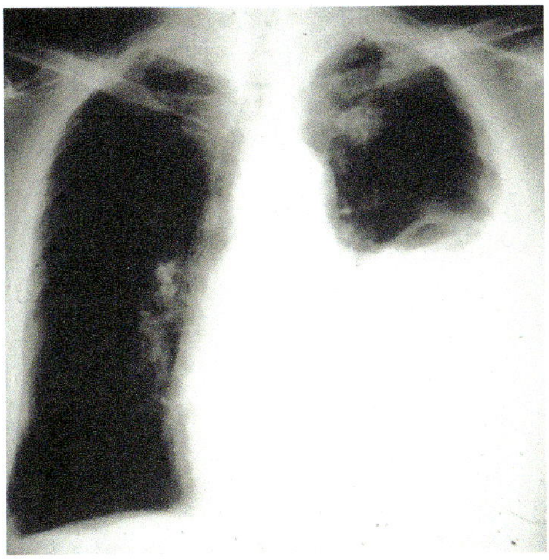

Figure 11. Unilateral large left pleural effusion attributable to tuberculosis. (Figure reprinted from Fuehner et al. 2007 with permission, from Springer, © 2007.)

exudative fluid is, in the majority of cases, predominantly lymphocytic, although in ~10%, mainly polymorphonuclear leukocytes are found (Bielsa et al. 2013).

Several laboratory and microbiological tests have been developed during recent years, including nucleic acid amplification and detection, markers of specific and nonspecific immune response such as adenosine deaminase (ADA), and IGRA. These may help in diagnosing TB as the cause of pleural effusion and have a reasonable high sensitivity and specificity (Trajman et al. 2008; Light 2010). However, at least in countries with a low TB prevalence, the accuracy may not be sufficient in individual cases (Hooper et al. 2009, 2010). The diagnostic yield of closed-needle pleural biopsies, especially under ultrasound guidance, is up to 80% (Diacon et al. 2003; Koegelenberg et al. 2010).

The accuracy of medical thoracoscopy (pleuroscopy) is almost 100%, as the pathologist is provided with multiple biopsies selected under direct vision (Figs. 12 and 13). Culture is therefore more often positive (78% in one study) (Fig. 14), which in turn enables drug susceptibility testing to be performed (Loddenkemper 1998; Loddenkemper et al. 2011).

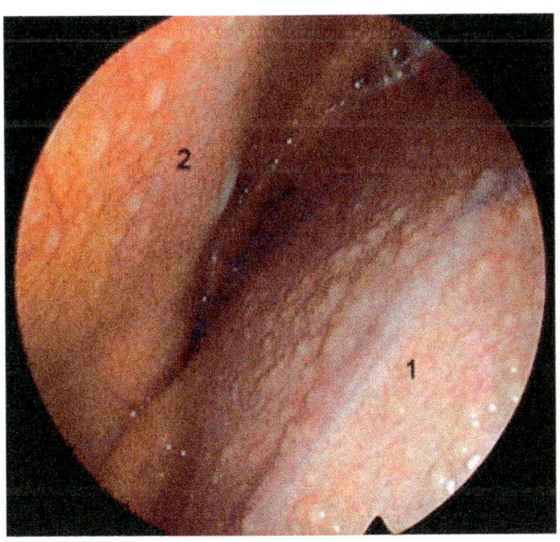

Figure 12. Thoracoscopic image of early TB pleural effusion. Following drainage of 800 mL of serous effusion, typical miliary sago-like nodules in all parts of the right parietal pleura can be seen (1) on the diaphragm and (2) the anterior chest wall. (Figure reprinted from Loddenkemper et al. 2011, with permission, from Thieme, © 2011.)

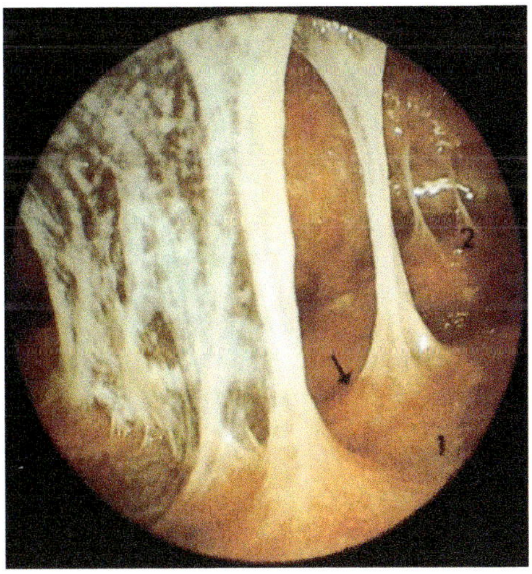

Figure 13. Thoracoscopic image of established TB pleural effusion. Following drainage of 2000 mL of serous effusion, inflamed and hyperemic visceral and parietal pleura covered with fibrinous patches is evident. The posterior costovertebral region is shown with the diaphragm (1) and the chest wall (2). The lung cannot be visualized as it is fibrin-covered. The fibrinous adhesions pull the diaphragm cranially, producing tenting, and show vascularization at their base (arrows). (Figure reprinted from Loddenkemper et al. 2011, with permission, from Thieme, © 2011.)

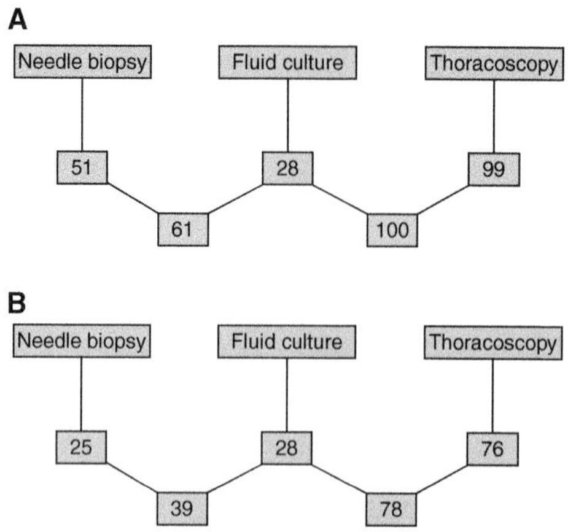

Figure 14. (*A*) Combined histological and bacteriological yield (%) of standard techniques in diagnosis of TB-related pleural effusion. (*B*) Cultural yield (%) of standard techniques in diagnosis of TB-related pleural effusion. (Figure reprinted from Loddenkemper et al. 2011, with permission, from Thieme, © 2011.)

Once again, it cannot be overemphasized that clinicians need to think of TB as a possible cause of pleural effusions—and hence perform appropriate investigations if they wish to make the diagnosis. This is particularly important given that effusions often spontaneously resolve, although the patient is at high risk of recurrence or more widespread disease if they do not receive anti-TB treatment at that stage.

Pleural thickening, trapped lung, and chronic empyema are potential sequelae of tuberculous pleural effusion. However, extensive fibrous pleural changes and tuberculous empyema (Fig. 15) are rare if an early diagnosis is made and appropriate treatment started (Sahn 2002). There are insufficient data to support evidence-based recommendations regarding the use of adjunctive corticosteroids in the treatment of tuberculous pleurisy (Engel et al. 2007; Light 2010). The early removal of pleural fluid may also reduce the long-term impact of residual pleural fibrosis (Chung et al. 2008; Light 2010).

Bone/Joints

TB affecting the bones and/or joints is one of the most frequent EPTB manifestations in adults. In Germany, skeletal TB accounts for 8% of EPTB cases (Forssbohm et al. 2008), although in high-incidence countries, it is much more common. It presents usually several (5–7) years after the primary pulmonary infection (Wallgren 1948).

The spine is involved in almost half of skeletal TB cases (Pott's disease). This starts as inflammation of the intervertebral disk, most often in the lower thoracic and upper lumbar vertebrae, and later involves typically two adja-

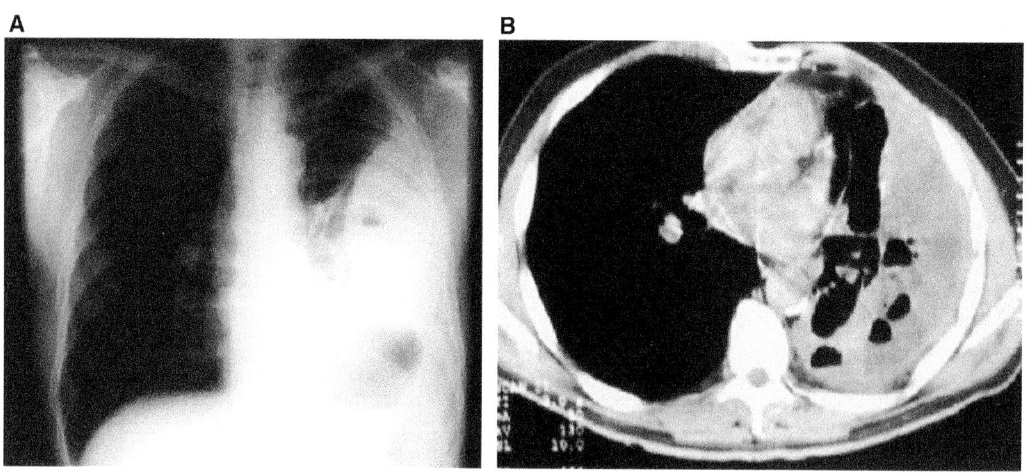

Figure 15. Tuberculous pleural empyema. (Figure reprinted from Siemon 2007, with permission, from Springer, © 2007.)

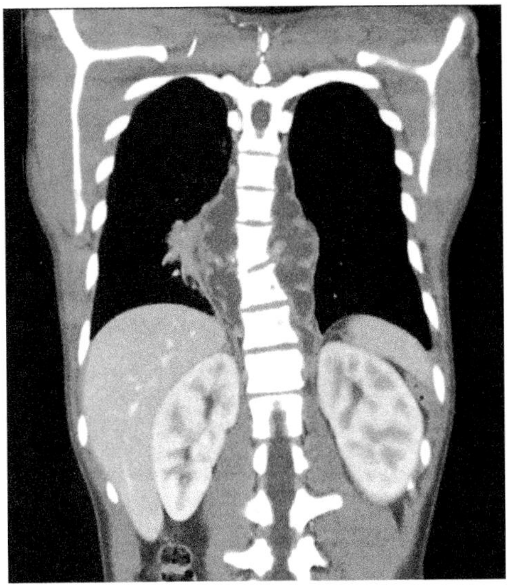

Figure 16. Coronal CT image of young male with back pain, fever, and weight loss with tuberculous paraspinal abscess secondary to vertebral involvement. (Figure provided by Marc Lipman.)

cent vertebrae and the intervertebral disk (Jain and Dhammi 2007). The most common first symptom is slowly progressive, often over weeks and months, back pain with occasionally associated abdominal pain. Local tenderness on palpation may be present. At later stages, kyphoscoliosis or even a gibbus may develop. Spinal cord or nerve root compression with sensory or motor symptoms, even paraplegia, can occur. A paraspinal abscess may develop within the psoas muscle and cause pain in the groin, in particular, on hip flexion. However, paraspinal collections can be seen at any site within the vertebral column (Fig. 16). Modern imaging techniques such as CT, MRI, and bone scan have considerably enhanced the diagnostic work up. Whole-spine imaging is recommended as multiple vertebral sites are involved in up to 50% of cases (Fig. 17). The differential diagnosis includes other infectious etiologies such as chronic bacterial infection, NTM, and malignancy (lymphoma, [lung] cancer). The diagnosis is established by open surgical or needle biopsy for both culture and cytology/histology. Surgical treatment may be indicated (e.g., using external fixation) if there is clear vertebral collapse or destruction or increasing pain suggesting imminent risk of spinal cord or nerve root compression (Fig. 18).

In other bones and joints, the metaphyses of long bones are the most common sites of TB, but hips, knees, shoulders, elbows (Fig. 19), ankles, wrists, or any other bone or joint may be involved (Watts and Lifeso 1996). The diagnosis is established by open surgical or needle biopsy with culture and histology.

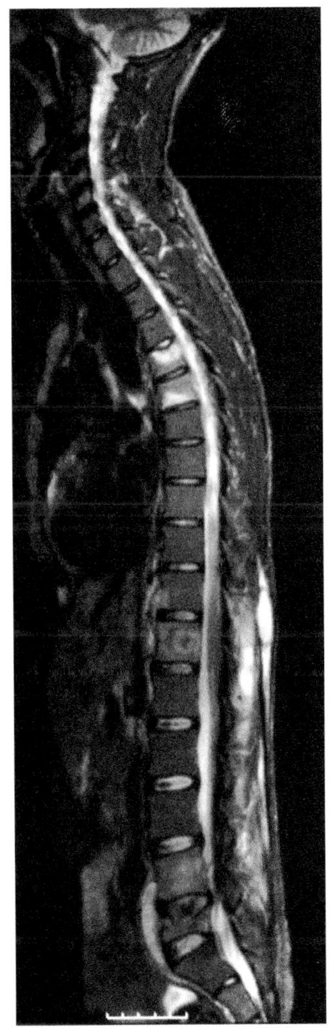

Figure 17. Spinal tuberculosis. Whole-spine MRI showing abnormal signal at multiple vertebral levels within cervical, thoracic, and lumbar spine, plus anterior paraspinal collections at sites of disease. (Figure provided by Marc Lipman.)

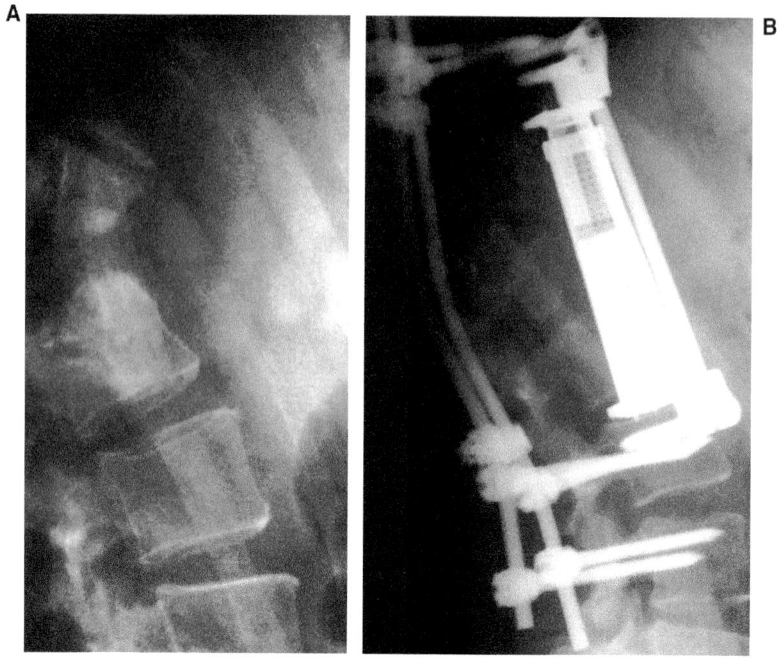

Figure 18. Spinal tuberculosis. (*A*) Destruction of vertebrae after tuberculous spondylitis; (*B*) treatment with external fixator. (Figure reprinted from Siemon 2007, with permission, from Springer, © 2007.)

Genitourinary System

Genitourinary system disease includes TB of the kidney, ureter, bladder, and the male and female genital tract (Cek et al. 2005; Kulchavenya 2013). In Germany, it is a frequent extrapulmonary manifestation in adults and accounts for 17% of such cases (Forssbohm et al. 2008). This is in marked contrast to the United Kingdom, where it is responsible for ~3% (Public Health England 2014). A variety of local symptoms can develop depending on the involved organ, usually many years after the primary infection. Systemic symptoms are less common. Many patients are asymptomatic, and TB may only be detected by urinalysis of pyuria with no apparent bacterial growth. This occurs in >90% of cases. Around 50% will have evidence of previous or active TB present on the chest radiograph (Wilberschied et al. 1999).

Urological TB can cause destruction of the involved kidney, usually unilateral, perinephric or psoas abscess, and/or may lead to stenosis of the ureter and/or involvement of the bladder with cystitis, often accompanied by hematuria.

TB of the female genital system presents as tubal or endometrial involvement (endometritis) causing pelvic pain and/or menorrhagia and may cause infertility. The ovaries (adnexitis) can be involved also, and this may mimic an ovarian cancer (Fig. 20). The diagnosis is established by image-guided needle biopsy, laparoscopy, or open surgical biopsy. TB of the vulva is uncommon.

TB of the male genital system presents mainly as involvement of the scrotum (epididymitis, orchitis), but the prostate may be affected as well. The diagnosis is established by image-guided needle biopsy or open surgical biopsy.

In some patients, mostly caused by late diagnosis, medical treatment may not result in the resolution of symptoms. Thus, additional surgical intervention and reconstruction may be indicated (Kulchavenya 2013).

Abdomen

Abdominal TB includes involvement of the peritoneum with ascites or any intra-abdominal

 Cite this article as *Cold Spring Harb Perspect Med* doi: 10.1101/cshperspect.a017848

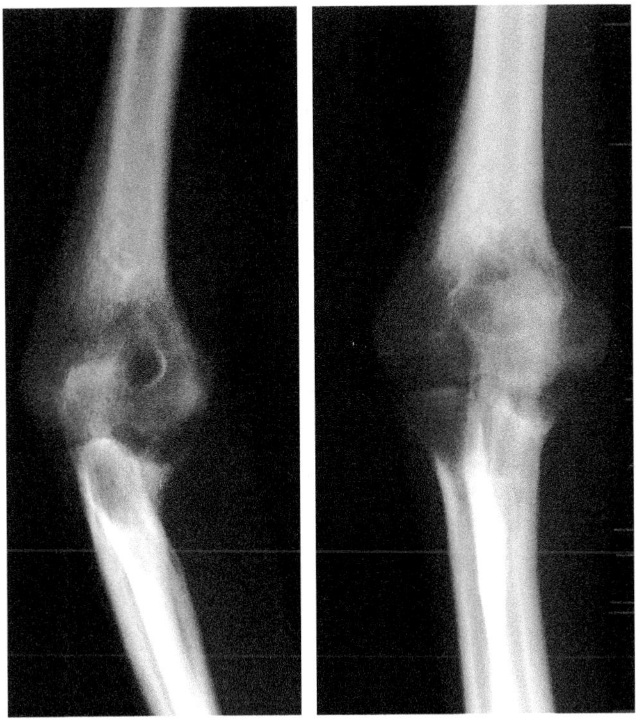

Figure 19. Tuberculosis of the elbow joint. Bone loss is present at the distal humerus, its epidondyles, and also the olecranon and coronoidal process of the ulna. (Figure reprinted from Siemon 2007, with permission, from Springer, © 2007.)

organ (Tan et al. 2009). This has become rare in low-incidence countries; in Germany, it accounts for 2% of EPTB cases (Forssbohm et al. 2008). Although elsewhere, such as the Indian subcontinent and countries (e.g., the United Kingdom) that see TB relatively frequently in these populations, it is more common. Infection can result from swallowing sputum or nonpasteurized milk (*Mycobacterium bovis*) or by hematogenous spread. In the gut, TB may occur in any location from the mouth to the anus, although is most often in the ileum and cecum.

Abdominal pain occurs frequently, sometimes mimicking acute appendicitis. Other presentations include small bowel obstruction or gastrointestinal bleeding. The liver, spleen (Fig. 21), pancreas, and adrenal glands may all be involved. In the latter case, the presentation can be one of insidious adrenal insufficiency, in which patients report lethargy or are noted to have metabolic derangements on blood testing.

The differential diagnosis (Khan et al. 2006) depends on the organs involved and includes other infectious etiologies, malignancy (Fig. 22), and inflammatory bowel disease (Almadi et al. 2009). Tuberculous peritonitis with ascites results in abdominal swelling often accompanied by acute symptoms of fever, anorexia, and weight loss. The final diagnosis is established by investigation of the ascitic fluid, which apart from cytology and mycobacterial smear, molecular diagnostics, and culture, may be tested for adenosine deaminase (Shen et al. 2013) and using IGRA (Chou et al. 2011). Laparoscopy, open surgical biopsy, or colonoscopy (Sanai and Bzeizi 2005) may need to be performed, and the diagnosis of TB of other abdominal organs is often made following surgical biopsy or tissue sampling guided by ultrasound or CT.

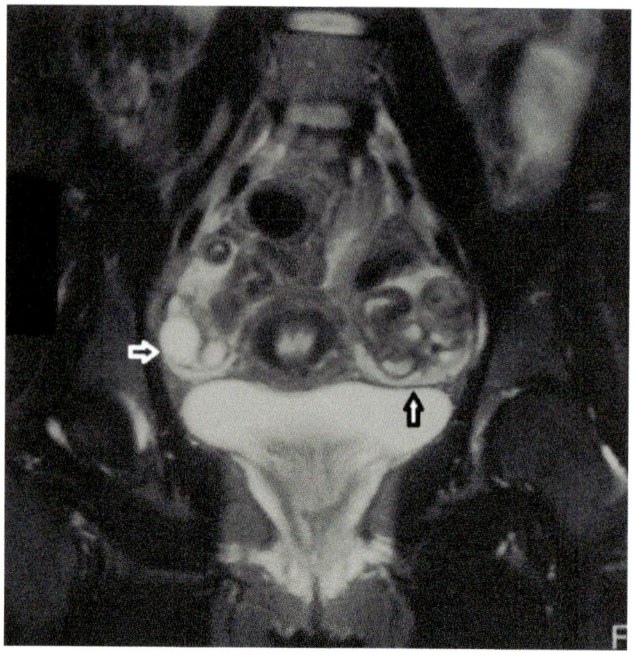

Figure 20. Coronal MRI showing TB of the left ovary (black arrow from caudal). Right ovary (white arrow from lateral) with cystic enlarged follicles. (Figure reprinted from Siemon 2007, with permission, from Springer, © 2007.)

Central Nervous System

TB of the central nervous system (CNS) includes tuberculous meningitis (TBM) (the most common manifestation) and encephalitis with or without cerebral tuberculomas (Fig. 23). CNS disease is often seen as part of a disseminated illness, with radiological evidence of, for example, miliary TB on chest imaging (see below). It has become rare in low-TB-incidence countries, and in Germany, it accounts for 2% of EPTB cases in adults (Forssbohm et al. 2008). Headache is the predominant local symptom. Others include a decreased level of consciousness, sei-

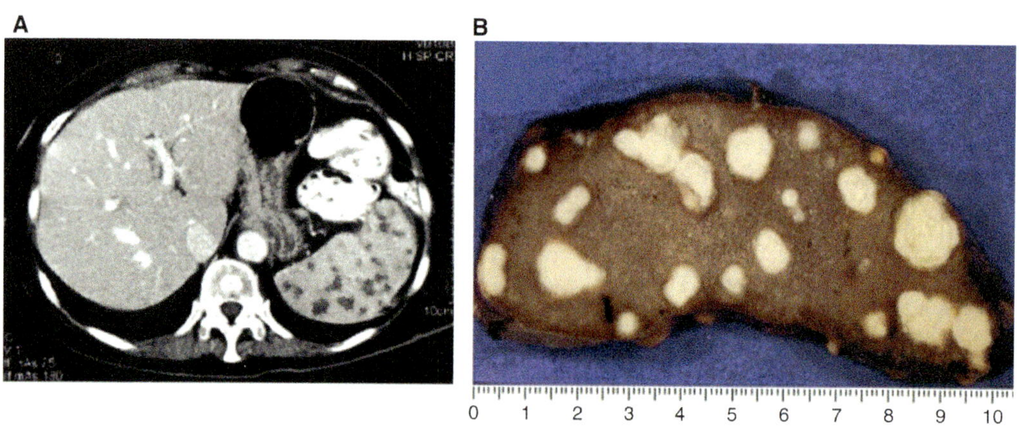

Figure 21. Splenic tuberculomas. (Figure reprinted from Siemon 2007, with permission, from Springer, © 2007.)

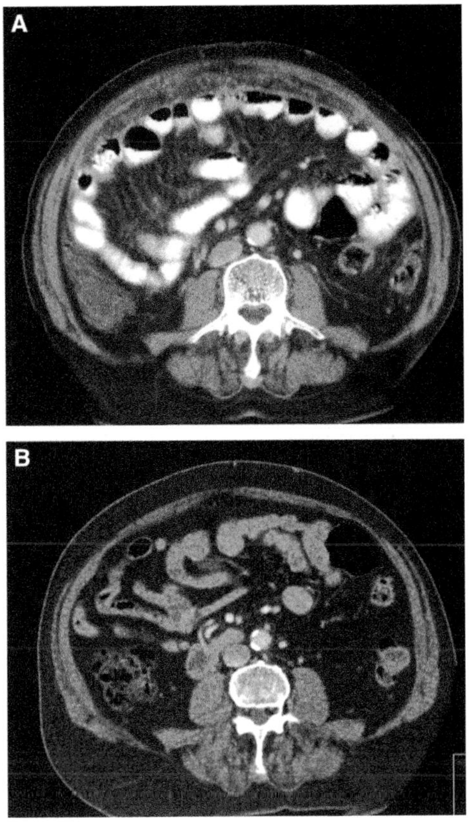

Figure 22. Abdominal TB attributable to TB. Pain and weight loss in an Indian male initially considered to result from disseminated abdominal malignancy. CT abdomen: (*A*) Pretreatment peritoneal and mesenteric thickening leading to omental "cake" (note oral contrast given); (*B*) posttreatment normal peritoneum and mesentery (no oral contrast given). (Figure provided by Marc Lipman.)

zures, neck stiffness, vomiting, and those attributable to involvement of cranial nerves. Spinal meningitis with involvement of the peripheral nerves and even paraplegia can occur (Thwaites et al. 2009). The severity of TBM at presentation is strongly associated with prognosis. Various factors and scoring models have been developed to predict the outcomes of TBM, and these are used in the evaluation of different treatment regimens (Chou et al. 2010).

Severe complications include cerebral and spinal cord infarction from granulomatous arteritis, midbrain and the brain stem involvement with loss of automatic, involuntary function, as well as the development of hydrocephalus requiring short- and long-term intervention. The pressure effects of an abscess or granuloma in the CNS may be catastrophic. This should be considered during both investigation and subsequent treatment of patients with "high-risk" lesions in, for example, the brain substance or spinal cord (Thwaites et al. 2009).

The differential diagnosis includes other infectious etiologies of meningitis. The diagnosis is established by lumbar puncture and investigation of the spinal fluid (Thwaites et al. 2009). Highly suspicious is a cerebrospinal fluid (CSF) leucocytosis (predominantly lymphocytes) and raised protein and low-glucose values. The diagnosis is hampered by its paucibacillary nature, but it may be enhanced by simple modification of the Ziehl-Neelsen stain and an ESAT-6 intracellular stain (Feng et al. 2014). The sensitivity is improved using the Xpert MTB/RIF (Nhu et al. 2014). Rapid techniques based on nucleic acid amplification such as polymerase chain reaction (PCR) are more sensitive and specific as they detect specific DNA sequences of the organism (Thwaites et al. 2004a; Galimi 2011; Nhu et al.

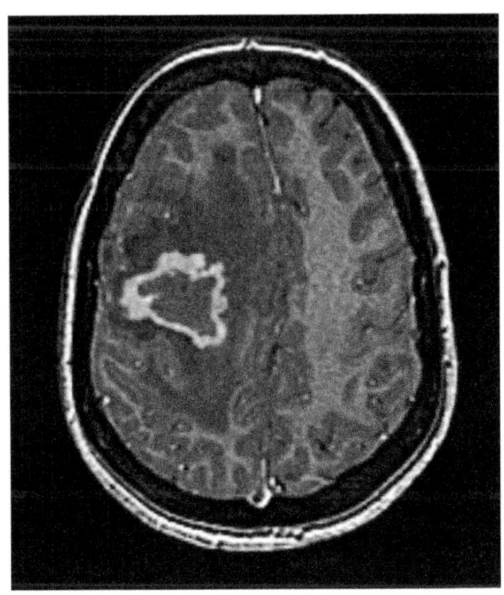

Figure 23. CNS tuberculoma. MRI brain with contrast shows enhancing lesion with associated edema and mass effect in a Somali female presenting with headache and a seizure. Biopsy-cultured *Mtb* (Figure provided by Marc Lipman.)

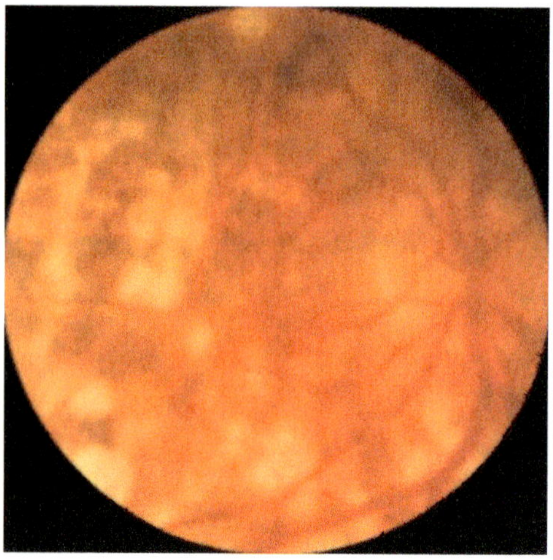

Figure 24. Retinal tuberculous lesions. (Figure reprinted from Siemon 2007, with permission, from Springer, © 2007.)

2014). CT-guided needle biopsies or open surgery may be needed for the diagnosis of tuberculomas (DeLance et al. 2013). MRI will show generally more lesions than CT (Bernaerts et al. 2003), although in many parts of the world, access to MRI is restricted and, although there is a greater radiation exposure, CT may be preferable if serial imaging is required during follow up.

Fundoscopic examination of the eye can reveal evidence of both anterior and posterior chamber disease (Gupta et al. 2007). Apart from presumed inflammatory responses to mycobacterial antigen (e.g., phlyctenular conjunctivitis, episcleritis, and anterior uveitis), papilloedema may be present in patients with CNS involvement. Choroidal tubercles can be visualized—and are helpful in the diagnosis of disseminated TB (Fig. 24).

Apart from specific anti-TB therapy, adjunctive corticosteroids (either dexamethasone or prednisolone) should be given to all patients with TBM, regardless of disease severity and HIV status (Thwaites et al. 2004b). Surgical shunting should be considered early in the patient with hydrocephalus and symptoms of raised intracranial pressure. Other neurosurgical operations may be indicated in patients with seizures or brain or spinal cord compression (DeLance et al. 2013).

Miliary TB

Disseminated TB can involve any number of organs (Zumla et al. 2013). Hematogenous spread, when it includes the lungs, is often characterized by the radiological feature of a "miliary" pattern on imaging. This was first described in chest radiographs (where the numerous granulomas were felt to resemble millet seed, i.e., 1–4-mm rounded opacities scattered throughout both lungs), although is also applicable to CT imaging (Fig. 25). In Germany, it

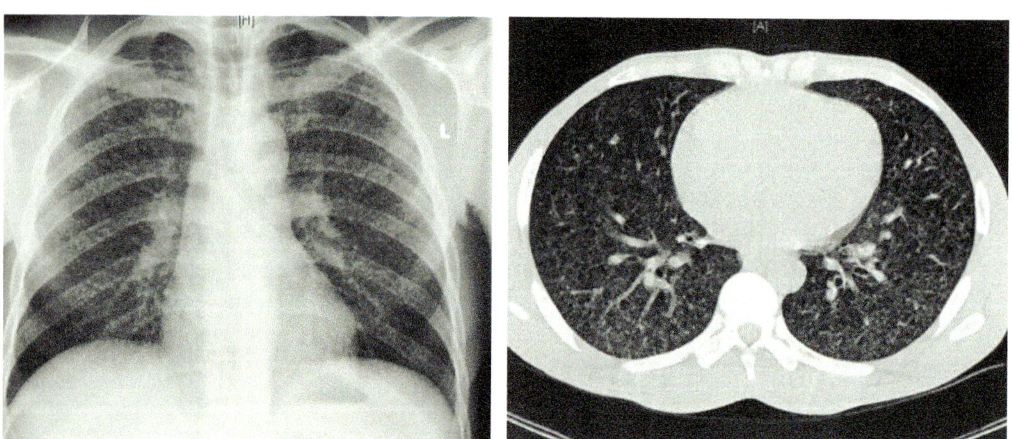

Figure 25. Miliary TB on chest radiograph and CT. (Figure reprinted from Fuehner et al. 2007, with permission, from Springer, © 2007.)

accounts for 3% of EPTB cases (Forssbohm et al. 2008).

The differential diagnosis of this radiographic appearance includes other infections (e.g., fungi, nocardia and healed varicella pneumonia) as well as malignancy (in particular, thyroid, breast, and renal cancers, plus melanoma and osteosarcoma) and conditions that result in granulomas) (e.g., sarcoidosis). Hence, clinicians must ensure that a diagnosis of miliary TB is based on as much laboratory information as possible (Ray et al. 2013) and that patients who are started on anti-TB treatment are carefully monitored for response and/or the development of new symptoms and signs. Patients may develop an acute respiratory distress syndrome (ARDS) associated with a high mortality despite intensive care (Erbes et al. 2006; Lee et al. 2011). The benefit of adjunctive corticosteroid administration in patients with miliary TB is unclear (Ray et al. 2013).

OTHER TB MANIFESTATIONS

TB can present at any body site. Therefore, clinicians should consider sending samples for mycobacterial molecular analysis, smear, and culture, as well as histo- or cytopathology. This situation occurs most frequently when patients present either with cutaneous disease (typically nonhealing lesions that have been treated for some time with standard antibacterials) (Fig. 26) or to breast, or ear, nose, and throat surgeons. In Germany, other TB manifestations account for 9% of all extrapulmonary TB cases (Forssbohm et al. 2008).

TB pericarditis is a globally important condition with a distinctly poor prognosis if not diagnosed promptly (Fig. 27). It is usually seen as an active acute or subacute condition associated with systemic features plus a pericardial effusion, which may lead to tamponade (Syed and Mayosi 2007). Adjunctive treatment with corticosteroids is recommended (Evans 2008). Constrictive pericarditis secondary to pericardial calcification can also occur (Fig. 28). Here, the initial (primary) infection is thought to have occurred several years earlier and was often asymptomatic. Over time, the patient notices increasing exercise limitation, yet even then may present to health-care services with apparent acute clinical decompensation.

The calcification associated with TB is generally thick, confluent, and irregular, although these features cannot be relied on. CT or MRI are useful investigations but should not detract from efforts to isolate or detect an organism (which may be from other sites including the lung). This may be unsuccessful (particularly with the chronic presentation). The patient will often have a history of exposure to TB, usually from having spent time as a child in a TB-endemic country. Anti-TB treatment should be given, in addition to cardiac and sur-

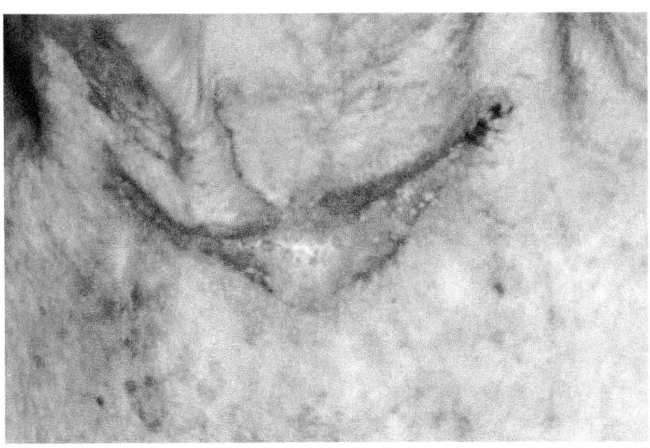

Figure 26. Tracheo-cutaneous fistula with scrofuloderma. (Figure reprinted from Siemon 2007, with permission, from Springer, © 2007.)

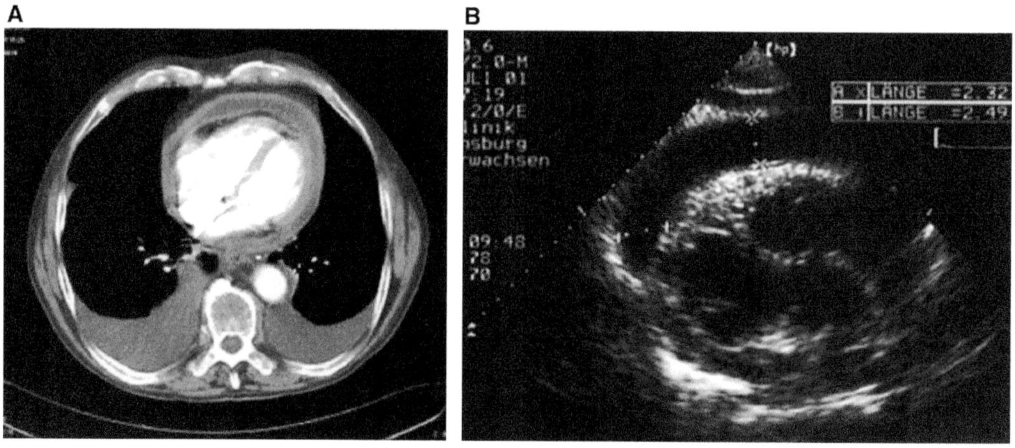

Figure 27. Tuberculous pericarditis with bilateral pleural effusions. (*A*) CT; (*B*) echocardiography. (Figure reprinted from Siemon 2007, with permission, from Springer, © 2007.)

gical management as needed (Syed and Mayosi 2007).

TREATMENT OF TB

The diagnosis of active TB (and hence the decision to start anti-TB drug therapy without which the great majority of cases will not be cured) uses information derived from the mycobacteria (e.g., positive AFB smear, molecular diagnostic test or culture), a compatible host response (e.g., cavitation on a chest radiograph), and environmental factors (e.g., a history of contact with TB in a person with consistent clinical features, or acquisition of HIV infection leading to altered [and impaired] immunity).

Prompt initiation of treatment will reduce morbidity and mortality for the affected indi-

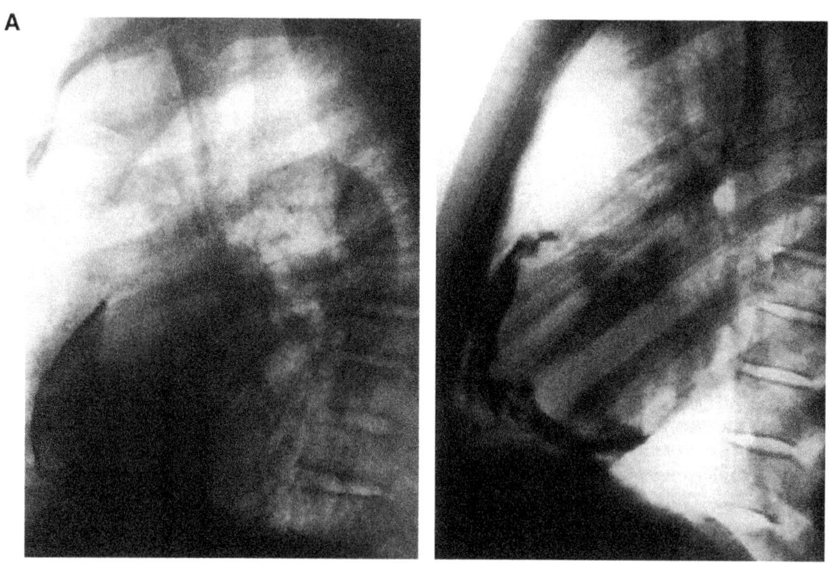

Figure 28. Calcification after tuberculous pericarditis. (Figure reprinted from Uehlinger et al. 1959, with permission, from EMH Schweizer Ärzteverlag, © 1959.)

vidual and also break the cycle of onward transmission that sustains TB. However, treatment is not without its complications. This is most evident in the management of HIV-associated TB (Khan et al. 2010; Schutz et al. 2010), in which there are considerable drug–drug interactions between antiretrovirals and anti-TB medication, and an increased risk of the intense inflammatory response provoked by concurrent use of these drugs (IRIS) (Meintjes et al. 2008). This means that in practice, the relative timing of introduction of these agents also needs to be factored (Blanc et al. 2011; Török et al. 2011).

Drug treatment is dealt with in more detail in other sections of this book. However, some of the key principles are described in brief here. Effective treatment is one that enables the individual to complete therapy and results in a very high cure rate and minimal risk of relapse owing to the original infection. Thus, drug therapy needs to be efficacious and have few adverse events (Breen et al. 2006). Both of these will maximize adherence to treatment regimens. However, factors such as duration of treatment, pill burden, cost of therapy, and even ensuring that the patient can access a sustained and secure supply of medication (Capstick et al. 2011) will impact on treatment effectiveness. Hence, at both a personal and a societal level, high-quality treatment programs must ensure that safe and effective drug supplies are available and that a TB service can provide regular monitoring with facilities that optimize the patient's ability to adhere to the prescribed regimen.

Therapeutic combinations should, if at all possible, be based on known sensitivity of the organism to the selected drugs (World Health Organization 2011). The increasing prevalence of drug resistance (World Health Organization 2013) and the ease of global travel mean that no longer can clinicians assume that the infecting organism is likely to be drug-sensitive. This emphasizes the importance of obtaining pretreatment samples for rapid molecular diagnostics and culture, both of which can indicate likely drug sensitivity and hence guide early and ongoing treatment (Mooreet al. 2011).

In presumed drug-sensitive disease, treatment should commence with a minimum of three effective drugs. In practice, this means a four-drug therapy with a rifamycin plus isoniazid as well as pyrazinamide and ethambutol for the first 2 mo (by which point, drug susceptibility should be known for any positive *Mtb* cultures). It can never be assumed that prescribing medication equates to the patient actually taking it, and arrangements must be in place to ensure that adequate treatment support and supervision are available for the duration of therapy.

On-treatment monitoring of individual response may use strategies such as directly observed therapy (Okanurak et al. 2007), pill counts, and urine tests, plus measures of patient characteristics that reflect disease alleviation, e.g., weight gain (Khan et al. 2006) and health status (Kruijshaar et al. 2010).

People on treatment for pulmonary TB can be followed with serial sputum cultures. However, in resource-rich environments, individuals often stop producing sputum within a few weeks of starting an effective treatment regimen (Hales et al. 2013). In cases in which there is doubt regarding adherence with medication or possible treatment failure, it is recommended that the patient be evaluated for therapeutic compliance, pharmacodynamics (e.g., is there any possibility of malabsorption?), drug resistance, or an alternative diagnosis.

The importance of close liaison with other experienced clinicians and microbiologists, as well as public health officials within the setting of a multidisciplinary team meeting or through the use of regular cohort reviews (Anderson et al. 2014), cannot be overemphasized. These provide optimal care for the individual and strengthen public health management of TB and are also an excellent method of education and training for all individuals involved in TB care (Migliori et al. 2012).

The diagnosis of TB enables health-care services to provide more than just treatment for TB. HIV testing should be routinely offered—with studies showing that "opt out" testing in TB clinics is a simple method of achieving this (Roy et al. 2013). Screening for other blood-borne viruses such as hepatitis B and C, as well as assessing nutritional status, blood pressure, blood sugar, and encouraging smoking cessation, can also be highlighted during clinical care as part of a package of person-related health management.

CONCLUSION

Given the generally excellent response to treatment if therapy is started early, there is now little excuse for "missed diagnoses" and "late presentations" of TB. It remains a condition that in many parts of the world is common and hence usually promptly diagnosed. Here, the clinical issues often center on the need to ensure that correct, effective medication is prescribed and adverse events are minimized. However, in environments where TB is less frequently seen, the recognition that it can present in multiple ways and that TB must be considered early (by both the patient and their health-care provider) within the clinical diagnostic algorithm are of paramount importance. This is made more complex by the increasing numbers of immunocompromised individuals (through, e.g., HIV infection and medical treatments) at risk of developing active TB who, by virtue of their altered host response, will often have a modified presentation of TB disease. Strategies to combat the loss of familiarity with TB in low TB burden areas include the use of clinical networks and multidisciplinary and multiprofessional team working, plus on-going, relevant education in at-risk communities, the general public, and health-care workers.

REFERENCES

Aït-Khaled N, Alarcón E, Armengol R, Bissell K, Boillot F, Caminero JA, Chiang C-Y, Clevenbergh P, Dlodlo R, Enarson DA, et al. 2010. Management of tuberculosis: A guide to the essentials of good practice. Paris, France, *International Union Against Tuberculosis and Lung Disease (The Union)* http://www.theunion.org/what-we-do/publications/technical/english/pub_orange-guide_eng.pdf

Almadi MA, Ghosh S, Aljebreen AM. 2009. Differentiating intestinal tuberculosis from Crohn's disease: A diagnostic challenge. *Am J Gastroenterol* **104:** 1003–1012.

Anderson C, White J, Abubakar I, Lipman M, Tamne S, Anderson SR, deKoningh J, Dart S. 2014. Raising standards in UK TB control: Introducing cohort review. *Thorax* **69:** 187–189.

Bernaerts A, Vanhoenacker FM, Parizel PM, Van Goethem JW, Van Altena R, Laridon A, De Roeck J, Coeman V, De Schepper AM. 2003. Tuberculosis of the central nervous system: Overview of neuroradiological findings. *Eur Radiol* **13:** 1876–1890.

Bhat VK, Latha P, Upadhya D, Hegde J. 2009. Clinicopathological review of tubercular laryngitis in 32 cases of pulmonary Kochs. *Am J Otolaryngol* **30:** 327–330.

Bielsa S, Palma R, Pardina M, Esquerda A, Light RW, Porcel JM. 2013. Comparison of polymorphonuclear- and lymphocyte-rich tuberculous pleural effusions. *Int J Tuberc Lung Dis* **17:** 85–89.

Blanc FX, Sok T, Laureillard D, Borand L, Rekacewicz C, Nerrienet E, Madec Y, Marcy O, Chan S, Prak N, et al. 2011. Earlier versus later start of antiretroviral therapy in HIV-infected adults with tuberculosis. *N Engl J Med* **365:** 1471–1481.

Blasi F, Matteelli A. 2013. Indicator condition-guided HIV testing in Europe: A step forward to HIV control. *Eur Respir J* **42:** 572–575.

Boehme CC, Nicol MP, Nabeta P, Michael JS, Gotuzzo E, Tahirli R, Tarcela Gler M, Blakemore R, Worodria W, Gray C, et al. 2011. Feasibility, diagnostic accuracy, and effectiveness of decentralised use of the Xpert MTB/RIF test for diagnosis of tuberculosis and multidrug resistance: A multicentre implementation study. *Lancet* **377:** 1495–1505.

Borgdorff MW, Nagelkerke NJ, Dye C, Nunn P. 2000. Gender and tuberculosis: A comparison of prevalence surveys with notification data to explore sex differences in case detection. *Int J Tuberc Lung Dis* **4:** 123–132.

Breen RAM, Smith CJ, Cropley I, Johnson MA, Lipman MCI. 2005. Does immune reconstitution syndrome promote active tuberculosis in patients receiving HAART? *AIDS* **19:** 1201–1206.

Breen RAM, Miller RF, Gorsuch T, Smith CJ, Schwenk A, Holmes W, Ballinger J, Swaden L, Johnson MA, Cropley I, et al. 2006. Adverse events and treatment interruption in tuberculosis patients with and without HIV co-infection. *Thorax* **61:** 791–794.

Breen RAM, Leonard O, Perrin FMR, Smith CJ, Bhagani S, Cropley I, Lipman MCI. 2008a. How good are systemic symptoms and blood inflammatory markers in detecting individuals with active tuberculosis? A prospective UK cohort study. *Int J Tuberc Lung Dis* **12:** 44–49.

Breen RA, Barry SM, Smith CJ, Shorten RJ, Dilworth JP, Cropley I, McHugh TD, Gillespie SH, Janossy G, Lipman MC. 2008b. Clinical application of a rapid lung-orientated immunoassay in individuals with possible tuberculosis. *Thorax* **63:** 67–71.

Brown M, Varia H, Bassett P, Davidson RN, Wall R, Pasvol G. 2007. Prospective study of sputum induction, gastric washing, and bronchoalveolar lavage for the diagnosis of pulmonary tuberculosis in patients who are unable to expectorate. *Clin Infect Dis* **44:** 1415–1420.

Cain KP, McCarthy KD, Heilig CM, Monkongdee P, Tasaneeyapan T, Kanara N, Kimerling ME, Chheng P, Thai S, Sar B, et al. 2010. An algorithm for tuberculosis screening and diagnosis in people with HIV. *N Engl J Med* **362:** 707–716.

Capstick T, Laycock D, Lipman M. 2011. Treatment interruptions and inconsistent supply of anti-TB drugs in the UK. *Int J Tuberc Lung Dis* **15:** 754–760.

Caws M, Thwaites G, Dunstan S, Hawn TR, Lan NT, Thuong NT, Stepniewska K, Huyen MN, Bang ND, Loc TH, et al. 2008. The influence of host and bacterial genotype on the development of disseminated disease with *Mycobacterium tuberculosis*. *PLoS Pathog* **4:** e1000034.

Cek M, Lenk S, Naber KG , Bishop MC, Johansen TE, Botto H, Grabe M, Lobel B, Redorta JP, Tenke P. 2005. Members of the Urinary Tract Infection (UTI) Working Group of the European Association of Urology (EAU) Guidelines Office. EAU guidelines for the management of genitourinary tuberculosis. *Eur Urol* **48:** 353–362.

Chegou NN, Walzl G, Bolliger CT, Diacon AH, van den Heuvel MM. 2008. Evaluation of adapted whole-blood interferon-γ release assays for the diagnosis of pleural tuberculosis. *Respiration* **76:** 131–138.

Chou CH, Lin GM, Ku CH, Chang FY. 2001. Comparison of the APACHE II, GCS and MRC scores in predicting outcomes in patients with tuberculous meningitis. *Int J Tuberc Lung Dis* **14:** 86–92.

Chou OH, Park KH, Park SJ, Kim SM, Park SY, Moon SM, Chong YP, Kim MN, Lee SO, Choi SH, et al. 2011. Rapid diagnosis of tuberculous peritonitis by T cell-based assays on peripheral blood and peritoneal fluid mononuclear cells. *J Infect* **62:** 462–471.

Chowdhury AM, Bhuiya A, Chowdhury ME, Rasheed S, Hussain Z, Chen LC. 2013. The Bangladesh paradox: Exceptional health achievement despite economic poverty. *Lancet* **382:** 1734–1745.

Chung HS, Lee JH. 2000. Bronchoscopic assessment of the evolution of endobronchial tuberculosis. *Chest* **117:** 385–392.

Chung CL, Chen CH, Yeh CY, Sheu JR, Chang SC. 2008. Early effective drainage in the treatment of loculated tuberculosis pleurisy. *Eur Respir J* **31:** 1261–1267.

Courtwright A, Turner AN. 2010. Tuberculosis and stigmatization: Pathways and interventions. *Public Health Rep* **125:** 434–442.

Craig SE, Bettinson H, Sabin CA, Gillespie SH, Lipman MC. 2009. Think TB! Is the diagnosis of pulmonary tuberculosis delayed by antibiotics? *Int J Tuberc Lung Dis* **13:** 208–213.

Crump JA, Ramadhani HO, Morrissey AB, Saganda W, Mwako MS, Yang LY, Chow SC, Njau BN, Mushi GS, Maro VP, et al. 2012. Bacteremic disseminated tuberculosis in sub-Saharan Africa: A prospective cohort study. *Clin Infect Dis* **55:** 242–250.

DeLance AR, Safaee M, Oh MC, Clark AJ, Kaur G, Sun MZ, Bollen AW, Phillips JJ, Parsa AT. 2013. Tuberculoma of the central nervous system. *J Clin Neurosci* **20:** 1333–1341.

de la Rua-Domenech R. 2006. Human *Mycobacterium bovis* infection in the United Kingdom: Incidence, risks, control measures and review of the zoonotic aspects of bovine tuberculosis. *Tuberculosis (Edinb)* **86:** 77–109.

Dhasmana DJ, Ross C, Bradley CJ, Connell DW, George PM, Singanayagam A, Jepson A, Craig C, Wright C, Molyneaux PL, et al. 2014. Performance of Xpert MTB/RIF in the diagnosis of tuberculous mediastinal lymphadenopathy by endobronchial ultrasound. *Ann Am Thorac Soc* **11:** 392–396.

Dhillon J, Fourie PB, Mitchison DA. 2014. Persister populations of *Mycobacterium tuberculosis* in sputum that grow in liquid but not on solid culture media. *J Antimicrob Chemother* **69:** 437–440.

Diacon AH, Van de Wal BW, Wyser C, Smedema JP, Bezuidenhout J, Bolliger CT, Walzl G. 2003. Diagnostic tools in tuberculous pleurisy: A direct comparative study. *Eur Respir J* **22:** 589–591.

Diel R, Loddenkemper R, Zellweger JP, Sotgiu G, D'Ambrosio L, Centis R, van der Werf MJ, Dara M, Detjen A, Gondrie P, et al. 2013. Old ideas to innovate TB control: Preventive treatment to achieve elimination. *Eur Respir J* **42:** 785–801.

Dooley SW Jr, Castro KG, Hutton MD, Mullan RJ, Polder JA, Snider DE Jr. 1990. Guidelines for preventing the transmission of tuberculosis in health-care settings, with special focus on HIV-related issues. *MMWR Recomm Rep* **39:** 1–29.

Elliott AM, Hayes RJ, Halwiindi B, Luo N, Tembo G, Pobee JO, Nunn PP, McAdam KP. 1993. The impact of HIV on infectiousness of pulmonary tuberculosis: A community study in Zambia. *AIDS* **7:** 981–987.

Engel ME, Matchaba PT, Volmink J. 2007. Corticosteroids for tuberculous pleurisy. *Cochrane Database Syst Rev* **17:** CD001876.

Erbes R, Oettel K, Raffenberg M, Mauch H, Schmidt-Ioanas M, Lode H. 2006. Characteristics and outcome of patients with active pulmonary tuberculosis requiring intensive care. *Eur Respir J* **27:** 1223–1228.

Evans DJ. 2008. The use of adjunctive corticosteroids in the treatment of pericardial, pleural and meningeal tuberculosis: Do they improve outcome? *Respir Med* **102:** 793–800.

Fernando SL, Saunders BM, Sluyter R, Skarratt KK, Goldberg H, Marks GB, Wiley JS, Britton WJ. 2007. A polymorphism in the P2X7 gene increases susceptibility to extrapulmonary tuberculosis. *Am J Respir Crit Care Med* **175:** 360–366.

Feng GD, Shi M, Ma L, Chen P, Wang BJ, Zhang M, Chang XL, Su XC, Yang YN, Fan XH, et al. 2014. Diagnostic accuracy of intracellular *Mycobacterium tuberculosis* detection for tuberculous meningitis. *Am J Respir Crit Care Med* **189:** 475–481.

Forssbohm M. 2004. Studie des DZK zur Epidemiologie der Tuberkulose. Abschlussbericht 1996–2000 (22.333 Fälle) [Study of the German Central Committee against Tuberculosis on the epidemiology of tuberculosis. Final report 1996-2000 (22.333 cases)]. In *28. Informationsbericht des DZK* (ed. Loddenkemper R), pp. 66–78. DZK, Berlin.

Forssbohm M, Zwahlen M, Loddenkemper R, Rieder HL. 2008. Demographic characteristics of patients with extrapulmonary tuberculosis in Germany. *Eur Respir J* **31:** 99–105.

Fuehner T, Stoll M, Bange FC, Welte T, Pletz MW. 2007. Klinik der Lungentuberkulose. *Pneumologe* **4:** 151–162.

Galimi R. 2011. Extrapulmonary tuberculosis: Tuberculous meningitis new developments. *Eur Rev Med Pharmacol Sci* **15:** 365–386.

Gopi A, Madhavan SM, Sharma SK, Sahn SA. 2007. Diagnosis and treatment of tuberculous pleural effusion in 2006. *Chest* **131:** 880–889.

Gupta V, Gupta A, Rao NA. 2007. Intraocular tuberculosis—An update. *Surv Ophthalmol* **52:** 561–587.

Hales CM, Heilig CM, Chaisson R, Leung CC, Chang KC, Goldberg SV, Gordin F, Johnson JL, Muzanyi G, Saukkonen J, et al. 2013. The association between symptoms and microbiologically defined response to tuberculosis treatment. *Ann Am Thorac Soc* **10:** 18–25.

Heyderman RS, Makunike R, Muza T, Odwee M, Kadzirange G, Manyemba J, Muchedzi C, Ndemera B, Gomo ZA, Gwanzura LK, et al. 1998. Pleural tuberculosis in Harare, Zimbabwe: The relationship between human immunodeficiency virus, CD4 lymphocyte count, granuloma formation and disseminated disease. *Trop Med Int Health* **3:** 14–20.

Honeyborne I, McHugh TD, Phillips PJ, Bannoo S, Bateson A, Carroll N, Perrin FM, Ronacher K, Wright L, van Helden PD, et al. 2011. Molecular bacterial load assay, a culture-free biomarker for rapid and accurate quantification of sputum *Mycobacterium tuberculosis* bacillary load during treatment. *J Clin Microbiol* **49:** 3905–3911.

Hooper CE, Lee YC, Maskell NA. 2009. Interferon-γ release assays for the diagnosis of TB pleural effusions: Hype or real hope? *Curr Opin Pulm Med* **15:** 358–365.

Hooper C, Lee YCG, Maskell N, on behalf of the BTS Pleural Guideline Group. 2010. Investigation of a unilateral pleural effusion in adults: British Thoracic Society pleural disease guideline 2010. *Thorax* **65:** i4–ii17.

Horsburgh CR Jr. 2004. Priorities for the treatment of latent tuberculosis infection in the United States. *N Engl J Med* **350:** 2060–2067.

Hu HY, Wu CY, Huang N, Chou YJ, Chang YC, Chu D. 2014. Increased risk of tuberculosis in patients with end-stage renal disease: A population-based cohort study in Taiwan, a country of high incidence of end-stage renal disease. *Epidemiol Infect* **142:** 191–199.

Huang CC, Tchetgen ET, Becerra M, Cohen T, Hughes KC, Zhang Z, Calderon R, Yataco R, Contreras C, Galea J, et al. 2014. The effect of HIV-related immunosuppression on the risk of tuberculosis transmission to household contacts. *Clin Infect Dis* **58:** 765–774.

Jain AK, Dhammi IK. 2007. Tuberculosis of the spine: A review. *Clin Orthop Relat Res* **460:** 39–49.

Khan A, Sterling TR, Reves R, Vernon A, Horsburgh CR. 2006. Lack of weight gain and relapse risk in a large tuberculosis treatment trial. *Am J Respir Crit Care Med* **174:** 344–348.

Khan FA, Minion J, Pai M, Royce S, Burman W, Harries AD, Menzies D. 2010. Treatment of active tuberculosis in HIV-coinfected patients: A systematic review and meta-analysis. *Clin Infect Dis* **50:** 1288–1299.

Koegelenberg CF, Bollinger CT, Theron, Walzl G, Wright CA, Louw M, Diacon AH. 2010. A direct comparison of the diagnostic yield of ultrasound-assisted Abrams and Tru-Cut needle biopsies for pleural tuberculosis. *Thorax* **65:** 857–862.

Kroot EJ, Hazes JM, Colin EM, Dolhain RJ. 2007. Poncet's disease: Reactive arthritis accompanying tuberculosis. Two case reports and a review of the literature. *Rheumatology (Oxford)* **46:** 484–489.

Kruijshaar ME, Lipman M, Essink-Bot ML, Lozewicz S, Creer D, Dart S, Sadler H, Maguire H, Abubakar I. 2010. Health status of UK patients with active tuberculosis. *Int J Tuberc Lung Dis* **14:** 296–302.

Kulchavenya E. 2013. Best practice in the diagnosis and management of urogenital tuberculosis. *Ther Adv Urol* **5:** 143–151.

Lamm DL. 1992. Complications of bacillus Calmette-Guerin immunotherapy. *Urol Clin North Am* **19:** 565–572.

Lawn SD, Zumla AI. 2011. Tuberculosis. *Lancet* **378:** 57–72.

Lawn SD, Kerkhoff AD, Vogt M, Wood R. 2013. HIV-associated tuberculosis: Relationship between disease severity and the sensitivity of new sputum-based and urine-based diagnostic assays. *BMC Med* **11:** 231.

Lee JY, Yi CA, Kim TS, Kim H, Kim J, Han J, Kwon OJ, Lee KS, Chung MJ. 2010. CT scan features as predictors of patient outcome after bronchial intervention in endobronchial TB. *Chest* **138:** 380–385.

Lee K, Kim JH, Lee JH, Lee WY, Park MS, Kim JY, Kim KC, Lee MG, Jung KS, Kim YS, et al. 2011. Acute respiratory distress syndrome caused by miliary tuberculosis: A multicentre survey in South Korea. *Int J Tuberc Lung Dis* **15:** 1099–1103.

Light RW. 2010. Update on tuberculous pleural effusion. *Respirology* **15:** 451–458.

Loddenkemper R. 1998. Thoracoscopy—State of the art. *Eur Respir J* **11:** 213–221.

Loddenkemper, Praveen, Noppen, Pyng. 2011. Medical Thoracoscopy/Pleuroscopy: Manual and Atlas. Georg Thieme, New York.

Mase SR, Ramsay A, Ng V, Henry M, Hopewell PC, Cunningham J, Urbanczik R, Perkins MD, Aziz MA, Pai M. 2007. Yield of serial sputum specimen examinations in the diagnosis of pulmonary tuberculosis: A systematic review. *Int J Tuberc Lung Dis* **11:** 485–495.

Meintjes G, Lawn SD, Scano F, Maartens G, French MA, Worodria W, Elliott JH, Murdoch D, Wilkinson RJ, Seyler C, et al. 2008. Tuberculosis-associated immune reconstitution inflammatory syndrome: Case definitions for use in resource-limited settings. *Lancet Infect Dis* **8:** 516–523.

Menzies D, Fanning A, Yuan L, FitzGerald JM. 2003. Canadian Collaborative Group in Nosocomial Transmission of Tuberculosis. Factors associated with tuberculin conversion in Canadian microbiologiy and pathology workers. *Am J Respir Crit Care Med* **167:** 599–602.

Migliori GB, Zellweger JP, Abubakar I, Ibraim E, Caminero JA, De Vries G, D'Ambrosio L, Centis R, Sotgiu G, Menegale O, et al. 2012. European Union standards for tuberculosis care. *Eur Respir J* **39:** 807–819.

Millen SJ, Uys PW, Hargrove J, van Helden PD, Williams BG. 2008. The effect of diagnostic delays on the drop-out rate and the total delay to diagnosis of tuberculosis. *PLoS ONE* **3:** e1933.

Möller M, de Wit E, Hoal EG. 2010. Past, present and future directions in human genetic susceptibility to tuberculosis. *FEMS Immunol Med Microbiol* **58:** 3–26.

Moure R, Muñoz L, Torres M, Santin M, Martín R, Alcaide F. 2011. Rapid detection of *Mycobacterium tuberculosis* complex and rifampin resistance in smear-negative clinical samples by use of an integrated real-time PCR method. *J Clin Microbiol* **49:** 1137–1139.

Navani N, Molyneaux PL, Breen RA, Connell DW, Jepson A, Nankivell M, Brown JM, Morris-Jones S, Ng B, Wickremasinghe M, et al. 2011. Utility of endobronchial ultrasound-guided transbronchial needle aspiration in patients with tuberculous intrathoracic lymphadenopathy: A multicentre study. *Thorax* **66:** 889–893.

Nhu NT, Heemskerk D, Thu do DA, Chau TT, Mai NT, Nghia HD, Loc PP, Ha DT, Merson L, Thinh TT, et al. 2014 Evaluation of GeneXpert MTB/RIF for diagnosis of tuberculous meningitis. *J Clin Microbiol* **52:** 226–233.

Okanurak K, Kitayaporn D, Wanarangsikul W, Koompong C. 2007. Effectiveness of DOT for tuberculosis treatment outcomes: A prospective cohort study in Bangkok, Thailand. *Int J Tuberc Lung Dis* **11:** 762–768.

Parimon T, Spitters CE, Muangman N, Euathrongchit J, Oren E, Narita M. 2008. Unexpected pulmonary involvement in extrapulmonary tuberculosis patients. *Chest* **134:** 589–594.

Public Health England. 2014. http://www.hpa.org.uk/Topics/InfectiousDiseases/InfectionsAZ/Tuberculosis/TBUKSurveillanceData/EnhancedTuberculosisSurveillance/nTBEnhanced11site/ (accessed 18 April 2014).

Ray S, Talukdar A, Kundu S, Khanra D, Sonthalia N. 2013. Diagnosis and management of miliary tuberculosis: Current state and future perspectives. *Ther Clin Risk Manag* **9:** 9–26.

Rice B, Elford J, Yin Z, Kruijshaar M, Abubakar I, Lipman M, Pozniak A, Kall M, Delpech V. 2013. Decreasing incidence of tuberculosis among HIV diagnosed heterosexuals in England and Wales. *AIDS* **27:** 1151–1157.

Rieder HL, Watson JM, Raviglione MC, Forssbohm M, Migliori GB, Schwoebel V, Leitch AG, Zellweger JP. 1996. Surveillance of tuberculosis in Europe. Working Group of the World Health Organization (WHO) and the European Region of the International Union Against Tuberculosis and Lung Disease (IUATLD) for uniform reporting on tuberculosis cases. *Eur Respir J* **9:** 1097–1104.

Roy A, Anaraki S, Hardelid P, Catchpole M, Rodrigues LC, Lipman M, Perkins S, Roche A, Stagg H, Figueroa J, Abubakar I. 2013. Implementing universal HIV testing in London tuberculosis clinics: A cluster randomised controlled trial. *Eur Respir J* **41:** 627–634.

Sahn SA. 2002. Pleural thickening, trapped lung, and chronic empyema as sequelae of tuberculous pleural effusion: Don't sweat the pleural thickening. *Int J Tuberc Lung Dis* **6:** 461–464.

Sanai FM, Bzeizi KI. 2005. Systematic review: Tuberculous peritonitis—Presenting features, diagnostic strategies and treatment. *Aliment Pharmacol Ther* **22:** 685–700.

Schoch OD, Rieder P, Tueller C, Altpeter E, Zellweger JP, Rieder HL, Krause M, Thurnheer R. 2007. Diagnostic yield of sputum, induced sputum, and bronchoscopy after radiologic tuberculosis screening. *Am J Respir Crit Care Med* **175:** 80–86.

Schutz C, Meintjes G, Almajid F, Wilkinson RJ, Pozniak A. 2010. Clinical management of tuberculosis and HIV-1 co-infection. *Eur Respir J* **36:** 1460–1481.

Shen YC, Wang T, Chen L, Yang T, Wan C, Hu QJ, Wen FQ. 2013. Diagnostic accuracy of adenosine deaminase for tuberculous peritonitis: A meta-analysis. *Arch Med Sci* **9:** 601–607.

Siemon G. 2007. Extrapulmonale tuberkulose. *Pneumolog* **4:** 163–174.

Syed FF, Mayosi BM. 2007. A modern approach to tuberculous pericarditis. *Prog Cardiovasc Dis* **50:** 218–236.

Tan KK, Chen K, Sim R. 2009. The spectrum of abdominal tuberculosis in a developed country: A single institution's experience over 7 years. *J Gastrointest Surg* **13:** 142–147.

TB CARE I. 2014. International standards for tuberculosis care. 3rd ed. TB CARE I, The Hague, Netherlands.

Thwaites GE, Caws M, Chau TT, Dung NT, Campbell JI, Phu NH, Hien TT, White NJ, Farrar JJ. 2004a. Comparison of conventional bacteriology with nucleic acid amplification (amplified mycobacterium direct test) for diagnosis of tuberculous meningitis before and after inception of antituberculosis chemotherapy. *J Clin Microbiol* **42:** 996–1002.

Thwaites GE, Nguyen DB, Nguyen HD, Hoang TQ, Do TT, Nguyen TC, Nguyen QH, Nguyen TT, Nguyen NH, Nguyen TN, et al. 2004b. Dexamethasone for the treatment of tuberculous meningitis in adolescents and adults. *N Engl J Med* **351:** 1741–1751.

Thwaites G, Fisher M, Hemingway C, Scott G, Solomon T, Innes J, British Infection Society. 2009. British Infection Society guidelines for the diagnosis and treatment of tuberculosis of the central nervous system in adults and children. *J Infect* **59:** 167–187.

Török ME, Yen NT, Chau TT, Mai NT, Phu NH, Mai PP, Dung NT, Chau NV, Bang ND, Tien NA, et al. 2011. Timing of initiation of antiretroviral therapy in human immunodeficiency virus (HIV)—Associated tuberculous meningitis. *Clin Infect Dis* **52:** 1374–1383.

Trajman A, Pai M, Dheda K, van Zyl Smit R, Zwerling AA, Joshi R, Kalantri S, Daley P, Menzies D. 2008. Novel tests for diagnosing tuberculous pleural effusion: What works and what does not? *Eur Respir J* **31:** 1098–1106

Uehlinger A, Schaub F, Bühlmann A. 1959. Zur klinik und pathophysiologie der pericarditis constrictiva. *Schweiz Med Wochenschr* **89:** 853–862.

Wallgren A. 1948. The time-table of tuberculosis. *Tubercle* **29:** 245–251.

Watts HG, Lifeso RM. 1996. Tuberculosis of bones and joints. *J Bone Joint Surg Am* **78:** 288–298.

Wilberschied LA, Kaye K, Fujiwara PI, Frieden TR. 1999. Extrapulmonary tuberculosis among foreign-born patients, New York City, 1995 to 1996. *J Immigr Health* **1:** 65–75.

World Health Organization. 2011. *Guidelines for the programmatic management of drug-resistant tuberculosis—2011 update*, 6th ed. WHO/HTM/TB/2011. WHO, Geneva.

World Health Organization. 2013. *Global tuberculosis report*

Zumla A, Raviglione M, Hafner R, von Reyn CF. 2013. Tuberculosis. *N Engl J Med* **368:** 745–755.

Tuberculosis in Children

Ben J. Marais[1] and H. Simon Schaaf[2]

[1]Marie Bashir Institute for Infectious Diseases and Biosecurity (MBI) and The Children's Hospital at Westmead, University of Sydney, Westmead, New South Wales 2145, Australia

[2]Desmond Tutu TB Centre, Department of Paediatrics and Child Health, Faculty of Medicine and Health Sciences, Stellenbosch University, Tygerberg, 7505, South Africa

Correspondence: ben.marais@health.nsw.gov.au

Many clinicians regard tuberculosis as an adult pulmonary disease, but tuberculosis (TB) is a major cause of disease, both pulmonary and extrapulmonary, and death in young children from TB-endemic countries, especially in areas affected by poverty, social disruption, and human immunodeficiency virus (HIV) infection. This article reviews the disease burden and the natural history of disease in children with TB. It also provides guidance regarding the diagnosis, treatment, and prevention of TB in children.

DISEASE BURDEN

Tuberculosis (TB) is a major cause of disease, both pulmonary and extrapulmonary, and death in children from TB-endemic areas (Bates et al. 2013; Graham et al. 2014), but is also seen in nonendemic areas because of increased international travel, population migration, and refugee resettlement. Although overdiagnosis does occur in some settings, underdiagnosis is the rule in most TB-endemic areas, where young children can only access TB care via referral hospitals. Table 1 summarizes key differences between adults and children with TB. Poor case ascertainment and incomplete recording and reporting limit the accuracy of disease burden estimates in children (Newton et al. 2008; Du Preez et al. 2011; Rose et al. 2013). According to the most recent estimates, nearly 1 million children develop TB every year (Jenkins et al. 2014); this is nearly double World Health Organization (WHO) estimates of 530,000 cases for 2012, causing 74,000 deaths, which exclude deaths in human immunodeficiency virus (HIV)–infected children (World Health Organization 2013).

HIV coinfection has had a major impact on the epidemiology of TB, especially in sub-Saharan Africa (Källenius 2014). In addition to a massive increase in the absolute number of TB patients, HIV induced a pronounced shift in the age and gender profile of TB patients, with more young adults and women of child-bearing age being affected (Lawn et al. 2006). This demographic shift implies increased TB exposure of young and vulnerable children living in HIV-affected households, as illustrated by high rates of TB exposure within the first 6 months of life in babies born to HIV-infected mothers (irrespective of their HIV status) (Cotton et al. 2008), and high disease rates among HIV-infected infants (Hesseling et al. 2009). Routine

Cite this article as *Cold Spring Harb Perspect Med* doi: 10.1101/cshperspect.a017855

Table 1. Tuberculosis: Differences between adults and children

Aspect	Adults[a]	Children[a]
Epidemiology	Massive global disease burden that is well quantified; excellent awareness	Massive global disease burden that is poorly quantified; minimal awareness
TB control	Main focus of TB control programs	Not recognized as a TB control priority
Pathogenesis	Usually "adult-type" lung disease	Usually intrathoracic lymph node disease, but extrapulmonary disease common
Infection control	Multibacillary; high infection risk	Paucibacillary; low infection risk, unless cavities or extensive lung involvement; epidemiologic marker of transmission
Drug resistance	Difficult to differentiate acquired from primary drug resistance	Nearly always primary drug resistance indicating recent transmission
Exposure history	Important, but often neglected[b]	Essential part of diagnostic work up
Risk of progression to disease	Relatively low risk of progression to disease following TB exposure/infection unless immune-compromised	Highly variable risk of progression to disease following TB exposure/ infection—greatest in the very young and/or immune-compromised
Preventive therapy	Limited value, except in immune-compromised adults	Definite value in young (<5 yr of age) and/ or immune-compromised children
Imaging studies	Chest radiographs (CXRs) not routinely required, unless sputum negative for mycobacterial investigations	CXRs (with both anteroposterior and lateral views, of good quality, and competently read) are the most informative study to perform
Disease classification	Pulmonary versus extrapulmonary distinction Postprimary TB is a confusing concept[c]	Diverse spectrum of pathology that requires accurate classification
Microbiological studies	Relatively easy to collect adequate respiratory specimen and confirm presence of mycobacteria	Difficult to collect adequate respiratory specimens (young children cannot expectorate); smear microscopy has very low yield
Treatment (drug-susceptible TB)	With four drugs in intensive phase	With three or four drugs depending on likely organism load and severity of disease in intensive phase
Prognosis	Excellent outcomes achievable with timely and appropriate treatment	Excellent outcomes achievable; potentially grave outcome with delayed diagnosis of especially tuberculous meningitis

Data adapted from supplementary material in Perez-Velez and Marais 2012.

[a]Typical characteristics in the absence of HIV infection and/or severe immune compromise.

[b]Taking a careful contact history is often neglected in adults, but it has particular relevance to identify drug-resistant TB suspects.

[c]The distinction between primary and postprimary TB obscures the fact that adult-type (postprimary) TB frequently results from recent reinfection and may also occur within months of documented primary infection (particularly in adolescents).

HIV testing in pregnancy, together with optimal prevention of mother-to-child transmission and early initiation of antiretroviral therapy (ART) in HIV-infected infants, is essential to reduce overall mortality and TB risk in HIV-infected infants (Violari et al. 2008).

The emergence of drug-resistant (DR)-TB poses a major threat to global TB control (Abubakar et al. 2013; Seung et al. 2014). For a long time, DR-TB strains, especially isoniazid-resistant strains, were considered to be less virulent and therefore less transmissible than drug-susceptible strains, with failure to appreciate the risk for global epidemic spread. However, pediatric TB cases provide a valuable epidemiological perspective because they reflect ongoing transmission within communities. The development of multidrug-resistant (MDR)-TB (i.e., resistance to at least isoniazid and rifampicin) in child contacts of infectious adult cases present confirmation that clinical MDR strains are transmissible and cause disease (Schaaf et al. 2007; Amanullah et al. 2014). This has been corroborated by molecular epidemiology studies that confirmed transmission from adult source cases to child contacts (Schaaf et al. 2000) and by high rates of clustering and multiple clusters with clear transmission chains among newly identified MDR-TB cases (Marais et al. 2013b). In settings with relevant surveillance data, rates of DR-TB in children were found to be similar to those in adults from the same community (Zignol et al. 2013), especially among treatment-naïve patients (Jenkins et al. 2004). Therefore, although the incidence of DR-TB in children is poorly quantified, the fact that WHO estimated MDR-TB to occur in 3.6% of newly diagnosed TB cases in 2012 (World Health Organization 2013) implies a similar burden among children.

NATURAL HISTORY OF DISEASE

Understanding the natural history of TB is fundamental to appreciate the variable vulnerability and the diverse spectrum of disease observed in children. Meticulous disease descriptions from the prechemotherapy literature provide unique insight into events following primary *Mycobacterium tuberculosis* infection, summarized as the so-called "timetable of childhood TB" (Fig. 1) (Marais et al. 2004a; Perez-Velez and Marais 2012). Pulmonary infection occurs when a few bacilli reach a terminal airway and establish infection. A localized inflammatory process occurs within the lung, referred to as the primary (Ghon) focus, from where bacilli drain via lymphatics to the regional lymph nodes. The primary focus together with affected regional lymph nodes (with/without overlying pleural reaction) is referred to as the primary (Ghon) complex. Before acquired immune responses contain disease progression, bacilli may enter the systemic circulation via the regional lymph nodes with occult hematogenous spread. Bacilli may survive in target organs for prolonged periods depending on dynamic pathogen–host interactions at the site of deposition; Figure 2 provides an overview of factors that influence disease risk.

The rate of progression is highly variable, with the youngest children experiencing the greatest risk and the most rapid disease progression. Table 2 provides an overview of clinical syndromes associated with primary *M. tuberculosis* infection in children; summarized in the following phases.

- *Phase 1* occurs 3–8 wk after primary infection and may be heralded by prolonged fever, the formation of a visible primary complex on chest radiograph (CXR), and hypersensitivity reactions such as erythema nodosum and tuberculin skin test (TST) conversion.
- *Phase 2* occurs 1–3 mo after primary infection and follows occult hematogenous

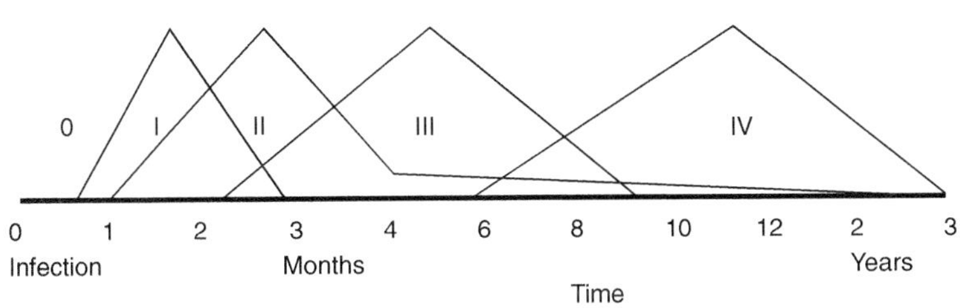

Figure 1. Schematic time line following primary pulmonary infection with *M. tuberculosis*. Data of time line of tuberculosis is adapted from Marais et al. (2005a), first described by Wallgren (1948). 0, Incubation; I, tuberculin skin test conversion; II, Ghon focus and/or disseminated (miliary) disease; III, lymph node disease (<5 yr of age)/pleural effusion (>5 yr of age); IV, adult-type disease (>10 yr of age).

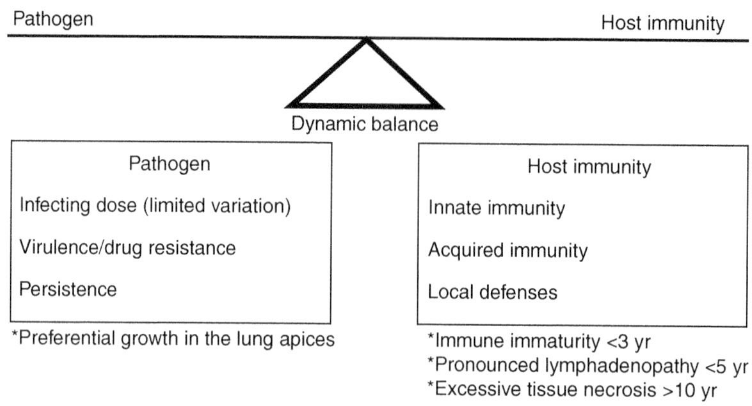

Figure 2. Factors that influence the dynamic balance between *M. tuberculosis* and host immunity in children. (Adapted from Marais et al. 2005a.)

spread. This represents the period of highest risk for the development of tuberculous meningitis (TBM) and disseminated (miliary) TB in young children. However, these disease entities may occur after any time interval; hematogenous dissemination frequently acted as the final terminal pathway following uncontrolled disease progression in the absence of treatment.

- *Phase 3* occurs 3–7 mo after primary infection and may manifest as airway involvement caused by diseased lymph nodes in young children (<5 yr of age) and reactive pleural effusions in older children.

- *Phase 4* lasts until the primary complex is calcified, 1–3 yr after primary infection. It represents the period of osteoarticular TB in children of <5 yr of age and adult-type disease in adolescents. As a general rule the risk of disease progression following primary infection had passed by the time calcification appeared, although adult-type disease may have a delayed presentation in adolescent children.

- *Phase 5* occurs after calcification is complete, >3 yr after primary infection. By this time the highest risk period has passed, although late manifestations of TB, including pulmonary reactivation, may be observed.

DISEASE SPECTRUM

Intrathoracic Disease

Pulmonary involvement in children presents with a diverse spectrum of pathology that can be visualized on CXR. Appreciating the mechanism of disease is helpful because a CXR is merely a two-dimensional reflection of the underlying pathology. Accurate disease classification has important clinical relevance for prognosis and management; it also facilitates scientific communication (Marais et al. 2004b).

Primary (Ghon) Focus

The primary focus describes the parenchymal involvement associated with recent primary infection. It is usually single, transient, and visualized as part of the primary complex. Primary foci are variable in size and may show an overlying pleural reaction. Rarely more than one primary foci may be seen or parenchymal involvement may progress. Complications include local parenchymal destruction with cavity formation, which may result in intrabronchial spread with bronchopneumonic consolidation (Marais et al. 2004b). Figures 3 and 4 illustrate uncomplicated and complicated Ghon foci, respectively.

Lymph Node Disease

Involvement of the intrathoracic lymph nodes (perihilar and/or paratracheal) is considered

Table 2. Different clinical syndromes associated with tuberculosis in children

Pathological classification	Disease phase (time period)	Clinical syndromes	Risk groups	Pathogenesis	Imaging manifestations
Primary *Mtb* infection	Incubation (0–6 wk)	Asymptomatic	All ages	No adaptive immunity TST(−); IGRA(−)	None
	Infection (1–3 mo)	Self-limiting symptoms (mild, viral-like)		Adaptive immunity IGRA(+); TST(+)	Transient hilar or mediastinal lymphadenopathy (50%–70% of cases), rarely visible transient Ghon focus
		Hypersensitivity reactions (fever; erythema nodosum. phlyctenular conjunctivitis)		No test to register reinfection	
Early disease progression >90% of disease occur within 12 months of primary infection	Very early (2–6 mo)	Uncomplicated lymph node (LN) disease	<10 years	Inadequate innate and/or adaptive immunity TST(+); IGRA(+)	Hilar or mediastinal lymphadenopathy without airway or parenchymal involvement
		Progressive Ghon focus	<1 yr	May be negative with immune compromise or extensive disease, cannot be used as "rule out" tests	Ghon focus with visible cavitation
		Disseminated disease:	<3 yr		
		Miliary disease			Discrete lung nodules (1–2 mm) on CXR; hepatosplenomegaly
		TB meningitis			Hydrocephalus; basal enhancement; brain infarcts and/or tuberculomas
	Early (4–12 mo)	Complicated LN disease:	<5 yr		
		Airway compression			Hyperinflation or atelectasis/ collapse
		Expansile caseating pneumonia			Expansile consolidation of a segment or lobe
		Infiltration of adjacent anatomic structures (esophagus, phrenic nerve, pericardium)			Tracheo-/bronchoesophageal fistula; pericardial effusion; hemidiaphragmatic palsy

Continued

Table 2. *Continued*

Pathological classification	Disease phase (time period)	Clinical syndromes	Risk groups	Pathogenesis	Imaging manifestations
		Pleural disease: Exudative effusion (rarely empyema; or chylothorax)	>3 yr		Effusion usually unilateral; some pleural thickening and loculations (attributable to fibrinous strands)
		Lymphadenitis: Most common extra-thoracic manifestation; usually cervical	1–10 yr		Usually not needed, matting and edema of adjacent soft tissue
Late disease progression Generally rare apart from adult-type disease in adolescents	Late (1–3 yr)	Adult-type pulmonary disease: Difficult to differentiate primary infection; reactivation and reinfection disease	≥8 yr	"Overagressive" innate and/or adaptive immunity	Apical cavities; may be bilateral; minimal or no LN enlargement (previously referred to as postprimary TB)
		Osteoarticular disease: Spondylitis/Arthritis/ Osteomyelitis	≥5 yr	Inadequate local control; usually local manifestations only, but can disseminate from any active focus	Periarticular osteopenia, subchondral cystic erosions, joint space narrowing
	Very late (>3 yr)	Urinary tract (renal, ureter, bladder) disease	>5 yr		Renal calcifications; hydronephrosis, calyceal dilation and/or ureter stricture

Data adapted from Perez-Velez and Marais 2012 and based on detailed disease descriptions provided by Wallgren 1948 and Lincoln and Sewell 1963.

Age ranges, risk groups, and time lines specified provide general guidance only. HIV-infected children are particularly vulnerable and may present with atypical features.

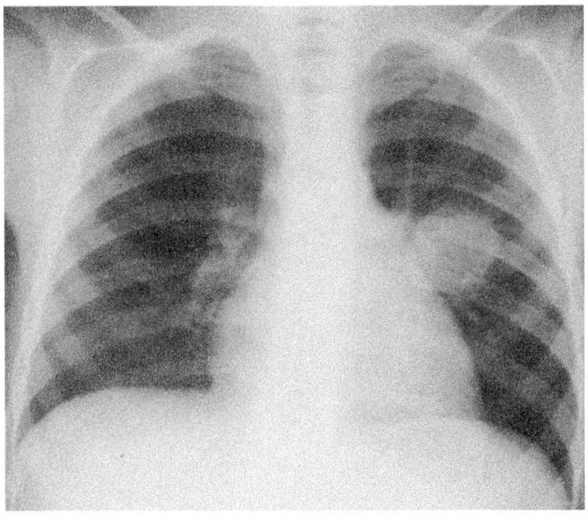

Figure 3. Uncomplicated Ghon focus—apex of the left lower lobe (Gie 2003; Marais et al. 2004b). Place where the "eagle has landed," rarely seen because it is usually transient.

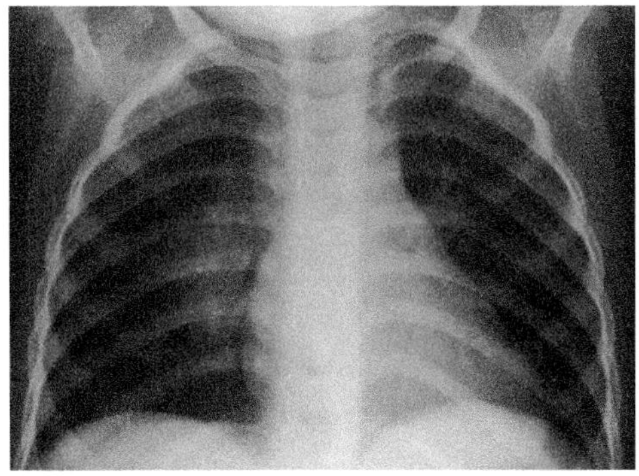

Figure 5. Intrathoracic lymph node disease (anteroposterior view) (Gie 2003; Marais et al. 2004b). Lymph nodes are part of the Ghon complex and the main site of disease; however, they are often difficult to visualize with certainty.

the radiological hallmark of primary infection. Both anteroposterior (AP) and lateral views are required for optimal lymph node visualization (Figs. 5 and 6). Lymph node disease may be complicated by airway involvement and/or penetration into adjacent anatomical structures. Complicated lymph node disease occurs most commonly in children <5 yr of age, probably because of exuberant lymph node responses and the small caliber of their airways.

Large airway compression results when the trachea or a main bronchus is surrounded and fixated by diseased lymph nodes and associated inflammation and this may be best visualized on a high-kilovolt (overpenetrated) CXR. Various disease presentations include partial airway obstruction with a check-valve effect and alveolar hyperinflation (Fig. 7) or total airway obstruction with alveolar collapse. When a diseased lymph node erupts into an airway, caseous material may be aspirated, and the resulting pathology may range from pure hypersensitivity-induced inflammation (dead bacilli and/or "toxins") to destructive caseating pneumonia (virulent bacilli), depending on the bacterial load and viability of the bacilli aspirated. Caseating pneumonia often causes an expansile (bulging against their anatomical boundaries) pneumonic process with visible parenchymal breakdown (Fig. 8). Penetration into adjacent anatomical structures may involve the phrenic nerve with unilateral diaphragmatic palsy, the esophagus with the formation of a broncho- or tracheoesophageal fistula, and/or the thoracic (lymphatic) duct with the formation of a unilateral chylothorax.

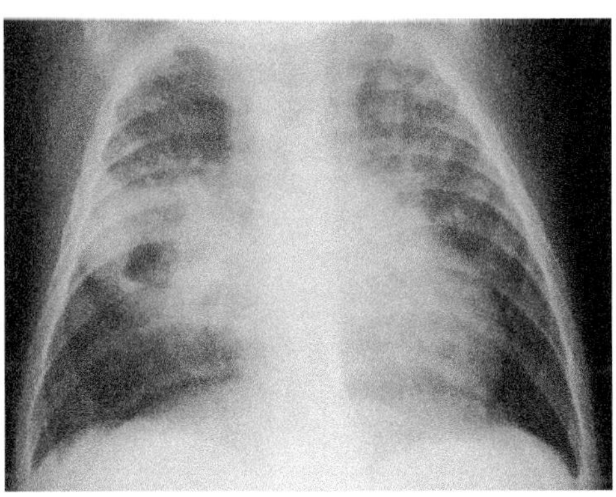

Figure 4. Complicated Ghon focus (Gie 2003; Marais et al. 2004b). This image reflects poor disease containment at the point of entry; infants and severely immune-compromised individuals are particularly vulnerable.

Pleural or Pericardial Effusion

The accumulation of the typical lymphocyte-rich, straw-colored fluid represents a hypersensitivity response (Fig. 9). Isolated pleural effu-

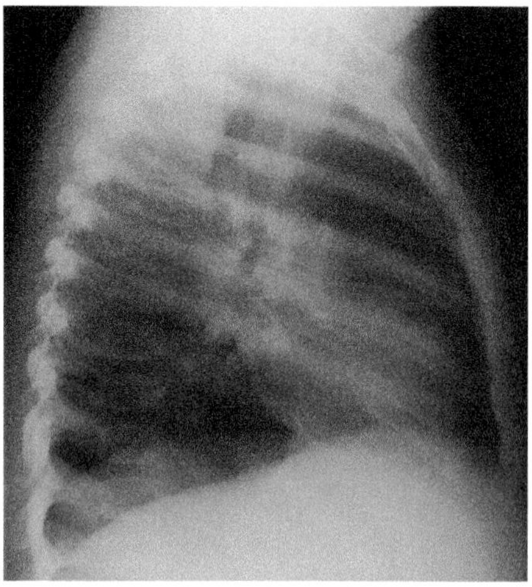

Figure 6. Intrathoracic lymph node disease (lateral view) (Gie 2003; Marais et al. 2004b). It is essential to perform good quality AP and lateral views. One can see density behind and below the carina, which is not the area where normal physiological structures occur. Also, some fluid in the horizontal and transverse fissures indicates some inflammatory response (not indicative of TB). The dense circular ring around the hilum (so-called doughnut sign) is indicative of perihilar lymph node involvement.

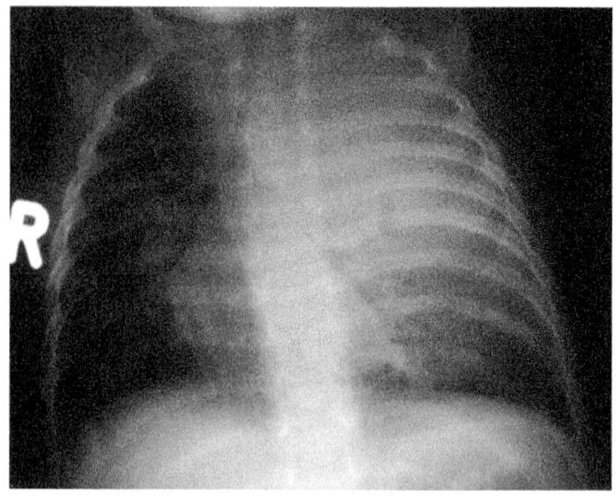

Figure 8. Caseating (expansile) pneumonia (Gie 2003; Marais et al. 2004b). TB lymph nodes cause airway narrowing (almost pathognomonic), because, unlike other mass lesions, it traps and compresses the airway. Lymph nodes can also "rupture" (with sinus formation) into the airway (as occurs with scrofula), which may result in aspiration of caseous material and development of dense (expansile) caseating pneumonia. If this was any other organism, the child would have been in the intensive care unit. Always think of TB when there is this dichotomy between the radiological severity of disease and the clinical signs and symptoms (children often chronically ill, but rarely hyperacute—probably because of reduced V/Q [ventilation/perfusion ratio] mismatch).

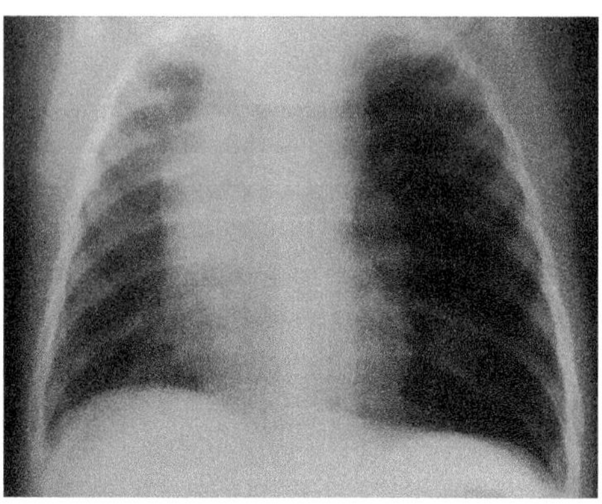

Figure 7. Airway obstruction with "check valve" effect (Gie et al. 2003; Marais et al. 2004b). The enlarged lymph nodes frequently cause airway complications, especially in young children with small and pliable airways. Hyperinflation (ball valve effect) of left lung. See remnant of Ghon focus and large left-sided perihilar nodes.

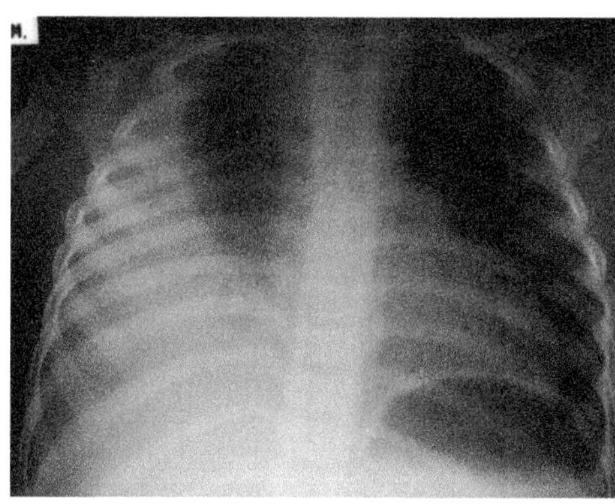

Figure 9. Pleural effusion (Gie 2003; Marais et al. 2004b). Uncommon in children of $<$6–8 yr. Usually a hypersensitivity response (may develop TB empyema) with typical presentation, well localized chest pain with intermittent fever, and the child otherwise remarkably well. Unilateral dullness on percussion. Fluid characteristically clear with yellow discoloration; TST (tuberculin skin text) very reactive $>$15–20 mm.

Cite this article as *Cold Spring Harb Perspect Med* doi: 10.1101/cshperspect.a017855

sions are unusual in children <3 yr of age and tend to develop soon (within the first 3–9 mo) after primary infection. A loculated fluid collection may indicate TB empyema that results when bacilli actively multiply within the pleural space. Pericardial effusion usually develops when a subcarinal lymph node erupts into the pericardial space. Cardiac ultrasound is the most sensitive test to confirm or exclude the presence of a pericardial effusion; long-term sequelae include constrictive pericarditis.

Disseminated (Miliary) Disease

Dissemination represents a condition of infinite gradation. Occult dissemination is common following primary infection; however, it rarely progresses to disseminated disease except in very young (<2–3 yr of age) and immune-compromised children. Typical radiologic signs include the presence of even-sized miliary lesions (<2 mm) that are distributed bilaterally into the very periphery of the lung (Fig. 10). Diagnostic confusion often exists in HIV-infected children in whom lymphocytic interstitial pneumonitis (LIP), malignancies, and opportunistic infections such as *Pneumocystis jiroveci* pneumonia (PCP) may present with a similar radiological picture. In these instances, response to treatment and/or bacteriologic confirmation may be the only way to establish a definitive diagnosis.

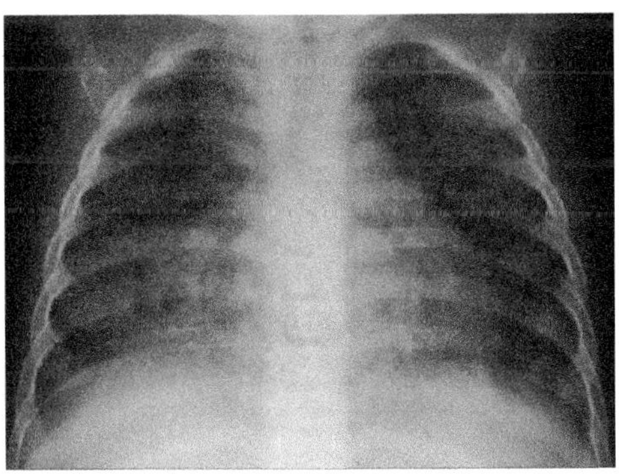

Figure 10. Disseminated (miliary) disease (Gie 2003; Marais et al. 2004b). Usually in very young children (<2–3 yr of age) or severely immune-compromised within 6 mo after primary infection. Incidence proven to be reduced by BCG vaccination in HIV-uninfected/unexposed children (not in HIV-infected). *Mtb* spreads via the bloodstream; therefore, tubercles are not restricted to the lungs, but also affect other organs (e.g., liver, spleen) and is frequently associated with TB meningitis (consider lumbar puncture to exclude TBM—management the same).

Adult-Type Disease

Adult-type disease first appears around puberty (8–10 yr of age) and becomes the dominant disease manifestation during adolescence. As with pulmonary TB in adults, the apical and posterior segments of the upper lobes and the apical segment of the lower lobes are most commonly affected (Fig. 11). Complications include progressive cavity formation and bronchial spread.

Extrathoracic Disease

Cervical Lymphadenitis

The most common extrathoracic manifestation of TB in children is cervical lymphadenitis (Marais et al. 2006a) (Table 3). The cervical mass is usually painless and includes matted nodes with considerable periadenitis. A cold abscess results when the caseous material liquefies. This is signified by a soft fluctuant node with violaceous discoloration of the overlying skin; spontaneous drainage and sinus formation may follow. Untreated, the natural course of TB lymphadenitis follows a prolonged and relapsing course, often interrupted by transient lymph node enlargement, fluctuation, and/or sinus formation.

Table 4 reflects the clinical characteristics of children diagnosed with TB lymphadenitis (Marais et al. 2006b). A simple clinical algorithm that identifies children with persistent (>4 wk) cervical adenopathy, without a visible local cause or response to first-line antibiotics, and a cervical mass of $\geq 2 \times 2$ cm showed excellent diagnostic accuracy, but would be far less accurate in nonendemic areas and in areas where alternative diagnoses, such as Burkitt's lymphoma, are more common. Establishing a

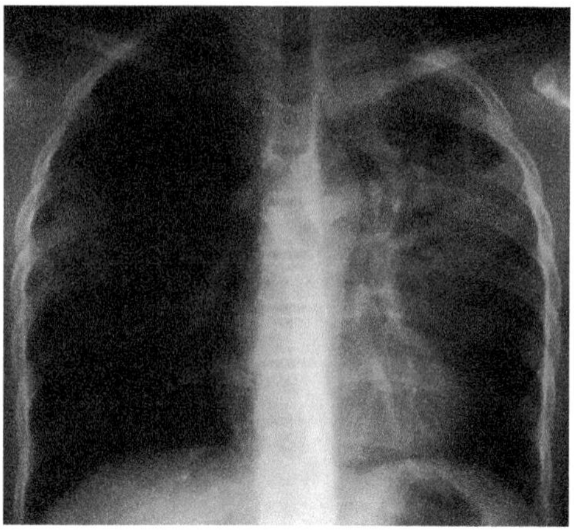

Figure 11. Adult-type disease (Gie 2003; Marais et al. 2004b). This type of disease manifestation is not seen in young children, emerges with the onset of puberty at ~8–10 yr of age, and seems to be associated with an excessive and poorly regulated immune response (excessive hypersensitivity type response). Any child with cavitary disease is infectious (as infectious as an adult sputum smear-positive case) and should be regarded as a potential source case.

definitive tissues and/or culture diagnosis remains preferable and this can be performed in a minimally invasive fashion using fine needle aspiration biopsy (FNAB). In areas where the control of bovine TB is poor and milk is not routinely pasteurized, *Mycobacterium bovis* might cause similar disease, whereas nontuberculosis mycobacteria should be considered in areas where both human and bovine TB are well controlled.

Tuberculous Meningitis (TBM)

TBM is the most severe manifestation of childhood TB. Bacille Calmette–Guérin (BCG) vaccination provides some degree of protection against the severe forms of TB (miliary disease and TBM) (Trunz et al. 2006), but despite universal BCG vaccination in most TB-endemic areas, severe disease manifestations still occur. TBM is most common in young children (<3 yr of age) who frequently present with nonspecific symptoms before more advanced disease becomes apparent. This requires clinical vigilance and careful assessment of potential TB exposure, because early diagnosis is essential to ensure an optimal outcome. Symptoms and signs of early disease include fever, listlessness, apathy, anorexia, and/or failure to thrive and headache (in older children). As the disease progresses, localizing neurological signs with/without a suppressed level of consciousness and/or convulsions develop. Most clinical features can

Table 3. Disease spectrum documented in children treated for TB in a highly endemic area

TB manifestation	Total (%) $N = 439$
Not TB	**85 (19.4)**
Intrathoracic TB	**307 (69.9)**
Ghon focus	
Uncomplicated (with/without hilar adenopathy)	16/307 (5.2)
Complicated	3/307 (1.0)
Lymph node disease	
Uncomplicated	147/307 (47.9)
Complicated	
Compression	25/307 (8.1)
Consolidation	62/307 (20.6)
Pleurisy	24/307 (7.8)
Pericarditis	1/307 (0.3)
Disseminated (miliary) disease	15/307 (4.9)
Adult-type disease	14/307 (4.6)
Extrathoracic TB	**72 (16.4)**
Peripheral lymphadenitis	
Cervical	35/72 (48.6)
Other	1/72 (1.4)
Central nervous system TB	
Meningitis	14/72 (19.4)
Tuberculoma	2/72 (2.8)
Abdominal TB	1/72 (1.4)
Osteoarticular TB	
Vertebral spondylitis	4/72 (5.6)
Other	7/72 (9.7)
Skin	8/72 (11.1)
Intra- + Extrathoracic TB	**[25 (5.7)]**

Data adapted from Marais et al. 2006a.

TB, tuberculosis; Not TB, chest radiograph not suggestive of TB (confirmed by two independent child TB experts), no bacteriologic or histologic proof and no extrathoracic TB recorded; Intra- + extrathoracic TB, intra- and extrathoracic TB, included in both groups.

Table 4. Clinical characteristics of children with TB lymphadenitis

Lymph node characteristics	Total (%) N = 35
Persistence (present for >4 wk, no response to antibiotics)	35 (100)
Size	
<2 × 2 cm	4 (11.4)
(2–4) × (2–4) cm	25 (71.5)
>4 × 4 cm	6 (17.1)
Character	
Single	5 (14.3)
Multiple	
discrete	14 (40.0)
matted	16 (45.7)
Solid	28 (80.0)
Fluctuant	
without secondary bacterial infection	5 (14.3)
with secondary bacterial infection (red and warm)	2 (5.7)
Associated findings	
Tuberculin skin test	
0 mm	2 (5.7)
1–9 mm	0
≥10 mm	33 (94.3)
≥15 mm	32 (91.4)
Constitutional symptoms	
Any symptom	21 (60.0)
Fever	7 (20.0)
Cough	9 (25.7)
Night sweats	8 (22.8)
Fatigue	19 (54.3)
Failure to thrive	10 (28.6)
Chest radiograph	
Suggestive of tuberculosis	13 (37.1)
Lymph node disease	
uncomplicated	8 (22.8)
with airway compression	1 (2.9)
with parenchymal consolidation	4 (11.4)

Data adapted from Marais et al. 2006b.

Size, transverse diameter of the largest cervical mass; Fatigue, less playful and active since the mass was first noted; Failure to thrive, crossing at least one weight-for-age centile line in the preceding 3 mo or having lost >10% of body weight (≥1 kg) over any time interval.

be explained by the combined effects of raised intracranial pressure and cerebral vasculitis with brain ischemia/infarction. Together with a dense basal exudate these are the key findings suggestive of TBM on brain imaging (Thwaites et al. 2013).

Perinatal TB

Newborn babies may acquire TB in multiple ways, but generally experience rapid disease progression that requires early diagnosis and treatment (Schaaf et al. 2010). Congenital TB infection is acquired via the placenta, with the primary (Ghon) focus located in the liver or during birth by aspiration of infected amniotic fluid, in which case primary lung involvement usually follows. This occurs when the mother develops hematogenous dissemination during pregnancy, which may be overt (as a result of advanced maternal disease) or occult following recent primary infection of the mother, sometimes signified by a pleural effusion in pregnancy. Alternatively, if mothers or other close contact have infectious pulmonary TB, the baby may inhale the bacillus after delivery (postnatal TB rather than congenital TB).

Other TB Manifestations

TB can affect nearly every organ system as a result of disease progression that occurs at sites where the TB bacillus was deposited during the initial phase of occult dissemination.

Immune Reconstitution

The clinical syndrome was first documented in the prechemotherapy era, following nutritional rehabilitation and/or the termination of high-dose steroid treatment. Recently immune reconstitution inflammatory syndrome (IRIS) has emerged as an important complication to consider shortly after the introduction of combination antiretroviral therapy (cART) in HIV-infected patients with severe immune compromise, usually within the first 6–12 wk. This may manifest as "unmasking IRIS" if mycobacterial disease was undetected before ART initiation or as "paradoxical IRIS" if preexisting disease deteriorates after ART initiation (Meintjes et al. 2009). Radiologic signs may include airway compression caused by increased inflammation surrounding diseased lymph nodes or dense alveolar consolidation caused by excessive inflammation in areas of previous "subclinical" TB infiltration. This temporary exacerbation of TB symptoms and signs is mainly ascribed to the effects of improved immune function, although a "hypersensitivity" reaction to antigens released by killed TB bacilli may also contribute. Although temporary, central nervous system IRIS (resulting from TBM) is associated with rapid clinical deterioration and poor outcomes (Marais et al. 2013c). Care should also be taken to differentiate IRIS from superimposed infections, poor adherence, and drug-resistant disease (Marais et al. 2013c).

DIAGNOSIS

Differentiating infection from disease is critically important because infection is a common event and the management of the two conditions is very different. Disease progression is usually indicated by the onset of persistent nonremitting symptoms. Children may be evaluated for TB following presentation with symptoms or signs suggestive of TB (passive case finding) or as a result of contact investigation or during routine immigrant screening (active case finding). The clinical presentation of children detected by active case finding differs from those detected by passive case finding, with the former often having *M. tuberculosis* infection only or disease in a very early phase. *M. tuberculosis* infection detected in young children or following recent TB exposure implies a higher risk of disease progression. In nonendemic areas, the pretest probability is highly dependent on the child's TB exposure status, which influences the positive predictive value of all subsequent investigations (Perez-Velez and Marais 2012).

Clinical Evaluation

Taking a careful history is essential to explore possible TB exposure and to perform adequate symptom characterization. The variable presentation and the nonspecific nature of most symptoms complicate the diagnosis. Common constitutional symptoms include failure to thrive (documented deviation of the growth curve trajectory) and reduced playfulness; low-grade or intermittent fever is less common (Marais et al. 2004a). With airway involvement, the usual presenting symptom is a persistent nonremitting cough or wheeze, unresponsive to treatment of likely alternative causes (Marais et al. 2006c). However, clinical signs may be fairly acute or more subtle. Scoring systems, of which there are many, often make use of clinical symptoms, signs, contact history, and basic investigations, but no diagnostic scoring system has been adequately validated (Hesseling et al. 2002); sensitivity and specificity is particularly poor in HIV-infected children (Edwards et al. 2007). Despite these limitations a combination of clinical, radiological, and/or laboratory findings consistent with TB disease, together with epidemiological evidence of TB exposure or immunological evidence of *M. tuberculosis* infection, allow for an accurate diagnosis in most cases (Perez-Velez and Marais 2012).

Imaging Studies

In clinical practice, chest radiography, if adequately performed and read, is one of the most useful studies to perform. Both anteroposterior and lateral views should be taken; lateral views assist assessment of the mediastinum and hilar areas. The International Union Against Tuberculosis and Lung Disease (The Union) compiled an atlas of illustrative cases that provides a wonderful resource for clinicians (Gie 2003). Ultrasound is useful to confirm pericardial or pleural effusions and abdominal lymphadenopathy, solid organ involvement, or ascites. High-resolution computed tomography (CT) offers excellent anatomical visualization (Andronikou et al. 2009), but its use should be reserved for complicated intrathoracic cases caused by high radiation exposure and cost. CT and/or magnetic resonance imaging (MRI) are particularly helpful to visualize intracranial pathology. MRI is more sensitive for detecting brain-stem lesions or early perfusion defects in patients with TBM, and also provides better evaluation of the spine and soft tissues (Pienaar et al. 2009).

 Cite this article as *Cold Spring Harb Perspect Med* doi: 10.1101/cshperspect.a017855

Laboratory Studies

Table 5 summarizes available diagnostic investigations. Sputum smear microscopy provides the cornerstone of TB diagnosis in most countries, but it has limited utility in young children with paucibacillary disease who are unable to expectorate. Although sensitivity remains suboptimal in children, the Xpert-MTB/RIF assay is rapid and highly specific. Using two sputum samples. it detects three times more cases than microscopy and ~70% of the cases detected by liquid culture (Nicol et al. 2011; Rachow et al. 2012). Both immunological assays, the traditional TST and newer interferon-γ release assays (IGRAs), fail to differentiate *M. tuberculosis* infection from TB disease. WHO recommends that IGRAs should not replace the TST for the detection of *M. tuberculosis* infection in low- or middle-income countries (World Health Organization 2011a), although they may be complementary by improving sensitivity and/or specificity in specific clinical situations (MMWR 2010).

Collecting expectorated sputum in young children is problematic; gastric aspirates and

Table 5. Summary of investigations to diagnose tuberculosis in children

Investigation	Uses	Strengths and limitations
Microbiological studies		
Microscopy	Diagnosis of TB	Strengths: Specificity high; useful in all specimen types; rapid (<1 h) detection; low cost. Limitations: Sensitivity very low, especially in young children; highly operator-dependent; labor intensive; unable to distinguish viable and dead bacilli.
Culture	Diagnosis of TB; drug susceptibility testing	Strengths: Specificity high. Limitations: Sensitivity moderate to low in young children; slow turnaround time; need proper laboratory facilities.
DNA detection (PCR)		Strengths: Specificity high; fully automated; rapid turnaround. Limitations: Sensitivity moderate to low in young children; unable to distinguish viable from dead bacilli.
Histopathological studies		
Stained tissue samples	Diagnosis of TB	Allows exclusion of other diagnoses (such as malignancy).
Immune-based studies		
TST; IGRA (e.g., Quantiferon Gold)	Diagnosis of *Mtb* infection	Neither test can differentiate *Mtb* infection from TB disease; careful evaluation of discordant results. TST: Affected by BCG vaccination; requires a second visit after 48–72 h. IGRAs: Unaffected by BCG vaccination; single visit; reduced sensitivity in very young and/or immune-compromised children; collecting adequate volume of blood and indeterminate results problematic.
Imaging		
Radiography CT and MRI Ultrasonography	Diagnosis of TB	Chest radiography (AP and lateral views) most helpful; CT or MRI useful in uncertain or complicated cases; ultrasonography useful to identify intraabdominal/retroperitoneal lymphadenopathy or pleural/pericardial effusions, highly operator-dependent.

Data adapted from Perez-Velez and Marais 2012.

TST, tuberculin skin test; IGRA, interferon-γ release assay; CT, computed tomography; MRI, magnetic resonance imaging.

induced sputa offer feasible alternatives (Nicol and Zar 2011). Table 6 provides an overview of specimen collection techniques (Marais and Pai 2006). The string test works well in sputum-scarce adults and preliminary results in children seem promising (Perez-Velez et al. 2010), although administration is difficult in young children who are unable to swallow the string-containing capsule. With adequate DNA extraction protocols, stool also offers promise as a diagnostic specimen (Nicol et al. 2013). FNAB has a high utility in children with a peripheral lymph node mass (Wright et al. 2009). The Union developed a pragmatic desk guide-to-guide TB diagnosis and management in resource-limited settings (IUTLD 2010).

MANAGEMENT

Although bacteriological confirmation of TB remains the ideal, yields are low and treatment initiation is a clinical decision in most instances once all appropriate tests have been completed.

Table 6. Bacteriologic specimen collection methods—perceived problems and/or benefits

Specimen collection method	Problems/Benefits	Potential clinical application
Sputum	Not feasible in very young children; assistance and supervision may improve the quality of the specimen	Routine sample to be collected in children >7 yr of age (all children who can produce a good quality specimen)
Induced sputum	Comparable yield to gastric aspirate; no age restriction; specialized technique, which requires nebulization and suction facilities; potential transmission risk	To be considered in the hospital setting on an in- or out-patient basis
Gastric aspirate	Unpleasant procedure, but not difficult to perform; requires fasting; sample collection advised on 3 consecutive days	Routine sample to be collected in hospitalized who cannot produce a good quality sputum specimen
Nasopharyngeal aspiration	Less invasive than gastric aspirate; no fasting required; comparable yield to gastric aspirate	To be considered in primary health care clinics or on an outpatient basis
String test	Less invasive than gastric aspirate; tolerated well in children >4 yr; bacteriologic yield and feasibility requires further investigation	Potential to become the routine sample collected in children who can swallow the capsule but cannot produce a good quality sputum specimen
Bronchoalveolar lavage	Extremely invasive	Only for use in patients who are intubated or who require diagnostic bronchoscopy
Stool	Culture not practical, DNA extraction difficult; not invasive; *M. tuberculosis* excretion well documented	Reasonable yield using Gene Xpert
Urine	Not invasive; excretion of *M. tuberculosis* components	Lipoarabinomannan (LAM) assay has poor sensitivity; unreliable in children
Blood/Bone marrow	Good sample sources to consider in the case of probable disseminated TB	To be considered for the confirmation of probable disseminated TB in hospitalized patients
Cerebrospinal fluid (CSF)	Fairly invasive; bacteriologic yield low	To be considered if signs of tuberculous meningitis
Fine needle aspiration (FNA)	Minimally invasive using a fine 23G needle; excellent bacteriologic yield; minimal side effects	Procedure of choice in children with superficial lymphadenopathy

Data adapted from Marais and Pai 2006.

Young children rarely experience serious adverse events with first-line TB drugs and are at low risk of acquiring or transmitting DR-TB. TB treatment aims to cure the individual patient, whereas the public health aim is to terminate transmission and prevent the emergence of drug resistance. Actively metabolizing bacilli are rapidly killed by bactericidal drugs, improving clinical symptoms, terminating transmission, and providing protection to companion drugs. Sterilizing drugs are required to eradicate persistent subpopulations of bacilli to establish long-term cure. Pragmatic disease classification should guide individual case management (Fig. 12).

The most important disease variables to consider are bacillary load and anatomical location. Drug resistance should be considered in children from settings with a high prevalence of DR-TB or following documented contact with a drug-resistant source case—someone who died while on TB treatment without known drug susceptibility test results, is poorly adherent to therapy, or is a retreatment case. Young children with uncomplicated disease, from settings with a low prevalence of isoniazid resistance, can be treated with three drugs (isoniazid, rifampicin, and pyrazinamide) during the 2-mo intensive phase, followed by isoniazid and rifampicin during the 4-mo continuation phase.

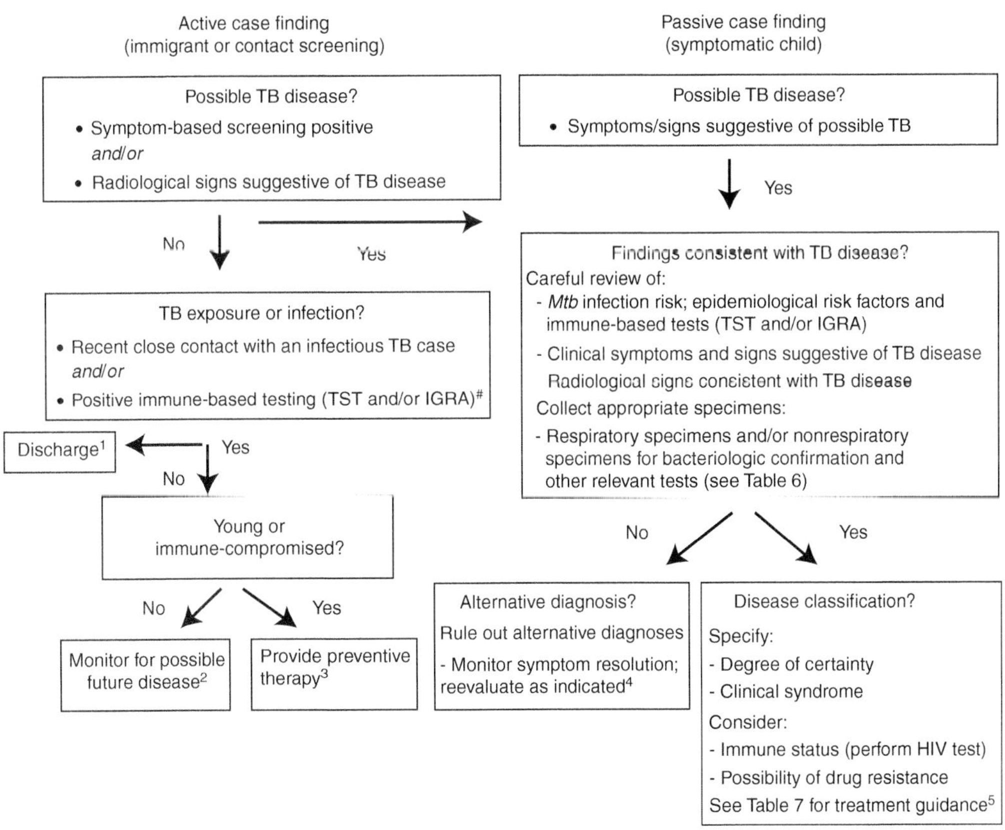

Figure 12. Algorithm for diagnosis and classification of tuberculosis in children. HIV, human immunodeficiency virus; TST, tuberculin skin test; IGRA, interferon-γ release assay; *Mtb*—*Mycobacterium tuberculosis*. #None of the immune-based tests (TST/IGRA) can "rule out" TB disease with confidence and conversion may be delayed for 2–3 mo after documented exposure. Diagnostic labels: [1]No TB exposure or infection; [2]TB exposure/infection with low risk of progression to disease; [3]TB exposure/infection with high risk of progression to disease; [4]unlikely TB disease; [5]TB disease. (Data adapted from Perez-Velez and Marais 2012.)

However, children with extensive and/or cavitary lung disease (implying a high organism load) or from settings with a high prevalence of isoniazid resistance, should receive a fourth drug (ethambutol, which is safe in children of all ages within the recommended dosage range) during the 2-mo intensive phase (WHO Press 2014). Table 7 summarizes the mechanism of action, main adverse effects, and recommended pediatric dosages of first-line TB drugs.

The most likely cause of poor response to treatment, in the absence of drug resistance, is nonadherence. All TB medications should preferably be given as directly observed therapy (DOT). Standard first-line treatment is appropriate in the absence of exposure to a source case with likely DR-TB or clinical and radiological deterioration while receiving adherent first-line therapy. Use of an escalated retreatment regimen that includes only streptomycin is not indicated; TB recurrence >12 mo after treatment completion most likely represents a new disease episode (reinfection) and should be treated as such. Poor clinical response to adherent treatment requires critical reevaluation of the diagnosis, including consideration of IRIS and drug resistance. Practice-based recommendations on the management of children with DR-TB were recently published (Seddon et al. 2012) and excellent treatment outcomes can be achieved with optimal management (Ettehad et al. 2012).

Immune recovery following ART initiation or nutritional rehabilitation may unmask existing subclinical disease or induce paradoxical deterioration despite adequate TB treatment. IRIS does not indicate treatment failure and treatment should usually not be interrupted; severe cases may require a course of corticosteroids. Despite the risk of IRIS, adult data indicate that ART is best initiated within 8 wk of starting TB treatment and within 2–4 wk in the severely immune-compromised (Blanc et al. 2011). The only exception for stopping ART would be patients with central nervous system TB, where IRIS could have devastating consequences (e.g., CSF outflow obstruction due to new tuberculomas or brain abscesses with increasing intracranial pressure) (Török et al. 2011). With HIV-associated TB, treatment should be daily and the total duration may require extension depending on the level of immune compromise and extent of disease (Siberry et al. 2013).

PREVENTION

Transmission within health-care facilities is a particular concern in settings where very young or immune-compromised children may be exposed. Careful consideration should be given to patient flows and air exchange in hospitals and clinics, considering that symptomatic parents or caregivers pose a transmission risk (Muñoz et al. 2002). Although BCG vaccination reduces the risk of disseminated (miliary) disease and TBM in young children, it offers no consistent protection against adult-type TB (Trunz et al. 2006). No benefit has been established in HIV-infected children, in whom BCG vaccination is contraindicated because of the risk of disseminated BCG disease (Hesseling et al. 2007; World Health Organization 2007). However, with good prevention of mother-to-child transmission of HIV (PMTCT) the risk of not giving BCG in the 97% infants of HIV-infected mothers who will be HIV-negative outweighs the benefit of not giving it to the few who might become HIV-infected (Rabie et al. 2011). In addition, early ART initiation prevents disseminated BCG disease and BCG IRIS that has been observed with delayed ART initiation (Rabie et al. 2001). The development of a safe and effective vaccine remains a top global health research priority.

With good adherence, isoniazid preventive therapy (IPT) for 6–9 mo provides excellent protection against TB disease (Marais et al. 2009), but implementation remains poor with a pronounced policy-practice gap (Hill et al. 2011). Parents are often reluctant to provide "treatment" to an otherwise well child and the long duration of preventive therapy provides further discouragement. Isoniazid and rifampicin for 3 mo provides equivalent efficacy and improved adherence compared with 9 mo of isoniazid (Spyridis et al. 2007). A regimen of 12 doses of weekly rifapentine and isoniazid was effica-

Table 7. Summary of first-line TB drugs and dosage recommendations in children

First-line drugs	Mode and mechanism of action	Main toxicities[a]	Daily dose mg/kg (range) [maximum dose][b]
Isoniazid (INH)	Bactericidal—inhibits cell wall synthesis; most potent early bactericidal activity offering the best protection to companion drugs Contributes mainly by rapidly killing actively metabolizing extracellular bacilli; contributes to sterilization if given for a prolonged period	Hepatitis; peripheral neuropathy	10 (7–15) [300 mg]
Rifampicin (RMP)	Bactericidal and sterilizing—inhibits RNA synthesis; contributes by killing extracellular and slower growing intracellular bacilli; important contribution to sterilization	Hepatitis; orange discoloration of secretions; drug–drug interactions	15 (10–20) [600 mg]
Pyrazinamide (PZA)	Sterilizing—disrupts energy metabolism; contributes by specifically killing bacilli that persist within the acidic centers of caseating granulomas	Hepatitis; arthralgia	35 (30–40) [2000 mg]
Ethambutol (EMB)	Bacteriostatic—inhibits cell wall synthesis; contributes mainly by offering some additional protection against drug-resistant mutants	Visual disturbance (acuity, color vision)	20 (15–25) [1200 mg]

Suggested treatment regimens

Disease category	Treatment regimen	Rationale
Uncomplicated intrathoracic disease	INH, RMP, PZA (2-mo intensive phase) INH, RMP (4-mo continuation phase)	Organism load low; drug penetration good
Extensive lung infiltrates and/or cavities	Add EMB during 2-mo intensive phase	Organism load high; drug penetration good
Tuberculous meningitis (TBM)[c]	Add fourth drug—at least during 2-mo intensive phase. Prolong continuation phase to 10 months (WHO recommendation) Add steroids for 1 mo	Organism load low; drug penetration variable; risk of severe immune mediated sequelae
Severe airway compression	Three- or four-drug regimen depending on extent of lung infiltration/cavities Consider adding steroids for 1 mo	Organism and drug penetration variable[d]; inflammation may worsen airway compression
Recent exposure/ infection	Preventive therapy	
No active disease	INH (6–9 mo) INH, RMP (3 mo)	Organism load very low; drug penetration good

Data adapted from Perez-Velez and Marais 2012.

[a]Hypersensitivity reactions and drug rashes may occur with any drug.

[b]WHO dosage recommendations for children.

[c]Recommendations around fourth drug and duration of therapy vary.

[d]Drug penetration into large cold abscesses may be limited, requiring surgical drainage.

cious in adults (Sterling et al. 2011), but is not yet recommended in children of <12 yr of age awaiting safety data. All rifampicin- and rifapentine-containing regimens interact with protease inhibitor-containing ART; this is less with rifabutin, but its use in preventive therapy regimens has not been evaluated. WHO recommends IPT for 6-36 mo after completion of TB treatment in all HIV-infected individuals, including children, who live in settings with a high TB prevalence (World Health Organization 2011b). However, ongoing TB exposure screening and meticulous postexposure prophylaxis following every documented TB exposure event, together with early ART initiation in all HIV-infected children, seem adequate (Schaaf et al. 2013). Preventive therapy has benefit in vulnerable children following exposure to DR-TB, but this should be tailored to the drug susceptibility test result of the source case or known drug resistance profiles in the region (Seddon et al. 2013).

Ultimately, the burden of childhood TB within a community reflects the underlying variables that sustain the TB epidemic, because pediatric cases reflect ongoing *M. tuberculosis* transmission (Fig. 13) (Marais et al. 2005b). Whereas ultimate epidemic control require these factors to be addressed at a population level, much can be done to alleviate the TB disease burden in children by offering adequate prevention, considering TB in the differential diagnosis, and providing appropriate treatment.

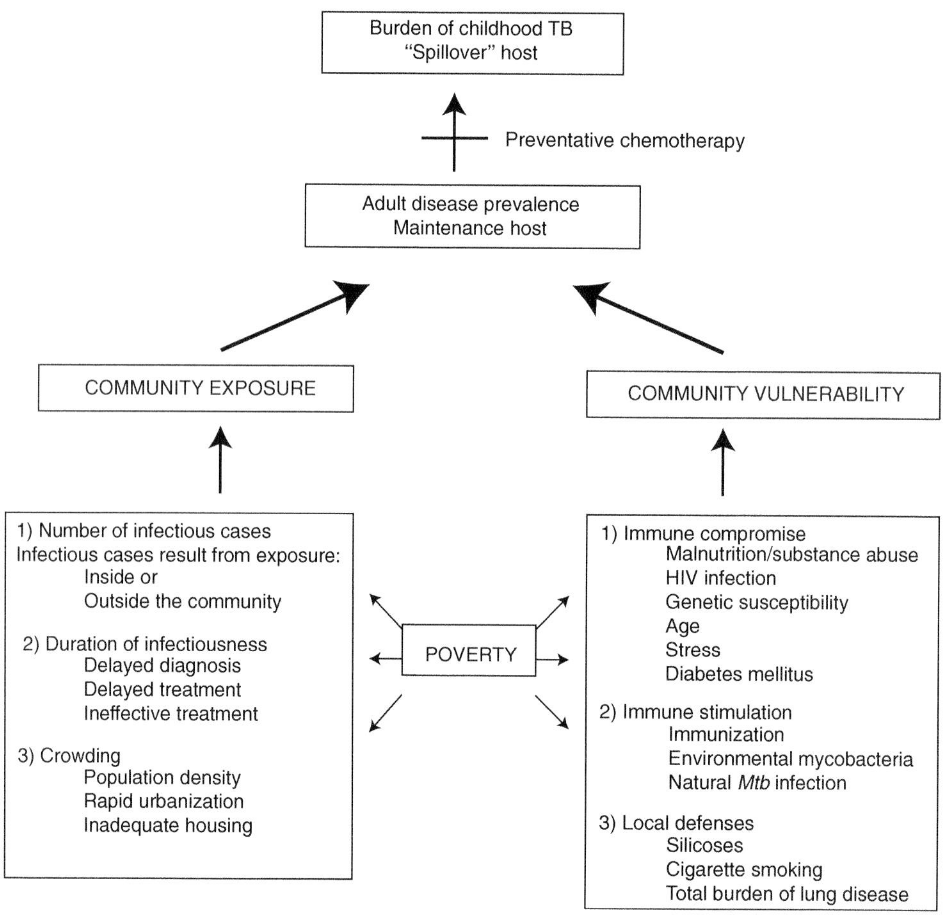

Figure 13. The main variables that contribute to the burden of childhood TB in a particular community. (Data adapted from Marais et al. 2005b.)

Cite this article as *Cold Spring Harb Perspect Med* doi: 10.1101/cshperspect.a017855

REFERENCES

*Reference is also in this subject collection.

Abubakar I, Ford N, Cox H. 2013. The rising tide of drug-resistant tuberculosis—Time for visionary political leadership. *Lancet Infect Dis* **13:** 529–539.

Amanullah F, Ashfaq M, Khowaja S, Parekh A, Salahuddin N, Lotia-Farrukh I, Khan A, Becerra MC. 2014. High tuberculosis prevalence in children exposed at home to drug-resistant tuberculosis. *Int J Tuberc Lung Dis* **18:** 520–527.

Andronikou S, van Hoenacker FM, de Backer AI. 2009. Advances in imaging chest tuberculosis: Blurring-of-differences-between-children-and-adults. *Clin Chest Med* **30:** 717–744.

Bates M, Mudenda V, Mwaba P, Zumla A. 2013. Deaths due to respiratory tract infections in Africa: A review of autopsy studies. *Curr Opin Pulm Med* **19:** 229–237.

Blanc FX, Sok T, Laureillard D, Borand L, Rekacewicz C, Nerrienet E, Madec Y, Marcy O, Chan S, Prak N, et al. 2011. Earlier versus later start of antiretroviral therapy in HIV-infected adults with tuberculosis. *N Engl J Med* **365:** 1471–1481.

Cotton MF, Schaaf HS, Lottering G, Wever HL, Coetzee J, Nachman S. 2008. Tuberculosis exposure in HIV-exposed infants in a high-prevalence setting. *Int J Tuberc Lung Dis* **12:** 225–227.

Du Preez K, Schaaf HS, Dunbar R, Swartz A, Bissell K, Enarson DA, Hessling AC. 2011. Incomplete registration and reporting of culture-confirmed childhood tuberculosis diagnosed in hospital. *Public Health Action* **1:** 19–24.

Edwards DJ, Kitelele F, van Rie A. 2007. Agreement between clinical scoring systems used for the diagnosis of tuberculosis in the HIV era. *Int J Tuberc Lung* **11:** 263–269.

Ettehad D, Schaaf HS, Seddon JA, Cooke G, Ford N. 2012. Treatment outcomes for children with multi-drug resistant tuberculosis: A systematic review and meta-analysis. *Lancet Infect Dis* **12:** 449–456.

Gie RP. 2003. *Diagnostic atlas of intrathoracic tuberculosis in children: A guide for low income countries.* IUATLD, Paris. http://www.theunion.org/download/clh/diagnostic_atlas_intrathoraric_tuberculosis_child.pdf.

Graham SM, Sismanidis C, Menzies HJ, Marais BJ, Detjen AK, Black RE. 2014. Importance of tuberculosis control to address child survival. *Lancet* **383:** 1605–1607.

Hesseling AC, Schaaf HS, Gie RP, Starke JR, Beyers N. 2002. A critical review of diagnostic approaches used in the diagnosis of childhood tuberculosis. *Int J Tuberc Lung Dis* **6:** 1038–1045.

Hesseling AC, Marais BJ, Gie RP, Schaaf HS, Fine PEM, Godfrey-Faussett P, Beyers N. 2007. The risk of disseminated bacilli Calmette–Guérin (BCG) disease in HIV-infected children. *Vaccine* **25:** 14–18.

Hesseling AC, Cotton MF, Jennings T, Whitelaw A, Johnson LF, Eley B, Roux P, Godfrey-Faussett P, Schaaf HS. 2009. High incidence of tuberculosis among HIV-infected infants: Evidence from a South African population-based study highlights the need for improved tuberculosis control strategies. *Clin Infect Dis* **48:** 108–114.

Hill PC, Rutherford ME, Audas R, van Crevel R, Graham SM. 2011. Closing the policy-practice gap in the management of child contacts of tuberculosis in developing countries. *PLoS Med* **8:** e10001105.

IUATLD. 2010. Desk-guide for the diagnosis and management of TB in children. www.theunion.org/index.php/en/resources/scientific-publications/tuberculosis/item/193-desk-guide-for-diagnosis-and-management-of-tb-in-children.

Jenkins HE, Tolman AW, Yuen CM, Parr JB, Keshavjee S, Perez-Velez CM, Pagano M, Becerra MC, Cohen T. 2014. Incidence of multidrug-resistant tuberculosis disease in children: Systematic review and global estimates. *Lancet* **383:** 1572–1579.

* Källenius G. 2014. Tuberculosis and HIV coinfections. *Cold Spring Harb Perspect Med* doi: 10.1101/cshperspect.a017871.

Lawn SD, Bekker LG, Middelkoop K, Myer L, Wood R. 2006. Impact of HIV infection on the epidemiology of tuberculosis in a peri-urban community in South Africa: The need for age-specific interventions. *Clin Infect Dis* **42:** 1040–1047.

Lincoln EM, Sewell EM. 1963. Tuberculosis in children. McGraw-Hill, New York.

Marais BJ, Pai M. 2006. Specimen collection methods in the diagnosis of childhood tuberculosis. *Indian J Med Microbiol* **24:** 249–251.

Marais BJ, Gie RP, Schaaf HS, Hesseling AC, Obihara CC, Starke JJ, Enarson DA, Donald PR, Beyers N. 2004a. The natural history of childhood intra-thoracic tuberculosis: A critical review of literature from the pre-chemotherapy era. *Int J Tuberc Lung Dis* **8:** 392–402.

Marais BJ, Gie RP, Schaaf HS, Starke JR, Hesseling AC, Donald PR, Beyers N. 2004b. A proposed radiologic classification of childhood intra-thoracic tuberculosis. *Pediatr Rad* **33:** 886–894.

Marais BJ, Donald PR, Gie RP, Schaaf HS, Beyers N. 2005a. Diversity of disease manifestations in childhood pulmonary tuberculosis. *Ann Trop Paed* **25:** 79–86.

Marais BJ, Obihara CC, Warren RM, Schaaf HS, Gie RP, Donald PR. 2005b. The burden of childhood tuberculosis: A public health perspective. *Int J Tuberc Lung Dis* **9:** 1305–1313.

Marais BJ, Gie RP, Schaaf HS, Hesseling AC, Enarson DA, Beyers N. 2006a. The spectrum of disease in children treated for tuberculosis in a highly endemic area. *Int J Tuberc Lung Dis* **10:** 732–738.

Marais BJ, Wright CA, Schaaf HS, Gie RP, Hesseling AC, Enarson DA, Beyers N. 2006b. Tuberculous lymphadenitis as a cause of persistent cervical lymphadenopathy in children from a tuberculosis-endemic area. *Pediatr Inf Dis J* **25:** 142–146.

Marais BJ, Gie RP, Hesseling AC, Schaaf HS, Lombard C, Enarson DA, Beyers N. 2006c. A refined symptom-based approach to diagnose pulmonary tuberculosis in children. *Pediatrics* **118:** e1350–e1359.

Marais BJ, Ayles H, Graham SM, Godfrey-Faussett P. 2009. Screening and preventive therapy for tuberculosis. *Chest Clin N Am* **30:** 827–846.

Marais B, Graham S, Maeurer M, Zumla A. 2013a. Progress and challenges in childhood tuberculosis. *Lancet Infect Dis* **13:** 287–289.

Marais BJ, Mlambo CK, Rastogi N, Zozio T, Duse AG, Victor TC, Marais E, Warren RM. 2013b. Epidemic spread of multidrug-resistant (MDR) tuberculosis in Johannesburg, South Africa. *J Clin Microbiol* **51:** 1818–1825.

Marais S, Meintjes G, Pepper DJ, Dodd LE, Schutz C, Ismail Z, Wilkinson KA, Wilkinson RJ. 2013c. Frequency, severity, and prediction of tuberculous meningitis immune reconstitution inflammatory syndrome. *Clin Infect Dis* **56:** 450–460.

Meintjes G, Rabie H, Wilkinson RJ, Cotton MF. 2009. Tuberculosis-associated immune reconstitution inflammatory syndrome and unmasking of tuberculosis by antiretroviral therapy. *Clin Chest Med* **30:** 797–810.

MMWR. 2010. Updated guidelines for using interferon gamma release assays to detect Mycobacterium tuberculosis infection—United States. *MMWR* **59:** 1–25.

Muñoz FM, Ong LT, Seavy D, Medina D, Correa A, Starke JR. 2002. Tuberculosis among adult visitors of children with suspected tuberculosis and employees at a children's hospital. *Infect Control Hosp Epidemiol* **23:** 568–572.

Newton SM, Brent AJ, Anderson S, Whittaker E, Kampmann B. 2008. Paediatric tuberculosis. *Lancet Infect Dis* **8:** 499–510.

Nicol MP, Zar HJ. 2011. New specimens and laboratory diagnostics for childhood pulmonary TB: Progress and prospects. *Paediatr Respir Rev* **12:** 16–21.

Nicol MP, Workman L, Isaacs W, Munro J, Eley B, Boehme CC, Zemanay W, Zar HJ. 2011. Accuracy of the Xpert MTB/RIF test for the diagnosis of pulmonary tuberculosis in children admitted to hospital in Cape Town, South Africa: A descriptive study. *Lancet Infect Dis* **11:** 819–824.

Nicol MP, Spiers K, Workman L, Isaacs W, Munro J, Black F, Zemanay W, Zar HJ. 2013. Xpert MTB/RIF testing of stool samples for the diagnosis of pulmonary tuberculosis in children. *Clin Infect Dis* **57:** e18–e21.

Perez-Velez CM, Marais BJ. 2012. Tuberculosis in children. *N Engl J Med* **367:** 348–361.

Perez-Velez CM, Wilches-Luna EC, Hernández-Sarmiento JM, Casanova-Reynolds AL, Hernández N, Moreno-Ortega SP, Atehortúa-Muñoz SL, Rozo-Anaya JC, Mejía GI, Gómez V, et al. 2010. Preliminary results of a comparative yield study of induced sputum, string test, and gastric aspirate for the microbiological diagnosis of pulmonary tuberculosis in children. *Am J Respir Crit Care Med* **181:** A1775.

Pienaar M, Andronikou S, van Toorn R. 2009. MRI to demonstrate diagnostic features and complications of TBM not seen with CT. *Child Nerv Syst* **25:** 941–947.

Rabie H, Violari A, Duong T, Madhi SA, Josipovic D, Innes S, Dobbels E, Lazarus E, Panchia R, Babiker AG, et al. 2011. Early antiretroviral treatment reduces risk of bacille Calmette–Guérin immune reconstitution adenitis. *Int J Tuberc Lung Dis* **15:** 1194–1200.

Rachow A, Clowes P, Saathoff E, Mtafya B, Ntinginya EN, Kowour D, Rojas-Ponce G, Kroidl A, Maboko L, Heinrich N, et al. 2012. Increased and expedited case detection by Xpert MTB/RIF assay in childhood tuberculosis: A prospective cohort study. *Clin Infect Dis* **54:** 1388–1396.

Rose PC, Schaaf HS, du Preez K, Seddon JA, Garcia-Prats AJ, Zimri K, Dunbar R, Hesseling AC. 2013. Completeness and accuracy of paediatric electronic drug-resistant tuberculosis registration in Cape Town, South Africa. *Public Health Action* **3:** 214–219.

Schaaf HS, Van Rie A, Gie RP, Beyers N, Victor TC, Van Helden PD, Donald PR. 2000. Transmission of multidrug resistant tuberculosis. *Pediatr Infect Dis J* **19:** 695–699.

Schaaf HS, Marais BJ, Whitelaw A, Hesseling AC, Eley B, Hussey GD, Donald PR. 2007. Culture-confirmed childhood tuberculosis in Cape Town, South Africa: A review of 596 cases. *BMC Infect Dis* **7:** 140.

Schaaf HS, Collins A, Bekker A, Davies PDO. 2010. Tuberculosis at the extremes of age. *Respirology* **15:** 747–763.

Schaaf HS, Cotton MF, Boon GPG, Jeena PM. 2013. Isoniazid preventive therapy in HIV-infected and uninfected children (0–14 years). *S Afr Med J* **103:** 714–715.

Seddon JA, Furin JJ, Gale M, Del Castillo Barrientos H, Hurtado RM, Amanullah F, Ford N, Starke JR, Schaaf HS, Sentinel Project on Pediatric Drug-Resistant Tuberculosis. 2012. Caring for children with drug-resistant tuberculosis: Practice-based recommendations. *Am J Respir Crit Care Med* **186:** 953–964.

Seddon JA, Hesseling AC, Finlayson H, Fielding K, Cox H, Hughes J, Godfrey-Faussett P, Schaaf HS. 2013. Preventive therapy for child contacts of multidrug-resistant tuberculosis: A prospective cohort study. *Clin Infect Dis* **57:** 1676–1684.

* Seung KJ, Rich M, Keshavjee S. 2014. MDR and XDR tuberculosis. *Cold Spring Harb Perspect Med* doi: 10.1101/cshperspect.a017863.

Siberry GK, Abzug MJ, Nachman S, the Panel on Opportunistic Infections in HIV-Exposed and HIV-Infected Children. 2013. Guidelines for the prevention and treatment of opportunistic infections in HIV-exposed and HIV-infected children: Recommendations from the National Institutes of Health, Centers for Disease Control and Prevention, the HIV Medicine Association of the Infectious Diseases Society of America, the Pediatric Infectious Diseases Society, and the American Academy of Pediatrics. *Pediatr Infect Dis J* **32.**

Spyridis NP, Spyridis PG, Gelesme A, Sypsa V, Valianatou M, Metsou F, Gourgiotis D, Tsolia MN. 2007. The effectiveness of a 9-month regimen of isoniazid alone versus 3- and 4-month regimens of isoniazid plus rifampin for treatment of latent tuberculosis infection in children: Results of an 11-year randomized study. *Clin Infect Dis* **45:** 715–722.

Sterling TR, Villarino ME, Borisov AS, Shang N, Gordin F, Bliven-Sizemore E, Hackman J, Hamilton CD, Menzies D, et al. 2011. Three months of rifapentine and isoniazid for latent tuberculosis infection. *N Eng J Med* **365:** 2155–2166.

Thwaites GE, van Toorn R, Schoeman J. 2013. Tuberculous meningitis: More questions, still too few answers. *Lancet Neurol* **12:** 999–1010.

Török ME, Yen NT, Chau TT, Mai NT, Phu NH, Mai PP, Dung NT, Chau NV, Bang ND, Tien NA, et al. 2011. Timing of initiation of antiretroviral therapy in human immunodeficiency virus (HIV)-associated tuberculous meningitis. *Clin Infect Dis* **52:** 1374–1383.

Trunz BB, Fine P, Dye C. 2006. Effect of BCG vaccination on childhood tuberculous meningitis and miliary tuberculosis worldwide: A meta-analysis and assessment of cost-effectiveness. *Lancet* **367:** 1173–1180.

Violari A, Cotton MF, Gibb DM, Babiker AG, Steyn J, Madhi SA, Jean-Philippe P, McIntyre JA,CHER Study Team. 2008. Early antiretroviral therapy and mortality among HIV-infected infants. *N Engl J Med* **359:** 2233–2244.

Wallgren A. 1948. The time-table of tuberculosis. *Tubercle* **29:** 245–251.

WHO Press. 2014. *Guidance for national tuberculosis programmes on the management of tuberculosis in children*, 2nd ed. Geneva, Switzerland (WHO/HTM/TB/2014.03).

World Health Organization. 2007. Revised BCG vaccination guideline for infants at risk of HIV infection. *Wkly Edimiol Rev* **82:** 193.

World Health Organization. 2011a. Use of tuberculosis interferon-γ release assays (IGRAs) in low- and middle-income countries: Policy statement. Geneva, WHO Press.

World Health Organization. 2011b. Guidelines for intensified TB case-finding and INH preventive therapy for people living with HIV in resource-constrained settings: Annexes. WHO Press, Geneva. http://whqlibdoc.who.int/publications/2011/9789241500708_annexes_eng.pdf.

World Health Organization. 2013. Global Tuberculosis Report 2013. World Health Organisation, Geneva. WHO/HTM/TB/2013.

Wright CA, Warren RW, Marais BJ. 2009. Fine needle aspiration biopsy: An undervalued diagnostic modality in pediatric mycobacterial disease. *Int J Tuberc Lung Dis* **13:** 1467–1475.

Zignol M, Sismanidis C, Falzon D, Glaziou P, Dara M, Floyd K. 2013. Multidrug-resistant tuberculosis in children: Evidence from global surveillance. *Eur Respir J* **42:** 701–707.

Multidrug-Resistant Tuberculosis and Extensively Drug-Resistant Tuberculosis

Kwonjune J. Seung[1,2,3], Salmaan Keshavjee[1,2,3], and Michael L. Rich[1,2,3]

[1]Division of Global Health Equity, Brigham and Women's Hospital, Boston, Massachusetts 02115

[2]Department of Global Health and Social Medicine, Harvard Medical School, Boston, Massachusetts 02115

[3]Partners In Health, Boston, Massachusetts 02215

Correspondence: kjseung@pih.org

The continuing spread of drug-resistant tuberculosis (TB) is one of the most urgent and difficult challenges facing global TB control. Patients who are infected with strains resistant to isoniazid and rifampicin, called multidrug-resistant (MDR) TB, are practically incurable by standard first-line treatment. In 2012, there were approximately 450,000 new cases and 170,000 deaths because of MDR-TB. Extensively drug-resistant (XDR) TB refers to MDR-TB strains that are resistant to fluoroquinolones and second-line injectable drugs. The main causes of the spread of resistant TB are weak medical systems, amplification of resistance patterns through incorrect treatment, and transmission in communities and facilities. Although patients harboring MDR and XDR strains present a formidable challenge for treatment, cure is often possible with early identification of resistance and use of a properly designed regimen. Community-based programs can improve treatment outcomes by allowing patients to be treated in their homes and addressing socioeconomic barriers to adherence.

EPIDEMIOLOGY

Even though tuberculosis (TB) is a treatable infectious disease, an estimated 1.3 million people died from TB in 2012 (WHO 2013a). One of the major reasons is that TB continues to evolve resistance to drugs. For patients with drug-susceptible TB, standard treatment based on isoniazid and rifampicin, the two most powerful drugs, results in excellent cure rates. Patients who are infected with strains resistant to isoniazid and rifampicin, called multidrug-resistant (MDR) TB, are practically incurable by standard first-line treatment (Fig. 1).

Today, the continuing spread of MDR-TB is one of the most urgent and difficult challenges facing global TB control. In 2012, there were approximately 450,000 new cases of MDR-TB and 170,000 deaths. Globally, MDR-TB is present in 3.8% of new TB patients and 20% of patients who have a history of previous treatment. The highest MDR rates are found in countries of Eastern Europe and central Asia, where MDR strains threaten to become as common as pan-susceptible strains. In some countries, MDR strains account for up to 20% of new TB cases and well over 50% of patients with a history of previous TB treatment. In

Cite this article as *Cold Spring Harb Perspect Med* doi: 10.1101/cshperspect.a017863

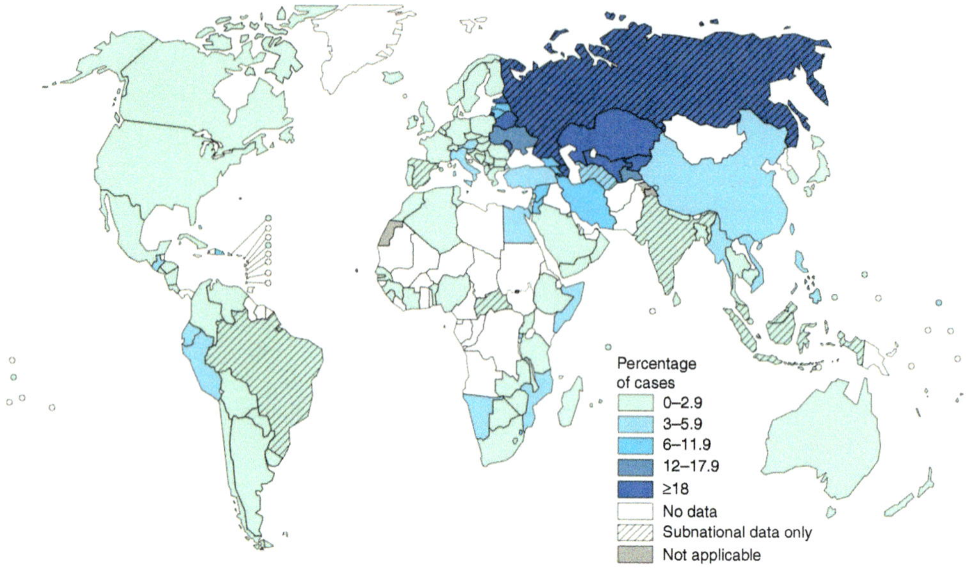

Figure 1. Percentage of new TB cases with MDR-TB (WHO 2013a).

2011, Minsk, Belarus reported that 35% of new patients had MDR-TB, as did 75% of those who had been treated previously for TB (Skrahina et al. 2012).

Equally worrisome rates have emerged from China and India, which have the highest and second-highest number of MDR-TB patients in the world. In 2012, the China Centers for Disease Control and Prevention reported that 10% of China's 1.4 million TB patients had MDR-TB, and the great majority of MDR-TB patients had never been treated for TB—evidence of unfettered human-to-human transmission (Zhao et al. 2012). MDR-TB is also a growing problem in South Africa, where high rates of HIV (human immunodeficiency virus) have exacerbated both the spread and deadliness of MDR-TB, raising the specter of a "perfect storm" of MDR-TB/HIV coinfection (Wells et al. 2007). In clinical practice today, the possibility of unsuspected drug resistance must always be considered when evaluating a TB patient in any country (Box 1).

In 2006, the term extensively drug-resistant TB (XDR-TB) was coined to describe strains of MDR-TB resistant to fluoroquinolones and second-line injectable drugs. It is estimated that 9.6% of MDR-TB cases worldwide have XDR-

BOX 1. TYPES OF DRUG-RESISTANT TB (WHO 2013b) (TYPES ARE NOT MUTUALLY EXCLUSIVE)

Monoresistance: Resistance to one first-line anti-TB drug only.
Polydrug resistance: Resistance to more than one first-line anti-TB drug, other than both isoniazid and rifampicin.
Multidrug resistance (MDR): Resistance to at least both isoniazid and rifampicin.
Rifampicin resistance (RR): Resistance to rifampicin detected using phenotypic or genotypic methods, with or without resistance to other anti-TB drugs. It includes any resistance to rifampicin, whether monoresistance, multidrug resistance, polydrug resistance, or extensive drug resistance.
Extensive drug resistance (XDR): Resistance to any fluoroquinolone, and at least one of three second-line injectable drugs (capreomycin, kanamycin, and amikacin), in addition to multidrug resistance.

TB (WHO 2013a). Because access to second-line drug susceptibility testing (DST) is poor in many areas of the world, XDR-TB often goes unrecognized. Although patients harboring MDR and XDR strains present a formidable challenge for treatment, cure is often possible with early identification of resistance and use of a properly designed regimen.

CAUSES OF DRUG RESISTANCE

Drug resistance is a biological phenomenon that has been observed in *Mycobacterium tuberculosis* since the discovery of the first anti-TB drug, streptomycin. Many patients who were injected with streptomycin were brought from the brink of death and their sputum became temporarily clear of *M. tuberculosis*. But despite continuing to receive treatment, they soon began to excrete bacilli that were resistant to streptomycin in the laboratory (Pyle 1947).

With the advent of new drugs—thioacetazone and para-aminosalicylic acid in 1948 and isoniazid in 1952—it became clear that combination chemotherapy was the key to preventing the development of resistance. Initial combination regimens required 18 mo of treatment, but the invention of rifampicin in 1957, the most powerfully sterilizing anti-TB drug, paved the way for development of the shorter and more effective isoniazid- and rifampicin-containing regimens known as short-course chemotherapy. As part of the global TB control strategy called DOTS (directly observed treatment, short-course), these regimens became the standard of care even in resource-limited settings starting in 1993.

Outbreaks of MDR-TB were initially thought to be driven by nosocomial transmission, particularly among HIV-positive patients. One of the largest and best-documented outbreaks occurred in New York in the late 1980s and early 1990s (Frieden et al. 1993; Frieden et al. 1995). As DST laboratory capacity improved in resource-limited settings and global drug-resistant TB surveillance efforts grew, it became clear that MDR-TB was increasingly common throughout the world and a growing threat to the general public health. The causes of the global spread of MDR-TB include the following:

- *Chaotic treatment.* Before the late 1980s, many countries were not using standard protocols for the treatment of TB and did not have systems in place to support patients. Furthermore, in many settings, TB treatment was not provided for free, contributing to poor adherence. Even today, drug-resistant TB can be created very quickly during times of socioeconomic instability if there are stockouts of anti-TB drugs or other structural weaknesses in the health care system.
- *Amplifier effect of short-course chemotherapy.* Once drug resistance has been created, the DOTS strategy can paradoxically exacerbate the problem. In Figure 2, the initial strain has polydrug resistance, but, as a result of repeated use of short-course chemotherapy, it becomes resistant to all first-line anti-TB drugs (Seung et al. 2004). Amplification of drug resistance patterns through repeated courses of DOTS short-course chemotherapy continues to be a major driving force of the epidemic in many parts of the world that do not have the resources to diagnose or treat drug-resistant TB correctly (Keshavjee and Farmer 2012).
- *Community transmission.* In the early 2000s, it was believed that resistance mutations conferred a loss of fitness, so the transmission of resistant strains would be self-limited (Dye et al. 2002; Cegielski 2010). This has not turned out to be the case. Current models indicate that in most countries, the majority of MDR-TB patients were infected initially with an MDR-TB strain, rather than slowly acquiring resistance caused by inadequate or irregular treatment (Lin et al. 2011).
- *Facility-based transmission.* Nosocomial transmission in busy, crowded hospitals and health centers is likely an important driver of the epidemic, especially in high HIV prevalence settings. This can result in the spread of drug-resistant strains among patients receiving therapy for drug-susceptible TB as well as to the health workers (Gelmanova et al. 2007).

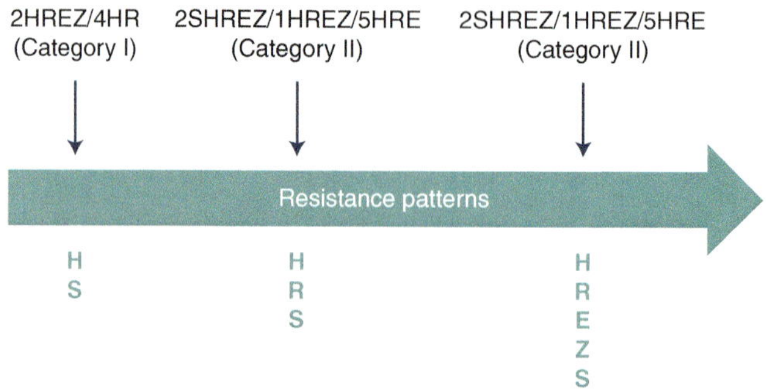

Figure 2. Amplifier effect of short-course chemotherapy. H, isoniazid; R, rifampicin; E, ethambutol; Z, pyrazinamide; S, streptomycin.

DIAGNOSIS OF MDR-TB AND XDR-TB

DST is required for the definitive diagnosis of MDR-TB or XDR-TB. The traditional way to do this is through phenotypic (or culture-based) methods. *M. tuberculosis* is isolated from patient sputum and then tested for growth in the presence of anti-TB drugs. Culture-based methods can take weeks to months. They are also expensive and difficult to master, making them mostly unavailable in resource-limited settings.

Genotypic (or molecular) methods have revolutionized the diagnosis of MDR-TB. These methods generally use polymerase chain reaction techniques to detect the genetic mutations that are known to confer resistance to drugs. Commercially available systems include GeneXpert System (Xpert MTB/RIF, Cepheid, USA), GenoType MTBDRplus and MTBDRsl assays (Hain Lifescience GmbH, Germany), and INNO-LiPA Rif.TB line probe assay (Innogenetics Inc., Belgium), but there are other systems in development. Molecular methods of DST give results much faster than culture-based methods. Some commercially available systems are almost fully automated and require little training. For these reasons, these systems are increasingly the method of choice for DST in resource-limited settings.

There is no "gold standard" for the diagnosis of drug resistance. Molecular testing may detect mutations that confer low levels of resistance that are not detected by culture-based testing but are still clinically significant. Molecular testing also cannot detect all of the mutations that are known to confer resistance to a drug. Nevertheless, it is not necessary to routinely confirm the results of molecular DST with culture-based DST, even though clinicians may choose to do so if the clinical picture warrants it. Specifically, a positive molecular test for rifampicin resistance can be considered diagnostic for MDR-TB, because in most countries, greater than 90% of rifampicin-resistant strains are also resistant to isoniazid.

A public health strategy of "universal DST," meaning testing all patients with active TB disease for drug resistance at the start of therapy, is certainly feasible in the near future because of the increasing availability of molecular DST. A WHO analysis determined that this would be a lifesaving and cost-effective strategy for any country with greater than 1% MDR-TB in new patients (WHO 2011a).

At the current time, however, DST is not widely available in many countries so patients with risk factors for MDR-TB are prioritized for testing. Empiric treatment for MDR-TB can be considered if there is clear bacteriological evidence of failure to respond to treatment, such as persistently positive sputum smears after 4 mo of regular treatment with a first-line DOTS regimen (Chavez Pachas et al. 2004; Satti et al. 2013). Household contacts of MDR-TB patients should also be started empirically on treatment if any delay in DST is anticipated (Box 2).

All patients diagnosed with MDR-TB should be tested for XDR-TB. This includes testing for resistance to the three second-line injectable drugs (kanamycin, amikacin, and

BOX 2. RISK FACTORS FOR MDR-TB

- Failure to respond to a first-line DOTS regimen (WHO Category I or II)
- Relapse after a full course of treatment with a first-line regimen
- Treatment after defaulting from treatment with a first-line regimen
- Exposure to a known case of MDR-TB
- Exposure to TB in institutions with high prevalence of MDR-TB, such as a prison or hospital
- Living in areas or countries with high prevalence of MDR-TB
- HIV coinfection

capreomycin) and at least one fluoroquinolone. Laboratories with a capacity for second-line DST, however, are even less common than those with capacity for first-line DST. Patients who should be prioritized for second-line DST include those who have failed to respond to an MDR-TB treatment regimen containing an injectable and fluoroquinolone, and close contacts with an individual with documented XDR-TB or with an individual for whom treatment with a regimen including second-line drugs is failing or has failed.

The GenoType MTBDRsl assays (Hain Lifescience GmbH, Germany) test for mutations in the *gyrA* gene, which confers resistance to fluoroquinolones, and in the *rrs* gene, which confers resistance to injectable drugs. This assay can be considered a "rule-in" test for second-line drug resistance, although it cannot reliably rule out XDR-TB when no genetic mutations are detected. Because the sensitivity and specificity of this assay are not well characterized, culture-based DST should be used as a confirmatory test.

TREATMENT

MDR-TB treatment is difficult because the second-line TB drugs are mostly weak and toxic. Most of these drugs were developed decades ago but hardly ever used because of poor side effect profiles. Because of the weak sterilizing activity of the second-line TB drugs, MDR-TB treatment generally takes 18–24 mo. In the best treatment programs, which address socioeconomic barriers and aggressively manage side effects, cure rates of 60%–80% have been reported (Mitnick et al. 2003; Shin et al. 2006). Globally, however, the cure rate for MDR-TB is much lower. In 2013, the WHO reported that only 48% of MDR-TB patients were cured. The global cure rate for XDR-TB is even lower: Only 20% are cured, and 44% die (WHO 2013a).

Anti-TB drugs have traditionally been divided into first- and second-line anti-TB drugs with isoniazid, rifampicin, pyrazinamide, ethambutol, and streptomycin being the primary first-line anti-TB drugs. In this review, we use the WHO system, which classifies the drugs into five different groups based on efficacy, experience of use, safety, and drug class. Drugs in the same group do not always come from the same drug class nor do they have the same safety profile or efficacy. Table 1 provides detailed information on each drug including the WHO group, dosage, side effects, and monitoring requirements.

In recent years, there has been considerable research devoted to developing new anti-TB drugs, with the goal of improving TB treatment. There are now two new purpose-built anti-TB drugs, the first in over 40 yr. Bedaquiline was conditionally approved by the U.S. FDA for the treatment of MDR-TB in December 2012. Delamanid was conditionally approved by the European Medicines Agency in November 2013. At least three additional new TB drugs are in late-phase clinical testing. These new drugs are likely to revolutionize the treatment of MDR-TB and XDR-TB.

Table 1. Anti-TB drugs and their side effects

Drug name (abbreviation)	Description and adult dose	Side effects	Monitoring requirements and comments
Group 1: First-line oral drugs			
Isoniazid (H)	**Description:** Bactericidal; inhibits mycolic acid synthesis most effectively in dividing cells; hepatically metabolized. **Dose:** 300 mg daily or 900 mg twice or thrice weekly.	**Common:** Hepatitis (10%–20% have elevated transaminases), peripheral neuropathy (dose-related; increased risk with malnutrition, alcoholism, diabetes, concurrent use of aminoglycosides, or ethionamide). **Less common:** Gynecomastia, rash, psychosis, seizure.	**Monitoring:** Consider baseline and monthly liver enzymes, especially if age >50 yr. **Comments:** Give with pyridoxine 50 mg/d if using large dose or if patient is at risk for peripheral neuropathy (diabetes, alcoholism, HIV, etc.).
Rifamycins Rifampicin (R) Rifabutin (Rfb) Rifapentine (Rpt)	**Description:** Bactericidal; inhibits protein synthesis by blocking mRNA transcription and synthesis; hepatically metabolized. **Dose:** rifampicin 600 mg/d; rifabutin 300 mg/d.	**Common:** Orange-colored bodily secretions, transient transaminitis, hepatitis, gastrointestinal distress. **Less common:** Cholestatic jaundice.	**Monitoring:** Consider baseline liver enzymes, repeat if symptoms (jaundice, fatigue, anorexia, weakness, or nausea and vomiting) appear.
Pyrazinamide (Z)	**Description:** Bactericidal; mechanism unclear; effective in acidic milieu (e.g., cavitary disease, intracellular organisms); hepatically metabolized, renally excreted. **Dose:** 15–40 mg/kg daily.	**Common:** Arthritis/arthralgias, hepatotoxicity, hyperuricemia, abdominal distress. **Less common:** Impaired diabetic control, rash.	**Monitoring:** Baseline liver enzymes; uric acid can be measured if arthralgias, arthritis, or symptoms of gout are present. **Comments:** Usually given once daily, but can split dose initially to improve tolerance.
Ethambutol (E)	**Description:** Bacteriostatic at conventional dosing (15 mg/kg); inhibits lipid and cell wall metabolism; renally excreted. **Dose:** 15–25 mg/kg.	**Common:** Generally well-tolerated. **Less common:** Optic neuritis, gastrointestinal distress, arthritis/arthralgia.	**Monitoring:** Baseline and monthly visual acuity and red/green color vision test when dosed at greater than 15 mg/kg daily (>10% loss is considered significant); regularly question patient about visual symptoms.

Continued

Table 1. *Continued*

Drug name (abbreviation)	Description and adult dose	Side effects	Monitoring requirements and comments
Group 2: Injectable drugs			
Aminoglycosides Amikacin (Amk) Kanamycin (Km) Streptomycin (S) *Polypeptides* Capreomycin (Cm)	**Description:** Bactericidal; aminoglycosides inhibit protein synthesis through disruption of ribosomal function; less effective in acidic, intracellular environments; polypeptides appear to inhibit translocation of the peptidyl-tRNA and the initiation of protein synthesis; renally excreted. **Dose:** 15–20 mg/kg daily.	**Common:** Pain at injection site; proteinuria; electrolyte wasting (more common with capreomycin); cochlear ototoxicity (hearing loss, dose-related to cumulative and peak concentrations, increased risk with renal insufficiency, may be irreversible). **Less common:** Nephrotoxicity (dose-related to cumulative and peak concentrations, increased risk with renal insufficiency, often irreversible); peripheral neuropathy; rash; vestibular toxicity (nausea, vomiting, vertigo, ataxia, nystagmus); eosinophilia; ototoxicity potentiated by certain diuretics, especially loop diuretics.	**Monitoring:** Baseline and then monthly creatinine, urea, and serum potassium; more frequently in high-risk patients; if potassium is low, check magnesium and calcium; baseline audiometry and monthly monitoring in high-risk patients (high-risk patients: elderly, diabetic, or HIV-positive patients, or patients with renal insufficiency). **Comments:** Increase dosing interval or reduce dose and monitor serum drug concentrations as needed to control side effects.
Group 3: Fluoroquinolones			
Levofloxacin (Lfx) Moxifloxacin (Mfx)	**Description:** Bactericidal; DNA-gyrase inhibitor; renally excreted. **Dose:** levofloxacin 750–1000 mg/d; moxifloxacin 400 mg/d.	**Common:** Generally well-tolerated, well-absorbed. **Less common:** Diarrhea, dizziness, gastrointestinal distress, headache, insomnia, photosensitivity, rash, vaginitis, tendonitis, psychosis, seizure (CNS effects seen almost exclusively in elderly).	**Monitoring:** No laboratory monitoring requirements. **Comments:** Do not administer with antacids, sucralfate, iron, zinc, calcium, or oral potassium and magnesium replacements; levofloxacin, moxifloxacin have the most activity against *M. tuberculosis.*
Group 4: Oral bacteriostatic drugs			
Cycloserine (Cs)	**Description:** Bacteriostatic; alanine analog; interferes with cell-	**Common:** Neurologic and psychiatric disturbances, including headaches, irritability, sleep	**Monitoring:** Consider serum drug monitoring to establish optimal dosing.

Continued

Table 1. *Continued*

Drug name (abbreviation)	Description and adult dose	Side effects	Monitoring requirements and comments
	wall proteoglycan synthesis; renally excreted. **Dose:** 500–1000 mg/d.	disturbances, aggression, and tremors. **Less common:** Psychosis, peripheral neuropathy, seizures (increased risk of CNS effects with concurrent use of ethanol, isoniazid, ethionamide, or other centrally acting medications), hypersensitivity.	**Comments:** Give 50 mg of pyridoxine for every 250 mg of cycloserine (to lessen neurologic adverse effects).
Thiamides **Ethionamide (Eto)** **Prothionamide (Pto)**	**Description:** May be bactericidal or bacteriostatic depending on susceptibility and concentrations attained at the infection site; the carbothioamide group, also found on thiacetazone, and the pyridine ring, also found on isoniazid, appear essential for activity; hepatically metabolized, renally excreted. **Dose:** 500–1000 mg/d.	**Common:** Gastrointestinal distress (nausea, vomiting, diarrhea, abdominal pain, loss of appetite); dysgeusia (metallic taste); hypothyroidism (especially when taken with PAS). **Less common:** Arthralgias, dermatitis, gynecomastia, hepatitis, impotence, peripheral neuropathy, photosensitivity.	**Monitoring:** Consider baseline liver enzymes. **Comments:** May split dose or give at bedtime to improve tolerability; ethionamide and prothionamide efficacies are considered similar; prothionamide may cause fewer gastrointestinal adverse effects.
Para-aminosalicylic acid (PAS)	**Description:** Bacteriostatic; disrupts folic acid metabolism (thought to inhibit the biosynthesis of coenzyme F in the folic acid pathway); hepatic acetylation, renally excreted. **Dose:** Depends on specific formulation.	**Common:** Gastrointestinal distress (nausea, vomiting, diarrhea); hypersensitivity; hypothyroidism (especially when taken with ethionamide). **Less common:** Hepatitis, electrolyte abnormalities. **Drug interactions:** Decreased isoniazid acetylation; decreased rifampicin absorption in nongranular preparation; decreased vitamin B_{12} uptake.	**Monitoring:** No laboratory monitoring requirements. **Comments:** PASER consists of enteric coated granules that need to be administered with an acidic food or beverage (e.g., yogurt or acidic juice); PASER is stable for up to 8 wk at 40°C and 75% humidity, and therefore can be distributed to the patient on a monthly basis in most environments with no cold chain; if storage of

Continued

 Cite this article as *Cold Spring Harb Perspect Med* doi: 10.1101/cshperspect.a017863

Table 1. *Continued*

Drug name (abbreviation)	Description and adult dose	Side effects	Monitoring requirements and comments
			>8 wk is needed, refrigeration below 15°C is required.
Group 5: Drugs with limited data on efficacy or long-term safety			
Bedaquiline (Bdq)	**Description:** A diarylquinoline antimycobacterial drug that inhibits ATP synthesis. **Dose:** 400 mg once daily for 2 wk, followed by 200 mg three times per week for 22 wk with food; the drug has a 5.5-mo half-life.	**Common:** Gastrointestinal distress (nausea, vomiting, abdominal pain, loss of appetite); joint pain; headache. **Less common:** QT prolongation, hyperuricemia, phospholipidosis (the accumulation of phospholipids in the body's tissues), elevated aminotransferases, chest pain, hemoptysis (coughing up blood). Possibly an increased risk of pancreatitis. **Drug Interactions:** All CYP3A4 inhibitors or inducers. Rifampicin (a CYP3A4 inducer) reduces bedaquiline in blood by half; drugs that prolong the QT interval (e.g., clofazimine, moxifloxacin, antifungals, and many others) may result in additive cardiac toxicity—their use is only indicated when there are no other alternatives; more frequent ECG monitoring is required.	**Monitoring:** Monitor QT interval with ECG at baseline, 2, 12, and 24 wk (more often if risk of QT prolongation is present); discontinue if significant ventricular arrhythmia or a QTcF interval >500 msec develops; monitor liver enzymes every month. **Comments:** A significant imbalance in fatalities was noted in Trial C208 Stage 2, with a higher number of deaths in the bedaquiline group (10 vs. 2 in the placebo group; RR = 5.1; $P = 0.017$). There was no sudden death reported in the study. There was no discernible pattern for cause of deaths, and the reason for the imbalance in deaths is not clear.
Linezolid (Lzd)	**Description:** Oxazolidinone; inhibits protein synthesis; increasingly used for treatment of XDR-TB. **Dose:** 600 mg/d (reduce to 300 mg/d if serious side effects	**Common:** Diarrhea and nausea. **Less common:** Myelosuppression (decreased level of white blood cells, and/or anemia); lactic acidosis; optic and peripheral neuropathy (may be irreversible, and linezolid	**Monitoring:** Monitor for peripheral neuropathy and optic neuritis. Monitor with a complete blood count (CBC) weekly during the initial period, then monthly. If symptoms of lactic acidosis develop, a medical evaluation

Continued

Table 1. *Continued*

Drug name (abbreviation)	Description and adult dose	Side effects	Monitoring requirements and comments
	or intolerance develops).	should be considered for suspension weighed against the risk of permanent blindness or disabling permanent neuropathy).	including a lactic acid blood test should be performed. **Comments:** All patients should receive pyridoxine while receiving linezolid (child: 5–10 mg/d; adult: 50 mg/d); do not use with patients taking serotonergic drugs, such as monoamine oxidase inhibitors (MAOIs), selective serotonin reuptake inhibitors (SSRIs, e.g., fluoxetine, sertraline, paroxetine), lithium, etc., as it may cause serotonin syndrome; avoid or monitor closely with tricyclic antidepressants.
Clofazimine (Cfz)	**Description:** Riminophenazine; has activity in vitro but limited clinical evidence of efficacy. **Dose:** 100 to 200 mg/d (oral) has been used. A regimen of 200 mg/d for 2 mo, followed by 100 mg/d has been used.	**Common:** Orange/red discoloration of skin, conjunctiva, cornea, and body fluids; dry skin, pruritus, rash, ichthyosis, xerosis; gastrointestinal intolerance; photosensitivity. **Less common:** Retinopathy, severe abdominal symptoms, bleeding, and bowel obstruction; QT prolongation.	**Monitoring:** Symptomatic monitoring only. **Comments:** Discolors skin and body secretions orange, red, or brownish-black; this should go away after stopping the medicine, but may take a long time; avoid sun; use strong sunscreens.
Amoxicillin/ clavulanic acid (Amx/Clv)	**Description:** Penicillin/ β-lactam inhibitor; very limited clinical evidence of efficacy. **Dose:** 80 mg/kg daily in two divided doses.	**Common:** Diarrhea and abdominal discomfort are most common; nausea and vomiting. **Less common:** Hypersensitivity and rash; rare side effects have been reported in other organ systems.	**Monitoring:** Symptomatic monitoring only. **Comments:** Best tolerated and well absorbed when taken at the start of a standard meal.
Imipenem/ cilastatin (Imp/Cln)	**Description:** β-lactam/ carbapenem (related to the penicillin/	**Common:** Diarrhea, nausea, or vomiting. **Less common:** Seizure (noted with CNS infection), palpitations,	**Monitoring:** Symptomatic monitoring only. **Comments:** Meropenem is preferred in children as fewer seizures have been

Continued

Table 1. *Continued*

Drug name (abbreviation)	Description and adult dose	Side effects	Monitoring requirements and comments
	cephalosporin family of antibiotics but classified as belonging to the carbapenem class); very limited clinical experience. Given that imipenem is rapidly degraded by renal proximal tubule dipeptidases, it is used in combination with the dipeptidase inhibitor cilastatin. **Dose:** 1000 mg IV every 12 h.	pseudomembranous colitis.	associated with it; consider adding clavulanate (available as Amx/Clv) 125 mg every 8–12 h.
Meropenem (Mpm)	**Description:** β-lactam/ carbapenem (related to the penicillin/ cephalosporin family of antibiotics but classified as belonging to the carbapenem class); very limited clinical experience. **Dose:** 1000 mg IV every 8 h.	**Common:** Diarrhea, nausea, or vomiting. **Less common:** Seizure (but less is seen than with imipenem), palpitations, pseudomembranous colitis.	**Monitoring:** Symptomatic monitoring only. **Comments:** Consider adding clavulanate (available as amoxicillin/ clavulanate) 500/ 125 mg every 8–12 h.
High-dose isoniazid (High-dose H)	**Description:** May be bactericidal or bacteriostatic depending on susceptibility and concentrations attained at the infection site; the carbothioamide group, also found on Thz, and the pyridine ring, also found on H, appear essential for activity; hepatically metabolized, renally excreted. **Dose:** 500–1000 mg/d.	**Common:** Gastrointestinal distress (nausea, vomiting, diarrhea, abdominal pain, loss of appetite); dysgeusia (metallic taste); hypothyroidism (especially when taken with PAS). **Less common:** Arthralgias, dermatitis, gynecomastia, hepatitis, impotence, peripheral neuropathy, photosensitivity.	**Monitoring:** Consider baseline and monthly liver enzymes, especially if age >50 yr. **Comments:** Give with pyridoxine 50 mg/d.

Continued

Table 1. *Continued*

Drug name (abbreviation)	Description and adult dose	Side effects	Monitoring requirements and comments
Clarithromycin (Clr)	**Description:** More active against nontuberculous mycobacteria, especially MAC, but some isolates of TB are susceptible in vitro; does not have proven value for the treatment of TB in humans, and in vitro data are not particularly encouraging (*M. tuberculosis* is intrinsically resistant to macrolides, a characteristic associated with expression of the *ermB* gene). **Dose:** 500 mg twice daily.	**Common:** Diarrhea, nausea, abnormal taste, dyspepsia, abdominal pain/discomfort, headache, rare allergic skin reactions, liver toxicity, QT prolongation, pseudomembranous colitis, hearing loss.	**Monitoring:** No routine laboratory monitoring is indicated. **Comments:** This medication may be taken with or without food; contraindicated in patients taking cisapride, pimozide, astemizole, terfenadine, ergotamine, or dihydroergotamine.
Thioacetazone (T)	**Description:** Known to be active against TB (by inhibiting cyclopropanation of cell wall mycolic acids in mycobacteria), but its role in MDR-TB treatment is not well-established; cross-resistance with some of the other anti-TB drugs (isoniazid, ethionamide, PAS) and overall is a weakly bacteriostatic drug; prevents the emergence of resistance when used with other first-line drugs. **Dose:** 150 mg once daily.	**Common:** Nausea, vomiting, diarrhea, loss of appetite, skin rashes, aching joints and muscles, neuropathy. **Rare:** Severe cutaneous hypersensitivity (including Stevens–Johnson syndrome), seizures, mood changes, hepatitis, bone marrow suppression.	**Monitoring:** No routine laboratory monitoring is indicated. **Comments:** Contraindicated in HIV-infected individuals because of a risk of serious adverse reactions (Stevens–Johnson syndrome and death); persons of Asian descent also have a higher incidence of Stevens–Johnson syndrome; rarely used in MDR-TB treatment.

From Seung and Rich 2010; Curry International Tuberculosis Center & California Department of Public Health 2012; Partners In Health 2013.

CNS, central nervous system; ECG, electrocardiogram; RR, relative risk; IV, intravenously; MAC, *Mycobacterium avium* complex.

REGIMEN DESIGN

One of the most important steps in designing an MDR-TB regimen is taking a detailed history of past TB treatment. This is particularly important in patients who have received multiple treatment courses with first- or second-line anti-TB drugs, as there may be omissions or errors in the written medical record. As a general rule, any drug that has been used in a regimen that did not cure the patient should be considered unlikely to still be effective, even if a recent DST indicates that the patient's strain is still susceptible. For example, if the patient previously used ethambutol or pyrazinamide as part of a failed first-line regimen, neither of these drugs should be considered likely to be effective.

All DST results should be compared carefully with the clinical history; DST can be incorrect like any laboratory test. Only DST to first-line anti-TB drugs, injectables, and fluoroquinolones is considered reliable. Laboratory resistance to pyrazinamide, ethionamide, or PAS, combined with a history of use in a failing regimen, however, strongly suggests the drug is ineffective.

At least four second-line anti-TB drugs likely to be effective should be included in the MDR regimen. All regimens should include a later-generation fluoroquinolone such as levofloxacin or moxifloxacin (Johnson et al. 2006; Peloquin et al. 2008), a second-line injectable drug, and other oral second-line drugs as shown in Figure 3 (Mukherjee et al. 2004). Pyrazinamide may also be included unless there is a contraindication (such a history of a drug allergy) or evidence that it is not likely to be effective against the patient's strain (a clear history of failing to respond to a pyrazinamide-including regimen and DST indicating resistance) (Mitnick et al. 2003). Pyrazinamide is often routinely included in MDR regimens in resource-limited settings because DST to pyrazinamide is often not available. These recommendations are supported by a large meta-analysis of individual data from more than 9000 patients (Ahuja et al. 2012).

Dosing of anti-TB drugs is based on the weight of the patient. For simplicity, commonly used dosing tables use only a few weight bands. When adults gain weight or move into a higher weight band, drug doses should be adjusted. Even though anti-TB drugs are generally administered once a day to improve peak-dependent killing, many of the second-line anti-TB drugs have severe side effects that can be reduced by twice-daily divided dosing. For example, ethionamide and cycloserine are traditionally given in two divided doses to reduce side effects, but once-daily dosing is acceptable if tolerated.

In the case of XDR-TB, the same approach for designing a regimen may be used, with some important caveats. In chronic patients with a history of multiple failed courses of treatment, a minimum of four likely effective second-line anti-TB drugs may not be available. The XDR regimen may then include drugs that are resistant on DST but have never been used or drugs that have been used but are still susceptible on DST. Many clinicians will use a later-generation fluoroquinolone such as moxifloxacin despite documented resistance to an early generation fluoroquinolone such as ofloxacin.

If there is an injectable drug that is still likely to be effective, many clinicians will try to use it for a longer duration, such as 12 mo or even the entire duration of treatment. New drugs with demonstrated efficacy such as bedaquiline or delamanid should be strongly considered, as well as resective surgery in patients with localized disease.

According to provisional guidance from the United States Centers for Disease Control and Prevention (CDC) and WHO, bedaquiline may be used for MDR-TB patients in whom treatment options are limited (CDC 2013; WHO 2013c). Bedaquiline should be added to a conventional MDR or XDR regimen designed as above. There are still many uncertainties about the risks and benefits of bedaquiline (Table 1). Bedaquiline may be used to treat strains with XDR or fluoroquinolone resistance. Bedaquiline may also have a role when the injectable drug is causing toxicity (such as ototoxicity or nephrotoxicity) that requires its suspension or when there is resistance to all second-line injectable drugs. Bedaquiline should be administered within a program that has the capacity to closely monitor for side effects. Delamanid has

Step 1	**Choose an injectable drug** **Group 2:** Kanamycin (or amikacin) Capreomycin	Choose a drug based on DST and treatment history. Streptomycin is generally not used because of high rates of resistance in patients with MDR-TB.
Step 2	**Choose a fluoroquinolone** **Group 3:** Levofloxacin Moxifloxacin	Add a later-generation fluoroquinolone. If Ofx resistance is suspected or documented, use Mfx.
Step 3	**Plus at least two Group 4 drugs** **Group 4:** Ethionamide (or prothionamide) Cycloserine Para-aminosalicylic acid	Add Group 4 drugs until the regimen has at least four second-line drugs likely to be effective (all three may be needed). Choice is based on treatment history and side effect profile. DST is not fully reliable for the drugs in this group.
Step 4	**Add Group 1 drugs** **Group 1:** Pyrazinamide Ethambutol	Z is routinely added except if the patient is intolerant or if resistance is highly likely based on history and DST. If the criteria of being a "likely effective drug" for E are met, it can be added to the regimen (but not counted as a core drug in the regimen).
Step 5	**Consider Group 5 drugs** **Group 5:** Bedaquiline Linezolid Clofazimine Amoxicillin/clavulanic acid High-dose isoniazid Imipenem/cilastatin	If there are not four second-line anti-TB drugs that are likely to be effective from Groups 2–4, add at least two Group 5 drugs.

Figure 3. Designing an MDR-TB regimen. (Created from data in Varaine and Rich 2013.)

no international recommendations or published drug insert at the time of this writing.

DURATION AND MONITORING OF TREATMENT

The injectable should be continued for at least 8 mo and at least 4 mo after the patient becomes culture-negative, whichever is longer. Clinicians may use an individualized approach that reviews the cultures, smears, X-rays, and clinical status to decide how long to continue the injectable. With respect to the duration of the injectable, however, the limiting factor is often toxicity. One option is intermittent dosing of the injectable. Many patients have less nephrotoxicity or ototoxicity if the injectable is given three times a week (e.g., Monday, Wednesday, and Friday) compared with daily. For this reason, some clinicians routinely choose to switch to an intermittent schedule after the patient becomes culture-negative even if there is no toxicity.

MDR-TB treatment should continue for a minimum of 20 mo and at least 18 mo after the patient becomes culture-negative, whichever is longer. Chronic patients with extensive pulmonary disease may require MDR-TB treatment for 24 mo or longer, but there is limited evidence about the optimal length of treatment for patients with XDR-TB.

The previous recommendations about the duration of the injectable and of treatment are supported by the meta-analysis of individual data from more than 9000 patients, but there is controversy about the optimal length of treatment. One study showed that a 9-mo treatment regimen was sufficient to affect cure in a small cohort of patients in Bangladesh (Van Deun et al. 2010). This particular regimen is currently the subject of a multisite clinical trial.

Sputum cultures should be performed monthly during treatment. Other symptoms and signs are important, but they cannot be relied on to determine treatment failure or cure. Programs with very limited culture capacity may consider doing smears monthly and cultures every other month after the injectable has been discontinued, but this may delay identification of treatment failure.

MANAGEMENT OF SIDE EFFECTS

Second-line anti-TB drugs have many more side effects than first-line anti-TB drugs. Side effects are expected as part of the normal course of treatment, and it is the responsibility of the clinician to diagnose and manage them. Mismanagement of side effects is the major reason why patients do not adhere or continue to take MDR-TB treatment.

Even before starting treatment, the patient should receive education regarding potential side effects. During treatment, patients should be evaluated regularly by a clinician. Community health workers can be trained to screen for side effects between clinical evaluations. Laboratory testing can be helpful in screening for some side effects; a typical monitoring schedule is shown in Table 2.

Table 2. Follow-up schedule for uncomplicated MDR-TB patients

Month	Clinical consult	Weight	Smear	Culture	DST	Chest X-ray	LFT	Cr, K	TSH
0 (baseline)	√	√	√	√	√	√	√	√	
1	Every 2 wk	√	√	√				√	
2	Every 2 wk	√	√	√				√	
3	Every 2 wk	√	√	√				√	√
4	√	√	√	√	If culture pos			√	
5	√	√	√	√				√	
6	√	√	√	√	If culture pos			√	√
7	√	√	√	√				√	
8	√	√	√	√	If culture pos			√	
9	√	√	√	√				If on inj.	
10	√	√	√	√	If culture pos			If on inj.	
11	√	√	√	√				If on inj.	
12	√	√	√	√	If culture pos			If on inj.	√
Until completion	√	Monthly	Monthly	Monthly	If culture pos			If on inj.	Every 6 mo

From Partners in Health 2013.

DST, drug susceptibility testing; pos, positive; LFT, liver function test; Cr, creatinine, K, potassium; TSH, thyroid-stimulating hormone; inj., injectable.

Mild side effects are common, and can be managed symptomatically with ancillary drugs without altering the treatment regimen. Side effects often diminish or disappear with time, allowing patients to finish their treatment without further problems. A number of second-line anti-TB drugs have highly dose-dependent side effects. With cycloserine and ethionamide, for example, a patient may be completely intolerant at one dose and completely tolerant at a slightly lower dose. Unfortunately, given the narrow therapeutic margins of these drugs, lowering the dose may also affect efficacy. Reducing the dose of these drugs should be performed only in cases in which the reduced dose is still expected to produce adequate serum levels and not compromise the regimen.

A poorly tolerated drug may be temporarily suspended. In patients with highly resistant TB, however, a satisfactory replacement drug may not be available. In such cases, permanent discontinuation of the drug should be avoided if possible. The decision to suspend any drug should be made by weighing the risk of continued side effects against the chances of curing a deadly disease.

- Gastrointestinal distress is a common side effect of MDR-TB treatment, caused by PAS and ethionamide. Nausea and vomiting are common in early weeks of therapy but usually improve over time and with supportive therapy.
- Nephrotoxicity is a known complication of the aminoglycosides and capreomycin. Because symptoms of acute renal failure can be nonspecific, serum creatinine monitoring is recommended. Patients with advanced age or a history of renal disease (including comorbidities such as HIV and diabetes) should be monitored more closely, particularly at the start of treatment.
- Electrolyte wasting with similar characteristics to Fanconi's Syndrome can be induced by all of the injectable drugs. It is reversible once the injectable is suspended, but it may take weeks or months to be resolved completely. Because electrolyte wasting is generally managed with electrolyte replacement therapy, serum potassium should be checked at least monthly in all patients during the initial injectable phase.
- Hypothyroidism can be induced by prolonged exposure to PAS or ethionamide/prothionamide. The exact incidence of hypothyroidism during MDR-TB treatment is unknown, but rates of up to 80% have been reported in some patient populations. Because symptoms are nonspecific, all patients should be screened for hypothyroidism starting after the third month of MDR-TB treatment.
- Neurotoxic effects such as psychosis or depression can be caused by cycloserine. Clinicians should screen patients for abnormal behavior and symptoms of depression, anxiety, and agitation on a regular basis.
- Ototoxicity can be caused by the injectables, which can cause damage to cranial nerve VIII. This may result in hearing loss, tinnitus (ringing in the ear), or other vestibular symptoms such as nystagmus, ataxia, and disequilibrium. Hearing loss is generally not reversible on discontinuation of therapy. Hearing and balance should be assessed at least monthly while the patient is receiving the injectable. Where available, audiometry should be performed monthly and is an excellent way of detecting early hearing loss.

RESECTIVE SURGERY

Lung resection was once a mainstay of TB treatment but disappeared almost completely once effective chemotherapy was discovered. There has been a resurgence of interest in resective surgery as an adjunct to MDR-TB chemotherapy, which is much less effective. For patients with localized disease, resection of a lobe or a lung can significantly improve outcome (Pomerantz et al. 2001; Somocurcio et al. 2007). Experienced thoracic surgeons, stringent infection control measures, and excellent pre- and post-operative care are necessary; resective surgery

 Cite this article as *Cold Spring Harb Perspect Med* doi: 10.1101/cshperspect.a017863

for TB is often more complicated than for other diseases.

The most important indication for resective surgery is lack of a sustained bacteriological response to chemotherapy. Computerized tomography (CT) is the best way to assess if there is a localized lesion that is amenable to resection. Patients with bilateral cavitary disease, for example, would not be good surgical candidates. Pulmonary function testing with predicted postoperative forced expiratory volume in one second (FEV1) can be helpful to evaluate if the patient has sufficient pulmonary reserve postresection.

Another type of surgical candidate is those who have experienced culture conversion through chemotherapy, but who are thought to have a high probability of future failure or relapse caused by a high level of resistance. Surgical resection can also be considered for complications of MDR-TB, such as massive hemoptysis, empyema, or aspergilloma.

In patients who are smear- or culture-positive at the time of surgery, treatment is continued for minimum of 18 mo of negative sputum cultures, and generally includes an extended period of injectable. In patients who are smear- and culture-negative at the time of surgery, treatment should be continued for a minimum of 18 mo after culture conversion and no less than 6 mo after surgery.

SPECIAL SITUATIONS

Extrapulmonary MDR-TB

There is limited evidence about treatment of extrapulmonary MDR-TB. In general, every effort should be made to obtain tissue or fluid samples to confirm the diagnosis of MDR-TB, as the clinical or radiological picture may be deceptive. The length of therapy has not been clearly defined but should likely be at least as long as treatment for pulmonary MDR-TB.

- *MDR-TB lymphadenitis.* Lymph node aspiration followed by culture-based or molecular DST is a simple way to confirm the diagnosis and can be useful in guiding therapy.
- *MDR-TB osteomyelitis and spondylitis.* Bone biopsy or sampling of paravertebral fluid collections should be attempted to obtain material for DST. Persistent or increasing fluid collections on CT despite treatment with first-line anti-TB drugs may be sufficient evidence for empiric MDR-TB treatment in some patients with other bacteriological evidence of TB. Operative intervention, either through open debridement or by percutaneous drainage of fluid collections, is often required in combination with drug therapy.
- *MDR-TB meningitis.* Diagnosis of MDR-TB meningitis may be difficult because mycobacterial concentration in cerebrospinal fluid can be very low. Treatment of a patient with MDR-TB meningitis is complicated because many second-line drugs do not have good penetration into the cerebrospinal fluid.

Children

Most children with MDR-TB have been infected by someone in the same household (Becerra et al. 2013). For this reason, careful investigation of family members is crucial. If it is difficult to collect a specimen from the child for laboratory analysis for whatever reason, the regimens can be designed based on the DST of the index case in the same household. Otherwise, the basic principles of regimen design for children with MDR-TB are no different than those for adults. Children generally tolerate second-line anti-TB drugs well. Pediatric formulations, however, do not exist for most drugs, and it is often necessary prepare adult formulations, for example, by splitting tablets (The Sentinel Project 2012; Garcia-Prats et al. 2013; Varaine and Rich 2013).

Pregnant Women

Some second-line anti-TB drugs are known to cause birth defects. For this reason, all women of childbearing age should be strongly advised to use a reliable method of contraception during MDR-TB treatment. For pregnant women who are diagnosed with MDR-TB, the benefit of treating MDR-TB in pregnancy in most circumstances outweighs the risks. Most patients should start treatment as soon as the diagnosis is made. Aminoglycosides can be particularly toxic to the developing fetal ear. Capreomycin may also carry a risk of ototoxicity but may be used if an injectable is absolutely necessary. Ethionamide is also usually avoided as it can increase the risk of nausea and vomiting associated with pregnancy, and teratogenic effects have been observed in animal studies. MDR regimens for pregnant women may be designed with three or four oral second-line anti-TB drugs plus pyrazinamide. The regimen can then be reinforced with an injectable and other drugs immediately postpartum. The risk of birth defects in MDR-TB treatment is highest in the first trimester of pregnancy, so the gestational age of the fetus should be carefully confirmed, preferably by dating using ultrasound. In rare cases, in which the mother does not accept the risks of the treatment and is clinically stable, treatment can be delayed until the second trimester.

HIV Coinfection

People living with HIV are vulnerable to MDR-TB infection and are at high risk of developing active MDR-TB once infected. HIV-positive patients often die while waiting for laboratory confirmation of MDR-TB and before starting effective therapy. This was best illustrated by the rapid and deadly spread of XDR-TB among HIV-positive patients in South Africa (Gandhi et al. 2006). The WHO currently recommends Xpert MTB/RIF as the initial diagnostic test in settings with high prevalence of HIV-associated TB or MDR-TB (WHO 2011b).

Early identification and prompt initiation of appropriate treatment can reduce mortality among HIV-infected patients infected with MDR-TB. ART improves survival in MDR-TB patients infected with HIV and should be started as soon as possible, as early as the first week after starting MDR-TB treatment. Stavudine and tenofovir are often avoided because of overlapping toxicities (neuropathy and nephrotoxicity, respectively) with second-line anti-TB drugs; nonetheless, cotreatment with ART is still challenging in most patients because of side effects and the high pill burden. HIV-positive patients seem to experience a higher incidence of side effects with second-line anti-TB drugs (Seung et al. 2009).

COMMUNITY-BASED CARE FOR MDR-TB

MDR-TB may be hospital-, clinic-, or community-based. These approaches may not be mutually exclusive, and in fact, they may all be used within the same program. In some settings, patients are hospitalized at the beginning of treatment to allow for more intensive monitoring of side effects, especially for patients who are physically debilitated. But in many countries, the lack of MDR-TB hospital beds becomes a bottleneck to scale-up. Mandatory hospitalization may also exacerbate nosocomial transmission of MDR-TB because in many settings, infection control measures are not adequate.

Many countries have moved to decentralize MDR-TB treatment to increase access. One common method is to provide DOT at a primary care clinic. This strategy can be quite physically and economically burdensome to the patient because it requires daily travel to the clinic, sometimes twice daily. This is especially true in rural areas where primary care systems are weak.

Community-based MDR-TB treatment allows patients to be treated in their homes. By providing a flexible and convenient solution, it promotes patient adherence and reintegration into family, social, and work life. It can be fully supervised by a nurse or community health worker during daily home visits. Community-based care reduces cost in the health system and can be more cost-effective than hospital care, but in many ways, it is more challenging to implement. Each dose is administered under DOT, often through a system of a compensated, trained, and well-supervised nurse or community health workers.

Another important aspect of MDR-TB treatment is addressing socioeconomic determinants of health. Socioeconomic problems, including hunger, homelessness, and unemployment, are common among MDR-TB patients. These problems have been successfully tackled through socioeconomic interventions that include the use of provisions in the form of "incentives" and "enablers." Incentives are rewards that encourage patients to adhere to treatment, such as food packages, whereas enablers are goods or services that make it easier for patients to adhere to treatment, such as transportation vouchers. Addressing socioeconomic barriers to adherence is a crucial part of successful MDR-TB treatment (USAID 2011).

CONCLUSION

The continuing spread of MDR-TB is one of the most urgent and difficult challenges facing global TB control. The main causes of the increasing spread of resistant TB strains are weak medical systems, amplification of resistance through incorrect treatment, and ongoing transmission in communities and facilities. New molecular methods of DST have revolutionized the diagnosis of MDR-TB, but they are still not widely available in resource-limited settings. Although patients harboring MDR and XDR strains present a formidable challenge for treatment, cure is often possible with early identification of resistance and use of a properly designed regimen. Community-based programs can improve treatment outcomes by allowing patients to be treated in their homes and addressing socioeconomic barriers to adherence.

REFERENCES

Ahuja SD, Ashkin D, Avendano M, Banerjee R, Bauer M, Bayona J, Becerra M, Benedetti A, Burgos M, Centis R, et al. 2012. Multidrug resistant pulmonary tuberculosis treatment regimens and patient outcomes: An individual patient data meta-analysis of 9,153 patients. *PLoS Med* **9:** e1001300.

Becerra M, Franke MF, Appleton SC, Joseph JK, Bayona J, Atwood SS, Mitnick CD. 2013. Tuberculosis in children exposed at home to multidrug-resistant tuberculosis. *Pediatr Infect Dis J* **32:** 115–119.

Cegielski JP. 2010. Extensively drug-resistant tuberculosis: "There must be some kind of way out of here". *Clin Infect Dis* **50:** S195–S200.

Centers for Disease Control and Prevention (CDC). 2013. Provisional CDC guidelines for the use and safety monitoring of bedaquiline fumarate (Sirturo) for the treatment of multidrug-resistant tuberculosis. *MMWR Recomm Rep* **62:** 1–12.

Chavez Pachas AM, Blank R, Fawzi Smith MC, Bayona J, Becerra M, Mitnick CD. 2004. Identifying early treatment failure on category I therapy for pulmonary tuberculosis in Lima Ciudad, Peru. *Int J Tuberc Lung Dis* **8:** 52–58.

Curry International Tuberculosis Center, California Department of Public Health. 2012. *Tuberculosis Drug Information Guide*, 2nd ed. Curry International Tuberculosis Center, San Francisco, California.

Dye C, Williams BG, Espinal MA, Raviglione MC. 2002. Erasing the world's slow stain: Strategies to beat multidrug-resistant tuberculosis. *Science* **295:** 2042–2046.

Frieden TR, Sterling T, Pablos-Mendez A, Kilburn JO, Cauthen GM, Dooley SW. 1993. The emergence of drug-resistant tuberculosis in New York City. *New Engl J Med* **328:** 521–526.

Frieden TR, Fujiwara PI, Washko RM, Hamburg MA. 1995. Tuberculosis in New York City—Turning the tide. *New Engl J Med* **333:** 229–233.

Gandhi NR, Moll A, Sturm AW, Pawinski R, Govender T, Lalloo U, Zeller K, Andrews J, Friedland G. 2006. Extensively drug-resistant tuberculosis as a cause of death in patients co-infected with tuberculosis and HIV in a rural area of South Africa. *Lancet* **368:** 1575–1580.

Garcia-Prats AJ, Donald PR, Hesseling AC, Schaaf HS. 2013. *Second-Line antituberculosis drugs in children: A commissioned review for the World Health Organization 19th Expert Committee on the Selection and Use of Essential Medicines.* World Health Organization, Geneva.

Gelmanova IY, Keshavjee S, Golubchikova VT, Berezina VI, Strelis AK, Yanova GV, Atwood S, Murray M. 2007. Barriers to successful tuberculosis treatment in Tomsk, Russian Federation: Non-adherence, default and the acquisition of multidrug resistance. *Bull World Health Organ* **85:** 703–711.

Johnson JL, Hadad DJ, Boom WH, Daley CL, Peloquin CA, Eisenach KD, Jankus DD, Debanne SM, Charlebois ED, Maciel E, et al. 2006. Early and extended early bactericidal activity of levofloxacin, gatifloxacin and moxifloxacin in pulmonary tuberculosis. *Int J Tuberc Lung Dis* **10:** 605–612.

Keshavjee S, Farmer PE. 2012. Tuberculosis, drug resistance, and the history of modern medicine. *New Engl J Med* **367:** 931–936.

Lin H, Shin S, Blaya JA, Zhang Z, Cegielski P, Contreras C, Asencios L, Bonilla C, Bayona J, Paciore CJ, et al. 2011. Assessing spatiotemporal patterns of multidrug-resistant and drug-sensitive tuberculosis in a South American setting. *Epidemiol Infect* **139:** 1784–1793.

Mitnick C, Bayona J, Palacios E, Shin S, Furin J, Alcántara F, Sánchez E, Sarria M, Becerra M, Fawzi MC, et al. 2003. Community-based therapy for multidrug-resistant tuberculosis in Lima, Peru. *New Engl J Med* **348:** 119–128.

Mukherjee JS, Rich ML, Socci AR, Joseph JK, Virú FA, Shin SS, Furin JJ, Becerra MC, Barry DJ, Kim JY, et al. 2004. Programmes and principles in treatment of multidrug-resistant tuberculosis. *Lancet* **363:** 474–481.

Partners In Health. 2013. *The PIH guide to the medical management of multidrug-resistant tuberculosis*, 2nd ed. Partners In Health, Boston.

Peloquin CA, Hadad DJ, Molino LP, Palaci M, Boom WH, Dietze R, Johnson JL. 2008. Population pharmacokinetics of levofloxacin, gatifloxacin, and moxifloxacin in adults with pulmonary tuberculosis. *Antimicrob Agents Chemother* **52:** 852–857.

Pomerantz BJ, Cleveland JC, Olson JK, Pomerantz M. 2001. Pulmonary resection for multi-drug resistant tuberculosis. *J Thorac Cardiovasc Surg* **121:** 448–453.

Pyle M. 1947. Relative number of resistant tubercle bacilli in sputa of patients before and during treatment with streptomycin. In *Proceedings of the staff meetings Mayo Clinic* **22:** 465–473.

Satti H, McLaughlin MM, Seung KJ, Becerra MC, Keshavjee S. 2013. High risk of drug-resistant tuberculosis when first-line therapy fails in a high HIV prevalence setting. *Int J Tuberc Lung Dis* **17:** 100–106.

Seung KJ, Rich ML. 2010. Diagnosis and treatment of drug-resistant tuberculosis. In *Tuberculosis: The essentials*, 4th ed. (ed. Raviglione MC), pp. 170–214. Informa Healthcare, New York.

Seung KJ, Gelmanova IE, Peremitin GG, Golubchikova VT, Pavlova VE, Sirotkina OB, Yanova GV, Strelis AK. 2004. The effect of initial drug resistance on treatment response and acquired drug resistance during standardized short-course chemotherapy for tuberculosis. *Clin Infect Dis* **39:** 1321–1328.

Seung KJ, Omatayo DB, Keshavjee S, Furin JJ, Farmer PE, Satti H. 2009. Early outcomes of MDR-TB treatment in a high HIV-prevalence setting in Southern Africa. *PloS ONE* **4:** e7186.

Shin S, Pasechnikov AD, Gelmanova IY, Peremitin GG, Strelis AK, Mishustin S, Barnashov A, Karpeichik Y, Andreev YG, Golubchikova VT, et al. 2006. Treatment outcomes in an integrated civilian and prison MDR-TB treatment program in Russia. *Int J Tuberc Lung Dis* **10:** 402–408.

Skrahina A, Hurevich H, Zalutskaya A, Sahalchyk E, Astrauko A, van Gemert W, Hoffner S, Rusovich V, Zignol M. 2012. Alarming levels of drug-resistant tuberculosis in Belarus: Results of a survey in Minsk. *Eur Respir J* **39:** 1425–1431.

Somocurcio JG, Sotomayor A, Shin S, Portilla S, Valcarcel M, Guerra D, Furin J. 2007. Surgery for patients with drug-resistant tuberculosis: Report of 121 cases receiving community-based treatment in Lima, Peru. *Thorax* **62:** 416–421.

The Sentinel Project for Pediatric Drug-Resistant Tuberculosis. 2012. *Management of multidrug-resistant tuberculosis in children: A field guide.* The Sentinel Project for Pediatric Drug-Resistant Tuberculosis, Boston.

USAID TB CARE II. 2011. *Community-based care for drug-resistant tuberculosis: A guide for implementers.* Partners In Health, Boston.

Van Deun A, Maug AK, Salim MA, Das PK, Sarker MR, Daru P, Rieder HL. 2010. Short, highly effective, and inexpensive standardized treatment of multidrug-resistant tuberculosis. *Am J Respir Crit Care Med* **182:** 684–692.

Varaine F, Rich ML. 2013. *Tuberculosis: Practical guide for clinicians, nurses, laboratory technicians and medical auxiliaries.* Médecins San Frontières and Partners in Health, Paris.

Wells CD, Cegielski JP, Nelson LJ, Laserson KF, Holtz TH, Finlay A, Castro KG, Weyer K. 2007. HIV infection and multidrug-resistant tuberculosis: The perfect storm. *J Infect Dis* **196:** S86–S107.

World Health Organization (WHO). 2011a. *Guidelines for the programmatic management of drug-resistant tuberculosis, 2011 update.* World Health Organization, Geneva.

World Health Organization (WHO). 2011b. *Policy Statement: Automated real-time nucleic acid amplification technology for rapid and simultaneous detection of tuberculosis and rifampicin resistance: Xpert MTB/RIF system.* World Health Organization, Geneva.

World Health Organization (WHO). 2013a. *Global tuberculosis report 2013.* World Health Organization, Geneva.

World Health Organization (WHO). 2013b. *Definitions and reporting framework for tuberculosis—2013 revision.* World Health Organization, Geneva.

World Health Organization (WHO). 2013c. *The use of bedaquiline in the treatment of multidrug-resistant tuberculosis: Interim policy guidance.* World Health Organization, Geneva.

Zhao Y, Xu S, Wang L, Chin DP, Wang S, Jiang G, Xia H, Zhou Y, Li Q, Ou X, et al. 2012. National survey of drug-resistant tuberculosis in China. *New Engl J Med* **366:** 2161–2170.

Tuberculosis and HIV Coinfection

Judith Bruchfeld[1,5], Margarida Correia-Neves[2,3,5], and Gunilla Källenius[4,5]

[1]Unit of Infectious Diseases, Institution of Medicine Solna, Karolinska Institutet and Karolinska University Hospital, Stockholm SE-171 77, Sweden

[2]Life and Health Sciences Research Institute (ICVS), School of Health Sciences, University of Minho, Braga 4710-057, Portugal

[3]ICVS/3B's, PT Government Associate Laboratory, Braga/Guimarães 4710-057, Portugal

[4]Karolinska Institutet, Department of Clinical Science and Education, Stockholm SE-118 83, Sweden

Correspondence: gunilla.kallenius@ki.se

Tuberculosis (TB) and human immunodeficiency virus/acquired immunodeficiency syndrome (HIV/AIDS) constitute the main burden of infectious disease in resource-limited countries. In the individual host, the two pathogens, *Mycobacterium tuberculosis* and HIV, potentiate one another, accelerating the deterioration of immunological functions. In high-burden settings, HIV coinfection is the most important risk factor for developing active TB, which increases the susceptibility to primary infection or reinfection and also the risk of TB reactivation for patients with latent TB. *M. tuberculosis* infection also has a negative impact on the immune response to HIV, accelerating the progression from HIV infection to AIDS. The clinical management of HIV-associated TB includes the integration of effective anti-TB treatment, use of concurrent antiretroviral therapy (ART), prevention of HIV-related comorbidities, management of drug cytotoxicity, and prevention/treatment of immune reconstitution inflammatory syndrome (IRIS).

Tuberculosis and HIV/AIDS (acquired immunodeficiency syndrome) constitute the main burden of infectious disease in resource-limited countries. In the individual host, the two pathogens, *Mycobacterium tuberculosis* and HIV, potentiate each other, accelerating the deterioration of immunological functions and resulting in premature death if untreated.

EPIDEMIOLOGY OF HIV AND HIV-TB

The Global Burden of HIV Infection

At the end of 2012, an estimated 34.5 million adults and children worldwide were living with HIV (WHO 2013). There were 2.3 (1.9–2.7) million estimated new HIV infections globally the same year, showing a 33% decline in the number of new infections from 3.4 (3.1–3.7) million in 2001. At the same time, the estimated number of AIDS deaths was also declining with 1.6 (1.4–1.9) million AIDS deaths in 2012, down from 2.3 (2.1–2.6) million in 2005, in part because of the increasing number of people receiving antiretroviral therapy. The HIV/AIDS epidemic affects all parts of the world, but the global burden of infection with HIV is highest in developing countries, among which the sub-Saharan Africa remains most severely affected. It is esti-

[5]These authors contributed equally to this work.

Cite this article as *Cold Spring Harb Perspect Med* doi: 10.1101/cshperspect.a017871

mated that nearly 5% (1 in every 20) of adults in sub-Saharan Africa live with HIV and account for 69% of the people living with HIV worldwide (UNAIDS 2012). Whereas the great proportion of HIV infection is attributable to HIV-1, HIV-2 is responsible for limited epidemics in specific countries in West Africa, such as Cape Verde, Guinea-Bissau, Gambia, Ivory Coast, and Senegal, and is also present in European countries with historical long connections with these African countries like Portugal and France (Camacho 2012).

The Epidemiology of Dual TB-HIV Infection

Some 14 million individuals worldwide are estimated to be dually infected with HIV and *M. tuberculosis* (Getahun et al. 2010), and TB remains the leading cause of death among people living with HIV. HIV infection is estimated to increase the risk of TB 20-fold compared with HIV-seronegative individuals in high HIV-prevalence countries (WHO 2013).

Of the estimated 8.7 million people who developed TB globally in 2012, 1.1 million (13%) were estimated to be HIV-coinfected. Of the 2.8 million people with TB who actually were screened for HIV in 2012, 20% tested HIV-positive, including 42% of people with TB in sub-Saharan Africa. More than 75% of the estimated HIV-positive incident TB cases live in just 10 countries (Ethiopia, India, Kenya, Mozambique, Nigeria, South Africa, United Republic of Tanzania, Uganda, Zambia, and Zimbabwe) (WHO 2013).

In sub-Saharan Africa, the age-distribution in the population is strongly skewed toward the younger age groups, and more than half of the population aged 15–49 yr are estimated to be infected with *M. tuberculosis* and also develop active TB more frequently (Styblo 1989; Nunn et al. 1994). These young adults are also at greatest risk for HIV infection, thus resulting in overlapping epidemics in this age range (Girardi et al. 2000; Martinson et al. 2011a).

The increased incidence of active TB in HIV-infected individuals can be attributed to at least two mechanisms: the increased reactivation of latent TB or increased susceptibility to *M. tuberculosis* infection. The increased risk of active TB among HIV-infected persons was initially mainly attributed to an increased risk of reactivation of a latent infection (Selwyn et al. 1989; Girardi et al. 2000); however, a growing body of evidence suggests that both situations are present and should be carefully analyzed for different countries/populations. Studies performed in urban settings in the United States indicated that almost two-thirds of *M. tuberculosis* isolates from HIV-infected patients appeared in clusters, suggesting increased recent infections (Small et al. 1994; Allwood et al. 1997). Further support for this suggestion was provided by DNA fingerprinting of nosocomial TB outbreaks, including transmission of multidrug-resistant (MDR) strains (Beck-Sague et al. 1992; Daley et al. 1992; Edlin et al. 1992; Coronado et al. 1993). These studies showed rapid progression to symptomatic disease in immunosuppressed HIV-infected individuals after de novo infection. In India, a TB-endemic country, most recurrences after successful treatment of TB are attributable to exogenous reinfection in HIV-infected persons but endogenous reactivation in HIV-uninfected persons (Narayanan et al. 2010). In a study of a general population cohort from Malawi, HIV infection increased the rate of recurrent TB by increasing the rate of diseases due to reinfection and not to relapse (Crampin et al. 2010), and in HIV-infected South African gold miners, recurrences were more often caused by reinfection (69%) than relapse (Charalambous et al. 2008). A recent review of epidemiological TB studies using molecular fingerprinting showed that HIV status was linked to *M. tuberculosis* clustering, suggesting that recent *M. tuberculosis* infection is the main cause of TB disease rather than reactivation of latent TB in areas endemic for TB and HIV (Houben et al. 2011). In line with early reports from nosocomial spread of MDR-TB, exogenous reinfection has been identified as an important mechanism for the development of MDR and extensively drug-resistant (XDR) TB in HIV patients in Tugela Ferry, KwaZulu Natal, South Africa (Andrews et al. 2008). Thus, both increased risk of reactivation of latent TB and increased susceptibility to de novo TB infection or reinfection are factors to be taken into consideration in the strategies for prevention and treatment of TB including MDR- and XDR-TB in HIV-TB-endemic settings (Cohn and O'Brien 1998; Kato-Maeda and Small 2000).

INCREASED SUSCEPTIBILITY OF HIV PATIENTS TO DEVELOP ACTIVE TB

As described in the literature, the great majority of individuals infected with *M. tuberculosis* do not develop active TB. This scenario is distinct for individuals who are coinfected with HIV (Pawlowski et al. 2012). In high-burden settings, HIV coinfection is the most important risk factor to develop active TB, which dramatically increases the susceptibility to primary infection or reinfection and also the risk of TB reactivation for patients with latent *M. tuberculosis* infection (Kwan and Ernst 2011). The main feature of immunosuppression in AIDS patients is the manifest loss of $CD4^+$ T cells, in the blood, lymphoid tissues, and mucosa, which is obviously an important contributor to the increased risk of developing active TB (Moir et al. 2011). However, susceptibility to TB increases soon after HIV infection, far before the decrease of the $CD4^+$ T-cell counts below 500 cells/μL (Sonnenberg et al. 2005), clearly showing that the mechanisms underlying the increased susceptibility of HIV-infected individuals to active TB goes beyond the $CD4^+$ T-cell drop. In fact, the World Health Organization (WHO) recommends the initiation of antiretroviral therapy for any HIV-infected individual who develops TB, regardless of the $CD4^+$ T-cell counts (WHO 2013). However, the modifications induced in the immune system by HIV infection that underlie the recognized increased susceptibility to TB are far from being understood.

Besides the inability to eradicate the virus from the infected host, a strong and sustained immune response against HIV is established on infection (Sauce et al. 2013). Innate and acquired components of the immune system become activated and fight viral infection. In the context of the acquired immune response, both HIV-specific B and T lymphocytes, and among these, both $CD4^+$ and $CD8^+$ T cells, become activated. HIV-2 infection also causes the activation of both B and T lymphocytes, although at a much slower pace, and as a consequence also causes a slower loss of $CD4^+$ T cells and progression to AIDS (Sousa et al. 2002). The activation of the T-cell population is such an important component of the HIV infection that it is recognized as a hallmark of pathogenic HIV infection. In fact, the level of immune activation is considered the best predictor of progression from HIV infection to AIDS and even to death, independently of HIV viral load (Sousa et al. 2002; Deeks et al. 2004).

Although the hallmark of the HIV infection is the loss of $CD4^+$ T cells, different cell populations are preferentially deleted at distinct periods of the HIV infection. During the initial period, the effector memory $CD4^+$ T cells in the gut mucosa are preferentially depleted (Mehandru et al. 2004; Brenchley and Douek 2008; Moir et al. 2011), followed by the progressive generalized loss of naïve T cells. The $CD4^+$ T cells are initially reconstituted through the production of new T cells by the thymus, the increased homeostatic proliferation of the peripheral naïve T cells, and the extension of the half-life of the $CD4^+$ T cells (Corbeau and Reynes 2011). However, the pool of peripheral naïve T cells tends to become progressively exhausted, and thymic production of new naïve T cells also becomes impaired as the infection progresses (Moir et al. 2011). Factors such as direct death of thymocytes, depletion of T-cell precursors within the bone marrow, and disruption of the thymic epithelia have been proposed to explain thymic failure (Ho Tsong Fang et al. 2008). In addition to the loss of T cells, the continuous stimulation renders T cells dysfunctional (Moir et al. 2011), and the desired balance between distinct T-cell populations, necessary to maintain the immune system's homeostasis, such as the proportion between naïve/effector/activated, Th17/regulatory T cells (Treg), is progressively lost (Kanwar et al. 2010; Hartigan-O'Connor et al. 2011).

Activation of the immune system in chronically HIV-infected individuals is also characterized by the increased expression of several proinflammatory cytokines and other biomarkers associated with the activation of the immune system (Neaton et al. 2010; Nixon and Landay 2010). Several studies have been performed attempting to correlate the expression of some of these markers with progression to AIDS, development of opportunistic diseases, and ultimately death (Neaton et al. 2010; Nixon and Landay 2010).

Distinct mechanisms have been proposed to explain the sustained immune activation in HIV-infected individuals. One of the most studied hypotheses is the translocation of bacterial products from the gut to the blood stream. However, to which extent this is necessary and the contribution of the mature T-cell depletion from the gut mucosa are controversial (Douek 2007; Vassallo et al. 2012). It has also been suggested that sustained immune activation, even in virus-suppressed individuals, is caused by continuous replications of HIV (Allavena et al. 2013). The excessive production of type-1 interferon (IFN) by hyperresponsive plasmacytoid dendritic cells during the primary infection, and the following chronic activation of these cells, may contribute to the general immune activation (Fitzgerald-Bocarsly and Jacobs 2010). Some authors have also suggested that a dysregulation of Treg cells would be responsible for the sustained immune activation in HIV-infected individuals (Chevalier and Weiss 2013).

An important question addressed in the most recent years is—What are the alterations of the immune system induced by the HIV infection that precede and are potentially maintained during $CD4^+$ T-cell depletion that renders the HIV-infected individuals so susceptible to develop active TB? Although general alterations of the immune system have been proposed, some authors have added the possibility that HIV infection perturbs specifically the *M. tuberculosis*-specific T cells. In fact, a selective depletion of *M. tuberculosis* antigen-specific $CD4^+$ T cells was shown to occur before generalized $CD4^+$ T-cell depletion in HIV-infected individuals (Geldmacher et al. 2008, 2010). This increased depletion of the *M. tuberculosis*–specific $CD4^+$ T cells has been associated with increased susceptibility to productive HIV-1 infection of cells producing interleukin-2 (IL-2). An increasing body of evidence suggests that cells expressing a specific set of cytokines simultaneously, referred to as polyfunctional T cells (expressing INF-γ, IL-2, tumor necrosis factor [TNF], and/or IL-17), are essential for a protective immune response to *M. tuberculosis*. In accordance, one study comparing the number of these cells in the lung of TB individuals showed that they are present in quite reduced numbers in HIV-coinfected patients (Kalsdorf et al. 2009).

$CD8^+$ T cells have been shown to play a relevant role for the control of latent TB (Behar 2013; Nunes-Alves et al. 2014). Disrupted $CD8^+$ T-cell function in HIV-infected individuals might occur because of direct dysfunction of these cells or because of the abrogated activity of the $CD4^+$ T cells in general and/or the specific loss of *M. tuberculosis*–specific $CD4^+$ T cells (Haas et al. 2011).

An increased production of TNF has been suggested to cause increased susceptibility to active TB (Roca and Ramakrishnan 2013). This has been shown in the context of individuals that naturally produce increased levels of TNF in response to *M. tuberculosis* infection (Roca and Ramakrishnan 2013). HIV infection has been shown to impair TNF-mediated macrophage apoptosis upon infection with *M. tuberculosis* (Patel et al. 2007). Decreased apoptosis and increased necrosis of infected macrophages have been shown to assist infection and to delay the establishment of antigen-specific immune responses (Behar et al. 2010). In accordance, it is reasonable to consider that the general activation of the immune system, characteristic of HIV infection, renders the hosts more susceptible to develop active TB.

Regarding potential alterations on the innate immune response, several studies have addressed the ability of macrophages to control the growth and/or kill intracellular *M. tuberculosis*. However, data in this respect have been quite controversial with some reports showing decreased ability of the macrophages from HIV-infected patients to control *M. tuberculosis* growth (Pathak et al. 2010), whereas others suggest no effect of HIV infection on the ability of the macrophages to control *M. tuberculosis* (Kalsdorf et al. 2009).

The IFN-γ/IL-12 axis is central for the interaction between the initially infected innate cells and the activation of antigen-specific T cells. The suppressor of cytokine signaling 1 (SOCS1) and IL-27 have been shown to impair the immune response against *M. tuberculosis* through down-regulating this axis (Carow et al. 2011; Pearl et al. 2004). T-cell exhaustion is a common alteration found in chronic HIV-infected patients. Markers of T-cell exhaustion such as programmed-death 1 (PD-1) and T-cell immunoglobulin and mucin domain 3 (Tim-3) (Day et al. 2006; Jones et al. 2008) both involved in the down-regulation of host immune responses, have been associated with chronic progressive HIV infection (Jones et al. 2008) and progression to active TB (Wang et al. 2011), indicating that similar inhibitory receptor/ligand interactions play a role in modulating host immunity to both HIV and *M. tuberculosis* infections in humans.

Other alterations of the immune system among HIV-infected individuals reported to promote *M. tuberculosis* infection and active TB are the up-regulation of *M. tuberculosis* entry receptors on macrophages (Rosas-Taraco et al. 2006), HIV manipulation of macrophage bactericidal pathways (Spear et al. 1990), deregulated chemotaxis (Wahl et al. 1989), and a tipped Th1/Th2 balance (Havlir and Barnes 1999).

IRIS

The introduction of antiretroviral therapy (ART) drastically reduced the mortality of HIV-infected patients. By effectively suppressing the replication of HIV, most patients under ART present a reduced viral load and a concomitant raise in the number of peripheral $CD4^+$ T cells, especially evident during the first months of treatment (Autran et al. 1997). Unfortunately, this rapid $CD4^+$ T-cell reconstitution leads, in some patients, to the phenomenon known as immune reconstitution inflammatory syndrome (IRIS) also referred to as immune restoration disease (Pearl et al. 2004). IRIS develops shortly after the initiation of ART and is associated with an exacerbated immune response to a coinfecting pathogen. Whereas IRIS can occur because of coinfection with several pathogens, and even be associated with autoimmune diseases (French et al. 2004; Lawn et al. 2005a), it has been estimated to be because of coinfection with *M. tuberculosis* in ~15.7% of the cases (Lawn et al. 2005b; Muller et al. 2010). This exacerbated immune response might be presented in one of two distinct forms, defined as paradoxical IRIS, when it occurs as the result of recurrent, new, or worsening symptoms of coinfection under treatment, and referred to as unmasking IRIS when associated with a subclinical infection. Because of the lack of distinctive biomarkers or definitive diagnostic tests, the definition of IRIS in TB-HIV-coinfected patients is difficult. A consensus clinical case definition for TB-IRIS has been defined (Meintjes et al. 2008a). Studies on patients that developed TB-IRIS led to the determination of the most obvious risk factors for the development of this syndrome, although the underlying mechanisms responsible for IRIS are still not clearly defined. Low $CD4^+$ T lymphocyte counts before ART initiation (<50–100 cells/μL) followed by a successful $CD4^+$ T-cell raise is one of the most important risk factors to develop IRIS (Olalla et al. 2002; Breton et al. 2004; Ratnam et al. 2006; Bourgarit et al. 2009). Another important risk factor is the initiation of TB treatment shortly after initiation of ART (Navas et al. 2002; Tansuphasawadikul et al. 2007). Extrapulmonary TB has also been reported to be associated with a higher risk of TB-IRIS (Manosuthi et al. 2006; Burman et al. 2007).

It has been extremely difficult to determine the mechanisms responsible for IRIS because of the difficulty in defining and making use of all necessary control groups (Lai et al. 2013) and to a certain extent also to the lack of a satisfactory animal model. Both alterations in the acquired and the innate immune response associated with ART have been proposed as being potentially responsible for TB-IRIS. One of the most explored mechanisms has been the expansion of antigen-specific Th1 $CD4^+$ T cells shortly after ART initiation. Although several studies propose these $CD4^+$ T cells as a causal link for IRIS (Bourgarit et al. 2006), it is far from being consensual because several other studies showed similar development of Th1-CD4$^+$ T-cell expansions in the absence of IRIS (Lai et al. 2013). A defect on the CD4$^+$ Treg cells has been investigated as a potential mechanism responsible for the CD4$^+$ T-cell exacerbated response. Because Treg cells are essential to maintain T-cell homeostasis, this hypothesis sounded obvious; however, data are contradictory (Meintjes et al. 2008b; Seddiki et al. 2009).

In addition to a potential defect directly on the T cells, it has been reported that TB-HIV-coinfected patients with IRIS had significantly lower levels of specific antibodies to the phenolic glycolipid (PGL-TB1) antigen from *M. tuberculosis*, compared with patients without TB-IRIS (Simonney et al. 2008).

Elevated production of pro- and anti-inflammatory cytokines has been consistently associated with TB-IRIS, although a casual effect has not been shown (Lim et al. 2008; Worsley et al. 2010; Tadokera et al. 2011; Skolimowska et al. 2012). Interestingly, some of the cytokines that have been implicated are produced exclusively by cells of the innate immune systems, strongly suggesting that innate immune cells play an important part in the pathogenesis of TB-IRIS (Jones et al. 2008). Among the cells of the innate immune system, it is of relevance that ART has been shown to lead to macrophage hyperactivation in response to *M. tuberculosis* antigens (Van den Bergh et al. 2006). Higher numbers of IFN-γ producing γδ T cells lacking the expression of the killer immunoglobulin-related receptor (KIR$^-$) were also shown (Seddiki et al. 2009). Recent studies add to the list of potential candidates the NK cells (Conradie et al. 2011) and the neutrophils (Marais et al. 2013).

TB EXACERBATES PROGRESSION FROM HIV INFECTION TO AIDS

In the HIV/*M. tuberculosis* dual interplay not only does HIV affect the progression of TB, but *M. tuberculosis* infection also has a negative impact on the immune response to HIV, accelerating the progression from HIV infection to AIDS (Pape et al. 1993; Whalen et al. 1995). Research on the potential mechanisms underlying this effect is, however, quite scarce.

M. tuberculosis and HIV share anatomical reservoirs such as the lung (Costiniuk and Jenabian 2014), and it has been suggested that TB patients have a microenvironment that facilitates HIV infection. In fact, active TB has been associated with accelerated loss of CD4$^+$ T cells and increased risk of opportunistic infections (Badri et al. 2001). The ongoing immune response against *M. tuberculosis* has been shown to increase the replication of HIV-1 in the blood (Goletti et al. 1996; Toossi et al. 2001) and at sites of *M. tuberculosis* infection in the lung (Nakata et al. 1997; Collins et al. 2002) and within activated cells including lymphocytes and CD14$^+$ macrophages of the pleural space in the case of tuberculous pericarditis (Lawn et al. 2001; Matthews et al. 2012). *M. tuberculosis* induces the production of proinflammatory cytokines and chemokines, including TNF (Rosas-Taraco et al. 2006), that activate signal transduction pathways in CD4$^+$ T cells and monocytic cells that also result in transcriptional activation of the long terminal repeats (LTRs) of HIV (Israel-Biet et al. 1991; Garrait et al. 1997; Hoshino et al. 2002).

In addition, in vitro experiments using *M. tuberculosis* have been shown to up-regulate HIV-1 replication in infected T cells, macrophages (Shattock et al. 1993; Zhang et al. 1995), and dendritic cells, as well as ex vivo in alveolar macrophages and lymphocytes from HIV-infected patients (Toossi et al. 1997; Goletti et al. 1998). Multiple mechanisms have been implicated, including cytokine- and chemokine-mediated mechanisms (Toossi et al. 2001; Hoshino et al. 2004), and loss of an inhibitory transcription factor CCAAT/enhancer-binding protein β (C/EBPb) (Hoshino et al. 2007). These mechanisms cause transcription activation of HIV genes, resulting in enhanced viral replication, spread to uninfected cells, and their subsequent depletion. Terminal differentiation of CD4$^+$ T cells at TB disease sites leads the CD4$^+$ T cells to express CCR5, an HIV coreceptor, rendering these cells more susceptible to HIV infection (Matthews et al. 2012).

 Cite this article as *Cold Spring Harb Perspect Med* doi: 10.1101/cshperspect.a017871

Both HIV and *M. tuberculosis* infect macrophages (Landay et al. 1993; Sierra-Madero et al. 1994; Nakata et al. 1995) and trigger production of host inflammatory mediators (Kedzierska et al. 2003; Ansari et al. 2013) that subsequently regulate the immune response and disease pathogenesis. These inflammatory mediators can impose beneficial or detrimental effects on each pathogen and eventually on the host. In vitro studies have shown that *M. tuberculosis* infection can increase both HIV infection and replication within macrophages and the efficiency of virus transmission from infected macrophages to T cells (Mancino et al. 1997). Upregulation of the coreceptors CXCR4 and CCR5 (Hoshino et al. 2004; Rosas-Taraco et al. 2006), SOCS1, which is stimulated by infection with *M. tuberculosis* (Rosas-Taraco et al. 2006), has been shown to facilitate the late replication pathways of HIV infection (Ryo et al. 2008) and mediate viral evasion of type-1 IFN antiviral signaling (Fenner et al. 2006). The transcription factors NF-κB and NFAT5 are required for *M. tuberculosis*–induced HIV-1 replication in macrophages (Ranjbar et al. 2012).

Although the major cell targets of HIV are $CD4^+$ T cells, dendritic cells have multiple roles at different stages of HIV infection (Manchez, Trends in Immunology, in press). In this context, it is suggested that *M. tuberculosis* increases HIV transinfection and induces viral sequestration within surface-accessible compartments suppressing major histocompatibility complex class II antigen processing by dendritic cells (Reuter et al. 2010) and that mycobacteria-infected bystander macrophages trigger maturation of dendritic cells and enhance their ability to mediate HIV transinfection (Mazurek et al. 2012).

Clinical Handling of TB Patients with HIV, Including IRIS

The current management of patients with HIV-associated TB includes provision of effective anti-TB treatment, use of concurrent ART, prevention of HIV-related comorbidities, management of drug cytotoxicity and prevention/treatment of IRIS (Lawn et al. 2013).

TB treatment in concomitant HIV infection follows the same principles as in non-HIV-infected individuals (for more details on TB treatment, see Sotgiu et al. 2014). However, caution is advocated because of interactions between anti-TB and -HIV drugs, such as protease inhibitors and rifamycins, in particular rifampicin. The clinical entity IRIS and the phenomenon of "unmasking TB" are now well-known complications on institution of ART in TB disease.

Drug-susceptible TB in low-incidence settings is usually treated with a 2-mo intensive phase of the four standard drugs (Sotgiu et al. 2014), followed by a 4-mo continuation phase if rifamycins and INH (isoniazid) are used. Intermittent dosing is not recommended in HIV patients during the intensive phase because it has been associated with an increased risk of treatment failure or relapse with acquired drug resistance to rifamycins (IDSA 2013) (see http://www.idsociety.org/uploadedFiles/HIVMA/Guidelines_Patient_Care/HIVMA_Standards_Practice_Guidelines/HIV_Guidelines/Guidelines_Content/adult_oi.pdf) (Nettles et al. 2004; Li et al. 2005; Swaminathan et al. 2010). During the follow-up phase, daily or a minimum of thrice weekly intermittent dosing should be used (IDSA 2013), the latter has not been associated with increased risk of relapse, treatment failures, or acquired drug resistance (Khan et al. 2010). Treatment of drug susceptible disease in coinfected patients in high endemic settings follow the same principles as in low-endemic settings; however, the optimal duration of treatment has been debated as higher frequencies of recurrent TB has been observed in 6-mo regimens compared with 9- and 12-mo regimens (Perriens et al. 1995). However, as previously described, recurrences in standard length treatment were mainly caused by reinfection episodes (Charalambous et al. 2008; Crampin et al. 2010; Narayanan et al. 2010).

Important Interactions between Anti-TB and -HIV Drugs

Recommended first-line anti-HIV regimens are based on nonnucleoside reverse transcriptase inhibitors (NNRTI) with efavirenz as the drug of choice and nevirapine as an alternative (Lawn et al. 2013) (IDSA 2013). A summary of recommended anti-HIV regimens and their interactions with anti-TB drugs are shown in Table 1. As new HIV drugs are entering the market and more recently new TB drugs, updated information can be retrieved (see http://www.hiv-druginteractions.org). For cotoxicity of TB and HIV drugs see IDSA (2013).

Treatment of IRIS

In mild cases of IRIS, specific treatment is usually not necessary and both anti-HIV and anti-TB treatment should be continued (Lawn et al.

Table 1. Approaches to cotreatment for HIV-infected patients with rifampicin-susceptible tuberculosis

Combined regimes	Treatment recommendations	Drug–drug interactions
Efavirenz + rifampicin-based TB treatment	No dose adjustments TDF + 3TC/FTC + EFV (WHO-recommended optimum regimen) AZT + 3TC + EFV (alternative WHO regimen)	Rifampicin induces CYP2B6 but inhibition of CYP2A6 by isoniazid might account for increased efavirenz concentrations during TB treatment in those patients with slow CYP2B6 metabolizer genotype.
Nevirapine + rifampicin-based TB treatment	Omit 14 d lead-in phase of once daily dose of NVP TDF = 3TC/FTC = NVP (alternative WHO regimen) AZT + 3TC + NVP (alternative WHO regimen)	Rifampicin induces CYP2B6 and CYP3A4. Although TB treatment reduces nevirapine concentrations, toxicity concerns curtail increasing the dose and outcomes are acceptable (but inferior to EFV) on standard doses.
Lopinavir/ritonavir + rifampicin-based TB treatment	Double-dose lopinavir/ritonavir (800/200 mg every12 h) or superboost lopinavir (lopinavir/ritonavir 400/400 mg every 12 h). Monitor alanine transaminase (ALT) closely.	Ritonavir counteracts this effect and adjusted doses of ritonavir or lopinavir/ritonavir are used to compensate, but lopinavir concentrations may be more variable. Increased risk of hepatotoxicity and gastrointestinal side effects.
PI/ritonavir + rifabutin-based TB treatment	Reduce rifabutin dose to 150 mg daily or thrice weekly. Monitor closely for rifabutin toxicity.	Ritonavir-boosted PIs markedly increase rifabutin concentrations and reduce its clearance necessitating reduction in the dose of rifabutin by 50% to 75%. Toxicity (neutropenia, uveitis, hepatoxicity, rash, gastrointestinal symptoms) and suboptimal rifamyin exposures with reduced dose are concerns.
Triple nucleoside/nucleotide regime + rifampicin-based TB treatment	No dose adjustments. A triple nucleoside/nucleotide regimen should include tenofovir or abacavir. Monitor viral load.	Triple nucleoside/nucleotide regimens may perform adequately in patients with viral suppression who have not failed a first line regimen and provide alternative ART regimens in patients with contraindications to efavirenz or nevirapine, in which other options are unavailable. TB treatment has minimal effect on tenofovir concentrations. Although rifampicin induces the enzymes responsible for glucuronidation of abacavir and zidovudine, this effect is not thought to be clinically important.

Data adapted from Lawn et al. 2013.

3TC, 2′,3′-dideoxy-3′-thiacytidine; ART, antiretroviral therapy; CYP, cytochrome P450; EFV, efavirenz; FTC, emtricitabine; OATP, organic anion-transporting polypeptide; NNRTI, nonnucleoside reverse transcriptase inhibitor; NVP, nevirapine; PI, protease inhibitor; TB, tuberculosis; TDF, tenofovir; WHO, World Health Organization.

2013). If symptoms are more pronounced, high-dose corticosteroids are indicated, in particular for IRIS of the central nervous system (Lawn et al. 2013; Lee et al. 2013).

STRATEGIES FOR PREVENTION OF THE LINKED EPIDEMICS OF HIV INFECTION AND TB

Treatment of HIV to Prevent TB

Focused efforts to deliver ART to all HIV-infected individuals with *M. tuberculosis* infection would reduce the number of people who develop active TB and are vital to prevent the two epidemics fueling each other. Numerous cohort studies have shown that in HIV-infected persons, ART reduces TB risk in adults (Lawn et al. 2010) as well as in children (Lawn et al. 2005a). There is recent evidence that earlier initiation of ART in HIV-infected patients with newly diagnosed TB reduces mortality significantly (Martinson et al. 2011b).

The Three Is Strategy

The WHO Three Is strategy—*Intensified* case finding, *Isoniazid* preventive therapy, and *Infection* control in clinical settings—must be effectively implemented.

Intensified Case Finding

It is recommended that people living with HIV who live with or are close contacts of active cases of TB should be prioritized for clinical evaluation of TB. Those who, after an appropriate clinical evaluation, are found not to have active TB should be treated for presumed latent TB with isoniazid preventive therapy (WHO 2013). More intensive TB screening, both for active and latent TB, with broader definitions of target populations and expanded indications for screening in high HIV prevalence settings would further improve the control of TB (Corbett and MacPherson 2013). Lack of better and adequate diagnostic methods are, however, still a barrier (Corbett and MacPherson 2013).

Isoniazid Preventive Therapy

In 2012, 42 countries provided isoniazid preventive therapy to nearly 520,000 people living with HIV. Although the trend toward increased uptake of preventive therapy is encouraging, the number of individuals currently receiving isoniazid preventive therapy is believed to represent a small fraction of the number of people living with HIV who could benefit from the intervention. Among 30 countries reporting both denominator and numerator for preventive therapy, 30% of those newly registered in care received isoniazid preventive therapy (WHO 2013, see http://www.unaids.org/en/media/unaids/contentassets/documents/epidemiology/2013/gr2013/UNAIDS_Global_Report_2013_en.pdf). Isoniazide preventive treatment has been shown to have an additive effect combined with ART on active TB prevention.

Infection Control

As discussed earlier, people living with HIV are very vulnerable to the risk of *M. tuberculosis* infection if exposed, and there is also an excess in the occupational risk of TB including MDR- and XDR-TB in sub-Saharan Africa compared with that of the general population (Kompala et al. 2013; Rothe et al. 2013). WHO recommends that TB infection control practices should be in place in all congregate settings and in health facilities providing HIV care. TB infection control practices include personal, administrative, and environmental controls as well as health worker surveillance. Informing communities and the general public about these practices will also help to reduce the spread of TB to people living with HIV (WHO 2013, see http://whqlibdoc.who.int/publications/2009/9789241598323_eng.pdf).

Vaccination

Ultimately, the most cost-effective approach to combat the two diseases would be vaccination. Presently, there is no effective vaccine, neither against TB nor HIV. Vaccination against TB and the need for and design of new TB vaccine(s) are discussed in Andersen and Kaufmann (2014).

However, even if we have a good TB vaccine, HIV infection will most probably reduce the efficacy of this vaccine because HIV has been suggested to eliminate preferentially *M. tuberculosis*–specific T cells (Geldmacher et al. 2008, 2010).

One approach that has been suggested would be to construct a combined TB-HIV vaccine (Kaufmann and McMichael 2005), such as a recombinant BCG (Bacillus Calmette–Guérin) vaccine as a vehicle for combinations of mycobacterial and HIV antigens (Hiroi et al. 2001; Kawahara et al. 2002; Yu et al. 2007). However, the interaction of the immunomodulatory role of individual antigens of the two pathogens needs further elucidation as, for example, the major HIV antigen gp120 (Del Corno et al. 2001) and mycobacterial compounds such as glycolipids of the cell wall, particularly LAMs, PIMs, and phenolic glycolipids (Portevin et al. 2011), that play a crucial role in modulating immune responses. It is also increasingly apparent that these compounds may differ in biologic activity depending on strain lineages of the two pathogens (Locher et al. 2005; Carow et al. 2011; Portevin et al. 2011). Because both pathogens enter the host through mucosal surfaces, a combination vaccine given at mucosal sites would probably be optimal (Hiroi et al. 2001; Kawahara et al. 2002; Yu et al. 2007). However, for this end, further research in the biology of concurrent *M. tuberculosis* and HIV infections is urgently needed.

An integrated approach to the two diseases should thus lead to novel concepts and correlates of protection and to the identification of antigen targets useful for new therapies to overcome the rapidly increasing drug resistance of both diseases, as well as for vaccination (Pawlowski et al. 2012).

REFERENCES

*Reference is also in this subject collection.

Allavena C, Rodallec A, Secher S, Reliquet V, Baffoin S, André-Garnier E, Billaud E, Raffi F, Ferré V. 2013. Evaluation of residual viremia and quantitation of soluble CD14 in a large cohort of HIV-infected adults on a long-term non-nucleoside reverse transcriptase inhibitor-based regimen. *J Med Virol* **85:** 1878–1882.

Allwood MDM, Lee YC, Salaniponi FM, Nyangulu DS, Kuppysamu I, et al. 1997. Case-finding with a single sputum smear and household bleach (abstract). *Int J Tuberc Lung Dis* **1:** S144.

* Andersen P, Kaufmann SHE. 2014. Novel vaccination strategies against tuberculosis. *Cold Spring Harb Perspect Med* **4:** a018523.

Andrews JR, Gandhi NR, Moodley P, Shah NS, Bohlken L, Moll AP, Pillay M, Friedland G, Sturm AW, Tugela Ferry Care Research Collaboration. 2008. Exogenous reinfection as a cause of multidrug-resistant and extensively drug-resistant tuberculosis in rural South Africa. *J Infect Dis* **198:** 1582–1589.

Ansari AW, Kamarulzaman A, Schmidt RE. 2013. Multifaceted impact of host C-C chemokine CCL2 in the immunopathogenesis of HIV-1/co-infection. *Front Immunol* **4:** 312.

Autran B, Carcelain G, Li TS, Blanc C, Mathez D, Tubiana R, Katlama C, Debré P, Leibowitch J. 1997. Positive effects of combined antiretroviral therapy on CD4$^+$ T cell homeostasis and function in advanced HIV disease. *Science* **277:** 112–116.

Badri M, Ehrlich R, Wood R, Pulerwitz T, Maartens G. 2001. Association between tuberculosis and HIV disease progression in a high tuberculosis prevalence area. *Int J Tuberc Lung Dis* **5:** 225–232.

Beck-Sague C, Dooley SW, Hutton MD, Otten J, Breeden A, Crawford JT, Pitchenik AE, Woodley C, Cauthen G, Jarvis WR. 1992. Hospital outbreak of multidrug-resistant *Mycobacterium tuberculosis* infections. Factors in transmission to staff and HIV-infected patients. *JAMA* **268:** 1280–1286.

Behar SM. 2013. Antigen-specific CD8(+) T cells and protective immunity to tuberculosis. *Adv Exp Med Biol* **783:** 141–163.

Behar SM, Divangahi M, Remold HG. 2010. Evasion of innate immunity by *Mycobacterium tuberculosis*: Is death an exit strategy? *Nat Rev Microbiol* **8:** 668–674.

Bourgarit A, Carcelain G, Martinez V, Lascoux C, Delcey V, Gicquel B, Vicaut E, Lagrange PH, Sereni D, Autran B. 2006. Explosion of tuberculin-specific Th1-responses induces immune restoration syndrome in tuberculosis and HIV co-infected patients. *AIDS* **20:** F1–F7.

Bourgarit A, Carcelain G, Samri A, Parizot C, Lafaurie M, Abgrall S, Delcey V, Vicaut E, Sereni D, Autran B, et al. 2009. Tuberculosis-associated immune restoration syndrome in HIV-1-infected patients involves tuberculin-specific CD4 Th1 cells and KIR-negative γδ T cells. *J Immunol* **183:** 3915–3923.

Brenchley JM, Douek DC. 2008. HIV infection and the gastrointestinal immune system. *Mucosal Immunol* **1:** 23–30.

Breton G, Duval X, Estellat C, Poaletti X, Bonnet D, Mvondo Mvondo D, Longuet P, Leport C, Vildé JL. 2004. Determinants of immune reconstitution inflammatory syndrome in HIV type 1-infected patients with tuberculosis after initiation of antiretroviral therapy. *Clin Infect Dis* **39:** 1709–1712.

Burman W, Weis S, Vernon A, Khan A, Benator D, Jones B, Silva C, King B, LaHart C, Mangura B, et al. 2007. Frequency, severity and duration of immune reconstitution events in HIV-related tuberculosis. *Int J Tuberc Lung Dis* **11:** 1282–1289.

Camacho RJ. 2012. Special aspects of the treatment of HIV-2-infected patients. *Intervirology* **55:** 179–183.

Carow B, Ye X, Gavier-Widen D, Bhuju S, Oehlmann W, Singh M, Sköld M, Ignatowicz L, Yoshimura A, Wigzell H, et al. 2011. Silencing suppressor of cytokine signaling-1 (SOCS1) in macrophages improves *Mycobacterium tuberculosis* control in an interferon-γ (IFN-γ)-dependent manner. *J Biol Chem* **286:** 26873–26887.

Charalambous S, Grant AD, Moloi V, Warren R, Day JH, van Helden P, Hayes RJ, Fielding KL, De Cock KM, Chaisson RE, et al. 2008. Contribution of reinfection to recurrent tuberculosis in South African gold miners. *Int J Tuberc Lung Dis* **12:** 942–948.

Chevalier MF, Weiss L. 2013. The split personality of regulatory T cells in HIV infection. *Blood* **121:** 29–37.

Cohn DL, O'Brien RJ. 1998. The use of restriction fragment length polymorphism (RFLP) analysis for epidemiological studies of tuberculosis in developing countries. *Int J Tuberc Lung Dis* **2:** 16–26.

Collins KR, Quinones-Mateu ME, Toossi Z, Arts EJ. 2002. Impact of tuberculosis on HIV-1 replication, diversity, and disease progression. *AIDS Rev* **4:** 165–176.

Conradie F, Foulkes AS, Ive P, Yin X, Roussos K, Glencross DK, Lawrie D, Stevens W, Montaner LJ, Sanne I, et al. 2011. Natural killer cell activation distinguishes *Mycobacterium tuberculosis*-mediated immune reconstitution syndrome from chronic HIV and HIV/MTB coinfection. *J Acquir Immune Defic Syndr* **58:** 309–318.

Corbeau P, Reynes J. 2011. Immune reconstitution under antiretroviral therapy: The new challenge in HIV-1 infection. *Blood* **117:** 5582–5590.

Corbett EL, MacPherson P. 2013. Tuberculosis screening in high human immunodeficiency virus prevalence settings: Turning promise into reality. *Int J Tuberc Lung Dis* **17:** 1125–1138.

Coronado VG, Beck-Sague CM, Hutton MD, Davis BJ, Nicholas P, Villareal C, Woodley CL, Kilbum JO, Crawford JT, Frieden TR, et al. 1993. Transmission of multidrug-resistant *Mycobacterium tuberculosis* among persons with human immunodeficiency virus infection in an urban hospital: Epidemiologic and restriction fragment length polymorphism analysis. *J Infect Dis* **168:** 1052–1055.

Costiniuk CT, Jenabian MA. 2014. The lungs as anatomical reservoirs of HIV infection. *Rev Med Virol* **24:** 35–54.

Crampin AC, Mwaungulu JN, Mwaungulu FD, Mwafulirwa DT, Munthali K, Floyd S, Fine PE, Glynn JR. 2010. Recurrent TB: Relapse or reinfection? The effect of HIV in a general population cohort in Malawi. *AIDS* **24:** 417–426.

Daley CL, Small PM, Schecter GF, Schoolnik GK, McAdam RA, Jacobs WR Jr, Hopewell PC. 1992. An outbreak of tuberculosis with accelerated progression among persons infected with the human immunodeficiency virus. An analysis using restriction-fragment-length polymorphisms. *N Engl J Med* **326:** 231–235.

Day CL, Kaufmann DE, Kiepiela P, Brown JA, Moodley ES, Reddy S, Mackey EW, Miller JD, Leslie AJ, DePierres C, et al. 2006. PD-1 expression on HIV-specific T cells is associated with T-cell exhaustion and disease progression. *Nature* **443:** 350–354.

Deeks SG, Kitchen CM, Liu L, Guo H, Gascon R, Narvaez AB, Hunt P, Martin JN, Kahn JO, Levy J, et al. 2004. Immune activation set point during early HIV infection predicts subsequent $CD4^+$ T-cell changes independent of viral load. *Blood* **104:** 942–947.

Del Corno M, Liu QH, Schols D, de Clercq E, Gessani S, Freedman BD, Collman RG. 2001. HIV-1 gp120 and chemokine activation of Pyk2 and mitogen-activated protein kinases in primary macrophages mediated by calcium-dependent, pertussis toxin-insensitive chemokine receptor signaling. *Blood* **98:** 2909–2916.

Douek D. 2007. HIV disease progression: Immune activation, microbes, and a leaky gut. *Top HIV Med* **15:** 114–117.

Edlin BR, Tokars JI, Grieco MH, Crawford JT, Williams J, Sordillo EM, Ong KR, Kilburn JO, Dooley SW, Castro KG, et al. 1992. An outbreak of multidrug-resistant tuberculosis among hospitalized patients with the acquired immunodeficiency syndrome. *N Engl J Med* **326:** 1514–1521.

Fenner JE, Starr R, Cornish AL, Zhang JG, Metcalf D, Schreiber RD, Sheehan K, Hilton DJ, Alexander WS, Hertzog PJ. 2006. Suppressor of cytokine signaling 1 regulates the immune response to infection by a unique inhibition of type I interferon activity. *Nat Immunol* **7:** 33–39.

Fitzgerald-Bocarsly P, Jacobs ES. 2010. Plasmacytoid dendritic cells in HIV infection: Striking a delicate balance. *J Leukoc Biol* **87:** 609–620.

French MA, Price P, Stone SF. 2004. Immune restoration disease after antiretroviral therapy. *AIDS* **18:** 1615–1627.

Garrait V, Cadranel J, Esvant H, Herry I, Morinet P, Mayaud C, Israël-Biet D. 1997. Tuberculosis generates a microenvironment enhancing the productive infection of local lymphocytes by HIV. *J Immunol* **159:** 2824–2830.

Geldmacher C, Schuetz A, Ngwenyama N, Casazza JP, Sanga E, Saathoff E, Boehme C, Geis S, Maboko L, Singh M, et al. 2008. Early depletion of *Mycobacterium tuberculosis*-specific T helper 1 cell responses after HIV-1 infection. *J Infect Dis* **198:** 1590–1598.

Geldmacher C, Ngwenyama N, Schuetz A, Petrovas C, Reither K, Heeregrave EJ, Casazza JP, Ambrozak DR, Louder M, Ampofo W, et al. 2010. Preferential infection and depletion of *Mycobacterium tuberculosis*-specific CD4 T cells after HIV-1 infection. *J Exp Med* **207:** 2869–2881.

Getahun H, Gunneberg C, Granich R, Nunn P. 2010. HIV infection-associated tuberculosis: The epidemiology and the response. *Clin Infect Dis* **50:** S201–S207.

Girardi E, Raviglione MC, Antonucci G, Godfrey-Faussett P, Ippolito G. 2000. Impact of the HIV epidemic on the spread of other diseases: The case of tuberculosis. *AIDS* **14:** S47–S56.

Goletti D, Weissman D, Jackson RW, Graham NM, Vlahov D, Klein RS, Munsiff SS, Ortona L, Cauda R, Fauci AS. 1996. Effect of *Mycobacterium tuberculosis* on HIV replication. Role of immune activation. *J Immunol* **157:** 1271–1278.

Goletti D, Weissman D, Jackson RW, Collins F, Kinter A, Fauci AS. 1998. The in vitro induction of human immunodeficiency virus (HIV) replication in purified protein derivative-positive HIV-infected persons by recall antigen response to *Mycobacterium tuberculosis* is the result of a balance of the effects of endogenous interleukin-2 and proinflammatory and anti-inflammatory cytokines. *J Infect Dis* **177:** 1332–1338.

Hartigan-O'Connor DJ, Hirao LA, McCune JM, Dandekar S. 2011. Th17 cells and regulatory T cells in elite control over HIV and SIV. *Curr Opin HIV AIDS* **6:** 221–227.

Haas A, Zimmermann K, Oxenius A. 2011. Antigen-dependent and -independent mechanisms of T and B cell hyperactivation during chronic HIV-1 infection. *J Virol* **85:** 12102–12113.

Havlir DV, Barnes PF. 1999. Tuberculosis in patients with human immunodeficiency virus infection. *N Engl J Med* **340:** 367–373.

Hiroi T, Goto H, Someya K, Yanagita M, Honda M, Yamanaka N, Kiyono H. 2001. HIV mucosal vaccine: Nasal immunization with rBCG-V3J1 induces a long term V3J1 peptide-specific neutralizing immunity in Th1- and Th2-deficient conditions. *J Immunol* **167:** 5862–5867.

Hoshino Y, Nakata K, Hoshino S, Honda Y, Tse DB, Shioda T, Rom WN, Weiden M. 2002. Maximal HIV-1 replication in alveolar macrophages during tuberculosis requires both lymphocyte contact and cytokines. *J Exp Med* **195:** 495–505.

Hoshino Y, Tse DB, Rochford G, Prabhakar S, Hoshino S, Chitkara N, Kuwabara K, Ching E, Raju B, Gold JA, et al. 2004. *Mycobacterium tuberculosis*-induced CXCR4 and chemokine expression leads to preferential X4 HIV-1 replication in human macrophages. *J Immunol* **172:** 6251–6258.

Hoshino Y, Hoshino S, Gold JA, Raju B, Prabhakar S, Pine R, Rom WN, Nakata K, Weiden M. 2007. Mechanisms of polymorphonuclear neutrophil-mediated induction of HIV-1 replication in macrophages during pulmonary tuberculosis. *J Infect Dis* **195:** 1303–1310.

Ho Tsong Fang R, Colantonio AD, Uittenbogaart CH. 2008. The role of the thymus in HIV infection: A 10 year perspective. *AIDS* **22:** 171–184.

Houben RM, Crampin AC, Ndhlovu R, Sonnenberg P, Godfrey-Faussett P, Haas WH, Engelmann G, Lombard CJ, Wilkinson D, Bruchfeld J, et al. 2011. Human immunodeficiency virus associated tuberculosis more often due to recent infection than reactivation of latent infection. *Int J Tuberc Lung Dis* **15:** 24–31.

ISDA. 2013. Primary care guidelines for the management of persons infected with human immunodeficiency virus: Update by the HIV Medicine Association of the Infectious Diseases Society of America. *Clin Infect Dis* **39:** 609–629.

Israel-Biet D, Cadranel J, Beldjord K, Andrieu JM, Jeffrey A, Even P. 1991. Tumor necrosis factor production in HIV-seropositive subjects. Relationship with lung opportunistic infections and HIV expression in alveolar macrophages. *J Immunol* **147:** 490–494.

Jones RB, Ndhlovu LC, Barbour JD, Sheth PM, Jha AR, Long BR, Wong JC, Satkunarajah M, Schweneker M, Chapman JM, et al. 2008. Tim-3 expression defines a novel population of dysfunctional T cells with highly elevated frequencies in progressive HIV-1 infection. *J Exp Med* **205:** 2763–2779.

Kalsdorf B, Scriba TJ, Wood K, Day CL, Dheda K, Dawson R, Hanekom WA, Lange C, Wilkinson RJ. 2009. HIV-1 infection impairs the bronchoalveolar T-cell response to mycobacteria. *Am J Respir Crit Care Med* **180:** 1262–1270.

Kanwar B, Favre D, McCune JM. 2010. Th17 and regulatory T cells: Implications for AIDS pathogenesis. *Curr Opin HIV AIDS* **5:** 151–157.

Kato-Maeda M, Small PM. 2000. How molecular epidemiology has changed what we know about tuberculosis. *West J Med* **172:** 256–259.

Kaufmann SH, McMichael AJ. 2005. Annulling a dangerous liaison: Vaccination strategies against AIDS and tuberculosis. *Nat Med* **11:** S33–S44.

Kawahara M, Hashimoto A, Toida I, Honda M. 2002 Oral recombinant *Mycobacterium bovis* bacillus Calmette-Guerin expressing HIV-1 antigens as a freeze-dried vaccine induces long-term, HIV-specific mucosal and systemic immunity. *Clin Immunol* **105:** 326–331.

Kedzierska K, Crowe SM, Turville S, Cunningham AL. 2003. The influence of cytokines, chemokines and their receptors on HIV-1 replication in monocytes and macrophages. *Rev Med Virol* **13:** 39–56.

Khan FA, Minion J, Pai M, Royce S, Burman W, Harries AD, Menzies D. 2010. Treatment of active tuberculosis in HIV-coinfected patients: A systematic review and meta-analysis. *Clin Infect Dis* **50:** 1288–1299.

Kompala T, Shenoi SV, Friedland G. 2013. Transmission of tuberculosis in resource-limited settings. *Curr HIV/AIDS Rep* **10:** 264–272.

Kwan CK, Ernst JD. 2011. HIV and tuberculosis: A deadly human syndemic. *Clin Microbiol Rev* **24:** 351–376.

Lai RP, Nakiwala JK, Meintjes G, Wilkinson RJ. 2013. The immunopathogenesis of the HIV tuberculosis immune reconstitution inflammatory syndrome. *Eur J Immunol* **43:** 1995–2002.

Landay AL, Schade SZ, Takefman DM, Kuhns MC, McNamara AL, Rosen RL, Kessler HA, Spear GT. 1993. Detection of HIV-1 provirus in bronchoalveolar lavage cells by polymerase chain reaction. *J Acquir Immune Defic Syndr* **6:** 171–175.

Lawn SD, Pisell TL, Hirsch CS, Wu M, Butera ST, Toossi Z. 2001. Anatomically compartmentalized human immunodeficiency virus replication in HLA-DR$^+$ cells and CD14$^+$ macrophages at the site of pleural tuberculosis coinfection. *J Infect Dis* **184:** 1127–1133.

Lawn SD, Bekker LG, Miller RF. 2005a. Immune reconstitution disease associated with mycobacterial infections in HIV-infected individuals receiving antiretrovirals. *Lancet Infect Dis* **5:** 361–373.

Lawn SD, Badri M, Wood R. 2005b. Tuberculosis among HIV-infected patients receiving HAART: Long term incidence and risk factors in a South African cohort. *AIDS* **19:** 2109–2116.

Lawn SD, Wood R, De Cock KM, Kranzer K, Lewis JJ, Churchyard GJ. 2010. Antiretrovirals and isoniazid preventive therapy in the prevention of HIV-associated tuberculosis in settings with limited health-care resources. *Lancet Infect Dis* **10:** 489–498.

Lawn SD, Meintjes G, McIlleron H, Harries AD, Wood R. 2013. Management of HIV-associated tuberculosis in resource-limited settings: A state-of-the-art review. *BMC Med* **11:** 253.

Lee SS, Meintjes G, Kamarulzaman A, Leung CC. 2013. Management of tuberculosis and latent tuberculosis infection in human immunodeficiency virus-infected persons. *Respirology* **18:** 912–922.

Li J, Munsiff SS, Driver CR, Sackoff J. 2005. Relapse and acquired rifampin resistance in HIV-infected patients with tuberculosis treated with rifampin- or rifabutin-based regimens in New York City, 1997–2000. *Clin Infect Dis* **41:** 83–91.

Lim A, D'Orsogna L, Price P, French MA. 2008. Imbalanced effector and regulatory cytokine responses may underlie mycobacterial immune restoration disease. *AIDS Res Ther* **5:** 9.

Locher CP, Witt SA, Kassel R, Dowell NL, Fujimura S, Levy JA. 2005. Differential effects of R5 and X4 human immunodeficiency virus type 1 infection on $CD4^+$ cell proliferation and activation. *J Gen Virol* **86:** 1171–1179.

Manches O, Frieta D, Bhardwaj N. 2013. Dendritic cells in progression and pathology of HIV infection. *Trends Immunol* **35:** 114–122.

Mancino G, Placido R, Bach S, Mariani F, Montesano C, Ercoli L, Zembala M, Colizzi V. 1997. Infection of human monocytes with *Mycobacterium tuberculosis* enhances human immunodeficiency virus type 1 replication and transmission to T cells. *J Infect Dis* **175:** 1531–1535.

Manosuthi W, Kiertiburanakul S, Phoorisri T, Sungkanuparph S. 2006. Immune reconstitution inflammatory syndrome of tuberculosis among HIV-infected patients receiving antituberculous and antiretroviral therapy. *J Infect* **53:** 357–363.

Marais S, Meintjes G, Pepper DJ, Dodd LE, Schutz C, Ismail Z, Wilkinson KA, Wilkinson RJ. 2013. Frequency, severity, and prediction of tuberculous meningitis immune reconstitution inflammatory syndrome. *Clin Infect Dis* **56:** 450–460.

Martinson NA, Barnes GL, Moulton LH, Msandiwa R, Hausler H, Ram M, McIntyre JA, Gray GE, Chaisson RE. 2011a. New regimens to prevent tuberculosis in adults with HIV infection. *N Engl J Med* **365:** 11–20.

Martinson NA, Hoffmann CJ, Chaisson RE. 2011b. Epidemiology of tuberculosis and HIV: Recent advances in understanding and responses. *Proc Am Thorac Soc* **8:** 288–293.

Matthews K, Ntsekhe M, Syed F, Scriba T, Russell J, Tibazarwa K, Deffur A, Hanekom W, Mayosi BM, Wilkinson RJ, et al. 2012. HIV-1 infection alters $CD4^+$ memory T-cell phenotype at the site of disease in extrapulmonary tuberculosis. *Eur J Immunol* **42:** 147–157.

Mazurek J, Ignatowicz L, Kallenius G, Jansson M, Pawlowski A. 2012. Mycobacteria-infected bystander macrophages trigger maturation of dendritic cells and enhance their ability to mediate HIV transinfection. *Eur J Immunol* **42:** 1192–1202.

Mehandru S, Poles MA, Tenner-Racz K, Horowitz A, Hurley A, Hogan C, Boden D, Racz P, Markowtiz M. 2004. Primary HIV-1 infection is associated with preferential depletion of $CD4^+$ T lymphocytes from effector sites in the gastrointestinal tract. *J Exp Med* **200:** 761–770.

Meintjes G, Lawn SD, Scano F, Maartens G, French MA, Worodria W, Elliott JH, Murdoch D, Wilkinson RJ, Seyler C, et al. 2008a. Tuberculosis-associated immune reconstitution inflammatory syndrome: Case definitions for use in resource-limited settings. *Lancet Infect Dis* **8:** 516–523.

Meintjes G, Wilkinson KA, Rangaka MX, Skolimowska K, van Veen K, Abrahams M, Seldon R, Pepper DJ, Rebe K, Mouton P, et al. 2008b. Type 1 helper T cells and FoxP3-positive T cells in HIV-tuberculosis-associated immune reconstitution inflammatory syndrome. *Am J Respir Crit Care Med* **178:** 1083–1089.

Moir S, Chun TW, Fauci AS. 2011. Pathogenic mechanisms of HIV disease. *Annu Rev Pathol* **6:** 223–248.

Muller M, Wandel S, Colebunders R, Attia S, Furrer H, Egger M; IeDEA Southern, Central Africa. 2010. Immune reconstitution inflammatory syndrome in patients starting antiretroviral therapy for HIV infection: A systematic review and meta-analysis. *Lancet Infect Dis* **10:** 251–261.

Nakata K, Weiden M, Harkin T, Ho D, Rom WN. 1995. Low copy number and limited variability of proviral DNA in alveolar macrophages from HIV-1-infected patients: Evidence for genetic differences in HIV-1 between lung and blood macrophage populations. *Mol Med* **1:** 744–757.

Nakata K, Rom WN, Honda Y, Condos R, Kanegasaki S, Cao Y, Weiden M. 1997. *Mycobacterium tuberculosis* enhances human immunodeficiency virus-1 replication in the lung. *Am J Respir Crit Care Med* **155:** 996–1003.

Narayanan S, Swaminathan S, Supply P, Shanmugam S, Narendran G, Hari L, Ramachandran R, Locht C, Jawahar MS, Narayanan PR. 2010. Impact of HIV infection on the recurrence of tuberculosis in South India. *J Infect Dis* **201:** 691–703.

Navas E, Martin-Davila P, Moreno L, Pintado V, Casado JL, Fortún J, Pérez-Elías MJ, Gomez-Mampaso E, Moreno S. 2002. Paradoxical reactions of tuberculosis in patients with the acquired immunodeficiency syndrome who are treated with highly active antiretroviral therapy. *Arch Intern Med* **162:** 97–99.

Neaton JD, Neuhaus J, Emery S. 2010. Soluble biomarkers and morbidity and mortality among people infected with HIV: Summary of published reports from 1997 to 2010. *Curr Opin HIV AIDS* **5:** 480–490.

Nettles RE, Mazo D, Alwood K, Gachuhi R, Maltas G, Wendel K, Cronin W, Hooper N, Bishai W, Sterling TR. 2004. Risk factors for relapse and acquired rifamycin resistance after directly observed tuberculosis treatment: A comparison by HIV serostatus and rifamycin use. *Clin Infect Dis* **38:** 731–736.

Nixon DE, Landay AL. 2010. Biomarkers of immune dysfunction in HIV. *Curr Opin HIV AIDS* **5:** 498–503.

Nunes-Alves C, Booty MG, Carpenter SM, Jayaraman P, Rothchild AC, Behar SM. 2014. In search of a new paradigm for protective immunity to TB. *Nat Rev Microbiol* **12:** 289–299.

Nunn PP, Elliott AM, McAdam KP. 1994. Tropical respiratory medicine. 2. Impact of human immunodeficiency virus on tuberculosis in developing countries. *Thorax* **49:** 511–518.

Olalla J, Pulido F, Rubio R, Costa MA, Monsalvo R, Palenque E, Costa JR, Del PA. 2002. Paradoxical responses in a cohort of HIV-1-infected patients with mycobacterial disease. *Int J Tuberc Lung Dis* **6:** 71–75.

Pape JW, Jean SS, Ho JL, Hafner A, Johnson WD Jr. 1993. Effect of isoniazid prophylaxis on incidence of active tuberculosis and progression of HIV infection. *Lancet* **342:** 268–272.

Patel NR, Zhu J, Tachado SD, Zhang J, Wan Z, Saukkonen J, Koziel H. 2007. HIV impairs TNF-α mediated macrophage apoptotic response to *Mycobacterium tuberculosis*. *J Immunol* **179:** 6973–6980.

Pathak S, Wentzel-Larsen T, Asjo B. 2010. Effects of in vitro HIV-1 infection on mycobacterial growth in peripheral blood monocyte-derived macrophages. *Infect Immun* **78:** 4022–4032.

Pawlowski A, Jansson M, Skold M, Rottenberg ME, Kallenius G. 2012. Tuberculosis and HIV co-infection. *PLoS Pathog* **8:** e1002464.

Pearl JE, Khader SA, Solache A, Gilmartin L, Ghilardi N, deSauvage F, Cooper AM. 2004. IL-27 signaling compromises control of bacterial growth in mycobacteria-infected mice. *J Immunol* **173:** 7490–7496.

Perriens JH, St Louis ME, Mukadi YB, Brown C, Prignot J, Pouthier F, Portaels F, Williams JC, Mandala JK, Kaboto M, et al. 1995. Pulmonary tuberculosis in HIV-infected patients in Zaire. A controlled trial of treatment for either 6 or 12 months. *N Engl J Med* **332:** 779–784.

Portevin D, Gagneux S, Comas I, Young D. 2011. Human macrophage responses to clinical isolates from the *Mycobacterium tuberculosis* complex discriminate between ancient and modern lineages. *PLoS Pathog* **7:** e1001307

Ranjbar S, Jasenosky LD, Chow N, Goldfeld AE. 2012. Regulation of *Mycobacterium tuberculosis*-dependent HIV-1 transcription reveals a new role for NFAT5 in the toll-like receptor pathway. *PLoS Pathog* **8:** e1002620.

Ratnam I, Chiu C, Kandala NB, Easterbrook PJ. 2006. Incidence and risk factors for immune reconstitution inflammatory syndrome in an ethnically diverse HIV type 1-infected cohort. *Clin Infect Dis* **42:** 418–427.

Reuter MA, Pecora ND, Harding CV, Canaday DH, McDonald D. 2010. *Mycobacterium tuberculosis* promotes HIV trans-infection and suppresses major histocompatibility complex class II antigen processing by dendritic cells. *J Virol* **84:** 8549–8560.

Rieder HL. 1999. *Epidemiologic basis of tuberculosis control*. International Union against Tuberculosis and Lung Disease, Paris.

Roca FJ, Ramakrishnan L. 2013. TNF dually mediates resistance and susceptibility to mycobacteria via mitochondrial reactive oxygen species. *Cell* **153:** 521–534.

Rosas-Taraco AG, Arce-Mendoza AY, Caballero-Olin G, Salinas-Carmona MC. 2006. *Mycobacterium tuberculosis* upregulates coreceptors CCR5 and CXCR4 while HIV modulates CD14 favoring concurrent infection. *AIDS Res Hum Retroviruses* **22:** 45–51.

Rothe C, Schlaich C, Thompson S. 2013. Healthcare-associated infections in sub-Saharan Africa. *J Hosp Infect* **85:** 257–267.

Ryo A, Tsurutani N, Ohba K, Kimura R, Komano J, Nishi M, Soeda H, Hattori S, Perrem K, Yamamoto M, et al. 2008. SOCS1 is an inducible host factor during HIV-1 infection and regulates the intracellular trafficking and stability of HIV-1 Gag. *Proc Natl Acad Sci* **105:** 294–299.

Sauce D, Elbim C, Appay V. 2013. Monitoring cellular immune markers in HIV infection: From activation to exhaustion. *Curr Opin HIV AIDS* **8:** 125–131.

Seddiki N, Sasson SC, Santner-Nanan B, Munier M, van Bockel D, Ip S, Marriott D, Pett S, Nanan R, Cooper DA, et al. 2009. Proliferation of weakly suppressive regulatory $CD4^+$ T cells is associated with over-active $CD4^+$ T-cell responses in HIV-positive patients with mycobacterial immune restoration disease. *Eur J Immunol* **39:** 391–403.

Selwyn PA, Hartel D, Lewis VA, Schoenbaum EE, Vermund SH, Klein RS, Walker AT, Friedland GH. 1989. A prospective study of the risk of tuberculosis among intravenous drug users with human immunodeficiency virus infection. *N Engl J Med* **320:** 545–550.

Shattock RJ, Friedland JS, Griffin GE. 1993. Modulation of HIV transcription in and release from human monocytic cells following phagocytosis of *Mycobacterium tuberculosis*. *Res Virol* **144:** 7–12.

Sierra-Madero JG, Toossi Z, Hom DL, Finegan CK, Hoenig E, Rich EA. 1994. Relationship between load of virus in alveolar macrophages from human immunodeficiency virus type 1-infected persons, production of cytokines, and clinical status. *J Infect Dis* **169:** 18–27.

Simonney N, Dewulf G, Herrmann JL, Gutierrez MC, Vicaut E, Boutron C, Leportier M, Lafaurie M, Abgrall S, Sereni D, et al. 2008. Anti-PGL-Tb1 responses as an indicator of the immune restoration syndrome in HIV-TB patients. *Tuberculosis (Edinb)* **88:** 453–461.

Skolimowska KH, Rangaka MX, Meintjes G, Pepper DJ, Seldon R, Matthews K, Wilkinson RJ, Wilkinson KA. 2012. Altered ratio of IFN-γ/IL-10 in patients with drug resistant *Mycobacterium tuberculosis* and HIV-tuberculosis immune reconstitution inflammatory syndrome. *PLoS ONE* **7:** e46481.

Small PM, Hopewell PC, Singh SP, Paz A, Parsonnet J, Ruston DC, Schecter GF, Daley CL, Schoolnik GK. 1994. The epidemiology of tuberculosis in San Francisco. A population-based study using conventional and molecular methods. *N Engl J Med* **330:** 1703–1709.

Sonnenberg P, Glynn JR, Fielding K, Murray J, Godfrey-Faussett P, Shearer S. 2005. How soon after infection with HIV does the risk of tuberculosis start to increase? A retrospective cohort study in South African gold miners. *J Infect Dis* **191:** 150–158.

* Sotgiu G, Centis R, D'ambrosio L, Battista Migliori G. 2014. Tuberculosis treatment and drug regimens. *Cold Spring Harb Perspect Med* doi: 10.1101/cshperspect.a017822.

Sousa AE, Carneiro J, Meier-Schellersheim M, Grossman Z, Victorino RM. 2002. CD4 T cell depletion is linked directly to immune activation in the pathogenesis of HIV-1 and HIV-2 but only indirectly to the viral load. *J Immunol* **169:** 3400–3406.

Spear GT, Kessler HA, Rothberg L, Phair J, Landay AL. 1990. Decreased oxidative burst activity of monocytes from asymptomatic HIV-infected individuals. *Clin Immunol Immunopathol* **54:** 184–191.

Styblo K. 1989. Overview and epidemiologic assessment of the current global tuberculosis situation with an emphasis on control in developing countries. *Rev Infect Dis* **11:** S339–346.

Swaminathan S, Narendran G, Venkatesan P, Iliayas S, Santhanakrishnan R, Menon PA, Padmapriyadarsini C, Ramachandran R, Chinnaiyan P, Suhadev M, et al. 2010. Efficacy of a 6-month versus 9-month intermittent treatment regimen in HIV-infected patients with tuberculosis: A randomized clinical trial. *Am J Respir Crit Care Med* **181:** 743–751.

Tadokera R, Meintjes G, Skolimowska KH, Wilkinson KA, Matthews K, Seldon R, Chegou NN, Maartens G, Rangaka MX, Rebe K, et al. 2011. Hypercytokinaemia accompanies HIV-tuberculosis immune reconstitution inflammatory syndrome. *Eur Respir J* **37:** 1248–1259.

Tansuphasawadikul S, Saito W, Kim J, Phonrat B, Dhitavat J, Chamnachanan S, Pitisuttithum P. 2007. Outcomes in HIV-infected patients on antiretroviral therapy with tuberculosis. *Southeast Asian J Trop Med Public Health* **38:** 1053–1060.

Toossi Z, Nicolacakis K, Xia L, Ferrari NA, Rich EA. 1997. Activation of latent HIV-1 by *Mycobacterium tuberculosis* and its purified protein derivative in alveolar macrophages from HIV-infected individuals in vitro. *J Acquir Immune Defic Syndr Hum Retrovirol* **15:** 325–331.

Toossi Z, Johnson JL, Kanost RA, Wu M, Luzze H, Peters P, Okwera A, Joloba M, Mugyenyi P, Mugerwa RD, et al. 2001. Increased replication of HIV-1 at sites of *Mycobacterium tuberculosis* infection: Potential mechanisms of viral activation. *J Acquir Immune Defic Syndr* **28:** 1–8.

UNAIDS. 2012. *Report on the global AIDS epidemic.* United Nations, New York.

Van den Bergh R, Vanham G, Raes G, De Baetselier P, Colebunders R. 2006. Mycobacterium-associated immune reconstitution disease: Macrophages running wild? *Lancet Infect Dis* **6:** 2–3; author reply 4–5.

Vassallo M, Mercie P, Cottalorda J, Ticchioni M, Dellamonica P. 2012. The role of lipopolysaccharide as a marker of immune activation in HIV-1 infected patients: A systematic literature review. *Virol J* **9:** 174.

Wahl SM, Allen JB, Gartner S, Orenstein JM, Popovic M, Chenoweth DE, Arthur LO, Farrar WL, Wahl LM. 1989. HIV-1 and its envelope glycoprotein down-regulate chemotactic ligand receptors and chemotactic function of peripheral blood monocytes. *J Immunol* **142:** 3553–3559.

Wang X, Cao Z, Jiang J, Li Y, Dong M, Ostrowski M, Cheng X. 2011. Elevated expression of Tim-3 on CD8 T cells correlates with disease severity of pulmonary tuberculosis. *J Infect* **62:** 292–300.

Whalen C, Horsburgh CR, Hom D, Lahart C, Simberkoff M, Ellner J. 1995. Accelerated course of human immunodeficiency virus infection after tuberculosis. *Am J Respir Crit Care Med* **151:** 129–135.

WHO. 2013. *Global tuberculosis report.* WHO, Geneva.

Worsley CM, Suchard MS, Stevens WS, Van Rie A, Murdoch DM. 2010. Multi-analyte profiling of ten cytokines in South African HIV-infected patients with immune reconstitution inflammatory syndrome (IRIS). *AIDS Res Ther* **7:** 36.

Yu JS, Peacock JW, Jacobs WR Jr, Frothingham R, Letvin NL, Liao HX, Haynes BF. 2007. Recombinant *Mycobacterium bovis* bacillus Calmette-Guerin elicits human immunodeficiency virus type 1 envelope-specific T lymphocytes at mucosal sites. *Clin Vaccine Immunol* **14:** 886–893.

Zhang Y, Nakata K, Weiden M, Rom WN. 1995. *Mycobacterium tuberculosis* enhances human immunodeficiency virus-1 replication by transcriptional activation at the long terminal repeat. *J Clin Invest* **95:** 2324–2331.

Tuberculosis Comorbidity with Communicable and Noncommunicable Diseases

Matthew Bates[1,2], Ben J. Marais[3], and Alimuddin Zumla[4]

[1]University of Zambia-University College London Medical School (UNZA-UCLMS) Research and Training Project[5], University Teaching Hospital, Lusaka RW1X, Zambia

[2]Center for Clinical Microbiology, Department of Infection, Division of Infection and Immunity, University College London, London, United Kingdom

[3]Marie Bashir Institute for Infectious Diseases and Biosecurity (MBI) and The Children's Hospital at Westmead, Sydney Medical School, University of Sydney, Sydney, Australia

[4]National Institute of Health Research, Biomedical Research Centre, Royal Free Campus Rowland Hill St, University College London Hospitals, London NW3 2PF, United Kingdom

Correspondence: a.zumla@ucl.ac.uk

The 18th WHO Global Tuberculosis Annual Report indicates that there were an estimated 8.6 million incident cases of tuberculosis (TB) in 2012, which included 2.9 million women and 530,000 children. TB caused 1.3 million deaths including 320,000 human immunodeficiency virus (HIV)-infected people; three-quarters of deaths occurred in Africa and Southeast Asia. With one-third of the world's population latently infected with *Mycobacterium tuberculosis* (*Mtb*), active TB disease is primarily associated with a break down in immune surveillance. This explains the strong link between active TB disease and other communicable diseases (CDs) or noncommunicable diseases (NCDs) that exert a toll on the immune system. Comorbid NCD risk factors include diabetes, smoking, malnutrition, and chronic lung disease, all of which have increased relentlessly over the past decade in developing countries. The huge overlap between killer infections such as TB, HIV, malaria, and severe viral infections with NCDs, results in a "double burden of disease" in developing countries. The current focus on vertical disease programs fails to recognize comorbidities or to encourage joint management approaches. This review highlights major disease overlaps and discusses the rationale for better integration of tuberculosis care with services for NCDs and other infectious diseases to enhance the overall efficiency of the public health responses.

During the past two decades, health priorities in developing countries have been determined primarily by the epidemics of killer infectious diseases, particularly tuberculosis (TB), HIV/AIDS (acquired immunodeficiency syndrome), and malaria. The 2013 WHO Global TB report estimates that 8.6 million TB cases occurred in 2012, causing 1.3 million deaths of which 320,000 were in HIV-infected people (WHO 2013). Three-quarters of TB deaths oc-

[5]www.unza-uclms.org

Cite this article as *Cold Spring Harb Perspect Med* doi: 10.1101/cshperspect.a017889

curred in Africa and Southeast Asia, with South Africa and India accounting for one-third of all deaths. An estimated 3 million people with active TB were either not diagnosed or diagnosed but not reported. Copresentation of severely ill patients with other communicable and noncommunicable diseases (NCDs) is a major cause of TB-associated deaths (Bates et al. 2012; Geneau and Hallen 2012; Remais et al. 2013) (Table 1).

The global burden of NCDs, particularly cancer, cardiovascular disease, diabetes, and chronic respiratory disease, accounts for nearly half of all disability and two-thirds of deaths worldwide (Beaglehole et al. 2011; WHO 2011). The prevalence of NCDs is increasing the fastest in low- and middle-income countries and impacting disproportionately on disadvantaged communities. In 2010, more than 2 million deaths attributable to NCDs occurred in sub-Saharan Africa, a 46% (95% CI 41–59) increase from 1990 (Lozano et al. 2012). In developing countries, major demographic shifts, urbanization, changing environmental factors, economic empowerment, and accompanying lifestyle changes have led to a rapid increase in NCDs (Lim et al. 2012). Undernutrition, tobacco use, the growing diabetes epidemic, and indoor air pollution are also impacting TB control adversely in Southeast Asian nations. In the sub-Saharan African context, the impact of the HIV epidemic is more significant on TB. So prevention and treatment policy and programming have to take these factors into account.

Table 1. Key messages

TB comorbidity with noncommunicable diseases (NCDs) and other communicable diseases (CDs) is highly prevalent in TB endemic regions of the world. Population attributable TB risk estimates for diabetes, malnutrition, smoking, excessive alcohol use, and HIV infection are high.
Traditional vertical (disease-specific) approaches to health care services delivery often fail to recognize potential synergies. Wider integration of TB control activities present opportunities to explore commonalities and optimize synergies without sacrificing recent gains or eroding the functionality of existing programs.
The lethal bidirectional interaction between TB and HIV coinfection in sub-Saharan Africa exemplifies the need for well-integrated approaches to disease management and control.
The looming threat of diabetes mellitus (DM) and TB also calls for bidirectional screening and the need to tackle a broader range of overlapping diseases in resource-poor countries. High levels of TB comorbidity in patients admitted to hospital with CDs or NCDs and in pregnant women attending antenatal clinics are easily overlooked in TB endemic areas.
Efficient integration of TB services should be encouraged, while maintaining some vertical elements to secure essential functions such as drug supply, monitoring and evaluation, and national surveillance, to a point in which the national TB program may be limited to a small central team providing general oversight.

The convergence of certain NCDs with TB and other communicable diseases now poses concurrent health challenges, which requires a radical shift in emphasis toward multidisciplinary collaboration and integrated strategies. Health services in resource-limited countries are not tailored to deal with this double burden of disease, and thus simple and effective adjustments to health systems are required, which can significantly improve joint care (Adeyi and Robles 2007). In high comorbidity populations, it is critical that health ministries, and nongovernmental intervention and research organizations, appreciate the limitations of vertical approaches focused on individual diseases.

Table 2 illustrates synergies between TB and NCDs that could be explored in public health efforts, such as joint health promotion strategies, reciprocal screening programs, and coordinated treatment. Figure 1 provides absolute and attributable TB risk estimates for diabetes, malnutrition, smoking, excessive alcohol use, and HIV infection. A review of autopsies performed on patients who died with TB in London determined that 35 out of 46 cases had comorbidities, which were primarily hepatitis C virus and HIV infections, cancer, cardiovas-

Table 2. Differences, similarities, and potential synergies between tuberculosis (TB) and noncommunicable diseases (NCDs)

Differences and similarities	
Tuberculosis	**NCDs**
Transmissible	Not transmissible
Infection control important	No infection control issues
Need to prevent	Need to prevent
POC testing problematic	POC testing common
Curable	Rarely curable
Long-term treatment	Long-term management
Major adherence issues	Major adherence issues
Require lifestyle changes	Require lifestyle changes
Most cases can be managed at primary HC level	Most cases managed at primary HC level
Potential synergies	
Reciprocal screening for TB, other CDs (malaria, HIV) and NCDs	
Combined health messaging and communication strategies	
Coordinated human resource development/training opportunities	
Combined infrastructure development	
Cross-utilization of health care workers	
Unified point of care; avoids multiple clinic attendances	
Integrated recording/reporting systems	
Opportunities for community and user education/engagement	
Poverty alleviation strategies	
Creating an environment that sustains health and well-being	

POC, point of care.

cular disease, and chronic obstructive pulmonary disease (COPD) (Sbrana et al. 2011). This review describes the major comorbidities associated with active TB disease, describes key clinical and molecular interactions, and discusses the implications for disease control policy.

TUBERCULOSIS AND NONCOMMUNICABLE DISEASES

Diabetes

The epidemiological link between diabetes and TB is well established, but during the last half century, populations that have developed high rates of diabetes (wealthier, overnourished, more sedentary working environments) have been distinct from those still dogged by rampant TB (poorer, undernourished, persistence of grueling manual working environments). Increasing industrialization and urbanization in developing countries are leading to growth in rates of diabetes, leading to a potentially cataclysmic confluence of NCDs (of which diabetes is one of the most common) and CDs (of which TB is the most common). In parts of India and China, this has already become a reality, as swathes of the traditionally rural populous flock to overcrowded dwellings in urban centers to take up minimum wage employment in poorly ventilated factories and mines (Li et al. 2012; Lin et al. 2012; Viswanathan et al. 2012).

Several large case-controlled and longitudinal cohort studies have shown that the relative odds of developing active TB ranges from two to eight in diabetic patients versus nondiabetic controls (reviewed by Dooley and Chaisson 2009). These studies were in different populations globally, controlling for the particular risk factors, which predominate in each study population. A recent meta-analysis concluded that diabetes patients were 3.1× more likely to develop active TB than controls, although relative risk was lower in North American study populations (Jeon and Murray 2008). TB is also more likely in insulin-dependent versus non-insulin-dependent diabetes patients (Olmos et al. 1989; Swai et al. 1990; Leung et al. 2008).

Studies have shown a negative impact of diabetes on treatment outcomes including an up to fourfold increase in the risk of treatment failure (Mboussa et al. 2003; Morsy et al. 2003; Alisjahbana et al. 2007). Studies from Turkey and the United States following up patients for a shorter period suggest that diabetes is linked with modest delays in clearance (Guler et al. 2007; Restrepo et al. 2008), although one Indian study found that whereas diabetes patients were more likely to be smear-positive (which bodes well for diagnosis), they had higher smear conversion rates at 3 mo (Singla et al. 2006).

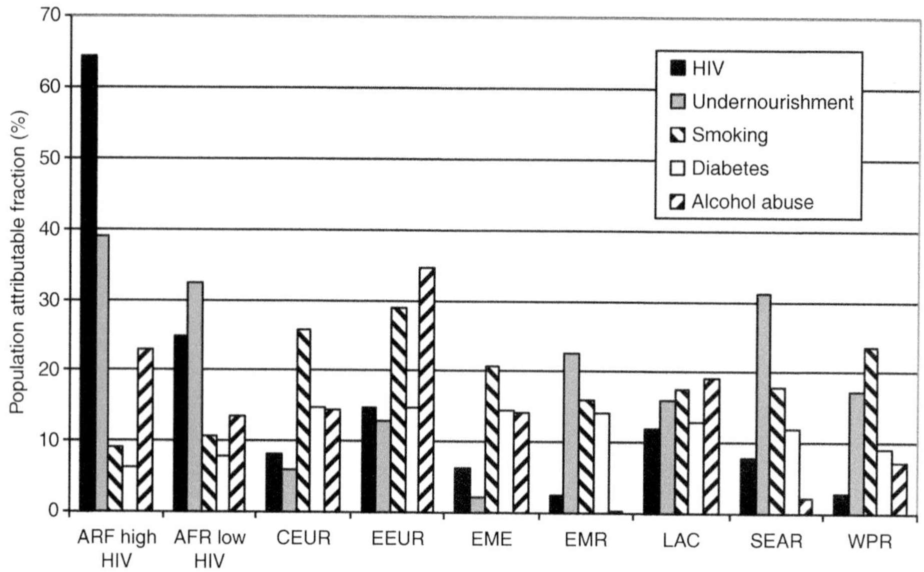

Figure 1. Estimates of population attributable to TB disease risk caused by HIV, undernutrition, smoking, diabetes, and alcohol abuse. AFR high HIV: African countries with high HIV prevalence. AFR low HIV: African countries with low/moderate HIV prevalence. CEUR: Central European countries. EEUR: Eastern European countries. EME: Established market economies. EMR: Eastern Mediterranean region. LAC: Latin American countries. SEAR: Southeast Asian region. WPR: Western Pacific region (except EME). Population attributable fraction (PAF) = [prevalence × (relative risk − 1)]/[prevalence × (relative risk − 1) + 1]. Point estimates of relative risk from systematic reviews were used. When prevalence was only available for adults, the prevalence in adults was adjusted for proportion of population under the age of 15 to estimate the total population PAF. *HIV (human immunodeficiency virus infection)*: Relative risk = 27. *Undernourishment (undernutrition):* Relative risk = 3.2 (for BMI 16 vs. BMI 25). *Diabetes (DM, diabetes mellitus)*: Relative risk = 3.1. *Alcohol abuse*: Relative risk = 2.9. Prevalence data: Average of prevalence of heavy drinking in China, Brazil, India, Nigeria, Pakistan, Russia, South Africa, and Thailand. *Smoking (cigarette smoking):* Relative risk = 2.0 (current vs. never smokers). (Adapted from Lönnroth et al. 2010 and Creswell et al. 2011.)

There are reports for and against an association between diabetes and drug-resistant tuberculosis (Dooley and Chaisson 2009), with possible explanations including delayed clearance resulting in routine switching to a two-drug regimen in patients who are still culture-positive or lowered rifampicin levels in diabetes patients (Nijland et al. 2006). Among TB patients, having diabetes is linked with a significant increase in the risk of death (Dooley et al. 2009; Ismail and Bulgiba 2013). Very little of the available data comes from sub-Saharan African populations, where diabetes prevalence will increase over the next decade (Dooley and Chaisson 2009) and where TB and diabetes treatment decisions for significant numbers of patients will have to frequently accommodate antiretroviral therapy, which itself is associated with increased risk of TB (Marais et al. 2013). Diabetes mellitus (DM) increases the risk of active TB by a factor of 2 to 3. In addition, people with TB, who have diabetes, have been found to have worse TB treatment outcomes. The WHO and The International Union Against Tuberculosis and Lung Disease Framework for Collaborative Activities recommend screening for TB and diabetes simultaneously. The recommended collaborative activities, outcome indicators, and research areas for guiding public health policies for joint TB and diabetes care recommend screening for active TB in patients with diabetes and for diabetes in patients with TB to make

 Cite this article as *Cold Spring Harb Perspect Med* doi: 10.1101/cshperspect.a017889

earlier diagnoses, which in turn may lead to better treatment outcomes and control of both diseases (Table 3) (WHO/IUATBLD 2011]).

Malnutrition

Malnutrition is a risk factor for all infectious diseases because it impairs immunity. Both protein calorie malnutrition (PCM) and micronutrient deficiencies can cause immune suppression through a variety of mechanisms, as reviewed in Bhaskaram (2002) and Schaible and Kaufmann (2007). Chronic malnutrition has a great impact on chronic infectious diseases such as HIV and TB, which require constant immune surveillance and control. The prevalence of malnutrition, generally defined by a BMI of <18.5 kg/m^2, among adult pulmonary TB patients can range from 42% to 80% (Kennedy et al. 1996; Zachariah et al. 2002; Dodor 2008; Mupere et al. 2012; Bhargava et al. 2013). In the African studies, the prevalence of malnutrition was lower among women, whereas in the Indian study, it was lower among men. These studies did not compare the prevalence of malnutrition among TB patients with that of the general population, but they did look at the effect of malnutrition on TB treatment outcomes. Three of these studies showed improvements in nutritional status with TB treatment, but weight gain did not correlate with microbiological response and significant numbers of patients cured of TB were still underweight at 12 mo, indicating the overriding influence of socioeconomic factors (Kennedy et al. 1996; Dodor 2008; Bhargava et al. 2013). A Korean study also found malnutrition to be associated with poorer outcomes in disseminated TB (Kim et al. 2008). One Tanzanian study identified TB as an important correlate of wasting, independent of HIV (Villamor et al. 2006), and Malawian, Ugandan, and Indian studies found that severe malnutrition on admission was independently linked with increased risk of early mortality (Zachariah et al. 2002; Mupere et al. 2012; Bhargava et al. 2013). A Latvian study found that being underweight was linked with worse outcomes and increased mortality in multidrug-resistant (MDR)-TB (Podewils et al. 2011).

Children primarily acquire active TB from adults with whom they live, and so one would expect the prevalence of malnutrition among children with TB to be similar if not higher than among adult TB patients, with households affected by malnutrition more likely to suffer transmission events from infected adults to children. A study from Pakistan found 51% of children initiating TB therapy to have PCM (Uddin Siddiqui et al. 2010), and there is a need for more research to evaluate possible interventions to cotreat malnutrition and tuberculosis and to assess to what degree nutritional interventions might be able to prevent the development of active TB in high-risk children (Jaganath and Mupere 2012).

TUBERCULOSIS AND OTHER COMMUNICABLE DISEASES

HIV/AIDS

In the early 1990s, researchers started to ask questions about the effect of HIV coinfection on TB prevalence, drug reactions, and treatment outcomes. A U.S. study of prisoners was the first paper in which the term "coinfection" was used with respect to HIV and TB (Salive et al. 1990). Subsequent studies in various patient groups showed significantly higher prevalence of HIV-1 infection in TB patients (Singh et al. 1993; Greenberg et al. 1994; Kivihya-Ndugga et al. 1994a), including children (Chintu et al. 1993), showing associations with more severe disease (Kivihya-Ndugga et al. 1994a), more advanced immune suppression (Kivihya-Ndugga et al. 1994b; Martin et al. 1995), and drug reactions (Pozniak et al. 1992).

In the subsequent two decades, the HIV epidemic has expanded dramatically in some countries, dragging both pulmonary and extrapulmonary TB in its wake, fueling a fivefold increase in TB notification rates between 1990 and 2010 in sub-Saharan Africa, which bears 80% of the global HIV disease burden. HIV increases TB risk by 20- to 40-fold and TB accounts for 25% of HIV-related deaths worldwide—the single largest cause. The WHO Global Tuberculosis Report 2013 states that 13%

Table 3. Recommended collaborative activities, outcome indicators, and research areas for guiding public health policies for joint TB and diabetes care

Area	Recommendation
A. Establish mechanisms for collaboration	
A.1. Setup means of coordinating diabetes and TB activities A.2. Conduct surveillance of TB disease prevalence among people with diabetes in medium and high TB burden settings A.3. Conduct surveillance of diabetes prevalence in TB patients in all countries A.4. Conduct monitoring and evaluation of collaborative diabetes and TB activities	*Recommendation 1:* Joint coordination should be established at regional, district, and/or local levels (sensitive to country-specific factors), with representation from all relevant stakeholders. A joint plan for diabetes and TB activities should be drawn up and reflected in national plans on noncommunicable diseases and TB, respectively. *Recommendation 2:* There should be TB surveillance among diabetes patients in settings with medium to high TB burden. *Recommendation 3:* There should be surveillance of diabetes among TB patients in all countries. *Recommendation 4:* Where diabetes and TB collaboration is being established, programs for both diseases should agree on a core set of indicators and data collection tools for the monitoring and evaluation of collaborative activities. Diabetes programs should explore the possibility of adapting the directly observed therapy (DOT) system to monitor and report cases and treatment outcomes.
B. Detect and manage TB in patients with diabetes	
B.1. Intensify detection of TB among people with diabetes B.2. Ensure TB infection control in health-care settings where diabetes is managed B.3. Ensure high-quality TB treatment and management in people with diabetes	*Recommendation 5:* At a minimum, people with diabetes should be asked about the presence of cough (lasting >2 wk) at the time of diabetes diagnosis, and if possible at each regular check-up for diabetes. Those with positive symptoms should be examined as per national guidelines. Other diagnostic procedures, such as those for extrapulmonary TB, should be pursued rigorously as per national guidelines. *Recommendation 6:* Screening for active TB on broader indications (e.g., in all people diagnosed with diabetes, regardless of symptoms) should be explored as part of the research agenda for improved TB diagnosis among people with diabetes. *Recommendation 7:* A referral system should be established so that patients with suspected TB are promptly sent to TB diagnostic and treatment centers and evaluated in accordance with the guidelines of the national TB control program. *Recommendation 8:* Tuberculosis case finding should be intensified by increasing the awareness and knowledge of the interactions between diabetes and TB, including joint risk factors, among health-care workers and populations they serve. *Recommendation 9:* Each health-care facility, including diabetes clinics, should have an infection control plan (including a plan for TB infection control), which includes administrative and environmental control

Continued

Table 3. *Continued*

Area	Recommendation
	measures to reduce transmission of TB within this setting. These measures should adhere to WHO's International guidelines for TB infection control. *Recommendation 10:* Treatment and case management of TB in people with diabetes should be provided in accordance with existing TB treatment guidelines and international standards. The same TB treatment regimen should be prescribed to people with diabetes as for people without diabetes.
C. Detect and manage diabetes in patients with TB C.1. Screen TB patients for diabetes C.2. Ensure high-quality diabetes management among TB patients	*Recommendation 11:* TB patients should be screened for diabetes at the start of treatment. Type of screening and diagnostic tests should be adapted to the context of local health systems and the availability of resources, while awaiting additional evidence on the best screening and diagnostic approach. *Recommendation 12:* Management of diabetes in TB patients should be provided in line with existing guidelines.
D. Key processes, outcome indicators, and research questions	1. Joint TB and diabetes plan in place 2. Number and proportion of people with diagnosed diabetes who have been screened for chronic cough 3. Number and proportion of people with diabetes who have been tested for TB (radiography, sputum smear microscopy, culture, Xpert MTB/Rif Assay, etc.) 4. Prevalence of TB among people with diabetes 5. Number and proportion of people with TB who have been screened for diabetes 6. Prevalence of diabetes among people with TB 7. TB treatment outcomes among people with diabetes

Data adapted from WHO/IUATBLD 2011.

(1.1 million) of 8.6 million people who developed TB in 2012 are coinfected with HIV (WHO 2013). With respect to HIV/TB, the report highlights some modest improvements—coverage of ART (antiviral therapy) and cotrimoxazole preventative therapy have improved among HIV-positive TB patients in recent years. Isoniazid preventive therapy (IPT) was provided to one-third of all new HIV cases diagnosed in 2012, although 50% are likely eligible. It remains unclear how appropriate this is in extremely high-burden settings.

As one of five key priority areas, the report highlights the need for improved coverage of dual HIV/TB testing, which in some countries approaches 100%, indicating what is possible. Low HIV burden countries have had more problems, or shown less initiative, in promoting HIV counseling and testing among newly diagnosed TB patients. In the Africa region, the epicenter of the HIV pandemic, up to 77% of TB patients are coinfected with HIV, and the rate of TB patients who have undergone HIV testing has increased dramatically in recent years. Seven high-burden countries, mainly from Eastern and Southern Africa, have HIV testing rates in TB clinics higher than 90%, lead by Zambia, the only country to test virtually all notified TB cases for HIV. Because HIV status may inform on treatment decisions in comorbid patients (e.g., toxicities and pharmacokinetic interactions of TB and ART or other drugs), Diagnostic Counseling and Testing (DCT) or "opt out" strategies have been instigated in some in-patient settings and high-risk groups. In recent years, WHO has invested in improved data collection systems for TB/HIV; however, in many countries, there is still a great need for improved data collection, with data from both HIV and TB programs irreconcilable in some cases. There are also still significant patient groups that go under the radar and are not captured. For example, data from Zambia shows that TB is frequently missed in a range of hospitalized patients, attributable to overriding symptoms indicative of one or more comorbid communicable or noncommunicable diseases (Bates et al. 2012). Those who are discharged should be referred back to their community TB treatment center, but there are no funds to follow up such cases, and the large number of missed TB patients who die shortly after admission are not reported to the National Tuberculosis Programmes (NTPs). Most importantly, rates of MDR-TB within this high morbidity and mortality, HIV-positive in-patient group may approach 10%, resulting in possible gross underestimation of MDR-TB cases in what are currently considered to be relatively low MDR-TB prevalence countries (Bates et al. 2012).

The treatment of HIV and TB in coinfected patients is potentially complicated by toxicities and pharmacokinetic interactions between the drugs used in anti-TB and ART, but because of the considerable number of drugs available, regimens can often be adjusted to reduce side effects and nonadherence (Arentz et al. 2012). HIV-infected TB patients initiated on ART benefit from increased survival and cure rates, whether on first-line (Gengiah et al. 2011) or second-line anti-TB therapy (Arentz et al. 2012). WHO recommend that ART should be commenced as soon as possible after initiating TB treatment, especially in patients with CD4 counts of <50 cells/mL, but early mortality remains a significant problem in patients initiating ART and trials are under way to evaluate the possible benefits of presumptive TB treatment in high-risk patients with very low CD4 counts (Zumla et al. 2013).

In sub-Saharan Africa, TB now supersedes obstetric causes of death in HIV-infected pregnant women, with vertical transmission of TB occurring in up to 15% of neonates born to mothers suffering from HIV/TB coinfection (Adhikari et al. 2011; Bekker et al. 2012). With HIV-infected persons living longer on ART (Volberding and Deeks 2010; Ullrich et al. 2011), and the huge success of interventions to reduce mother-to-child-transmission (MTCT) of HIV (Sturt et al. 2010), the number of children born to HIV/TB coinfected mothers is set to increase and so is the burden of neonatal TB. There is a need for more research into possible ways to prevent MTCT of TB and on how best to diagnose and treat TB in the HIV-exposed neonate, which compounds just about all diagnostic and treatment challenges seen in other patient groups.

Malaria

Although there is considerable literature on HIV/tuberculosis and HIV/malaria coinfections and comorbidity, there has been distinctly less attention given to both clinical and immunological interactions between TB and malaria. Unlike HIV, both *Mycobacterium tuberculosis* (*Mtb*) and *Plasmodium* species are ancient pathogens that have coevolved in the same human populations over millennia, with molecular evidence for coinfections shown in 2000–3000-yr-old mummified remains from lower Egypt (Lalremruata et al. 2013). When two chronic pathogens have coevolved in the same population, it is possible (if not highly likely) that they have evolved mutually beneficial "win–win" strategies, to aid their own persistence and transmission. Could there be molecular synergies between plasmodium and *Mtb* that contribute to each other's persistence in endemic regions (Enwere et al. 1999)?

Animal model studies suggest infection with malaria induces immune responses that impair host resistance to chronic TB infection, with exacerbated leukocyte infiltrates, tissue pathology, and hypercytokinemia accompanied by altered T-cell responses, pointing to malaria-induced dysregulation of innate and adaptive antimycobacterial defenses (Hawkes et al. 2010; Mueller et al. 2012). Other animal model studies have shown that coinfected mice were less able to inhibit *Mtb* growth in lungs, spleen, and liver (Scott et al. 2004) and that TB and malaria trigger similar innate immune responses such as the heme oxygenase 1 pathway, enhancing the efficiency of the liver stage in the *Plasmodium* life cycle (Sinnis and Ernst 2008). Conversely, it is also possible that under certain circumstances, coinfecting pathogens may possess competitive strategies, with one study showing *Mtb*-induced protective effects against lethal murine malaria (Page et al. 2005). Another study showed that murine malaria infection did not have any effect on vaccine-induced TB immunity (Parra et al. 2011).

There are few studies that document cross-sectional prevalence of malaria in TB patients, with rates ranging from 5% to 37%, because of differences in study location, population, and definitions used (Range et al. 2007; Valadas et al. 2013). Malaria infection can inhibit TB interferon-γ release assays (IGRAS) (Banfield et al. 2012), but this is mute, in that these diagnostics are not generally recommended for use in high-burden populations. There are also some potential drug interactions that should be considered when treating coinfected patients. Fluoroquinalones are contraindicated with other drugs that prolong ventricular repolarization, recorded as lengthening of the QT interval on an electrocardiogram (Murphy et al. 2012). Induction of the hepatic cytochrome P450 enzyme system by rifampicin results in a halving in the serum concentrations of artemisinin and its derivatives, complicating the concurrent management of TB and acute malaria. There is a case report in the literature of malaria and TB coinfection presenting as sepsis in a neonate (Thapa et al. 2010). This is of potential impact in that blood cultures from neonates with suspected sepsis are often negative, with testing for nonbacterial infections such as malaria and TB often overlooked.

Influenza

Data from the 1918 influenza epidemic suggested a clear association with increased risk for TB-related disease and death during this time period. Mouse models have shown that prior exposure to influenza A impairs immune responses to *Mtb* infection and decreases survival (Redford et al. 2014), possibly through down-regulated MHC (major histocompatibility complex) expression on dendritic cells and reduced activation of CD4 and CD8 T cells to clear mycobacteria (Florido et al. 2013). A similar murine study found influenza had little effect on mycobacterial load (Co et al. 2006). Clinical data from Southeast Asia does not support an association between influenza and TB (de Paus et al. 2013; Noh et al. 2013; Roth et al. 2013). Even studies from high HIV burden patient groups in South Africa have found TB coinfection in the 2009 H1N1 outbreak to be rare in influenza deaths (10%), with pregnancy being a more potent risk factor (Archer et al. 2009).

Other acute respiratory tract infections are also likely to increase patients' vulnerability to develop *Mtb* infection or disease, and may partially explain some of the seasonal variability observed in temperate regions. A randomized controlled trial to assess the impact of pneumococcal vaccination showed decreased rates of culture-confirmed and clinically diagnosed TB in vaccinated children (Moore et al. 2010). Case ascertainment bias could not be excluded, because unvaccinated children had more frequent respiratory illness warranting diagnostic workup, but it offers the intriguing possibility that pneumococcal coinfection may increase children's vulnerability to develop active TB.

Helminths

There is increasing recognition that a high exposure to pathogens in poor communities living in tropical and subtropical regions results in immunological profiles with different responses to TB infection (Black et al. 2002). A U.S. study of refugees from TB-endemic countries (free of any acute illness or recent treatment history) showed that among those latently infected with TB, those with concurrent helminth or *Helicobacter pylori* infections had raised levels of IFN-γ and other cytokines. *H. pylori* was associated with enhanced IFN-γ responses to TB (Perry et al. 2013). A recent review concluded that there is now strong evidence that helminth-induced T-cell responses impair defenses against *Mtb* infection, with consequences not only for disease prevalence and severity in different regions, but also with respect to TB vaccine efficacy (Rafi et al. 2012). However, there is murine data showing TB vaccine responses are unaffected by helminth-induced Th2 responses (Frantz et al. 2010) and that helminth infection does not exacerbate TB disease (Hubner et al. 2012). Another rodent model showed that prior helminth infections appear to illicit a macrophage response, which is protective during the early stages of mycobacterial infection (du Plessis et al. 2013).

Human studies in high- and low-burden helminth infection populations found no differences in tuberculin skin test responses in patients with and without helminth infections, or after treatment with albendazole (Pelly et al. 2005; Zevallos et al. 2010). Looking in more detail at components of the immune response, there is evidence for helminth-associated regulatory T cells suppressing responses to BCG (Bacillus Calmette-Guérin) vaccination in children (Wammes et al. 2010) and *Mtb*-specific Toll-like receptor expression in adults (Babu et al. 2009). Ex vivo studies in which monocytes differentiated into dendritic cells and macrophages, and then stimulated in vitro with live

Table 4. Social determinants and clinically observed associations with the development of tuberculosis

Social determinants	Clinically observed associations
Living conditions	***Other communicable diseases***
Poverty	HIV/AIDS
Crowded accommodation with poor ventilation (e.g., prisons, refugee camps, homeless shelters, mass gatherings, shanty towns)	Sexually transmitted infections
Under/malnutrition (including micronutrient deficiencies)	Infections linked to injection drug use
Poor health services	Acute lung infections (viral, bacterial, fungal)
Alcohol or substance misuse	Chronic helminth infestations
Cigarette smoking (active or passive)	***Noncommunicable diseases***
Indoor biomass fuel smoke exposure	Diabetes mellitus
Birth or residence in TB endemic country	Chronic lung disease (e.g., COPD, pneumoconiosis)
Visit to or regular close contact with people from TB endemic countries	Chronic kidney disease or end stage renal failure
High-risk work or living environment	Gut malabsorption or gastric bypass surgery
Mine workers	Skin disorders (e.g., psoriasis, alopecia areata)
Health care workers	Sarcoidosis
Laboratory personnel	Congenital and other immunodeficiencies
Residential care staff	Autoimmune diseases
Inpatients in hospitals	Solid organ transplants
Prisoners and prison staff	Cancers
Refugee camp workers	***Immunosuppressive therapy***
Homeless	Steroids (e.g., prednisone, methylprednisolone)
Migrants and nomads	Antimetabolites (e.g., methotrexate, azathioprine)
	T-cell inhibitors (e.g., cyclosporin, tacrolimus)
	Alkylating agents (e.g., cyclophosphamide)
	Biologicals (e.g., anti-TNF-α drugs, IL-2 blockers)
	Pregnancy and childbirth
	Extremes of age
	Elderly
	Very young

Table 5. Priorities for integration of tuberculosis care with that of other communicable and noncommunicable diseases (CDs and NCDs)

TB and HIV services

Joint services

Family clinics for family diseases

Optimized infection control

Pragmatic screening and active case-finding strategies

HIV patients regularly screened for TB and all TB patients routinely tested for HIV infection, especially where HIV prevalence exceeds 1%

Screening package to include weight and growth monitoring, blood pressure, blood sugar/HbA1c, and cholesterol if indicated

TB and diabetes programs

Pragmatic screening and active case-finding strategies

All diabetes patients regularly screened for TB, and TB patients routinely tested for diabetes (random glucose of HbA1c), especially in highly prevalent areas

Enhanced disease control

Shared treatment supervision (e.g., DOT for diabetes and TB)

TB, smoking cessation, and chronic respiratory care

Linking smokers diagnosed with TB to smoking cessation programs

Linking TB patients with chronic lung disease to ongoing respiratory care

Supporting and enhancing existing PAL projects

Regular TB screening in smokers/people with COPD (especially in TB endemic areas)

TB and alcohol/substance abuse care programs

Screening for harmful drinking and alcohol use disorder in TB patients

Linking TB patients with abuse problems to outreach and other care programs

Increasing TB risk awareness and symptom-identification in substance abuse program

Maternal and child health initiatives and services

Antenatal and obstetric services

Routine screening for HIV, TB, malaria (in endemic areas), DM, and hypertension

Routine STD screening

Administration of BCG vaccination to newborns

Child health

Routine administration of expanded EPI with hepatitus B, *Haemophilus influenza* type B, pneumococcal, rotavirus, and HPV vaccines

Regular monitoring and mapping of weight gain on a "Road to Health chart"

Inclusion of pediatric TB in integrated management of childhood illness (IMCI) approaches

Regular deworming

Public health and advocacy campaigns

Reduce poverty and deprivation

Promote healthy living

Reduce cigarette smoking (tobacco control), solid fuel use

Reduce excessive alcohol use/substance abuse

Improve health literacy

Modified and adapted from Marais et al. 2013, with permission.

microfilariae, resulted in cytokine and chemokine expression that would impair the immune response (Talaat et al. 2006). But do these cell responses translate to poorer clinical outcomes? One large well-controlled trial found that treatment of helminths did not affect vaccine responses in Ugandan children (Webb et al. 2011).

NEED FOR INTEGRATED STRATEGIES

With diminishing investment in global health, integrated solutions should seek to unlock latent synergies and optimize resource utilization. It is particularly important to encourage local ownership and increase equitable domestic investment in health and sustainable development. Rates of TB provide a useful barometer as an "indicator disease" of socioeconomic inequality and deprivation (see Table 4). However, meeting the social and medical care needs of vulnerable communities requires a cohesive response from multiple role players. Within the emerging post-2015 development framework, it is essential to emphasize the strong link between health and responsible development, with TB providing a classic example of two-way causality. Governments need to develop national health strategic plans that integrate surveillance, diagnostic, and treatment systems to meet the challenges posed by current CD and NCD epidemics including new epidemics and drug-resistant infections. Priorities for integration and alignment of TB care with that of other communicable and noncommunicable diseases (CDs and NCDs) are listed in Table 5. Wider integration of TB control activities presents opportunities to explore latent synergies and getting convergence for achieving universal health care within programs.

ACKNOWLEDGMENTS

Support from the European Commission FW7 Rid-RTI Project; European and Developing Countries Clinical Trials Partnership, The Hague, Netherlands (EDCTP grants REMOX, PANACEA, and TB-NEAT); UBS Optimus Foundation, Switzerland; NIHR Biomedical Research Centre, University College London Hospital, London, UK; and Australian NHMRC and the Centre for Research Excellence in Tuberculosis. We are grateful to Mr. Adam Zumla for technical and search strategy support and to Dr. Knut Lonroth, Global TB Department, WHO, Geneva for providing data and Figure 1.

REFERENCES

Adeyi OSO, Robles S. 2007. *Public policy and the challenge of chronic noncommunicable diseases.* World Bank, Washington, DC.

Adhikari M, Jeena P, Bobat R, Archary M, Naidoo K, Coutsoudis A, Singh R, Nair N. 2011. HIV-associated tuberculosis in the newborn and young infant. *Int J Pediatr* **2011:** 354208.

Alisjahbana B, Sahiratmadja E, Nelwan EJ, Purwa AM, Ahmad Y, Ottenhoff TH, Nelwan RH, Parwati I, van der Meer JW, van Crevel R. 2007. The effect of type 2 diabetes mellitus on the presentation and treatment response of pulmonary tuberculosis. *Clin Infect Dis* **45:** 428–435.

Archer B, Cohen C, Naidoo D, Thomas J, Makunga C, Blumberg L, Venter M, Timothy G, Puren A, McAnerney J, et al. 2009. Interim report on pandemic H1N1 influenza virus infections in South Africa, April to October 2009: Epidemiology and factors associated with fatal cases. *Euro Surveill* **14:** 19369.

Arentz M, Pavlinac P, Kimerling ME, Horne DJ, Falzon D, Schunemann HJ, Royce S, Dheda K, Walson JL, group ARTs. 2012. Use of anti-retroviral therapy in tuberculosis patients on second-line anti-TB regimens: A systematic review. *PloS ONE* **7:** e47370.

Babu S, Bhat SQ, Kumar NP, Anuradha R, Kumaran P, Gopi PG, Kolappan C, Kumaraswami V, Nutman TB. 2009. Attenuation of toll-like receptor expression and function in latent tuberculosis by coexistent filarial infection with restoration following antifilarial chemotherapy. *PLoS Negl Trop Dis* **3:** e489.

Banfield S, Pascoe E, Thambiran A, Siafarikas A, Burgner D. 2012. Factors associated with the performance of a blood-based interferon-γ release assay in diagnosing tuberculosis. *PloS ONE* **7:** e38556.

Bates M, O'Grady J, Mwaba P, Chilukutu L, Mzyece J, Cheelo B, Chilufya M, Mukonda L, Mumba M, Tembo J, et al. 2012. Evaluation of the burden of unsuspected pulmonary tuberculosis and co-morbidity with non-communicable diseases in sputum producing adult inpatients. *PloS ONE* **7:** e40774.

Beaglehole R, Bonita R, Alleyne G, Horton R, Li L, Lincoln P, Mbanya JC, McKee M, Moodie R, Nishtar S, et al. 2011. UN high-level meeting on non-communicable diseases: Addressing four questions. *Lancet* **378:** 449–455.

Bekker A, Du Preez K, Schaaf HS, Cotton MF, Hesseling AC. 2012. High tuberculosis exposure among neonates in a high tuberculosis and human immunodeficiency virus burden setting. *Int J Tuberc Lung Dis* **16:** 1040–1046.

Bhargava A, Chatterjee M, Jain Y, Chatterjee B, Kataria A, Bhargava M, Kataria R, D'Souza R, Jain R, Benedetti A, et al. 2013. Nutritional status of adult patients with pulmonary tuberculosis in rural central India and its association with mortality. *PloS ONE* **8:** e77979.

Bhaskaram P. 2002. Micronutrient malnutrition, infection, and immunity: An overview. *Nutr Rev* **60:** S40–S45.

Black GF, Weir RE, Floyd S, Bliss L, Warndorff DK, Crampin AC, Ngwira B, Sichali L, Nazareth B, Blackwell JM, et al. 2002. BCG-induced increase in interferon-γ response to mycobacterial antigens and efficacy of BCG vaccination in Malawi and the UK: Two randomised controlled studies. *Lancet* **359:** 1393–1401.

Chintu C, Bhat G, Luo C, Raviglione M, Diwan V, Dupont HL, Zumla A. 1993. Seroprevalence of human immunodeficiency virus type 1 infection in Zambian children with tuberculosis. *Pediatr Infect Dis J* **12:** 499–504.

Co DO, Hogan LH, Karman J, Heninger E, Vang S, Wells K, Kawaoka Y, Sandor M. 2006. Interactions between T cells responding to concurrent mycobacterial and influenza infections. *J Immunol* **177:** 8456–8465.

Creswell J, Raviglione M, Ottmani S, Migliori GB, Uplekar M, Blanc L, Sotgiu G, Lönnroth K. 2011. Tuberculosis and non-communicable diseases: Neglected links and missed opportunities. *Eur Respir J* **37:** 1269–1282.

de Paus RA, van Crevel R, van Beek R, Sahiratmadja E, Alisjahbana B, Marzuki S, Rimmelzwaan GF, van Dissel JT, Ottenhoff TH, van de Vosse E. 2013. The influence of influenza virus infections on the development of tuberculosis. *Tuberculosis* **93:** 338–342.

Dodor E. 2008. Evaluation of nutritional status of new tuberculosis patients at the Effia-Nkwanta Regional hospital. *Ghana Med J* **42:** 22–28.

Dooley KE, Chaisson RE. 2009. Tuberculosis and diabetes mellitus: Convergence of two epidemics. *Lancet Infect Dis* **9:** 737–746.

Dooley KE, Tang T, Golub JE, Dorman SE, Cronin W. 2009. Impact of diabetes mellitus on treatment outcomes of patients with active tuberculosis. *Am J Trop Med Hyg* **80:** 634–639.

du Plessis N, Kleynhans L, Thiart L, van Helden PD, Brombacher F, Horsnell WG, Walzl G. 2013. Acute helminth infection enhances early macrophage mediated control of mycobacterial infection. *Mucosal Immunol* **6:** 931–941.

Enwere GC, Ota MO, Obaro SK. 1999. The host response in malaria and depression of defence against tuberculosis. *Ann Trop Med Parasitol* **93:** 669–678.

Florido M, Grima MA, Gillis CM, Xia Y, Turner SJ, Triccas JA, Stambas J, Britton WJ. 2013. Influenza A virus infection impairs mycobacteria-specific T cell responses and mycobacterial clearance in the lung during pulmonary coinfection. *J Immunol* **191:** 302–311.

Frantz FG, Rosada RS, Peres-Buzalaf C, Perusso FR, Rodrigues V, Ramos SG, Kunkel SL, Silva CL, Faccioli LH. 2010. Helminth coinfection does not affect therapeutic effect of a DNA vaccine in mice harboring tuberculosis. *PLoS Negl Trop Dis* **4:** e700.

Geneau R, Hallen G. 2012. Toward a systemic research agenda for addressing the joint epidemics of HIV/AIDS and noncommunicable diseases. *AIDS* **31:** S7–S10.

Gengiah TN, Gray AL, Naidoo K, Karim QA. 2011. Initiating antiretrovirals during tuberculosis treatment: A drug safety review. *Expert Opin Drug Saf* **10:** 559–574.

Greenberg BL, Weisfuse IB, Makki H, Adler J, el-Sadr W, Clarke L, Gainey S, Alford T, McFarlane K, Thomas PA. 1994. HIV-1 seroprevalence in chest clinic and hospital tuberculosis patients in New York City, 1989–1991. *AIDS* **8:** 957–962.

Guler M, Unsal E, Dursun B, Aydln O, Capan N. 2007. Factors influencing sputum smear and culture conversion time among patients with new case pulmonary tuberculosis. *Int J Clin Pract* **61:** 231–235.

Hawkes M, Li X, Crockett M, Diassiti A, Liles WC, Liu J, Kain KC. 2010. Malaria exacerbates experimental mycobacterial infection in vitro and in vivo. *Microbes Infect* **12:** 864–874.

Hubner MP, Killoran KE, Rajnik M, Wilson S, Yim KC, Torrero MN, Morris CP, Nikonenko B, Blanco JC, Hemming VG, et al. 2012. Chronic helminth infection does not exacerbate *Mycobacterium tuberculosis* infection. *PLoS Negl Trop Dis* **6:** e1970.

Ismail I, Bulgiba A. 2013. Predictors of death during tuberculosis treatment in TB/HIV co-infected patients in Malaysia. *PloS ONE* **8:** e73250.

Jaganath D, Mupere E. 2012. Childhood tuberculosis and malnutrition. *J Infect Dis* **206:** 1809–1815.

Jeon CY, Murray MB. 2008. Diabetes mellitus increases the risk of active tuberculosis: A systematic review of 13 observational studies. *PLoS Med* **5:** e152.

Kennedy N, Ramsay A, Uiso L, Gutmann J, Ngowi FI, Gillespie SH. 1996. Nutritional status and weight gain in patients with pulmonary tuberculosis in Tanzania. *Trans R Soc Trop Med Hyg* **90:** 162–166.

Kim DK, Kim HJ, Kwon SY, Yoon HI, Lee CT, Kim YW, Chung HS, Han SK, Shim YS, Lee JH. 2008. Nutritional deficit as a negative prognostic factor in patients with miliary tuberculosis. *Eur Respir J* **32:** 1031–1036.

Kivihya-Ndugga LE, Ochola JJ, Otieno G, Muthami LN, Gathua S. 1994a. Clinical and immunological markers in Kenyan pulmonary tuberculosis patients with and without HIV-1. *East Afr Med J* **71:** 373–375.

Kivihya-Ndugga LE, Otieno G, Muthami LN, Gachihi G, Gathua S. 1994b. Markers in HIV associated tuberculosis in Kenya. *Afr J Health Sci* **1:** 122–125.

Lalremruata A, Ball M, Bianucci R, Welte B, Nerlich AG, Kun JF, Pusch CM. 2013. Molecular identification of falciparum malaria and human tuberculosis co-infections in mummies from the Fayum depression (Lower Egypt). *PloS ONE* **8:** e60307.

Leung CC, Lam TH, Chan WM, Yew WW, Ho KS, Leung GM, Law WS, Tam CM, Chan CK, Chang KC. 2008. Diabetic control and risk of tuberculosis: A cohort study. *Am J Epidemiol* **167:** 1486–1494.

Li L, Lin Y, Mi F, Tan S, Liang B, Guo C, Shi L, Liu L, Gong F, Li Y, et al. 2012. Screening of patients with tuberculosis for diabetes mellitus in China. *Trop Med Int Health* **17:** 1294–1301.

Lim SS, Vos T, Flaxman AD, Danaei G, Shibuya K, Adair-Rohani H, Amann M, Anderson HR, Andrews KG, Aryee M, et al. 2012. A comparative risk assessment of burden of disease and injury attributable to 67 risk factors and risk factor clusters in 21 regions, 1990–2010: A systematic analysis for the Global Burden of Disease Study 2010. *Lancet* **380:** 2224–2260.

Lin Y, Li L, Mi F, Du J, Dong Y, Li Z, Qi W, Zhao X, Cui Y, Hou F, et al. 2012. Screening patients with diabetes mellitus for tuberculosis in China. *Trop Med Int Health* **17:** 1302–1308.

Lönnroth K, Castro K, Chakaya JM, Chauhan LS, Floyd K, Glaziou P, Raviglione M. 2010. Tuberculosis control and elimination 2010–50: Cure, care, and social development. *Lancet* **375:** 1814–1829.

Lozano R, Naghavi M, Foreman K, Lim S, Shibuya K, Aboyans V, Abraham J, Adair T, Aggarwal R, Ahn SY, et al. 2012. Global and regional mortality from 235 causes of death for 20 age groups in 1990 and 2010: A systematic analysis for the Global Burden of Disease Study 2010. *Lancet* **380:** 2095–2128.

Marais BJ, Lonnroth K, Lawn SD, Migliori GB, Mwaba P, Glaziou P, Bates M, Colagiuri R, Zijenah L, Swaminathan S, et al. 2013. Tuberculosis comorbidity with communicable and non-communicable diseases: Integrating health services and control efforts. *Lancet Infect Dis* **13:** 436–448.

Martin DJ, Sim JG, Sole GJ, Rymer L, Shalekoff S, van Niekerk AB, Becker P, Weilbach CN, Iwanik J, Keddy K, et al. 1995. $CD4^+$ lymphocyte count in African patients co-infected with HIV and tuberculosis. *J Acquir Immune Defic Syndr Hum Retrovirol* **8:** 386–391.

Mboussa J, Monabeka H, Kombo M, Yokolo D, Yoka-Mbio A, Yala F. 2003. *Rev Pneumol Clin* **59:** 39–44. [Course of pulmonary tuberculosis in diabetics.]

Moore DP, Klugman KP, Madhi SA. 2010. Role of *Streptococcus pneumoniae* in hospitalization for acute community-acquired pneumonia associated with culture-confirmed *Mycobacterium tuberculosis* in children: A pneumococcal conjugate vaccine probe study. *Pediatr Infect Dis J* **29:** 1004–1099.

Morsy AM, Zaher HH, Hassan MH, Shouman A. 2003. Predictors of treatment failure among tuberculosis patients under DOTS strategy in Egypt. *East Mediterr Health J* **9:** 689–701.

Mueller AK, Behrends J, Hagens K, Mahlo J, Schaible UE, Schneider BE. 2012. Natural transmission of *Plasmodium berghei* exacerbates chronic tuberculosis in an experimental co-infection model. *PloS ONE* **7:** e48110.

Mupere E, Malone L, Zalwango S, Chiunda A, Okwera A, Parraga I, Stein CM, Tisch DJ, Mugerwa R, Boom WH, et al. 2012. Lean tissue mass wasting is associated with increased risk of mortality among women with pulmonary tuberculosis in urban Uganda. *Ann Epidemiol* **22:** 466–473.

Murphy ME, Singh KP, Laurenzi M, Brown M, Gillespie SH. 2012. Managing malaria in tuberculosis patients on fluoroquinolone-containing regimens: Assessing the risk of QT prolongation. *Int J Tuberc Lung Dis* **16:** 144–149, i-iii.

Nijland HM, Ruslami R, Stalenhoef JE, Nelwan EJ, Alisjahbana B, Nelwan RH, van der Ven AJ, Danusantoso H, Aarnoutse RE, van Crevel R. 2006. Exposure to rifampicin is strongly reduced in patients with tuberculosis and type 2 diabetes. *Clin Infect Dis* **43:** 848–854.

Noh JY, Lee J, Choi WS, Song JY, Seo YB, Kim IS, Cheong HJ, Kim WJ. 2013. Concurrent tuberculosis and influenza, South Korea. *Emerg Infect Dis* **19:** 165–167.

Olmos P, Donoso J, Rojas N, Landeros P, Schurmann R, Retamal G, Meza M, Martinez C. 1989. [Tuberculosis and diabetes mellitus: A longitudinal-retrospective study in a teaching hospital.] *Rev Med Chil* **117:** 979–983.

Page KR, Jedlicka AE, Fakheri B, Noland GS, Kesavan AK, Scott AL, Kumar N, Manabe YC. 2005. Mycobacterium-induced potentiation of type 1 immune responses and protection against malaria are host specific. *Infect Immun* **73:** 8369–8380.

Parra M, Derrick SC, Yang A, Tian J, Kolibab K, Oakley M, Perera LP, Jacobs WR, Kumar S, Morris SL. 2011. Malaria infections do not compromise vaccine-induced immunity against tuberculosis in mice. *PloS ONE* **6:** e28164.

Pelly TF, Santillan CF, Gilman RH, Cabrera LZ, Garcia E, Vidal C, Zimic MJ, Moore DA, Evans CA. 2005. Tuberculosis skin testing, anergy and protein malnutrition in Peru. *Int J Tuberc Lung Dis* **9:** 977–984.

Perry S, Chang AH, Sanchez L, Yang S, Haggerty TD, Parsonnet J. 2013. The immune response to tuberculosis infection in the setting of *Helicobacter pylori* and helminth infections. *Epidemiol Infect* **141:** 1232–1243.

Podewils LJ, Holtz T, Riekstina V, Skripconoka V, Zarovska E, Kirvelaite G, Kreigere E, Leimane V. 2011. Impact of malnutrition on clinical presentation, clinical course, and mortality in MDR-TB patients. *Epidemiol Infect* **139:** 113–120.

Pozniak AL, MacLeod GA, Mahari M, Legg W, Weinberg J. 1992. The influence of HIV status on single and multiple drug reactions to antituberculous therapy in Africa. *AIDS* **6:** 809–814.

Rafi W, Ribeiro-Rodrigues R, Ellner JJ, Salgame P. 2012. Coinfection-helminthes and tuberculosis. *Curr Opin HIVAIDS* **7:** 239–244.

Range N, Magnussen P, Mugomela A, Malenganisho W, Changalucha J, Temu MM, Mngara J, Krarup H, Friis H, Andersen AB. 2007. HIV and parasitic co-infections in tuberculosis patients: A cross-sectional study in Mwanza, Tanzania. *Ann Trop Med Parasitol* **101:** 343–351.

Redford PS, Mayer-Barber KD, McNab FW, Stavropoulos E, Wack A, Sher A, O'Garra A. 2014. Influenza A virus impairs control of *Mycobacterium tuberculosis* coinfection through a type I interferon receptor-dependent pathway. *J Infect Dis* **15:** 270–274.

Remais JV, Zeng G, Li G, Tian L, Engelgau MM. 2013. Convergence of non-communicable and infectious diseases in low- and middle-income countries. *Int J Epidemiol* **42:** 221–227.

Restrepo BI, Fisher-Hoch SP, Smith B, Jeon S, Rahbar MH, McCormick JB, Nuevo Santander Tuberculosis T. 2008. Mycobacterial clearance from sputum is delayed during the first phase of treatment in patients with diabetes. *Am J Trop Med Hyg* **79:** 541–544.

Roth S, Whitehead S, Thamthitiwat S, Chittaganpitch M, Maloney SA, Baggett HC, Olsen SJ. 2013. Concurrent influenza virus infection and tuberculosis in patients hospitalized with respiratory illness in Thailand. *Influenza Other Respir Viruses* **7:** 244–248.

Salive ME, Vlahov D, Brewer TF. 1990. Coinfection with tuberculosis and HIV-1 in male prison inmates. *Public Health Rep* **105:** 307–310.

Sbrana E, Grise J, Stout C, Aronson J. 2011. Co-morbidities associated with tuberculosis in an autopsy case series. *Tuberculosis* **91:** S38–S42.

Schaible UE, Kaufmann SH. 2007. Malnutrition and infection: Complex mechanisms and global impacts. *PLoS Med* **4:** e115.

Scott CP, Kumar N, Bishai WR, Manabe YC. 2004. Short report: Modulation of *Mycobacterium tuberculosis* infection by *Plasmodium* in the murine model. *Am J Trop Med Hyg* **70:** 144–148.

Singh NB, Singh EK, Singh HL, Singh YI. 1993. Tuberculosis/HIV co-infection in India's north-eastern states. *J Infect* **26:** 344–345.

Singla R, Khan N, Al-Sharif N, Ai-Sayegh MO, Shaikh MA, Osman MM. 2006. Influence of diabetes on manifestations and treatment outcome of pulmonary TB patients. *Int J Tuberc Lung Dis* **10:** 74–79.

Sinnis P, Ernst JD. 2008. CO-opting the host HO-1 pathway in tuberculosis and malaria. *Cell Host Microbe* **3:** 277–279.

Sturt AS, Dokubo EK, Sint TT. 2010. Antiretroviral therapy (ART) for treating HIV infection in ART-eligible pregnant women. *Cochrane Database Syst Rev*: CD008440.

Swai AB, McLarty DG, Mugusi F. 1990. Tuberculosis in diabetic patients in Tanzania. *Trop Doct* **20:** 147–150.

Talaat KR, Bonawitz RE, Domenech P, Nutman TB. 2006. Preexposure to live *Brugia malayi* microfilariae alters the innate response of human dendritic cells to *Mycobacterium tuberculosis*. *J Infect Dis* **193:** 196–204.

Thapa R, Mallick D, Biswas B. 2010. Perinatal malaria and tuberculosis co-infection: A case report. *Int J Infect Dis* **14:** e254–256.

Uddin Siddiqui E, Ejaz K, Lone S, Raza SJ. 2010. Investment in paediatric tuberculosis prevention in Pakistan: Loss or gain? *J Pak Med Assoc* **60:** 897–901.

Ullrich A, Ott JJ, Vitoria M, Martin-Moreno JM, Atun R. 2011. Long-term care of AIDS and non-communicable diseases. *Lancet* **377:** 639–640.

Valadas E, Gomes A, Sutre A, Brilha S, Wete A, Hanscheid T, Antunes F. 2013. Tuberculosis with malaria or HIV co-infection in a large hospital in Luanda, Angola. *J Infect Dev Ctries* **7:** 269–272.

Villamor E, Saathoff E, Mugusi F, Bosch RJ, Urassa W, Fawzi WW. 2006. Wasting and body composition of adults with pulmonary tuberculosis in relation to HIV-1 coinfection, socioeconomic status, and severity of tuberculosis. *Eur J Clin Nutr* **60:** 163–171.

Viswanathan V, Kumpatla S, Aravindalochanan V, Rajan R, Chinnasamy C, Srinivasan R, Selvam JM, Kapur A. 2012. Prevalence of diabetes and pre-diabetes and associated risk factors among tuberculosis patients in India. *PloS ONE* **7:** e41367.

Volberding PA, Deeks SG. 2010. Antiretroviral therapy and management of HIV infection. *Lancet* **376:** 49–62.

Wammes LJ, Hamid F, Wiria AE, de Gier B, Sartono E, Maizels RM, Luty AJ, Fillie Y, Brice GT, Supali T, et al. 2010. Regulatory T cells in human geohelminth infection suppress immune responses to BCG and *Plasmodium falciparum*. *Eur J Immunol* **40:** 437–442.

Webb EL, Mawa PA, Ndibazza J, Kizito D, Namatovu A, Kyosiimire-Lugemwa J, Nanteza B, Nampijja M, Muhangi L, Woodburn PW, et al. 2011. Effect of single-dose anthelmintic treatment during pregnancy on an infant's response to immunisation and on susceptibility to infectious diseases in infancy: A randomised, double-blind, placebo-controlled trial. *Lancet* **377:** 52–62.

WHO. 2011. Burden: Mortality, morbidity and risk factors. In *Global status report on noncommunicable diseases 2010* (ed. WHO). WHO, Geneva.

WHO. 2013. Global tuberculosis report 2013. 306. WHO Library Cataloging-in-Publication Data, Geneva, Switzerland.

WHO/IUATBLD. 2011. Collaborative framework for acre and control of tuberculosis and diabetes. WHO/HTM/2011.15. International Union Against Tuberculosis and Lung Disease 1–53. http://whqlibdoc.who.int/publications/2011/9789241502252_eng.pdf.

Zachariah R, Spielmann MP, Harries AD, Salaniponi FM. 2002. Moderate to severe malnutrition in patients with tuberculosis is a risk factor associated with early death. *Trans R Soc Trop Med Hyg* **96:** 291–294.

Zevallos K, Vergara KC, Vergara A, Vidal C, Garcia HH, Evans CA. 2010. Tuberculin skin-test reactions are unaffected by the severity of hyperendemic intestinal helminth infections and co-infections. *Am J Trop Med Hyg* **83:** 319–325.

Zumla A, Nahid P, Cole ST. 2013. Advances in the development of new tuberculosis drugs and treatment regimens. *Nat Rev Drug Discov* **12:** 388–404.

Transmission and Institutional Infection Control of Tuberculosis

Edward A. Nardell

Division of Global Health Equity, Brigham & Women's Hospital, Boston, Massachusetts 02115

Correspondence: ean@hsph.harvard.edu

Tuberculosis (TB) transmission control in institutions is evolving with increased awareness of the rapid impact of treatment on transmission, the importance of the unsuspected, untreated case of transmission, and the advent of rapid molecular diagnostics. With active case finding based on cough surveillance and rapid drug susceptibility testing, in theory, it is possible to be reasonably sure that no patient enters a facility with undiagnosed TB or drug resistance. Droplet nuclei transmission of TB is reviewed with an emphasis on risk factors relevant to control. Among environmental controls, natural ventilation and upper-room ultraviolet germicidal ultraviolet air disinfection are the most cost-effective choices, although high-volume mechanical ventilation can also be used. Room air cleaners are generally not recommended. Maintenance is required for all engineering solutions. Finally, personal protection with fit-tested respirators is used in many situations where administrative and engineering methods cannot assure protection.

HOW TUBERCULOSIS IS TRANSMITTED

Uncontrolled transmission is fueling the global tuberculosis (TB) epidemic (Bacaër et al. 2008). Although some transmission probably occurs out of doors, it is believed to be less likely primarily because of infinite dilution of infectious droplet nuclei in air. Transmission occurs more efficiently indoors where dilution is limited and occupants are concentrated. All indoor environments are potential sites of transmission, most importantly, homes and congregate settings such as hospitals, clinics, refugee camps, factories, homeless shelters, prisons, and many more, including most modes of transportation (Middelkoop et al. 2008; Johnstone-Robertson 2011a,b). Tuberculosis is almost exclusively airborne because initially it is usually an infection of the alveolar macrophage (Ordway et al. 2006; Orme 2014). To reach macrophages in the far reaches of the lung, inhaled particles in the 1 to 5 μm range are required—small enough to remain suspended indefinitely and to follow room air currents. Droplet nuclei are the dehydrated residua of larger respiratory droplets generated by patients with pulmonary or laryngeal TB who are coughing or otherwise generating aerosol (Riley 1974). These dried respirable particles are small enough to accommodate one or at most a few tubercle organisms (Riley 1957). Infectious aerosols are also generated in TB laboratories when concentrated specimens are processed, and occasionally by other means, such as the irrigation of wounds,

Cite this article as *Cold Spring Harb Perspect Med* doi: 10.1101/cshperspect.a018192

at autopsies, and in surgery (Hutton et al. 1990). It is believed that once impacted onto surfaces, microorganisms in droplet nuclei are extremely difficult to re-aerosolize again as respirable particles (Ko et al. 1998). Dust generated by sweeping or shaking bedclothes, for example, may contain viable *Mycobacterium tuberculosis* (*Mtb*) organisms, but predominantly attached to relatively large, nonrespirable particles, impacting on the relatively resistant upper airways if inhaled rather than the lower respiratory tract. In a comprehensive investigation of shipboard transmission on a United States Navy vessel, no evidence was found of person-to-person spread by direct contact with respiratory droplets as occurs in influenza, for example, nor was there evidence of transmission through dust or fomites (Houk et al. 1968). Shared air fully accounted for the patterns of transmission seen.

Normally intracellular pathogens, *Mtb* bacilli are believed to die off during airborne transport, but at an uncertain rate, with measured half-lives in air ranging from 20 min to 6 h according to two different artificial aerosol experiments under optimal conditions of light, humidity, and temperature (Loudon et al. 1969a; Lever et al. 2000). The exact length of survival of viable and infectious naturally aerosolized organisms in air is unknown, and likely varies with ambient conditions, but it is clearly long enough for propagation of the infection under a variety of conditions around the world. On the other hand, in almost all cases, transmission is believed to require the simultaneous presence of both source cases and exposed persons, suggesting that risk decreases rapidly once the source case leaves. Dilution in room air and ventilation account for much of the rapid reduction in concentration, but die-off is another less well-defined factor. Barer has recently shown that a portion of tubercle bacilli recovered from human airways assume a spore-like phenotype by turning off unnecessary metabolic processes and storing fat (Garton et al. 2008). These "fat and lazy" organisms, he suggests, may be adapting to airborne transport, increasing their resistance to environmental stresses, and possibly adapted to ingestion and reversion to a replicating phenotype once inside the macrophage.

Airborne *Mycobacterium tuberculosis*

Once airborne, dilution, removal, or disinfection of indoor air are the main ways that the risk of airborne tubercle bacilli is reduced indoors (Nardell 1993b). It is not possible to culture naturally generated *Mtb* organisms from room air by air sampling because of low concentrations and overgrowth of more rapidly growing environmental bacteria and fungi. Although molecular methods have detected *Mtb* nucleic acid, advanced methods are required to estimate viability, and no molecular methods are able to determine infectivity, which requires a vulnerable host (Nardell 1999). However, good estimates of the concentration of infectious doses, what Wells called "infectious quanta," have been made epidemiologically in a few outbreak situations in which it was assumed that each infected person represented one infectious dose or quanta (Catanzaro 1982; Nardell et al. 1991). It has also been measured experimentally using large numbers of guinea pigs as quantitative air samplers (Riley et al. 1962). Guinea pigs are exquisitely susceptible to human *Mtb* and respond to tuberculin skin testing in a similar way (Smith et al. 1970). There is evidence to suggest that a single deeply inhaled infectious droplet nucleus can infect a guinea pig—and probably a vulnerable human as well (Riley 1957). During a 4-yr period, for example, Riley estimated an average concentration of infectious quanta of 1 in 11,000 cf (311 m^3) and also calculated that this extremely low average concentration was sufficient to explain the rates of transmission to student nurses in hospitals during the prechemotherapy era (Riley 1957; Riley et al. 1962). This same approach, using guinea pigs to quantify infectious quanta, has been used to measure the impact of such interventions as ultraviolet air disinfection, electrostatic precipitators, surgical masks on patients, and, most importantly, effective treatment as discussed below (Escombe et al. 2009; Dharmadhikari et al. 2012, 2014).

 Cite this article as *Cold Spring Harb Perspect Med* doi: 10.1101/cshperspect.a018192

Dose and Risk of Infection

Assuming complete susceptibility of exposed persons, the risk of acquiring a TB infection depends entirely on the chance of inhaling an infectious dose or quanta, and its progression to an established infection. As noted, for the guinea pig, the infectious dose has been estimated experimentally to be just one colony forming unit, that is, one quanta equals one droplet nucleus (Wells 1955). For humans with highly variable resistance, the exact infectious dose likely varies with microbial strain virulence and from person to person depending on host defenses, including general immunocompetence, innate immunity, adaptive immunity attributable to Bacillus Calmette–Guérin (BCG) immunization and prior exposure to *Mtb*, leprosy, and related environmental mycobacteria. Contrary to common teaching, not all established TB infections persist (Nardell and Wallis 2006; Dharmadhikari et al. 2011). Because respirable particles cannot carry large numbers of organisms and are generally quite dilute in room air, the concept of dose is different from, for example, the dose of ingested food or waterborne organisms (Smith and Wiengeshaus 1989). Radiographs of children with primary TB indicate a random, mostly lower lung distribution of single foci of infection, not multiple foci—consistent with single implantations by chance caused by low average concentrations, as reported by Riley. It also seems likely that not every deeply inhaled droplet nucleus or "hit" containing TB organisms results in infection, or persistent infection (Nardell and Wallis 2006). This was the rationale for Wells' term "quanta" because the necessary number of inhaled droplet nuclei or hits necessary for one to result in a single infectious focus is not known (Wells 1955). Organisms can be nonviable, viable but not fully virulent, or by chance, encounter a particularly nonpermissive macrophage that halts progression. In natural human to guinea pig experiments similar to Riley's, we have described a range of outcomes following exposure, including transient tuberculin skin test responses that later revert without progression to disease, even following immunosuppression, and sometimes followed by a second or third tuberculin skin test response, suggesting reinfection (Dharmadhikari et al. 2011). Both humans and guinea pigs can show transient, self-limited immunological evidence of infection following exposure without progression and, ultimately, reversion of both immunological markers and risk (Friedman et al. 2006; Nardell and Wallis 2006). How often TB infections are transient is not known. Vaccination with BCG, the avirulent strain of *Mycobacterium bovis*, is the best-documented example of transient infection with reversion of tuberculin skin test over time in many, if not most, cases. Finally, with or without tuberculin reversion, exogenous reinfection commonly occurs with repeated exposure and has been postulated to be an essential pathogenic pathway to cavitary disease under endemic conditions (Smith and Wiengeshaus 1989).

Grzybowski et al. (1975) in British Colombia showed that children household contacts were more likely to get infected if the source case was both smear- and culture-positive rather than culture-positive only. Importantly, he also showed that contacts of smear-positive cases were more likely to progress to clinical disease given infection. This suggests a dose effect on progression from infection to disease. As noted above, this cannot be explained by larger numbers of organisms in individual droplet nuclei, but perhaps by multiple hits over time being more likely to overcome innate or adaptive immunity or impact in a vulnerable area of the lung. This is also consistent with many nonprogressive hits, or transient infections, before at least one that does progress (Smith and Wiengeshaus 1989).

Under steady-state conditions (however unlikely under real world conditions), the risk of infection (C) is a function of several factors: (1) the number of infectious persons (I) and source strength (q)—number of infectious quanta generated per hour or day; (2) the number of susceptible people breathing the same air (S); (3) the breathing rate of exposed persons (p); (4) the exposure time (t); and (5) the ventilation rate of the room or rooms where exposure occurs (Q). The relationship of these factors is captured by a mass balance relationship known as the Wells–Riley equation, adapted from an epidemiological model by Edward Riley, Richard's brother, an engineer, to explain measles transmission in a school (Riley et al. 1978):

$$C = S(1 - e^{-Iqpt/Q}).$$

More recently, Rudnick and Milton (2003) have argued that human-generated indoor CO_2 levels are a good surrogate of rebreathed air exposure, representing a more dynamic model of infection, accommodating the ever-changing non-steady-state conditions of real exposures.

Source Factors

There have been several outbreaks in which many of the essential transmission factors in the Wells–Riley equation were known or were estimated. In an office building TB exposure, in which building ventilation rates were known, one infectious source infected 27 of 67 susceptible occupants (40%) over a 1 mo period, and the calculated *q* was 13 quanta per hour. Other exposures have shown *q* values as high as 250 quanta per hour compared with Riley's ward average figure of 1.25 quanta per hour (Riley et al. 1962; Catanzaro 1982; Nardell et al. 1991). This leads to one of the clearest facts about TB transmission—that patients vary greatly in infectiousness. It has been estimated that only one in three TB patients infects any close contacts (Fennelly et al. 2004; Fennelly 2007). Furthermore, it appears that a minority of infectious cases, so called "disseminators," accounts for much of observed transmission. This is true of other respiratory infections as well (Sultan et al. 1960).

Variability in infectiousness is believed to relate to the source patient, the strain, the host, and environmental factors, but they are difficult to separate. The same source patient and strain will infect more contacts in a crowded, poorly ventilated environment with highly susceptible hosts. Frequency of cough, viscosity of respiratory secretions, presence of lung cavities or laryngeal disease, and duration of exposure are important variables (Loudon and Spohn 1969). Among potential interventions to reduce transmission, however, nothing is as rapidly and completely effective than treatment with the appropriate drug regimen, as will be discussed below (Rouillon et al. 1976).

ADMINISTRATIVE APPROACHES TO TB TRANSMISSION CONTROL

Known or Suspected versus Unsuspected Cases

Most interventions to prevent transmission focus on the known or suspected case, often on effective treatment, but there is ample evidence that unsuspected, untreated cases account for much more transmission (Jensen et al. 2005). Under high-burden conditions, TB is commonly missed in persons presenting with unrelated conditions (Willingham et al. 2001; Bates et al. 2012, 2013). Under low-burden conditions, the diagnosis is less likely to be considered even with classical symptoms. Studies in Peru and Africa have shown the prevalence of unsuspected TB in general medical settings, including smear-positive, drug-resistant cases (Willingham et al. 2001; Bates et al. 2012).

Interventions to Reduce Transmission

Breathing shared air is required for transmission, and separation or isolation of suspected infectious source is usually the first and most immediately effective administrative and environmental approach. However, much household transmission is likely to have occurred before symptoms lead patients to a diagnosis and treatment, at which point transmission normally stops abruptly, as discussed below. Contact tracing and active case finding in the community can find cases earlier but the latter, unless targeted to high-incidence populations, may not be cost-effective (Gilpin and Hammond 1987; Puisis et al. 1996; Zachariah et al. 2003; Gounder et al. 2011; Hoek et al. 2011; Lorent et al. 2014). Active case finding leading to rapid diagnosis and effective treatment may be highly effective in some congregate settings in identifying otherwise unsuspected cases, but it requires resources and a highly organized infrastructure and, ideally, the on-site availability of rapid molecular diagnostics tests. In theory, if all entrants to a general medical ward are screened for unexplained chronic cough, and all otherwise unsuspected pulmonary cases diagnosed and effectively treated, there would be few, if any, sources of transmission. Because of the power of drug susceptibility test (DST)-directed treatment to stop transmission, it will be discussed first, followed by environmental interventions and respiratory protection, which play secondary roles—unless administrative control is incompletely successful.

Impact of Treatment on Transmission

That effective treatment rapidly stops transmission was suspected soon after chemotherapy was introduced (Crofton 1962). Confidence that patients on effective treatment become quickly noninfectious was the basis for shifting to completely ambulatory treatment. In a review article on the impact of treatment on transmission among household contacts, Roullion and colleagues concluded that infectiousness ended well before sputum smear or culture conversion, "probably in less than two weeks" (Rouillon et al. 1976). Although the "two-week rule" has guided practice before the resurgence of drug-resistant TB, there is more direct evidence of an even faster impact of effective treatment on transmission. In his initial 2-yr human to guinea pig study in the late 1950s, Riley et al. (1995) found that transmission occurred primarily (21 of 22 infections) from chronic patients, on treatment, but resistant to one or more of the three available antibiotics at the time. In the second 2-yr study, treatment was delayed for one group of patients, but it started immediately on admission for another group. Among patients with drug-susceptible TB, there was an almost immediate 98% reduction in transmission in the treated group, adjusting for time on the ward (Riley et al. 1962). Therefore, the effect of chemotherapy on transmission appears to have been rapid, well before the 2-wk estimate based on epidemiological studies. For drug-resistant cases, the few remaining drugs also seemed to be promptly effective, but the numbers of such cases were too few, Riley felt, to be sure.

Using a similar human to guinea pig model in South Africa, preliminary observations suggest that even multidrug-resistant (MDR) TB appears to respond quickly to appropriate treatment (Dharmadhikari et al. 2014). Considering the three drugs available in Riley's studies, isoniazid (INH), streptomycin, and para-aminosalicylic acid (PAS), INH was most likely responsible owing to its early bactericidal activity. For MDR-TB, in which both INH and rifamycin are ineffective, we speculate that fluoroquinolones may be responsible for the rapid effect of treatment on transmission. Loudon speculated that it could be the high residual concentration of drug in droplet nuclei as they evaporate that accounts for the rapid effect on transmission, but he was unable to produce confirmatory evidence (Loudon et al. 1969b). The observed discordance on transmission by patients on effective treatment, with positive sputum smears and culture, in both household contact and guinea pig transmission studies, may reflect aerosolization stress and high local drug concentrations, but this discordance could also represent immediate stress effects of certain drugs on specific *Mtb* metabolic functions that are necessary for successful implantation in an immunocompetant host but not for growth of sputum samples in supportive culture media. Further basic research on the rapid effects of treatment is warranted.

FAST: An Intensified, Refocused Approach to TB Transmission

The advent and wide use of new rapid molecular diagnostics together with a renewed appreciation of the rapid impact of treatment on transmission has led us to a reformulated approach to TB infection control that we call FAST: find cases actively, separate safely, and treat effectively based on rapid DST (Nardell and Dharmadhikari 2010).

To reiterate, the FAST approach is based on four underlying principles: (1) That TB is spread in institutions predominantly by coughing patients with unsuspected TB or unsuspected drug resistance; (2) that most potentially infectious patients can be identified by cough surveillance; (3) that coughing TB patients most likely to be infectious can be diagnosed by rapid molecular sputum tests, including drug resistance (GeneXpert® MTB/RIF); and (4) that by dramatically reducing institutional exposure duration through effective treatment, transmission among patients and to health-care workers will be reduced proportionately (Boehme et al. 2010). Although these are solid principles, like most transmission control interventions, their efficacy in preventing transmission has yet to be proven, and there are many practical barriers to implementation.

In many high-burden settings, health-care workers are already overstretched. Who will do cough surveillance? Who will assure that sputum is promptly collected, delivered to the lab, results obtained, and effective treatment started? If these activities are as critical in stopping transmission as we contend, they cannot be assigned to volunteers or simply added to already full workloads. Where, then, are the sustainable funding sources for the additional human resources, GeneXpert MTB/RIF machines, and laboratory supplies? If the benefits in terms of secondary cases averted were obvious, the costs of prevention through rapid diagnosis and effective treatment might be easily justified, but they rarely are clear. On the other hand, diagnosing and treating active TB is a fundamental public health and personal health imperative—it must be performed sooner or later. The argument here is that the public health and personal health benefits of diagnosing and treating sooner through active surveillance, rapid diagnostic testing, and effective treatment will far outweigh the added costs, especially for MDR TB in which the costs, both human and financial, are staggering for each additional case transmitted (Fitzpatrick and Floyd 2012). Demonstrations of reduced transmission in clinical settings and formal cost–benefit analyses are needed.

Unlike hand washing to prevent droplet-spread infection, effective FAST implementation is fundamentally not an educational campaign for employees, although understanding its rationale is important for achieving its ambitious goals. FAST implementation requires an institutional investment in resources and specific personnel to introduce new policies and procedures (and streamline old ones) to achieve the goal of reduced exposure time. Although it has proven difficult to measure the impact of any TB infection control interventions in terms of reduced transmission, the process indicators entailed (time from admission to cough detection, time from cough detection to sputum submission, Xpert turnaround time, and time from admission to effective therapy) are measureable and logically closely tied to exposure duration. Performance goals for these process indicators should be set, and achieving those measurable goals should be considered by funding agencies as primary proof of impact. Improvements and slippage in performance process indicators can be tracked over time.

AMBULATORY VERSUS INPATIENT TB TREATMENT

The site of treatment, hospital versus clinic or home, has transmission control implications. As mentioned, when numerous household contact studies in the 1960s and 1970s suggested little additional risk of transmission in the home, ambulatory treatment became the norm around the world for uncomplicated, drug susceptible cases (Andrews et al. 1960). Many programs also treat MDR TB in the community or in clinics, but other programs continue to treat in hospital, at least for the period while daily injections are given. Community-based programs have been shown to have outcomes as good as or better than hospital-based programs, and the cost is much less in the community, and it is usually easier on patients and families (Fitzpatrick and Floyd 2012). Again, our human to guinea pig transmission studies suggest that MDR treatment is also rapidly effective in preventing transmission, so the risk in the community or hospital should not be an issue, although more vulnerable patients are concentrated in hospitals. Community-based MDR programs do require a developed community infrastructure. Experienced groups have published guidelines for community-based MDR programs (Mitnick et al. 2003).

ENVIRONMENTAL APPROACHES TO TB TRANSMISSION CONTROL

In the traditional industrial hygiene hierarchical approach to safety in the workplace, environmental controls come into play when administrative source controls cannot provide adequate protection, and respiratory protection is used when both administrative and environmental controls are inadequate. Common TB infection control practice has been to use all three approaches, implicitly indicating that none are fully effective (Jensen et al. 2005).

Crowding, Building Design, and Usage

Environmental control begins with the building. Occupancy rate (crowding) and building use are fundamental factors in TB transmission and control. Consider a hypothetical large room with 100 occupants with a 2% risk of TB. Simplistically, there would be two active cases and 98 other occupants exposed to them. Divide those same 100 occupants into 10 rooms of 10 occupants each and suddenly only two rooms (and possibly one) have a TB case and only eight to 18 others are exposed, an 82%–92% risk reduction simply by dividing up occupants into smaller clusters. Although hypothetical, the principle is broadly applicable, for example, to the design and use of hospital or clinic waiting rooms.

Space does not allow an exhaustive discussion of hospital design and engineering for airborne infection control. Courses are available for architects, engineers, and administrators to learn the principles. Application of these principles has resulted in award-winning designs around the world, but actual assessment of building designs from an airborne infection perspective remains elusive. Ventilation and space usage can be documented at specific rooms and times of day, but exposure is often in multiple rooms and 24/7. A more meaningful assessment of buildings must consider the degree to which occupants share air throughout the day and in different seasons (Rudnick and Milton 2003).

Ventilation

Buildings must be ventilated, defined for contagion purposes as replacing a portion of room/building air with a percentage of outside air, presumed free of airborne pathogens. In many high-burden, resource-limited settings in mild climates, natural ventilation is the common and essential means of air disinfection. In other less hospitable climates, especially in resource-rich settings, mechanical ventilation of hospitals and clinics may be the norm, although many (World Health Organization 2009) older buildings still depend on radiator heat and operable windows. Most ventilation systems are designed for comfort, not airborne infection control (Nardell et al. 1991). The difference is that levels of ventilation adequate for odor control are generally not adequate for infection control, depending on source strength and duration of exposure. Recommendations exist for both natural and mechanical ventilation for airborne infection control, but implementation and maintenance are often challenging (Jensen et al. 2005; Escombe et al. 2007; Atkinson et al. 2009).

Natural ventilation depends entirely on pressure differences created by wind or on temperature differences that cause warm air to rise and replacement air to enter (Atkinson et al. 2009). Buildings designed for natural ventilation need to have adequate openings and be properly sited for wind or use other specialized features such as wind catchers, solar heating stacks, or rooftop whirlybird ventilators. Simple rules of thumb, such as window open area being 10% or 20% of floor area can be highly misleading. The window area needed is entirely dependent on each situation. In windy locations, for example, moderate openings with cross-ventilation may be adequate, whereas in poorly sited buildings without cross-ventilation, even large openings may be inadequate. Ventilation estimates using CO_2 decay curves have been reported for hospitals in Peru at 60 or more air changes per hour (ACH), but ventilation experts have challenged the accuracy of CO_2 decay measurements, often taken at one location, at one time, and in one season (Escombe et al. 2007). Nonetheless, such measurements are usually good enough to be able to say with certainty that ventilation is adequate or not at that moment and in that location. Renovation of older buildings for new uses presents greater challenges than new construction from an airborne infection perspective. The necessary climatic conditions, building site, and structural features may not be present for effective use of this modality.

Where natural ventilation is the main mode, provisions need to be made to assure that windows and other openings stay open day and night and in all seasons. Occupants often close windows for security, to keep out vermin, or because of cold, and each of these concerns need to be addressed if natural ventilation is to remain effective.

Mechanical Ventilation

Mechanical and hybrid (or mixed-mode) mechanical-natural systems are less dependent on climatic conditions, but they are heavily dependent on the initial design, subsequent renovations, and, importantly, maintenance. For airborne infection control, six to 12 ACH outside air are commonly recommended (Jensen et al. 2005; World Health Organization 2009). In cold climates, and in warm climates in which cooling is provided, this can be extremely expensive in terms of energy use. Even six to 12 ACH can prove inadequate if the source strength is great or exposure prolonged. As a general rule, under well-mixed conditions, doubling the outdoor ventilation rate reduces the risk of infection by half. Doubling ventilation again reduces risk by half again, and so on for each doubling. Clearly, there are practical limits to increasing ventilation rates because of system capacity, comfort, cost, and noise (Nardell et al. 1991). Although not true outside air ventilation, two additional interventions can provide the equivalent of air changes per hour (EqACH) from an infection control perspective—upper-room ultraviolet germicidal irradiation (UVGI) and room air cleaners.

Upper Room UVGI

Air disinfection by UVGI is the least well-understood intervention by engineers and architects, but also among the most well-studied, effective, and cost effective of environmental interventions (First et al. 2007; Rudnick and First 2007). Special 254-nm wavelength germicidal lamps in wall or suspended fixtures provide an irradiated zone of air in the upper room, above the heads of occupants. Good air mixing, best assured by low-velocity ceiling fans, brings contaminated air to the upper room and returns disinfected air to the lower room. Because the entire upper room area is available as an air disinfection chamber, room air turnover rates through the upper room can be high, approaching 60 ACH in a recent study, using commercially available inexpensive ceiling fans. Both room testing and modeling suggest that neither fan velocity nor direction are critical factors, although some fan experts favor downward direction in rooms with high ceilings to avoid lower room stagnation (Escombe et al. 2009; Zhu et al. 2013, 2014). Low vertical air velocity results in longer but fewer passages of particles through the irradiated zone, whereas with higher vertical air velocities, particle exposure per pass is shorter, but passages are more frequent, with similar net exposure.

The fundamental factors determining the efficacy of upper-room UVGI are (1) well-designed wall or center-mounted fixtures generating a prescribed UV output to the upper room (usually louvered to produce low levels to the occupied space); (2) optimal ray length, that is, locating fixtures on walls to achieve maximum use of available germicidal energy; and (3) good vertical air mixing, as noted above. Based on a well-characterized study of UVGI efficacy in a South African TB hospital, new room dosing guidelines based on fixture output have been published. The basic recommendation is to provide ~20 mW total fixture output per cubic meter of room volume, with the additional requirement that wall fixtures be arranged for maximum average ray length. This dosing recommendation requires that the total fixture UV output of commercial fixtures be provided by manufacturers, which is currently not done.

Upper-room UVGI has a good safety record, with most eye or skin overexposure resulting from poor fixture design or placement (Nardell 1993b; Rudnick 2001; Nardell et al. 2008, 2013). Guidelines for evaluating UV fixture safety and for maintenance are available (First et al. 1999a,b). The threshold limit value (TLV) for UVGI is 6 mJ/cm^2 over any 8 h exposure period (ACGIH 1999). Occupant movement within rooms with UVGI greatly reduces exposure, and no single irradiance value should be used as a safety threshold. Depending on how the space is used, maximum eye level irradiance levels of 0.4 to 0.6 μW/cm^2 are routinely well-tolerated because eye and skin exposure is well within the TLV (First et al. 2005). The main maintenance requirement is to turn off and clean lamps with 70% alcohol periodically, the frequency based on the cleanliness of the environment, and the replacement of lamps, most cost-effectively when measured output drops by 30% from commissioning values when measured in a standard way.

Room air cleaners are rarely recommended, despite claims of sales personnel that they are the answer to TB infection control (Nardell 1993a). Their problem is that, although either HEPA (high-efficiency particulate air) filters or UVGI inside the box can readily remove or inactivate infectious organisms, rarely can these units provide effective clean air delivery (CADR) adequate for TB infection control (Miller-Leiden et al. 1996). Many units simply provide too few equivalent air changes per hour, and almost all are subject to "short circuiting" of air, reentrapment of air that just exited the unit. Faced with optimistic claims, hospital administrators often jump at the opportunity to solve TB infection control by plugging in a device. Considering short circuiting, many units provide less than 1 equivalent ACH, and rarely can they approach the air disinfection achievable by optimal natural ventilation or upper-room UVGI.

RESPIRATORY PROTECTION

Respirators are last in the hierarchy of interventions because they cannot be worn constantly and are likely not to be used for unsuspected, untreated TB patients, the greatest threat for transmission (NEHW Health Watch 1992; Centers for Disease Control and Prevention 1996; Coffey et al. 1998, 2004; Fennelly and Nardell 1998; Jensen et al. 2005; World Health Organization 2009). By convention, respirators refer to devices that cover the nose and mouth for the purpose of protecting the wearer, whereas masks, such as surgical masks, are intended to protect the environment, such as the surgical field. Respirators have several features to ensure a tight fit to prevent face seal leak, the main reason for incomplete protection. They normally have a pliable nose clip to allow a close fit around the nose and two elastic straps to assure adherence to the face. Respirators used for TB infection control are usually the disposable type (N95 or equivalent) with a filtering face piece, although reusable industrial elastomeric respirators can be used with the appropriate filter cartridges (Centers for Disease Control and Prevention 1996). All respirators require fit testing on the wearer at least once to assure that the anticipated protection factor is obtained. Normally, institutions have several sizes and styles of respirators available because no one size or style fits every face. More details on respirator use and fit testing are available on line (http://www.cdc.gov/niosh/npptl/topics/respirators/disp_part/) (Coffey et al. 2002). Surgical masks are sometimes recommended for patients who cannot cover their coughs or sneezes, they are less expensive in one study; however, they provided only a 53% reduction in infectious cough aerosol (Dharmadhikari et al. 2012). This is not insignificant, the equivalent reduction to doubling room ventilation, but it does not assure that transmission will not occur. Respirators are not normally used for infectious patients because only a barrier to stop respiratory droplets is required—not air filtration.

Health-Care Worker Surveillance

Periodic testing of health-care workers for latent TB infection (LTBI) or active disease is commonly performed in some countries, but not others. High rates of community-acquired infection and policies that do not include treatment for LTBI are among the reasons that many workers are not tested. Radiological screening of asymptomatic workers is generally not cost effective (Menzies et al. 2007; Cummings et al. 2009; de Perio et al. 2009). Worker education about TB and its symptoms can reduce the stigma of the disease, which sometimes is a barrier to workers seeking care. In low-burden settings, testing for LTBI by tuberculin skin testing or interferon-γ release assays is difficult because of test performance issues. In high-burden settings, it can also be difficult to interpret test results, but skin testing has been used effectively in medical and nursing students as a good indicator of institutional transmission (Silva et al. 2000). Unfortunately, although effective, treatment of latent TB infection is often incomplete because of nonadherence (MMWR Recomm Rep 2000).

REFERENCES

ACGIH. 1999. Documentation of the threshold limit values and biological exposure indices. American Conference of Governmental Industrial Hygienists, Cincinnati.

Andrews RH, Devadatta S, Fox W, Radhakrishna S, Ramakrishnan CV, Velu S. 1960. Prevalence of tuberculosis among close family contacts of tuberculous patients in South India, and influence of segregation of the patient on early attack rate. *Bull World Health Organ* **23:** 463–510.

Atkinson J, Chartier Y, Pessoa-Silva CL, Jensen P, Li Y, Seto WH. 2009. *Natural Ventilation for Infection Control in Health Care Settings.* WHO, Geneva.

Bacaër N, Ouifki R, Pretorius C, Wood R, Williams B. 2008. Modeling the joint epidemics of TB and HIV in a South African township. *J Math Biol* **57:** 557–593.

Bates M, O'Grady J, Mwaba P, Chilukutu L, Mzyece J, Cheelo B, Chilufya M, Mukonda L, Mumba M, Tembo J, et al. 2012. Evaluation of the burden of unsuspected pulmonary tuberculosis and co-morbidity with non-communicable diseases in sputum producing adult inpatients. *PloS ONE* **7:** e40774.

Bates M, Ahmed Y, Chilukutu L, Tembo J, Cheelo B, Sinyangwe S, Kapata N, Maeurer M, O'Grady J, Mwaba P, et al. 2013. Use of the Xpert® MTB/RIF assay for diagnosing pulmonary tuberculosis comorbidity and multidrug-resistant TB in obstetrics and gynaecology inpatient wards at the University Teaching Hospital, Lusaka, Zambia. *Trop Med Int Health* **18:** 1134–1140.

Boehme CC, Nabeta P, Hillemann D, Nicol MP, Shenai S, Krapp F, Allen J, Tahirli R, Blakemore R, Rustomjee R, et al. 2010. Rapid molecular detection of tuberculosis and rifampin resistance. *N Engl J Med* **363:** 1005–1015.

Catanzaro A. 1982. Nosocomial tuberculosis. *Am Rev Respir Dis* **125:** 559–562.

Centers for Disease Control and Prevention. 1996. NIOSH Guide to the selection and use of particulate respirators certified under 42 CFR 84.[*DHHS (NIOSH) Pub No. 96-101*]. National Institutes for Occupational Safety and Health, HHS, CDC. Cincinnati.

Coffey CC, Campbell DL, Myers WR, Zhuang Z. 1998. Comparison of six respirator fit-test methods with an actual measurement of exposure in a simulated health care environment: Part II—Method comparison testing. *Am Ind Hyg Assoc J* **59:** 862–870.

Coffey CC, Lawrence RB, Zhuang Z, Campbell DL, Jensen PA, Myers WR. 2002. Comparison of five methods for fit-testing N95 filtering-facepiece respirators. *Appl Occup Environ Hyg* **17:** 723–730.

Coffey CC, Lawrence RB, Campbell DL, Zhuang Z, Calvert CA, Jensen PA. 2004. Fitting characteristics of eighteen N95 filtering-facepiece respirators. *J Occup Environ Hyg* **1:** 262–271.

Crofton J. 1962. The contribution of treatment to the prevention of tuberculosis. *Bull Int Union Tuberc* **32:** 643–653.

Cummings KJ, Smith TS, Shogren ES, Khakoo R, Nanda S, Bunner L, Smithmyer A, Soccorsi D, Kashon ML, Mazurek GH, et al. 2009. Prospective comparison of tuberculin skin test and QuantiFERON-TB Gold In-Tube assay for the detection of latent tuberculosis infection among healthcare workers in a low-incidence setting. *Infect Control Hosp Epidemiol* **30:** 1123–1126.

de Perio MA, Tsevat J, Roselle GA, Kralovic SM, Eckman MH. 2009. Cost-effectiveness of interferon γ release assays vs tuberculin skin tests in health care workers. *Arch Intern Med* **169:** 179–187.

Dharmadhikari AS, Basaraba RJ, Van Der Walt ML, Weyer K, Mphahlele M, Venter K, Jensen PA, First MW, Parsons S, McMurray DN, et al. 2011. Natural infection of guinea pigs exposed to patients with highly drug-resistant tuberculosis. *Tuberculosis* **91:** 329–338.

Dharmadhikari AS, Mphahlele M, Stoltz A, Venter K, Mathebula R, Masotla T, Lubbe W, Pagano M, First M, Jensen PA, et al. 2012. Surgical face masks worn by patients with multidrug-resistant tuberculosis: Impact on infectivity of air on a hospital ward. *Am J Respir Crit Care Med* **185:** 1104–1109.

Dharmadhikari AS, Mphahlele M, Venter K, Stoltz A, Mathebula R, Masotla T, van der Walt M, Pagano M, Jensen P, Nardell E. 2014. Rapid impact of effective treatment on transmission of multidrug-resistant tuberculosis. *Int J Tuberc Lung Dis* **18:** 1019–1025.

Escombe AR, Oeser CC, Gilman RH, Navincopa M, Ticona E, Pan W, Martínez C, Chacaltana J, Rodríguez R, Moore DA, et al. 2007. Natural ventilation for the prevention of airborne contagion. *PLoS Med* **4:** e68.

Escombe AR, Moore DA, Gilman RH, Navincopa M, Ticona E, Mitchell B, Noakes C, Martínez C, Sheen P, Ramirez R, et al. 2009. Upper-room ultraviolet light and negative air ionization to prevent tuberculosis transmission. *PLoS Med* **6:** e43.

Fennelly KP. 2007. Variability of airborne transmission of *Mycobacterium tuberculosis*: Implications for control of tuberculosis in the HIV era. *Clin Infect Dis* **44:** 1358–1360.

Fennelly K, Nardell E. 1998. The relative efficacy of respirators and room ventilation in preventing occupational tuberculosis. *Inf Control Hosp Epidemiol* **19:** 754–759.

Fennelly KP, Martyny JW, Fulton KE, Orme IM, Cave IM, Heifets LB. 2004. Cough-generated aerosols of *Mycobacterium tuberculosis*: A new method to study infectiousness. *Am J Respir Crit Care Med* **169:** 604–609.

First M, Nardell EA, Chaisson W, Riley R. 1999a. Guidelines for the application of upper-room ultraviolet germicidal irradiation for preventing transmission of airborne contagion—Part II: Design and operations guidance. *ASHRAE Trans* **105:** 877–887.

First M, Nardell EA, Chaisson W, Riley R. 1999b. Guidelines for the application of upper-room ultraviolet germicidal irradiation for preventing transmission of airborne contagion—Part I: Basic principles. *ASHRAE Trans* **105:** 869–876.

First MW, Weker RA, Yasui S, Nardell EA. 2005. Monitoring human exposures to upper-room germicidal ultraviolet irradiation. *J Occup Environ Hyg* **2:** 285–292.

First M, Rudnick SN, Banahan KF, Vincent RL, Brickner PW. 2007. Fundamental factors affecting upper-room ultraviolet germicidal irradiation—Part I. Experimental. *J Occup Environ Hyg* **4:** 321–331.

Fitzpatrick C, Floyd K. 2012. A systematic review of the cost and cost effectiveness of treatment for multidrug-resistant tuberculosis. *Pharmacoeconomics* **30:** 63–80.

Friedman LN, Nash ER, Bryant J, Henry S, Shi J, D'Amato J, Khaled GH, Russi MB, O'Connor PG, Edberg SC, et al. 2006. High rate of negative results of tuberculin and QuantiFERON tests among individuals with a history of positive skin test results. *Infect Control Hosp Epidemiol* **27:** 436–441.

Garton NJ, Waddell SJ, Sherratt AL, Lee SM, Smith RJ, Senner C, Hinds J, Rajakumar K, Adegbola RA, Besra GS, et al. 2008. Cytological and transcript analyses reveal fat and lazy persister-like bacilli in tuberculous sputum. *PLoS Med* **5:** e75.

Gilpin TP, Hammond M. 1987. Active case-finding—For the whole community or for tuberculosis contacts only? *S Afr Med J* **72:** 260–262.

Gounder CR, Wada NI, Kensler C, Violari A, McIntyre J, Chaisson RE, Martinson NA. 2011. Active tuberculosis case-finding among pregnant women presenting to antenatal clinics in Soweto, South Africa. *J Acquir Immune Defic Syndr* **57:** e77–e84.

Grzybowski S, Barnett GD, Styblo K. 1975. Contacts of cases of active pulmonary tuberculosis. *Bull Int Union Tuberc* **50:** 90–106.

Hoek KG, Van Rie A, van Helden PD, Warren RM, Victor TC. 2011. Detecting drug-resistant tuberculosis: The importance of rapid testing. *Mol Diagn Ther* **15:** 189–194.

Houk VH, Kent DC, Baker JH, Sorensen K, Hanzel GD. 1968. The Byrd study. In-depth analysis of a micro-outbreak of tuberculosis in a closed environment. *Arch Environ Health* **16:** 4–6.

Hutton MD, Stead WW, Cauthen GM, Bloch AB, Ewing WM. 1990. Nosocomial transmission of tuberculosis associated with a draining abscess. *J Infect Dis* **161:** 286–295.

Jensen PA, Lambert LA, Iademarco MF, Ridzon R. 2005. Guidelines for preventing the transmission of *Mycobacterium tuberculosis* in health-care settings. *MMWR Recomm Rep* **54:** 1–141.

Johnstone-Robertson S, Lawn SD, Welte A, Bekker LG, Wood R. 2011a. Tuberculosis in a South African prison—A transmission modelling analysis. *S Afr Med J* **101:** 809–813.

Johnstone-Robertson SP, Mark D, Morrow C, Middelkoop K, Chiswell M, Aquino LD, Bekker LG, Wood R. 2011b. Social mixing patterns within a South African township community: Implications for respiratory disease transmission and control. *Am J Epidemiol* **174:** 1246–1255.

Joshi R, Reingold AL, Menzies D, Pai M. 2006. Tuberculosis among health-care workers in low- and middle-income countries: A systematic review. *PLoS Med* **3:** e494.

Ko G, Burge HA, Muilenberg M, Rudnick S, First M. 1998. Survival of mycobacteria on HEPA filter material. *Appl Biosaf* **3:** 65–78.

Lever MS, Williams A, Bennett AM. 2000. Survival of mycobacterial species in aerosols generated from artificial saliva. *Lett Appl Microbiol* **31:** 238–241.

Lorent N, Choun K, Thai S, Kim T, Huy S, Pe R, van Griensven J, Buyze J, Colebunders R, Rigouts L, et al. 2014. Community-based active tuberculosis case finding in poor urban settlements of Phnom Penh, Cambodia: A feasible and effective strategy. *PloS ONE* **9:** e92754.

Loudon RG, Spohn SK. 1969. Cough frequency and infectivity in patients with pulmonary tuberculosis. *Am Rev Respir Dis* **99:** 109–111.

Loudon RG, Bumgarner LR, Lacy J, Coffman GK. 1969a. Aerial transmission of mycobacteria. *Am Rev Respir Dis* **100:** 165–171.

Loudon RG, Bumgarner LR, Coffman GK. 1969b. Isoniazid and the survival of tubercle bacilli in airborne droplet nuclei. *Am Rev Respir Dis* **100:** 172–176.

Menzies D, Joshi R, Pai M. 2007. Risk of tuberculosis infection and disease associated with work in health care settings. *Int J Tuberc Lung Dis* **11:** 593–605.

Middelkoop K, Bekker LG, Myer L, Dawson R, Wood R. 2008. Rates of tuberculosis transmission to children and adolescents in a community with a high prevalence of HIV infection among adults. *Clin Infect Dis* **47:** 349–355.

Miller-Leiden S, Lobascio C, Nazaroff WW, Macher JM. 1996. Effectiveness of in-room air filtration and dilution ventilation for tuberculosis infection control. *J Air Waste Manag Assoc* **46:** 869–882.

Mitnick C, Bayona J, Palacios E, Shin S, Furin J, Alcántara F, Sánchez E, Sarria M, Becerra M, Fawzi MC, et al. 2003. Community-based therapy for multidrug-resistant tuberculosis in Lima, Peru. *N Engl J Med* **348:** 119–128.

MMWR Recomm Rep. 2000. Targeted tuberculin testing and treatment of latent tuberculosis infection. *MMWR Recomm Rep* **49:** 1–51.

Nardell E. 1993a. Fans, filters, or rays? Pros and cons of the current envirnonmental tuberculosis control technologies. *Infect Control Hosp Epidemiol* **14:** 681–685.

Nardell EA. 1993b. Environmental control of tuberculosis. *Med Clin North Am* **77:** 1315–1334.

Nardell EA. 1999. Air sampling for tuberculosis—Homage to the lowly guinea pig. *Chest* **116:** 1143–1145.

Nardell EA, Wallis RS. 2006. Here today—Gone tomorrow: The case for transient acute tuberculosis infection. *Am J Respir Crit Care Med* **174:** 734–735.

Nardell E, Dharmadhikari A. 2010. Turning off the spigot: Reducing drug-resistant tuberculosis transmission in resource-limited settings. *Int J Tuberc Lung Dis* **14:** 1233–1243.

Nardell EA, Keegan J, Cheney SA, Etkind SC. 1991. Airborne infection. Theoretical limits of protection achievable by building ventilation. *Am Rev Respir Dis* **144:** 302–306.

Nardell EA, Bucher SJ, Brickner PW, Wang C, Vincent RL, Becan-McBride K, James MA, Michael M, Wright JD. 2008. Safety of upper-room ultraviolet germicidal air disinfection for room occupants: Results from the Tuberculosis Ultraviolet Shelter Study. *Public Health Rep* **123:** 52–60.

Nardell E, Vincent R, Sliney DH. 2013. Upper-room ultraviolet germicidal irradiation (UVGI) for air disinfection: A symposium in print. *Photochem Photobiol* **89:** 764–769.

NEHW Health Watch. 1992. Particulate respirators and tuberculosis transmission. *NEHW Health Watch* **12:** 8–9.

Ordway D, Harton M, Henao-Tamayo M, Montoya R, Orme IM, Gonzalez-Juarrero M. 2006. Enhanced macrophage activity in granulomatous lesions of immune mice challenged with *Mycobacterium tuberculosis*. *J Immunol* **176:** 4931–4939.

Orme IM. 2014. A new unifying theory of the pathogenesis of tuberculosis. *Tuberculosis* **94:** 8–14.

Puisis M, Feinglass J, Lidow E, Mansour M. 1996. Radiographic screening for tuberculosis in a large urban county jail. *Public Health Rep* **111:** 330–334.

Riley R. 1957. Aerial dissemination of pulmonary tuberculosis—The Burns Amberson lecture. *Am Rev Tuberc Pulmon Dis* **76:** 931–941.

Riley RL. 1974. Airborne infection. *Am J Med* **57:** 466–475.

Riley RL, Mills CC, O'Grady F, Sultan LU, Wittstadt F, Shivpuri DN. 1962. Infectiousness of air from a tuberculosis ward. Ultraviolet irradiation of infected air: Comparative infectiousness of different patients. *Am Rev Respir Dis* **85:** 511–525.

Riley E, Murphy G, Riley R. 1978. Airborne spread of measles in a suburban elementary school. *Am J Epidemiol* **107:** 421–432.

Riley RL, Mills CC, Nyka W, Weinstock N, Storey PB, Sultan LU, Riley MC, Wells WF. 1995. Aerial dissemination of pulmonary tuberculosis: A two-year study of contagion in a tuberculosis ward: 1959. *Am J Epidemiol* **142:** 3–14.

Rouillon A, Perdrizet S, Parrot R. 1976. Transmission of tubercle bacilli: The effects of chemotherapy. *Tubercle* **57:** 275–299.

Rudnick SN. 2001. Predicting the ultraviolet radiation distribution in a room with multilouvered germicidal fixtures. *AIHAJ* **62:** 434–445.

Rudnick SN, First MW. 2007. Fundamental factors affecting upper-room ultraviolet germicidal irradiation—Part II. Predicting effectiveness. *J Occup Environ Hyg* **4:** 352–362.

Rudnick SN, Milton DK. 2003. Risk of indoor airborne infection transmission estimated from carbon dioxide concentration. *Indoor Air* **13:** 237–245.

Silva VM, Cunha AJ, Oliveira JR, Figueira MM, Nunes ZB, DeRiemer K, Kritski AL. 2000. Medical students at risk of nosocomial transmission of *Mycobacterium tuberculosis*. *Int J Tuberc Lung Dis* **4:** 420–426.

Smith D, Wiengeshaus E. 1989. What animal models can teach us about the pathogenesis of tuberculosis in humans. *Rev Infect Dis* **11:** S385–S393.

Smith DW, McMurray DN, Wiegeshaus EH, Grover AA, Harding GE. 1970. Host-parasite relationships in experimental airborne tuberculosis. IV. Early events in the course of infection in vaccinated and nonvaccinated guinea pigs. *Am Rev Respir Dis* **102:** 937–949.

Sultan L, Myka W, Mills C, O'Grady F, Wells W, Riley RL. 1960. Tuberculosis disseminators—A study of variability of aerial infectivity of tuberculosis patients. *Am Rev Respir Dis* **82:** 358–369.

Wells WF. 1955. *Airborne Contagion and Air Hygiene*. Harvard University Press: Cambridge, MA.

Willingham FF, Schmitz TL, Contreras M, Kalangi SE, Vivar AM, Caviedes L, Schiantarelli E, Neumann PM, Bern C, Gilman RH, et al. 2001. Hospital control and multidrug-resistant pulmonary tuberculosis in female patients, Lima, Peru. *Emerg Infect Dis* **7:** 123–127.

World Health Organization. 2009. WHO Policy on TB Infection Control in Health-Care Facilities, Congregate Settings and Households. WHO, Geneva.

Zachariah R, Spielmann MP, Harries AD, Gormani P, Graham SM, Bakali E, Humblet P. 2003. Passive versus active tuberculosis case finding and isoniazid preventive therapy among household contacts in a rural district of Malawi. *Int J Tuberc Lung Dis* **7:** 1033–1039.

Zhu S, Srebric J, Rudnick SN, Vincent RL, Nardell EA. 2013. Numerical investigation of upper-room UVGI disinfection efficacy in an environmental chamber with a ceiling fan. *Photochem Photobiol* **89:** 782–791.

Zhu S, Srebric J, Rudnick SN, Vincent RL, Nardell EA. 2014. Numerical modeling of indoor environment with a ceiling fan and an upper-room ultraviolet germicidal irradiation system. *Build Environ* **72:** 116–124.

 Cite this article as *Cold Spring Harb Perspect Med* doi: 10.1101/cshperspect.a018192

Index

H

I

J

K

L

M

Q

R

U

V

W

X

Z